A LANGE medical book

Pathology: A Modern Case Study

Howard M. Reisner, PhD
Professor
Department of Pathology and Laboratory Medicine
University of North Carolina
Chapel Hill, North Carolina

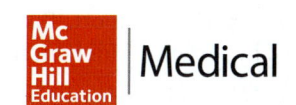

McGraw Hill Education | Medical

New York   Chicago   San Francisco   Athens   London   Madrid   Mexico City
Milan   New Delhi   Singapore   Sydney   Toronto

Pathology: A Modern Case Study

Copyright © 2015 by McGraw-Hill Education. All rights reserved. Printed in China. Except as permitted under the United States Copyright Act of 1976, no part of this publication may be reproduced or distributed in any form or by any means, or stored in a data base or retrieval system, without the prior written permission of the publisher.

1 2 3 4 5 6 7 8 9 0 CTP/CTP 19 18 17 16 15 14

ISBN 978-0-07-162156-4
MHID 0-07-162156-3

Notice

Medicine is an ever-changing science. As new research and clinical experience broaden our knowledge, changes in treatment and drug therapy are required. The authors and the publisher of this work have checked with sources believed to be reliable in their efforts to provide information that is complete and generally in accord with the standards accepted at the time of publication. However, in view of the possibility of human error or changes in medical sciences, neither the authors nor the publisher nor any other party who has been involved in the preparation or publication of this work warrants that the information contained herein is in every respect accurate or complete, and they disclaim all responsibility for any errors or omissions or for the results obtained from use of the information contained in this work. Readers are encouraged to confirm the information contained herein with other sources. For example and in particular, readers are advised to check the product information sheet included in the package of each drug they plan to administer to be certain that the information contained in this work is accurate and that changes have not been made in the recommended dose or in the contraindications for administration. This recommendation is of particular importance in connection with new or infrequently used drugs.

This book was set in Minion Pro by Aptara Inc.
The editors were Michael Weitz and Brian Kearns.
The production supervisor was Catherine Saggese.
Project management was provided by Amit Kashyap at Aptara Inc.
China Translation & Printing Services, Ltd. was printer and binder.

This book is printed on acid-free paper.

Library of Congress Cataloging-in-Publication Data

Pathology (2014)
  Pathology : a modern case study / [edited by] Howard M. Reisner.
    p. ; cm.
  ISBN-13: 978-0-07-162156-4 (pbk. : alk. paper)
  ISBN-10: 0-07-162156-3 (pbk. : alk. paper)
  I. Reisner, Howard M., editor.   II. Title.
  [DNLM: 1. Pathology—methods. QZ 4]
  RB113
  616.07–dc23

2014005370

International Edition ISBN 978-1-25-925251-8; MHID 1-25-925251-5. Copyright © 2015. Exclusive rights by McGraw-Hill Education, for manufacture and export. This book cannot be re-exported from the country to which it is consigned by McGraw-Hill Education.
The International Edition is not available in North America.

McGraw-Hill books are available at special quantity discounts to use as premiums and sales promotions, or for use in corporate training programs. To contact a representative please visit the Contact Us pages at www.mhprofessional.com.

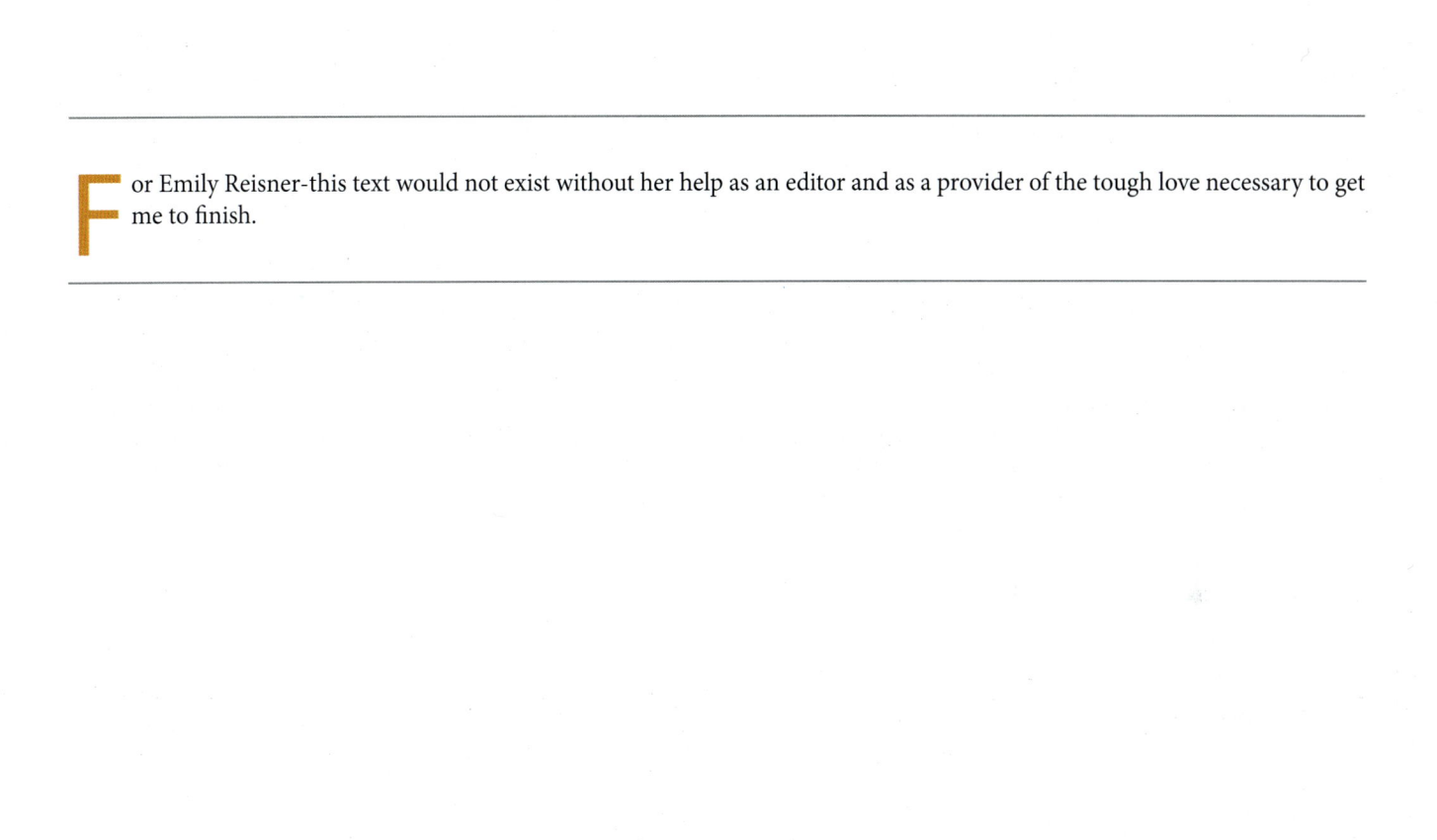

For Emily Reisner-this text would not exist without her help as an editor and as a provider of the tough love necessary to get me to finish.

Contents

Preface ix

1. Disease and the Genome: Genetic, Developmental, and Neoplastic Disease 1
2. Cell Injury, Cell Death, and Aging 21
   The Vascular Response to Injury 78
3. Environmental Injury 93
4. Clinical Practice: Anatomic Pathology 121
5. Clinical Practice: Molecular Pathology 129
6. Clinical Practice: Laboratory Medicine and Patient Care 137
7. The Vascular System 147
8. Pulmonary Pathology 217
9. Pathology of the Gastrointestinal Tract 241
10. Pathology of the Liver, Gallbladder, and Extrahepatic Biliary Tract 271
11. Pathology of the Pancreas 287
12. Pathology of Medical Renal Disease 297
13. Urologic Pathology of the, Lower Urinary Tract, Male GU System and Kidney 329
14. Hematopathology 357
15. Pathology of the Endocrine System 399
16. Breast Pathology 433
17. The Female Reproductive Tract 455
18. Soft Tissue and Bone Pathology 483
19. Neuromuscular Pathology 527
20. Pathology of the Skin 539
21. Pathology of the Nervous System 567

Index 595

Contents

Preface ix

1. Disease and the Genome: Genetic, Developmental and Neoplastic Disease 1
2. Cell Injury, Cell Death, and Aging 21
3. The Vascular Response to Injury 78
4. Environmental Injury 93
5. Clinical Practice Anatomic Pathology 121
6. Clinical Practice Molecular Pathology 126
7. Clinical Practice Laboratory Medicine and Patient Care 132
8. The Vascular System 152
9. Pulmonary Pathology 217
10. Pathology of the Gastrointestinal Tract 241
11. Pathology of the Liver, Gallbladder, and Extrahepatic Biliary Tract 273
12. Pathology of the Pancreas 287
13. Pathology of Medical Renal Disease 292
14. Urologic Pathology of the Lower Urinary Tract, Male GU System and Kidney 329
15. Hematopathology 357
16. Pathology of the Endocrine System 399
17. Breast Pathology 433
18. The Female Reproductive Tract 455
19. Soft Tissue and Bone Pathology 483
20. Neuromuscular Pathology 527
21. Pathology of the Skin 530
22. Pathology of the Nervous System 567

Index 595

Contributors

Diane M. Armao, MS, MD
Research Instructor
Department of Radiology
University of North Carolina at Chapel Hill
Chapel Hill, North Carolina

Natalie Banet, MD
Fellow (Gynecologic Pathology)
Johns Hopkins University
School of Medicine
Baltimore, Maryland

Thomas W. Bouldin, MD
Professor
Department of Pathology and Laboratory Medicine
University of North Carolina at Chapel Hill
Chapel Hill, North Carolina

John D. Butts, MD
Professor (Emeritus)
Department of Pathology and Laboratory Medicine
University of North Carolina at Chapel Hill
Chapel Hill, North Carolina

Nizar Chahin, MD
Assistant Professor
Department of Neurology
University of North Carolina at Chapel Hill
Chapel Hill, North Carolina

Frank C. Church, PhD
Professor
Department of Pathology and Laboratory Medicine
University of North Carolina at Chapel Hill
Chapel Hill, North Carolina

William B. Coleman, PhD
Professor
Department of Pathology and Laboratory Medicine
University of North Carolina at Chapel Hill
Chapel Hill, North Carolina

Cherie H. Dunphy, MD
Professor (Adjunct)
Medical Director of Hematopathology
Laboratory Corporation of America and Integrated Oncology
Department of Pathology and Laboratory Medicine
University of North Carolina at Chapel Hill
Chapel Hill, North Carolina

George Fedoriw, MD
Associate Professor
Department of Pathology and Laboratory Medicine
University of North Carolina at Chapel Hill
Chapel Hill, North Carolina

Karen J. Fritchie, MD
Assistant Professor
Department of Laboratory Medicine and pathology
Mayo Clinic
Rochester, Minnesota

William K. Funkhouser, MD, PhD
Professor
Department of Pathology and Laboratory Medicine
University of North Carolina at Chapel Hill
Chapel Hill, North Carolina

Adil M. Hussein Gasim, MBBS
Assistant Professor
Department of Pathology and Laboratory Medicine
University of North Carolina at Chapel Hill
Chapel Hill, North Carolina

Kevin G. Greene, MD
Assistant Professor
Department of Pathology and Laboratory Medicine
University of North Carolina at Chapel Hill
Chapel Hill, North Carolina

Margaret L. Gulley, MD
Professor
Department of Pathology and Laboratory Medicine
University of North Carolina at Chapel Hill
Chapel Hill, North Carolina

Catherine A. Hammett-Stabler, PhD, DABCC, FACB
Professor
Department of Pathology and Laboratory Medicine
University of North Carolina at Chapel Hill
Chapel Hill, North Carolina

J. Charles Jennette, MD
Kenneth M. Brinkhous Distinguished Professor and Chair
Department of Pathology and Laboratory Medicine
University of North Carolina at Chapel Hill
Chapel Hill, North Carolina

CONTRIBUTORS

Karen L. Kelly, MD
Associate Professor
Brody School of Medicine
East Carolina University
Greenville, North Carolina

Eric T. Lee, DO
Clinical Instructor
Department of Neurology
University of North Carolina at Chapel Hill
Chapel Hill, North Carolina

Ruth A. Lininger, MD, MPH
Associate Professor
Department of Pathology and Laboratory Medicine
University of North Carolina at Chapel Hill
Chapel Hill, North Carolina

Chad A. Livasy, MD
Professor (Adjunct)
Carolinas Pathology Group
Carolinas Medical Center
Charlotte, North Carolina (and)
Department of Pathology and Laboratory Medicine
University of North Carolina at Chapel Hill
Chapel Hill, North Carolina

Stephanie P. Mathews, MD
Assistant Professor
Department of Pathology and Laboratory Medicine
University of North Carolina at Chapel Hill
Chapel Hill, North Carolina

Susan J. Maygarden, MD
Professor
Department of Pathology and Laboratory Medicine
University of North Carolina at Chapel Hill
Chapel Hill, North Carolina

Jayson R. Miedema, MD
Resident (Dermatopathology)
Department of Dermatology
University of North Carolina at Chapel Hill
Chapel Hill, North Carolina

Chantelle M. Rein-Smith, PhD
Post-Doctoral Fellow
Department of Hematology and Oncology
University of North Carolina at Chapel Hill
Chapel Hill, North Carolina

Howard M. Reisner, PhD
Professor
Department of Pathology and Laboratory Medicine
University of North Carolina at Chapel Hill
Chapel Hill, North Carolina

Ashley G. Rivenbark, PhD
Assistant Professor
Department of Pathology and Laboratory Medicine
University of North Carolina at Chapel Hill
Chapel Hill, North Carolina

Christopher J. Sayed, MD
Assistant Professor
Department of Dermatology
University of North Carolina at Chapel Hill
Chapel Hill, North Carolina

Dimitri G. Trembath, MD, PhD
Assistant Professor
Department of Pathology and Laboratory Medicine
University of North Carolina at Chapel Hill
Chapel Hill, North Carolina

Daniel C. Zedek, MD
Assistant Professor
Department of Dermatology
University of North Carolina at Chapel Hill
Chapel Hill, North Carolina

Preface

In the first edition of *Textbook of Pathology with Clinical Applications* published in 1957, Stanley Robbins M.D., the founding author of perhaps the best known of all pathology textbooks, stated:

"Anyone who essays to predict the future of pathology tempts the fates. But it requires no prophet to appreciate that pathology stands on the threshold of great advances."

His statement is just as true today. For Dr. Robbins those advances involved the ultrastructure of disease assayed by electron microscopy. Today we study the molecular structure of disease using genomics and proteomics. About tomorrow, who can say?

Any textbook for medical students that attempts to provide an overview of pathology today must balance between the molecular nature of pathogenesis and well-established and clinically critical descriptions of the disease process at the organ, cellular, and ultrastructural levels. The balance is made more difficult by the fact that only a few percent of medical students will become pathologists. Those who do will use the traditional microscope as well as genomic and molecular tools to recognize and characterize disease. Even students who choose clinical and surgical specialties still must know the etiology and pathogenesis of the disorders they deal with in the setting of direct patient care and understand what the pathologist has to offer for that care.

For these reasons, the choice of what to include in a textbook aimed at undergraduate medical students is always a compromise. However, the editor and authors of this work firmly believe that whatever the scope of information chosen, such information must be tied to the patient's condition to be meaningful to the student as well as exemplifying the clinical practice of pathology.

Hence, we have centered our presentations around case studies designed to emphasize the role of the pathologist in the team that provides patient care, examining the role of anatomic, clinical, and molecular pathologists in that multi-membered group both in dedicated chapters and in descriptions of the pathology of specific organ systems. We have "tempted the fates" as did Dr Robbins by making predictions as to what areas of today's biomedical research might become tomorrow's standard of care.

Howard M. Reisner

Disease and the Genome: Genetic, Developmental, and Neoplastic Disease

CHAPTER 1

Ashley G. Rivenbark and William B. Coleman

INTRODUCTION

Through the ages, physicians and scientists have studied diseases of humans, describing the abnormal lesions (pathology) and their adverse effects on the patient (pathophysiology), seeking to identify risk factors (susceptibility) and causes (etiological agents), and pursuing a greater understanding of how diseases come to be (pathogenesis). With progress in these directions, some human diseases are now well understood from the perspective of risk and causal factors, and effective preventative and/or treatment strategies have been developed. For many other human diseases, investigation into the fundamental elements of the molecular and cellular pathogenesis represents an ongoing endeavor. Nevertheless, in the last several decades, the field of pathology has evolved to recognize that disease manifests in many cases as a direct reflection of changes in patterns of gene expression and often involves changes in the genome. There is also the recognition that gene expression patterns in a given lesion type (e.g., a certain form of cancer) will influence the clinical behavior of that lesion and its response to therapy. Hence, a great effort has been expended to characterize the genetic basis of various human diseases (molecular pathology), leading to a greater understanding of the contributions of genomic alterations to the development and progression of disease. Molecular pathology represents the application of the principles of basic molecular biology to the investigation of human disease processes. Our ever broadening insights into the molecular basis of disease provide opportunities for the development of new and novel approaches for diagnosis, classification, and prognostic assessment of human disease, and for expansion of treatments that are directed at specific molecular targets or pathways. In this chapter, we provide an overview of the role of the genomic alterations in genetic, developmental, and neoplastic diseases, with special emphasis on the role of mutations and epimutations in the pathogenesis of these disease states.

THE HUMAN GENOME

DNA is the Source of Genetic Information

Among the essential building blocks of living cells that were identified and characterized by chemists and early biochemists were nucleic acids—long-chain polymers composed of nucleotides. Nucleic acids were named based partly on their chemical properties and partly on the observation that they represent a major constituent of the cell nucleus. The critical realization that nucleic acids form the chemical basis for the transmission of genetic traits did not occur until about 65 years ago. Prior to that time, there was considerable disagreement among scientists as to whether genetic information was contained in and transmitted by proteins or nucleic acids. It was recognized that chromosomes contained deoxyribonucleic acid (DNA) as a primary constituent, but it was not known if this DNA carried genetic information or merely served as a scaffold for some undiscovered class of proteins that carried genetic information. However, the demonstration that genetic traits could be transmitted through DNA formed the basis for numerous investigations focused on elucidation of the nature of the genetic code. During the last 65 years, numerous investigators participated in the scientific revolution leading to modern molecular biology. Of particular significance were the elucidation of the structure of DNA, determination of structure-function relationships between DNA and RNA, and acquisition of basic insights into the processes of DNA replication, RNA transcription, and protein synthesis.

The Central Dogma of Molecular Biology

Molecular biology has developed into a broad field of scientific pursuit and, at the same time, has come to represent a basic component of most other basic research sciences. This has come about through the rapid expansion of our insights into numerous basic aspects of molecular biology and the development of an understanding of the fundamental interaction among the several major processes that comprise the larger field of investigation. A theory, referred to as the *central dogma*, describes the interrelationships among these major processes. The central dogma defines the paradigm of molecular biology that genetic information is perpetuated as sequences of nucleic acid and that genes function through their expression in the form of protein molecules. Individual DNA molecules serve as templates for either complementary DNA strands during the process of replication or complementary RNA molecules during the process of transcription. In turn, RNA molecules serve as blueprints for the ordering of amino acids by ribosomes during protein synthesis or translation. This simple representation of the complex interactions and interrelationships among DNA, RNA, and protein (Figure 1-1A) was proposed and commonly accepted shortly after the discovery of the structure of DNA. Nonetheless, this paradigm still holds more than 50 years later and continues to represent a guiding principle for molecular biologists involved in all areas of basic biological, biomedical, and genetic research.

With advances in our understanding of the molecular underpinnings of the eukaryotic cell, the concept of the central dogma remains largely the same, but we now recognize the importance of maintenance of genomic integrity through DNA repair mechanisms, multiple mechanisms and layers of regulation of gene expression (at the transcriptional and post-transcriptional levels), and modification of protein functionality through post-translational modification (Figure 1-1B). Numerous DNA repair mechanisms are expressed in eukaryotic cells to ensure the integrity of the primary structure of the DNA (the DNA sequence). These mechanisms function in conjunction with the processes of replication (to protect against replication errors) and transcription (to protect expressed regions of the genome). Major DNA repair pathways for damage to the primary sequence of the DNA include mismatch repair, nucleotide excision repair, and direct chemical reversal mechanisms. Eukaryotic cells also have DNA repair pathways that can correct strand breaks and other damage at the chromosomal level. Transcriptional regulation of gene expression is accomplished through balanced interactions of specific activating transcription factors and repressive gene expression inhibitors. In addition, transcriptional control of gene expression is heavily influenced by epigenetic factors, including methylation of the DNA sequence and remodeling of chromatin secondary to modification of histone proteins. Post-transcriptional regulation of gene expression is influenced by microRNAs (miRNAs) that function to direct the degradation of specific mRNAs. The proteins encoded by structural genes are often modified post-translationally through glycosylation, phosphorylation, acetylation, methylation, or through enzymatic cleavage, resulting in a polypeptide with new or modified functionality. This new concept of the central dogma more accurately describes the number and complexity of cellular functions that impinge on the genome and its expression (Figure 1-1B).

Structure and Organization of the Human Genome

Chemical Nature of DNA

DNA is a polymeric molecule that is composed of repeating nucleotide subunits. The order of nucleotide subunits contained in the linear sequence or primary structure of these polymers represents all of the genetic information carried by a cell. Each nucleotide is composed of (i) a phosphate group, (ii) a pentose (5 carbons) sugar, and (iii) a cyclic nitrogen containing compound called a base. In DNA, the sugar moiety is 2-deoxyribose. Eukaryotic DNA is composed of four different bases: adenine, guanine, thymine, and cytosine (Figure 1-2A). These bases are classified based on their chemical structure into two groups: adenine and guanine are double-ring structures termed purines and thymine and cytosine are single-ring structures termed pyrimidines (Figure 1-2A). Within the overall composition of DNA, the concentration of thymine is always equal to the concentration of adenine, and the concentration of cytosine is always equal to guanine. Thus, the total concentration of pyrimidines always equals the total concentration of purines. The constant ratio of purines to pyrimidines in DNA, and more specifically the equal concentrations of adenine/thymine and guanosine/cytosine, is known as Chargaff rule. Chargaff observations related to the

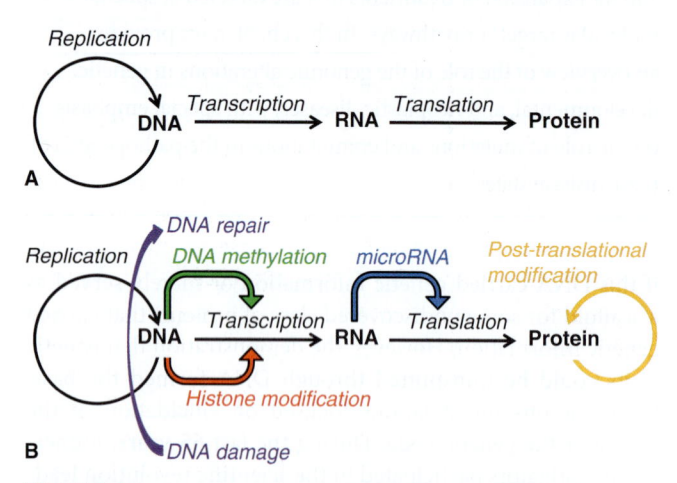

FIGURE 1-1 The central dogma. (A) The central dogma of molecular biology as originally described by Crick. This schematic illustrates the flow of genetic information from DNA to RNA and then to protein, as well as illustrates that DNA serves as its own template in replication. **(B)** The new central dogma reflects advances in our understanding of molecular processes that occur in normal cells. These processes include epigenetic regulation of gene expression by DNA methylation and histone modification, post-transcriptional regulation of gene expression by microRNAs, and modification of protein functionality by post-translational modification (which might include glycosylation, ubiquitination, phosphorylation, or other). This new central dogma also emphasizes the importance of DNA repair processes in the maintenance of genome integrity.

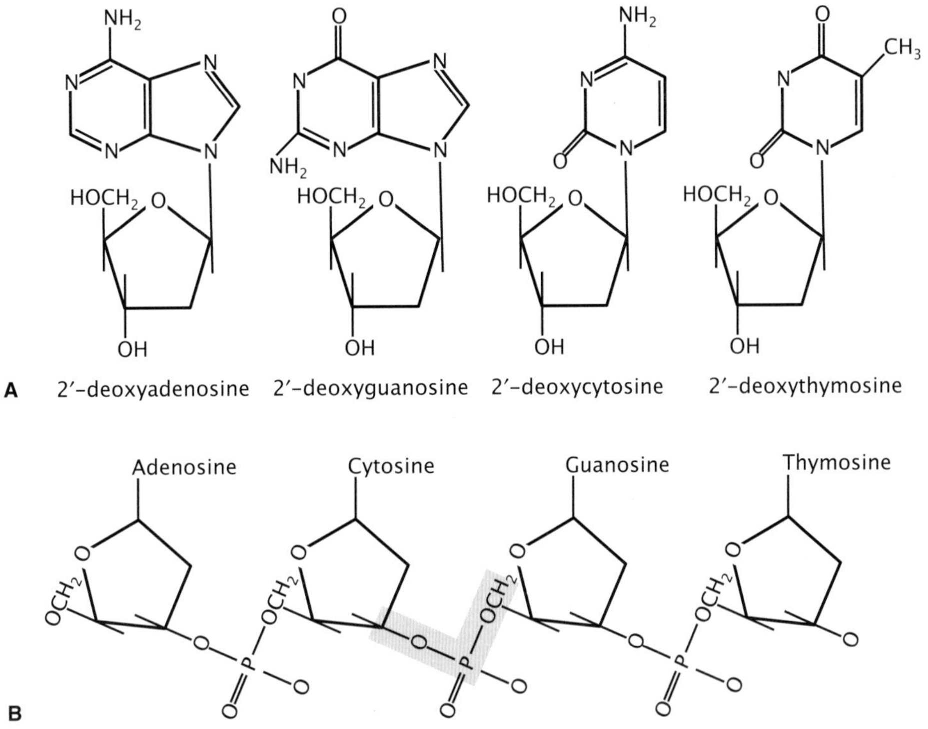

FIGURE 1-2 Building blocks of DNA. **(A)** The chemical structure of purine (2'-deoxyadenosie and 2'-deoxyguanosine) and pyrimidine (2'-deoxycytosine and 2'-deoxythymosine) deoxyribonucleosides. **(B)** The chemical structure of repeating nucleotide subunits in DNA. The shaded area highlights a 3'-5' phosphodiester bond.

purine/pyrimidine composition of DNA was validated when it was recognized that adenine/thymine (A:T) and guanosine/cytosine (G:C) are specifically hydrogen bond in the structure of DNA. Adenine–thymine pairs are linked in the structure of DNA by double hydrogen bonding, and guanosine–cytosine pairs are linked by triple hydrogen bonding. The extensive hydrogen bonding between strands of DNA in the double helical structure of the molecule confers great stability under physiological conditions. The monomeric nucleotide units are linked together into the polymeric structure of DNA by 3',5'-phosphodiester bonds (Figure 1-2B). Natural DNAs display widely varying sizes depending on the source. Relative molecular weights range from 1.6×10^6 daltons for bacteriophage DNA to 1×10^{11} daltons for a human chromosome.

Structure of DNA

The structure of DNA is a double helix, composed of two polynucleotide strands that are coiled about one another in a spiral. Each polynucleotide strand is held together by phosphodiester bonds linking adjacent deoxyribose moieties (Figure 1-2B). The two polynucleotide strands are held together by a variety of noncovalent interactions, including lipophilic interactions between adjacent bases and hydrogen bonding between the bases on opposite strands. The sugar-phosphate backbones of the two complementary strands are antiparallel—that is, they possess opposite chemical polarity. Moving along the DNA double helix in one direction, the phosphodiester bonds in one strand are oriented 5'-3', whereas in the complementary strand, the phosphodiester bonds are oriented 3'-5'. This configuration results in base pairs being stacked between the two chains perpendicular to the axis of the molecule. The base pairing is always specific: adenine is always paired to thymidine, and guanine is always paired to cytosine. This specificity results from the hydrogen-bonding capacities of the bases themselves. Adenine and thymine form two hydrogen bonds, and guanine and cytosine form three hydrogen bonds. The specificity of molecular interactions within the DNA molecule allows one to predict the sequence of nucleotides in one polynucleotide strand if the sequence of nucleotides in the complementary strand is known. Although the hydrogen bonds themselves are relatively weak, the number of hydrogen bonds within a DNA molecule results in a very stable molecule that does not spontaneously separate under physiological conditions. There are many possibilities of hydrogen bonding between pairs of heterocyclic bases. Most important are the hydrogen bonded base pairs A:T and G:C that were proposed by Watson and Crick in their double-helix structure of DNA. However, other forms of base pairing have been described. In addition, hydrophobic interactions between the stacked bases in the double helix lend additional stability to the DNA molecule. Three helical forms of DNA are recognized to exist: A, B, and Z. The B conformation is the dominant form under physiological conditions. In B DNA, the base pairs are stacked 0.34 nm apart, with 10 base pairs per turn of the right-handed double helix and a diameter of approximately 2 nm. Like B DNA, the A conformer is also a right-handed helix. However,

A DNA exhibits a larger diameter (2.6 nm), with 11 bases per turn of the helix, and the bases are stacked closer together in the helix (0.25 nm apart). Careful examination of space-filling models of A and B DNA conformers reveals the presence of a major groove and a minor groove. These grooves (particularly the minor groove) contain water molecules that interact favorably with the amino and keto groups of the bases. In these grooves, DNA-binding proteins can interact with specific DNA sequences without disrupting the base pairing of the molecule. In contrast to the A and B conformers of DNA, Z DNA is a left-handed helix. Z DNA possesses a minor groove but no major groove, and the minor groove is sufficiently deep that it reaches the axis of the DNA helix. The natural occurrence and potential physiological significance of Z DNA in living cells has been the subject of much speculation, but is now gaining recognition. Additional non-B DNA structures have been described, some of which may contribute to the genetic basis of human disease.

Sequence of the Human Genome

The diploid genome of the typical human cell contains approximately 3×10^9 base pairs of DNA that is subdivided into 23 pairs of chromosomes (22 autosomes and sex chromosomes X and Y). For many years, it was suggested that discernment of the complete sequence of the human genome would enable the genetic causes of and contributions to human disease to be investigated. However, early molecular biology techniques and approaches to DNA cloning and sequencing were slow and cumbersome. Nevertheless, practical methods for DNA sequencing appeared in the mid to late 1970s, and numerous reports of DNA sequences corresponding to segments of the human genome began to appear. In the mid-1980s, a project to sequence the complete human genome was proposed, and this project began in the later years of that decade. The development of automated methods for DNA sequencing made the ambitious goals of the Human Genome Project attainable. Subsequently, detailed genetic and physical maps of the human genome appeared, expressed sequences were identified and characterized, and gene maps of the human genome were constructed. Efforts by several consortiums using differing approaches to large-scale sequencing of human DNA and sequence contig assembly culminated in 2001 with the publication of a draft sequence of the human genome. Several years later, a more complete sequence of the human genome was released. Today, the human genome is thought to contain approximately 21,000 distinct protein-coding genes. Analysis of the human genome sequence reveals considerable variability between individuals, including in excess of 1.1–1.4 million single-nucleotide polymorphisms (SNPs) distributed throughout the genome. Refinement of the sequence of the human genome, identification and characterization of the genes contained, and description of the features of the genome (SNPs and other variations) continue at a rapid pace (www.genome.gov). The implications for knowing the sequence of the human genome in the context of understanding the impact of genetic factors on human disease are enormous.

Organization of the Human Genome

Human genomic DNA is packaged into discreet structural units that vary in size and genetic composition. The structural unit of DNA is the chromosome, which is a large continuous segment of DNA. A chromosome represents a single genetically specific DNA molecule to which a large number of protein molecules are attached that are involved in the maintenance of chromosome structure and regulation of gene expression. Genomic DNA contains both coding and noncoding sequences. Noncoding sequences contain information that does not lead to the synthesis of an active RNA molecule or protein. This is not to suggest that noncoding DNA serves no function within the genome. On the contrary, noncoding DNA sequences have been suggested to function in DNA packaging, chromosome structure, chromatin organization within the nucleus, and/or in the regulation of gene expression. A portion of the noncoding sequences represent intervening sequences that split the coding regions of structural genes. However, the majority of noncoding DNA falls into several families of repetitive DNA whose exact functions have not been entirely elucidated. Coding DNA sequences give rise to all of the transcribed RNAs of the cell, including mRNAs that encode for protein products. The organization of transcribed structural genes consists of coding regions that are interrupted by intervening noncoding regions of DNA. Thus, primary RNA transcripts contain both coding and noncoding sequences, and the noncoding sequences must be removed from the primary RNA transcript during processing to produce a functional mRNA molecule appropriate for translation.

DNA Function

DNA serves two essential functions with respect to cellular homeostasis: (i) storage of genetic information and (ii) transmission of genetic information. The DNA molecule serves as a template to fulfill each of these general functions. During cell division, DNA serves as a template for the faithful replication of genetic information that is ultimately passed into daughter cells. Likewise, the DNA molecule serves as a template for restoration of normal DNA sequence during DNA repair processes. During normal cellular operations, DNA serves as a template for the transcription of RNA. Transcribed RNA molecules may function directly (as is the case for ribosomal RNAs and transfer RNAs), may function after processing (as is the case of miRNAs), or may function as the template for synthesis of cellular proteins (as in the case of mRNAs).

Replication of DNA

Discovery of the double-stranded structure of DNA led rapidly to the suggestion that DNA replication could be accomplished in a semiconservative manner. In semiconservative DNA replication, each strand of the DNA helix serves as a template for the synthesis of the complementary strand. The result is the formation of two complete copies of the DNA molecule, each consisting of one strand from the parent DNA molecule and one newly synthesized strand. Utilization of the DNA strands as templates for the synthesis of complimentary DNA strands ensures the faithful reproduction of the genetic material for transmission into daughter cells.

Transcription of RNA

Contained within the linear nucleotide sequence of DNA is the information necessary for the synthesis of all protein constituents of a cell, as well as numerous species of functional RNA molecules. Transcription is the process by which RNA molecules are synthesized with a sequence complimentary to the transcriptional unit of DNA. Hence, the mRNA that encodes a specific protein is complimentary to the DNA sequence of that specific gene. In similar fashion, rRNAs, tRNAs, and various other RNA species are transcribed. The correct start and end points for transcription of a particular gene are determined by the promoter sequence upstream of the coding sequence of the gene and by termination signals downstream. Various other regulatory elements are present in the human genome in association with transcribed sequences. Some of these regulatory elements are enhancers of transcription, while others provide for negative regulation (repression) of gene expression in response to specific physiological signals. In contrast to DNA replication where both strands of the molecule serve as templates for synthesis of complementary DNA strands, in RNA transcription, only one strand of the DNA serves as template. This strand is referred to as the *sense* strand. Transcription of the sense strand ultimately yields an mRNA molecule that encodes the proper amino acid sequence for a specific protein.

Genetic Recombination

Genetic recombination represents one mechanism for the generation of genetic diversity through the exchange of genetic material between two homologous nucleotide sequences. Such an exchange of genetic material often results in alterations of the primary structure (nucleotide sequence) of a gene and alteration of the primary structure (amino acid sequence) of the encoded protein product. In organisms that reproduce sexually, recombination is initiated by formation of a junction between similar nucleotide sequences carried on the same chromosome from two different parents. The junction is able to move along the DNA helix through branch migration resulting in an exchange of the DNA strands (sister chromatid exchange).

DNA Damage and Mutagenesis

Overview of DNA Damaging Agents

The DNA contained in each of the cells of the human body is assaulted on a daily basis by various endogenous and exogenous DNA damaging agents, and some of this damage leads to mutation. DNA damage can result from spontaneous alteration of the DNA molecule or from the interaction of numerous chemical and physical agents with the structural DNA molecule. Spontaneous lesions can occur during normal cellular processes, such as DNA replication, DNA repair, or gene rearrangement, or through chemical alteration of the DNA molecule itself as a result of hydrolysis, oxidation, or methylation. In most cases, DNA lesions create nucleotide mismatches that lead to point mutations. Nucleotide mismatches can result from the formation of apurinic or apyrimidinic sites following depurination or depyrimidination reactions, nucleotide conversions involving deamination reactions, or in rare instances, from the presence of a tautomeric form of an individual nucleotide in replicating DNA. Deamination reactions result in the conversion of cytosine to uracil, adenine to hypoxanthine, and guanine to xanthine. However, the most common nucleotide deamination reaction involves methylated cytosines, which can replace cytosine in the linear sequence of a DNA molecule in the form of 5-methylcytosine. The 5-methylcytosine residues are always located next to guanine residues on the same chain, a motif referred to as a CpG dinucleotide. The deamination of 5-methylcytosine results in the formation of thymine. This particular deamination reaction accounts for a large percentage of spontaneous mutations in human disease. Interaction of DNA with physical agents, such as ionizing radiation, can lead to single-strand or double-strand breaks as a result of scission of phosphodiester bonds on one or both polynucleotide strands of the DNA molecule. Ultraviolet (UV) light can produce different forms of photoproducts, including pyrimidine dimers between adjacent pyrimidine bases on the same DNA strand. Other minor forms of DNA damage caused by UV light include strand breaks and cross-links. Nucleotide base modifications can result from exposure of the DNA to various chemical agents, including N-nitroso compounds and polycyclic aromatic hydrocarbons. DNA damage can also be caused by chemicals that intercalate the DNA molecule and/or cross-link the DNA strands. Bifunctional alkylating agents can cause both intrastrand and interstrand cross-links in the DNA molecule.

Types of DNA Mutation

Mutation is simply defined as any permanent change to the DNA molecule. The various forms of spontaneous and induced DNA damage give rise to a plethora of different types of molecular alterations to the DNA molecule, leading to stable mutations. These various types of mutation include both gross alteration of chromosomes and more subtle alterations to specific gene sequences in otherwise normal chromosomes.

Chromosomal Alterations

Gross chromosomal aberrations include large deletions, additions (reflecting amplification of DNA sequences), translocations (reciprocal and nonreciprocal), and other forms of chromosomal rearrangement. All of these forms of chromosomal abnormality can be distinguished through standard karyotype analyses of G-banded or R-banded chromosomes. However, currently employed chromosomal analysis methodologies typically rely on fluorescence in situ hybridization (FISH) and derived techniques. FISH can be utilized to address questions related to a single genetic locus or region (to score for amplification or deletion), or might be applied more broadly as a means for karyotypic analysis. Spectral karyotyping (or SKY) is a method where FISH probes paint individual chromosomes a distinct color, enabling easy and straightforward enumeration of chromosome numbers and identification of structural rearrangements.

The major consequence of chromosomal deletion is the loss of specific genes that are located in the deleted chromosomal region, resulting in changes in the copy number of the affected genes. For instance, deletion of certain classes of genes, including tumor suppressor genes or genes encoding the proteins involved in DNA repair, leads to predisposition of affected cells to neoplastic transformation. Likewise, amplification of chromosomal regions results in an increase in gene copy numbers, which can lead to the same circumstance if the affected region contains genes for dominant proto-oncogenes or other positive mediators of cell cycle progression and proliferation. The direct result of chromosomal translocation is the movement of some segment of DNA from its natural location into a new location within the genome, which can result in altered expression of the genes that are contained within the translocated region. If the chromosomal breakpoints utilized in a translocation are located within structural genes, then new hybrid genes can be generated. Likewise, some chromosomal rearrangements cause loss of structural genes due to the presence of a breakpoint within the gene itself.

Nucleotide Sequence Alterations

The most common forms of mutation involve single-nucleotide alterations, small deletions, or small insertions into specific gene sequences. Unlike chromosomal alterations, these molecular changes to the genome can only be detected through DNA sequencing or other sensitive molecular analyses that employ sequence-specific PCR primers.

Single-nucleotide alterations that involve a change in the normal coding sequence of the gene are referred to as point mutations. The consequence of most point mutations is an alteration in the amino acid sequence of the encoded protein. However, some point mutations are silent and do not affect the structure of the gene product. Silent mutations (also known as synonymous mutations) are possible because most amino acids are encoded by more than one triplet codon. Silent mutations represent one mechanism for introduction of genetic variability, but are without functional consequence. The remaining point mutations fall into two classes: (i) missense mutations and (ii) nonsense mutations. Missense mutations involve nucleotide base substitutions that alter the translation of the affected codon triplet, very often with a nonconservative amino acid change. Missense mutations are frequently classified as transitions or transversions based on the nature of the nucleotide change in the sequence of the DNA. A transition is the replacement of a nucleotide by another nucleotide of the same chemical class (i.e., purine for purine or pyrimidine for pyrimidine). Transition point mutations include A to G, G to A, C to T, and T to C. In contrast, a transversion is the substitution of a nucleotide from one chemical class with one from the other chemical class (i.e., purine for pyrimidine or pyrimidine for purine). Transversion point mutations include A to T, A to C, G to C, G to T, T to A, T to G, C to A, and C to G. Nonsense mutations differ from missense mutations in that they involve nucleotide base substitutions that modify a triplet codon that normally encodes for an amino acid into a translational stop codon. This results in the premature termination of translation and the production of a truncated protein product. In some cases, the truncated protein product resulting from a missense mutation lacks functionality and is rapidly degraded. In other cases, the truncated protein may retain some function or may gain new functionality (like freedom from normal regulatory mechanisms).

Small deletions and insertions usually give rise to frameshift mutations because the deletion or insertion of a single nucleotide (for instance) alters the reading frame of the gene on the 3′ side of the affected site. This results in the synthesis of a polypeptide product that does not resemble the normal gene product. In addition, small insertions or deletions can result in the premature termination of translation resulting from the presence of a stop codon in the new reading frame of the mutated gene. Deletions or insertions that occur involving multiples of three nucleotides will not result in a frameshift mutation, but will alter the resulting polypeptide gene product, which will exhibit either loss of specific amino acids or the presence of additional amino acids within its primary structure. These types of alteration can also lead to a loss of protein function.

Somatic Mutations Versus Germ-Line Mutations

All cellular DNA is subject to mutation through spontaneous mechanisms or in response to mutagenic agents. When DNA damaging and mutational events affect the DNA of a somatic cell, the resulting mutations are referred to as somatic mutations. Somatic cells represent the cells that compose all of the tissues in the organism outside of the germ line. Somatic mutations have been implicated in numerous disease types, particularly those that are characterized by clonal proliferation of altered cells (like in the case of cancer). Some somatic mutations occur during development, resulting in specific kinds of localized developmental abnormalities. Somatic mutations are not heritable. In contrast, DNA damaging and mutational events affecting the DNA of cells in the germ line produce mutations that are referred to as germ-line mutations. This distinction is biologically and clinically significant. The cells of the germ line are responsible for the genesis of oocytes (in the female) and spermatocytes (in the male). Hence, transmission of a germ-line mutation introduces a nucleotide sequence alteration into the fertilized egg. If that egg produces a viable organism, the mutation will be found in every cell in the organism. Germ-line mutations account for numerous genetic diseases, which can manifest systemic or organ-system-specific diseases (single organ or multiorgan). In addition, the germ-line mutation is found in the germ line of the affected individual, meaning that their offspring might also inherit the mutation.

THE HUMAN EPIGENOME

Conrad Waddington coined the term epigenetics in 1942 and defined it as "...the causal interactions between genes and their products, which bring the phenotype into being..." Today epigenetics refers to heritable alterations in gene expression patterns that are due to mechanisms other than changes in the nucleotide sequence of the genomic DNA. Epigenetic alterations differ from genetic alterations in that they arise more frequently, are reversible, and occur at defined regions of specific genes. Epigenetics explains how the same genotype can produce different phenotypes, such as in the case of monozygotic twins. Epigenetic information is stored as chemical modifications to (i) the histone proteins that package the genome and (ii) cytosines within the sequence of the DNA. These chemical changes regulate DNA accessibility and directly influence how the genome is expressed throughout different developmental stages, across different tissue and cell types, and in various disease states. Many epigenomic modifications affect DNA, RNA, and protein, but DNA methylation, histone modifications, chromatin remodeling factors, and noncoding RNAs are among the most well-studied epigenetic mechanisms. Numerous epigenomic processes function together to establish and preserve the global or site-specific open or closed chromatin states that ultimately determine whether a gene is active or inactive.

DNA Methylation

DNA methylation is regarded as the hallmark of epigenetic modifications. This chemical modification on cytosine bases provides heritable epigenetic information that is transmitted during DNA replication. DNA methylation is found in various bacteriophages, bacteria (without chromatin), fungi, plants, and mammals. However, DNA methylation is not found in model organisms such as *Caenorhabditis elegans* (worms) and *Saccharomyces cerevisiae* (budding yeast). Most of these organisms appear to survive when their genomic DNA methylation is dramatically decreased, but when DNA methylation is completely lost in mice embryonic lethality during organ development ensues. DNA methylation is a well-studied epigenetic mechanism that contributes to genetic instability and to the silencing of specific genes.

CpG Islands

DNA methylation occurs almost exclusively on cytosines within CpG dinucleotides, which are found in the genome at approximately 20% of the predicted frequency, and the majority (>70%) of CpG dinucleotides are methylated. However, regions of CpG density, termed CpG islands, occur in the promoter regions of numerous genes proximal to their transcription start site, and/or in sequences adjacent to the promoter region (like exon 1). It has been suggested that up to 50% of all human genes may contain a promoter CpG island (Figure 1-3). These CpG islands are conventionally defined as ≥200 base pairs with ≥50% G+C and ≥0.6 CpG observed/CpG expected, although a more rigorous definition (≥200 base pairs with ≥60% G+C and ≥0.7 CpG observed/CpG expected) has been proposed. Some studies have suggested that large CpG islands are not required for sensitivity of gene promoters to methylation-dependent silencing. Rather, other regions of CpG density can behave like classically defined CpG islands. Most promoter CpG islands are unmethylated in normal tissues, but may become methylated in various pathological conditions. Distinct patterns of DNA methylation are found in the genomes of cells under different physiological conditions and in development. During most developmental stages DNA is heavily methylated. However, promoters and other regulatory regions of housekeeping genes are largely unmethylated in most cell types, and tissue-specific expressed genes are unmethylated only in the cell types where these genes are transcriptionally active.

DNA Methyltransferase Enzymes

There are three active DNA methyltransferase (DNMT) enzymes, which catalyze the addition of methyl groups to cytosine within a CpG dinucleotide including the maintenance methyltransferase DNMT1 and de novo methyltransferases DNMT3a and DNMT3b (Figure 1-4A). Human DNMT1 cDNA was cloned in 1992 and mapped to chromosome 19p13.2. DNMT1 function is coordinated with the processes of

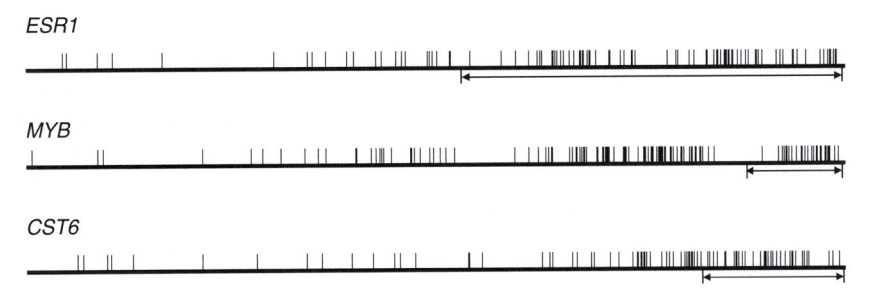

FIGURE 1-3 CpG island containing genes. The distribution of CpG dinucleotides proximal to the transcription start site in the promoter and exon 1 (black arrow) of estrogen receptor 1 (*ESR1*), myeloblastosis viral oncogene (*MYB*), and cystatin (*CST6*) are depicted schematically (vertical lines indicate the relative position of individual CpG dinucleotides). CpG islands are found in all representative genes. The CpG island is found in exon 1 of *ESR1*. In *MYB* and *CST6*, the CpG island is located in the proximal promoter and exon 1, spanning the transcriptional start site.

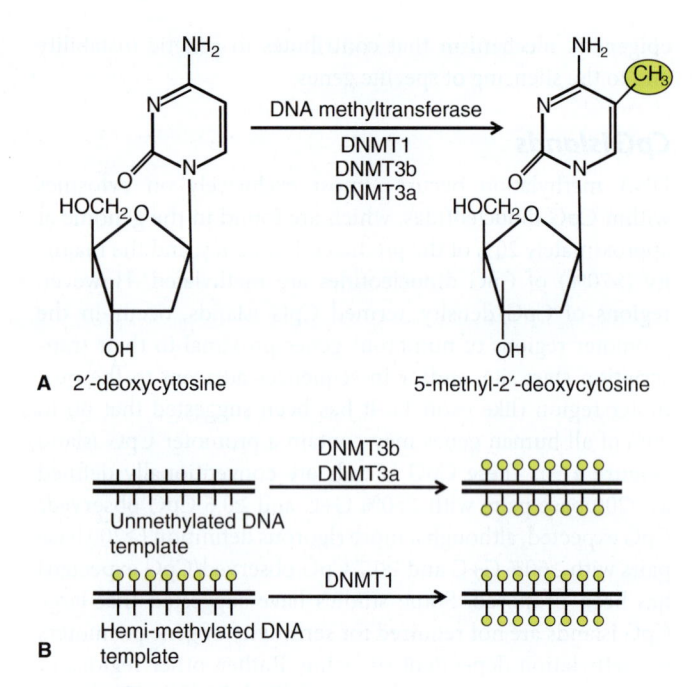

FIGURE 1-4 DNA methylation. (A) Chemical structural representation of the addition of a methyl group by DNMTs, yielding a 5-methyl-cytosine. **(B)** Schematic of DNA methylation (yellow circles) on a representative gene promoter by de novo methyltransferases (DNMT3b and DNMT3a) and a methyltransferase (DNMT1) involved in DNA replication.

density and gene expression levels, and multiple molecular mechanisms for DNA methylation-mediated regulation of gene expression have been proposed (Figure 1-5). However, the relationship between CpG methylation and gene expression status only holds for CpG methylation affecting gene promoters and their proximal sequences (such as intron 1), and not methylation that occurs in transcribed portions of the gene sequence. DNA methylation can take place in certain known transcription factor binding sites that include a CpG within their recognition sequence, thereby blocking the transcription machinery from binding to the site and inhibiting gene transcription (Figure 1-5B). Additionally, methyl-CpG-binding proteins are recruited to some sites of DNA methylation and can form a blockade inhibiting the transcriptional complex from transcribing along the promoter of a gene (Figure 1-5C). Methyl-CpG-binding (MBD) proteins have been identified to bind to either a single CpG site or multiple CpG sites to repress transcription. MBD proteins include MBD1, MBD2, MBD3, MBD4, MeCP1, and MeCP2. In some cases,

DNA replication in many cell types. DNMT1 lacks the ability to efficiently methylate unmethylated DNA (de novo methylation) and preferentially methylate hemi-methylated DNA (Figure 1-4B). During replication, hemi-methylated CpG sites are produced reflecting a lack of methylation in the newly synthesized daughter strand when the parental DNA was methylated. DNMT1 methylates the daughter strand CpG sites opposite of methylated CpGs in the parent strand (Figure 1-4B). In 1999, the genes for DNMT3a and DNMT3b were discovered and mapped to chromosome 2p23 and 20q22.3, respectively. DNMT3a binds relatively nonspecifically and preferentially to unmethylated DNA substrates compared with hemi-methylated DNA substrates (Figure 1-4B). DNMT3a may only methylate the CpG sites on one strand of DNA, leaving the complementary strand unmethylated. DNMT3b exhibits de novo methylation capability and is the accepted source of new methylation in mammalian cells (Figure 1-4B). De novo methylation through the action of DNMT3b establishes new DNA methylation at sequence targets that lack CpG methylation. DNMT3b along with DNMT1 works together to establish and maintain genome-wide DNA methylation patterns especially in densely methylated or repetitive sequences. The mechanisms that govern most of these processes are not yet well understood.

DNA Methylation-Mediated Regulation of Transcription

There is a strong inverse correlation between the methylation status of promoter CpG islands and/or regions of CpG

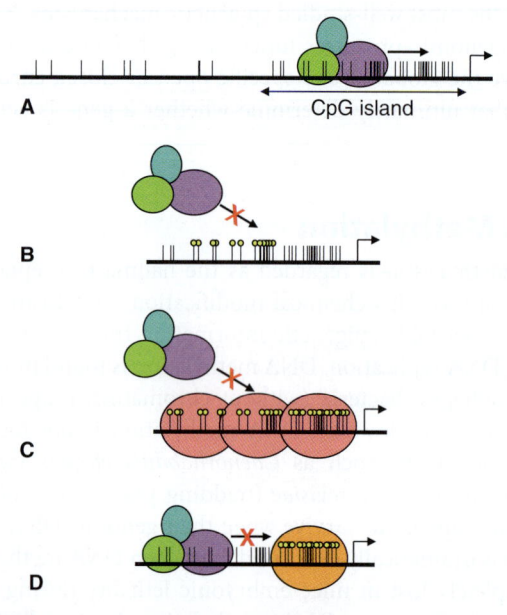

FIGURE 1-5 Methylation-dependent epigenetic regulation of gene expression. The distribution of CpG dinucleotides proximal to the transcription start site (indicated by the bent arrow) is depicted schematically (vertical lines indicate the relative position of individual CpG dinucleotides) for theoretical genes with variable promoter CpG density. Yellow circles correspond to methylated CpG dinucleotides. Genes with CpG islands are subject to both regional and discrete methylation events. **(A)** Lack of CpG island methylation leads to transcriptional activation by the transcriptional machinery (represented as associated green, blue, and purple circles) and subsequent gene expression. **(B)** Regional and discrete methylation events at transcription factor binding sites lead to transcriptional inactivation and subsequent lack of gene expression. **(C)** Regional methylation can affect transcription through recruitment of methylated DNA-binding proteins (pink circles). **(D)** Likewise, focal methylation within a larger CpG island may attract methylated DNA-binding proteins (orange circle) that may inhibit transcription by blocking the procession of the transcription machinery to the transcriptional start site.

methyl-CpG-binding proteins bind to promoter sequences impairing the ability of the transcription machinery to recognize and bind to the promoter sequence (Figure 1-5C). In other cases, the transcriptional complexes form but are impeded from movement along the gene sequence by the binding of methyl-CpG-binding proteins to a discrete region of the promoter (Figure 1-5D).

Genomic Imprinting

Parentally determined traits are typically the result of genetic imprinting, which is defined as the restricted epigenetic modification of specific chromosomal domains related to the parental origin of the allele (i.e. both maternal or paternal alleles are present by are not equally expressed). Small subsets of genes are known to be epigenetically modified in this manner. These genes are termed imprinted genes and are characterized by differential DNA methylation marks at specialized sequence elements called imprinting control regions (ICRs). These methylation patterns occur in one or the other of the parental germ lines where male and female individuals establish opposite methylation states (either methylated or unmethylated) at the ICRs in their respective germ line. This process depends on epigenetic reprogramming, erasing the preexisting methylation pattern and establishment of a new methylation pattern according to the sex of the individual. Once established, these germ line patterns are then passed into the next generation to regulate the expression status of imprinted genes that are essential for proper embryonic development. The first imprinted gene (*IGF2*) was identified in 1991 and now more than 100 imprinted genes have been identified. Major disease-associated genes that are subject to genetic imprinting include *IGF2* (paternal allele expressed), *WT1* (maternal allele expressed), *INS* (paternal allele expressed), *SNRPN* (paternal allele expressed), and *IGF2R* (maternal allele expressed).

Histone Proteins and Histone Modifications

Eukaryotic genomic DNA is packaged into chromatin within the nucleus of a cell through its interaction with histone proteins. The nucleosome core particle is the basic unit of chromatin, and it consists of 147 bp of DNA wrapped around an octamer of four core histones that include H3, H4, H2A, and H2B. The properties of histones can be altered by more than 100 different post-translational modifications to their N-terminal tails, which are rich in the basic amino acids arginine and lysine. Although many of these modifications remain poorly understood, in recent years there has been considerable progress made in the understanding of lysine acetylation and methylation. Many reports in the literature have substantiated an important role for these histone tails in regulating chromatin organization and gene transcription.

The Histone Code

The N-terminal amino acid tails of the various histone proteins are subject to numerous different modifications that reflect the addition of methylation, acetylation, phosphorylation, and ubiquitination marks to individual amino acid residues (Figure 1-6), all of which have been linked to variation in gene activity. The totality of these modifications led to the hypothesis that a *histone code* regulates chromatin structure and DNA packaging contributing directly to the regulation of gene expression. This histone code exerts its control on gene regulation through combinations of histone modifications that dictate the recruitment of specific proteins that elicit biological outputs. Understanding how histone modifications regulate gene expression and transcription will be integral in elucidation of the transcriptional control of cellular development and function, and how disruption of these processes can lead to disease.

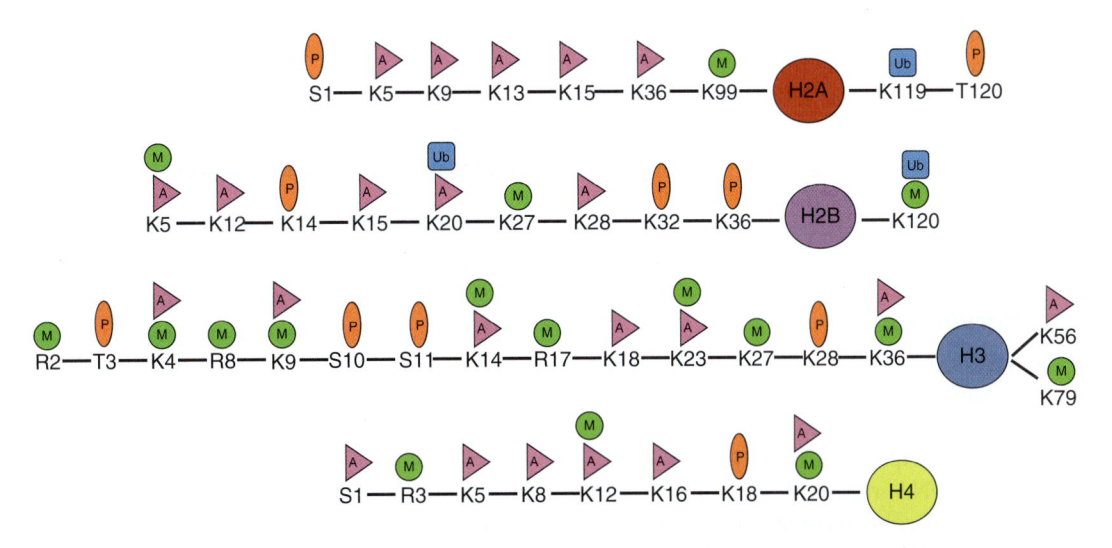

FIGURE 1-6 **The histone code.** This schematic depicts the main histone modifications including phosphorylation (P), acetylation (A), methylation (M), and ubiquitination (Ub) of the four core histones (H2A, H2B, H3, H4) in normal cells. Most of the known histone modifications occur on the N-terminal tails of the histones (shown on left of large colored circles) with few exceptions.

Histone Methylation

Histone methylation occurs on both lysine (Lys) and arginine (Arg) amino acid residues (Figure 1-6). While arginine residues can receive two methyl groups, in either *cis-* or *trans-*configuration, lysine residues can either be mono-methylated, di-methylated, or tri-methylated. Highly conserved methylation sites are found on histone H3 at lysine 4 (Lys4), Lys9, Lys27, Lys36, and Lys79, as well as on histone H4 at Lys20. Histone methylation has different effects on gene transcription depending on which amino acid residue is modified. Methylation of H3 Lys4 (H3K4) and H3 Lys36 (H3K36) is associated with active gene transcription. However, methylation of H3 Lys9 (H3K9), H3 Lys27 (H3K27), or H4 Lys20 (H4K20) is typically associated with inactive transcription. Lysine methyltransferases have enormous specificity and usually modify a single lysine on an individual histone. The most well-studied gene activation mark is H3K4, which can be methylated by the MLL complex of methyltransferases consisting of MLL1-MLL5. When present, this mark is localized to the 5′ end of active genes and is found associated with the transcription machinery (RNA polymerase II). Methylation of H3K9 can be produced by several methyltransferases including SUV39H, G9a, SETDB1, GLP, and RIZ1. The methylation of H3K9 forms silent heterochromatin, which involves the recruitment of HP1 to the promoter of repressed genes to further stabilize gene repression.

Histone Acetylation

Histone acetylation occurs on lysine amino acid residues (Figure 1-6). Acetylation sites are found on histone H3 at Lys9, Lys14, Lys18, Lys23, and Lys27, as well as on histone H4 Lys5, Lys8, and Lys16. These acetylation marks are associated with transcriptional activation. Acetyltransferases are divided into three main families, GNAT, MYST, and CBP/p300. The enzymes that compose these families can modify more than one lysine; for example, CBP/p300 modifies H3K14, H3K18, H4K5, and H4K8. Repression of transcription activity occurs with the removal of acetylation marks from histones H3 and H4 by histone deacetylase enzymes (HDACs) and HDAC inhibitors (HDACi) can inhibit this process. The effect of acetylation in terms of opening or closing chromatin leading to gene activation/inactivation reflects the neutralization of the charge interaction between the DNA backbone and the histone tails.

Histone Phosphorylation

Histone phosphorylation occurs on serine, threonine, histidine, and tyrosine amino acid residues (Figure 1-6). Histone phosphorylation is associated with a number of cellular processes including transcriptional regulation, apoptosis, cell cycle progression, DNA repair, developmental gene regulation, and chromatin condensation. Phosphorylation sites are found on histone H3 at threonine 3 (Thr3), Thr10, Thr11, and Thr45, serine 10 (Ser10), Ser28, and tyrosine 41 (Tyr41); on histone H4 Ser1, histidine 18 (His18), and His75; on histone H2B Ser32 and Ser36; and on histone H2A Ser1 and Ser119. One of the most extensively studied phosphorylation sites is H3Ser10 that is targeted by the MSK1/2 and RSK2 kinases. Phosphorylation of histones is not as well studied as methylation or acetylation because distinct signaling pathways need to be activated to observe these events.

Post-Transcriptional Regulation of Gene Expression

Noncoding RNAs provide another level of epigenetic control given that they can establish other epigenetic marks and control gene expression. miRNAs are small noncoding RNAs (19–25 nucleotide long) that regulate gene expression post-transcriptionally through sequence-specific targeting of mRNAs, producing either translational repression or degradation of the target mRNA. miRNAs are expressed in a tissue-specific manner and have been implicated in the regulation of several biological processes, including cellular proliferation, apoptosis, and development. Many miRNA species are encoded by genes that are contained within the intronic sequences of structural genes encoding proteins. The functional miRNA (mature) is released from the intronic sequences of the structural gene through the process of RNA processing, secondary to specific splicing events. It follows that regulation of expression of this class of miRNA gene is coordinated with the regulation (positive and negative) of the structural gene that contains the pre-miRNA sequence. Additional processing of pre-miRNAs is required for the generation of a functional miRNA that can target a specific mRNA sequence. These processing events typically reflect nuclease cleavage by various enzymes including Dicer and Drosha. Recent studies have identified miRNAs as both regulators of DNMT expression and targets of aberrant DNA methylation in various tissue types. These observations suggest that direct interactions and cross talk between the DNA methylation machinery and miRNAs occur in the regulation of gene expression.

GENETIC DISEASES

Major Forms of Genetic Disease

Genetic diseases can be classified into three major groupings: (i) chromosomal disorders, (ii) monogenic disorders, and (iii) polygenic disorders. Chromosomal disorders are the end result of the loss, gain, or abnormal rearrangement of one or more chromosomes, resulting in deficiencies of genetic material or excessive genetic material. Monogenic disorders are the result of a single mutant gene and display typical Mendelian inheritance patterns (autosomal dominant, autosomal recessive, and X linked). Polygenic or multifactorial disorders result from multiple genetic and/or epigenetic factors that do not conform to typical Mendelian inheritance patterns.

Single Gene Disorders

Single gene disorders involve mutation of one gene that accounts for the phenotype observed in the affected individual. These disorders typically follow one of three patterns of inheritance: (i) autosomal dominant, (ii) autosomal recessive, or (iii) X linked. The overall frequency of monogenic disorders among the general population is approximately 10 per 1000 live births.

Autosomal Dominant Disorders

Autosomal dominant disorders are those in which the presence of a single copy of a mutant gene (allele) results in disease. Hence, both homozygous and heterozygous individuals express the disease phenotype, males and females are equally affected, and any affected individual can transmit the condition to their offspring. In most cases, individuals affected by one of these disorders have at least one parent that is also affected. The autosomal dominant pattern of inheritance is characterized by vertical transmission of the disease from generation to generation, equal expressivity among males and females, lack of affected children from unaffected parents, a 50% chance of affected offspring from affected parents, and most affected individuals have an affected parent (Figure 1-7A). Individuals with an autosomal dominant disorder but without an affected parent typically have a founder mutation in the disease gene. Founder mutations are not found in the germ line of the parents, but occurred in either the sperm or the egg prior to fertilization. Hence, the affected offspring carries the mutated gene in their germ line and can pass the mutation to their offspring. The siblings of individuals with founder mutations are unaffected and have no increased risk of development of disease.

The expression of the disease state reflected in the clinical features among individuals affected by autosomal dominant disorders can vary due to reduced penetrance and variable expressivity. Likewise, the age of disease onset can vary, ranging from early childhood to late adulthood. Some individuals who inherit a mutant gene will be phenotypically normal (no evidence of disease). This reflects incomplete penetrance of the mutation-associated disease state. Penetrance is a measure of how often patients with a mutant allele express the mutation-related disease. Hence, a mutation that displays 100% penetrance will produce disease in every individual who carries the mutation. In contrast, a mutation that displays 50% penetrance will produce disease in only 50% of mutation carriers. Variable expressivity refers to the observation that among a cohort of individuals with a mutation-associated disease, the manifestation of disease can be different (differences in severity, differences in disease phenotype). The mechanisms that account for reduced penetrance and variable expressivity are not well understood. However, it is thought that the effects of other genes or environmental factors might influence the expression of disease-causing mutations. Differences in the age of onset of disease reflect the observation that some mutation-associated diseases develop early in life and others develop in adults or later in life. This phenomenon is likely related to the developmental and physiological context in which disease-causing genes are expressed.

Autosomal dominant disorders affect numerous organ systems, including the nervous system (Huntington disease, neurofibromatosis, myotonic dystrophy, tuberous sclerosis), urinary system (polycystic kidney disease), gastrointestinal system (familial polyposis coli), the hematopoietic system (von Willebrand disease), and the skeletal system (Marfan syndrome, osteogenesis imperfecta, achondroplasia, and others). In addition, some autosomal dominant disorders represent metabolic diseases (such as familial hypercholesterolemia). This listing of examples is intended to be representative and not comprehensive.

Autosomal Recessive Disorders

Autosomal recessive disorders are those in which two copies of the mutant gene are required for expression of the disease phenotype. Hence, heterozygous individuals are indistinguishable from individuals who carry two normal copies of the disease-associated gene. However, it should be noted that in some heterozygous individuals, there are subtle alterations in various biochemical measures that are not readily detectable because they cause no discernible symptoms. These heterozygous individuals (which carry one normal gene and one mutant gene) are termed *carriers*. The offspring of two carriers with the same mutant disease gene will have a 25% chance of developing the disease (due to homozygous inheritance

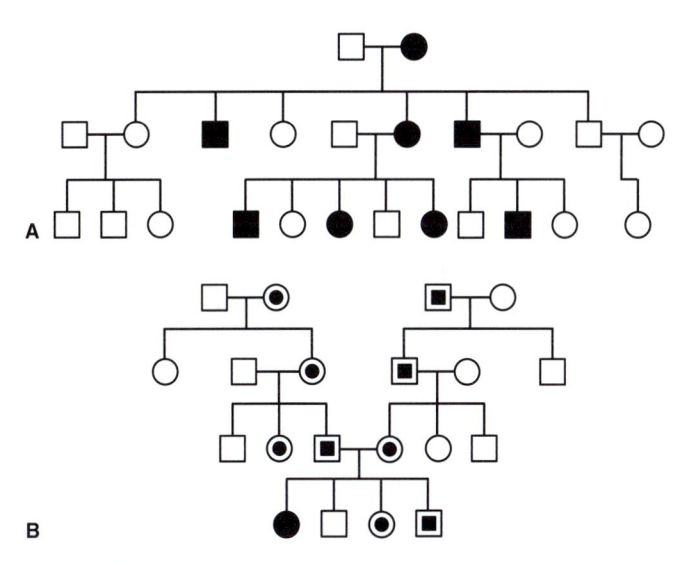

FIGURE 1-7 Inheritance patterns associated with autosomal dominant and autosomal recessive monogenic disorders. (A) Family pedigree depicting autosomal dominant inheritance pattern of a genetic disease. This is the pattern associated with diseases like Huntington disease, neurofibromatosis, myotonic dystrophy, familial hypercholesterolemia, and numerous others. Circle, female; square, male; open, unaffected; solid, affected. **(B)** Family pedigree showing autosomal recessive inheritance pattern of a genetic disease. This is the pattern associated with diseases like cystic fibrosis, Tay–Sachs disease, sickle cell anemia, and several metabolic disorders. Circle, female; square, male; open, unaffected; solid, affected; partially filled, carrier.

of the mutant disease gene), and a 50% chance of becoming carriers (due to heterozygous inheritance of the mutant disease gene). In contrast to autosomal dominant disorders, autosomal recessive disorders demonstrate a more uniform expression of the defect, complete penetrance is common, and disease onset typically occurs early in life. Hence, the pattern of autosomal recessive inheritance is characterized by horizontal penetrance, affected homozygous individuals have unaffected heterozygous parents, and heterozygous parents (mother and father) have a 25% chance of producing an affected offspring (Figure 1-7B).

Autosomal recessive disorders include the majority of inborn errors of metabolism. Metabolic autosomal recessive disorders include cystic fibrosis, phenylketonuria, galactosemia, homocystinuria, various lysosomal storage diseases, α1-antitrypsin deficiency (several forms), Wilson disease, hemochromatosis, and glycogen storage diseases. Other autosomal recessive disorders affect specific organ systems, including the hematopoietic system (sickle cell anemia, thalassemias), endocrine system (congenital adrenal hyperplasia), skeletal system (alkaptonuria), and nervous system (neurogenic muscular atrophies, spinal muscular atrophy, Friedreich ataxia). This listing of examples is intended to be representative and not comprehensive.

X-Linked Disorders

Genes responsible for X-linked disorders are carried on the X chromosome. The risk of development of X-linked disorders and the severity of the disorders that develop varies between males and females related to the fact that males have one X chromosome and females have two. Hence, females can be either heterozygous or homozygous for a mutant X-linked gene, and the associated trait can be expressed in either a dominant or recessive fashion. In contrast, males express the mutant X-linked gene whenever it is inherited. There is an absence of male-to-male transmission of X-linked disorders and all daughters of affected males inherit the mutant disease gene. X-linked recessive disorders primarily affect males. In the case of X-linked dominant disorders, all daughters of affected males are also affected. X-inactivation results in the expression of X-linked genes from only one X chromosome. Thus, the expression of an X-linked disorder in a female will depend on the presence of the mutant gene as well as its location on an active X chromosome.

X-linked recessive inheritance accounts for a small number of well-defined clinical conditions. Some of these X-linked disorders affect specific organ systems, including the musculoskeletal system (Duchenne muscular dystrophy), the blood (hemophilia A, hemophilia B, chronic granulomatous disease, glucose-6-phosphate dehydrogenase deficiency), immune system (agammaglobulinemia), or nervous system (fragile X syndrome). In addition, some metabolic disorders are X-linked diseases, including Lesch–Nyhan syndrome and diabetes insipidus. This listing of examples is intended to be representative and not comprehensive.

Mitochondrial Disorders

The human (and other mammalian) mitochondrion contains its own approximately 17 kb DNA molecule that contains a number of genes that encode proteins associated with mitochondrial function and specifically with energy metabolism (encoding some of the proteins of the electron transport chain enzyme complexes and the mitochondrial ATP synthase enzyme). Each mitochondrion may contain multiple copies of the mitochondrial chromosome, and each cell contains numerous (and perhaps hundreds) mitochondria. Mutations in genes encoded by the mitochondrial DNA are associated with various diseases. However, expression of a disease state requires accumulation of sufficient numbers of copies of mutated mitochondrial DNA (by random drift and cytoplasmic segregation) to result in mitochondrial dysfunction at the cellular level. Inheritance of mitochondrial-associated disorders is strictly maternal. Hence, females transmit mitochondrially determined traits to all their offspring. In rare instances, affected mothers will produce an unaffected child. This phenomenon probably reflects cytoplasmic segregation of mutant mitochondria in the gamete-forming tissue.

Mitochondrial disorders include myoclonic epilepsy and ragged red fiber disease, Leber hereditary optic neuropathy, neurogenic muscle weakness/ataxia/retinitis pigmentosum, Kearns–Sayre syndrome, maternally inherited Leigh syndrome, progressive ophthalmoplegia, and several others. This listing of examples is intended to be representative and not comprehensive. It is notable that many of these mitochondrial diseases manifest with muscular defects, reflecting the large energy consumption of muscle tissues and the fact that most of these mitochondrial diseases are characterized by compromised energy metabolism.

Polygenic Diseases

Polygenic or multifactorial disorders result from multiple genetic and/or epigenetic factors (mutations or gene silencing events) and do not conform to traditional Mendelian patterns of inheritance. Hence, polygenic diseases represent pathologies where no single gene or mutational event will ever definitively diagnose or predict risk. Polygenic disorders include chronic diseases of adulthood, congenital malformations, and dysmorphic syndromes. In some cases, broad classes of disease reflect polygenic molecular pathogenesis; for instance, cancer (in nearly all cases) is a multiple gene disorder. Other examples of polygenic diseases include hypertension, ischemic heart disease, Alzheimer disease, and diabetes mellitus. In all of these cases, the manifestation of disease is related to the interactions of numerous altered genes and environmental factors. Given the complexity of these diseases (and families of diseases), there is a lack of understanding of the genetic complexities of most polygenic diseases, and elucidation of the molecular pathogenesis of multifactorial disorders remains poorly understood.

Cytogenetic Disorders

Cytogenetic disorders are diseases that are associated with chromosomal alterations. In some cases, these diseases are characterized by karyotypic abnormalities involving abnormal numbers of chromosomes (losses or gains), while in other cases, these diseases are associated with abnormal rearrangement of one or more chromosomes. Irrespective of the molecular manifestation of the chromosomal abnormality, all of these disorders result in deficiencies of genetic material or excessive genetic material. The normal chromosome compliment of a female is 46XX (referring to 22 pairs of autosomes and the XX sex chromosomes), and the normal chromosome compliment of a male is 46XY (referring to 22 pairs of autosomes and the XY sex chromosomes). Monosomy involving an autosome is typically embryonic lethal, reflecting the loss of too much genetic information for viability of developing fetus. However, some numerical abnormalities involving trisomy of autosomes permit live birth. However, with rare exception (Down Syndrome), these autosomal trisomies lead to severely handicapped infants that die at an early age. In contrast, several chromosomal disorders affecting the number of sex chromosomes have been characterized.

Cytogenetic Disorders Involving Autosomes

Down syndrome is the most common autosomal chromosomal disorder and is characterized by trisomy of chromosome 21. This disorder occurs with an incidence of 1 in 700 live births in the United States, and is a major cause of mental retardation. These individuals have a chromosome count of 47 (reflecting 44 autosomes and 2 sex chromosomes, plus the extra copy of chromosome 21). The extra copy of chromosome 21 in Down syndrome individuals originates from a meiotic nondisjunction event. The parents of Down syndrome children are karyotypically and phenotypically normal. While the actual cause of meiotic nondisjunction resulting in trisomy 21 is not known, it has long been suggested that maternal age plays a major role in this disease—most Down syndrome babies are born to older mothers. The frequency of Down syndrome among mothers <20 years of age is 1 in 1550 live births, compared with 1 in 25 live births for women over age 45. Individuals with Down syndrome are affected by mental retardation that can vary in severity. In addition, these individuals tend to have congenital heart disease, are at risk of development of acute leukemias, and most have immune system compromise that puts them at risk of severe infections. Congenital heart problems are responsible for most Down syndrome deaths in infancy or early childhood. Older Down syndrome individuals develop neurodegenerative symptoms and neuropathologic changes characteristic of Alzheimer disease.

Cytogenetic Disorders Involving Sex Chromosomes

Genetic diseases associated with altered sex chromosomes are more common than those involving autosomes, perhaps reflecting that imbalance of sex chromosomes (excess or loss) is better tolerated than imbalances involving autosomes. Klinefelter syndrome and Turner syndrome represent two common cytogenetic disorders involving sex chromosomes.

Klinefelter syndrome is characterized by the presence of two or more X chromosomes and one or more Y chromosomes. All affected individuals are male and the condition manifests as hypogonadism. The majority (>80%) of Klinefelter syndrome individuals are associated with a 47XXY karyotype. Abnormalities associated with this disorder are related to the presence of the extra X chromosome, and the origin of this chromosome (maternal versus paternal) does not affect the nature of the disorder. This condition occurs in 1 in 500 live male births. Klinefelter syndrome is rarely diagnosed prior to puberty. Affected individuals tend to have a lower IQ than normal, but mental retardation is uncommon. Reduced spermatogenesis and male infertility are common among Klinefelter syndrome men.

Turner syndrome is characterized by monosomy of the X chromosome. All affected individuals are female and the condition manifests as hypogonadism. The majority (>55%) of Turner syndrome individuals are associated with a 45X karyotype. Others with Turner syndrome have structural abnormalities of the X chromosome. This condition occurs in 1 in 2000 live female births. The presentation of abnormalities in Turner syndrome may be related to the degree of mosaicism in the individual, but the most severely affected patients present with symptoms in infancy. Turner syndrome individuals commonly have congenital heart disease and fail to develop secondary sex characteristics.

Epigenetic Mechanisms in Familial Disease

Epigenetic modifications of DNA and histones play critical roles in the molecular pathogenesis of complex familial diseases. Epigenetic factors exhibit plasticity and are reactive to cues from the internal and external environments. By definition, epigenetics refers to heritable regulation of genomic functions that can be potentially reversible, which includes DNA methylation (methylation of cytosines) and histone modifications (such as histone acetylation, methylation, or phosphorylation). Epigenetic regulation or misregulation represents core unifying molecular mechanisms of complex, non-Mendelian, traits and diseases. Therefore, epigenetically regulated (or misregulated) genes carrying no mutations or predisposing polymorphisms may have harmful consequences if not expressed in the correct amount, at the right time in the cell cycle, or in the right location within the cell. Increasing evidence indicates that cells can operate normally only if both DNA sequence and epigenetic components of the cellular genome function properly. The role of epigenetics has been investigated in various rare pediatric syndromes, like Prader–Willi syndrome, Angelman syndrome, Beckwith–Wiedemann syndrome, and Rett syndrome, as well as in Alzheimer disease, Parkinson disease, and fragile X syndrome.

Alzheimer disease is the most common age-dependent neurodegenerative disorder and is linked to family history. Pathological pathways of Alzheimer disease include aberrant processing of amyloid precursor protein (APP), the Aβ precursor, and hyperphosphorylation of tau. The APP gene is constitutively methylated under normal conditions and becomes hypomethylated with age. Alzheimer disease has more recently been associated with modified histone acetylation profiles as well as elevated levels of phosphorylated histone H3. Therefore, it seems likely that epigenetic mechanisms are a marker of disease and triggers signaling cascades linked with a number of pathological mechanisms in Alzheimer disease.

Parkinson disease affects 1–2% of the population over the age of 65 and 4% of those over the age of 85. A family history of Parkinson disease occurs in approximately 20% of cases and studies of families with Parkinson disease have identified 15 Parkinson disease loci (PARK1-15) that are associated with the disease. There is some evidence that five of those genes (α-*synuclein, parkin, PTEN, DJ-1,* and *leucine-rich repeat kinase 2*) cause typical Parkinson disease and mutations in *ATP13A2* cause a form of autosomal recessive Parkinson disease (Kufor–Rakeb disease). Two of these genes (α-*synuclein* and *leucine-rich repeat kinase 2*) cause autosomal forms of Parkinson disease, where *parkin, PTEN, DJ-1,* and *ATP13A2* are inherited in an autosomal recessive fashion. A number of studies have shown α-*synuclein* to be misregulated in Parkinson disease due to aberrant DNA methylation patterns. However, no differences in the percentage of DNA methylation between Parkinson disease patients and normal individuals have been noted for any other Parkinson Disease-associated genes. α-*synuclein* interacts with histones and inhibits histone acetylation and HDACis have been shown to be neuroprotective against toxicity associated with aberrant regulation of α-*synuclein*.

Fragile X syndrome is an X-linked disorder and the most common inherited form of mental retardation. Fragile X syndrome affects an estimated 1 in 4000 males and 1 in 6000 females, and approximately 1 in 100–250 women in the general population is fragile X carriers. Fragile X is caused by a CGG trinucleotide repeat expansion in the 5′-untranslated region of the folate-sensitive fragile site (*FMR1*) gene. *FMR1* is involved in regulating translation at synapses and mRNA transport. Normally, 6–52 copies of the CGG trinucleotide repeat are present. However, patients with fragile X syndrome typically have >200 repeats. Affected individuals show DNA hypermethylation of the repeat region leading to *FMR1* silencing. DNMT inhibitors have been successful at reactivating *FMR1* transcription.

DEVELOPMENTAL DISEASES

Developmental diseases represent a broad category of diseases that are driven by genetic and epigenetic alterations in the genome. Many developmental diseases are also considered to be diseases of childhood or pediatric diseases. This is primarily because the developmental abnormalities manifest in the developing fetus, the neonate, or in early childhood. These congenital abnormalities generally represent structural defects that are present at birth, although some do not present until later in development. For instance, cardiac and renal abnormalities may not present for several years after birth.

Major Forms of Developmental Disease

Developmental diseases primarily reflect errors in morphogenesis. These diseases include (i) malformations, (ii) disruptions, and (iii) deformations. In addition, secondary abnormalities can result from primary manifestations of developmental disease. Some of these are sequence abnormalities and others are considered malformation syndromes.

Malformations are the manifestation of intrinsic abnormalities of the developmental processes. Hence, these represent primary errors of morphogenesis. Malformations are typically the result of multiple factors rather than a single gene defect or single chromosomal abnormality. In some cases, malformations are restricted to a single organ system (like the heart), and in others, several organ systems may be involved. Furthermore, malformations vary in severity. Some are cosmetic, and others cause functional consequences that can be tolerated, while others are lethal. Examples of less severe malformations include polydactyly (the presence of extra digits) and syndactyly (fusion of multiple digits). Malformations of functional consequence include cleft lip, which requires surgical correction, but can be tolerated. More severe malformations include those that affect proper formation of the brain and nervous system, which usually result in stillbirth.

Disruptions result from secondary destructive processes impinging on a tissue or body region that was previously normal in development. Hence, disruptions arise from extrinsic disturbances to morphogenesis. A variety of environmental agents have been suggested to cause disruptions. Given the nature of this form of congenital anomaly, disruptions are not heritable. Amniotic bands represent one example of a disruption. Amniotic bands refer to the rupture of the amnion resulting in the formation of a band that encircles, compresses, or attaches to parts of the developing fetus.

Deformations are similar to disruptions in that they represent the end result of an extrinsic disturbance to development rather than an intrinsic error of morphogenesis. Deformations are very common, affecting approximately 2% of live births. The pathogenesis of deformations involves localized or generalized compression of the growing fetus by abnormal biomechanical forces. The compression of the fetus leads to a variety of structural abnormalities. The most common cause of deformation is uterine constraint that can result from an imbalance in the growth of the fetus and the uterus late in gestation. A number of maternal factors can contribute to this phenomenon, including first pregnancy, small uterine size, malformed uterus, or presence of leiomyomas. Likewise, several fetal factors can contribute to deformation, including the presence of multiple fetuses, abnormal fetus presentation, or lack of sufficient amniotic fluid.

Gene Alterations and Developmental Disease

Genes that directly regulate morphogenesis are thought to be targets of teratogens. Hence, exposure of the mother (and developing fetus) to such agents can affect specific developmental processes. Likewise, genes that regulate patterns of gene expression in fetal development may also be targets of the action of teratogens. For instance, the *Hox* family of transcriptional regulators control the expression of numerous genes that govern development. Agents that alter *Hox* gene function produce malformations in experimental model systems. One such agent that targets *Hox* gene function is retinoic acid. Infants born to mothers that have been exposed to retinoic acid (as a treatment for severe acne) tend to display retinoic acid embryopathy (characterized by CNS and heart defects, as well as craniofacial abnormalities). In animal models, *Hox* disruptors cause fetal abnormalities that are similar to those seen in retinoic acid embryopathy.

Chromosomal Abnormalities and Developmental Disease

Angelman syndrome is an example of a developmental disease whose molecular pathogenesis frequently involves a chromosomal abnormality. The Angelman syndrome gene (*UBE3A*) is located on chromosome 15 (at 15q12). In the majority of cases, a large deletion encompassing 15q12 (and the *UBE3A* locus) results in a deficiency for the *UBE3A* gene product and Angelman syndrome ensues. In some cases, loss of *UBE3A* expression/function is attributed to uniparental disomy or inactivating gene mutation. Children with Angelman syndrome display developmental delays that are typically evident by 6–12 months of age. In affected children, language comprehension and nonverbal skills develop, but spoken language is rudimentary. Angelman syndrome children also have difficulties with movement/balance, hand flapping movements, hyperactive behavior, and short attention span, as well as some other physical features and functional deficits (including sleep and feeding issues).

Epigenetic Mechanisms and Developmental Diseases

Environmental signals that occur early during development may produce epigenetic modifications that are inherited along with potential long-term consequences. Epigenetic modifications depict a memory of environmental exposures such as inadequate or inappropriate chemical or nonchemical (nutrition) exposures that can influence early development. Studies of monozygotic twins have shown epigenetic alterations in a number of developmental diseases such as bipolar disorder, Silver–Russell syndrome, Beckwith–Wiedemann syndrome, and transient neonatal diabetes mellitus. For example, Beckwith–Wiedemann syndrome is a maternally transmitted disorder that leads to a predisposition of embryonic tumors, such as Wilms tumor. The Beckwith–Wiedemann syndrome locus is found at chromosomal location 11p15.5 and spans approximately 1 Mb, including several imprinted genes (*IGF2*, *H19*, *KCNQ1*, and *ICR2*). Aberrant hypomethylation affects *ICR2* and *KCNQ1*. However, the molecular mechanism of epigenetic regulation is not fully understood.

NEOPLASTIC DISEASES

Classification of Neoplastic Diseases

The word neoplasia is derived from the Greek word meaning "condition of new growth." The term tumor is commonly used to refer to a neoplasm. Tumor literally means "a swelling." In the early 1950s, R.A. Willis provided a description of neoplasm that we still utilize today: "… A neoplasm is an abnormal mass of tissue the growth of which exceeds and is uncoordinated with that of the normal tissues and persists in the same manner after the cessation of the stimuli which evoked the change…" More recently, other investigators described tumors as the result of a disease process in which a single cell acquires the ability to proliferate abnormally (clonal growth), resulting in an accumulation of progeny cells, and define cancers as tumors that have acquired the ability to invade the surrounding normal tissues. This definition highlights one of the most important distinguishing factors in the overall classification of neoplasms—the distinction between benign and malignant tumors. The division of neoplastic diseases into benign and malignant categories is extremely important, both for understanding the biology of these neoplasms and for recognizing the potential clinical challenges for treatment. At the most basic level, neoplasms are classified as benign or malignant. Benign neoplasms exhibit no invasive characteristics and are deemed to have low probability of invasion and spread. In contrast, malignant neoplasms exhibit invasive behaviors and/or are deemed to be high risk of metastatic spread. Further subclassification of malignant neoplasms draws distinctions to (i) cancers of childhood versus cancers that primarily affect adults, (ii) solid tumors versus hematopoietic neoplasms, and (iii) hereditary cancers versus sporadic neoplasms. Both benign and malignant neoplasms are composed of neoplastic cells that form the parenchyma, and the non-neoplastic stroma that is composed of connective tissue, blood vessels, and other cells that support the tumor parenchyma. The tumor stroma serves a critical function in support of the growth of the neoplasm by providing a blood supply for oxygen and nutrients. In nearly all cases, the parenchymal cells determine the biologic behavior (and clinical course) of the neoplasm. Further, the parenchymal cell type of the neoplasm determines how the lesion is named.

Genetic Predisposition of Neoplastic Disease

Cancer is not a single disease, but is a myriad collection of diseases with as many different manifestations as there are tissues and cell types in the human body. All of these disease states share in common certain biological properties of the cells that compose the tumors, including unregulated (clonal) cell growth, impaired cellular differentiation, invasiveness, and metastatic potential. It is now recognized that cancer, in its simplest form, is a genetic disease. More precisely, cancer is a disease of abnormal gene expression. The molecular mechanisms governing uncontrolled cellular proliferation in neoplastic disease involve loss, mutation, or dysregulation of genes that positively and negatively regulate cell proliferation, migration, and differentiation. Carcinogenesis is the multistep process through which cancer develops in response to changes in gene expression driven by chromosomal alterations, gene mutations, and epigenetic alterations of DNA. The idea that carcinogenesis is a multistep process is supported by morphologic observations of the transitions between premalignant (benign) cell growth and malignant tumors. In colorectal cancer (and some other cancer systems), the transition from benign lesion to malignant neoplasm can be easily documented and occurs in discernible stages, including benign adenoma, carcinoma in situ, invasive carcinoma, and eventually local and distant metastasis. Moreover, specific genetic alterations have been shown to correlate with each of these well-defined histopathologic stages of tumor development and progression. However, it is important to recognize that it is the accumulation of multiple genetic alterations in affected cells (and associated abnormal gene expression patterns), and not necessarily the order in which these changes accumulate that determines cancer formation and progression.

Familial Cancer Syndromes

A number of familial cancer syndromes and hereditary cancers have been recognized and characterized. Familial cancers have been described for most major organ systems, including colon, breast, ovary, and skin. These cancers are associated with genetic predisposition to development of disease. Hereditary cancers are typically characterized by (i) early age at onset (or diagnosis), (ii) neoplasms arising in first-degree relatives of the index case, and (ii) in many cases multiple or bilateral tumors. For example, epidemiologic evidence has consistently pointed to family history as a strong and independent predictor of breast cancer risk. Thus, women with a first-degree relative (mother or sister) who have been diagnosed with breast cancer are at elevated risk of development of the disease themselves. This same relationship is observed in other hereditary cancers.

Inherited Mutations in Cancer Susceptibility Genes

The Li–Fraumeni syndrome was initially characterized among several kindreds with excess cancer incidence. Patients with Li–Fraumeni syndrome develop various types of neoplasms, including breast cancer, soft tissue sarcomas and osteosarcomas, brain tumors, and various forms of leukemia, among others. Cancer susceptibility among individuals with Li–Fraumeni syndrome follows an autosomal dominant pattern of inheritance and is highly penetrant (90% by age 70), but many neoplasms develop early in life. It is now known that Li–Fraumeni syndrome is associated with germ-line mutations in the $p53$ tumor suppressor gene.

It is well known that approximately 5–10% of breast cancers are related to genetic predisposition. These breast cancers are typically associated with a strong family history of breast cancer development. A substantial amount of research has led to the discovery of several breast cancer susceptibility genes, including $BRCA1$, $BRCA2$, and $p53$, which may account for the majority of inherited breast cancers. In some cases, families at increased susceptibility for breast cancer also show elevated rates of ovarian cancer. Patients that are affected by familial breast and ovarian cancer syndrome tend to have germ-line mutation of $BRCA1$.

Familial melanoma is associated with (i) a family history of melanoma, (ii) the presence of large numbers of common or atypical nevi, (iii) a history of primary melanoma or other (nonmelanoma) skin cancers, (iv) immunosuppression, (v) susceptibility to sunburn, and/or (vi) a history of blistering sunburn. Given the linkage between excess exposure to sunlight and development of skin cancers (including melanoma), it is not surprising that susceptibility to sunburn (sensitivity to sunlight) would confer an increased risk of melanoma. This susceptibility is particularly pronounced in individuals with fair complexion characterized by freckling, blue eyes, red hair, and skin that burns readily in response to sunlight and/or fails to tan. Two highly penetrant melanoma susceptibility genes have been identified: $CDKN2A$ (which encodes cyclin-dependent kinase inhibitor 2A) and $CDK4$ (which encodes cyclin-dependent kinase 4). $CDKN2A$ is found on chromosome 9p21 and $CDK4$ resides on 12q13. Germ line inactivating mutations of the $CDKN2A$ gene are the most common cause of inherited susceptibility to melanoma, while mutations of $CDK4$ occur much more rarely. Nevertheless, germ-line mutations of $CDKN2A$ are rare and many account for a very small proportion of melanoma susceptibility among the general population. The $CDKN2A$ gene encodes two important cell cycle regulatory proteins: $p16^{INK4A}$ and $p14^{ARF}$. While other melanoma susceptibility loci have been mapped through genome-wide linkage analysis, the gene targets that contribute to familial melanoma predisposition remain undiscovered for a large proportion of recognized kindreds. Ongoing research is focused on the identification of low-penetrance melanoma susceptibility genes that confer a lower melanoma risk with more frequent variations. For instance, specific variants of the $MC1R$ and the $OCA2$ genes have been demonstrated to confer an increase in melanoma risk.

As the prototypic tumor suppressor gene, the mechanism of inactivation and loss of function associated with the $Rb1$ gene are illustrative of the whole class of tumor suppressor genes. The inactivation of both alleles of the $Rb1$ gene is required for development of retinoblastoma, an eye malignancy that usually occurs at a very young age. Two mutations are required for development of retinoblastoma and these mutations are inactivating mutations. Thus, the loss of both functional copies of the *Rb1* gene is necessary for neoplastic transformation and cancer formation. The *Rb1* gene has been found to be associated with many human neoplasms, usually through a genetic mechanism involving mutations or deletions.

Familial cancers affecting a number of other tissues and organs have been described or suggested. Familial cancer of the pancreas has been reported and suggested to follow an autosomal dominant inheritance pattern. A familial form of gastric cancer has been suggested to represent approximately 10% of all gastric cancers and is associated with the *CDH1* gene on chromosome 16q22.1. A genome-wide scan of 66 high-risk prostate cancer families produced evidence of disease linkage to chromosome 1q24-25. Subsequently, the chromosome 1q24-25 susceptibility locus was connected to the *HPC1* gene.

Cancer Associated with Faulty DNA Repair Mechanisms

Colorectal cancer is a fairly common disease worldwide, and particularly in populations from Western nations. A substantial fraction of colorectal cancers exhibit a genetic component, and several familial colorectal cancer syndromes are recognized, including familial adenomatous polyposis (FAP) and hereditary nonpolyposis colon cancer (HNPCC). Genes associated with each of these conditions have been identified and characterized. Of these familial colorectal cancer syndromes, HNPCC has been determined to be related to defective DNA repair. HNPCC is characterized by the occurrence of predominately right-sided colorectal carcinoma with an early age of onset and an increased risk of the development of certain extracolonic cancers, including cancers of the endometrium, stomach, urinary tract, and breast. Tumors associated with HNPCC exhibit a unique form of genomic instability, which represents a unique mechanism for a genome-wide tendency for instability in short repeat sequences (microsatellites), which was originally termed the replication error phenotype. The molecular defect responsible for microsatellite instability in HNPCC involves the genes that encode proteins required for normal mismatch repair.

Two additional familial cancer syndromes have been described that exhibit clinical features similar to that of HNPCC or FAP. The Muir–Torre syndrome is defined by the development of at least one sebaceous gland neoplasm and a minimum of one internal cancer, which is frequently colorectal carcinoma. This syndrome shares several features with HNPCC syndromes Lynch I and Lynch II, including the occurrence of microsatellite instability in a subset of cancers. This observation suggests the possible involvement of abnormal mismatch repair mechanisms in the genesis of a subset of Muir–Torre syndrome tumors. Turcot syndrome is defined by the occurrence of a primary brain tumor and multiple colorectal adenomas. The molecular basis for this syndrome has been suggested to involve mutation of the *APC* gene or mutation of a mismatch repair gene in tumors exhibiting microsatellite instability.

Chromosomal Instability and Cancer Susceptibility

The observation that most cancer cells contain discernible genetic abnormalities (chromosomal aberrations and/or DNA sequence abnormalities) suggests that all neoplastically transformed cells have sustained genetic damage and may have experienced some form of genomic instability during their development. Cancer cells from patients with HNPCC exhibit progressive genomic instability, which is manifest as alterations in microsatellite sequences.

Gene Mutations and Other Molecular Alterations in Nonfamilial Neoplastic Disease

Nonfamilial Cancers

Research efforts have revealed that different forms of cancer share common molecular mechanisms governing uncontrolled cellular proliferation, involving loss, mutation, or dysregulation of genes that positively and negatively regulate cell proliferation, migration, and differentiation (generally classified as proto-oncogenes and tumor suppressor genes). The majority of human cancers are classified as solid tumors (grouped as carcinomas or sarcomas). The major types of solid tumors include lung, colorectal, liver, skin, prostate, breast, ovarian, brain, and cervical. The exceptions to this classification include the malignant neoplasms of hematopoietic origin, including lymphoma, myeloma, and leukemia.

Gene Mutations in Nonfamilial Neoplastic Diseases

Several cellular proto-oncogenes have been shown to be activated through point mutation. However, the c-*ras* family of proto-oncogenes represents the most important subset of proto-oncogenes that are activated through this mechanism. This family includes the cellular homologs of the Harvey-*ras* (H-*ras*) and Kirsten-*ras* (K-*ras*) retroviral oncogenes. The activated form of c-*ras* (oncogenic) exhibits markedly different properties from that of the normal c-*ras* proto-oncogene. The activated form consistently and efficiently induces neoplastic transformation in cultured cells, whereas the normal proto-oncogene does not. The critical molecular difference between the two forms of c-*ras* was found in the nucleic acid sequence—the activated form of c-*ras* harbors a point mutation in codon 12 of exon 1, which results in a glycine to valine amino acid substitution. Up to 30% of all human neoplasms are now known to harbor c-*ras* mutations, and mutations in c-H-*ras*, c-K-*ras*, and N-*ras* reflect specific alterations affecting only codon 12 (most mutations), codon 13, or codon 61. An additional mutation in an intron of c-H-*ras* has been shown to upregulate production of the structurally normal gene product, resulting in increased transforming activity. A common theme of c-*ras* mutations is that a single point mutation is capable of drastically altering the biological activity of a normal protein product into one with efficient transforming properties. Mutations of c-*ras* are found in a large number of human tumor types, including thyroid, gastrointestinal tract, uterus, lung, myelodysplastic syndromes, and leukemias.

Abnormal DNA Repair Mechanisms in Nonfamilial Neoplastic Diseases

Several rare genetic disorders involving dysfunctional DNA repair pathways are associated with elevated risk of cancer development. These disorders include xeroderma pigmentosum, ataxia telangiectasia, and Fanconi anemia. Individuals affected by these conditions are prone to development of various malignancies when exposed to specific DNA damaging agents. Patients with xeroderma pigmentosum display hypersensitivity to UV light and increased incidence of several types of skin cancer, including basal cell carcinoma, squamous cell carcinoma, and malignant melanoma. Patients with ataxia telangiectasia exhibit hypersensitivity to ionizing radiation and chemical agents, and are predisposed to the development of B-cell lymphoma and chronic lymphocytic leukemias, and affected women demonstrate an increased risk of developing breast cancer. Patients with Fanconi anemia demonstrate sensitivity to DNA cross-linking agents and are predisposed to malignancies of the hematopoietic system, particularly acute myelogenous leukemia.

Bloom syndrome is a rare genetic disorder that involves dysfunctional DNA repair pathways. Patients with Bloom syndrome demonstrate an increased incidence of several forms of cancer, including leukemia, skin cancer, and breast cancer. These patients exhibit chromosomal instability that manifest as abnormally high levels of sister chromatid exchange. The molecular defect in Bloom syndrome has been suggested to involve faulty regulation of DNA repair enzymes. The candidate Bloom syndrome gene product is an enzyme with helicase activity.

Chromosomal Alterations in Nonfamilial Neoplastic Diseases

The majority of human cancers (including solid tumors, leukemias, and lymphomas) contain chromosomal abnormalities, consisting of either numerical changes (aneuploidy) and/or structural aberrations. These two general types of chromosomal damage may reflect two distinct mechanisms of chromosomal instability: (i) chromosome number instability and (ii) chromosome structure instability. In some forms of cancer, chromosomal instabilities predominate over nucleotide sequence instabilities, suggesting that these mechanisms of genetic instability may not significantly overlap. It is generally accepted that many (if not the majority) of the alterations of chromosome structure occurring in cancer cells confer some selective advantage to the evolving tumor. Thus, accumulation of a critical number of chromosomal aberrations or development of specific chromosomal abnormalities may represent essential steps in the process of neoplastic transformation. Three general forms of chromosomal structural alterations are observed in cancer cells: gene amplifications, rearrangements and translocations, and large-scale deletions. The p53 tumor suppressor protein has long been suggested to play significant roles in cell cycle progression and cell cycle checkpoint function in response to DNA damage. The p53 gene is commonly mutated in human cancers, and these same cancers frequently exhibit abnormalities of chromosome number. Therefore, it has been suggested that the loss of normal p53 function may contribute significantly to chromosomal instability in certain forms of cancer.

Epigenetics of Cancer

In cancer cells, epigenetic alterations occur within the larger context of extensive changes to chromatin structure related to altered patterns of histone modification, and methylation gains and losses on CpG dinucleotides within DNA sequences. The most studied and best-understood mechanism of epigenetic regulation is DNA methylation, which can transcriptionally silence tumor suppressor genes (and other negative mediators of neoplastic growth) resulting in selective growth advantages for emergent neoplastic cells. Neoplastic transformation associated with alterations in DNA methylation includes both global loss of methylation (hypomethylation) and gene-specific gain of methylation (hypermethylation). Hypomethylation takes place mostly at DNA-repetitive regions and hypermethylation at promoter regions of tumor suppressor genes.

DNA Hypomethylation in Cancer

In the early 1980s, global DNA hypomethylation events in human cancer were discovered. Hypomethylation of cancer cell genomes is associated with loss of methylation in CpG-depleted regions where most CpG dinucleotides would be expected to be methylated. This loss of methylation in these regions of the genome is possibly associated with aberrant or inappropriate expression of some genes that could contribute to neoplastic transformation, tumorigenesis, or cancer progression. In addition, genome-wide demethylation can contribute to chromosomal instability by destabilizing pericentromeric regions of certain chromosomes.

DNA Hypermethylation in Cancer

Gains in DNA methylation in cancer cells typically reflect hypermethylation of CpG islands in gene promoter regions, which can lead to gene silencing. The identification of CpG island promoter hypermethylation of tumor suppressor genes in cancer cells occurred in the mid-1990s. Methylation-dependent gene silencing is a normal mechanism for regulation of gene expression. However, in cancer cells methylation-dependent epigenetic gene silencing represents a mutation-independent mechanism for inactivation of tumor suppressor genes. A significant number of cancer-related genes have been identified that are subject to methylation-dependent silencing, and many of these genes contribute to the hallmarks of cancer.

Histone Modifications in Cancer

Aberrant lysine methyltransferase activity on histones is associated with a number of pathological states including various genetic diseases and cancer. Interestingly, lysine residues can either be mono-methylated, di-methylated, or tri-methylated, and each of these modifications is performed by a histone methyltransferase (HMT) that is responsible for a particular methylation mark that is dispersed throughout the genome. The aberrant regulation of HMTs results in loss or overexpression of the methylation mark that the enzyme is responsible for, which leads to abnormal gene expression and can ultimately lead to tumorigenesis. In addition, the metabolism of converting S-adenosylmethionine (SAM) to S-adenosylhomocysteine (SAH) by HMTs can be influenced by diet, and aberrant regulation of this process can contribute to carcinogenesis. The Rb pathway consists of the cooperative interplay of HDACs and HMTs, and is mutated in the majority (90%) of human solid tumors, an observation that may explain why Rb1 is a favored target of mutations in cancer. Histone H3 lysine 9 (H3K9) methylation by the HMT, G9a, or SETDB1, is critical for gene repression and the formation of heterochromatin in both fission yeast and mammals. In contrast, the methylation of histone H3 lysine 4 (H3K4) by the methyltransferase, SET7/9 is linked to transcriptional activation. The HMT responsible for methylating histone H3 lysine 27 (H3K27) is EZH2 and has been found to be involved in the progression of prostate cancer. There are two HMTs that have been found to methylate H3K36 in humans, NSD1 and HYPB, and both have been implicated in genetic disorders. NSD1 was found to be essential for embryo development in mice, and gene mutations have been associated with cerebral gigantism, called Sotos syndrome [171,173]. HYPB was identified as a huntingtin-interacting protein, and is implicated in the development of Huntington disease.

Recent work has shown that H4K20 methylation is lost in cancer cells. Furthermore, when the SUV4-20H enzyme responsible for H4K20 methylation is knocked out in mice, they are prone to develop cancer. This result indicates that HMTs for H4K20 methylation could function as tumor suppressor genes. In addition, the H3K4 methyltransferase, MLL, is translocated in hematological malignancies. In a recent study, the HMT associated with H3K79, hDOT1L, interacts with a MLL fusion partner involved in acute myeloid leukemia, and direct fusion of these two proteins results in leukemic transformation, indicating the mistargeting of hDOT1L can lead to leukemia. In addition to aberrant HMTs, there have also been several lines of evidence that acetyltransferases (HATs) are involved in carcinogenesis. The H4K16 HATs, MOZ, MOF, and MORF are recruited to repeat sequences in cancer cells, and leukemias and uterine myomas carry translocations that generate fusion proteins such as CREB-binding protein (CBP)-MOZ and MORF-CBP that associate with global loss of H4K16 acetylation.

Interplay Between Genetics and Epigenetics in Cancer

Whole genome sequencing has revealed that a high frequency of cancer-specific mutations in genes known to direct and participate in epigenetic processes occurs in multiple cancer types. These genes include enzymes that are required for DNA methylation (DNMTs), histone lysine methylation (EZH2, MLL), and chromatin remodeling (SMARCB1). Hence, aberrant epigenetic events may lie downstream of genetic abnormalities. The phenotypic consequences of the mutations are not well understood. Additionally, the inheritance of certain genetic alterations or mutations can increase the probability of DNA methylation targeting to key genes such as *MLH1* and could possibly contribute to familial cancers and early onset disease.

Cell Injury, Cell Death, and Aging

Howard M. Reisner, Ph.D.

The Vascular Response to Injury

Chantelle M. Rein-Smith, Ph.D., Frank C. Church, Ph.D.

GENERAL INTRODUCTION

A long tradition defines the scope of pathology as both a clinical specialty and an area of biomedical research. Although rooted in the correlation of anatomical and histological changes with clinically apparent disease (and hence the iconic images of autopsy and microscope), modern pathology studies the causes of disease (**etiology**) and the expression/evolution of such (**pathogenesis**) at the molecular level using the tools of molecular genetics and biochemical analysis as well as at the cellular and organ system levels. Because (as is apparent to the clinician) the first symptoms and signs of disease are often those of the body's response to injury, the pathologist is acutely interested in characterizing this response since, more often than not, such provides critical clues as to the etiological agent and likely mode of pathogenesis.

As a clinical endeavor, pathology is both a diagnostic and prognostic specialty, which by defining and classifying the disease process, hopes to suggest (and help evaluate) therapeutic approaches to the physician. But in a broad sense, pathology seeks to understand the basis of the disease process. At times, this broad scope of interest leads to a "pathocentric" view of medicine **(Figure 2-1)**.

This chapter will present an overview of how the pathologist views mechanisms of irreversible cell injury (cell death), reversible cell injury, and the organism's response to both. Oxygen deprivation to tissue (**ischemia**) leading to a form of tissue damage termed an **infarct** is of notable clinical significance (e.g., in **myocardial infarcts**, "heart attacks") and will serve as an important model. Second, this chapter will briefly consider injury resulting from the process of host defense, either as appropriately targeted to tissue injury or inappropriately directed toward self-components either as "bystander effects" or "autoimmunity." Finally, the chapter will consider changes due to the aging process. A simplistic, but nevertheless useful overview of this chapter is presented in **Figure 2-2**.

CELL INJURY AND CELL DEATH: AN INTRODUCTION

An interest in the effects of disease and trauma is nothing new. People have been pathologists observing the effects of disease since the dawn of recorded history, likely before. Egyptian medical texts described infectious diseases (tetanus is an often quoted example). The Tanach (Hebrew Bible) tells of a disease visited upon the Philistines that may well have been bubonic plague. The Iliad describes the surgeon Machaon treating Menaleus' arrow wound. Egyptian physicians described the host reaction to such wounds (suppuration, inflammation) as early as the third millennium BC and may have treated such wounds with antiseptic agents. Pathologists now study the cause (etiology), progression (pathogenesis), and host reaction to disease as a career in order to diagnose the illness, prognosticate, help suggest the best therapy, and ultimately discover the cause of death.

Death at the level of the organism (**somatic death**) would seem easy to define but it is not. This uncertainty has been historically expressed as fear of premature burial, a likely source of the custom of wakes and attendance on the recently dead. In 18th century, France brass pins under finger and toenails was a test for death, but the odor of decay was held more certain (a reasonable sign of postmortem change). Currently, brain death (irreversible coma) is generally accepted as the legal/clinical definition of somatic death. In a multicellular organism, cells die at different rates (depending in part on their particular requirement for oxidative metabolism). With the cessation of heartbeat, cerebral neurons, lacking oxygen, die within minutes, muscle, skin, and bone cells may survive for days. "Cessation of all life at the cellular level is not a necessary criterion for determination of death" (World Medical Association Declaration on Death). Hence, the medical determination of death relies on clinical judgment supplemented by a variety of neurological, physiological, and imaging

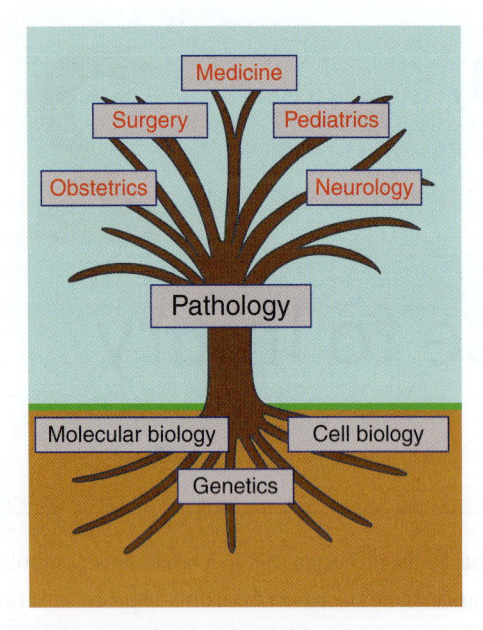

FIGURE 2-1 "Pathocentric" view of medicine.

techniques aimed at defining the cause and irreversibility of coma. Brain-dead individuals are respirator dependent, are areflexive and lack deep intracranial electrical activity. Removed from the respirator blood pressure collapses, oxidative metabolism ceases, and postmortem changes begin. ATP-dependent cellular processes such as the calcium transporting ATPases in muscle sarcomeres fail. The diffusion of calcium inward produces unrelieved muscle contraction termed rigor mortis ceasing only with the onset of decomposition of cells by cellular enzymes and bacteria.

Many societies have tried to prevent or slow postmortem decomposition. Mummification, the drying or embalming of the corpse as practised in pharaonic Egypt for reasons of religion, led to the understanding that the root of decomposition was the gut, which was removed prior to the application of chemical drying agents and preservatives. Observations made during the process of mummification led Egyptian concepts of disease to center around the anus, presumably because of what we now know to be the role of colonic bacterial flora in early decomposition. Based on these observations, an Egyptian pathologist might have considered rot as the etiological agent of disease, pathogenesis as the spread of rot from its source (the anus) through the body.

Contemporary pathologists maintain an interest in somatic death and injury, although as will be discussed in this chapter the focus has shifted to **cellular** death and injury and the **molecular** mechanisms associated with such. Nevertheless, the forensic pathologist interested in force injury still must deal with the manner and cause of death in cases of trauma where much or all of the body is affected. From the 14th century forward, the increasing popularity of anatomical dissection in Europe focused interest on abnormalities of organs and organ systems. The process of correlation of visible abnormality with disease continued through the 19th century and continues even today. The perfection of the microscope combined with the development of histological procedures for the fixation, sectioning, and staining of tissue by the late 19th century established our current emphasis on the expression of disease in tissue and cells, an emphasis now combined with genomic and proteomic pathology.

This chapter will discuss the visible signs of cell injury and death and the consequent host response using the well-established tools of the surgical pathologist who examines biopsy material (tissue taken from the living patient) to establish diagnosis or autopsy material to establish or confirm the cause of death. But the chapter will also summarize the molecular mechanisms associated with cell injury, death, and the host response to demonstrate how knowledge of basic mechanisms may translate into a better understanding of etiology and pathogenesis and improved patient care and perhaps a better understanding of the inevitable process of aging.

An all too common clinical scenario will serve to introduce many of the concepts presented in this chapter (see Case 2-1).

REVERSIBLE CELL INJURY

It is convenient to divide the effects of cell injury as being irreversible (lethal) or potentially reversible. However, there is no well-defined "point of no return" separating the two. Although pathologists most commonly use the morphological pattern of tissue injury to divide reversible from lethal injury, biochemical and molecular analysis is increasingly useful. Case 2-1 notes the use of blood-based tests indicative of the death of specific cell populations (cardiac myocytes and hepatocytes being commonly used examples). Evidence for loss of nuclear DNA, either as noted by histological signs of nuclear fragmentation and loss (**karyorrhexis** and **karyolysis**) or biochemical analysis indicating DNase-mediated

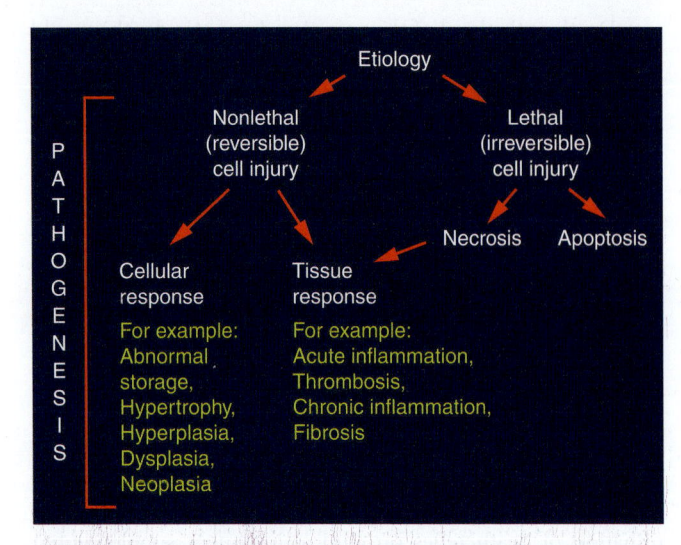

FIGURE 2-2 A simplified but useful overview.

CASE 2-1

John Doe, a 63-year-old obese man with a long history of cardiovascular disease, was drinking a double mocha frappe with extra whipped cream at his favorite coffee shop when he turned to the barista while clutching his left upper chest. He complained of crushing pain, was obviously **diaphoretic** (sweaty), and rapidly collapsed. The emergency response team arrived in 10 minutes, at which time Mr. Doe was unconscious and had no detectable pulse or heartbeat. Attempts to restore cardiac function at the scene and subsequently in the emergency room were unsuccessful and Mr. Doe was pronounced dead by the attending emergency room physician.

Given the frequency of occurrence of this particular mechanism of unattended sudden, presumably cardiac death (and Mr. Doe's prior medical history), it is unlikely that the medical examiner/forensic pathologist would have interest in requesting an autopsy (see Chapter 3). However, because this common scenario demonstrates many important principles discussed in this chapter, let us examine the temporal progression, etiology, and pathogenesis that led to Mr. Doe's pattern of irreversible cardiac myocyte injury (cellular necrosis) and ultimately somatic death.

John Doe at age 40 was diagnosed as having moderate hypertension. He was advised to lose weight, exercise, and prescribed a regimen of antihypertensive drugs (which he ignored claiming they made him feel tired and dizzy).

At age 50 Mr. Doe complained of intermittent chest pain on exertion that subsided on rest. His physician noted an enlarged left ventricular profile on plain chest film. Mr. Doe submitted to a supervised stress test. Resultant chest pain subsided on administration of a vasodilator (sublingual nitroglycerin). Mr. Doe was diagnosed with **left ventricular hypertrophy** subsequent to untreated hypertension and **stable angina pectoris** (chest pain resulting from reversible cardiac muscle ischemia most often related to compromise of blood flow in the coronary arteries). The angina was presumed to result from coronary vascular disease, **atherosclerosis**. Mr. Doe was placed on an aggressive course of antihypertensive and blood lipid reducing agents and provided with nitroglycerin tabs. He refused all invasive procedures aimed at evaluating the extent of, and possibly treating, his coronary vascular disease. If one were able to biopsy Mr. Doe's left ventricle, we would likely have observed the following (Figure 2-3).

Figure 2-3A demonstrates normal cardiac myocytes; and Figure 2-3B shows **hypertrophic** cardiac myocytes taken from the heart of an individual with left ventricular hypertrophy. Both views are at the same magnification. In response to physiological stress, cells may either divide and increase in total number (**hyperplasia**) or, in the case where cell division cannot occur (as in cardiac myocytes), cells may increase in size alone (**hypertrophy**). In the case of Mr. Doe, the ventricle had to pump against a significantly elevated systemic blood pressure increasing the cardiac workload. Cardiac myocytes compensated by increasing in size. Note that although cardiac myocytes do not divide, they undergo endomitosis in which the average ploidy of the cells increases in the absence of cell division. The resultant increased nuclear size (so-called "boxcar" nuclei) is striking.

At age 58 Mr. Doe suffered from an episode of crushing chest pain that was unrelieved by nitroglycerine. He was taken to the hospital emergency room where blood tests for **cardiac biomarkers troponin I** and **CK-MB** indicated elevated levels consistent with cardiac myocyte cell death (**necrosis**). Such markers are proteins with specificity for cardiac muscle cells whose release into the systemic circulation is indicative loss of myocyte cell integrity. A severe myocardial infarct was diagnosed and treated. Mr. Doe survived his cardiac injury. If a series of biopsies were available during the time course of the infarct, they would have shown the following (Figure 2-4).

Figure 2-4A (about 12 hours) shows **coagulative necrosis** of cardiac myocytes. Some cells are eosinophilic and show

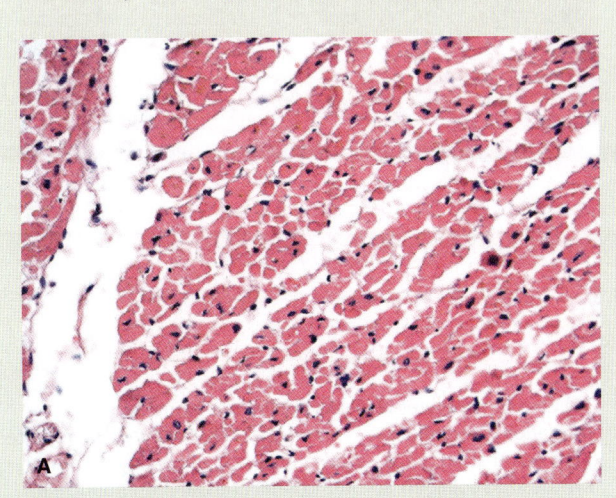

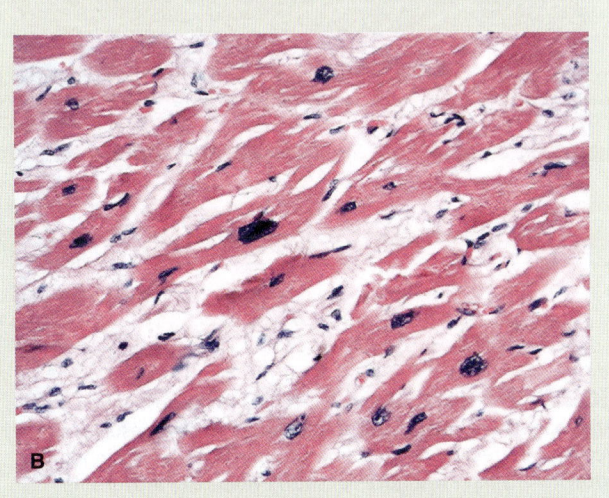

FIGURE 2-3 **(A)** Normal cardiac myocytes and **(B)** hypertrophic cardiac myocytes: Although cardiac myocytes do not divide, they compensate for the additional workload by increasing in size. The cells undergo endomitosis (increasing in ploidy without divison), resulting in large often rectangular nuclei ("boxcar nuclei").

evidence of nuclear changes ranging from partial dissolution to total loss. This is a result of irreversible injury resultant from local ischemia. Figure 2-4B (about 2 days) shows a marked infiltration of the infarct by **polymorphonuclear leukocytes** (**PMNs neutrophils**). This is characteristic of the **acute inflammatory response** to tissue injury. By about 2 weeks (Figure 2-4C) most necrotic debris has been removed from the site of the infarct by mononuclear cells, the presence of **granulation tissue**, consisting of fibroblasts, newly synthesized collagen, and sprouting capillaries, indicates a transition between **chronic inflammation** and **repair**. By 5 months, the area of the infarct has been replaced by **fibrosis** (scaring), an acellular patch consisting of compacted collagen (Figure 2-4D). Mr. Doe has survived his myocardial infarct but has been left with a compromised heart in which a collagenous scar has replaced the normal cardiac myocytes. *The pattern of necrosis, acute, and than chronic inflammation in response to cell necrosis followed by repair by fibrosis (scarring) is typical of injury to most organs and will be discussed below in detail*. Complete restitution of function (**regeneration**) is limited to only exceptional circumstances where replicative cell populations suffice to repair tissue injury in the absence of injury to the framework (stromal component) of the organ. Superficial epidermal wounds are a common example.

Between age 58 and death at age 63, Mr. Doe suffered from increasing loss of cardiac function because of recurrent cardiac ischemia (and his unwillingness to consider invasive modes of therapy). By age 63, at the time of his death, My Doe had great difficulty in walking to his favorite coffee shop and required oxygen supplementation. His sudden death was likely the result of an additional major ischemic event. His scarred heart was particularly susceptible to conduction defects and ventricular arrhythmia was also likely to have played a role (see Chapter 7).

The etiology and pathogenesis is complex involving multiple genetic, nutritional, and behavioral factors summarized as progressive ischemic cardiovascular disease.

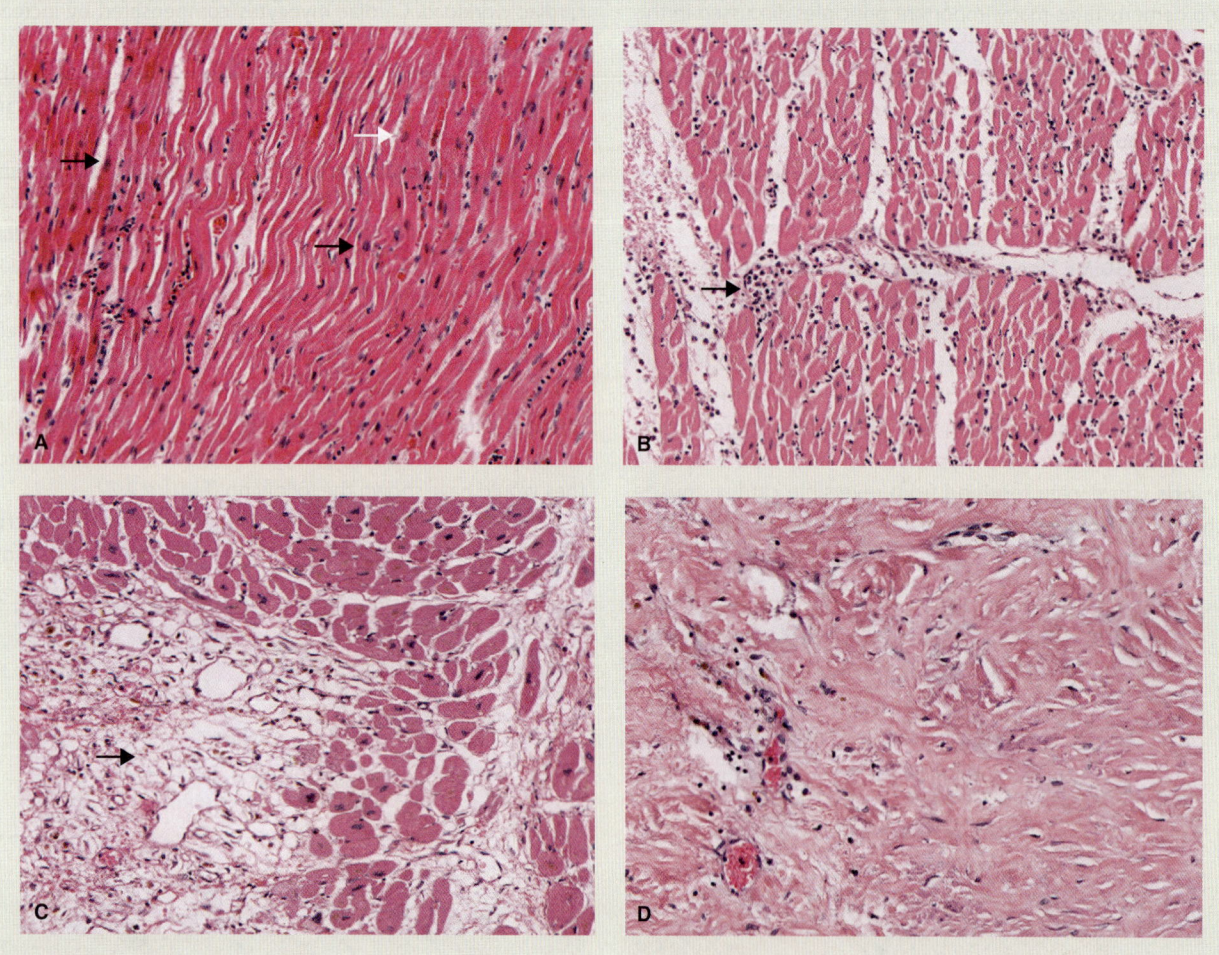

FIGURE 2-4 (**A**) Cardiac myocytes (12 hours postinfarct, early coagulative necrosis): Fibers are "wavy" (a likely result of mechanical stress on necrotic fibers). Some fibers are eosinophilic (arrow). Many have lost nuclei or show evidence of irreversible nuclear injury (smudging white arrow). (**B**) Cardiac myocytes (2 days postinfarct neutrophil infiltration acute inflammation): All fibers show evidence of necrosis and lack nuclei. Infiltration of neutrophils into tissue from vasculature is evident (arrow). (**C**) Cardiac myocytes (2 weeks postinfarct granulation tissue formation): Necrotic myocytes are partially removed and replaced with granulation tissue (arrow) consisting of fibroblasts, newly synthesized collagen, sprouting capillaries, and mononuclear cells. (**D**) Residual cardiac myocytes and scar (5 months postinfarct fibrosis): Essentially all cardiac myocytes are replaced by acellular collagenous scar. Scant mononuclear cells remain.

cleavage of DNA, would be obvious evidence of irreversible cell injury.

At the tissue level, the pathologist recognizes signs of cellular stress and injury that are potentially reversible to some degree. These patterns are often considered as normative elements of the response to increased physiological stress and hence may (or may not) be indicators of pathogenesis. These are defined as follows:

- **Hyperplasia** is the increase in *number* of cells in an organ or tissue (which may, as a result, increase in size) **(Figure 2-5)**.
- **Hypertrophy** is the increase in *size* of cells in an organ or tissue (which hence increases in size). Hyperplasia and hypertrophy often coexist (Figure 2-3).
- **Atrophy** is the decrease in the mass of an organ or tissue related to loss of cell number and/or cell size **(Figure 2-6)**.
- **Metaplasia** is the presumptively reversible change of one differentiated adult cell type to another. Most often this involves the change of one type of epithelial cell to another such as the change of ciliated mucosal epithelial cells to squamous in the bronchi of a smoker. Metaplasia can be pathogenetic and indicative of a "precancerous" change **(Figure 2-7)**.

Another cellular adaption that, unlike those above, is clearly associated with disease is **dysplasia**, an *abnormal* change in the size, shape, and pattern of growth of cells. It can be thought of as an abnormal (or atypical) form of hyperplasia/hypertrophy and as a precursor lesion to neoplasia (see Chapter 1). Dysplasia is often associated with (and often follows) metaplasia. Hence, squamous cell cancer of the lung may begin with the above-mentioned metaplasia of the bronchus **(Figure 2-8)**.

Hyperplasia and Hypertrophy

The cells of some tissues can proliferate and/or enlarge to share workload (see Case 2-1). This often serves a beneficial function in the physiological adaptation of organs to stress. For example, the athlete "pumping iron" will experience hyperplasia of the exercised skeletal muscle and possibly skin callous formation

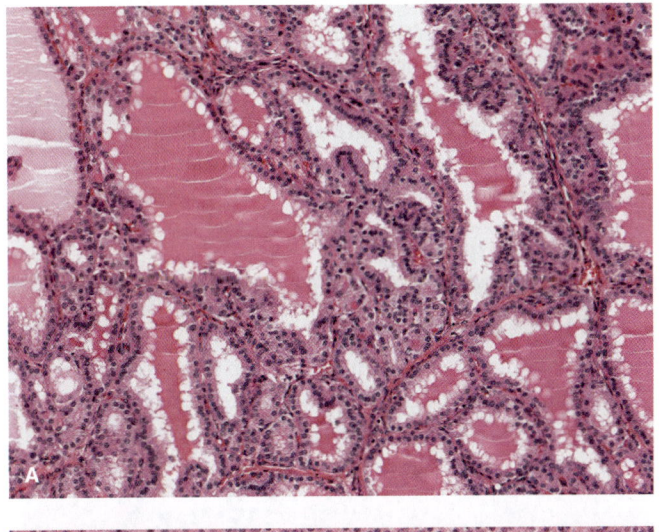

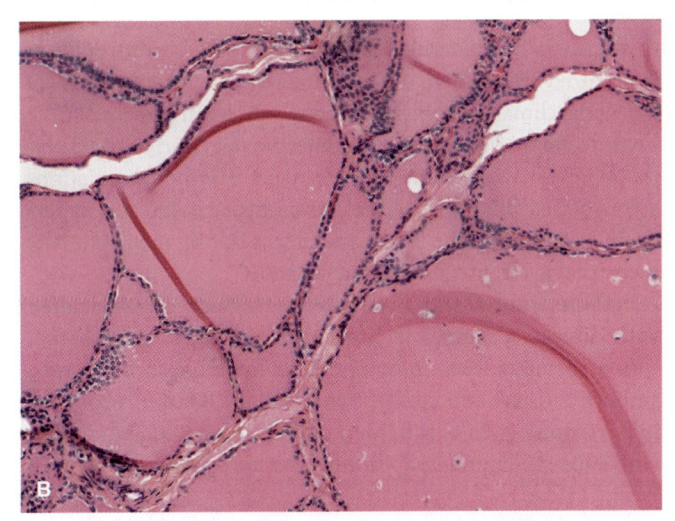

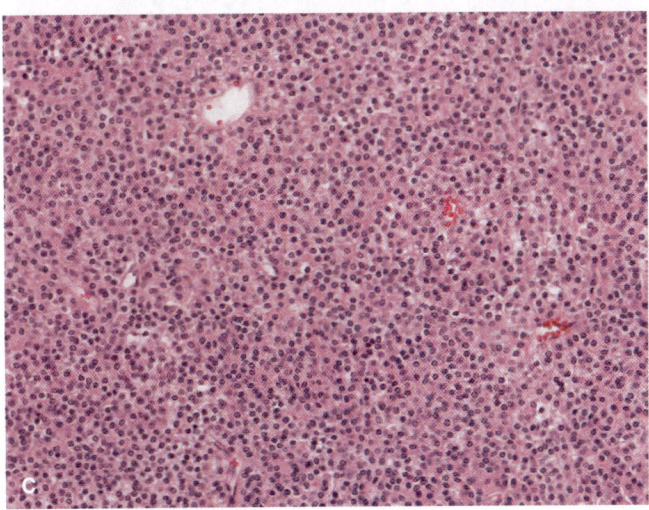

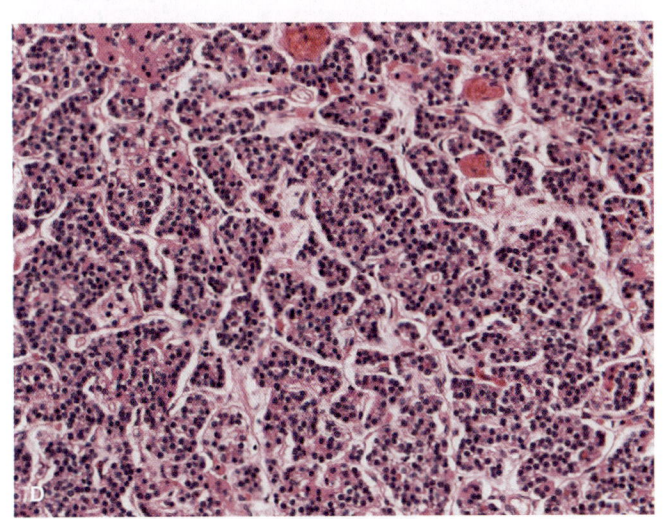

FIGURE 2-5 Two examples of endocrine gland hyperplasia: (**A**) Hyperplastic thyroid gland. Note the large number of follicular cells and small, highly active follicles as compared with (**B**) normal thyroid gland. (**C**) Hyperplastic parathyroid gland. The lobe is so packed with chief cells (principal cells) that connective tissue septae are not visible. This should be compared with (**D**) Normal parathyroid gland, which has a much lower density of cells and clearly visible septae.

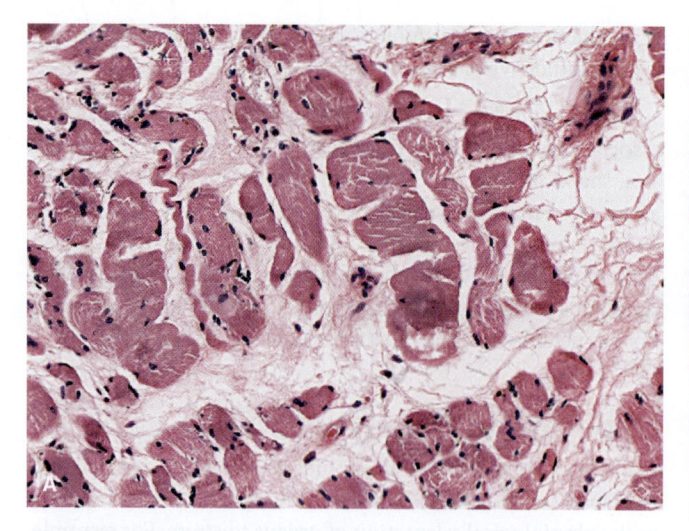

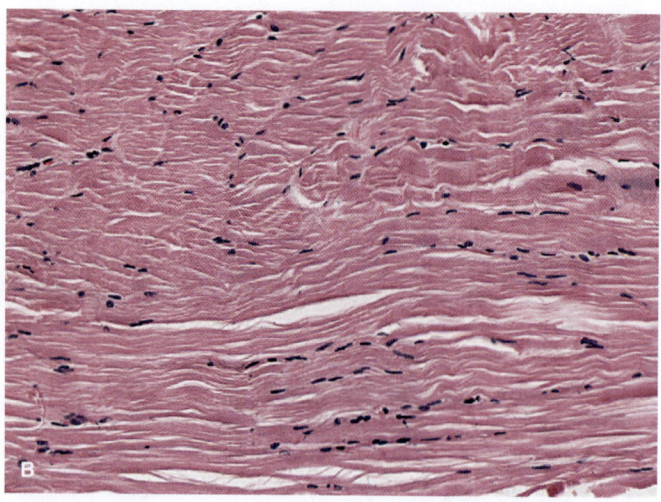

FIGURE 2-6 Denervation atrophy of skeletal muscle:
(A) Denervation of skeletal muscle leads to a characteristic form of atrophy. Myofibers loose mass and the contractile apparatus becomes disorganized until little is left but residual nuclei. The atrophic fibers become angulated on cross section. Cell necrosis ultimately occurs and the myofibers are replaced by connective tissue. **(B)** Normal skeletal myofibers.

(hyperplasia of epidermal/epithelial cells and hypertrophy of keratinized cells) where she grips the weights. Anoxic stress (of the nonacclimated to high altitudes) results in hyperplasia of erythrocyte marrow precursors; infection can lead to hyperplasia of bone marrow white cell precursors. Hormonal variations are associated with well-characterized hyperplastic and hypertrophic changes in the breast and uterus during menarche, the menstrual cycle, pregnancy, and lactation.

Hypertrophy and hyperplasia can also be associated with disease. Changes in hormones and other growth factors associated with aging result in hyperplasia of glands, smooth muscle, and connective tissue in "benign" **prostatic hypertrophy** (which is benign only in its lack of association with cancer). Human papilloma virus infection can result in impressive hypertrophy and hyperplasia of epithelial cells of the skin (warts). As noted above, (see Case 2-1) hypertension can result in ventricular hypertrophy that is initially physiological but can progresses to pathological ultimately resulting in heart failure and sudden cardiac death.

> **QUICK REVIEW**
> **Molecular Mechanisms of Hyperplasia and Hypertrophy**
> The molecular mechanisms of cardiac hypertrophy are of particular clinical significance because of their association with the most common disease among our aging population.

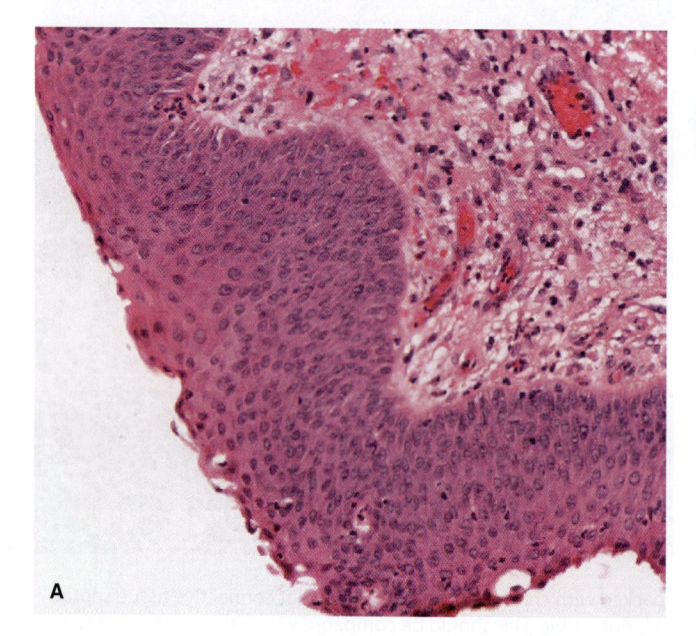

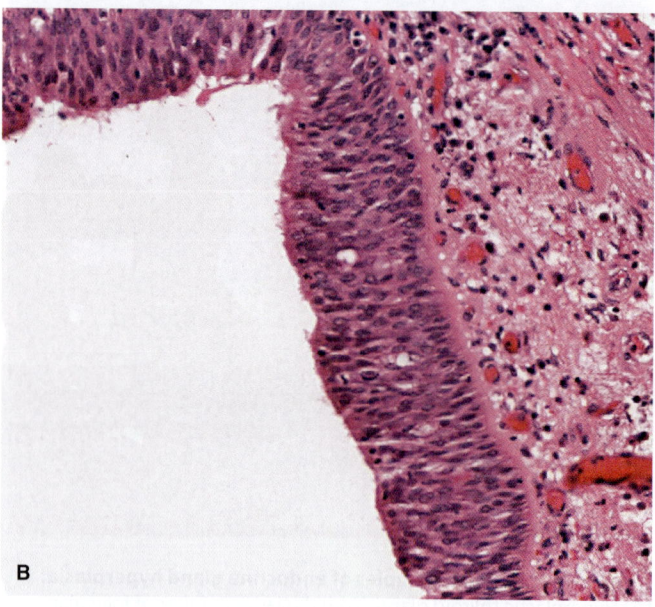

FIGURE 2-7 Metaplasia (bronchus): Two areas of the bronchus of a smoker **(A)** demonstrates squamous metaplasia and **(B)** a more normal area showing ciliated columnar epithelium.

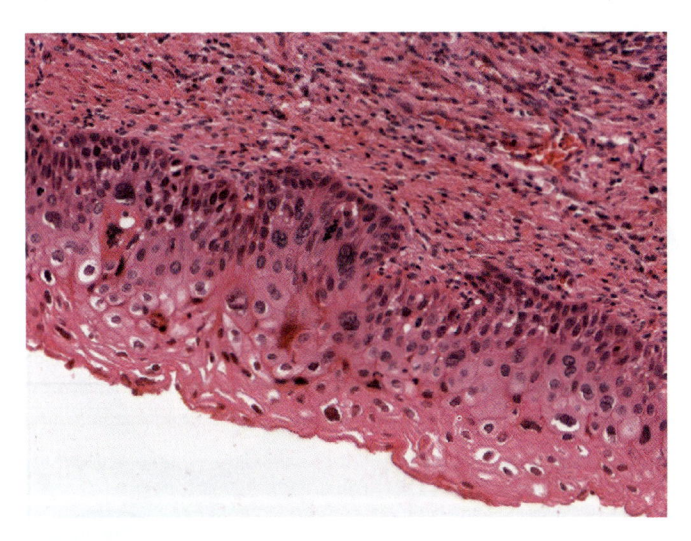

FIGURE 2-8 Dysplasia (cervix): This example of severe full thickness dysplasia is taken from the transition zone of the cervix (an area demonstrating squamous metaplasia). Cells have marked abnormality in size and shape. Nuclei are pleomorphic (differing in size and shape) and demonstrate abnormal mitoses.

The initial signals of physiological cardiac myocyte hypertrophy are biomechanical stress sensors involving integrin-mediated connections between sarcomeres and the extracellular matrix (ECM) and neurohormonal factors (such as adrenalin, angiotensin II, and endothelin) that serve to increase cardiac output in response to increased workload. Initially such signals result in compensatory increase in the expression of those genes involved in sarcomere functions, notably α-myosin heavy chain and cardiac α-actin. This increase in protein expression is associated with the addition of sarcomeres in parallel to each other and an increase in cardiomyocyte width to length ratio. Ongoing exposure of the heart to stress leads to cardiac injury and the resulting cellular response. With increased cardiac hypertrophy decreased force production occurs, vascularization is impaired, and changes in the ECM and deposition of collagen (fibrosis) occur. These nonadaptive responses are associated with induction of a distinctive array of genes:

- **Immediate early genes** involved in the rapid and transient response of cells to stimuli, resulting in changes in gene expression profiles and new protein synthesis. These include the proto-oncogenes c-jun, c-fos, and c-myc.
- **Heat shock protein genes** such as hsp70 that has both a protective role in stressed cells and aids in degrading damaged, misfolded proteins.
- **Fetal genes** normally expressed in the developing heart. These include the genes for β-myosin heavy chain, skeletal α-actin, and natriuretic factors [atrial natriuretic factor (ANF) and brain natriuretic peptide (BNP)]. BNP is of note because of its utility as a convenient biomarker for ventricular dysfunction.

A multiplicity of signaling pathways such as ligands, cellular receptors, and intracellular signal transduction pathways are involved in the hypertrophic response. Of particular importance are the following (Figure 2-9):

- **Phosphoinositide 3 kinase (PI3K)/Akt pathway:** Akt plays a crucial role in mediating many of the adaptive processes involved in the hypertrophic response, serving as the major effector of the **PI3K** signaling pathway. PI3K is activated by receptor tyrosine kinases including the insulin-like growth factor (IGF), fibroblast growth factor (FGF), and transforming growth factor (TGF) receptors. Akt *inactivates* glycogen synthetase kinase 3 beta (GSK-3-β) that *negatively* regulates cardiac size. Inactivation of this kinase leads to cardiomyocyte hypertrophy. In addition, the PI3K/Akt pathway mediates hypertrophy through the **mTOR** protein, a major regulator of cell growth and sensor of nutrient status. Cardiac hypertrophy is *opposed* by **FoxO** nuclear transcription factors. Akt phosphorylates and inactivates FoxO within the nucleus. The inactive phosphorylated FoxO is transported to the cytoplasm, ubiquinated and degraded in the proteasome.
- **G protein-coupled response (GPCR) signaling:** Adrenergic factors, angiotensin II and endothelin mediate their effects via G protein-coupled receptors (GPCRs) and the Gα (q) G protein subunit and result in activation of the PI3K pathway (see above).
- **Calcineurin signaling:** Increased Ca^{2+} released from the sarcoplasm in response to neurohormonal and mechanical stimuli leads to the activation of calcineurin by phosphorylation. Activated calcineurin in turn dephosphorylates nuclear factor of activated T cells (**NFATs**), which translocates to the nucleus where it serves to activate transcription factors important in the hypertrophic response.
- **Mitogen-activated protein kinase (MAPK) cascades:** The MAPK pathway is a complex system of protein kinase cascades that couple external stimuli (and in particular the stress response and GPCR agonists) to nuclear responses via phosphorylation. This ultimately results in the activation of multiple transcription factors including activation transcription factor 2 (**ATF-2**) and myocyte enhancer factor-2 (**MEF-2**). Of the complex family of MAPKs, **p38 kinases** and **c-jun** NH_2-terminal kinases (**JNKs**) are of particular importance in the pressure drive hypertrophic response.
- **Cytokine-mediated signaling:** Members of the interleukin 6 (**IL-6**) family of cytokines play a role in hypertrophy by binding to the gp130 containing class of cytokine receptors followed by signal transduction using the MAPK, PI3K, and JAK/STAT. The latter pathway involves the cytoplasmic phosphorylation of **STAT** proteins by **Janus kinases** (JK). Phosphorylated STAT proteins translocate to the nucleus leading the transcription of multiple genes involved in the hypertrophic response.

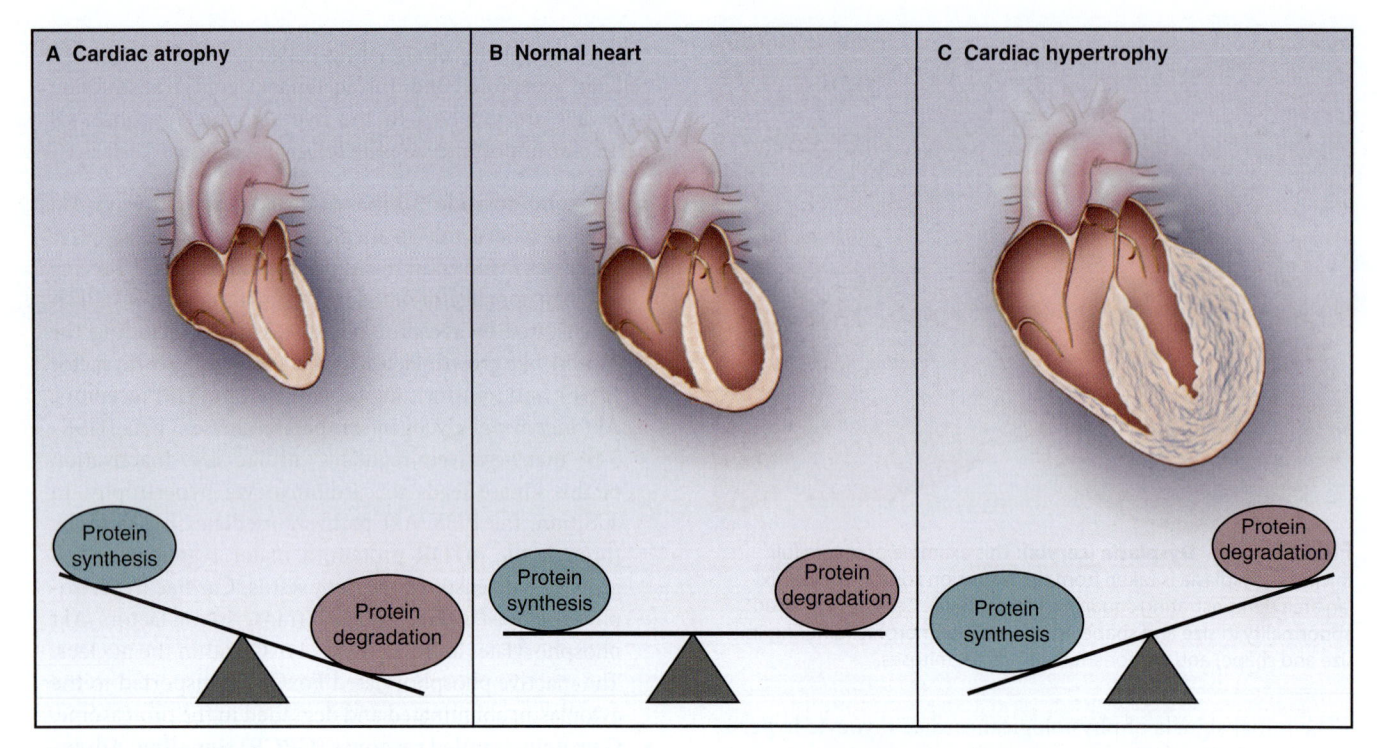

FIGURE 2-9 Factors in the development of cardiac atrophy and hypertrophy: **(A)** The development of cardiac atrophy involves both the inhibition of protein synthesis and a simultaneous increase in the rates of protein degradation resulting in shorter half-lives of individual cardiac proteins as compared with **(B)** when the half-lives of proteins are in a steady state, when protein synthesis and degradation are balanced. **(C)** The development of cardiac hypertrophy involves both an increased fractional synthesis of proteins and suppression of protein degradation, resulting in longer half-lives of cardiac proteins. Source: From NEJM, Willis MS, Patterson C, Proteotoxicity and Cardiac Dysfunction – Alzheimer's Disease of the Heart?, Vol. 368, 455–464. Copyright © 2013 Massachusetts Medical Society. Reprinted with permission from Massachusetts Medical Society.

The above pathways, although discussed in relation to cardiac myocyte hypertrophy, also function in the regulation of skeletal muscle hyperplasia induced by exercise. Signaling pathways important in promoting hyperplasia and hypertrophy are summarized in Figure 2-10.

Epidermal response to mechanical stress is mediated through stretch-induced Ca^{2+} ion channels that when triggered allow an influx of ion into the cytoplasm. This activates phospholipase C and protein kinase C and triggers the MAPK kinase pathways, ultimately resulting in a hyperplastic response. Of more general significance, the mTOR protein-mediated pathway (see above) serves a central role in controlling cell size and cell division in its role as a major nexus for cellular sensing of nutrient and energy status and by responding to systemic growth signals.

Atrophy

Atrophy, a decrease in organ size, is the result of a decrease in cell size (and in some cases, cell number), which like hypertrophy/hyperplasia can be either physiological or associated with disease states. Physiological atrophy is often associated with changes in hormone level (the postmenopausal breast, endometrium, vaginal epithelium, and the postparturition uterus). Aging may be associated with loss of muscle mass and "senile" atrophy of the brain and neurodegenerative disease (Figures 2-11 and 2-12).

Pathological atrophy is demonstrated by muscles with decreased workload following immobilization or after loss of innervation. **Cachexia**, characterized by generalized weight loss, body wasting, and loss of muscle mass, is associated with several chronic diseases including cancer, renal disease, chronic obstructive pulmonary disease, and chronic heart failure. **Marasmus**, a result of severe malnutrition in children as a result of caloric deficit, is likewise associated with muscle atrophy and general failure of growth. **Kwashiorkor**, severe childhood malnutrition resulting from a diet that is very low in protein but high in carbohydrates, is both associated with growth failure and muscle wasting and also specific changes including edema, anemia changes in skin and hair pigment, excessive fat storage in the liver (fatty liver see Chapter 10), and apathy.

QUICK REVIEW
Molecular Mechanisms of Atrophy

The regulation of cell (and hence organ) size requires a balance between the synthesis and breakdown of cellular proteins and other cellular components. It is not surprising that the atrophy of skeletal and cardiac muscle is associated

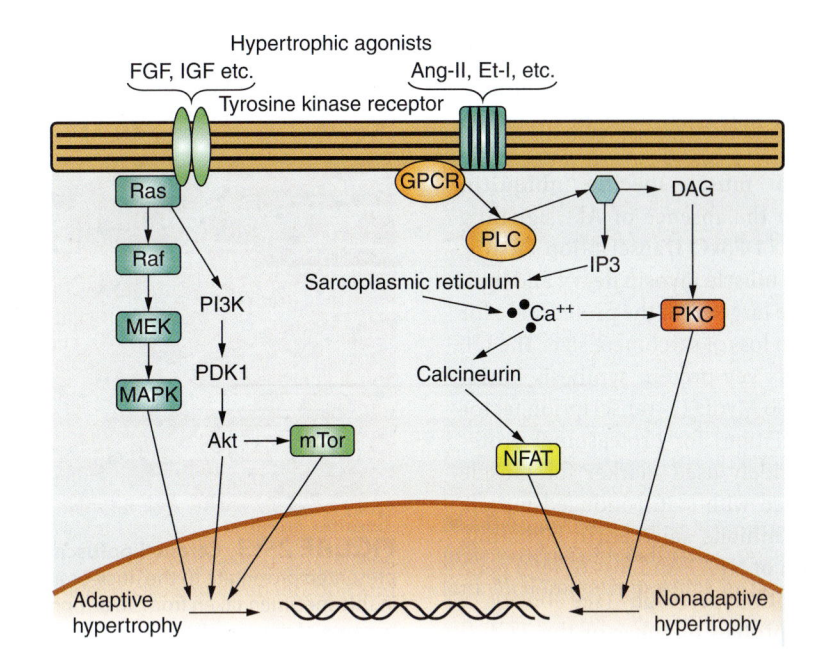

FIGURE 2-10 **Major pathways activated in response to hypertrophic signals.** Ang-II, angiotensin-II; DAG, diacylglycerol; Et-1, endothelin-1; FGF, fibroblast growth factor; GPCR, G protein coupled receptor; IGF, insulin-like growth factor; IP3, inositol 1,4,5-trisphosphate; MAPK, mitogen-activated protein kinase; NFAT, nuclear factor of activated T cells; PDK1; phosphoinositol-dependent kinase 1; PI3K, phosphoinositol-3-kinase; PKC, protein kinase C; PLC, phospholipase C; mTOR, mammalian target of rapamycin. Source: Reprinted from Agrawal Rohini, Neeraj Agrawal, Chintan N. Koyani, Randhir Singh. Molecular targets and regulators of cardiac hypertrophy. Pharmacological Research, Vol. 61, Issue 4, April 2010, Pages 269–280. Copyright 2010, with permission from Elsevier.

with specific proteolytic events mediated by the ubiquitination and targeting of proteins to the 26S proteasome for degradation. Some of the key steps in the atrophic pathway can be seen as the converse of those responsible for hypertrophy/hyperplasia as follows:

- **Diminished systemic progrowth factors** (notably IGF-1) lead to reduction in Akt activity and through additional downstream mediators, reduction in the activity of mTOR. As the central cellular sensor of

FIGURE 2-11 Uterine involution following childbirth: Uterus sectioned at level of placental attachment.

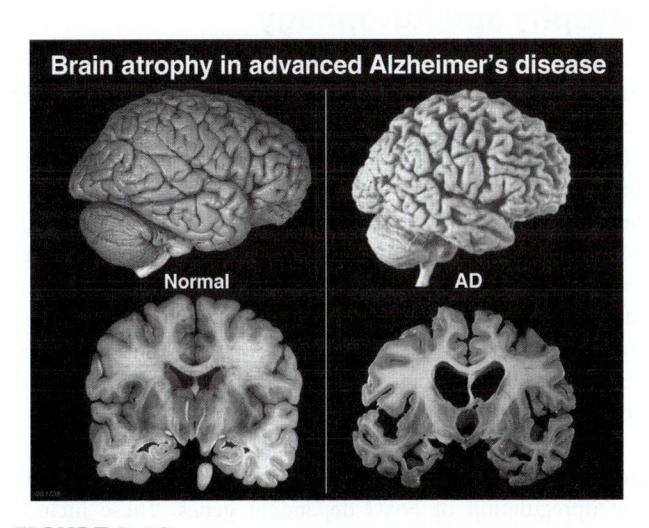

FIGURE 2-12 Brain atrophy in neurodegenerative disease.

pro-growth signals, mTOR plays a role in atrophy, analogous to its role in hypertrophy. Hence, *lack* of growth factors (or deficit in cell nutrients) leads to decreased protein synthesis and organ atrophy.
- **Upregulation of two muscle-specific ubiquitin ligases (ULs)** occurs in the absence of Akt signaling as a result of activation of FoxO transcription factors. UL **MuRF1** ubiquitinates muscle myosin heavy and light chains that as a result are targeted to the proteasome for degradation, resulting in loss of sarcomere size. The UL **atrogin1/MAFbx** targets key protein synthesis initiation factor eIF3-f and also MyoD (a transcription factor key in muscle differentiation) for proteasomal proteolysis. **Atrogin1** is a widely used marker for muscle wastage and is associated with statin-induced muscle disease. Atrogin1 also inhibits calcineurin signaling, resulting in inactivation of NFAT and loss of fetal gene expression associated with hypertrophy (see above).
- **Myostatin** (a secreted protein member of the TGF-β family) expression is increased in skeletal and heart muscle under conditions promoting atrophy. This results in downregulation of genes important in muscle differentiation including MyoD. In addition, myostatin may promote synthesis of atrogin-1 by activating FoxO.
- **Cytokines** including **TNFα**, and **IL-6** and **glucocorticoids** enhance the ubiquitin-proteasomal degradative pathway by upregulating the NF-κB transcription factor. In this regard, the inflammatory cytokine tumor necrosis factor-like weak inducer of apoptosis (**TWEAK**) signals through a cellular receptor (Fn-14) that is a member of the TNF receptor superfamily. TWEAK has an important role in mediating muscle atrophy, notably in conditions of denervation and immobilization. Under such conditions, TWEAK promotes MuRF1 expression leading to muscle proteolysis.

Atrophy and Autophagy

The physiological conditions that result in atrophy, most notably aging and lack of nutrients, result in an increase in recycling of cellular components via **autophagy**; the process of "self-eating", a lysosomal-dependent degradative process. In macroautophagy, organelles and portions of cytoplasm become enclosed by double membrane-bound **autophagosomes** that fuse with lysosomes to form **autophagolysosomes** (also termed "late" autophagic vacuoles). Some proteins contain a specific targeting sequence (KFERQ) that is recognized by a member of the Hsp70 family of heat shock proteins (Hsc70), which act as a lysosomal-targeting molecular chaperone (**Chaperone-mediated autophagy**).

As discussed in the quick review of hyperplasia (above), diminished pro-growth signaling through mTOR results in the upregulation of FoxO-dependent genes. These include several autophagy-related proteins including **atg6** (**Beclin-1**),

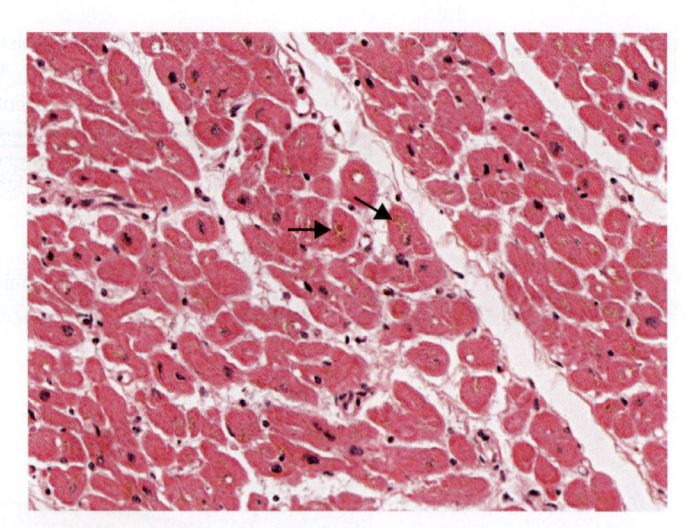

FIGURE 2-13 Ceroid (lipofuscin): Brown granular pigment is presented proximate to the nucleus in many cardiac myocytes (arrow) in this specimen taken from an atrophic heart. "Brown atrophy" because of the overall tint lent to the tissue by the pigment.

atg8, and **atg12** that are required for autophagosome membrane formation. Starvation and the molecular mechanisms associated with it, prolong longevity in organisms as diverse as *Drosophila* and mammals as well as promoting atrophy and autophagy. Hence, it has been hypothesized that autophagy, by removing damaged cellular constituents and allowing recycling of limiting nutrients, may also be critical for prolongation of life (see Aging and Nutrition, this chapter).

Under conditions demonstrating significant atrophy, that is, aging and in certain neurodegenerative diseases, cells accumulate a distinctive pigment termed **lipofuscin**, **ceroid**, or "wear and tear" pigment. The material forms within autophagolysosomes and represents oxidized and cross-linked proteins and lipid peroxidation products (derived, in part, from damaged mitochondria) that are resistant to further lysosomal degradation. Using standard H&E-stained tissue, lipofuscin appears as yellow to brown granules in a perinuclear distribution (although it is more commonly detected using its autofluorescent properties) (**Figure 2-13**).

Metaplasia

Metaplasia is a reversible change in which one adult cell type is replaced by another as a response to stress. Areas demonstrating metaplasia are often those in which neoplasia occurs, presumably because continuing stress is associated with loss of protective mechanisms and promotion of genetic instability. If the stressor is removed, the metaplastic cell population can return to its original state, although restoration of the initial tissue type is often incomplete. For example, the intestinal columnar metaplasia seen in Barrett esophagus as a result of chronic GERD (see **Case 2-2**) can completely revert to squamous epithelium that appears identical to normal following therapy when only limited areas of the esophagus are affected.

Another common example of metaplasia is seen in the change of ciliated columnar epithelium to squamous in

CASE 2-2

John Smith is a 47-year-old obese man who has had a history of heartburn for the past 12 years. He states that about 8 years ago he visited a gastroenterologist complaining of burning pain in his epigastric region, particularly when recumbent. Endoscopy at that time showed mild mucosal inflammatory changes consistent with gastroesophageal reflux disease (**GERD**) with no evidence of metaplastic or dysplastic change as confirmed by biopsy. The physician prescribed Prilosec 20 mg twice a day and elevation of the head of his bed. Five years prior to this visit, he noted increasing symptoms of reflux not always controlled by medication. He reported symptoms to be related to diet and alcohol consumption. At that time he did not complain of weight loss, **dysphagia** (difficulty in swallowing), or abdominal pain. Repeat endoscopy demonstrated mucosal changes consistent with **Barrett esophagus**, that is, the occurrence of metaplastic change within the esophagus related to GERD. Biopsy results disclosed normal esophagus (see **Figure 2-14**) and regions demonstrating significant metaplasia, definite low-grade dysplasia, and one localized area of concern for high-grade dysplasia (see **Figure 2-15A**). Because of the increased risk of developing adenocarcinoma, areas of metaplasia/dysplasia were treated by endoscopic radio frequency ablation. Mr Smith was advised to return in 3 months for potential additional therapy. At that time, he was scheduled to undergo periodic endoscopic surveillance but did not return to the clinic.

Figure 2-14 demonstrates a normal area of Mr. Smiths esophageal biopsy. The mucosa is lined with nonkeratinized squamous epithelium. The dark staining basal cells show occasional mitoses and subtend about 15–20% of the epithelial layer. Connective tissue papillae extend into the epithelial layer (arrow) and typical mucosal glands are evident (white arrow). The tissue shows hyperemia of blood vessels, likely a result of biopsy trauma. Figure 2-15A is taken from an area of the biopsy demonstrating metaplasia. The normal squamous epithelium (left margin of figure) is replaced by specialized columnar epithelium with scattered goblet cells similar to that seen in the intestine (at arrow). Other areas show cardiac type mucosa similar to that observed in the gastric cardia (at short arrow). Areas of the biopsy show evidence of dysplasia with hyperchromatic-stacked nuclei both in surface mucosa and within glands (at line) (Figures 2-14 and 2-15).

Mr. Smith now returns to the clinic with complaint of increasing dysphagia, hoarseness, and 15 pound weight loss over the last month. He states that his symptoms of GERD had worsened and are only poorly controlled by medication. Endoscopy discloses a flat lesion in the lower quarter of the esophagus adjacent to an area of Barrett metaplasia. Evaluation of biopsy discloses poorly differentiated adenocarcinoma (see Figure 2-15B short arrow) invading through the submucosa adjacent to an area showing metaplasia (Figure 2-15B arrow).

The great majority of esophageal adenocarcinomas occur in individuals with Barrett esophagus subsequent to GERD. An area of metaplastic/dysplastic change adjacent to adenocarcinoma is a common finding.

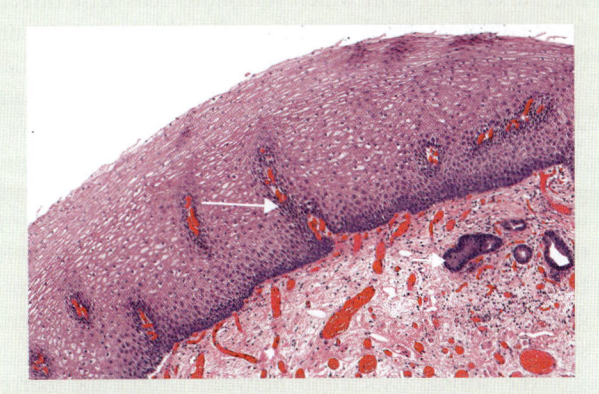

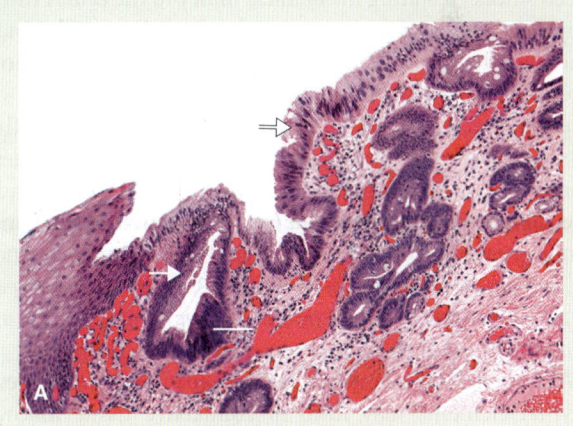

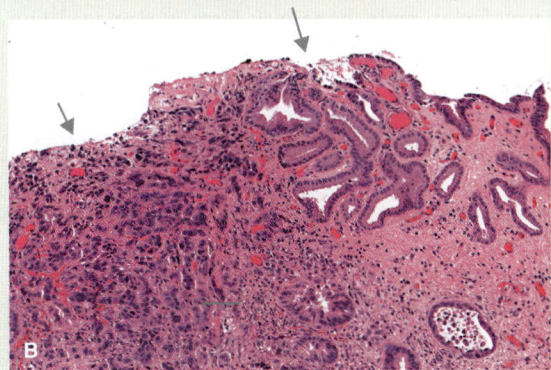

FIGURE 2-14 **Region of normal esophagus:** The mucosa is lined with nonkeratinized squamous epithelium. The dark staining basal cells show occasional mitoses and subtend about 15–20% of the epithelial layer. Connective tissue papillae extend into the epithelial layer (arrow), and typical mucosal glands are evident (short arrow). The tissue shows hyperemia of blood vessels, which is likely a result of biopsy trauma.

FIGURE 2-15 **(A)** Region of esophagus demonstrating Barrett esophagus: The normal squamous epithelium (left margin of figure) is replaced by specialized columnar epithelium with scattered goblet cells similar to that seen in the intestine (arrow). Other areas show cardiac type mucosa similar to that observed in the gastric cardia (white arrow). Areas of the biopsy show evidence of dysplasia with hyperchromatic-stacked nuclei both in surface mucosa and within glands (line). **(B)** Region of esophagus demonstrating adenocarcinoma: The biopsy specimen discloses poorly differentiated adenocarcinoma (short arrow) invading through the submucosa (line) adjacent to an area showing metaplasia (arrow).

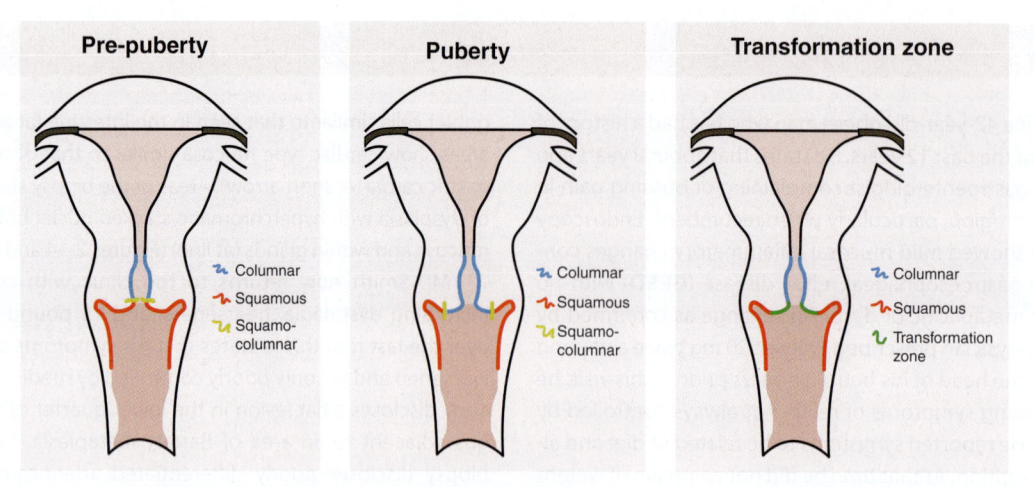

FIGURE 2-16 Formation of the transformation zone in the postpubertal cervix. Source: Image with permission from Tom Leach at Almost a Doctor. http://almostadoctor.co.uk/content/systems/obstetrics-and-gynaecology/cervical-cancer-and-cin.

the bronchus of a smoker demonstrated in Figure 2-7. The stressor is clearly a pyrolysis product contained in inhaled tobacco smoke, resulting in chemical injury to the cell. A third example can be found in the cervix where mucinous columnar epithelium frequently changes to squamous at the junction between the two types of epithelia (transformation zone of the cervix) (see Figure 2-16). The transformation zone of the cervix is located above the cervical os in prepubertal females. At puberty, the transition zone everts toward the exterior face of the cervix where it is exposed to the acid environment and potentially other proinflammatory agents found in the vaginal vault. *In both cases (as well as in Barrett esophagus), the area of metaplasia is associated with chronic inflammation and has an increased propensity to develop cancer* (Figure 2-17).

Although less commonly recognized, unexpected mesenchymal elements may form in connective tissue following injury, for example, bone may form in damaged muscle (termed **myositis ossificans**). The relationship of this to epithelial metaplasia is unclear.

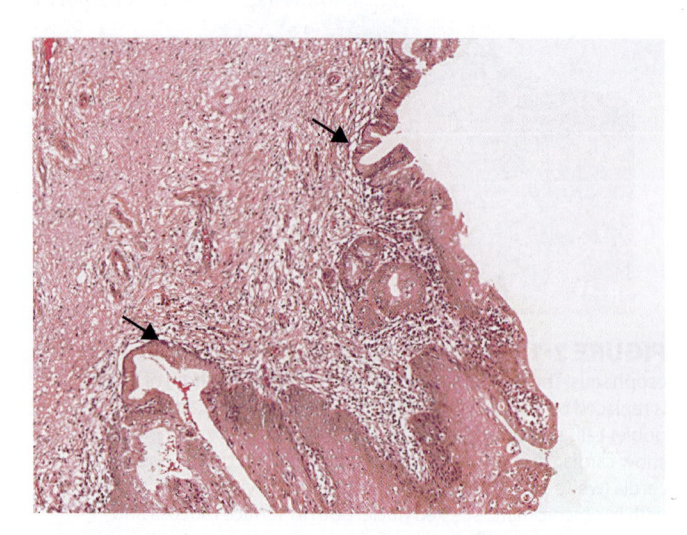

FIGURE 2-17 Cervical metaplasia: A large area of squamous metaplasia occurs between areas of nonmetaplastic columnar epithelium (arrows) in the transformation zone of the cervical biopsy specimen.

> ### QUICK REVIEW
> **Molecular Mechanisms of Metaplasia**
>
> The striking association between metaplasia and the development of adenocarcinoma in Barrett esophagus has spurred study of the molecular changes that occur in the latter disease process. There is a 30-125-fold increase in risk of adenocarcinoma in patients diagnosed with Barrett metaplasia. This represents a 1 in 20 lifetime risk. The metaplasia in Barrett will progress to cancer at a rate of 0.5–1% per year.
>
> The cell type in which Barrett metaplasia originates is in dispute. Stratified squamous epithelium might directly give rise to columnar, a process termed **transdifferentiation.** Such occurs during normal development of the murine esophagus in which squamous cells arise directly from columnar basal epithelial cells without intervening cell division. During this process, individual cells share cellular markers (**cytokeratins**) characteristic of both pathways of cellular differentiation. A more likely alternative is that an esophageal stem cell changes its developmental program to give rise to cells committed to the intestinal pathway of differentiation. Such stem cells may reside either in the esophageal mucosal interpapillary basal zone or derive from cuboidal epithelium lining the ducts of submucosal glands. Evidence gathered from patient biopsy material supports the latter source.
>
> The strong association between GERD and Barrett metaplasia suggests that refluxed bile salts, stomach acid, and the chronic inflammation they produce are important in the etiology of the disease. The nuclear transcription factor **NF-κB**, key in the regulation of inflammation, is (not unexpectedly) found in increased levels in Barrett metaplasia. Two caudal-related homeobox transcription factor

genes, *Cdx1* and *Cdx2*, important in the development and maintenance of the intestine, are expressed in the normal adult gut from the duodenum through the colon *but not in the esophagus or stomach. However, Cdx1 and 2 are overexpressed in areas of metaplasia in Barrett disease.* Inflammation can stimulate the expression of the two genes through NF-κB, suggesting a causative link between inflammation and metaplasia induced by the ectopic expression of genes important in maintenance of adult organ patterning.

Dysplasia

Dysplasia is not generally considered a normative response to cell and tissue injury. At the light microscopic level, it is characterized by a disordered pattern of growth in which cells show variation in size and shape and nuclear changes (Figures 2-8 and 2-15). As noted in Case 2-2, dysplasia is often found in epithelia showing metaplasia. At a molecular level, dysplasia is associated with an increasing number of mutations in genes associated with the control of cellular growth and DNA integrity, the same genetic changes that characterize neoplastic transformation. The line between neoplasia and dysplasia (if any) is exceedingly thin. In fact, what a pathologist would have called mild dysplasia of the cervix several years ago could now be called cervical intraepithelial neoplasia (CIN) grade 1. Dysplasia represents another (possibly reversible) step in the continuum of molecular changes that result in frank neoplasia and ultimately cancer.

Abnormal Intracellular Accumulations

As noted under atrophy, stressed cells may demonstrate the accumulation of abnormal amounts of substances produced locally or at other sites (Figure 2-13). The above-mentioned lipofuscin (ceroid) pigment represents residual nondegradable material predominantly within the autophagolysosomes of atrophic or aging cells. The accumulations may, in themselves, be harmless but (as is the case with lipofuscin) be indicative of a process of pathological significance. Several other common examples are as follows:

- **Fatty change in the liver** is most often associated with excess alcohol (ethanol) consumption (**alcoholic steatosis**) where it represents the excess deposition of triglycerides because of both increased synthesis and reduced release as a result of disordered hepatocyte metabolism. The fat accumulation is not, of itself, damaging and is completely reversible with decreased alcohol intake. However, alcoholic steatosis may become associated with the serious consequences of alcoholic liver disease with continuing consumption.
- **Anthracotic pigment in the lung** represents the accumulation of inhaled carbon particles in the lung alveolar macrophages. The presence of such pigment is universal in smokers as well as those living in urban environments or other areas with high levels of particulate air pollution. Carbon accumulation is not harmful but other agents found in combination with carbon (such as silica from anthracite coal production) can cause severe fibrotic lung disease.
- **Hemosiderosis** is an abnormal intracellular accumulation of hemosiderin (a breakdown product of ferritin, the major iron storage protein in the body). The accumulation may result from genetic defects in iron metabolism or, excess hemoglobin-derived iron, as a result of hemorrhage, red cell lysis, or multiple transfusions. Excess iron may result in cellular injury via iron-mediated free radical generation (see below) **(Figure 2-18)**.

Many additional abnormal intracellular accumulations of metabolically derived or exogenous substances occur some of which are discussed in the subsequent chapters.

MECHANISMS OF CELL INJURY: NECROSIS

Introduction

Although there is no clear-cut point at which cellular adaptations fail and cell injury becomes irreversible, the molecular mechanisms involved in cell injury and the histologically detectable cellular changes associated with it are well defined. Essentially all injurious agents act by disrupting one of four cellular pathways:

1. Aerobic respiration, mitochondrial oxidative phosphorylation, and the production of ATP,
2. Protein synthesis,
3. Maintenance of cell membrane integrity
4. Maintenance of the integrity of the genome (including DNA replication and repair).

Obviously, the four are interrelated; failure of any one pathway will ultimately lead to failure of the others. Of these, the first two pathways are associated with potentially reversible injury. For example, temporary impairment of blood flow to the kidneys (such as caused by a sudden decrease in blood pressure due to trauma and hemorrhage) will reduce perfusion to the renal tubules and result in local ischemia. Renal tubular cells depend, in large part, on oxidative metabolism. Much of the ATP produced is required to permit normal functioning of the Na^+, K^+ ATPase, the transmembrane ion pump responsible for maintaining a low intracellular Na^+ concentration (and a high intracellular K^+ concentration). With loss of ATP generation, the Na^+, K^+ ion pump fails, resulting in an influx of Na^+ and water into the tubular epithelial cells causing cell swelling. Such swelling is reversible given rapid restoration of perfusion and maintenance of an intact cytoskeleton. Hence, cell swelling (sometimes called **hydropic swelling**) is a visible sign of reversible injury that may be seen in many organs. However, loss of or damage to the nucleus (**pyknosis**, nuclear condensation; **karyorrhexis**, nuclear fragmentation or **karyolysis**, nuclear loss) is considered as a sign of irreversible cell injury and, for the last, cell death **(Figure 2-19)**.

As noted in the myocardial infarct example presented in Case 2-1, tissue ischemia is an extremely common form of cell injury associated with cardiovascular disease. Essentially

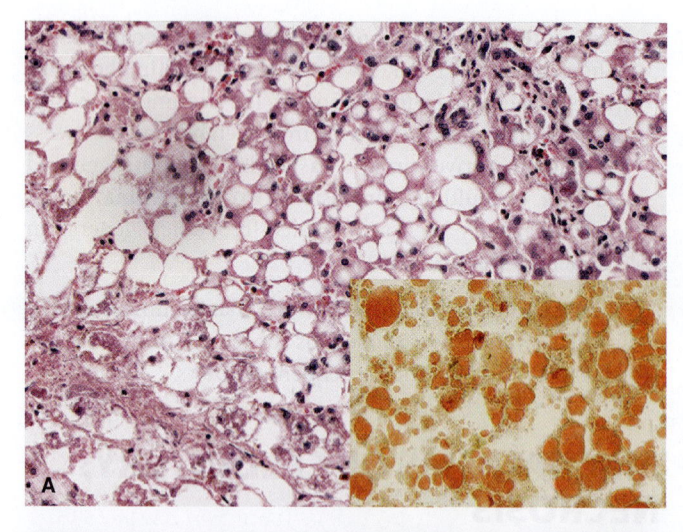

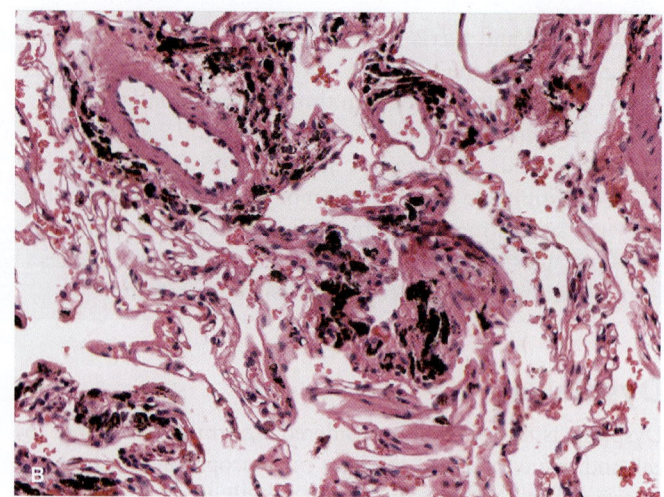

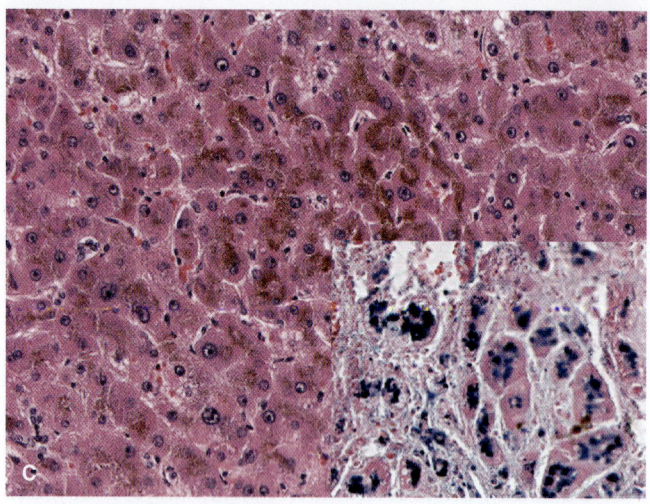

FIGURE 2-18 Abnormal intracellular accumulations: **(A)** Fatty change in liver (alcoholic steatosis): Tissue processed for H&E staining (lipid extracted). (Inset): Frozen section stained for fat. **(B)** Anthracotic pigment (carbon) in lung. **(C)** Hemosiderosis in lung. Note granular brown pigment in cells. (Inset): Iron-specific stain (Perls stain). Specimen is from a case of congenital hemochromatosis.

every organ system is susceptible to ischemic injury, resulting from impaired circulation. Hence, the mechanisms of ischemic injury are of clinical significance and have been extensively investigated. Ischemic cell death is the model for the process termed necrosis. *Necrosis is defined as cell and tissue death in an otherwise viable organism that occurs as a result of an "accidental" injury to the cell [examples being ischemia, environmental insults (such as heat, cold or physical force) and cell membrane destruction by chemical or biological agents].* Necrotic cell death is associated with early loss of internal and external membrane integrity, and release of autolytic lysosomal enzymes. Leakage of cellular contents to the tissue environment triggers multiple danger-associated molecular pattern (**DAMP**) sensing systems, notably pattern (or pathogen) recognition receptors (**PRRs**) and provokes the host response broadly termed **inflammation**, which will be discussed in detail in subsequent sections.

In contrast to necrosis is the process of **apoptosis**, or programmed cell death. *Apoptosis depends on a program of complex molecular processes within the cell initiated by specific molecular triggers. Triggering of apoptosis results in a distinctive mode of cell death that is, in part, designed to minimize the host response.*

Although often presented as mutually exclusive processes, mechanisms of cell death interact and overlap. A number of terms are used to better account for the complexity. For example, **necroptosis** is best understood as a form

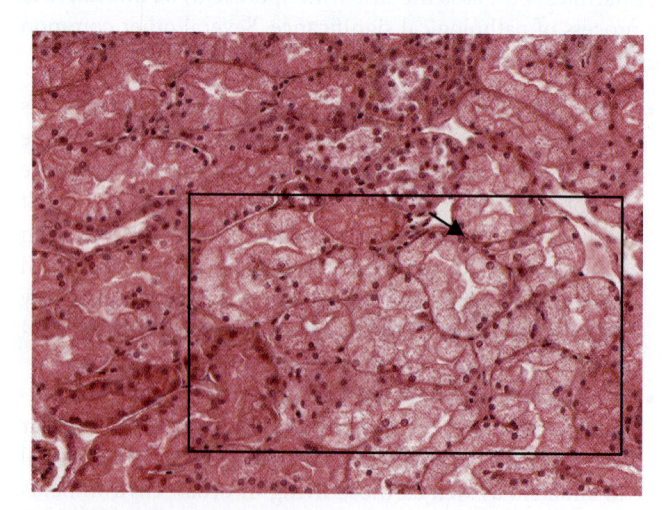

FIGURE 2-19 Cell swelling (hydropic change): Renal tubular cells show marked cellular swelling (boxed area). Many nuclei show signs of damage including varying degrees of karyolysis (arrow).

of receptor-mediated necrosis that shares many of the lethal mechanisms of necrosis but *unlike necrosis is triggered by cytokine/receptor interaction* (notably tumor necrosis factor receptor 1(TNFR1) and TNF. **Pyroptosis** is a form of cell death most commonly triggered by microbial pathogens but also associated with endogenous DAMPs. Like necrosis, pyroptosis results in cell swelling, lysis, and stimulation of the inflammatory reaction but unlike necrosis, pyroptosis depends on the activation of the protein **caspase 1** by cytoplasmic PRRs termed "nod-like receptors" (**NLRs**) that will be discussed later. Activated caspase 1 forms plasma membranes pores leading to cell lysis.

Molecular Mechanisms of Necrosis

It has been suggested that a better term for necrosis might be **oncosis** (derived from the Greek word for swelling). Cell swelling resulting from failure of ATP-dependent ion pumps is one of the earliest evidences of ischemic cell injury. Although many critical cellular systems are deranged by ischemia, the inability of metabolically active cells to produce sufficient ATP by glycolysis alone suggests that failure of mitochondrial oxidative phosphorylation is central to the process of necrosis. For example, about 25% of ATP produced in renal tubular cells is used by the Na^+, K^+ ATPase ion pump. Complete renal ischemia reduces ATP levels by 70–90% in 10 minutes, most notably in the cortex. The brain, which accounts for 2% of body mass, consumes about 20% of inspired oxygen. About 70% of the energy produced in the brain is consumed by the Na^+, K^+ ion pump. To compensate for decreasing ATP under ischemic conditions, cells deplete glucose and stored glycogen via relatively inefficient anaerobic glycolysis, which leads to a lactic acidosis in tissue and a drop in cellular pH. Derangement of oxidative phosphorylation leads to a cascade of interacting metabolic alterations that ultimately result in cell death. These include the following (Figure 2-20):

- **Damage to the electron transport chain:** Ischemia-induced damage to mitochondrial components leads to

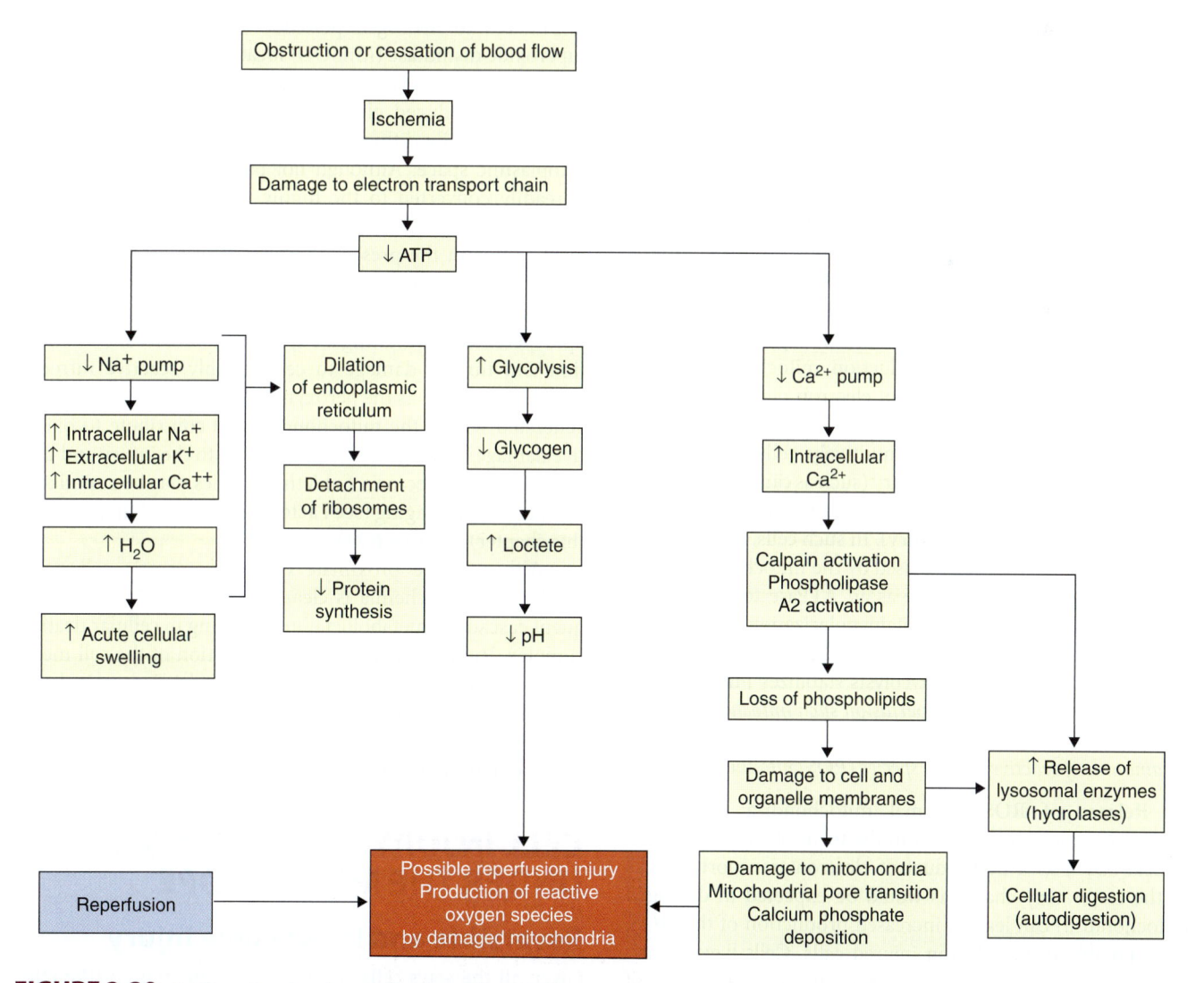

FIGURE 2-20 Outline of molecular mechanisms of necrosis.

hydrolysis of ATP and increases in free phosphate. This serves to further reduce energy for ion pump activity.

- **Increased intracellular Ca^{2+}:** Under physiological conditions, there is a 10,000-fold excess in calcium concentration external to cells. Failure of the plasma membrane Ca^{2+} ATPase (**PMCA**, the major Ca^{2+} ion efflux pump in nonexcitable cells) results in increased intracellular levels of Ca^{2+}. *Increased cytoplasmic Ca^{2+} activates a number of effectors of necrosis including calpains and phospholipases and has a critical role in promoting mitochondrial damage.*
- **Calpain activation:** Calpains are Ca^{2+} requiring neutral cysteine proteases that have a broad range of intracellular targets. Cleavage of actin-associated proteins (including talin, vinculin, and α-actinin) can lead to membrane damage associated with cell swelling and cytoplasmic blebbing, both characteristic of necrosis. Calpains are a major factor in the disruption of lysosomal membranes leading to the release of **cathepsins** a family of degradative proteases normally active within the acidic environment of the lysosome, potentially a terminal event in necrosis leading to cell lysis.
- **Phopholipase activation:** Phospholipases hydrolyze phospholipids thereby affecting the stability of cell and organelle membranes. The hydrolytic products (free fatty acids and lysophopholipids) may also damage membranes through a detergent-like activity. Many phospholipases including cytoplasmic phospholipase A2 are activated by Ca^{2+}.
- **Mitochondrial damage:** Increased cellular levels of Ca^{2+} result in increasing levels of mitochondrial calcium. Although initially tolerated, excess levels will lead to mitochondrial injury mediated by a process termed mitochondrial permeability transition (**MPT**). During MPT, the mitochondrial inner membrane forms pores leading to mitochondrial depolarization, uncoupling of electron transport, failure of ATP production, mitochondrial swelling (often with the presence of electron dense deposits of calcium phosphate), and lysis.
- **Reperfusion injury:** Contraintuitively, cells that are relatively *resistant* to ischemic injury (such as cardiac myocytes) suffer additional injury and necrosis upon resumption of perfusion (**reperfusion injury**). In such cells, residual ATP (produced by glycolysis) is used by the mitochondrial ATP synthetase acting in reverse as an ATPase to allow damaged mitochondria to maintain polarization and resume function when perfusion recommences. The low intracellular pH resulting from glycolysis stabilizes mitochondria and retards MPT. *Upon reperfusion such mitochondria continue to accumulate Ca^{2+} and, significantly, release elevated amounts of reactive oxygen species (ROS) into the cytoplasm.*

Release of ROS: Normal mitochondria leak small amounts of molecular oxygen in the form of superoxide free radical ($O_2^{\bullet-}$) as a by-product of electron transport. Blocks in the respiratory chain (as would be expected in damaged mitochondria) can lead to increased production of this ROS, most notably in reperfusion injured cells. Cells have a variety of protective antioxidants to cope with ROS, but a lack of balance between protective mechanisms and ROS production

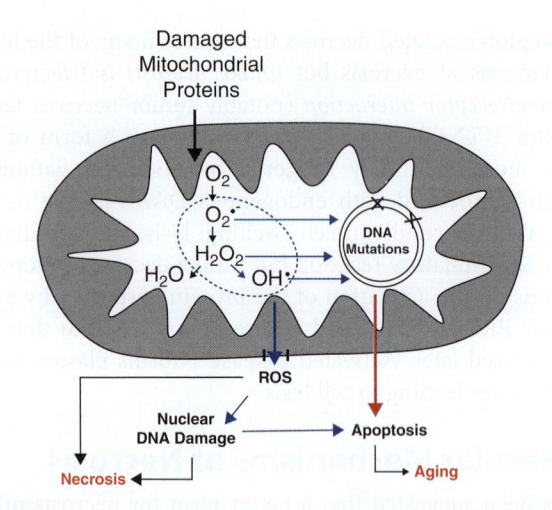

FIGURE 2-21 Reactive oxygen species and mitochondrial damage. Source: Modified from Loeb, LA. The mitochondrial theory of aging and its relationship to reactive oxygen species damage and somatic mtDNA mutations. Proc. Nat Acad Sci (USA) 102:18769–18770. Copyright (2005) National Academy of Sciences, U.S.A

leads to **oxidative stress** within the cell. Superoxide is rapidly dismutated to hydrogen peroxide (H_2O_2) by a manganese superoxide dismutase (**MnSOD**) located within the mitochondrial matrix. H_2O_2 is enzymatically detoxified to water in the presence of reduced glutathione. However, unlike superoxide, H_2O_2 readily diffuses through lipid membranes into the cytoplasmic space. Although not particularly reactive, H_2O_2 is readily converted to the highly reactive hydroxyl radical (HO•) either by reaction with superoxide (the Haber–Weiss reaction) or in the presence of ferrous iron (Fe^{2+}) (the Fenton reaction). Lysosomes contain abundant Fe^{2+}, are unable to detoxify H_2O_2, and are the major source of HO•, an effective lipid peroxidant resulting in lysosomal membrane destruction and further damage to cells. Highly reactive nitrogen compounds (such as the peroxynitrite anion $ONOO^-$) are also generated within the mitochondria and contribute to oxidative damage. Damage may be proximate to the injury and ultimately result in necrosis. Sublethal injuries may be cumulative and play a role in aging (see Factors in Aging and their Targets, this chapter) **(Figure 2-21)**.

Although the proximate cause of necrotic cell death resulting from ischemia is clearly tissue hypoxia, the subsequent cascade of metabolic failure resulting in cellular death is complex. Rupture of lysosomes, destruction of the cell membrane, or irreparable damage to mitochondria is terminal outcome but the relative roles of Ca^{2+} increase, ROS and failure of ATP generation by oxidative phosphorylation depend on the tissue and extent of the injury.

CELL INJURY AND NECROSIS UNDER THE MICROSCOPE

Reversible and Irreversible Injury

Given all the ways cells and tissues can be injured [the etiological agents of disease are immortalized in the mnemonic

CELL INJURY, CELL DEATH, AND AGING 37

CASE 2-3

A 22-year-old woman presents to the emergency room following a 3-day history of fever, **dysuria** (pain on urination) and right-sided flank pain. She has an elevated temperature. Significant examination findings include suprapubic tenderness and pain in the right costovertebral angle (the triangular area below the 12th rib and spinal column; the area above the right kidney). Rapid urine testing is indicative of bacteremia (confirmed to be positive for *Escherichia coli*). She is admitted to the hospital with suspected **pyelonephritis** (disease of the renal pelvis and kidney associated with an infectious process in the tubulointerstitial compartment.) Such infections are most commonly "ascending" and associated with fecal bacteria that have traveled up the urinary tract via the urethra. They are more common in females because of their short urethral length. She is treated with intravenous ampicillin and gentamicin and is discharged after 4 days on continued home IV therapy.

Two Weeks Later

She returns for follow-up and denies any continued complaints. Her physical examination is normal. However, urinalysis shows dark brown **casts** (material expressed from the renal tubules by the urinary stream, which contain cells and debris held together by protein secreted by the tubular cells). Her blood urea nitrogen (BUN) and serum creatinine are both elevated. Such results are suggestive of nephrotoxic tubular injury consistent with aminoglycoside antibiotic therapy-induced renal toxicity.

Although it is unlikely that a renal biopsy would be ordered, this is a well-understood disease process **Figure 2-22** is consistent with the patient's disease.

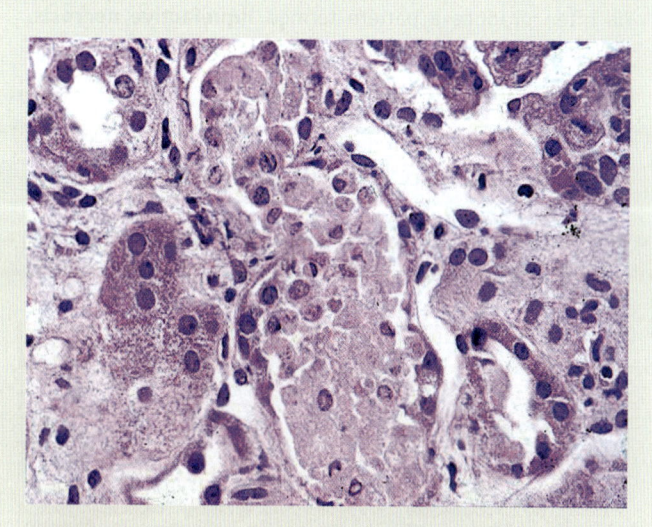

FIGURE 2-22 **Nephrotoxic acute tubular necrosis:** Tubular lumens are filled with necrotic debris and detached tubular epithelial cells.

VINDICATE (**V**ascular, **I**mmune, **N**eoplastic, **D**rug (toxicity), **I**nfectious, **C**ongenital, **A**llergic (autoimmune), **T**rauma, **E**ndocrine (metabolic, nutritional)], there are many visual clues that suggest cellular injury (which may be reversible) or necrotic cell death (irreversibly injured cells extant in a living organism). Examples can include vascular injury resulting in tissue ischemia, or the effect of toxic agents (aminoglycoside antibiotics as in Case 2-3).

Visual clues associated with **reversible injury** are cellular swelling (so-called **hydropic swelling**), an increase in intracellular swelling associated with failure of the ATP-dependent Na/K ion pump. In addition, plasma membrane blebbing, disaggregation of ribosomes and dilation of the endoplasmic reticulum, aggregation of cytoskeletal elements, and variable changes in mitochondria such as swelling and formation of internal calcium phosphate precipitates may variably occur. **Irreversible** injury is histologically defined by loss or disruption of the nucleus. Hence, nuclear loss or disruption of cells observed microscopically is a useful feature indicating necrosis (as opposed to reversible injury). Changes such as increased cytoplasmic staining with eosin (likely resulting from loss of mRNA), defects in the cell membrane, the formation of large densities in mitochondria, and rupture of lysosomes can be difficult to evaluate at the light microscopy level. Of course, gross enzymatic digestion of cells or tissue (**autolysis** when a product of the cell's own enzymes, as might be seen in postmortem tissue samples, **heterolysis** if the enzymes are produced by another source, as in certain tissue destructive bacterial infections) is unequivocal. **Figure 2-24** provides examples drawn from clinical material.

Types of Necrosis

As noted above, pathologists recognize patterns of necrosis that may be tissue specific or provide suggestions as to the etiology of injury. The names associated with such patterns although "traditional" are descriptive and useful.

- **Coagulative necrosis:** This form of necrosis occurs when enzymatic digestion/liquefaction of tissue by autolysis is retarded and coagulation (protein denaturation) predominates. The remnants of cells remain in place in tissue for some time as a necrotic area containing "cell ghosts." Lack of nuclei and nuclear disruption is obvious. Areas may show eosinophilia (as long as cytoplasmic proteins remain intact) or simply show reduced overall intensity of staining. This pattern of necrosis is commonly associated with vascular lesions that produce tissue ischemia and not only result in **infarcts** as in the heart (myocardial infarct; "heart attack") but also in other organs (kidney and spleen being common sites) (**Figure 2-25**).

WHAT WE DO

The ability of the pathologist to distinguish the histopathological signs of cell and tissue injury and death is of practical importance. At a minimum, it will direct attention to areas requiring further analysis. Different patterns of injury and necrosis may provide clues as to the etiology of injury and the pathogenetic process involved. For example, bacteria often produce a pattern termed **liquefactive necrosis**. An isolated or encapsulated area of liquefactive necrosis (an **abscess**) suggests a nidus of bacterial infection. **Coagulative** necrosis leaves the resistant structural architecture of tissue intact and is often described as "leaving in the ghostly remains of tissue intact." It is characteristic of ischemic necrosis. **Caseating granulomatous necrosis** is a strong indicator of infection by *Mycoplasma tuberculosis*. Particular patterns of necrosis are associated with specific tissues; **enzymatic fat necrosis** is associated with tissue rich in fat cells, most commonly the peripancreatic area, occasionally the breast and buttock. It is important to consider that these distinctions predated our knowledge of causation; hence, terminology does not always fit the biochemical facts. (Caseating necrosis is so called because German pathologists in the 19th century thought the tissue lesion looked like crumbly cheese-Käse.) Nevertheless, the ability to visually identify these types of necrosis in tissue is of continuing clinical utility and the terms frequently appear in surgical pathology reports. Consider a 2 cm indurated lesion on a woman's breast. On biopsy will it be an abscess demonstrating liquefactive necrosis within, or will it be a clonal proliferation of neoplastic cells, cancer? Obviously the difference is significant in terms of therapy and prognosis. Pathologists sitting at their microscopes help make the distinction **(Figure 2-23)**.

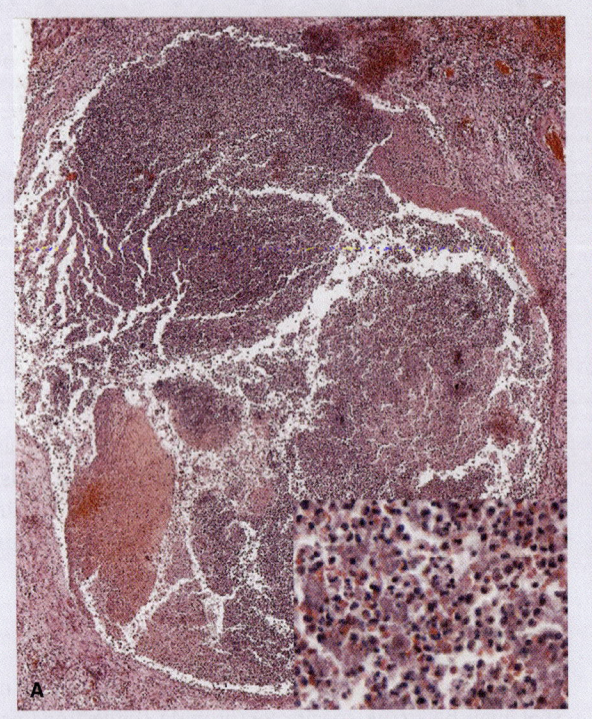

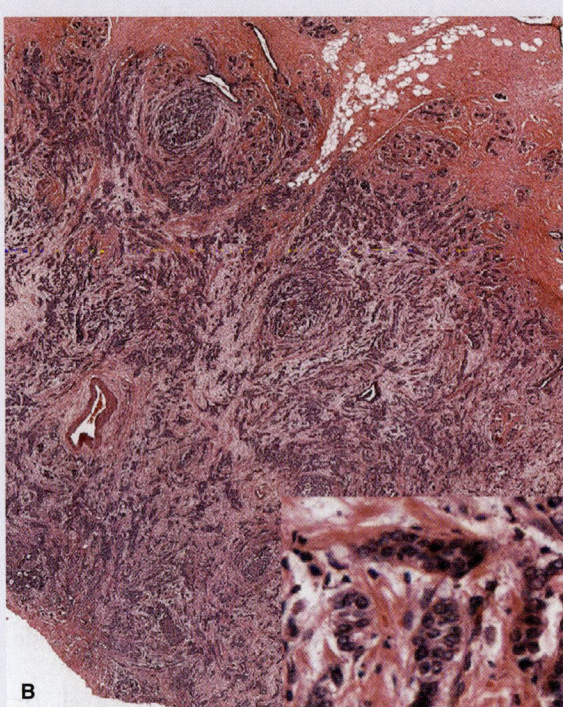

FIGURE 2-23 "Consider a 2 cm indurated lesion on a woman's breast" Two example of lesions: **(A)** Lesion 1 infectious (inset high power) **(B)** Lesion 2 neoplastic (inset high power).

- **Coagulative necrosis and hemorrhage and (incorrectly hemorrhagic necrosis):** Infarcts in organs that have dual blood supplies such as the lung and occasionally the liver may result in coagulative necrosis in the presence of sufficient residual circulation (from an alternate source) so as to demonstrate massive tissue hemorrhage. This is best demonstrated in the lung where pulmonary infarcts resulting from pulmonary embolic disease (**PEs** in clinical jargon) are a common problem, resulting in significant mortality **(Figure 2-26)**.

- **Liquefactive necrosis:** This form of necrosis commonly occurs in abscesses resulting from a bacterial infection where cellular enzymes are released from polymorphonuclear neutrophils (**PMN**) reacting as part of the acute inflammatory response release hydrolytic and other enzymes, resulting in tissue liquefaction. The resultant mixture of cells and debris is termed **pus**. Liquefactive necrosis also occurs in neural tissue in the case of infarcts. This ultimately results in a fluid-filled cyst (e.g., in the brain following an ischemic event, a stroke) **(Figure 2-27)**.

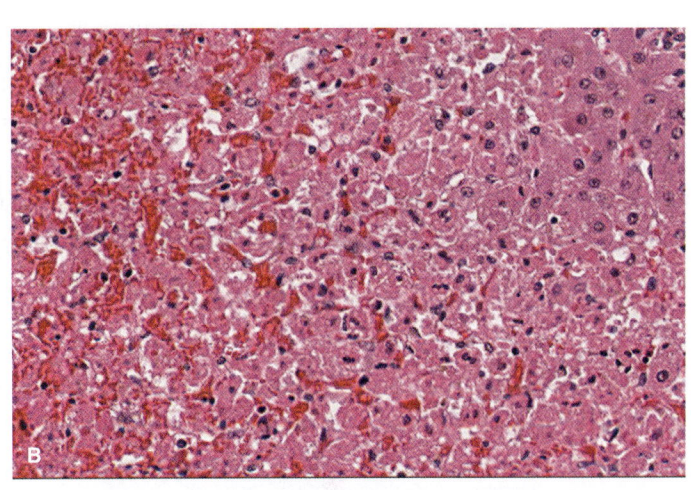

CELL INJURY, CELL DEATH, AND AGING   39

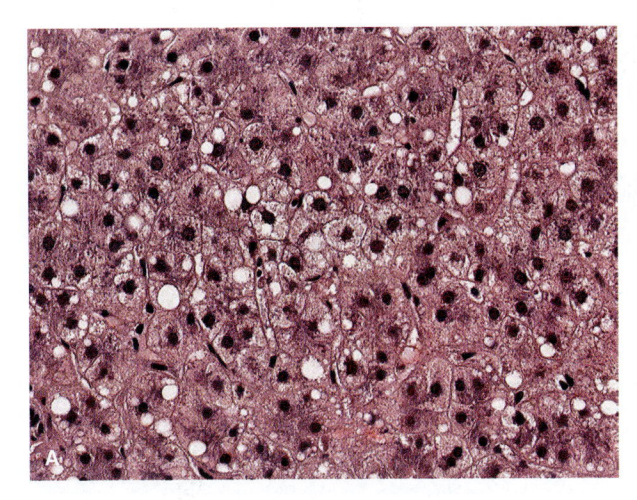

FIGURE 2-24 Reversible and irreversible injury. Two examples from the liver: **(A)** Potentially reversible cell swelling in a liver damaged by ethanol consumption. **(B)** Irreversible injury in a neonatal liver infected with *herpes simplex*. Hepatocytes have undergone varying degrees of nuclear damage and in many cells total loss. Some hemorrhage is evident.

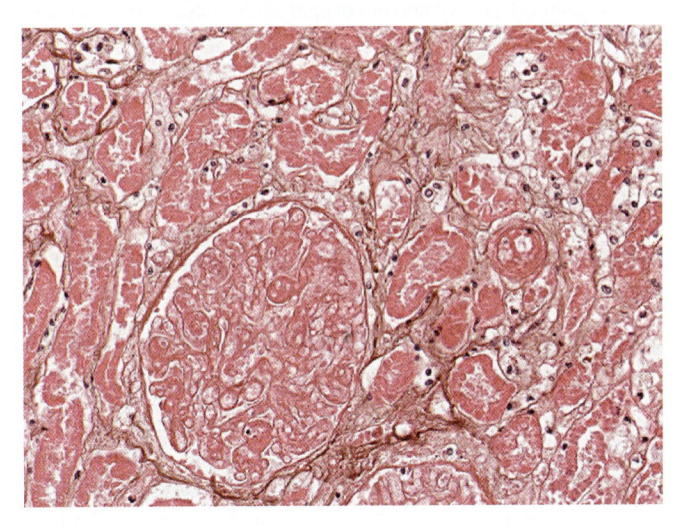

FIGURE 2-25 Renal infarct: The image demonstrates coagulative necrosis in the renal cortex. Structural details of glomeruli and tubules are retained but cells are necrotic and lack nuclei.

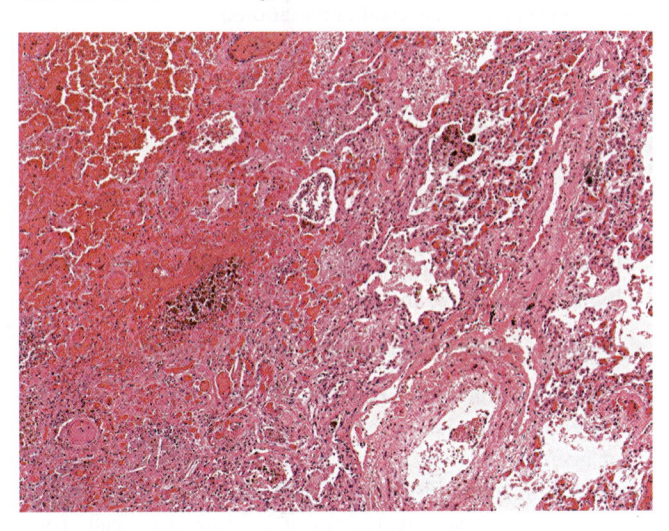

FIGURE 2-26 Coagulative necrosis and hemorrhage: The result of a recent pulmonary infarct that resulted in coagulative necrosis of alveoli and subsequent hemorrhage from extant circulation. The left side of the image is hemorrhagic with some anthracotic pigment visible (black punctate material). The right side shows necrotic alveoli and vasculature.

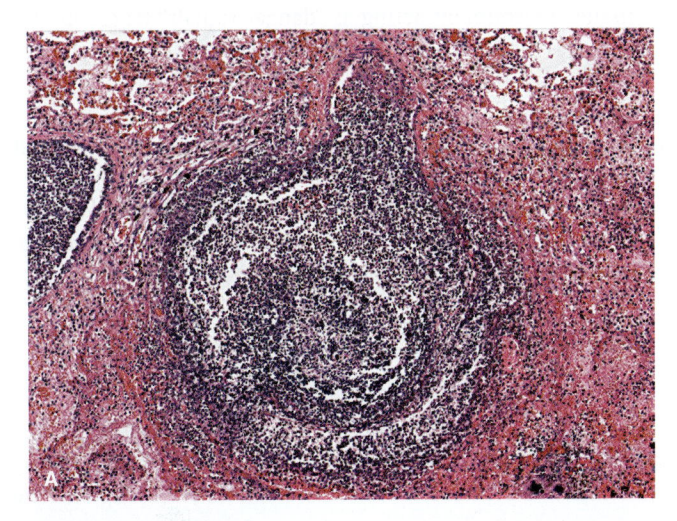

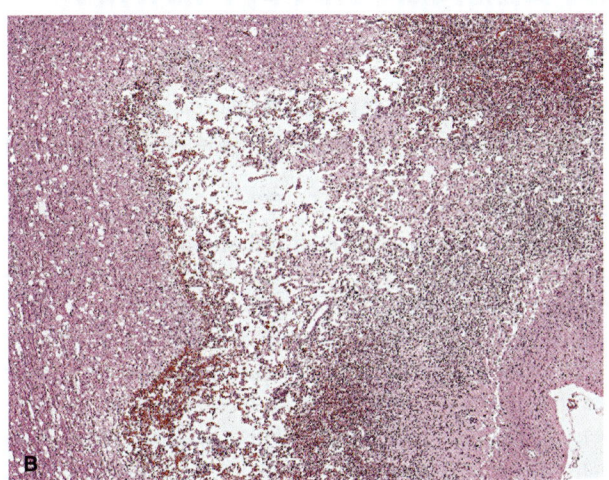

FIGURE 2-27 Liquefactive necrosis: (A) Pulmonary abscess: a "lake" of inflammatory cells with destruction of pulmonary parenchyma. **(B)** An ischemic infarct of the brain.

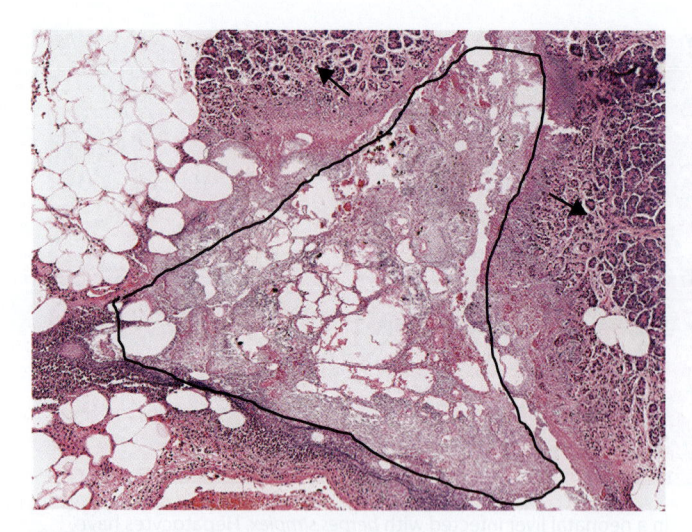

FIGURE 2-28 **Enzymatic fat necrosis:** The image shows an area of saponified pancreatic fat (outline) surrounded by an inflammatory reaction and damaged pancreatic acini (arrows).

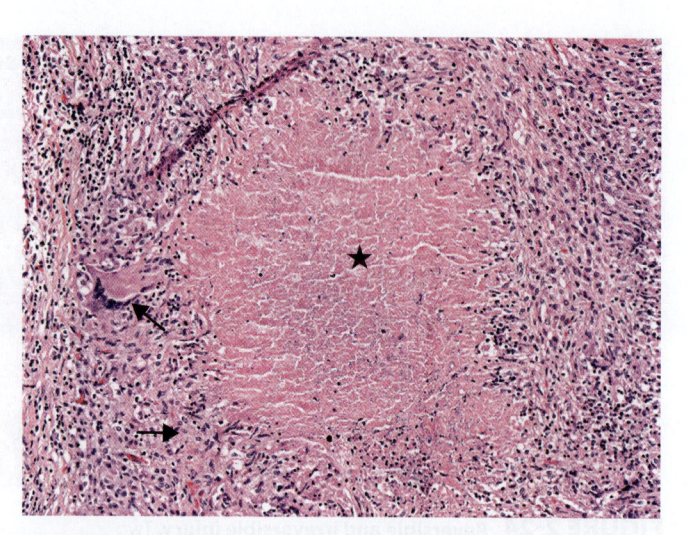

FIGURE 2-29 **Caseous necrosis:** The center of this image of a tuberculous granuloma (tubercule) shows typical caseous necrosis (star). A giant cell (arrow) and rim of epithelioid cells (short arrow) are also present.

- **(Enzymatic) fat necrosis:** As mentioned above, this process occurs in tissues with many adipocytes. Destruction of such cells releases triglycerides. Lipases (also released from damaged cells, particularly pancreatic acinar cells) convert the triglycerides into free fatty acids, which combine with tissue calcium to form soaps. The soaps are basic, highly destructive, and irritating. Enzymatic fat necrosis is a serious and potentially life-threatening complication of pancreatitis and surgical or other accidents damaging the pancreas and its exocrine ducts **(Figure 2-28)**.
- **Caseous necrosis:** As briefly discussed above, this form of necrosis is characteristic of the host response to infections with tuberculosis and will be discussed later. In this response, compact aggregates of inflammatory cells (primarily macrophages termed **epithelioid cells**) called **granulomas** have central areas of characteristic "cheesy" necrosis, hence are termed **caseating granulomas (Figure 2-29)**.

MECHANISMS OF CELL INJURY: APOPTOSIS

Necrosis versus Apoptosis

Necrosis is disorderly; apoptosis is highly programmed and orderly. Necrosis results in the release of cellular components into the tissue environment where they stimulate a vascular and cellular response termed **inflammation**. As shall be discussed, the inflammatory response may, of itself, provoke additional tissue injury (such as abscess formation). Most often, necrosis is provoked by results external to the cell itself such as tissue ischemia, physical injury produced by heat or force injury, and in some cases bacterial products. In such cases, energy production by the cell may cease abruptly. Given the specifics of injury, cells may or may not be able to survive, for a time, using anaerobic metabolism.

Apoptosis (from the Greek for "a falling off") is a highly programmed and orderly form of cellular suicide that may be provoked by *specific* external or internal cellular signals. It has been referred to as "controlled demolition at the cellular level." Although viewed by pathologists in the context of cellular injury, apoptosis is critical for normal embryogenesis and in the adult, for hormonally dependent loss of cell mass such as regression of the lactating breast and endometrial breakdown during menses.

Importantly, apoptosis is an energy requiring process that can only occur in cells that maintain some degree of metabolic integrity. Apoptotic cells shrink, while organelles remain relatively normal. Very early in the process of apoptosis a specific DNase is activated that results in a characteristic "ladder pattern" of DNA fragments. The degraded chromatin condenses, forming aggregates. The cells show extensive surface blebbing and (with a few exceptions) proceed to fragment into membrane-bound **apoptotic bodies**. These are neatly packaged cellular contents that otherwise would spill into the tissue environment acting as "danger signals" triggering host defenses (and particularly **innate immunity**). Apoptotic bodies display the membrane phospholipid phosphatidylserine (PTS) and other molecules on their surface that act as ligands for phagocytic cells thus promoting tidy disposal. *To reiterate, the key utility of the process of apoptosis is to provide cells with the ability to suicide without provoking (potentially damaging) host responses. Necrosis, on the other hand, serves to provoke such responses* **(Figure 2-30)**.

> **QUICK REVIEW**
> **Molecular Mechanisms of Apoptosis**
> Although apoptosis is now understood in great detail, initial understanding of the system grew from a simple observation in the nematode worm *Caenorhabditis elegans*. The

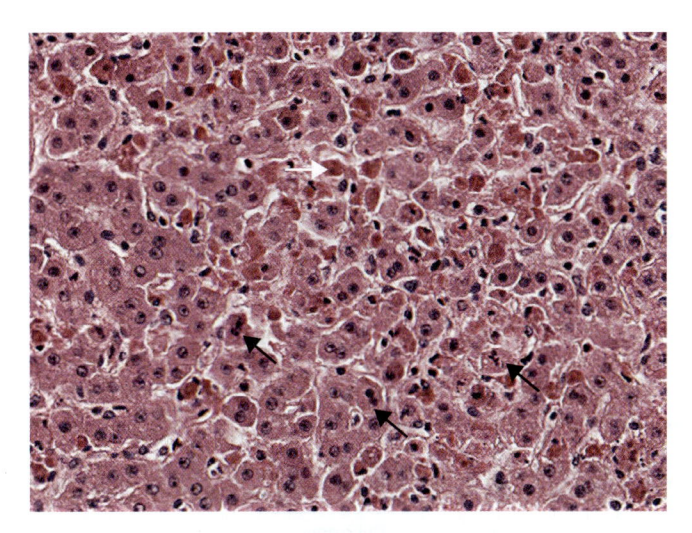

FIGURE 2-30 Apoptotic bodies: Hepatocytes in the liver from a case of yellow fever. Many of the cells are in various stages of apoptosis. For example, some cells (arrows) demonstrate a condensed fragmented nucleus. The eponymous term "Councilman body" refers to an anucleate eosinophilic remnant of a hepatocyte that has undergone apoptosis (apoptotic body) (white arrow).

worm has an absolutely fixed pattern of development that features 1090 somatic cells, 131 of which must die for normal body formation. Three highly conserved genes regulate this process. One of the genes (CED3) is homologous to the initially characterized caspase in humans (**caspase 1**).

The caspases are key to apoptosis, the result of a complex series of cascading enzyme interactions. The **caspases** are unique proteases containing an active site cysteine, which cleaves target proteins after aspartic acid residues. Caspases normally exist in an inactive form and must be proteolytically cleaved to become active. This is often accomplished by another active caspase. Hence, a critical issue is what are the initial triggers that start the process. A reasonable approach to this is to divide apoptotic caspase activation into three pathways: (1) extrinsic, (2) intrinsic, and (3) granzyme B mediated. (The third pathway is sometimes referred to using different names such as "cytotoxic T lymphocyte (CTL) mediated.). The three pathways utilize specific **initiator caspases** capable of autoactivation to start the apoptotic process. All three pathways converge on the activation of the **effector caspases** 3, 6, and 7, which are responsible for most, if not all, of the cellular changes (demolition) mentioned above. [Parenthetically not all caspases are involved in apoptosis. Several of them (including the prototypical caspase 1) are involved in innate immunity.] **(Figure 2-31)**.

Extrinsic Pathway

- Activation commences with the engagement of an extracellular ligand by **death receptors** on the surface of the cell. Receptors are members of the tumor necrosis factor receptor family (TNFr) and have an intracytoplasmic **death domain (DD)**, which couples cell surface signals to the intracellular environment. Examples of receptor/ligand pairs are Fas (CD95)/Fas ligand (CD95L) and TNF receptor 1/TNFα.
- Death receptor ligand engagement results in receptor trimerization and recruitment of DD containing **adaptor proteins** (FADD Fas-associated death domain) to form a death-inducing signaling complex (DISC).
- The DISC promotes oligomerization and autoactivation of **initiator caspase 8**.
- Activated caspase 8 may directly activate **executioner caspases** such as **caspase 3** or feed into (and be amplified by) the mitochondrial-dependent **intrinsic pathway** by cleaving a member of the Bcl-2 homology group of proteins, **Bid**.
- Cleaved Bid relocates to the mitochondria where it triggers the intrinsic apoptotic pathway by cleaving the Bcl-2 proteins, **Bak and Bax**.

Intrinsic Pathway

- The entry of a cell into the intrinsic pathway depends on the balance between pro- and antiapoptotic members of the Bcl-2 family of proteins that are defined by the presence of BH homology domains.
- The antiapoptotic proteins (such as **Bcl-2**) bind to and inhibit the polymerization of proapoptotic members of the family. An additional class of BCL-2 proteins (**BH-3 only proteins**) promotes apoptosis when expression levels are increased and serve to integrate a variety of cellular signals into the triggering of apoptosis. For example, levels of **Noxa** and **Puma** are upregulated by the p53 system and leading to apoptotic death of cells with irreparable DNA damage. As noted above, Bid integrates the extrinsic apoptotic pathway into the intrinsic.
- Once activated, Bak and Bax cause permeabilization of the mitochondrial outer membrane (**MOMP**) and subsequent cytosolic release of intramembrane mitochondrial proteins, notably **cytochrome c.**
- Released cytochrome c binds to the cytoplasmic protein **Apaf-1**, which together with dATP oligomerizes to serve as a scaffold for the binding and activation of the initiator caspase 9.
- The cytochrome c, Apaf-1 caspase 9 complex (the **apoptosome**) activates executioner caspase 3 and (directly or indirectly) activates executioner caspases 6 and 7.

Granzyme B (CTL) Pathway

- CTLs and NK cells mediate cell killing by inducing the formation of **perforin** pores in targets allowing for the entry of the caspase-like protease **granzyme B**.
- Granzyme B can either directly activate executioner caspase 3 or cleave Bid triggering the intrinsic apoptotic pathway.

Proteolysis of cellular components by executioner caspases is either directly or indirectly responsible for

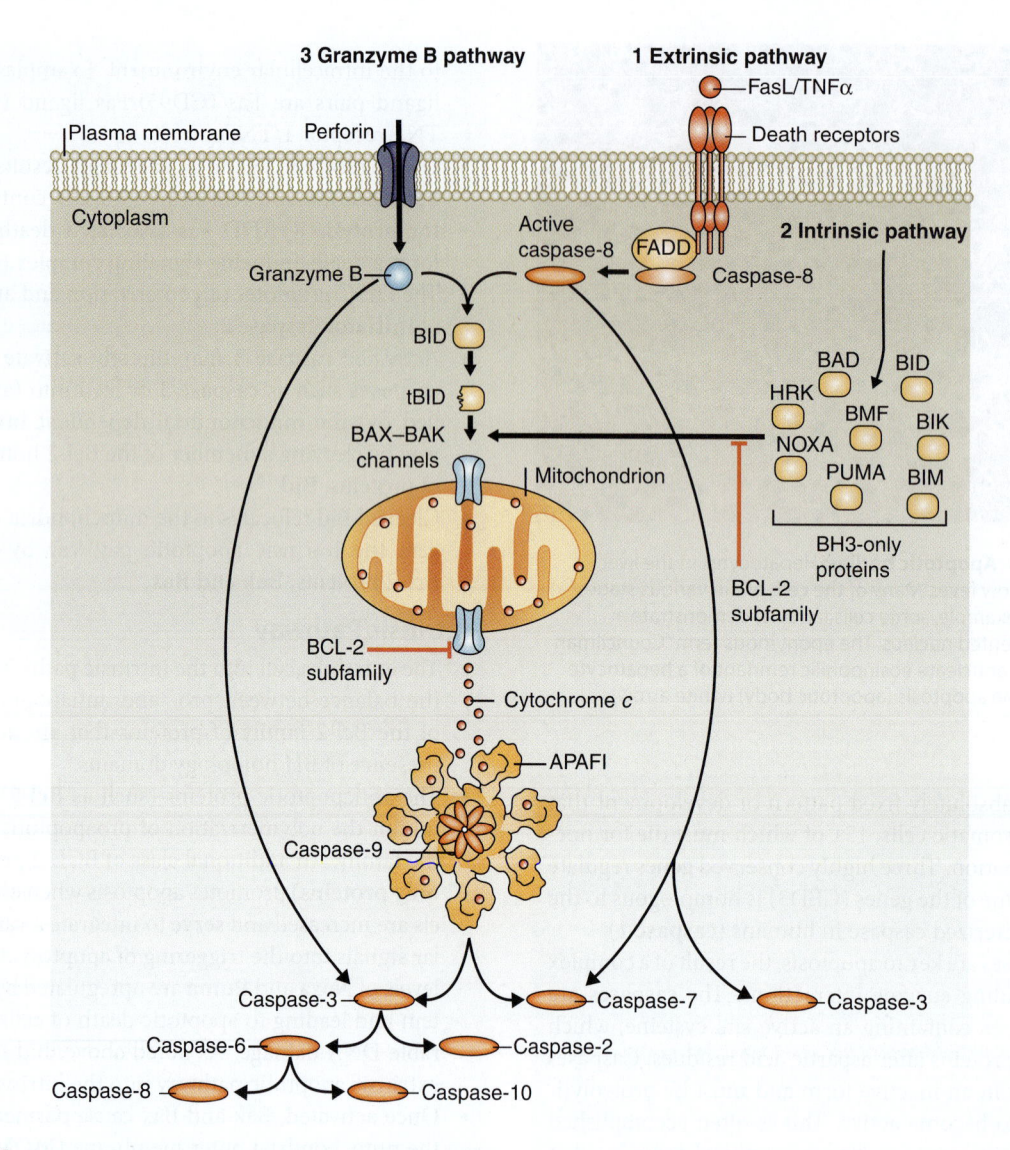

FIGURE 2-31 Apoptotic pathways in brief: Refer to text for details. Source: Reprinted by permission from Macmillan Publishers Ltd: Taylor RC, et al, Apoptosis: controlled demolition at the cellular level, Nature Reviews Molecular Cell Biology 9:231–240, Copyright 2008.

the events that characterize apoptosis. For example, production of the characteristic 180 bp DNA ladder during apoptosis (an often used biochemical indicator of the process) is the result of cleavage of DNA by a specific caspase 3 activated DNase (**CAD**). Caspase 3 cleaves an inhibitor of CAD (iCAD) activating the nuclease. Although seen as pathophysiology by the pathologist, active caspase 3 is necessary for cell differentiation. During development, caspase 3/CAD-induced DNA strand breaks are required for normal myogenesis.

IN TRANSLATION
Significance of Cell Death Scenarios

The four different mechanisms of cell death mentioned (necrosis, necroptosis, pyroptosis, and apoptosis) demonstrate several recurrent themes. The first three trigger host responses to injury (inflammation or, more broadly, innate immunity) either specifically (necroptosis and pyroptosis) or nonspecifically (necrosis) The fourth uses multiple mechanisms to prevent (and in some cases suppress) the host response.

The significance of these cell death scenarios for the future physician involves the fact that inflammation can be destructive as well as protective. Inflammation can rapidly exceed its protective role and produce cellular injury, resulting in systemic shock and multiorgan failure syndromes (**systemic multiorgan response syndrome**) with their significant morbidity and mortality. At the same time, anti-inflammatories are major therapeutic agents. However, many of these agents are directed at specific classes of inflammatory mediators such as arachidonic acid (AA) metabolites [predominantly prostaglandins (PGs)] or specific cytokines (such as TNFα or IL-1). Excessive stimulation of inflammation may result in a storm of interacting mediators, which no one drug, or group of drugs, can effectively suppress. Thus, understanding the initial triggering events of proinflammatory cellular processes would (at least in theory) provide a way of modulating the degree of inflammation. For example, modulation of caspase 1 activation would control pyroptosis, a critical event provoking the inflammatory reaction to a wide variety of pathogens. Hence, new classes of therapeutic agents controlling the initial events that trigger innate immunity are an area of great interest to the pharmaceutical industry.

Although physicians have an interest in being able to "turn off" or at least might wish to modulate, those modes of cell death that lead to inflammation, there is also an interest in being able to turn on apoptosis. Suppression of apoptosis by inactivation of components of the p53 pathway (e.g., by mutation of the *TP53* gene) is associated with increased malignancy in many forms of cancer. The p53 system that initiates apoptosis in cells which have irrecoverable genomic damage is important both in the progression of cancer and in mediating the effects of many cytotoxic chemotherapeutic agents, which act by inducing DNA damage. Hence, cells with defective p53 function may rapidly accumulate additional somatic mutations furthering tumor growth while also becoming resistant to chemotherapy. The ability to induce apoptosis in such malignant cells is an attractive potential approach in treating malignancies currently undergoing clinical trials. Agents, which inactivate antiapoptotic proteins (such as BCL2) or mimics of proapoptotic BH3 proteins, have shown promise in a number of cancers. Cancer cells are particularly sensitive to activation of the extrinsic apoptotic pathway via the TNF-related apoptosis inducing ligand (**TRAIL**). The use of TRAIL or antibodies directed toward the TRAIL receptor is also being evaluated as for clinical utility.

HOST RESPONSE TO INJURY

Triggers of Inflammation

The major threats to the human organism, that is, the etiological agents of disease and death, have remained constant during our evolutionary history. The specific array of pathogens, be they viral, bacterial, fungal or parasitic, changes with time, but their overall challenge to our survival does not. Force injury (physical or thermal) currently kills far more children in the United States than do pathogens, which are the major challenge to childhood survival in most of the underdeveloped world. Although the balance of threats alters, responding to temporal and geographic change, the nature of the threats does not. Thus, evolution provides us with an array of damage sensors that recognize characteristic molecular patterns associated with pathogens and cell injury, the pattern/pathogen recognition receptors (**PRRs**) that recognize DAMPs. The first result of triggering PRRs is the initiation of **innate immunity**, defined as host protective responses that do not involve variable region-dependent immunity. Innate immunity is preprogrammed to quickly respond to specific DAMPs, which are presumed to have presented a continuing challenge to the organism during evolution. Innate immunity includes what pathologists define as the acute inflammatory response with emphasis on triggering events. Adaptive immunity, traditionally the purview of the immunologist (and immunopathologist), deals with cellular and humoral responses that have the ability to adapt to new challenges and improve with continuing exposure. Such challenges need not have been present during evolution, but can be new to the species (such as synthetic organic molecules). Adaptive immunity tends to be slower than innate but with time the two systems interact and amplify each other. For example, chronic inflammation as defined by pathologists involves elements of both systems.

The response to infectious agents most often involves such interplay.

Sterile/Force Injury

Force injuries do not, of necessity, involve pathogens foreign to the injured host. Although the sites of injury may rapidly become infected with exogenous agents, the immediate host defense to "sterile injury" relies on the sensing of endogenous molecules (sometimes termed **alarmins**) released from injured cells and not normally present in the tissue environment.

High-mobility group box 1 (**HMGB1**) protein is a well-characterized prototypical alarmin that may be passively released from sterilely injured necrotic cells as well as actively released from immune and epithelial cells following either stress or exposure to proinflammatory cytokines (IL-1, TNFβ, IFN-γ). Actively secreted HMGB1 is important as a late acting mediator in systemic inflammation such as that resulting from severe sepsis. However, HMGB1 is also important in the early innate immune response since passively released HMGB1 binds to a number of receptors important in that response (toll-like receptors TLR-2 and -4 of myeloid cells and RAGE, discussed below). This results in activation of the NF-κB pathway and synthesis of a wide variety of inflammatory and chemotactic cytokines (such as CXCL12) from dendritic cells and monocyte/macrophages and promotes the early migration of leukocytes to the site of sterile injury. Other molecules that are predominantly released by necrotic cells and show alarmin-like stimulation of innate immunity include IL-1α, heat-shock proteins, uric acid, and hyaluronan.

During apoptosis, IL-1α is sequestered in the nucleus and not released. However, the molecule is readily released by necrotic cells and induces macrophages and neutrophils to release numerous cytokines (such as IL-6 and TNFα) and promotes accumulation of such cells at the site of injury. Released IL-1α is a major alarmin and crucial for the initiation of inflammation under such conditions.

Mitochondrial DNA and N-formyl peptides synthesized and released by damaged mitochondria also trigger PRRs (possibly because of the prokaryotic ancestry of mitochondria). Mitochondrial derived alarmins specifically trigger neutrophil PRRs and induce migration and degranulation of these cells in response to injury. Hence, mitochondrial damage is important in triggering the early cellular phase of acute inflammation (discussed below).

Sensing Pathogens: Pathogen Recognition Receptors

Pathogen-associated molecular patterns (often termed **PAMPs**) are molecules associated with pathogens foreign to self (with the exception of damaged mitochondrial products noted above). In general, PAMPs are essential for pathogen survival and unlikely to be lost by selection. A long and non-exhaustive list includes (1) microbial membrane components (notably lipopolysaccharide **LPS**, peptidoglycans, and other molecules), (2) surface glycoproteins, (3) bacterial flagella, (4) mannose containing polymers, (5) bacterial N-formylmethionyl containing peptides, and (6) nucleic acids (such as viral double-stranded and single-stranded RNA, and bacterial DNA characterized by unmethylated CpG motifs). The list of PRRs sensing PAMPs is equally long and includes cell membrane bound, intracellular, and secreted molecules specialized to deal with particular classes of molecules and pathogens. For example, intracellular PRRs deal with viral or intracellular bacterial threats. PRRs are germ line encoded and are often expressed constitutively (although upregulation may occur during pathogen challenge). The best-known set of receptors are the cell membrane located toll-like receptors (**TLRs**) predominantly expressed on normal macrophages and dendritic cells (but also on other specialized cell populations such as enteroendocrine cells of the intestine and in colonic epithelial cells).

Toll-Like Receptors

Although TLRs were first characterized in *Drosophila*, homologous proteins exist throughout the animal kingdom where they play a role in host defense. Hence, they represent what is likely to be the earliest host defense PRR to evolve. TLRs are expressed as integral membrane glycoproteins present on either the cell surface (TLRs-1, -2, -4, -5, -6) or within intracellular vesicles such as endosomes, endoplasmic reticulum, or lysosomes (TLRs-3, -7, -8, -9). Humans have 10 functional TLRs that are type I transmembrane proteins each of which has a differing specificity based on their leucine-rich repeat (LRR) containing ectodomains. Downstream signaling is mediated via an intracellular toll interleukin-1-like receptor (**TIR**) domain. The downstream signaling via TIR is dependent on sets of specific signaling molecules that yield responses that differ depending on the nature of the PAMP sensed and the cell bearing the receptor. Adapter **MyD88** is used by all TLRs except TLR3 and ultimately stimulates the production of proinflammatory cytokines via NF-κB and MAP kinases. Adaptor **TRIF** is active in TLRs-3, -4, -7, and -9 and results in downstream induction of type I interferons with antiviral activity in addition to proinflammatory cytokines stimulated via Myd88 (Figure 2-32).

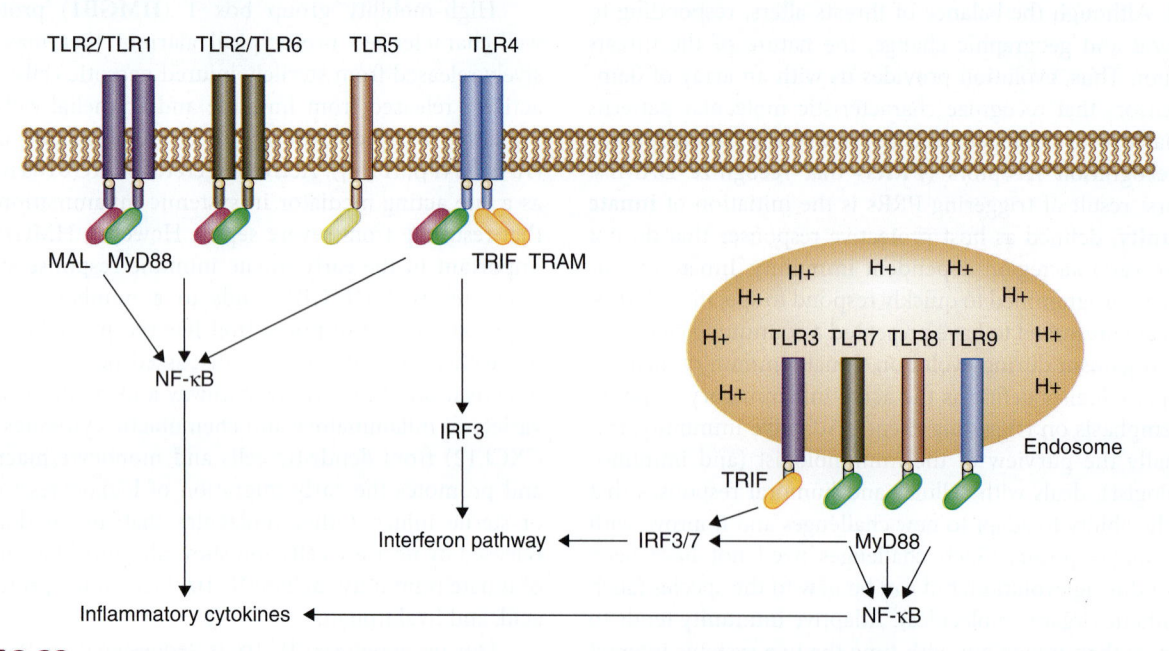

FIGURE 2-32 Localization and signaling pathways of TLRs: Note TLR-2 forms functional heterodimers with TLRs-1 and -6. MAL MyD88 adaptor like proteins; TRAM, TRIF-related adaptor molecule. See text for additional details. Source: This research was originally published in Clinical Science. Vallejo J. Role of toll-like receptors in cardiovascular disease. Clin Sci. 2011; 121:1–10, © copyright the Biochemical Society.

The PAMP specificity of particular TLRs has been clarified using murine knockouts. In general, the intracellular TLRs (3,7,8 and 9) are nucleic acid sensors detecting the products of bacterial and viral pathogens, whereas the cell surface TLRs sense a wide array of bacterial, fungal, and parasitic structural components. TLRs-1, -2, and -6 recognize bacterial-derived lipids and are important in sensing gram-positive bacteria; TLR-4 (in complexes with another protein, MD-2) recognizes the bacterial LPS of Gram-negative bacteria, which is responsible for septic shock. TLR-5 binds bacterial flagellin and is heavily expressed on epithelial cells of the gut and respiratory tree where it is important in localized host defense.

Cytoplasmic Receptors

An ever-increasing set of cytoplasmic PRRs is being defined. They detect bacteria that escape into the cytoplasm (e.g., *Shigella*, *Listeria*, and invasive *E. coli*). These include nuclear-binding and oligomerization domain (NOD)-like receptors (**NLRs**) and retinoid acid-inducible gene-I (RIG-1)-like receptors (**RLRs**).

Nod-Like Receptors (NLRs)

There are over 20 NLR genes in the human genome, which are organized into groups based on their amino-terminal protein–protein interaction domain.

- **NLRCs** contain a caspase recruitment domain (CARD)
- **NLRPs** have a pyrin domain (PYD)
- **NAIPs** have a baculovirus inhibitor repeat domain (BIR)

Both CARD and PYD domains are members of the "death domain fold" superfamily so named because of their importance in mediating the formation of high molecular weight complexes via self-association that are important in caspase activation and apoptosis. The BIR is a zinc-finger domain characteristic of a number of antiapoptotic proteins. All NLRs have a characteristic NOD domain necessary for oligonucleotide binding and self-association and a C-terminal LRR region conferring PAMP specificity. Binding of PAMPs by the LRR permits the NOD regions to oligomerize and expose the effector domains allowing them to interact thereby promoting interactions with other CARD or PYD effector molecules (Figure 2-33).

NOD1 (NLRC1) and **NOD2 (NLRC2)** both recognize bacterial-derived peptidoglycan components. Upon PAMP binding, additional CARD containing effector molecules are recruited (RICK, CARD9) ultimately resulting in NF-κB and MAP-kinase activation and expression of proinflammatory gene products including IL-6, IL-10, TNFα, and IL-1β. NOD1 and NOD2 are important in defense against many cytoinvasive bacteria. NOD1 polymorphisms are associated with risk of asthma and atopic eczema with increased serum IgE levels. Common NOD2 mutations are risk factors for the development of Crohn disease. Nod1 is expressed in many cell types, whereas NOD2 expression is more limited, being found in macrophages, dendritic cells, and paneth and epithelial cells of the gut.

Inflammasomes and NLRs

PAMP-engaged NODs may associate with a CARD containing adaptor protein (ASC) promoting the formation of large multimolecular complexes termed **inflammasomes** (in a manner analogous to apoptosomes). The interaction domains of the inflammasome than associate with and promote the activation

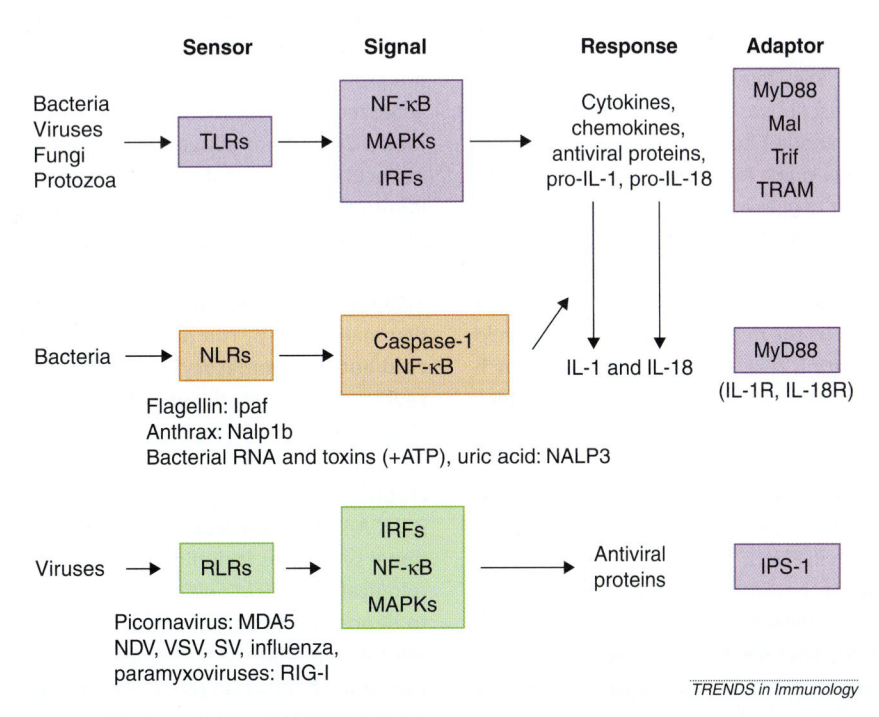

FIGURE 2-33 Families of pathogen receptors, TLRs, NLRs, and RLRs: Additional details in text. Source: Reprinted from Creagh E, O'Neil L. TLRs, NLRs and RLRs: a trinity of pathogen sensors that co-operate in innate immunity. Trends in Immunology, 2006, 27(8), 352–357. Copyright 2006, with permission from Elsevier.

of CARD containing caspase-1. Active caspase-1 results in (1) the formation of active IL-1β and IL-18 from precursor molecules by caspase-mediated proteolysis, (2) promotion of the release of IFN-γ, and (3) activation a number of cells important in the inflammatory process (some T cells, NK cells).

- **Ipaf (NLRC4)** inflammasomes sense bacterial flagellin and are important in the host defense against *Salmonella typhimurium* and *Legionella pneumophila*. NAIP NLRs appear to modify the specificity of this inflammasome.
- **Nalp1 (NLRP1) and cryopyrin (NLRP3)** inflammasomes are important in host defenses against bacterial toxins (and in particular anthrax lethal toxin in the case of NLRP1), and a wide variety of bacterial cell components, RNA, and uric acid crystals.

Macrophages infected with a number of pathogens associated with inflammasome formation and caspase-1 activation undergo a distinctive form of cell death termed **pyroptosis** characterized by rapid destruction of cell membrane integrity and production of large amounts of IL-1β (Figure 2-34).

Although cryopyrinopathies such as described in Case 2-4 are uncommon (FCAS is easily mistaken for classical urticaria, which is most often of allergic etiology), they are illustrative of the central importance of innate immunity and IL-1 in host defense. Many inherited autoinflammatory diseases exist and are associated with defects in the regulation of innate immunity. In fact, the most common of these **familial**

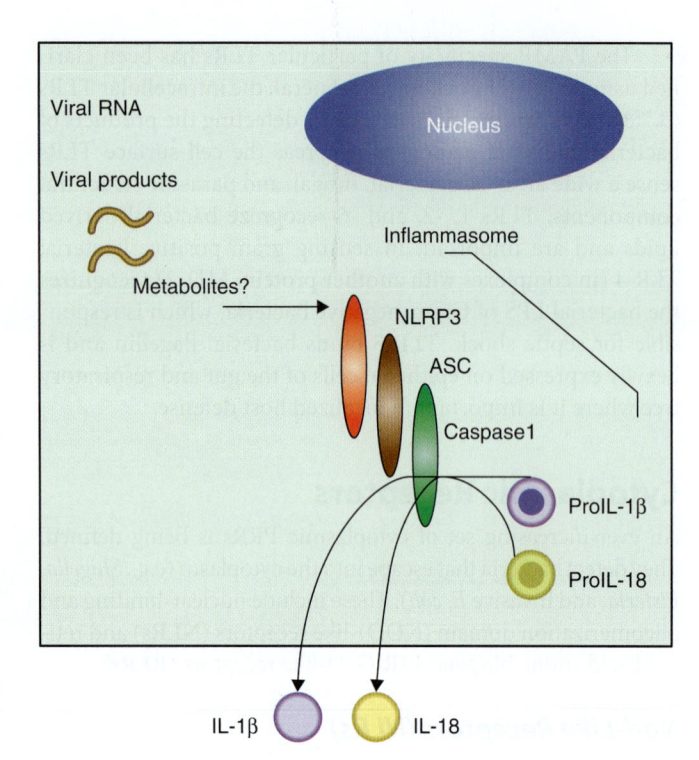

FIGURE 2-34 PRR signaling the inflammasome: A simplified model of NLRP3 signaling by viral RNA products. Source: Reprinted from Courtney Wilkins, Michael Gale Jr. Recognition of viruses by cytoplasmic sensors. Current Opinion in Immunology, 22(1), 41–47. Copyright 2010, with permission from Elsevier.

CASE 2-4

HUNTING FOR ZEBRAS

A 28-year-old primipara consults her pediatrician about her 3-month old male child. She states that the child develops a recurrent rash that she describes as "looking like hives" over different areas of his body about 2 hours after waking. The child becomes "fussy," has a low-grade fever, and sweats excessively. The rash and fever appear to peak in several hours, but the child becomes afebrile and rash free in 1 to 2 days. She states that she can prevent most such occurrences by keeping the child warm after waking. The pediatrician notes the occurrence of the symptoms described by the mother after keeping the child for 2 hours in a chilly waiting area. A blood sample and punch biopsy from an area of the rash are obtained from the child. An elevated erythrocyte sedimentation rate (ESR) and elevated C-reactive protein (CRP) level are reported by the laboratory. Both results are nonspecific indicators of systemic inflammation. The pathology report states the finding of perivascular dermal inflammation rich in PMNs.

On a return visit, the pediatrician questions the parent about the occurrence of similar symptoms in other members of her family. She states that her husband says he is "cold-sensitive" and has learned to bundle up to avoid unpleasant joint pains and rashes.

The pediatrician suspects an uncommon inherited autosomal dominant condition termed a **cryopyrinopathy**. Such are examples of **autoinflammatory** diseases, which are characterized by inappropriate and excessive systemic inflammation related to activation of the innate immune system. Molecular testing of the patient's (and father's) blood reveals identical mutations in the *NLRP3* gene that encodes the cryopyrin protein (see above). Such gain of function mutations lead to inappropriate activation of the NLRP3 (NALP3) inflammasome, resulting in excessive formation of proinflammatory IL-1β. The disease described is termed **familial cold autoinflammatory syndrome (FCAS)**. Two other more severe cryopyrinopathies related to *NLRP3* mutations are characterized (Muckle–Wells syndrome and neonatal-onset multisystem inflammatory disease [NOMID] also called chronic infantile neurological cutaneous articular syndrome [CINCA]). Both are associated with a constellation of additional symptoms including deafness, joint involvement, neurological complications, and ultimately renal disease related to deposition of amyloid protein, resulting from long-standing inflammation (see Chapter 12). Pharmacological inhibition of IL-1β results in rapid amelioration of symptoms in the more severe forms of the disease.

Mediterranean fever (**FMF**) is an autosomal recessive disease characterized by recurrent fevers, rashes, and serositis (sterile peritonitis) and ultimately renal failure from amyloidosis when untreated. The carrier rate may be greater than 1 in 5 among some ethnic groups. The disease results from inactivating mutations in the *MEFV* gene coding the protein pyrin (more poetically termed marenostrin in Latinophile Europe). Pyrin inhibits the activity of caspase 1 and hence, when functional, serves to limit IL-1β production.

ACUTE INFLAMMATION

Introduction

As discussed, the inflammatory response is triggered by tissue injury, either mediated by pathogens or more directly by trauma. Evolution has provided us (and our vertebrate and invertebrate relatives) with complex sensor systems designed to detect and trigger responses in order to diminish such injury. Such responses (as well as their lack) can, of themselves, cause tissue injury. The triggering of such early responses to injury is complex, depending on the production proinflammatory cytokines via NF-κB and MAP kinases and active IL-1β as a result of inflammasome activation. Although our understanding of such sensor systems is relatively recent, humankind has documented the physical effects of acute inflammation as early as 1000 BCE. Acute inflammation is defined as the rapid protective response of vascularized tissue so that humoral mediators and circulating cells (predominantly polymorphonuclear neutrophils, PMNs or neutrophils) are activated and move from the microvasculature (capillaries and postcapillary venules) into tissue toward the site of injury. The acute phase of inflammation lasts minutes to days and may result in **resolution** of the injury, wherein the source of injury is eliminated and tissue architecture and function are restored or may proceed to **chronic inflammation**. In addition to PMNs, endothelial cells of the microvasculature, tissue mast cells, and the hemostatic system play a major role in the acute response.

Chronic inflammation lasts days to years. Resolution is unlikely and fibrosis (scar formation) is likely to replace damaged parenchymal and stromal tissue. Hence, tissue architecture will not be restored and function is likely to be compromised. The major cellular players are the mononuclear cells (macrophages, lymphocytes, fibroblasts, and endothelial cells) along with noncellular tissue components. A specialized form of persistent chronic inflammation termed **chronic granulomatous inflammation** is associated with certain poorly degraded injurious agents such a mycobacteria, talc, and silica and in some cases with no defined etiological agent (the disease **sarcoidosis**). This form of chronic inflammation is associated with the formation of **granulomas**, compact aggregates of macrophages, which are flattened and often fused (**epithelioid cells**) sometimes into multinucleate **giant cells**. Such granulomas may have a necrotic center (**caseating granulomas**) and are associated with *Mycobacterium tuberculosis*. Granulomas are variably associated with mononuclear cells rims and fibroblastic activity producing fibrotic margins as will be discussed. In the case of a persistent irritant, an endogenous agent (such as in autoimmunity) or a defect in host defense, chronic inflammation may continue indefinitely. More often healing occurs, often in concert with abating chronic inflammation. During healing, the inflammatory cell exudate is replaced by a specialized **granulation tissue** that is rich in fibroblasts and developing capillaries, which ultimately restore damaged vasculature and form the mature scar (**Figure 2-35**).

Although acute and chronic inflammation are defined by time course and degree of persistence, particular etiological agents provoke particular patterns of inflammation in tissue.

- Bacteria generally provoke an acute pattern of inflammation. Some (predominantly intracellular) bacteria such as mycobacteria or listeria result in a chronic (or chronic granulomatous) pattern.
- Viruses and fungal agents provoke a chronic pattern of inflammation in which mononuclear cells predominate. The adaptive immune system is critical in defending against such agents.
- Sterile injury may also result in characteristic acute inflammation.

Certain anatomic sites may show unusual patterns of inflammation. Bacterial infections of the bone (osteomyelitis) may involve continuing acute inflammation without resolution. Inflammatory events in the lung result in a characteristic pattern of response termed **diffuse alveolar damage** (DAD), which results in the clinical syndrome termed **acute respiratory distress syndrome** (ARDS). Although the general principles of inflammation are maintained, the specific cellular response (involving elements of the pulmonary interstitium, pneumocytes and alveolar capillaries) is distinctive (**Figure 2-36**).

Termination of the immune response is of obvious importance in maintaining tissue homeostasis. Macrophages serve to inhibit its continuation, besides playing an important role in promoting early inflammation. Secretion of IL-10 and TGF-β by macrophages that have phagocytosed apoptotic bodies serves to limit ongoing inflammation and promote healing.

Acute inflammation is often divided into two components. The **vascular phase** is associated with changes in vascular permeability and leakage of soluble mediators into tissue with the subsequent production of tissue edema. The **cellular phase** initially involves the increasing interaction of neutrophils with endothelial cells near the site of tissue injury. This is followed by the transmigration of neutrophils through the vessel wall and their directed migration along a chemical gradient toward the site of injury (**chemotaxis**). At the site of injury, neutrophils ingest (**phagocytose**) and inactivate pathogens by release of granular contents containing a multiplicity of bioactive components. The release of such toxic components may be internal, into phagocytic vesicles containing the pathogen or injurious agent, or it may be external and into the tissue environment. The latter results in inflammation-related tissue injury. The two phases of acute inflammation are separable in terms of mechanism but often temporally overlap.

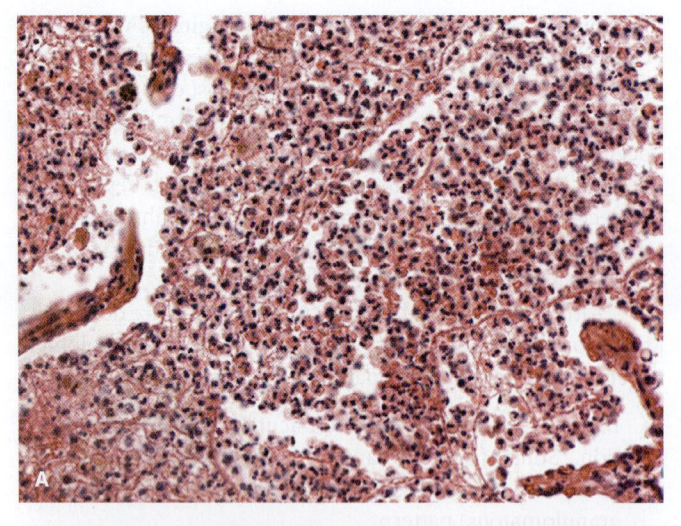

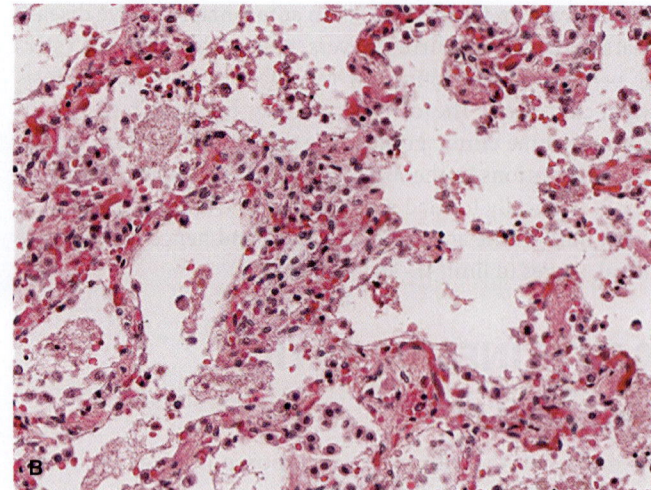

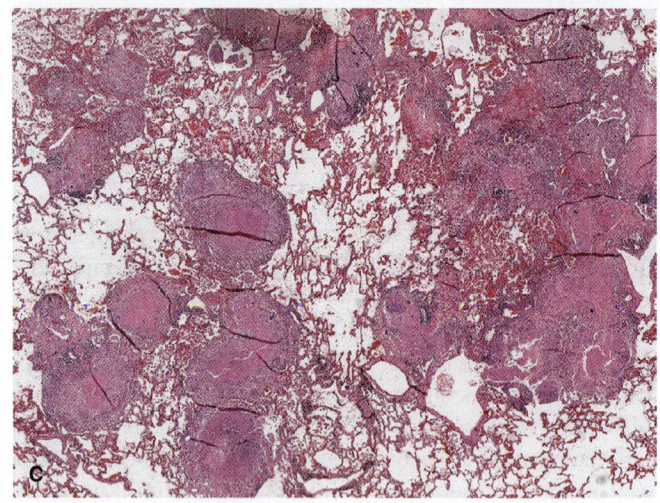

FIGURE 2-35 Patterns of inflammation in the lung: **(A)** Acute pattern of inflammation in bacterial pneumonia. Cells are predominantly (but not exclusively) neutrophils. **(B)** Chronic pattern of inflammation in viral (adenoviral) pneumonia. The process is predominantly interstitial. **(C)** Granulomatous pattern of inflammation in untreated tuberculosis (low power, see Figure 2-29 for high-power view).

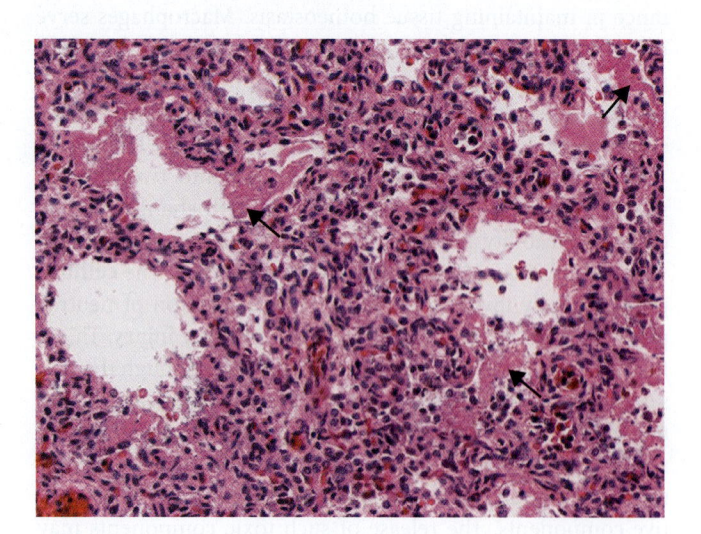

FIGURE 2-36 **DAD:** The exudative (acute) stage of DAD, resulting from a severe bacterial pneumonia. So-called "hyaline membranes" are the result of the leakage of plasma components into the alveolar space as a result of damage to type I pneumocytes (arrow). There is massive interstitial accumulation of mononuclear cells.

Vascular Phase of Inflammation

The vascular phase of acute inflammation is accompanied by obvious physical changes near the site of injury. The association of heat, redness, swelling, and pain with injury was codified by Celsus, a Roman encyclopedist as *calor, rubor, tumor, and dolor;* the four cardinal signs of inflammation, in the 1st century CE. Loss of function (*functio laesa*) was subsequently added (frequently misattributed to Galen in the 2nd century CE, most likely by German pathologists in the 19th century). In fact, the physical signs of inflammation, along with a specific term for such (lexigraphically related to heat), may be found in Egyptian medical texts by about 1000 BCE.

The four cardinal signs of inflammation are all related to the early vascular changes associated with acute inflammation.

- Initially there may be transient vasoconstriction of arterioles at the site of mild injury. This is likely to be of neurogenic origin.
- This is followed by vasodilation of precapillary arterioles increasing blood flow through capillaries in tissues

(**hyperemia**). The result is redness and heat. Likely mediators include PGs (prostacyclin) and nitric oxide.
- An increase in vascular permeability occurs (usually postcapillary venules and/or capillaries). The movement of fluid and proteins into the tissue is termed **exudation** and results in swelling and compromise of function. Mediators include histamine, serotonin, and **leukotrienes (LTs)**.
- The vasodilation and permeability changes are mediated by multiple mediators produced by cells and formed from plasma proteins. These chemical mediators also cause pain, and hence, additional compromise of function (notably **bradykinen** and PGs).

Resting endothelial cells produce basal levels of **nitric oxide**—the major mediator of inflammatory vasodilation. Nitric oxide synthase 3 (**NOS3**), the major endothelial cell isoform of NOS, is physiologically regulated by vascular shear stress to modulate vasodilation under physiological conditions and has anti-inflammatory actions (such as inhibiting platelet and neutrophil adhesion to the vascular wall). However, stimulation of endothelial cells by histamine, thrombin, and bradykinen leads to increased activity of NOS3, increased production of nitric oxide, and subsequent increased blood flow (rubor and calor) at the site of inflammation.

Mechanism of Tissue Edema

The hydrostatic pressure of blood tends to force fluid out of vessels into tissues. Intact capillaries present a barrier to the passage of plasma proteins (such as albumin) into the tissue. Increases in hydrostatic pressure in intact vasculature (such as might occur in hypertensive conditions) result in **transudation** of increased amounts of fluid, salt, and low molecular weight substances into the tissue space (but not high molecular weight proteins). At the arterial end of the capillary tree, there is a net loss of fluid into the tissue, that is, in part, balanced by the blood proteins' (mostly albumin's) oncotic pressure. The net result is a small loss of fluid into tissue. At the venous end of the capillary bed, there is reduced hydrostatic pressure within the vessels resulting from the pressure drop afforded by the capillary network. At this end of the bed, there is a net return of fluid into the circulation because of the oncotic pressure of the blood protein. In a normal vascular bed, net fluid loss is balanced or almost balanced by fluid reuptake. Any excess tissue fluid is channeled by the lymphatic system back to the circulation. However, if the level of plasma albumin falls (as can occur in hepatic disease), **ascites** (tissue edema) may occur. In the case of acute inflammation, the increase in vascular permeability allows escape of plasma proteins into the tissue, thereby reducing the plasma oncotic pressure, resulting in the characteristic exudative changes (tissue swelling). There are a number of technical terms used for types of exudates that may be encountered in clinical descriptions including the following (**Figure 2-37**):

- **Serous**, having few cells
- **Serosanguinous**, having red cells
- **Fibrinous**, containing fibrin
- **Purluent**, having prominent white cells (pus)

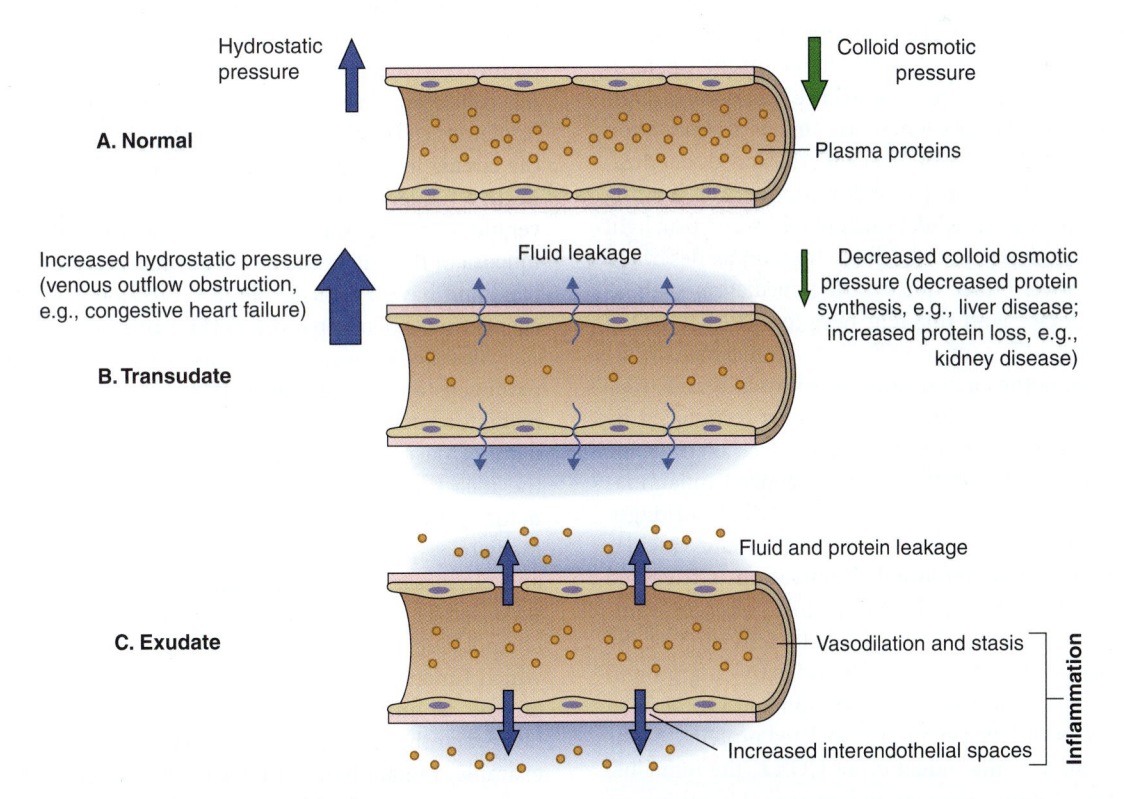

FIGURE 2-37 **Mechanism of transudation and exudation.** Source: Reprinted from Kumar V, et al. "Acute and Chronic Inflammation". In Robbins & Cotran Pathologic Basis of Disease 8E, (Saunders/Elsevier, 2009), pages 43–78. Copyright 2009, with permission from Elsevier.

> **QUICK REVIEW**
> **Molecular Mechanisms of Tissue Edema**
> The mechanism of increased vascular permeability relating to inflammation is complex and involves both the contraction of endothelial cells and the "unzipping" of the tight junctions between the cells. Mild injury produces a rapid and short-lived response (measured in minutes) predominantly in postcapillary venules. Mechanistically this relates to the interaction of humoral chemical mediators such as histamine with localized endothelial receptors. Such interactions produce **type I endothelial activation**, which does not depend on new gene expression. In such activating events, the ligand binds to a heterotrimeric GCPR. This leads to activation of two pathways:
>
> 1. Activation of phospholipase C beta (PLCβ) catalyses the release of inositol-1,45 triphosphate (InsP$_3$) from membrane lipid. Increases in released Ca^{2+} from endoplasmic reticulum activate cellular phospholipase A$_2$ (cPLA$_2$). The calcium-activated phospholipase cleaves membrane phosphatidylcholine yielding arachidonic acid (AA), the precursor molecule for the production of the important classes of PG and LT mediators discussed below.
> 2. GCPR activation also leads to activation of the small g protein **RHO** (RAS homologue) leading to contraction of actin filaments, resulting in cellular reorganization facilitating increased permeability and the adherence of inflammatory cells to the endothelial cell surface.
>
> Histamine binding to H1 endothelial receptors results in a site-specific tyrosine phosphorylation of the calcium-dependent VE-cadherin proteins whose homophilic interaction stabilizes adherens junctions. This phosphorylation results in internalization of VE-cadherin and destabilization of the endothelial permeability barrier. The binding event also leads to intracellular calcium release, myosin light chain kinase activation, and cell contraction as described under (2) above. Other quick acting mediators such as thrombin interact with different receptors (PAR-1 in the case of thrombin) but function by a similar mechanism.
>
> Type I endothelial activation is both rapid and transient lasting for tens of minutes and being terminated by receptor desensitization and subsequent lack of response to agents such as histamine. More prolonged inflammatory changes in the vasculature also contribute to ongoing changes including increased blood flow and vascular leakage. Such **type II endothelial activation** is triggered by agents such as IL-1 and TNF. Cellular receptor-binding triggers MAP kinases. This leads to activation of the nuclear transcription factor NF-κB and activating protein AP-1 resulting in increased transcription and synthesis of a large number of inflammation-associated proteins. Notable among these is the induction of **COX2** (the inducible form of this cyclooxygenase) and increased synthesis of prostaglandin **PGI$_2$** (prostacyclin), which acts as a potent vasodilator and inhibitor of platelet activation. In addition, reorganization of the endothelial cell actin network also occurs, leading to the formation of gaps. Type II activation does not resolve spontaneously and continues as long as stimulatory cytokines persist and with time may lead to endothelial cell injury and death, which is mediated via activation of apoptotic pathways.

Endothelial cell damage also triggers hemostatic and thrombotic pathways (see This Chapter "The Vascular Response to Injury") Such mechanisms and severe direct injury to endothelial cells in venules, arterioles, and capillaries may result in prolonged (hours to days) permeability changes visualized as endothelial cell blebbing and detachment from the basement membrane. This results in mechanical disruption of the permeability barrier. In some cases of direct injury, an initial rapidly resolving response (relating to chemical mediators such as histamine and thrombin) is followed by a second and prolonged increase in permeability caused by type II activation and/or direct endothelial injury.

Histamine and Mast Cells

Histamine, the prototype of an inflammatory mediator causing increased vascular permeability, is produced in vivo by degranulating **mast cells** or **basophils**. (Serotonin, a very similar mediator is secreted by platelets and is found in rodent mast cells.) Mast cells are derived from bone marrow hematopoietic stem cells via the common myeloid progenitor pathway, which gives rise to precursors of granulocytes and macrophages. Mast cell progenitors leave the bone marrow as immature cells and rapidly emigrate into tissue. After leaving the circulation, mast cells mature and are distributed in connective tissue of the skin and elsewhere around nerves and venules or as a distinct T-cell-dependent population found in mucosa of the gut and respiratory mucosa. The cells are long-lived and have a critical role in protection against infectious agents (in particular parasites) **(Figure 2-38)**.

Mast cells are early responders (seconds to minutes) to pathogens and tissue injury. Their cytoplasm is stuffed with mediator containing cytoplasmic granules that led to their name. (Mast was an Old German word for food based on the idea that the cytoplasmic granules were nutritional in nature.) Mast cell granules contain preformed inflammatory mediators, principally histamine and proteases (tryptases and chymases, which are bound to heparin and chondroitin sulphate, respectively) and TNF. Granules also contain chemotactic factor for eosinophils and released proteases, which function as chemotactic factors for neutrophils. Histamine is immediately available following degranulation; however, other granular components (proteases and TNF for example) remain bound to negatively charged carbohydrates as "nanoparticles," which are slowly released into the tissue environment.

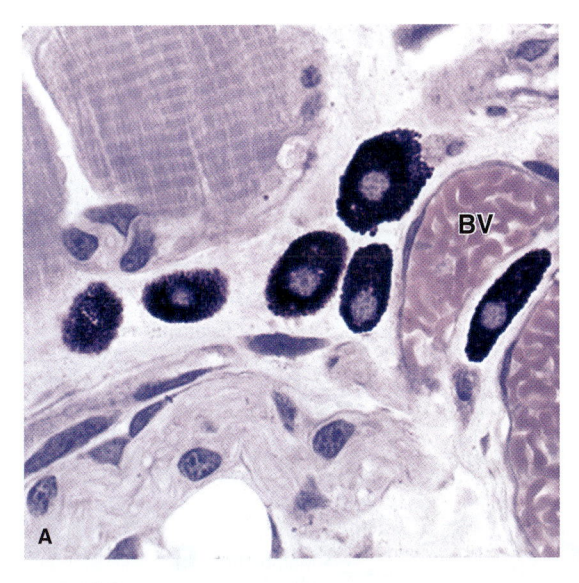

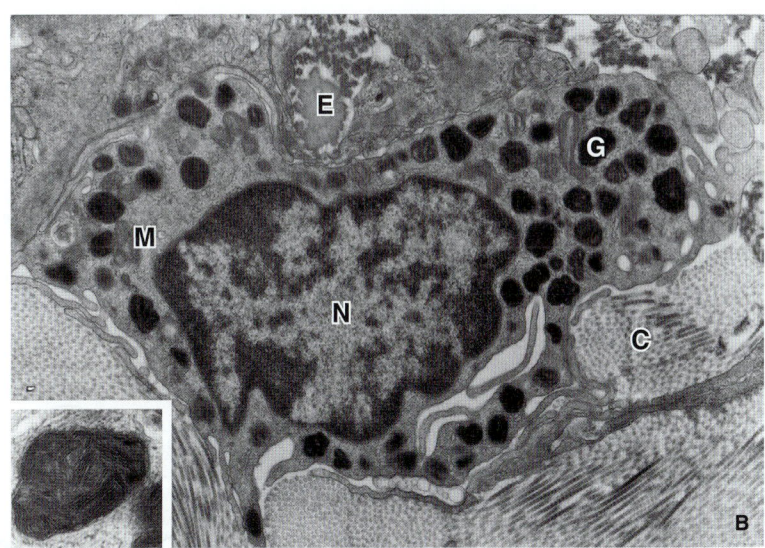

FIGURE 2-38 **Mast cells:** Mast cells are components of loose connective tissues, often located near small blood vessels (BV). **(A)** They are typically oval-shaped, with cytoplasm filled with strongly basophilic granules. ×400. PT. **(B)** Ultrastructurally mast cells show little else around the nucleus (N) besides these cytoplasmic granules (G), except for occasional mitochondria (M). The granule staining in the TEM is heterogeneous and variable in mast cells from different tissues; at higher magnifications, some granules may show a characteristic scroll-like substructure (inset) that contains preformed mediators such as histamine and proteoglycans. The ECM near this mast cell includes elastic fibers (E) and bundles of collagen fibers (C). Source: Mescher AL, Junqueira's Basic Histology text and Atlas 12th ed. McGraw Hill Lange New York, 2010:92, Chapter 5 Figure 5-5.

Mast cells are activated (and triggered to degranulate) by a variety of stimuli including.

- PRRs such as TLRs.
- Binding of Ig Fc to Fc receptors. Best characterized is the binding of IgE to FcεRI receptors. Cross-linking of such receptors by antigen results in allergic type 1 hypersensitive responses including allergic asthma and anaphylactic reactions as a result of mediator release.
- Physical and chemical stimuli such as heat, cold, trauma, and insect venoms.
- Products of inflammation, notably complement C5a via binding to a C5a receptor.

After degranulation, new granule synthesis occurs over a period of days.

In addition to release of preformed granular contents, activated mast cells initiate de novo synthesis of a variety of mediators of inflammation. Within minutes following degranulation, eicosanoids and other lipid mediators are generated and released.

- **Leukotrienes** predominantly aid in the recruitment of neutrophils, in part by their effect on the vascular endothelium. LTs also have vascular effects, including the promotion of dilation and increased permeability.
- The role of **Prostaglandins** is less well defined but may have similar vascular effects and be involved in pain production via neuronal stimulation.
- **Platelet activating factor** (PAF) is a phospholipid synthesized from phosphatidylcholine by the action of phospholipase A_2 followed by acetylation. In addition to being a potent platelet aggregator, PAF has vasodilating activity.

Cytokine and chemokine synthesis and release occurs over a period of hours and includes **TNF** (also present in granules), **IL-4** (important in the maturation of T_h2 cells and promotion of IgE production), **IL-5** (a potent activator of eosinophils and B cells), and CC-chemokine ligand 11 (**CCL11 also known as eotaxin**). The latter two are important in promoting the eosinophilia that often accompanies mast cell activation, parasitic, and allergic disease. Mast cells also play a critical role in activating endothelial cells, thus promoting the interaction of endothelium with circulating cells (predominantly neutrophils but also many other cell types). This will be discussed in greater detail under the cellular phase of acute inflammation. The secretion of IL-4 and IL-5 by mast cells suggests an additional role in adaptive immunity **(Figure 2-39)**.

Basophils

Blood basophils are an uncommon member of the granulocyte class that have many similarities to tissue mast cells. Both derive from a common bone marrow stem cell. However, basophils are released into the circulation as mature cells, can rapidly increase in number in response to inflammation, and have a short circulating life span. Basophils, in common with other granulocytes, migrate to sites of tissue injury where, in a manner similar to mast cells, they degranulate in response to a proinflammatory stimuli. The array and time course of mediator release is also similar to that of mast cells. However, LT C_4 is likely to be the only eicosanoid synthesized with no evidence of the production of PGs. PG D_2 secreted by mast cells is believed to be the major chemoattractant promoting basophil migration into inflamed tissue **(Figure 2-40)**.

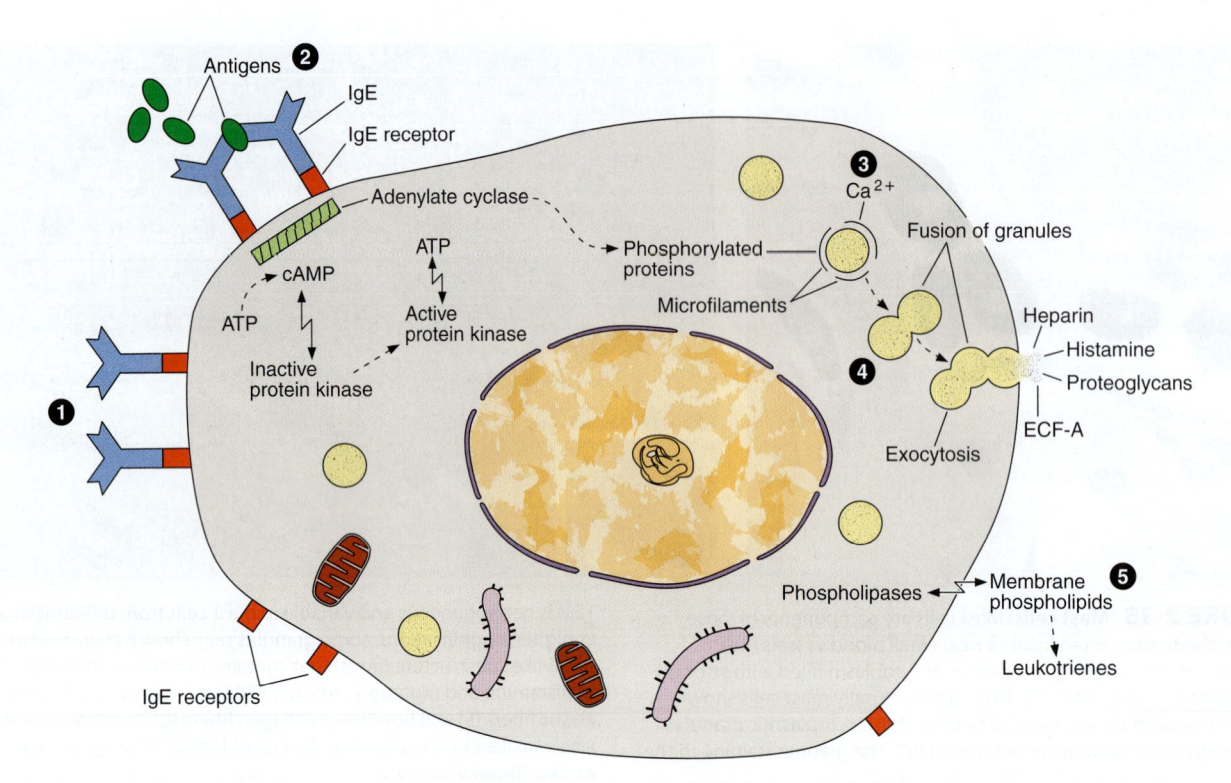

FIGURE 2-39 Function of mast cells: Mast cell secretion is triggered by re-exposure to certain antigens and allergens. Molecules of IgE antibody produced in an initial response to an allergen such as pollen or bee venom are bound to surface receptors for IgE **(1)**, of which 300,000 are present per mast cell. When a second exposure to the allergen occurs, IgE molecules bind this antigen and a few IgE receptors very rapidly become cross-linked **(2)**. This activates adenylate cyclase, leading to phosphorylation of specific proteins and **(3)** entry of Ca^{2+} and rapid exocytosis of some granules **(4)**. In addition, phospholipases act on specific membrane phospholipids, leading to production and release of leukotrienes **(5)**. The components released from granules, as well as the leukotrienes, are immediately active in the local microenvironment and promote a variety of controlled local reactions that together normally comprise part of the inflammatory process called the immediate hypersensitivity reaction. ECF-A, eosinophil chemotactic factor of anaphylaxis. Source: Mescher AL, Junqueira's Basic Histology text and Atlas 12th ed. McGraw Hill Lange New York, 2010:92, Chapter 5 Figure 5-6.

Platelets

Platelets store serotonin in dense granules. However, they lack the ability to synthesize the molecule. Over 90% of the body's serotonin is produced by gut enterochromaffin cells and released into the circulation. Serotonin is taken up from the plasma by a specific platelet transporter. Platelet serotonin release plays a major role in hemostasis and thrombosis by mediating platelet aggregation and may also play a role in the recruitment of neutrophils to the site of inflammation by promoting the interaction of circulating cells with the endothelium, platelets being similar to mast cells in this regard. Serotonin often induces vasoconstriction but causes vasodilation in some vascular beds (such as cerebral arterioles) depending on the serotonin receptors expressed on the endothelium (Figure 2-41).

Vascular Phase of Inflammation: Other Humoral Mediators

Arachidonic Acid Derivatives and Related Molecules

Arachidonic acid (AA) derivatives are eicosanoids (metabolites of 20 carbon unsaturated fatty acids) synthesized from cell membrane phospholipids following lipolysis by activated **phospholipase A_2**. Eicosanoids play a central role in both the vascular and cellular phases of inflammation by mediating changes in vascular tone and permeability, affecting platelet aggregation (and hence hemostatic and thrombotic mechanisms) and promoting migration of inflammatory cells toward the site of injury. In addition, AA products play a role in nociception and systemic effects of inflammation such as the febrile response. The production of the various AA derivatives differs with cell type and temporally during the course of inflammation. For example, during inflammation neutrophils switch from the production of predominantly proinflammatory AA derivatives to participating in the production of anti-inflammatory lipid derivatives (**lipoxins**, derived from AA, **resolvins** and **protectins** derived in an analogous manner from other lipid substrates). The switch in biosynthetic pathways heralds the onset of chronic inflammation with a suppression of neutrophils-mediated inflammation and an increasing role for macrophages (Figure 2-42).

Prostanoids

The biosynthesis of eicosanoids is complex, members of the class having different cellular sources and activities. **Prostaglandins** (PGs) and **thromboxane A_2** (TXA_2) (referred to

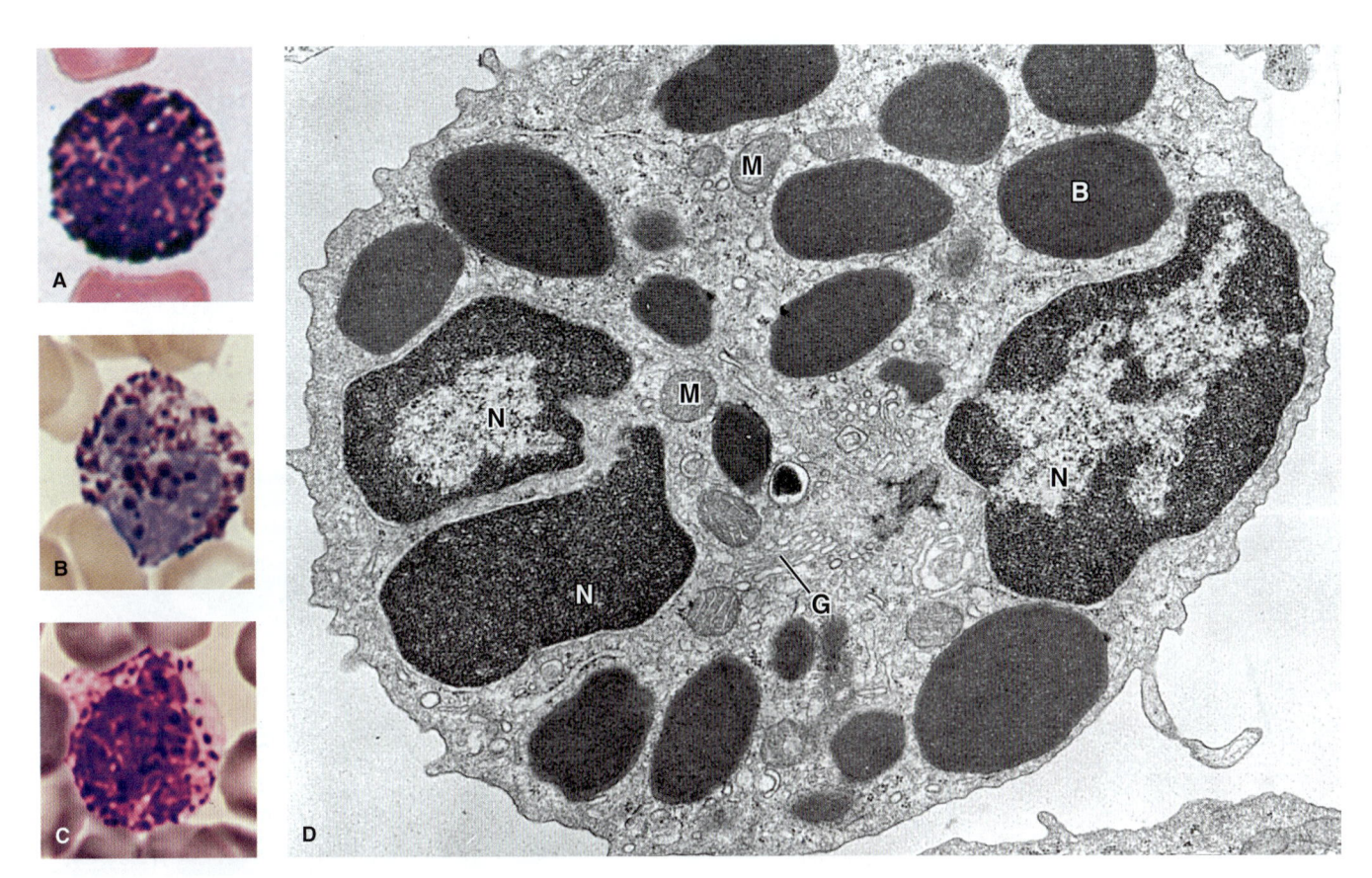

FIGURE 2-40 **Basophils:** Basophils are approximately the same size as neutrophils and eosinophils, but have large, strongly basophilic-specific granules that usually obstruct the appearance of the nucleus having two or three irregular lobes. **(A** and **B):** ×1500, Wright. **(C)** ×1500, Giemsa. **(D)** TEM of a sectioned basophil reveals the lobulated nucleus (N), appearing as three separated portions, the large specific basophilic granules (B), mitochondria (M), and Golgi complex (G). Basophils exert many activities modulating the immune response and inflammation and share many functions with mast cells, which are normal, longer term residents of connective tissue. ×16,000. Source: Mescher AL, Junqueira's Basic Histology text and Atlas 12th ed. McGraw Hill Lange New York 2010:211 (Figure 2-40D reproduced with permission from Terry RW et al. Lab Invest 1969;21:65, Chapter 12 Figure 12-10)

collectively as **prostanoids**) are produced by the action of COXs acting on AA followed by the action of a series of terminal **prostanoid synthetases**. COX occurs as two isoforms; **COX-1** is a widely expressed constitutive enzyme, which for example, produces cytoprotective gastrointestinal (GI) PGs. COX-1 is also responsible for the production of TXA_2 by the platelet, macrophage, and other leukocytes. *TXA_2 is a potent platelet aggregator and mediator of thrombosis.* **COX-2** is an inducible enzyme produced at the site of inflammation by macrophages and other cells stimulated by proinflammatory cytokines such as TNFα and IL-1β. **Prostaglandin E_2** (PGE_2) is a major product of COX-2 and is responsible for a variety of proinflammatory effects including fever, pain, and the vascular response (synergizing with other mediators to increase blood flow and increase vascular permeability) **(Figure 2-43)**.

> ### QUICK REVIEW
> #### Nonsteroidal Anti-Inflammatory Drugs
> The nonsteroidal anti-inflammatory drugs (NSAIDs) aspirin (and several other similar compounds such as ibuprofen and naproxen) function by inhibiting both COX isoforms and demonstrating in vivo anti-inflammatory activity consistent with their in vitro COX inhibiting activity. Such drugs have well recognized antithrombotic and anti-inflammatory activity. However, inhibition of COX-1-dependent GI protective PGs can result in mucosal ulceration and other damage to the GI system. Hence, careful titration of aspirin dose may be necessary. COX-1 inhibition by aspirin is the result of acetylation of a serine residue at the AA-binding site and produces irreversible inactivation. Aspirin has a somewhat different action on COX-2 in that the acetylated enzyme (ac-COX-2) is catalytically active but results in the production of a class of compounds (lipoxins) that are anti-inflammatory and inhibit neutrophil adhesion to, and emigration from, the vasculature. The quest for specific COX-2 inhibitors in an attempt to reduce GI toxicities is well known. However, COX-2-specific inhibitors reduce the production of prostaglandin I_2 (PGI_2) that is both antithrombotic (opposing the effects of thromboxane in the vasculature) and important in the regulation of the rennin-angiotensin system

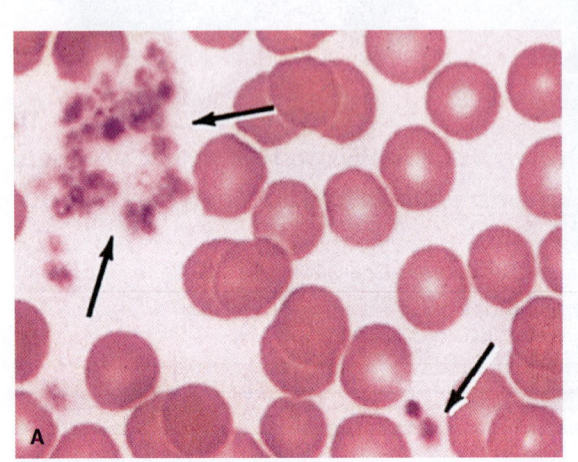

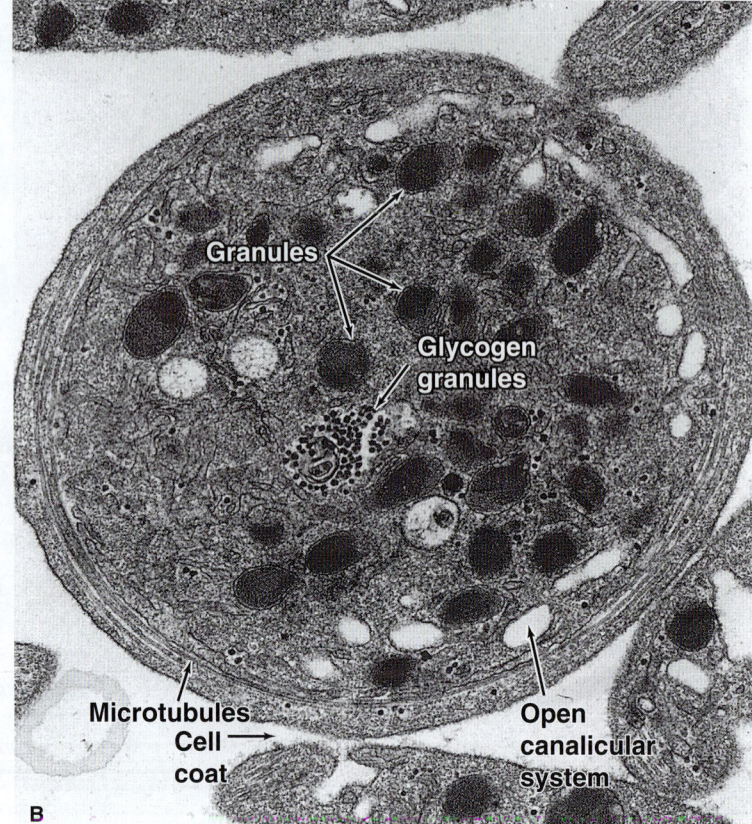

FIGURE 2-41 Platelets: Platelets are cell fragments 2–4 μm in diameter derived from megakaryocytes of bone marrow. Their primary function is to rapidly release the content of their granules upon contact with collagen (or other materials outside of the endothelium) to begin the process of clot formation and reduce blood loss from the vasculature. **(A)** In a blood smear, platelets (arrows) are often found as aggregates. ×1500. Wright. **(B)** Ultrastructurally a platelet typically shows a system of microtubules and actin filaments near the periphery to help maintain its shape and an open canalicular system of vesicles continuous with the plasmalemma. The central region contains glycogen and secretory granules of different types. ×40,000. Source: Mescher AL, Junqueira's Basic Histology text and Atlas 12th ed. McGraw Hill Lange New York 2010:214 (Figure 2-41B reproduced with permission from DR. MJG Harrison Middlesex Hospital and University College London, Chapter 12, Figure 12-13)

in the kidney. Concern remains about the cardiovascular safety of such COX-2-specific agents when used for extended periods of time.

PGs have both paracrine and autocrine roles in maintaining homeostasis in uninflamed tissue where production is generally at low levels. Induction of COX-2 during inflammation leads to much elevated synthesis. However, COX-1-dependent production of prostanoids may be significant early in inflammation, prior to COX-2 induction.

Prostaglandin H_2 is the source of the prostanoids (and is produced by both COX-1 and COX-2). A summary of major prostanoids important in inflammation, their action, and site of synthesis is as follows:

- **Prostaglandin E_2** (PGE_2) *plays a major role in acute inflammation producing both arteriolar dilation and increasing microvascular permeability*. It also plays a role in inflammatory pain production at both peripheral and central sites. PGE_2 activity is mediated by cellular receptors specific for the molecule (E prostanoid receptors) of which there are four major subtypes (EP1–EP4) that differ in cellular distribution and the signaling pathways they activate. In some cases, PGE_2 may oppose the action of other prostanoids and have an anti-inflammatory action. Major sources of PGE_2 in inflammation include platelets, vascular smooth muscle cells, and activated macrophages.
- **Prostacyclin** (PGI_2) is synthesized predominantly by vascular endothelial and smooth muscle cells where it acts locally and is rapidly inactivated. Although some PGI_2 is constitutively synthesized under the control of COX-1, COX-2 induced by inflammation or vascular stress is the major source. PGI_2 has anti-inflammatory activities by inhibiting platelet aggregation, leukocyte adhesion to the endothelium, and by acting as a vasodilator and opposing the action of TXA_2.
- **Prostaglandin D_2** (PGD_2) is produced predominantly by activated mast cells in peripheral tissues and also by cells important in the adaptive immune response (dendritic cells and T_h2 cells). This prostanoid is best known for it role in

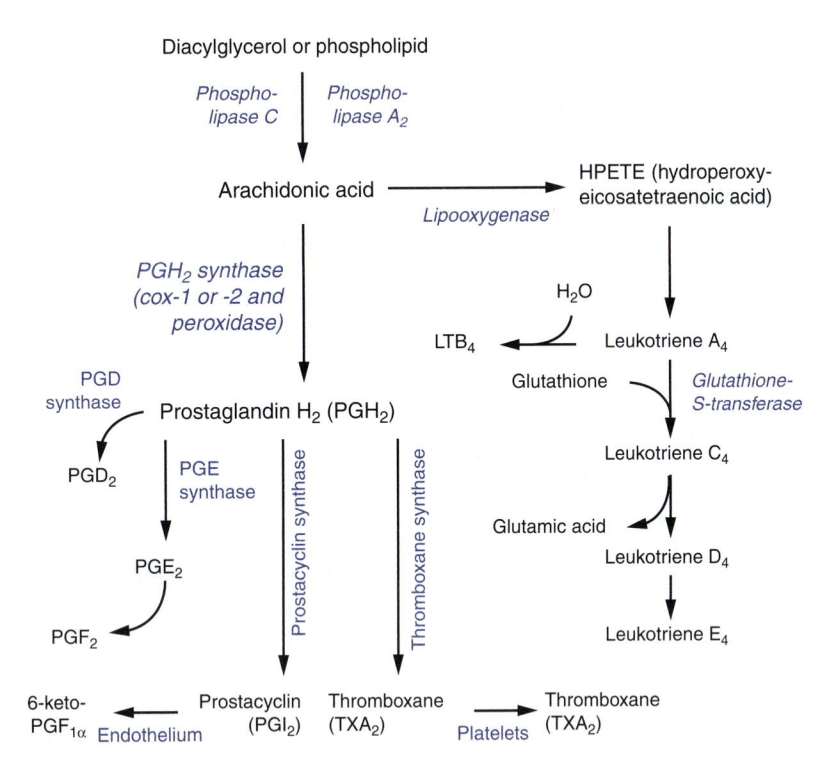

FIGURE 2-42 **Overview of eicosanoid synthesis:** Some anti-inflammatory eicosanoids use parallel pathways substituting dihomo-gamma-linolenic acid (DGLA), a derivative of linoleic acid or eicosapentaenoic acid (EPA) common in fish oils.

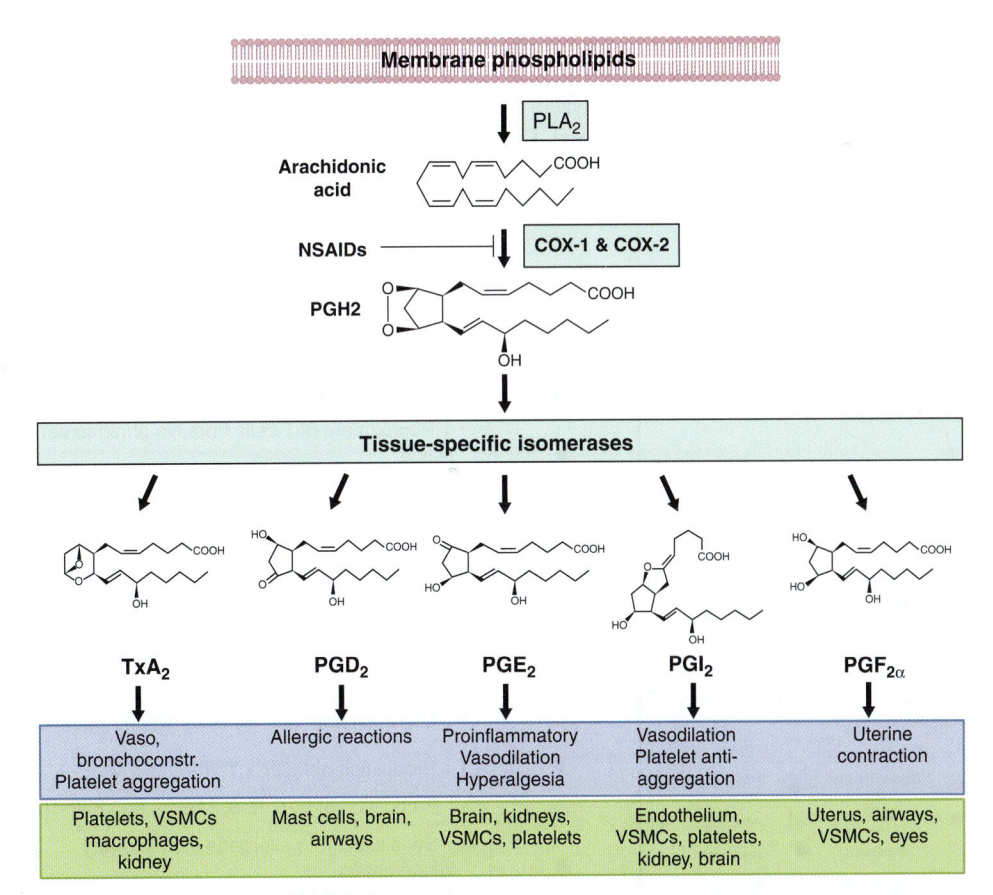

FIGURE 2-43 **Formation, biological effects, and tissue source of prostaglandins.** Source: Ricciotti, E, FitzGerald G. Prostaglandins and Inflammation Arterioscler Thromb Vasc Biol 2011 May;31(5):986–1000, Figure 1 Page 17) [modified with reference to Samuelsson B Role of Basic Science in the Development of New Medicines: Examples from the Eicosanoid Field. J Biol Chem. 2012 March 23; 287(13): 10070–10080, Figure 4 page 10074]

immune-mediated allergic disease where it is responsible for many of the symptoms associated with allergen-induced IgE-mediated asthma including bronchoconstriction and eosinophil and T_h2 cell accumulation in the bronchial tree.
- **Prostaglandin $F_{2\alpha}$** ($PGF_{2\alpha}$) has a major role in the regulation of the female reproductive system. The molecule is synthesized in endothelial cells and vascular smooth muscle cells and has a proinflammatory activity, which is not well defined but may be significant in chronic inflammatory conditions. It plays a particularly significant role in the umbilical cord where it is the major prostanoid synthesized in response to shear stress.
- **TXA_2** is a short-lived metabolite that is predominantly synthesized by platelet COX-1 but can also be produced by activated macrophages via COX-2. TXA_2 is a potent mediator of platelet adhesion and aggregation and vasoconstriction. It serves as a major stimulus for the response of the endothelial cell to inflammation.

Leukotrienes

The synthesis of **leukotirenes** (LTs) starts with the same AA molecule as does the synthesis of prostanoids. The initial stage of synthesis utilizes the enzyme **5-lipoxygense** (5-LO), hence LTs are referred to as products of the **5-LO pathway**. 5-LO is activated by Ca^{++} in tandem with PLA_2 and both active enzymes transit from the cytosol to the nuclear membrane. A 5-LO-activating protein (FLAP) located in the membrane interacts with 5-LO and furthers the production of the initial LT product LTA_4, which is than rapidly hydrolyzed to LTB_4 or glutathione conjugated to yield the **cysteinyl LTs** (**cyst-LT**) consisting of **LTC_4**, **LTD_4**, and **LTE_4**. LTs (as their name implies) are predominantly synthesized by bone-marrow-derived mature leukocytes. However, the predominant LT synthesized differs among cells. Neutrophils, dendritic cells and B lymphocytes secrete predominantly LTB_4. Eosinophils, basophils, and mast cells predominantly secrete cyst-LTs. Monocyte/macrophages secrete both classes of LT. Some cells unable to synthesize LTA_4 may nevertheless serve as an important source of LTs. For example, platelets do not contain 5-LO but can produce cyst-LT from exogenous sources. Platelet-derived cyst-LT (predominantly LTE_4) may play a role in asthma (**Figure 2-44**).

LT have both autocrine and paracrine effects on multiple cell targets mediated through a set of specific LT receptors. LTB_4 and the cyst-LT have differing sets of activities as summarized below.

- *LTB_4 is one of the most potent chemotactic factors known and has a critical role in the early phases of inflammation and innate immunity.* Neutrophils are a major source of LTB_4. This LT promotes the transit of such cells to the site of inflammation, activates the cells, and promotes degranulation. Notably, LTB_4 stimulates the release of the antimicrobial α-defensins and other neutrophil granule-derived antiviral and antibacterial proteins (see Chapter "Neutrophil Granules and Host Defense"). LTB_4 is also produced by monocyte/macrophages and similarly recruits and activates these cells. The molecule also recruits immature mast cell progenitors to tissue sites. Hence, LTB_4 synthesis is an important factor in promoting the increased number of inflammatory cells at the site of tissue injury.

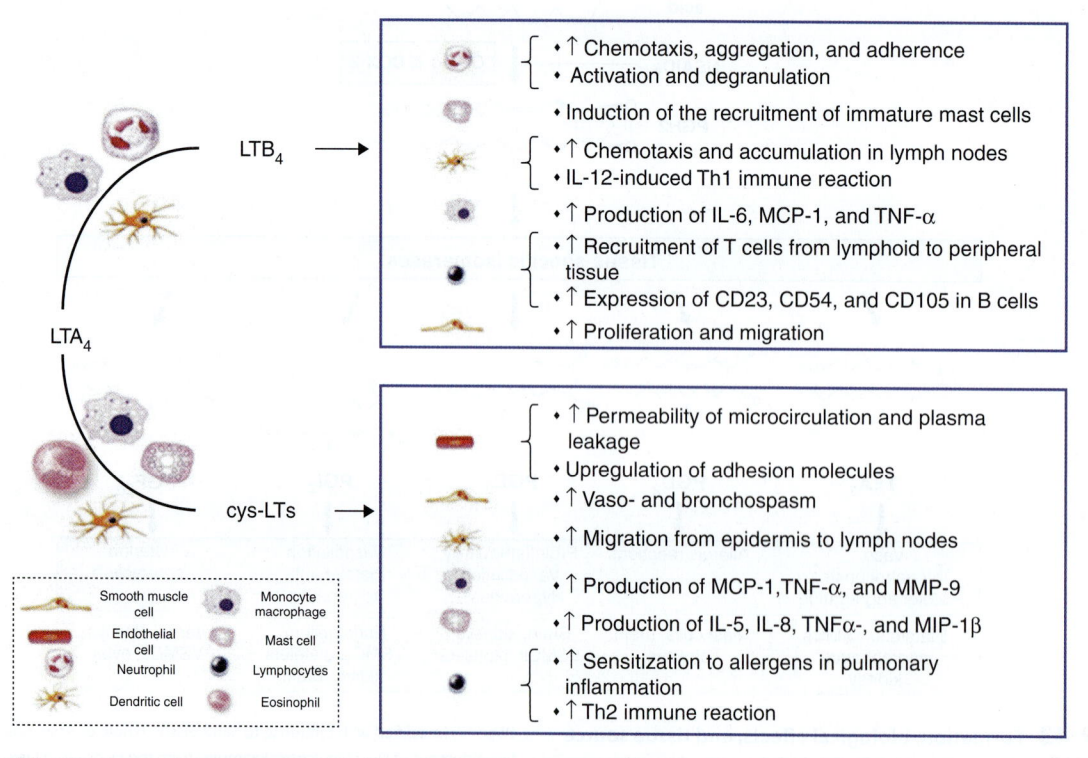

FIGURE 2-44 Formation, biological effects, and cellular source of leukotrienes.

- **Cyst-LT** as a group are potent bronchoconstrictors playing a major role in the pathogenesis of asthma including the bronchospasm, edema, eosinophilic infiltration, and goblet cell hyperplasia, which characterize the disease. Both eosinophils and mast cells, which play a major role in atopic allergy, are important sources of the molecules. There are subtle differences in the effects of the different cyst-LT. LTE_4 is the most long-lived and is of particular importance in some presentations of asthma, which are accompanied by high levels of this metabolite. Inhaled LTE_4 (but not LTC_4, or LTD_4) potentiates airway hyperresponsiveness on subsequent challenge with histamine and produces tissue eosinophilia and mast cell accumulation. Cyst-LT also constricts vascular smooth muscle cells. The molecules act on endothelial cells to promote upregulation of adhesive molecules and increase plasma leakage and tissue edema.

Platelet-Activating Factor

In response to inflammatory stimuli, **platelet-activating factor** (PAF) is rapidly synthesized through a so-called remodeling pathway in which membrane phosphatidylcholines are degraded to an intermediate alkyl-sn-glycero-phosphocholine (lyso-PAF). Lyso-PAF is than acetylated by lyso-PAF-acetyltransferase using acetyl CoA as a donor.

PAF has predominantly paracrine activity. The molecule has a short plasma half-life (minutes) and is degraded by a plasma acetylhydrolase. PAF acts through specific G-coupled protein receptor (PAFR) on target cells (Figure 2-45).

PAF is synthesized by endothelial cells stimulated by a variety of activators including locally produced thrombin. Much of the endothelial synthesized PAF remains surface bound directly interacting with PAFR on the juxtaposed neutrophil. Such PAF activates circulating neutrophils promoting their adhesion to the activated endothelium and ultimate transit into tissue toward sites of injury. PAF-activated neutrophils are primed for granule release and response to pathogens. PAF also activates monocytes/macrophages and platelets and enhances NF-κB-dependent expression of proinflammatory genes.

Nitric Oxide

Nitric oxide (NO) warrants brief discussion with the eicosanoids as there are similarities in the induction of both sets of molecules. Evidence suggests there may be some degree of coordinate regulation of the two pathways in that NO may serve to enhance eiconsanoid synthesis via COX-2 and nonenzymatic pathways. NO is synthesized from L-arginine through the action of NO synthetases (NOS) of which there are three isoforms. Neuronal NOS (nNOS) is found in the CNS where it participates in long-term memory formation and acts as an atypical neurotransmitter in the peripheral nervous system. Endothelial NOS (eNOS) has been described under the discussion of the cardinal signs of inflammation. Inducible NOS (iNOS) bears functional similarities to COX-2. iNOS is induced in cytokine-activated macrophages and neutrophils where it is essential in the killing of intracellular bacteria (such as *M. tuberculosis*). *In cases of severe systemic inflammatory*

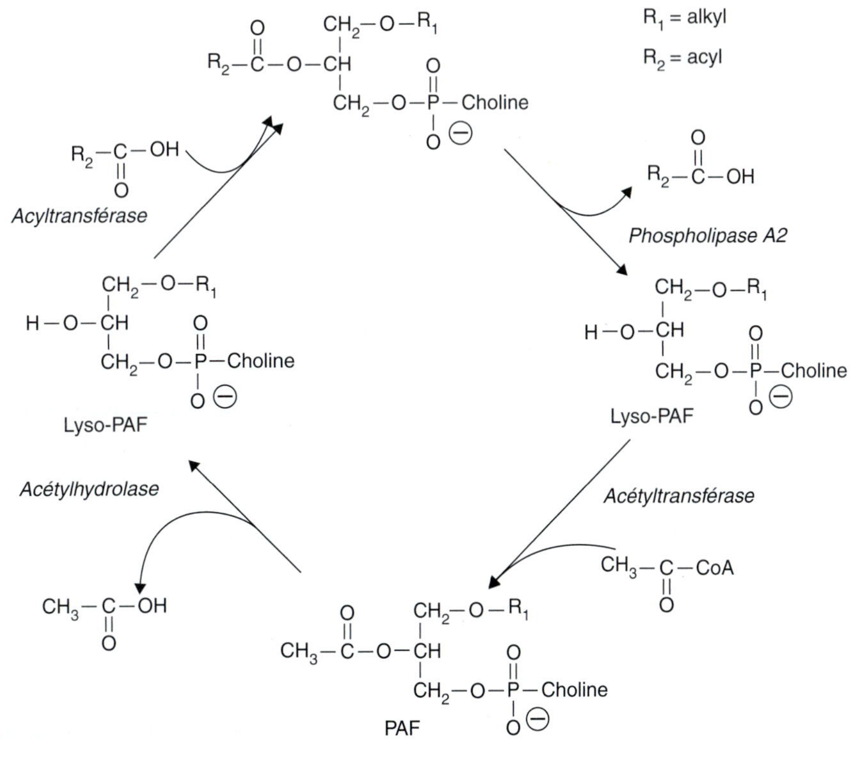

FIGURE 2-45 Synthetic and degradative pathways for PAF. Source: Image used with permission from www.pharmacorama.com. Source: http://www.pharmacorama.com/en/Sections/Eicosanoids_8.php.

disease (septic shock), NO produced as a result of iNOS induction is responsible for the severe hypotension observed. Eicosanoids such as TXA_2 along with other mediators also play a major role in the pathogenesis.

Plasma Contact System: Factor XII (Hageman Factor) and Related Molecules

Factor XII (FXII) acts in concert with **high molecular weight kininogen** (HMWK) and **plasma kallikrein** (PK) to initiate the **intrinsic pathway of coagulation** (termed contact activation). Individuals lacking any of the three factors are detected by an abnormal **activated partial thromboplastin time** (aPTT), a much used in vitro assay for this segment of the hemostatic pathway. Such individuals show normal hemostasis, even under conditions of trauma or surgery. However, based on both animal studies and epidemiological data in humans, a lack of FXII protects against pathological thrombosis. (Additional details about the intrinsic pathway of coagulation as related to hemostasis are found in This Chapter "The Vascular Response to Injury".) FXII circulates as an inactive zymogen, which upon contact with a negatively charged surface undergoes a change in conformation leading to limited autoactivation to FXIIa. FXIIa initiates a cascading reaction by activating PK to PKa, which in turn additionally produces FXIIa. The nature of the charged surface may be nonphysiological (kaolin is commonly used in the aPTT). Likely *in vivo* activators are collagen or basement membrane components of exposed in damaged vessels and, in the case of infection, the bacterial surface. Recently, release of platelet-derived polyphosphates and mast cell-derived heparin following activation of these cells have been demonstrated to be important physiological activators of contact activation, thus supporting the linkage of the hemostatic and inflammatory reactions. FXIIa may have a direct role in inflammation by activating the complement pathway and may also trigger the fibrinolytic system. The role of FXIIa in kinin generation is, however, significant. The major plasma inhibitor of FXIIa and PKa is the serpin **C1 esterase inhibitor** (C1NH). Lack of active C1NH is associated with the inherited disease **hereditary angioedema** (HAE). HAE is characterized by recurrences of acute life-threatening swelling of the oropharyngeal, laryngeal, and other mucosal sites related to inappropriate activation of the contact and complement systems (Figure 2-46).

Kinins

PKa releases the small active nonapeptide **bradykinin** (BK) and the closely related 10-mer lys-bradykinin (lys-BK, **kallidin**) from HMWK. The kinins have very short plasma half-lives (less than one minute) and are rapidly degraded by kininases (kininase II; angiotensin-converting enzyme, **ACE**). BK and lys-BK are also acted on by carboxypeptidases to yield the des-Arg[9] form of the molecules (des-BK, des-lys-BK) that have 10-fold increased half-lives.

BK is a potent inflammatory agent that produces endothelial cell-dependent vasodilation leading to production of nitric oxide, increases vascular permeability, and is involved in nociception. BK (and lys-BK) effects are mediated through interaction with two GPCRs. B_1R, which is sensitive to the des-ARG[9] kinins, is induced in tissues during inflammation by cytokines. B_2R, which is expressed constitutively in most tissues, responds to BK and lys-BK. Most of the proinflammtory action of the kinins is related to B_2R binding. However, kinin-dependent neutrophil recruitment is mediated via endothelial cell production of chemokine CXCL5 following B_1R stimulation.

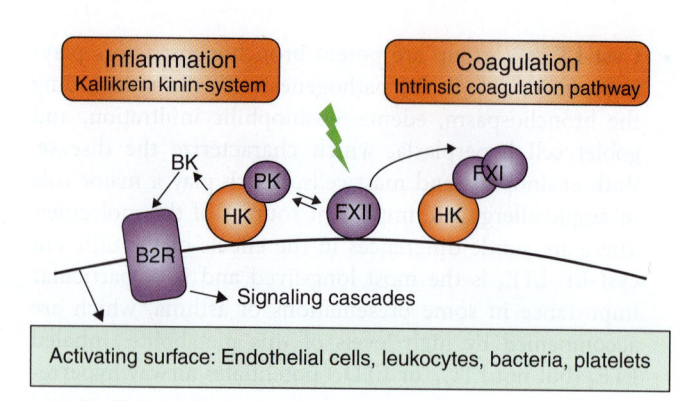

FIGURE 2-46 **Plasma contact system:** BK, bradykinen; B2R, bradykinen receptor 2; PK, plasma kallikrein; HK, high molecular weight kininogen.

Complement

The complement system is a complex series of cascading reactions involving at least 50 proteins. When triggered, these proteins interact to produce a multiplicity of inflammatory mediators including **anaphylotoxins**, **opsonins**, and the end-product of the cascade, the **membrane attack complex (MAC)**, which plays a critical role in defense against gram-negative bacteria (acting synergistically with lysozyme released from neutrophils) and certain protozoal pathogens by promoting pathogen cell lysis. MAC also plays a role in destroying virally infected cells. Three discreet pathways triggering complement activation are defined (Figure 2-47).

> **QUICK REVIEW**
> **Complement Pathways**
> **Pathways of Complement Activation**
>
> The **classical pathway** was the first to be defined and is often referred to as "antibody dependent" because closely spaced immunoglobulins (IgG and IgM) most often as part of antigen–antibody complexes were the first-recognized triggers for this pathway. Hence, the classical pathway is an effector mechanism for antibody-dependent adaptive immune responses. **C1q** (a component of C1) is the pattern recognition molecule for classical pathway and, as well as recognizing antigen–antibody complexes, it recognizes a numbers of PAMPs, that is, viral proteins and bacterial membranes and DAMPs including DNA, endogenous

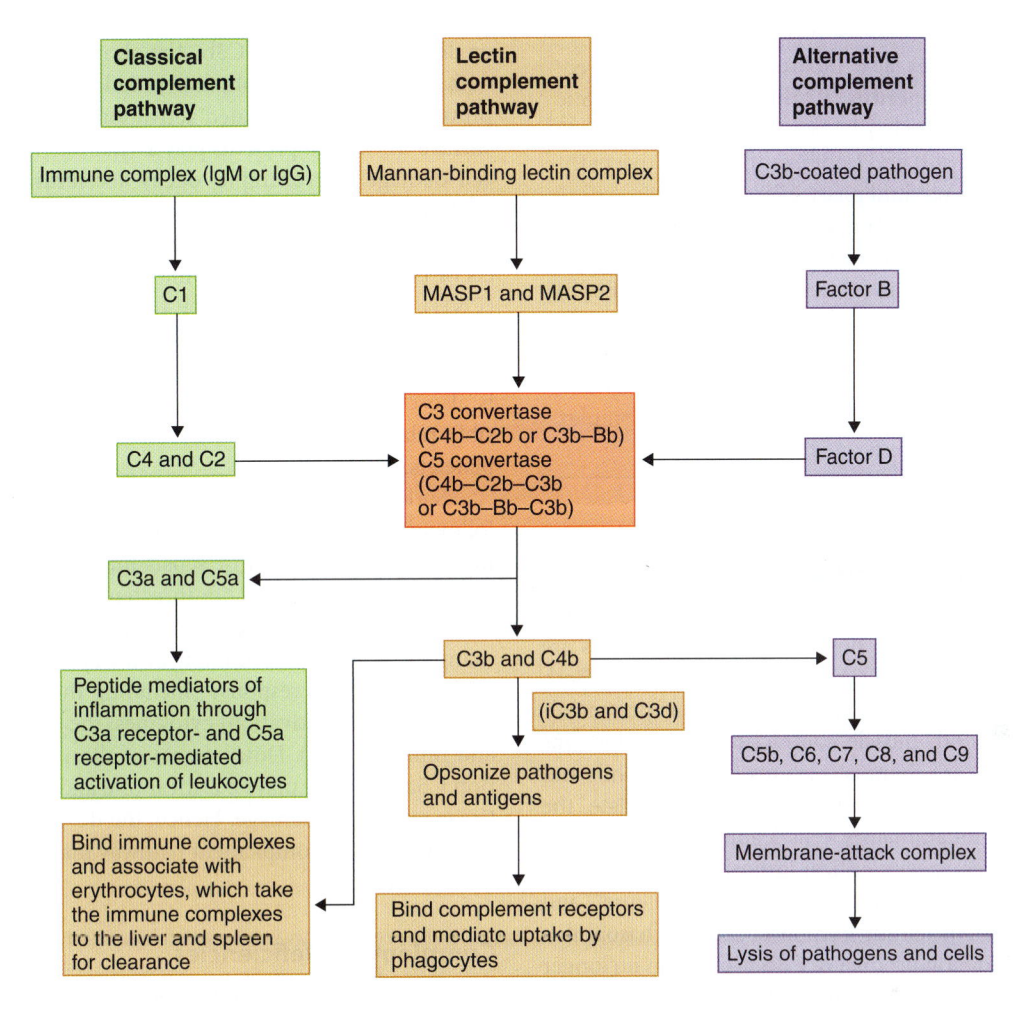

FIGURE 2-47 **Pathways of complement activation.** Source: Reprinted by permission from Macmillan Publishers Ltd. Carroll MC. A protective role for innate immunity in systemic lupus erythematosus. Nat Rev Immunol, 4:825–831, Copyright 2004.

proteins associated with ongoing inflammation such as CRP and β-amyloid peptide. Binding of C1q leads to activation of the endogenous protease activity of C1 (C1r that in turn activates C1s). C1s cleave C4 to C4b and C4a. C4b binds to an adjacent membrane surface (opsonization). Surface-bound C4b associates with C2. C1s cleave the bound C2 molecule removing a small peptide (C2b) forming a C4b2a **C3 convertase** that leads to the cleavage of C3 and the generation of multiple active peptides (as subsequently described) (Confusingly modern nomenclature has interchanged the designation of C2a and C2b so the C3 convertase is sometimes termed C4b2b, the same molecular complex with a different name.)

The **lectin pathway** of complement activation is similar to the classical pathway but does not use C1q as a pattern recognition molecule but rather relies on a **mannose-binding lectin** (MBL) or a group of similar acting carbohydrate binding **ficolins** to detect a variety of bacterial, fungal, and viral pathogens. The lectin-like PRM is associated with serine proteases (MBL-associated proteases MASP), which are activated by carbohydrate binding in an analogous manner to the activation of C1s in the classical pathway generating the identical C4b2a C3 convertase.

The **alternative pathway** of complement activation is a misnomer as it amplifies C3 conversion and can account for as high as 90% of total complement activity regardless of which pathway triggers activation. Unlike the C3 convertase generated by the classical or lectin pathway, the alternative pathway convertase acts in fluid phase, efficiently amplifying C3 activation. Although C3 has little activity, a small amount of spontaneous hydrolyses forms active $C3_{H2O}$. Hydrolysed $C3_{H2O}$ binds factor B protease (fB) that is subsequently cleaved by plasma factor D (into Ba and Bb peptides) generating a fluid phase $C3_{H2O}$ Bb convertase. The small amount of fluid phase convertase cleaves C3 into C3a and C3b forming an **alternative pathway C3 convertase** (AP convertase C3bBb). This convertase is unstable and is inhibited on host cells but amplified on foreign surfaces.

The alternative pathway also incorporates a pattern recognition molecule **properdin (P)** that binds to apoptotic and foreign cells by sensing PAMPs and DAMPs. Surface bound P associates with and stabilizes the alternative pathway C3 convertase and fluid phase C3b.

The continuing surface amplification of C3b leads to the addition of a second C3b molecule to either the classical or alternative pathway C3 convertases (C4b2a3b or C3bBb3b) forming **C5 convertases**. This results in the cleavage of C5 into C5a (a potent anaphylotoxin) and C5b. C5b associating with C6 and C7 inserts into cell membranes. C8 and C9 associate with the membrane inserted C5–C7 complex forming a membrane pore termed the MAC.

Activity of Complement Products

C3a and **C5a** are potent **anaphylotoxins** that have multiple roles in inflammation. The actions of the anaphylotoxins are mediated through GPCRs [C3aR and C5aR (CD88)]. Both molecules cause vasodilation, increase vascular permeability, and induce smooth muscle contraction. Anaphylotoxins (but especially C5a) are chemoattractants for neutrophils and monocyte/macrophages. The anaphylotoxins stimulate the oxidative burst in inflammatory cells leading to the production of active oxygen species critical in host defense (see This Chapter "Neutrophil NADPH Oxidase and Host Defense") and trigger the release of histamine from mast cells and basophils.

iC3b, a degradation product of **C3b**, which can no longer serve as a C3 convertase, and **C4b** function as **opsonins**, molecules that enhance the phagocytosis of pathogens or molecular complexes, that is, antigen–antibody complexes that have "fixed" complement components. A number of **complement receptors** on phagocytic cells function by binding the opsonins and promoting phagocytosis. For example, **CR1 (CD35)** binds both C3b and C4b and importantly, acting with plasma cofactors, promotes the degradation of C3b to iC3b. Hence, CR1 limits the production of additional active complement components, while liberating the opsonin iC3b, which can interact with several other complement receptors (CR2, CR3 and CR4) promoting opsonization, B cell-dependent immunity, and downregulating inflammation. Serum carboxypeptidases degrade anaphylotoxins to des-arginine forms with little or no proinflammatory activity.

Regulation of Complement Activity

The already-mentioned serpin **C1 esterase inhibitor (C1NH)** is the major regulator of both the classical and lectin pathway, acting to inhibit several of the active proteases of this pathway. As noted above, a lack of this inhibitor is associated with HAE and excessive production of active complement components expressed as low levels of intact C2 and C4 in the presence of normal C1q. The alternate pathway of activation in liquid phase is regulated by **factors H and I** and similarly by **C4b-binding protein**, which either inactivate the AP convertase or degrade fluid phase C3b. The above three factors interact with self-specific carbohydrates and glycosaminoglycans to prevent host cell-associated activation. A variety of other cell surface-associated proteins play a vital role in preventing host cell damage. For example, **decay accelerating factor** (DAF, CD55) is expressed on both erythrocytes and leukocytes and interferes with the activity of the AP convertase. Reduced levels of DAF occur in **paroxysmal nocturnal hemoglobinuria** (PNH). In PNH, lack of DAF [and a related inhibitor MAC inhibitory protein (CD59)] leads to inappropriate activation of complement on red cells and subsequent lysis. The disease is also characterized by life-threatening thrombophilia, possibly related in part to complement-dependent activation of platelets.

Sudden increases in DAMPs or PAMPs as may occur following trauma, burns, ischemia-reperfusion injury (in myocardial infarctions) or sepsis may overwhelm protective mechanisms and lead to life-threatening **systemic inflammatory response syndrome** (SIRS) associated with hyperinflammation and activation of many of the systems associated with the inflammatory response (including the alternate pathway of complement activation, cytokines, the coagulation system, and immune cells). Downstream of alternate pathway activation C5a signaling plays a critical role and is important in the tissue and organ damage. Hence, the development of specific inhibitors to the complement pathway may play an important therapeutic role.

Complement Deficiencies

Congenital complement deficiencies due to mutations leading to lack of functional protein result in defective host defense, primarily against bacterial pathogens and to a lesser extent fungi or parasites. Viral host defense is not affected. Defects in the classical pathway and in C3 are also associated with autoimmune disease, most commonly systemic lupus erythematosus (SLE) presumably because of defective clearance of immune complexes. Most defects are uncommon autosomal recessive diseases. Properdin deficiency is X-linked and C1-INH deficiency (discussed above as a cause of HAE) is an autosomal dominant. C2 deficiency is the most common seen in Caucasian populations with an incidence of 1 case per 10–20,000. Defects in MBL may approach several percent. Such defects are mild and may not result in disease, although some cases are associated with respiratory tract infections. Defects in C9 occur with a frequency as high as 1 per 1000 in Japan and Korea.

- **Defects in the classical pathway** are associated with increased susceptibility to infection with encapsulated bacteria such as *Sterptococcus pneumoniae, Haemophilus influenzae,* and *Neisseria meningitides*. Incidence rates of SLE are as high as 90% for C1q and C4 and with lower frequency (15%) for C2 deficiency.
- **Defects in the lectin-binding pathway** do not often appear to be associated with disease although (as noted above) such defects are frequent. Children and individuals with

additional defects in the immune system are at risk of infection with encapsulated bacteria. Autoimmune disease (SLE, rheumatoid arthritis) may occur with increased frequency and severity.

- **Defects in the alternative pathway (properdin, factors B and D)** are exceedingly rare and associated with a several hundred-fold increased risk of fulminant *Neisserial* disease and high mortality.
- **Defects in C3, Factors H and I deficiency** result in spectrum of infections similar to that seen in classical pathway defects. The low level of C3 (either intrinsic to the molecule or resulting from increased destruction in the absence of inhibitory factors H and I) results in defective bacterial opsonization and also defective adaptive immunity. Persistent reduced levels of C3 associated with factor H deficiency or caused by autoantibodies that result in chronic C3 consumption (nephritic antibodies) are strongly associated with membranoproliferative glomerulonephritis type II (dense deposit disease). Defects in complement factor H are also associated with increased risk of atypical hemolytic uremic syndrome and age-related macular degeneration.
- **Defects in the terminal pathway (C5-C9)** are associated with susceptibility to *Neisserial* infection, although disease may be somewhat milder than that seen with defects in the classical and alternative pathways. This is particularly true for C9 deficiency where an intact C5b-8 complex has some lytic activity.

Chemokines

The term chemokine is a portmanteau word derived from chemotactic cytokine. The term **cytokine** was initially applied to small signaling proteins important in either the intrinsic or adaptive immune response but is now more broadly used. Cytokine is most often used to refer to molecules produced by multiple cell types as opposed to hormones, whose synthesis is generally organ limited. However, the systemic (as well autocrine and paracrine) activity of many cytokines blurs this distinction. **Chemokines** represent a limited subset of cytokines, which are structurally related, low molecular weight (around 10 Kd) secreted peptides that play a major role in cell trafficking. Chemokines represent a family of about 50 proteins defined by conserved structure and the location of disulfide bridging cysteine residues. Current nomenclature defines four classes; **CC** having adjacent key cysteines, **CXC** and **CX₃** in which the cysteine residues are separated by one and three intervening amino acids respectively and **C** (or **XC**), which lack one of the pair of important cysteines. Chemokines signal through a set of about 25 seven-transmembrane domain GPCRs named by the class of chemokine they bind. The specificity of interaction between chemokine and receptor is complex and involves multiple combinations. Although chemokine names are now standardized, historical synonyms are common. CXCL8 originally termed IL-8 was defined by its potent ability to attract neutrophils. CXCL4 is better known as platelet factor 4, which is released from activated platelet granules. CXCL4 is chemotactic for inflammatory cells and plays a role in promoting coagulation. Chemokines bind to glycosaminoglycans such as chondroitin and heparin sulfate in tissue, thereby establishing chemoattractant gradients important in the directed migration of inflammatory cells toward sites of injury. Eosinophil, macrophage, mast cell, and, as noted, neutrophil homing all involve chemokine/chemokine receptor interactions. For example, CCL11 (eotaxin) and CCL5 (RANTES) interact with the CCR3 receptor on eosinophils to promote directed cell migration.

Cellular Phase of Inflammation

The increasing interaction of neutrophils and subsequently monocytes/macrophages with the endothelial cells of the microvasculature and the directed emigration of the circulating cells into the tissue marks the earliest phase of cellular inflammation. (Although this section refers specifically to neutrophils, macrophages use the same general mechanisms in mediating host defense and will be referred to specifically in the section on *chronic* **inflammation** a process in which macrophages play a leading role.) Initial emigration is followed by the directed migration of the cells toward PAMPs and DAMPs using pattern recognition molecules present on the migrating cells (**chemotaxis**). As noted in the section on cytokines, cells proximate to the site of injury may actively secrete molecules that form chemical gradients in tissue, thus acting as pathways for directed migration. Alternatively, the gradients may be associated with pathogen-specific molecules intrinsic to the damaged tissue (the PAMPs and DAMPs discussed above). Arriving at the scene of injury neutrophils and monocytes/macrophages are activated to engulf pathogens or damaged tissue (**phagocytosis**) and render them harmless, either using preformed or newly synthesized active chemical agents. Such agents are bioactive and capable of damaging tissue when released into the host environment, a common concomitant of inflammation.

To prevent systemic release of bioactive substances by activated neutrophils, which circulate through the vascular system, a complex series of ligand/receptor interactions occurs in the microvasculature (most often postcapillary venules) between neutrophil and endothelial cells. The necessity for mutual interactions between cells activated by the products of pathogens and cellular injury assures localization of the cellular aspects of acute inflammation to the vicinity of the target. The neutrophil–endothelial cell interaction is best described as a series of contacts of ever-increasing mutual affinity. This ultimately results in arrest of vascular flow-mediated movement of neutrophils, tangential movement of adherent neutrophils across flow to either endothelial cell junctions or selected areas of the endothelium through which the activated neutrophils exit the vasculature and migrate into tissues (**diapedesis**). Migration of neutrophils through junctions (**paracellular migration**) occurs most frequently, whereas migration through intact endothelial cells (**transcellular migration**), once considered controversial, also occurs during inflammation.

Endothelial Cell–Neutrophil Interactions

The ever-increasing interactions between neutrophil and endothelium are a series of steps each involving differing sets of interaction molecules on the two. In summary, the steps are described as tethering, rolling, neutrophil "inside-out" activation, adhesion, crawling, and transmigration (Figure 2-48).

- **Tethering:** Under normal conditions, up to half of all mature neutrophils are present as intravascular pools within several organs including the liver, spleen, and as a postmitotic bone marrow population. This **marginated pool** has a slow intravascular transit time and is not available as part of the normal circulating complement of cells as measured by determination of white cell counts in blood. A variety of stressors (including infection) results in liberation of marginated neutrophils in response to many different inflammatory mediators (IL-8 and other cytokines, LT B4, C5a, and TNFα for example) producing neutrophilia. Localization of neutrophils to areas of the vasculature adjacent to sites of injury results from the modification of the endothelial surface either as a result of exogenous inflammatory mediators or by triggering of PRRs on the endothelium itself. This results in rapid transit of preformed **P-selectin** from Weibel–Palade bodies to the endothelial surface followed by the surface expression of newly synthesized **E-selectin**. Selectins are adhesion molecules that bind to specific glycosylated ligands bearing the Sialyl LewisX carbohydrate moiety. **PSGL-1** expressed constitutively on neutrophils is the major binding partner of endothelial P- and E-selectins. It is the interaction between these molecules that is responsible for initial neutrophil tethering.

- **Rolling:** The strength of interaction between selectin and ligand is increased by shear stress under conditions of vascular flow. Rolling is mediated by the formation and breakage of bonds in a "step wise" peeling pattern in which new P-selectin PSGL-1 bonds form as prior bonds detach. Additional neutrophil endothelial cell interactions such as that between E-selectin and ESL-1 and CD44 on neutrophils contribute to reduction in the rate of rolling and eventual arrest.

- **Activation, adhesion, and crawling:** Slow rolling of neutrophils brings the leukocytes into proximity of the endothelial

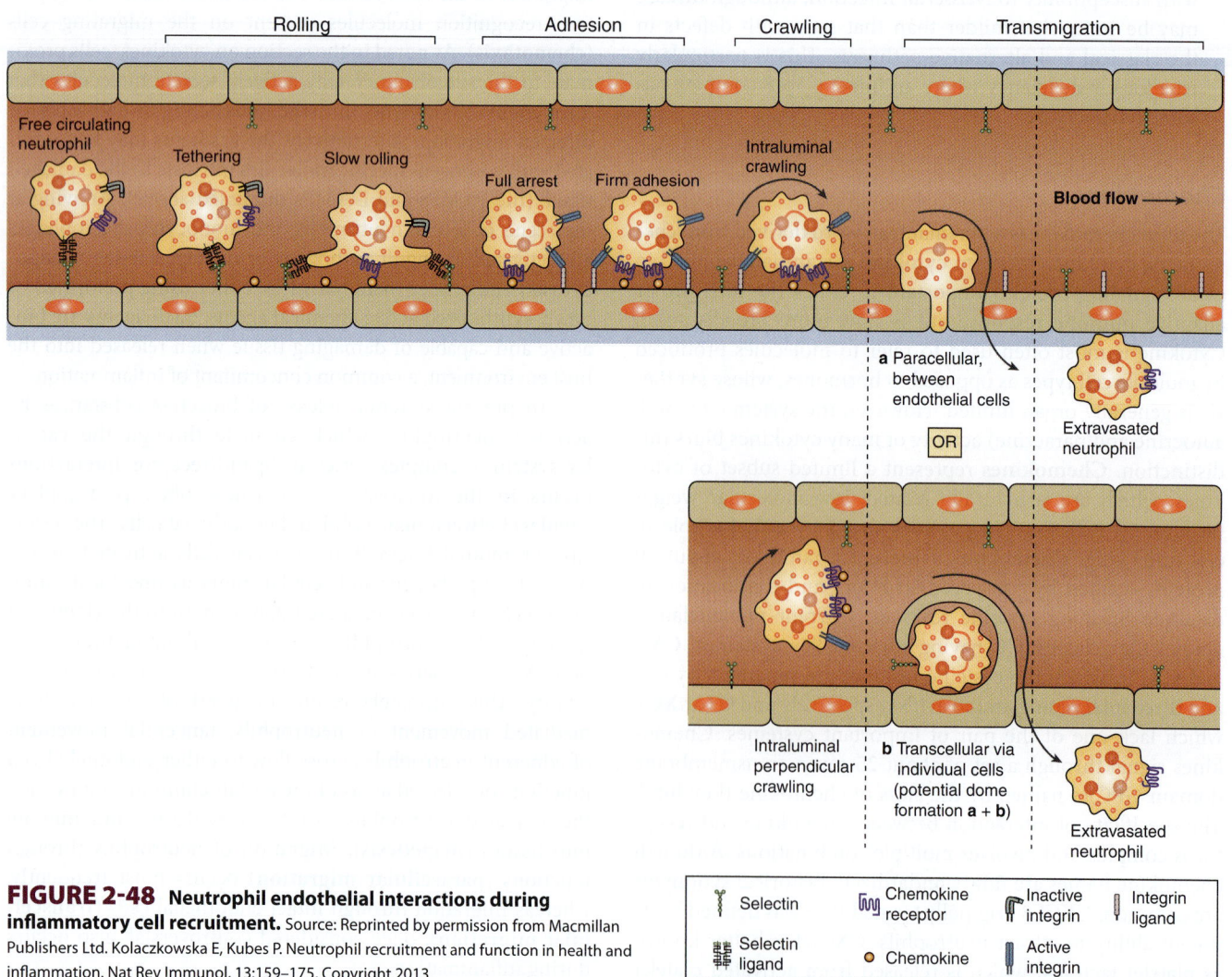

FIGURE 2-48 Neutrophil endothelial interactions during **inflammatory cell recruitment.** Source: Reprinted by permission from Macmillan Publishers Ltd. Kolaczkowska E, Kubes P. Neutrophil recruitment and function in health and inflammation. Nat Rev Immunol, 13:159–175, Copyright 2013.

surface, which bears a variety of stimulatory molecules. Most important is the chemokine IL-8 (CXCL8). As previously noted, chemokines bind to glycosaminoglycans such as chondroitin and heparin sulfate on the surface of cells, which produces fixed chemical gradients on the apical endothelial surface not disturbed by vascular flow. Endothelial-associated chemokine plays a critical role in the activation of neutrophils (1) priming them for subsequent synthesis and release of bioactive products but more immediately (2) promoting tight adhesion to the endothelial surface. Neutrophils constitutively express **integrin** molecules on their surface that bind to immunoglobulin-like cell adhesion molecules (**ICAMs**) on the endothelial surface. Integrin LFA1 (αLβ2 integrin, CD11a/CD18) binding to ICAM1 is primarily responsible for firm adhesion of neutrophils. MAC1 (αMβ2 integrin CD11b/CD18) binding to ICAM1 is necessary for the "crawling" of adherent neutrophils across vascular flow toward sites of transmigration.

Integrins, although constitutively expressed on the neutrophil surface, are not present in an active configuration allowing for firm cellular adhesion. Integrin activation requires stepwise exposure of the leukocyte to activating agents and so-called "inside-out" signaling. Neutrophil rolling on selectins initiates low-affinity activation of LFA-1 (extended configuration). However, adhesion and arrest requires chemokine-dependent activation of neutrophils and conversion of LFA-1 to an extended fully open form. This conformational change in the integrin is mediated by the interaction of **talin** 1 and **kindlin** 3 proteins that break salt bridges between the integrin α and β chains upon intracytoplasmic β chain binding. This leads to extension and opening of the extracytoplasmic integrin region.

- **Transmigration:** Paracellular transmigration of neutrophils is the preferred route through the endothelial layer. Both ICAM-1 and ICAM-2 are necessary for the process and are concentrated at endothelial cell junctions. Binding of neutrophil integrins to ICAM-1 results in signals that lead to loosening of endothelial cell junctions. Additional endothelial cell surface proteins including JAM family proteins, **PECAM-1** and CD99 serve to guide the neutrophil through the cell junction and are required for successful migration. PECAM-1 acts "upstream" to CD99. Blocking of the former prevents leukocytes from beginning transmigration. Blocking the later arrests the process midway. The three last-named molecules are also expressed on neutrophils. Homotypic binding between the molecules on the neutrophil and on the endothelial cell junction is likely to aid in the migratory process. Transcellular migration depends on the formation of **transmigratory cups** that move up the side of the neutrophil to form dome-like structures. The structures are rich in ICAM-1 and VCAM-1 (another ICAM) and depend on neutrophil LFA-1 and VLA4 (an α4β1 integrin) binding to their respective ligands. The endothelium covers over the neutrophil, which remains in an extracellular compartment as it transits the endothelial cell.

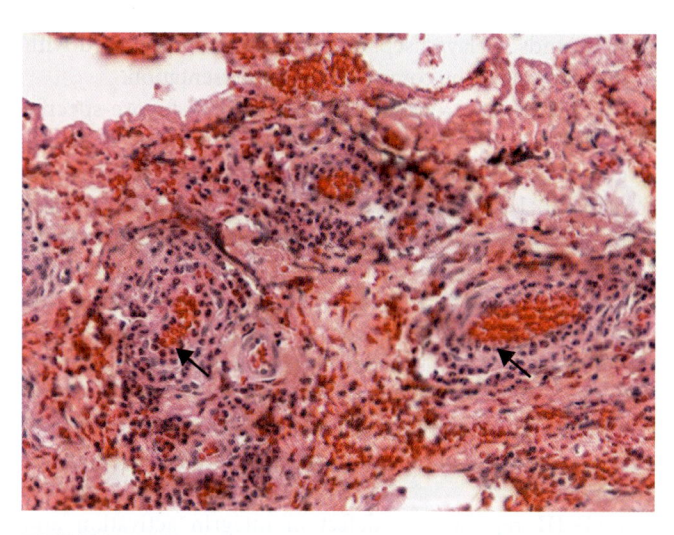

FIGURE 2-49 Early transmigration of neutrophils: The small vessels in this section of a hernia sack removed at surgery are surrounded by "cuffs" of neutrophils that are in the process of migrating into tissue. Some neutrophils remain adherent to the endothelium of the vessel (arrow). Others are in the vessel wall or proximate tissue.

The extravasated neutrophil must travel through the ECM of the vascular basement membrane to reach tissue. Endothelial cells rearrange their connections to the ECM adjacent to sites of migrating neutrophils easing the process. Neutrophils contain **matrix metallopeptidases (MMPs)** and enzymes such as neutrophil elastase that are active against ECM components, although the role of such enzymes versus selective migration of cells through areas of the basement membrane with decreased levels of ECM components (such as are found adjacent to gaps between pericytes) remains unclear **(Figure 2-49)**.

Leukocyte Adhesion Deficiency (LAD) Syndromes

The requirement of intact neutrophil/monocyte endothelial interactions in promoting the cellular phase of inflammation of host defense is emphasized by a number of uncommon autosomal recessive defects. In all cases, the affected individuals demonstrate a primary immunodeficiency characterized by leukocytosis in the absence of infection, recurring bacterial and fungal infections, and lack tissue accumulation of inflammatory cells (pus production) due to the failure of leukocytes to emigrate from the vascular compartment.

- **LAD-I** is the most common of the defects (although less than 500 cases are known). Individuals either lack or have much reduced levels of the common β2 chain of integrins as a result of mutations in the *ITGB2* gene and hence do not demonstrate leukocyte–endothelial adhesion. Individuals with severe disease die soon after birth in the absence of successful stem cell transplantation. Those with less severe disease show early onset gingivitis, recurrent bacterial infections of the skin and mucosa, and impaired healing of wounds. Delayed separation of the umbilical cord with neutrophilia is the common clinical presentation.

- **LAD-II** results from mutations of a GDP-fucose-specific transporter that results in defective glycosylation of oligosaccharides including the Sialyl LewisX carbohydrate of PSGL-1 and other selectin ligands. The defect results in defective leukocyte rolling and subsequent interactions with the endothelium. Host defense is less severely affected than in type I Lad since adhesion remains intact and some degree of leukocyte emigration occurs. Individuals with LAD-II have short stature, abnormal facies, mental retardation, and a defect in the ABO RBC antigen system resulting in the lack of H antigen (Bombay phenotype) as a result of defects in additional fucosylated glycoconjugates.
- **LAD-III** represents a defect in integrin activation and hence results in defective leukocyte adhesion. Although expression of leukocyte integrins is normal, a mutation in the *FERMT3* gene results in defective kindling-3 protein, which as noted above, binds to the integrin β subunit allowing it to assume a fully active configuration. The disease is similar to LAD-I but is also associated with a Glanzmann thrombasthenia-like bleeding diathesis related to a defect in platelet β3 integrin.

Neutrophils in Tissue

Chemotaxis

As reviewed above, PAMPs and DAMPs begin the process of inflammation by triggering PRRs, the sensors of tissue injury. PRR-mediated responses associated with tissue resident cells (macrophages and mast cells) secrete "intermediate" chemoattractant molecules [e.g. IL-8 (CXCL8) and LTB4] that function within and proximate to the vascular compartment to prime and activate leukocytes. Once within the tissue compartment, other chemotactic molecules override these "intermediate" chemoattractants. The bacterial products formyl methionyl leucyl phenylalanine (**fMLP**) and C5a act as "end-target" chemoattractants directing activated neutrophils (and subsequently monocyte/macrophages) to the site of tissue injury. Neutrophils themselves can either induce the release of chemoattractants from mesenchymal cells or produce agents (LTB4 and IL-8 for example) that recruit additional neutrophils to the site of tissue injury (Figure 2-50).

- **Signal prioritization:** The ability of "end-target" to override "intermediate" chemoattractants in orienting chemotactic cells is mediated by a complex signal processing system within the neutrophil. fMLP and other "end-target" molecules activate a **p38MAPK** pathway, whereas IL-8 and "intermediate" attractants activate the phosphatidylinositol 3-kinase (**PI3K**) pathway (see below). The phosphatase **PTEN**, which inactivates phosphatidylinositol-3,4,5-triphosphate [**Ptdins(3,4,5)P$_3$** [**PIP$_3$**]] by conversion to phosphatidylinositol-4,5-biphosphate [**Ptdins(4,5)P$_2$**], serves to integrate and prioritize chemotactic signals

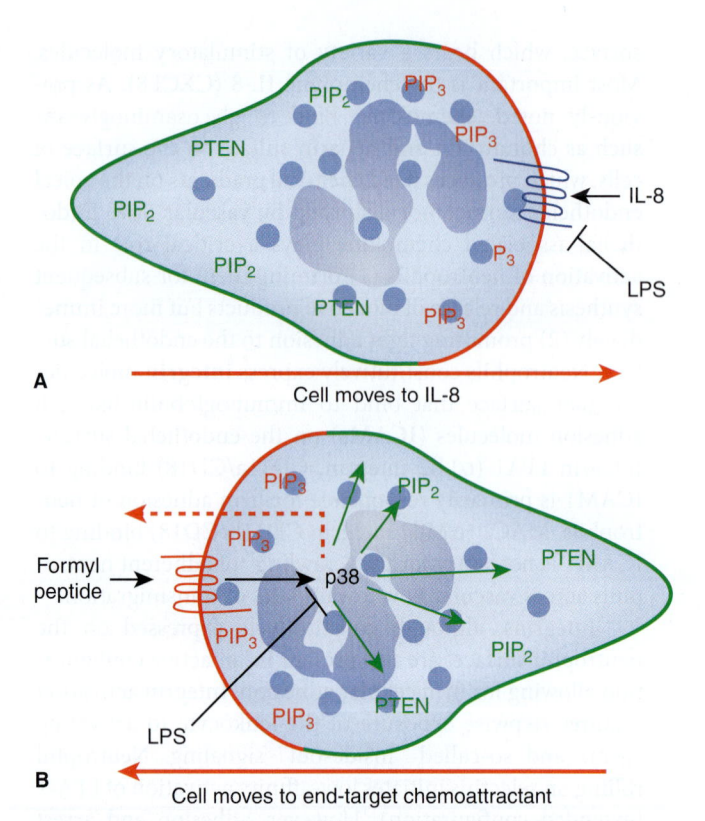

FIGURE 2-50 Neutrophil chemotaxis: Mechanism of orientation toward chemoattractants. The localizations of PIP3 are shown in red and the localizations of PTEN and PIP2 are shown in green. **(A)** Neutrophil is migrating toward an intermediate chemoattractant (IL-8). **(B)** Neutrophil is migrating toward an end-target chemoattractant (formyl peptide, FMLP). p38 MAPK mediates both PTEN localization (green arrows) as well as chemotaxis (dotted red arrow) toward end target chemoattractant. Source: Reprinted by permission from Macmillan Publishers Ltd. Phillipson M, Kubes P. The neutrophil in vascular inflammation. Nat Med, 17:1381–1390, Copyright 2011.

by inhibiting PI3K directed movement in the presence of fMLP p38MAPK signaling.
- **Directed migration:** Neutrophils have the ability to sense a 2% difference in chemoattractant concentration along their length, orient, and move up the gradient almost 50 times as rapidly as fibroblasts move in tissue. Thus, sensing, orientation, and directed movement toward the source of stimulus, the site of injury, define chemotaxis. The process is complex and many details remain hypothetical. On a surface neutrophils sensing a chemoattractant gradient polarize. They assume an elongated shape with a leading edge (**lamellipodium**) and a trailing end (**uropod**). Actin polymerization at the leading edge provides a forward push against transient surface contacts. Unlike the case in mesenchymal cells such as fibroblasts, strong, integrin-dependent surface adhesive contacts play little role in migration through three-dimensional substrates.
- At the leading edge, polymerization is dependent on localized presence of PIP$_3$ and on the Rho family small GTPase **Rac**. Rac localizes to the leading edge and plays a role in

CELL INJURY, CELL DEATH, AND AGING

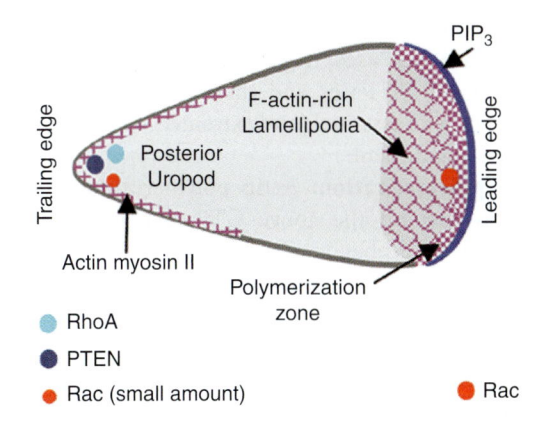

FIGURE 2-51 Mechanism of neutrophil polarization: Highly motile neutrophils develop marked polarity on stimulation. Only some of the proteins that show a polarized distribution are shown. Source: Reprinted by permission from Macmillan Publishers Ltd: Wu, D. Signaling mechanisms for regulation of chemotaxis. Cell Research, 15(1), pages 52–56. Copyright 2005.

The neutrophil has an array of granules containing a variety of bioactive mediators that fuse with the phagosome to produce a destructive internal environment. The fusion of phagosome and granule allows for the assembly of a membrane-bound NADPH oxidase that results in the synthesis of ROS toxic to most pathogens (the **respiratory burst**). Granule contents and ROS are also released into the local environment by activated neutrophils where they play not only a protective but also a tissue destructive role. The following section refers primarily to neutrophils but similar processes (albeit differing in several details) also occur in macrophages during chronic inflammation (Figure 2-52).

Phagocytosis is defined as an actin-dependent uptake of particles of 0.5 μm or greater that is triggered by a specific receptor. The best characterized neutrophil receptors for opsonized particles are (1) the **FcγR** family (FcγRIIA being the most important) that interact with the Fc region of IgG and mediating branched actin filament polymerization, which drives the cell forward. The phosphatase SHIP1 converts PIP_3 to inactive **Ptdins(3,4)P$_2$** and serves to regulate the process.

- At the trailing end, sites of neutrophil substrate attachment are dissolved and net movement occurs via actomyosin contraction. The small GTPase **RhoA**, which is excluded from the leading edge, acts through RhoA kinase (ROCK) to reorganize the actin cytoskeleton promoting detachment and contraction. Polarity is likely to be maintained by feedback loops such that Rac inhibits RhoA and RhoA inhibits Rac and recruits PTEN, which acts to inactivate PIP_3 at the sides and rear of the migrating cell (Figure 2-51).
- **Signal sensing:** Chemoattractants signal to neutrophils by interacting with cell surface **GCPRs**. On GCPR binding the Gβγ heterodimer, which is responsible for chemoattractant-mediated signaling, is released from the Gαl chain of the G-protein. As noted above downstream effectors stimulated by the active heterodimer include (1) PI3K producing active lipid second messages such as PIP_3, (2) Rho family GTPases, (3) protein kinase Cζ, (4) cytosolic tyrosine kinases, and (5) phopholipase A2.

Phagocytosis

Having reached the site of tissue injury using chemotaxis, neutrophils engage in a number of processes to contain the damaging agents. **Phagocytosis** is a receptor-mediated process whereby "debris" composed of fragments of endogenous damaged cells or exogenous pathogens become enclosed in the neutrophil cell membrane and are internalized as phagosomes. The receptors may recognize specific PAMPs and DAMPs intrinsic to the injurious agent but often rely on the presence of specific marker molecules such as immunoglobulins or complement components that become bound to the debris during inflammation, a process defined as **opsonization**.

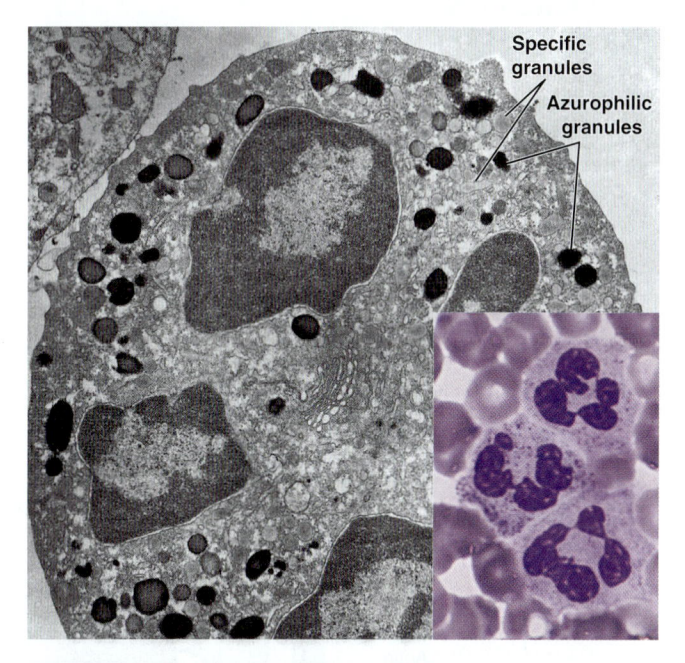

FIGURE 2-52 Neutrophils: Electron micrograph of a sectioned human neutrophil immunostained for peroxidase reveals the two types of cytoplasmic granules: the small, pale, peroxidase-negative-specific granules and the larger, dense, peroxidase-positive azurophilic granules. Specific granules undergo exocytosis during and after diapedesis, releasing many factors with various activities, including enzymes to digest ECM components and bacteriostatic factors. Azurophilic granules are modified lysosomes with components to kill engulfed bacteria. The nucleus is lobulated and the central Golgi apparatus is small. Rough ER and mitochondria are not abundant, because this cell utilizes glycolysis and is in the terminal stage of its differentiation. (Reproduced, with permission, from Bainton DF. Fed Proc. 1981;40:1443.). Inset: In blood smears, neutrophils can be identified by their multilobulated nuclei, with lobules held together by thin strands. Other identifying features of neutrophils include overall diameter of 12–15 μm, approximately twice that of the surrounding erythrocytes. The cytoplasmic granules are relatively sparse and heterogeneous in their staining properties, although generally pale and not obscuring the nucleus. Source: Mescher AL, Junqueira's Basic Histology text and Atlas 12th ed. McGraw Hill Lange New York 2010:214 (Figure 2-41B reproduced with permission from Bainton DF Fed. Proc. 1981;40:1443,Chapter 12 Figure 12-18)

(2) the integrin complement receptors **CR3** and **CR4** ($\alpha_m\beta_2$ and $\alpha_v\beta_2$) that bind to iC3b. In the group of receptors for non opsonized particles, **dectin 1**, which binds β1, 3-glucan in fungal cell walls, is well characterized. Nonspecific phagocytosis may be mediated by TLRs but such tend to augment phagocytosis produced by one of the "classical" receptors above. Phagocytic receptor activation requires clustering within the membrane so as to form multimeric aggregates. Hence, multivalent interaction of receptors with the particle to be engulfed is critical. The process of phagocytosis that results upon multimeric receptor binding is complex and differs for different receptors. In the case of FcγR-mediated phagocytosis, upward reaching pseudopod-like extensions of the cell membrane surround the particle forming a "cup-like" structure, which is eventually enclosed into the neutrophil as a membrane-bound **phagosome**.

> **QUICK REVIEW**
> **Cell Biology of Phagocytosis**
> A brief outline of the critical steps necessary for phagocytosis following FcγR engagement is as follows (Figure 2-53).
>
> - **Receptor clustering:** Upon receptor clustering unique domains in the cytoplasmic region of the receptors termed immunoreceptor tyrosine activation motifs (*ITAMs*) are phosphorylated by Src family kinases.
> - **Lipid signaling molecules:** $PI(4,5)P_2$ is transiently elevated in the vicinity of the forming phagocytic "cup" and then rapidly disappears. PIP_3 produced locally is necessary for the phagocytosis of large particles.
> - **Rho family GTPases:** As is the case in chemotaxis, Rho family small GTPases and their associated accessory factors play an essential (and extremely complex) role in particle engulfment.
> - **Actin polymerization:** Actin polymerization (dependent in part on the above GTPases) is an absolute requirement of phagocytosis. However, actin clearance at the base of the forming cup is necessary for phagosome closure.
> - **Myosin:** Myosin-mediated contraction is necessary for completion of particle engulfment.
> - **Membrane delivery:** Both plasma membranes and membranes from endosomes fuse with the developing phagocytic "cup." This is particularly important in the phagocytosis of large particles.
>
> Dectin-1 has a cytoplasmic ITAM-like region and appears to mediate phagocytosis in a manner similar to FcγR. However, complement receptor (CR3)-mediated phagocytosis differs. Unlike the above iC3b opsonized particles "sink" into the neutrophil cytoplasm without the formation of enveloping membrane pseudopods (so-called *sinking* as opposed to *reaching* phagocytosis). The mechanism is different from that used by FcγR and is dependent on RhoA activation mediated by integrin receptor binding. RhoA activation leads to recruitment of factors that attract microtubules and lead to both branched and unbranched actin polymerization. Although many of the steps necessary for effective phagocytosis via different receptors are defined, how the various processes effectively interact is still unclear.

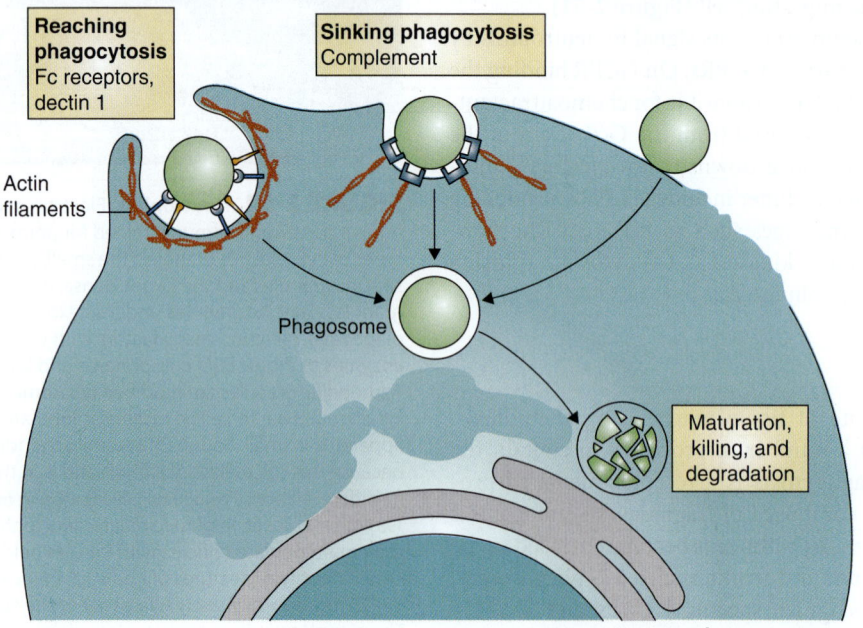

FIGURE 2-53 Modes of phagocytosis: Particles opsonized by Fc bearing molecules (immunoglobulins) or interacting bearing glucans interacting with dectin 1 undergo reaching phagocytosis. Particles opsonized by complement (iC3b) undergo sinking phagocytosis.

Phagosome Maturation

Significant differences exist in the fate of the developing phagosome in neutrophils and macrophages. (Although the most commonly presented schema is that of the latter.)

Macrophage Phagosome Maturation

Macrophage phagosomes show an orderly maturation process once internalization is complete.

- Early phagosomes fuse with endosomes and acquire specific GTP-bound Rab family small GTPases that are characteristic of the stage of phagosome maturation. For example, acquisition of Rab5 by the early phagosome leads to the accumulation of PIP_3 on the cytoplasmic side of the phagosome, which in turn leads to the accumulation of SNARE protein complexes that are critical mediators of membrane fusion. In addition, components of the NADPH oxidase system (to be discussed below) are recruited.
- Loss of Rab5 and acquisition of Rab7 marks the transition to late phagosome. This stage is characterized by lysosome/phagosome fusion and the gradual acidification of the maturing phagolysosome and the movement of phagosomes to a perinuclear position. Vacuolar ATPase (v-ATPase) is delivered by fusion with endosomes. V-ATPase is membrane bound and pumps H^+ inward, resulting in acidification of the phagolysosome interior.
- Phagolysome acidification has multiple functions: (1) Activation of proteolytic cathepsins (2) aiding in the outward transport of metals required by some bacteria for growth and (3) providing protons for the generation of ROS by the NADPH Oxidase system. The utility of the acidic phagolysome environment is supported by the multiple approaches used by bacteria to circumvent it. For example, *Helicobacter pylori* produces ammonium ions to buffer the phagolysosome aiding in its survival. *However, an acid environment is not a sine qua non for phagolysomes and host defense as the neutrophil phagolysome has a neutral to alkaline environment.*

Neutrophil Phagosome Maturation

As noted phagocytosis by neutrophils and the process of phagosome maturation show significant differences from that of macrophages. Although macrophage phagocytes undergo a well-ordered maturation process relying on fusion with endosomes and ultimately lysosomes, neutrophil phagosomes fuse with the preformed granules that define neutrophils as a member of the granulocytic class of white cells (Figure 2-52). Human neutrophils contain three types of granules that are produced by budding from the Golgi during cell maturation. In addition, **secretory vesicles**, which are produced by endocytosis in mature neutrophils, are often considered with granules. Granules differ in their content, which is determined in part by the temporal sequence in which they are produced starting at the myeloblast stage of development. Granules, as well as fusing with mature sealed phagosomes, may also fuse with phagosomes prior to closure and with the plasma membrane in sites not associated with phagocytic activity. Hence, neutrophils may actively secrete bioactive (and potentially damaging) substances into the tissue space. Neutrophils as the characteristic "first responder cell" defining sites of acute inflammation phagocytose more rapidly and have a much greater capacity to produce ROS via NADPH oxidase system than do macrophages. In macrophages, internalized plasma membranes serve as the sole source of NADPH oxidase, whereas neutrophil phagosomes obtain additional enzyme by granule fusion.

Pathogen Inactivation by Neutrophils

Two primary systems are responsible for the inactivation of pathogens and destruction of phagocytosed material by neutrophils, the bioactive mediators contained in granules and the products of the NADPH oxidase-mediated respiratory burst.

Neutrophil Granules and Host Defense

Neutrophil granules differ in the ease with which they are mobilized and either secreted into the tissue space or into the developing phagosome. Although there is significant overlap between the content of granules, each has characteristic components that delineate them. In the order of ease of mobilization, they are as follows:

- **Secretory vesicles:** Produced by endocytosis during the early phases of inflammation, secretory vesicles contain plasma proteins within membrane receptors that are characteristic of those used in endothelial attachment and chemotaxis as well as complement receptors and FcRs. They are the first to be released from activated neutrophils and by fusing with the cell membrane allow for continuing neutrophil activation. As such, secretory vesicle fusion provides the major source of cell surface receptors involved in endothelial cell binding and chemotaxis but do not release other bioactive mediators.
- **Gelatinase granules (tertiary granules):** Gelatinase granules are synthesized at the metamyelocyte and band stage of neutrophil development and are (not surprisingly) characterized by the presence of **gelatinase** (MMP9). Gelatinase plays a role in allowing the neutrophil passage through the basement membrane during emigration.
- **Specific granules (secondary granules):** Specific granules are synthesized only during the myelocyte stage of neutrophil development and are characterized by the presence of the transferrin-like protein **lactoferrin**, which has multiple antimicrobial roles. Lactoferrin binds free iron required by some pathogens and also binds to the LPS of gram-negative bacteria, resulting in damage to the bacterial cell wall by generation of free radicals. The granules also contain the membrane bound $gp91^{phox}$ (NOX2) and $p22^{phox}$ component of the NADPH oxidase system.
- **Azurophilic granules (primary granules):** Azurophilic granules (initially named because of their staining properties) are synthesized only during the promyelocytic stage

of neutrophil development and are characterized by containing the enzyme **myeloperoxidase**, which has a critical role in oxidative killing. In addition, the granules contain an array of additional bioactive components.

Secretory vesicles and gelatinase granules are easily exocytosed allowing for the process of emigration out of the vessel without release of the potentially damaging components contained within specific and azurophil granules, which require additional cell activation and are mobilized at the site of tissue damage and phagocytosis.

> **QUICK REVIEW**
> **Nonoxidative Host Defense Components of Neutrophil Granules**
>
> Neutrophils granules contain a variety of bioactive proteins that play a role in host defense. These can be subdivided as into several functional classes:
>
> - **Proteolytic enzymes:** The phagolysosome contains over 50 different acid hydrolases of lysosomal origin. This includes the cathepsin family that consists of serine, aspartyl, and cysteine proteases. Unlike the macrophage whose granules are acidic and represent an optimal environment for many lysosomal hydrolases, neutrophil granules are neutral in pH. Nevertheless, acid hydrolases play an active bactericidal role in the more acidic post-release tissue environment.
> - **Serprocidins:** Azurophilic granules contain three serine proteases with bactericidal properties including **proteinase 3** (PR3), **neutrophil elastase**, and **cathepsins G**. As well as having multiple activities against a variety of gram-positive and gram-negative, PR3 activates the cationic defense protein cathelicidin protein-18 (hCAP-18) found in specific granules. Elastase is capable of causing severe tissue injury (notably in the lung) and is inhibited by the plasma α1-antitrypsin.
> - **Azurocidin** is related to the serprocidins but lacks enzymatic activity. It is both bactericidal and chemotactic for macrophages.
> - **Lysozyme** is found in both azurophilic and specific granules and is active in cleaving the peptidoglycan polymers of gram-positive bacterial cell walls.
> - MMPs are zinc-dependent endopeptidases, which include the abovementioned MMP-9 (gelatinase) characteristic of tertiary granules and MMP-8 (collagenase) found in specific granules, which is active in degrading ECM.
> - **Cationic peptides:** Neutrophil granules contain a number of cationic proteins and peptides with activity against pathogens.
> - **Alpha-defensins:** They are a major component of azurophilic granules (making up a significant proportion of the neutrophils' protein content). There are four related small peptides (about 30 amino acids in length) termed HNP 1-4. Their exact function is in dispute but they appear to inhibit the synthesis of bacterial walls and show a very broad pattern of activity against bacteria fungi and enveloped viruses, possibly by disruption of membrane structure and function.
> - **Bactericidal permeability increasing (BPI) protein:** BPI is a full-length cationic protein found also found in azurophilic granules. It acts against gram-negative bacteria by binding to their LPS capsule and altering membrane permeability.
> - **Cathelicidins (hCAP-18):** hCAP-18 is the only human cathelicidin. It is found in an inactive preprotein form in specific granules. On degranulation, the protein is cleaved by azurophil PR-3 releasing a C-terminal peptide termed LL-37 that forms transmembrane pores in gram-positive and -negative bacteria. In addition, LL-37 has a variety of other effects important in host defense including endotoxin neutralization and wound healing.
> - **Metal chelating proteins: Lactoferrin** has been discussed as a characteristic protein of specific granules.

Neutrophil NADPH Oxidase and Host Defense

The generation of the products of the NADPH oxidase system plays a critical role in host defense. As noted below, inherited defects in the system result in **chronic granulomatous disease (CGD)**, a defect in the intrinsic immune defense system with potentially fatal consequences to the host. Although macrophages also utilize this mechanism, their response is much weaker than that of neutrophils and limited to the extracellular compartment. Upon degranulation, neutrophils show a rapid increase in oxygen consumption termed the **respiratory or oxidative burst** in which the hexose monophosphate pathway is used to generate NADPH. Upon activation, **NADPH oxidase**, a multicomponent enzyme system, transfers electrons from the cytosol generated NADPH across the neutrophil granule membrane to the acceptor molecular oxygen within the granule resulting in the production of superoxide radical ($O_2^{\bullet -}$) and subsequently, a variety of additional bioactive components (*see also Molecular Mechanisms of Necrosis* above) **(Figure 2-54)**.

Assembly of NADPH Oxidase and Its Molecular Products

Assembly of a functional membrane-associated NADPH-oxidase requires the interaction of both membrane bound and cytoplasmic components. The membrane-bound $gp91^{phox}$ (NOX2) and $p22^{phox}$ constitute flavocytochrome b_{558}, which is found predominantly in specific granule membranes with a smaller amount present in the cell surface membrane. Formation of active enzyme requires the association of three cytoplasmic components, $p40^{phox}$, $p47^{phox}$, and $p67^{phox}$ and the small GTPase RAC-GTP (mediated by the $p67^{phox}$ component). On activation of the neutrophil, $p47^{phox}$ is phosphorylated and allows for the interaction of the cytosolic complex with the $p22^{phox}$ domain of the membrane flavocytochrome to form the functional enzyme

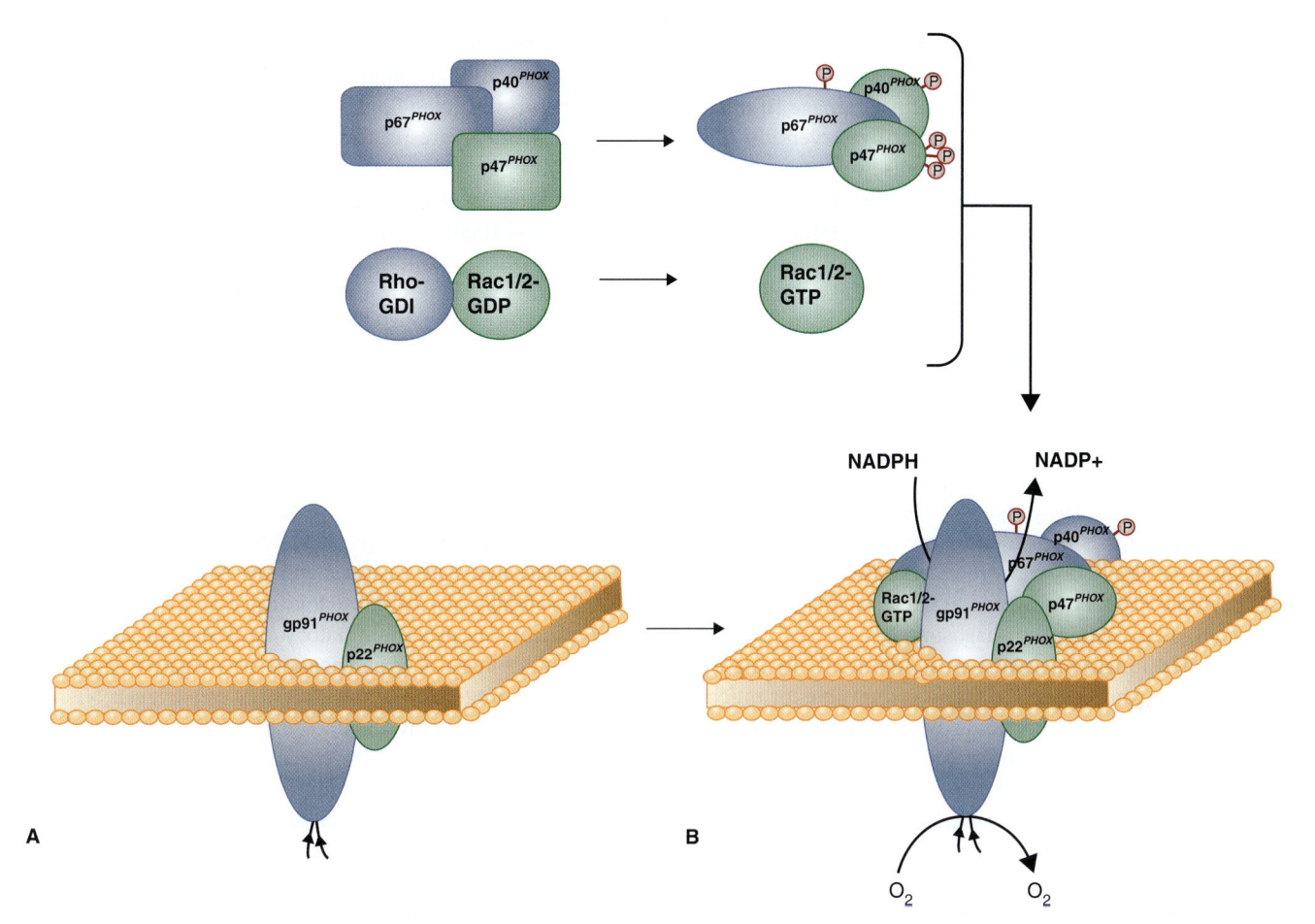

FIGURE 2-54 Assembly of the NADPH oxidase complex: **(A)** Resting cell. **(B)** Activated cell demonstrating assembly of cytosolic and membrane bound components of the NADPH oxidase complex. Labels as in text, Rho-GDI is inhibitor of Rac. Source: Priming of the neutrophil NADPH oxidase activation: role of p47phox phosphorylation and NOX2 mobilization to the plasma membrane. El-Benna J, et al. Seminars in Immunopathology. 2008, 30:279–289. With kind permission from Springer Science and Business Media.

bound NADPH–oxidase complex. Additionally, interaction of p40^{phox} with PIP$_3$ is associated with activation.

Superoxide radical ($O_2^{\bullet-}$), the initial product of the activated NADPH–oxidase complex, is cytotoxic but it is subsequent products that are most bioactive. Superoxide is rapidly dismutated to form the potent oxidant hydrogen peroxide (H_2O_2) and may also form other potent oxidants such as hydroxyl radicals and peroxinitrite (by reacting with nitric oxide). Of perhaps greater significance is the conversion of hydrogen peroxide and chloride ion into **hypochlorous acid** (HOCl, the active agent in laundry bleach) by the enzyme myeloperoxidase, derived from azurophilic granules. Hypochlorous acid is more active than superoxide radical and may also lead to the production of **chloramines** with bactericidal potential.

Defects in the Mechanism of Oxidative Killing

CGD results from either lack of or markedly diminished NADPH oxidase activity in neutrophils. Mutations in all of the five components of the oxidase have been associated with CGD as is an extremely rare mutation in Rac-2 small GTPase. The most common mutation accounting for 60–70% of all cases occurs in the gp91^{phox} (NOX2) component of flavocytochrome b$_{558}$. The *CYBB* gene that codes for the protein is on the X chromosome. Hence, the most common form of CGD exhibits sex-linked inheritance. Mutations in the *NCF1* gene coding for the p47^{phox} protein are responsible for the bulk of additional cases, which are inherited as autosomal recessives. Autosomal recessive mutations in the other three subunits account for 10% of cases with only a single case of mutations in p40^{phox} reported. The incidence of CGD is 1 in 200,000–250,000 live births but varies considerably from country to country.

Severity of disease is related to the level of residual enzymatic activity, and although the majority of CGD patient have essentially no activity, there are milder variants of the X-linked form of the disease in which significant enzymatic activity is retained. In such cases, CGD may not be diagnosed in childhood. In general, mutations in the p47^{phox} protein are associated with somewhat milder disease.

Prior to the development of modern prophylactic therapy with antibiotics and significantly, potent antifungal agents, CGD patients showed mortality in early childhood with only uncommon survival until the third and fourth decades. Currently, childhood survival is much improved with rates of over

90% in persons given optimal care and with many patients reaching age 40. However, prolonged survival comes at the cost of repeated infections, inflammatory damage to organs, and constant prophylactic and therapeutic intervention.

The disease most commonly presents by the age of 2 years with recurrent skin infections often resulting in perianal, axillary, or scalp abscesses. Recurrent deep abscessing infections of the liver, lung, and spleen occur. Granulomas in the GI and genitourinary tract are common and a third of patients develop a Crohn-like form of inflammatory bowel disease. Bacterial infections are generally from catalase-positive organisms including *Staphylococcus aureus, Serratia marcescens,* and members of the *Burkholderia cepacia* complex. In addition, a number of uncommon bacteria found in brackish water such as *Chromobacterium violaceum* have been reported to cause sepsis in CGD patients. The propensity for infection by catalase-positive organisms is explained by the ability of the bacteria to decompose the H_2O_2 they produce. In the absence of catalase, bacterial H_2O_2 is converted to bacteriocidal products by myeloperoxidase within the phagosome.

Repeated fungal infections most commonly by *Aspergillus* species are common in CGD and responsible for much of the morbidity and mortality of the disease. Fungal pneumonia may spread systemically to other organs including the bones producing a difficult to eradicate osteomyelitis. *The serious clinical consequences of CGD highlight the importance of oxidative killing in host defense.*

Given the above, one might speculate that absence of myeloperoxidase in the neutrophil would likewise result in serious impairment of host defense. Surprisingly, myeloperoxidase deficiency is common (about 1 case per 1500 persons in the United States) and generally benign. Infectious complications occur in less than 5% of cases, most often in persons who have diabetes. Such infections are of fungal and from a *Candida* species. Also unexpected is a strong association of myeloperoxidase deficiency and malignancy, suggesting a role for oxidative killing in tumor surveillance.

Neutrophil Extracellular Traps and the Resolution of Acute Inflammation

Although neutrophils have a short life span in tissue, signals at the site of inflammation prolong this. Phagocytosis, degranulation, and the production of ROS lead to neutrophil death. The process of neutrophil apoptosis is critical to the resolution of acute inflammation or transition into chronic inflammation. Chronic inflammation may be further divided into anti-inflammatory and pro-resolution phases (including the healing process). Neutrophil products such as azurocidin, LL37, and cathepsins G (see above) all serve to promote monocyte recruitment from circulation into tissue and the site of injury in a process analogous to that of neutrophil recruitment. Also critical to the process is a switch in the nature of lipid mediators produced by neutrophils. The production of inflammatory mediators such as LTB4 switches to the production of anti-inflammatory lipids such as **lipoxin A4**. This mediator both inhibits continued neutrophil migration and increases macrophage migration to the inflammatory site. The class of "pro-resolving lipid mediators" includes the resolvins, protectins, and maresin, the last being produced by macrophages. They are derived from omega-3 poly unsaturated fatty acids and their synthesis is potentiated in the presence of aspirin perhaps explaining, in part, the health benefits of both.

Apoptotic neutrophils produce "find me" signals that summon macrophages to the site of injury to remove the cellular remnants and debris from the site of injury and "eat me" signals that lead to the engulfment of apoptotic neutrophils by macrophages (a process sometimes termed **efferocytosis** see below).

In addition to apoptotic death, neutrophils (and other granulocytes) undergo an additional form of "active cell death" termed **NETosis** because the process leads to the formation of extracellular traps or **NETS** composed of chromatin fibers decorated with histones and the contents of cell granules. Essentially any of the many triggers of neutrophil activation including proinflammatory cytokines, sterile DAMPs, and a multiplicity of gram-positive or -negative organisms, pathogenic fungi, and some parasites can trigger NETosis. The factors influencing the choice of NETosis versus phagocytosis and degranulation by the cell are unclear, but NETosis is a slower process under many circumstances. It is clear that Rac2-mediated activation of the NADPH oxidase and generation of peroxide is necessary for NETosis as the neutrophils from CGD patients do not form NETS but restitution of function in such patients by gene therapy restores NET formation. The chromatin and histone structure of the net and the bioactive substances associated with it (including myeloperoxidase, neutrophil elastase, proteinase-3) are likely to play a role in the bactericidal properties of NETs. Chemical modification of NET histones (deimination leading to the formation of citrulline residues by the enzyme PAD4) is associated with NET formation and dispersion. Lack of the enzyme (in murine models) leads to poor NET formation and bacterial susceptibility. NETosis has been implicated as a factor in ANCA-mediated vasculitis (see Chapter 12) and several other inflammatory diseases. It may be of significance that autoantibodies to citrullinated proteins are associated with rheumatoid arthritis, suggesting a possible role for NETosis in the pathogenesis of this chronic inflammatory disease **(Figure 2-55)**.

Acute Phase Reactants

Acute phase reactants are circulating proteins whose level of synthesis is most often increased as a result of tissue injury, which may be acute or chronic. In general, this change in plasma levels represents increased hepatocyte synthesis in response to cytokines and in particular IL-6, Il-1β, and TNFα. The list is long but **C-reactive protein** (CRP), serum amyloid A (SAA), and fibrinogen are representative. The **erythrocyte sedimentation rate** (ESR), often used as a nonspecific indication of inflammation, is predominantly influenced by circulating fibrinogen levels. Fever, muscle pain and wasting, anorexia, and lethargy

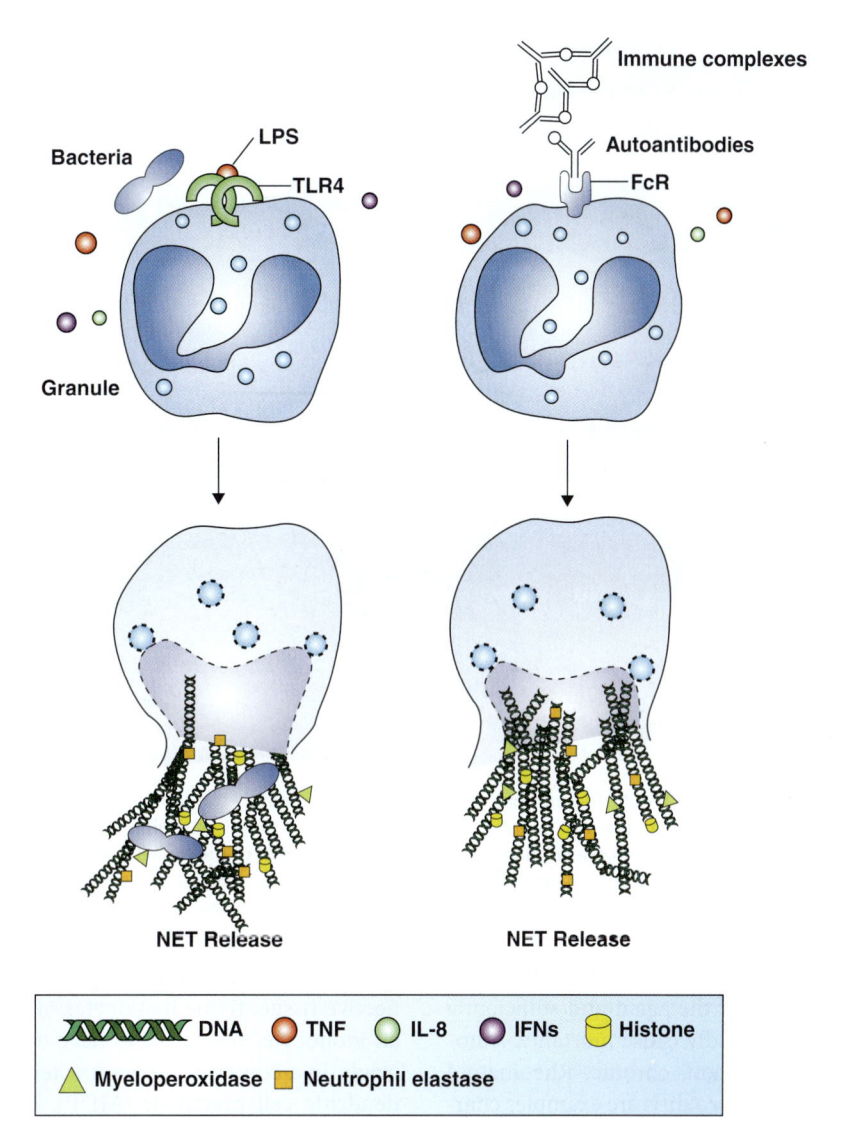

FIGURE 2-55 The generation of neutrophil nets: Potential mediators interacting with DNA of nets are indicated. Source: Kaplan MJ, Radic M. Neutrophil extracellular traps: double-edged swords of innate immunity. J Immunol. 2012 Sep 15;189(6):2689–2695 (Figure 2A page 15).

may also be regarded as nonspecific indicators of inflammation influenced by cytokine levels. The biological effect of acute phase reactants is manifold and it is often difficult to define their primary role. CRP not only activates the complement system but also plays a role in clearing apoptotic cells.

CHRONIC INFLAMMATION

Introduction

The transition of a principally neutrophilic population to one containing predominantly macrophages at the site of injury is the pathologist's tissue based hallmark of chronic inflammation. Chronic inflammation is characterized by the presence of mononuclear (as opposed to polynuclear) cells. With time, other mononuclear cells such as lymphocytes, marking the transition from intrinsic to adaptive immune responses, and fibroblasts, indicative of repair and the formation of new blood vessels (**angiogenesis**), will be found at the site of injury, their presence marking the stages of resolution and repair **(Figure 2-56)**.

Unlike acute inflammation that tends to be stereotyped, chronic inflammation is difficult to define with precision. It can be a sequel to acute inflammation in which inflammation and repair continue in a changing balance that may take months or longer to resolve. Chronic inflammation may also be a persistent response (often involving adaptive immunity) to an agent, which by its nature incites a mononuclear cell response. For example, persistent infections with the organisms that cause tuberculosis, syphilis, leprosy, some fungi, and parasites such as schistosomes are characterized by a chronic inflammatory response, which may be of a characteristic pattern (**chronic granulomatous inflammation** discussed below). Exogenous agents such as silica, cotton, and other organic dusts may

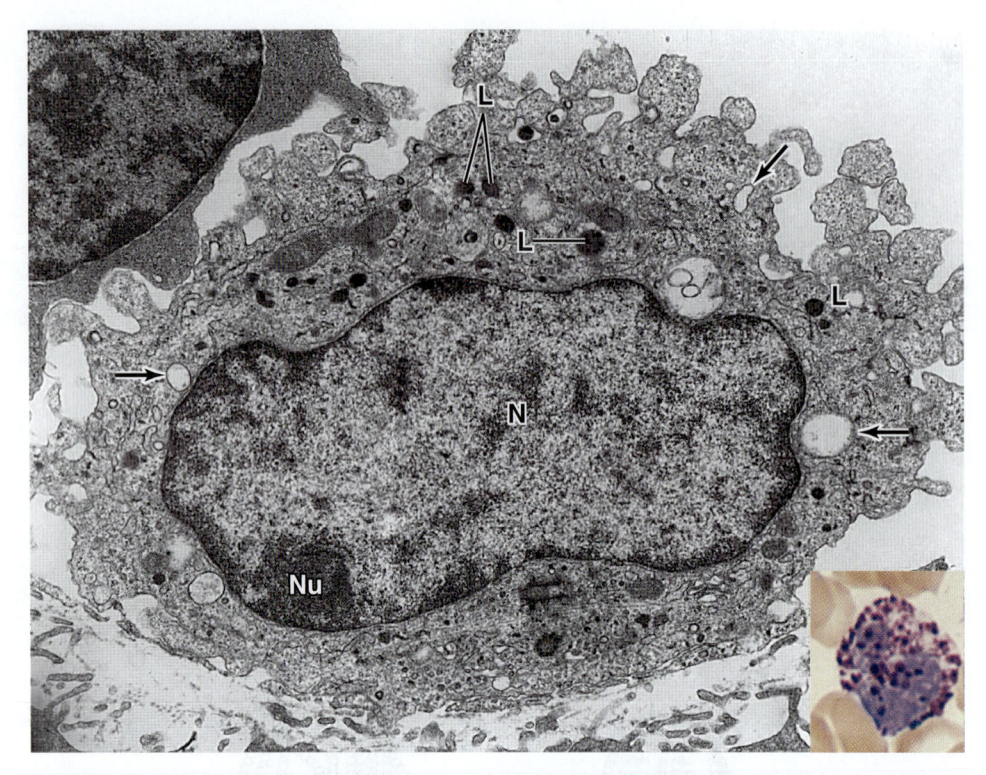

FIGURE 2-56 Mononuclear cells: Characteristic features of macrophages seen in this EM of one such cell are the prominent nucleus (N) and the nucleolus (Nu) and the numerous secondary lysosomes (L). The arrows indicate phagocytic vacuoles near the protrusions and indentations of the cell surface. Inset: Basophils are approximately the same size as neutrophils and eosinophils, but have large, strongly basophilic-specific granules that usually obstruct the appearance of the nucleus having two or three irregular lobes.
Source: Mescher AL, Junqueira's Basic Histology text and Atlas 12th ed. McGraw Hill Lange New York 2010, Chapter 5 Figure 5-4 Inset: Chapter 12 Figure 12-10

provoke chronic inflammatory lung disease. All of the above are characterized by persistence of the agent and sufficiently low pathogenicity so as to not rapidly cause mortality. Autoimmune responses are, by definition, chronic. Rheumatoid arthritis, SLE, and autoimmune thyroiditis are examples characterized by persistent chronic inflammation. Viruses and certain other pathogens may produce a cellular picture equivalent to other chronic inflammatory responses (but may show rapid resolution) by stimulating both innate and adaptive immune responses (Figure 2-57).

As previously noted, from a practical point of view, the histopathology of a lesion may provide evidence of the inciting agent. Most bacterial infections are characterized by the neutrophilic exudative picture of acute inflammation; viral infections show a mononuclear pattern characteristic of chronic inflammation. Tuberculosis produces a characteristic granulomatous chronic inflammation. Hence, a pathologist presented with a lung biopsy can rapidly make a reasonable estimate as to the nature of the infectious agent.

Macrophages in Chronic Inflammation
Macrophages Subtypes

To speak of macrophages as a single cell type is misleading, although they form a visually uniform population in blood as monocytes and in tissue as macrophages. Various organs have named resident macrophage populations (e.g., in the liver, Kupffer cells; in the lung, alveolar macrophages; in connective tissue, tissue histiocytes; in the brain, microglia) but all monocyte/macrophages have been believed to have their origin in a common progenitor termed the macrophage and dendritic cell precursor (MDP). However, recent evidence suggests that some populations of tissue resident macrophages (murine microglia being an example) may be derived from an independent early yolk sack-derived myeloid lineage. During inflammation, the bone marrow and the spleen serve as a store of mature monocyte/macrophages that transit through the circulation into tissue much as neutrophils. There are two major subtypes of monocyte/macrophages in many animal species and in humans that differ in function and expression of receptors and bioactive substances they produce and respond to. They are often referred to as "classical and alternative or "non-classical" monocyte/macrophages. However, based on analogy to T helper subsets they are best referred to as M1 and M2 subsets (or "polarizations"). This analogy has functional significance in the role that the monocyte/macrophage populations play in adaptive immunity, but this chapter will concentrate on their role in innate immunity, specifically inflammation and its resolution. The ontogeny of the M2 subset, as well as possible subdivisions of the M1 and M2 subsets, remains unclear. However, there is some evidence that M1 cells may convert to M2-like cells at the site of inflammation. *This is a significant finding as M1 cell function is proinflammatory, whereas M2 macrophages play a*

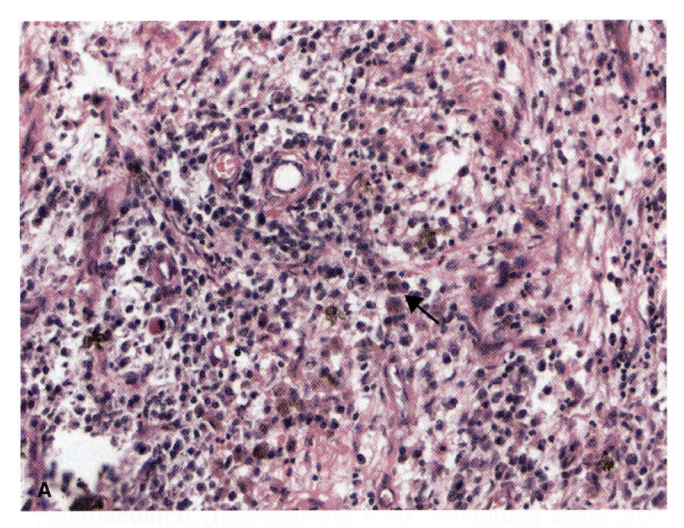

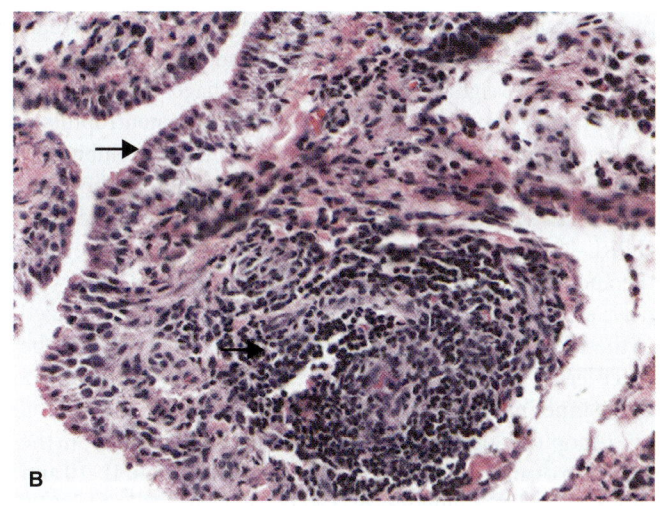

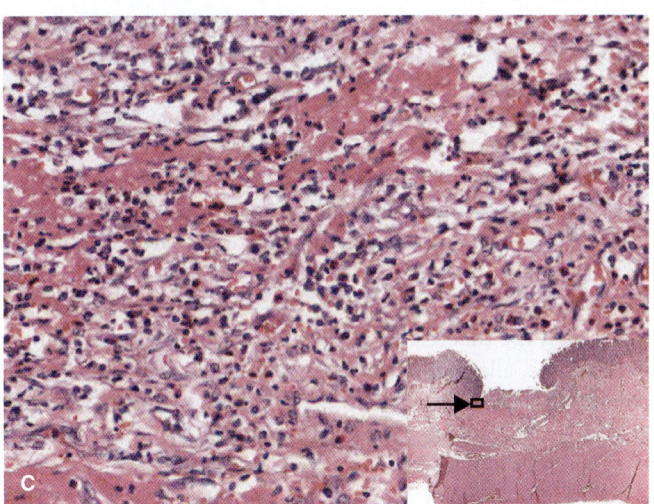

FIGURE 2-57 Examples of chronic inflammation: **(A)** Osteomyelitis: This is a long-standing infection of bone that is difficult to treat. Most of the cells are mononuclear and lymphocytic. Plasma cells are visible (arrow). **(B)** Rheumatoid arthritis: This is an example of chronic inflammation in an autoimmune disease. The image demonstrates an area of papillary synovium (synovial cells arrow) containing lymph node like aggregates of lymphocytes **(C)** Chronic peptic ulcer: The inset shows a low-power view of the ulcer. The area of higher magnification image is outlined and arrowed Ulcers represent a "balanced" and ongoing inflammatory process that may either heal or potentially perforate through the stomach wall. The inflammatory cells are mostly mononuclear. However, other areas of the ulcer will demonstrate a more acute picture of inflammation.

role in the dampening of inflammation, tissue remodeling, and angiogenesis.

- **M1 macrophages** are induced by IFNγ and microbial products such as LPS and cytokines such as TNF. They are characterized by having an IL-12^{high}, IL-23^{high}, and IL-10^{low} phenotype consistent with their proinflammatory polarization. M1 cells continue the production of inflammatory cytokines such as IL-1β, IL-6, and TNFα and actively produce products of the NADPH-oxidase system (albeit far less efficiently than the neutrophils they are replacing). Hence, they are active in tissue destruction and the killing of intracellular parasites. True to their name they induce and participate in Th1 adaptive responses (in which they play a critical role).
- **M2 macrophages** were initially defined by their "alternative mode" of polarization by IL-4, Il-13, and Il-33. M2 macrophages are characterized as IL-12^{low}, IL-23^{low}, and IL-10^{high} consistent with an anti-inflammatory function. They are rich in scavenger receptors, mannose and galactose receptors, and play a major role in clearing apoptotic neutrophils. Arginine metabolism via iNOS (yielding proinflammatory NO) is shifted toward the production of ornithine and polyamines (via induction arginase I expression necessary for collagen synthesis). Polyamines have an antiapoptotic role and are critical for cell division and protein synthesis needed in repair. M2 macrophages are present during early phases of wound healing and are required for the formation of the highly vascular **granulation tissue** critical in wound repair (see below). M2 cells produce profibrotic mediators that may play a role in both reparative (scar forming) and disease-related collagen deposition. Such cells play a role in the fibrotic encapsulation of some extracellular parasites and, as expected, play a role in T_h2 adaptive responses.
- **M2-like macrophage** is a term reserved for macrophages polarized to a cell with similarities to (but likely not identical to) M2 cells at the inflammatory site. They are induced by resolvins (important in the shift to inflammatory resolution as noted above), IL-1, glucocorticoids, and THFβ. Their functional properties are similar to M2 macrophages.

Macrophages and Neutrophil Apoptosis

As noted earlier phagocytosis and production of ROS by neutrophils trigger apoptotic death. Concomitant with these activities, the release of neutrophil components acts as monocyte/

macrophage attractants increasing the local influx of monocytes. Apoptotic neutrophils release "find me" and demonstrate "eat me" signals that attract macrophages and promote engulfment. Annexin A1 released by apoptotic neutrophils is a phospholipid-binding protein, which is a potent inhibitor of eicosanoids (PGs and LTs) via its ability to inhibit phospholipase A2. The released annexin A1 binds to the lipoxin A4 (FPRL-1) receptor on macrophages triggering phagocytosis of the apoptotic cell. Apoptotic neutrophils display a variety of new "eat me" signals on their surface. The best characterized of these is the expression of phosphatidyl serine (PTS) on the outer leaflet of the cell's membrane. Healthy cells restrict PTS to the inner membrane leaflet.

Apoptosis of neutrophils by macrophages results in the secretion of anti-inflammatory mediators TGFβ and IL-10 and suppresses the production of TNFα, IL-1, and IL-12 by LPS challenged macrophages. Hence, in addition to clearing apoptotic neutrophils at the site of injury, macrophages are polarized toward a noninflammatory M2-like phenotype. Failure of clearance of apoptotic debris is associated with autoimmune disease such as SLE and the production of autoantibodies.

Chronic Granulomatous Inflammation

As noted above, certain persistent pathogens, the most notable being *M. tuberculosis* but also a variety of exogenous agents, some organic (such as plant dusts) and others inorganic (such as silica and beryllium) all characterized by their persistence in the host, provoke a specialized form of chronic inflammation characterized by the presence of **granulomas** (chronic granulomatous inflammation). Although differing in details depending on the inciting agent, granulomas are defined as compact and organized aggregates of blood-derived macrophages surrounded by a collar of other mononuclear cells including T lymphocytes and sometimes fibroblasts. The macrophages in the granuloma are mature, large, and are often described as **epithelioid macrophages** because of their alleged resemblance to epithelial cells. That is, they appear large flat and have closely associated cell membranes that appear to be fused. The epithelioid cells may fuse into **multinucleated giant cells** (known as **Langhans giant cells** when the nuclei are arranged in a coronate pattern). Granulomas produced by *M. tuberculosis* (tubercles) are further defined by the presence of a **caseating** center, an acellular necrotic region. Formation of the tubercle is a complex process that is initially dependent on a T_H1 response driven by TNF and IFNγ. The mycobacterium furthers this process by the early secretion of products that induce the synthesis of matrix mataloproteinase-9 (MMP-9) from epithelial cells. MMP-9 is a potent chemoattractant for macrophages thus promoting the growth of the granuloma. The initial granuloma has a predominantly immune/inflammatory function containing M1 polarized macrophages, which serve to limit bacterial growth. However, the caseating center may serve as a protected haven for resistant bacteria. With time, the granuloma shifts to a predominantly M2 polarized pattern with reduced bactericidal activity through the induction of IL-10 synthesis within the granuloma. The type 2 granuloma becomes fibrotic and may house large numbers of persistent organisms. IL-4 production leads to enhanced e-cadherin expression and homotypic interaction between the macrophages promoting cell fusion and giant cell formation. Although the tubercle is, at least initially, a prototypic type 1 granuloma, allergens and parasites (in particular *Schistosoma mansoni* oocytes) produce predominantly type 2 granulomas that often become fibrotic. The mysterious disease **sarcoidosis** of currently unknown etiology produces granulomatous disease of lungs, lymph nodes, skin, and other organs. The disease is characterized by noncaseating granulomas, which are predominantly populated by M2 macrophages **(Figure 2-58)**.

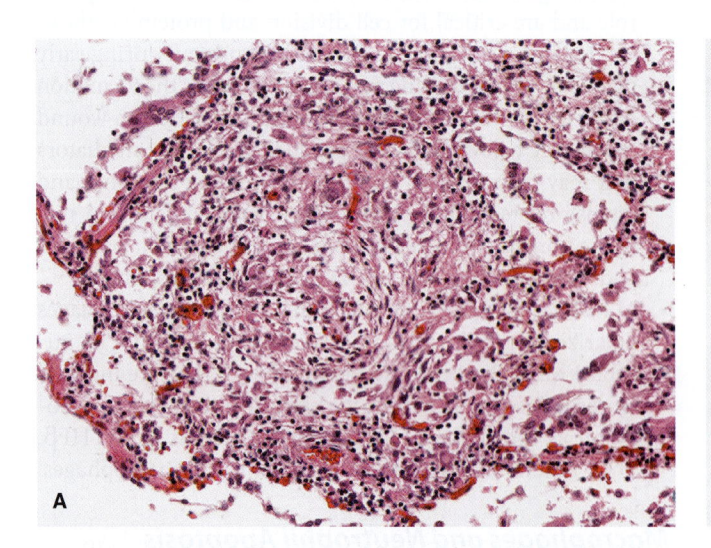

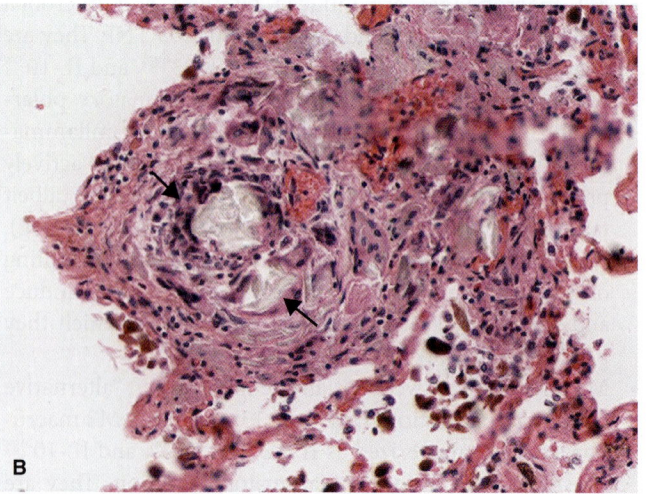

FIGURE 2-58 Granulomas: (A) Pulmonary sarcoidosis: A pathologist might note that this is a "poorly formed" granuloma, that is, it is not as compact as the caseating granuloma in Figure 2-29. Several giant cells are present. **(B)** Pulmonary foreign body granuloma: The foreign bodies are obvious crystalline deposits surrounded by encapsulating epithelioid macrophages and giant cells (foreign body giant cells arrow).

TISSUE REPAIR

Introduction

Since chronic inflammation as affected by M1 macrophages is associated with destruction of both parenchymal cells and the stromal framework, tissue repair is needed. In cases where parenchymal regeneration is possible, complete repair can (at least in theory) occur, for example, in tissues where parenchymal cells either represent a dividing population (**labile cells**) or where cell division may occur given the appropriate stimulus (**stabile cells**). An example of this is a minor wound to the epithelial layers of the skin. However, the process of repair is more often incomplete or defective. For example, although hepatocyte regeneration can occur in the liver, after extensive or repeated injury, repair leads to an abnormal structure consisting of regenerating hepatocyte nodules embedded in collagen. This abnormal deposition of collagen as part of the healing process is termed **fibrosis**, a non-normative and excessive deposition of ECM, predominantly collagen, which compromises organ function. In the liver, this abnormal repair defines the pathogenetic process termed **cirrhosis**. The fibrosis can isolate the incoming portal circulation from the venous return leading to portal hypertension, jaundice, and a constellation of other symptoms. Hence, the healing process when overly exuberant or defective may result in fibrosis, which can interfere with normal organ function (Figure 2-59).

Stages of Tissue Repair

Tissue repair occurs in a progression of stages starting with hemostasis and ending in the formation of a mature, predominantly acellular scar. Although repair differs in detail from organ to organ, the repair of epithelial injury to the skin is a well-studied model of obvious clinical importance. Effective healing is necessary to repair both functional integrity so as to provide host defense, thermoregulation, and control of fluid loss and also to maintain aesthetic value for the affected person and the beholder. In brief, the repair of skin injury proceeds as follows.

Hemostatic Phase

Although the details of hemostasis in relation to the immediate control of hemorrhage at the site of tissue injury are discussed in subsequently the fibrin clot and its components are also critical to the process of repair. Fibrin and associated fibronectin and vitronectin provide the **provisional matrix** that serves as the initial substrate for the inward migration of cells first including macrophages and later fibroblasts, keratinocytes and endothelial cells necessary for wound repair. **Factor XIII** (FXIII) is a two chain prototransglutaminase, which has important roles in both hemostasis and wound repair. Upon thrombin activation, the FXIII A chain acts as a transglutaminase and cross-links and stabilizes the fibrin clot. Additionally FXIII cross-links fibronectin and vitronection to fibrin in the provisional matrix thus providing the highway initially for macrophages and later in the process of wound healing for fibroblasts and endothelial cells to enter the site of repair. Individuals who are FXIII deficient show abnormal wound healing related in part to the reduced strength of the clot. Cells trapped within the provisional matrix, notably platelets, serve as a rich source of chemotactic factors and cytokines that play a role in the later phases of healing. **RANTES (ccl5)** is a monokine that plays a major role in attracting moncytes/macrophages to the site of injury. TGF-β and **platelet-derived growth factor** (PDGF) recruit additional cells into the matrix and subsequently play key roles in the activation of fibroblasts and also promote collagen synthesis. Additionally, IL-1 and IL-6 play a proinflammatory role and **fibroblast growth factor 2** (FGF2), **HIF-1α**, and **TGF-β** support the process of angiogenesis (and this list is far from exhaustive).

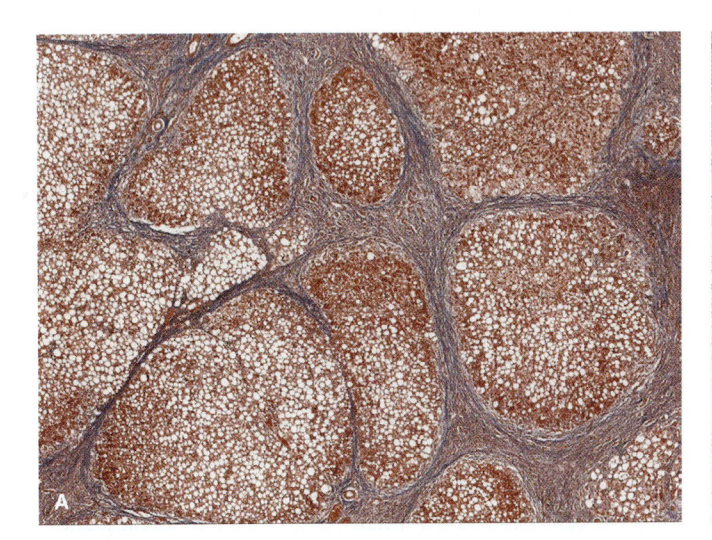

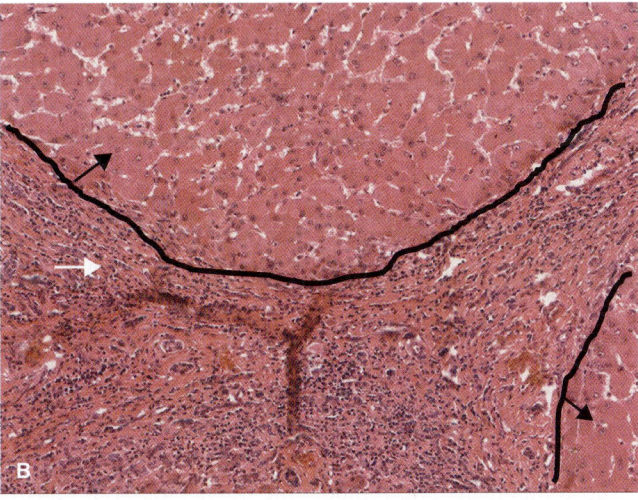

FIGURE 2-59 Cirrhosis: **(A)** Micronodular cirrhosis: A special stain has been used in this low-power view to stain the collagenous bands blue. **(B)** Micronodular cirrhosis: The high-power view of a similar specimen demonstrates two regenerating nodule of hepatocytes (arrow) and a portal triad area embedded in collagen showing mononuclear (chronic) inflammation (white arrow). Triad is outlined.

Thrombin, well known for its role in fibrin formation, is important in stimulating the release of proinflammatory cytokines from endothelial cells and blood monocytes. Such cytokines are important in the initial polarization of such cells as M1 macrophages. Hence, the hemostatic phase of wound healing can be seen as preparatory, providing a provisional matrix that serves as the initial scaffold for the cells playing a role in wound repair and as a reservoir for the bioactive molecules necessary to attract and activate such cells.

Inflammatory Phase

The chemoattractants released during hemostasis mark the beginning of the inflammatory phase of wound healing, initially by provoking the vascular and cellular phases of acute inflammation. Neutrophils appear in the wound bed within hours of injury, undergo apoptosis and are cleared by macrophages and also are shed into the **eschar** (scab) that serves to seal the wound surface. About 3 days after injury, macrophages become the predominant cell at the site of repair by exiting the vasculature in a manner analogous to that used by neutrophils. Initially macrophages are M1 polarized by IFNγ and microbial products such as LPS. These "inflammatory macrophages" (and residual neutrophils) have a role in host defense and removal of debris at the site of injury. With time (and most likely mediated by the process of scavenging apoptotic neutrophils) the macrophages in the provisional matrix shift to an M2 polarization. This is likely also influenced by the T cells present at the wound site. The polarization of macrophages to a profibrotic, and proangiogenic phenotype and the continued secretion of a multiplicity of growth factors and cytokines, is critical for the progression of wound healing from a phase marked by inflammation to one defined by cellular proliferation.

Proliferative Phase

The histological hallmark of tissue repair is the formation of **granulation tissue** that ultimately replaces the provisional matrix starting as early as 3–5 days after injury. Granulation tissue contains (1) many small new blood vessels as a result of the process of **angiogenesis**, (2) numerous mononuclear cells predominantly M2 macrophages but also lymphocytes, (3) fibroblasts responsible for synthesizing the components of the new ECM and also fibrosis, and (4) the new **ECM** containing collagen, glycoprotein, and proteoglycans. **Myofibroblasts** are defined by the presence of α-smooth muscle actin and are derived from resident fibroblasts and pericytes through the action of TGF-β1 and PDGF. Such cells, which can be considered as "activated" fibroblasts, produce large amounts of collagen I (changing with time to collagen III) and fibronectin. Later in wound healing they are responsible for wound contraction. Fibroblastic cells also secrete the additional components of the ECM and MMPs that help to remove damaged tissue components and remodel the developing scar. Fibroblast synthesis of ECM components starts 3–5 days after healing and is promoted by macrophage-derived TGF-β1, PDGF, FGF2, and IGF-1 **(Figure 2-60)**.

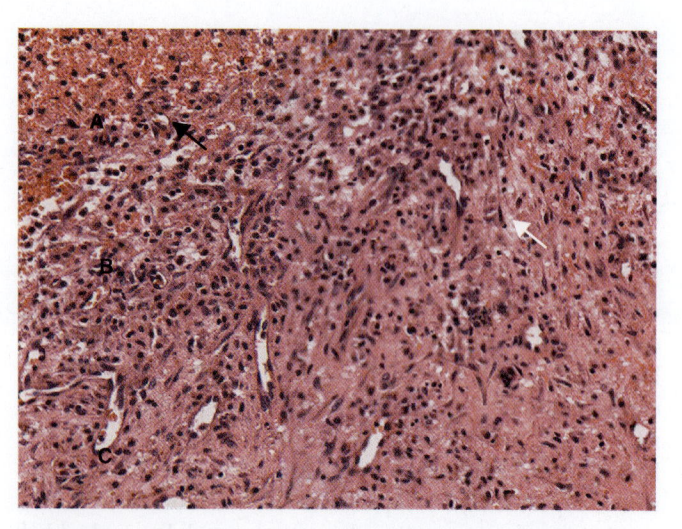

FIGURE 2-60 Granulation tissue: Organizing subdural hematoma demonstrates several stages of granulation tissue formation. Area A is a thrombus that is being organized. At the margin of the thrombus is a band of mononuclear cells and very early angiogenesis (arrow). In area B, one can observe more mature vascular channels and the beginning of synthesis of extracellular matrix. Spindle-shaped fibroblastic cells are present (white arrow). Area C is much less cellular consisting of extracellular matrix and many fibroblast like cells.

Angiogenesis: Angiogenesis is defined as the production of new capillaries from extant vessels predominantly by the process of "sprouting". Initially ECM proximate to the vessel is degraded by MMPs and other proteases produced by both macrophages and endothelial cells. Endothelial cells are activated to sprout off extant capillaries by TNFα and VEGF secreted by M2 macrophages activated by low O_2 tension, high concentrations of lactate and low tissue pH, all likely to be found at the site of injury. A variety of mediators play a role in the process. Endothelial cell migration into the healing wound and integrin receptor expression on the migrating cell are stimulated by VEGF, FGF, and TGF-β. VEGF is a key mediator in angiogenesis. Low O_2 tension is sensed by hypoxia inducing factor (HIF). HIF is stabilized under conditions of hypoxia and induces (by DNA binding) VEGF transcription and, ultimately angiogenesis, by binding to the VEGF receptor 2 on endothelial cells. During this process, new sprouts are oriented in the granulation tissue by M2 macrophage produced VEGF. The "sprouts" ultimately form small tubular channels that interconnect to form capillary loops, which with time remodel and differentiate into mature vasculature. The newly formed, immature capillaries are leaky and contribute to the edematous nature of the healing wound (Figure 2-60).

Reepithelialization: With the continued formation of granulation tissue in the wound bed, the wound surface is reepithelialized by local keratinocytes at the wound edge and by stem cells derived from hair shaft bulbs and sweat glands. The local keratinocytes, activated by any of a large number of cytokines and growth factors (EGF, IGF-1, NGF, and others), migrate across the surface and upper layers of the wound

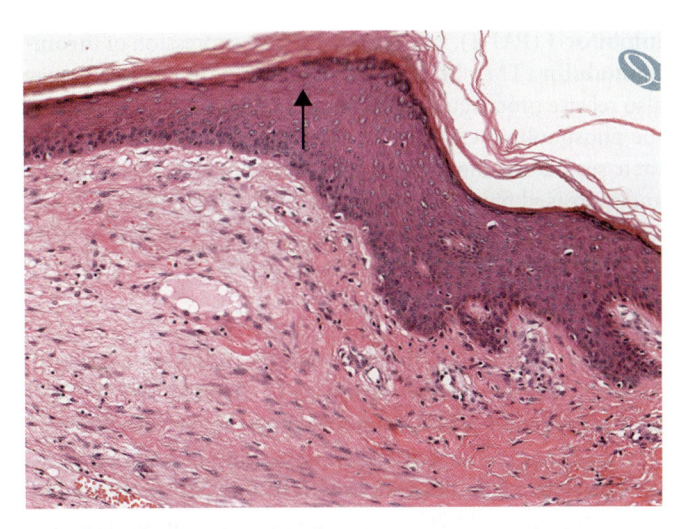

FIGURE 2-61 Reepithelialized surgical wound: The arrow indicates the margin of a healed surgical wound. The healed area on the left has a simplified epidermal layer that is thinner and lacks the rete pegs of the intact area on the right. The dermal connective tissue of the healed area shows much thinner fibers that are still separated by edema fluid.

centripetally, until the front of dividing cells touch each other (signaling covering of the wound) **(Figure 2-61)**.

Remodeling Phase

During the remodeling phase, granulation tissue is converted into a collagenous scar. Remodeling is the longest phase of wound healing and may last for months. This process involves changes in the organization of collagen from the fibrillar type I into type III fibrillar cross-linked collagen organized into small parallel bundles. The cross-linking is the product of lysyl oxidase secreted by fibroblasts in the wound. Although the wound never reaches the preinjury tensile strength, it may achieve 75% of that of uninjured tissue with continued maturation and contraction. During the remodeling process, tissue degradation mediated by MMPs is balanced by tissue inhibitor of metalloproteinase (TIMP). A lack of balance between MMPs and TIMPs may lead to excessive fibrosis and the presence of a **hypertrophic** scar or contrawise, a weak wound susceptible to dehiscence. Unlike hypertrophic scars, which although raised do not extend beyond the original site of damage, **keloids** are large, irregularly shaped scars that extend above and beyond the boundary of the original wound. They tend to be nodular and ridged. Hence, although not of clinical concern they may be unsightly. Keloids are predominantly composed of large disordered bundles of collagen. Keloids are associated with excessive fibroblast proliferation at the wound site. There is a genetic propensity for keloid formation and such are more common in people of African descent. Unfortunately, surgical removal is often accompanied by additional keloid formation **(Figure 2-62)**.

VASCULAR RESPONSE TO INJURY AND DISEASE

Introduction

Following injury or invasion by a pathogen, the body protects against the loss of blood and attempts to maintain hemostasis by activating the primary and secondary hemostatic pathways. The culmination of these events is the formation of a fibrin-rich platelet plug at the site of vessel damage. Along with its role in hemostasis, fibrin also plays roles in the inflammatory and wound healing processes that are occurring simultaneously following an injury. Fibrin deposition is seen frequently in areas of inflammation, whether vessel injury is present or not. Local fibrin deposition is able to induce adhesion molecule expression and chemokine expression in the endothelium, leading to recruitment of leukocytes and fibroblasts to the site of injury. Fibroblasts play a key role in the wound healing

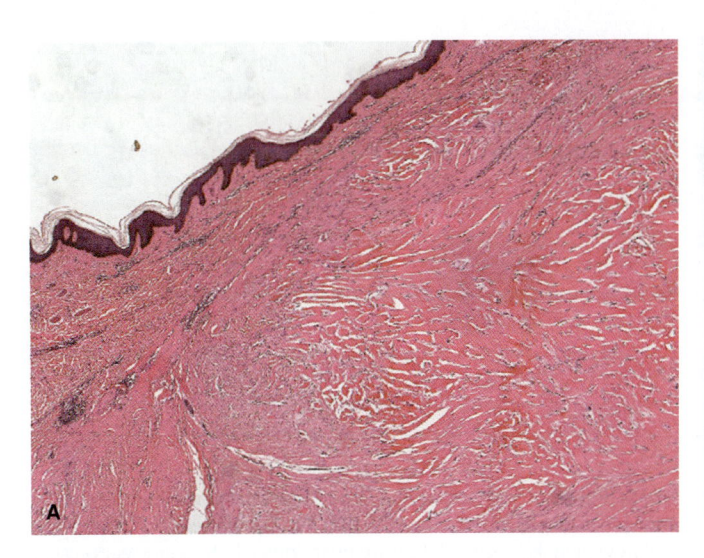

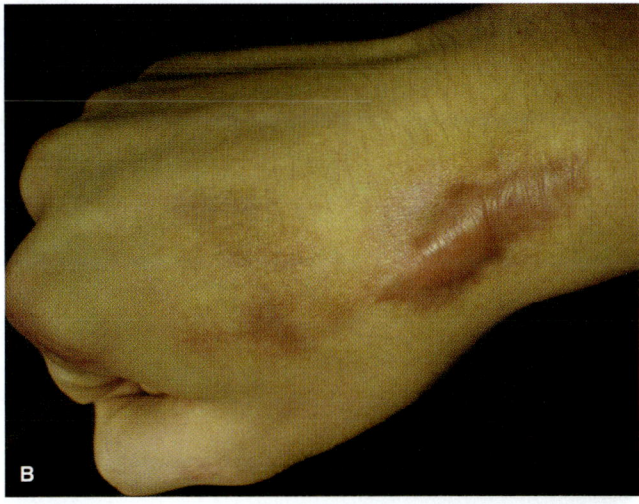

FIGURE 2-62 Keloid: (A) Note the irregularly organized large bundles of collagen most obvious on the right hand side of the image. **(B)** The gross photograph of a keloid scar demonstrated its raised and irregular contours.

processes, as they secrete matrix proteins, namely fibronectin and collagen. The foundation formed by this provisional matrix allows for reepithelialization of the injury, as local epithelial cells migrate to the wound and provide a protective covering. Finally, fibrin is able to directly interact with the integrin $\alpha_M\beta_2$ on the surface of leukocytes, leading to further recruitment of white blood cells to the site of injury.

The interplay between hemostasis and inflammation is a well-studied mechanism present in primitive organisms, such as the horseshoe crab, that have integrated coagulation and immune systems. Although more complex species have developed separate specialized hemostatic and inflammatory systems, the two have never become mutually exclusive. Inflammation triggers activation of coagulation and, conversely, coagulation triggers activation of inflammation. One of the earliest mediators of primary hemostasis, the platelet, secretes not only signaling molecules but also a barrage of inflammatory cytokines and chemokines from granules, leading to the recruitment of leukocytes to the site of injury.

In addition to being the most critical enzyme involved in the coagulation cascade, **thrombin** has many roles outside of hemostasis. It is able to activate several cell types to secrete proinflammatory mediators by binding to **protease-activated receptors** (PARs) on the surface of platelets, endothelial cells, fibroblasts, smooth muscle cells, and many other nonhemostatic cell types. The presence of inflammation can shift the endothelium from an anticoagulant surface, whose functions are detailed below, to a procoagulant surface by inducing expression of coagulation molecules such as **von Willebrand factor** (**vWF**), **tissue factor** (**TF**), and **plasminogen activator inhibitor-1** (**PAI-1**), and by reducing the expression of **thrombomodulin** (**TM**). These procoagulant endothelial cells may also release procoagulant microparticles containing both **PTS**, the phospholipid critical for thrombus formation, and TF on their surface, leading to increased amounts of circulating TF and increased fibrin formation.

Vascular Response to Injury

Primary Hemostasis

Platelets are a critical component of the initial vascular response to injury, termed **primary hemostasis**. Platelets, similar to all circulating blood cells, arise from precursors in the bone marrow. Hematopoietic stem cells are capable of responding to the signals of cytokines and growth factors, most importantly **thrombopoietin** (**TPO**), to become megakaryocytes. The mature megakaryocyte does not divide, and DNA synthesis occurs without the subsequent increase in cell cytoplasm and eventual division, leading to the formation of polyploid megakaryocytes containing multilobed nuclei. The megakaryocytes extend projections into the sinusoids of the bone marrow, and platelets are sheared off from these projections into flowing blood. Platelets formed from these projections are anucleate, granular fragments of cells capable of participating in the hemostatic process **(Figure 2-63)**.

Platelets have two types of granules; alpha and dense granules. **Alpha granules** contain chemokines and growth factors, such as PDGF, and proteins involved in primary and secondary hemostasis, including vWF, fibrinogen, and factor V. **Dense granules** contain mediators of primary hemostasis, such as ADP and ATP, serotonin, and calcium, the last of which is a required

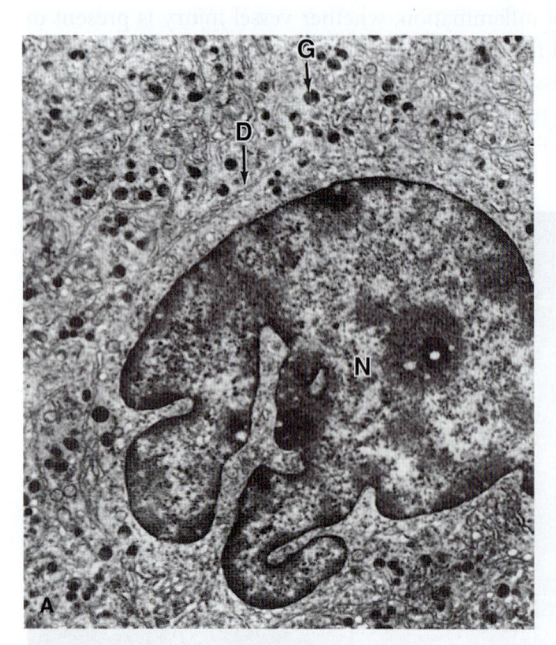

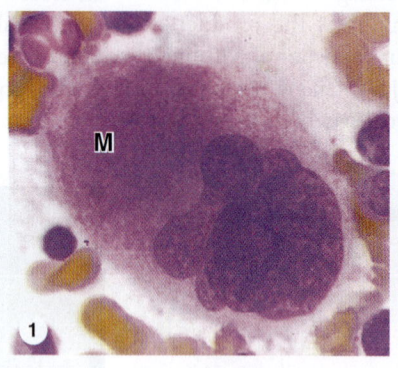

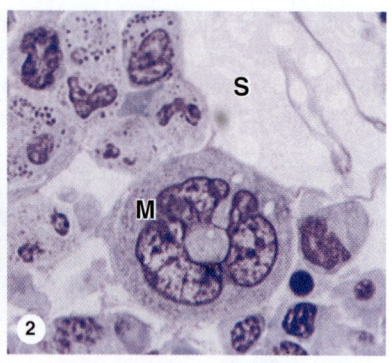

FIGURE 2-63 **Megakaryocytes: (A) Megakaryocyte ultrastructure.** Electron micrograph of a megakaryocyte during platelet formation showing a lobulated nucleus (N), numerous cytoplasmic granules (G), and an extensive system of demarcation membranes (D) through the cytoplasm. **(B1)** Megakaryocyte undergoes endomitosis (DNA replication without intervening cell divisions), becoming polyploid as they differentiate (M). **(B2)** Micrographic section of bone marrow megakaryocyte (M) shown near sinusoids (S). Source: Mescher AL, Junqueira's Basic Histology text and Atlas McGraw Hill Lange New York 2010, Chapter 13 Figure 13-12 Inset; Chapter 13 Figure 13-11 (modified)

cofactor for coagulation. The platelet surface harbors several glycoprotein receptors that are required for the proper function of platelets during primary hemostasis. Following injury, subendothelial proteins, namely type IV collagen, are exposed to flowing blood. Circulating vWF binds to collagen and tethers platelets to the site of injury by bridging exposed collagen and a specific platelet surface glycoprotein, the **glycoprotein (Gp) Ib/V/IX** complex. This binding, along with the binding of exposed collagen directly to the surface platelet via glycoprotein VI, adheres the platelet to the site of vessel injury to begin the formation of a hemostatic plug. Once bound at the site of injury, the platelet undergoes shape change and an activation characterized by the rearrangement of cytoskeletal elements, prominent filopodia formation, and the release of contents from both the alpha and dense granules.

The granule releasates contain several mediators, including ADP and serotonin, which recruit more platelets to the site of injury. Once activated, **glycoprotein IIbIIIa** (an integrin receptor), which binds to fibrinogen, becomes exposed at the platelet surface. Each bivalent fibrinogen molecule is capable of binding to two activated platelets, effectively bridging the activated platelets at the site of injury and increasing the area of the platelet plug. Phosphatidylserine exposure on the aggregated platelets then helps to catalyze the conversion of fibrinogen to fibrin through the coagulation pathway, termed **secondary hemostasis**.

Defects in Platelet Production

Normal platelet counts range from 150 to 440×10^9 cells/L (or 150–440,000/μL). Symptoms commonly seen in patients with low platelet numbers include epistaxis, mucocutaneous bleeding, bruising, petechiae, and heavy menses in females. Counts below 50,000 cells/μL are symptomatic, and below 20,000 cells/μL are life threatening (see What We Do, Tests of Hemostatic Function).

Drugs, chemotherapy, hematological malignancy, or vitamin deficiencies may inhibit production of platelets in the bone marrow. However, platelets may be produced normally but destroyed prematurely by an immune system malfunction as in the case of **immune thrombotic thrombocytopenia (ITP)** above (Table 2-1).

CASE 2-5

A 72-year-old woman was admitted four times in 1 year with **purpura** (small confluent patches of visible hemorrhage), epistaxis, hematuria, and **thrombocytopenia** (platelet count 35,000/μL; normal is 150,000–440,000/μL). Platelet count normalized after treatment with prednisone. Further review of her household revealed she took her husband's quinidine (quinine) tablets to treat nocturnal leg cramps. She was told to stop taking the quinidine. Without further treatment, her platelet count returned to the normal range within a few weeks. When tested for the presence of a drug-dependent antiplatelet antibody, activity was detected only in the presence of quinine with a resultant diagnosis of "quinine-induced" ITP. Recurrent ITP can be fatal, with intracerebral hemorrhage as a cause of death.

In ITP, antibodies are produced that are directed at platelet surface antigens or can result from the interaction of a drug with a platelet membrane component, as in Case 2-5. Either case leads to immune-mediated destruction of the platelets in the spleen. Treatment of ITP includes use of corticosteroids to increase platelet life span by inhibiting autoantibody formation and splenectomy to decrease platelet destruction (see Case 2-5).

Defects in the processing of vWF can also lead to thrombocytopenia, in this case **thrombotic thrombocytopenic purpura** (**TTP**) (Table 2-1). The etiology of most cases of **TTP** involves the protease **ADAMTS13**, whose function is to cleave ultra-long vWF (**ULVWF**) that is secreted from the endothelium into smaller, less adhesive fragments. Deficiency, dysfunction, or antibodies against ADAMTS13 lead to the presence of ULVWF in the circulation. The presence of ULVWF in plasma causes aberrant platelet adhesion and activation in the microvasculature, resulting in microvascular thrombosis and consumption of platelets. TTP is identified by the pentad of clinical symptoms including (1) thrombocytopenia,

TABLE 2-1 Thrombocytopenia due to peripheral destruction.

Platelet Dysfunction	Coagulation Tests (PT, Fibrinogen, FDPs)[a]	Treatment
ITP caused by antibodies to platelet surface protein	Normal	In children, may not require treatment; in adults, first-line treatment is corticosteroids (e.g., prednisone) or IVIg; if relapse, splenectomy; platelet transfusion generally not helpful unless patient is bleeding
TTP antibodies to metalloprotease, ADAMTS13, that processes vWF	Normal	Plasma exchange; do NOT transfuse platelets
DIC	Abnormal	Treat underlying cause, platelets and fresh frozen plasma may help

[a]Since there is peripheral platelet consumption (reduced number) in ITP, TTP, and DIC, there would be an abnormal PFA test, but typically a normal bone marrow.

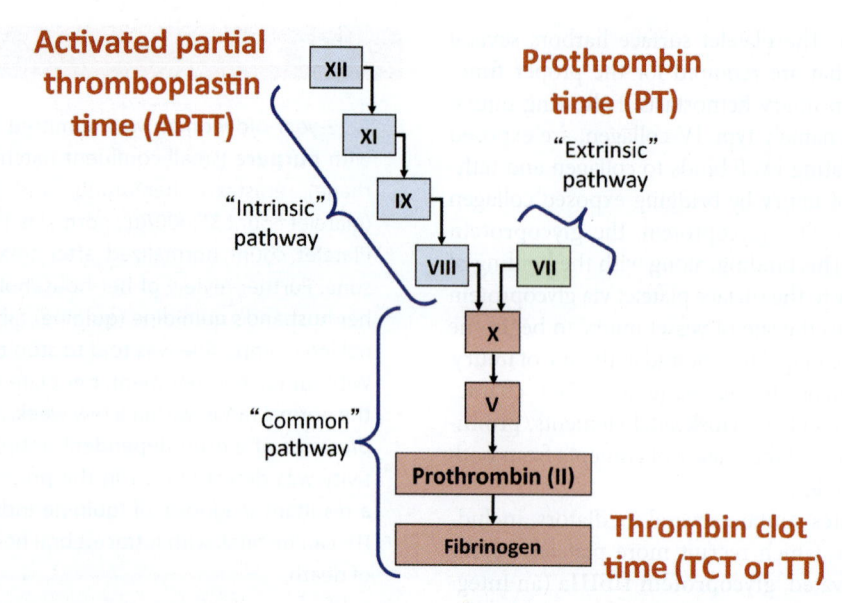

FIGURE 2-64 Canonical coagulation cascade.

(2) microangiopathic hemolytic anemia, (3) fever, (4) renal dysfunction, and (5) neurological abnormalities. Treatment of **TTP** is plasmapheresis to remove autoantibodies and the use of corticosteroids.

Defects in Platelet Function

Defects in platelet function are normally detected by **bleeding time** or **platelet function analysis** (**PFA**) when the platelet count is normal (see below What We Do, Tests of Hemostatic Function). Platelet dysfunction can resemble defects in platelet number, and symptoms include epistaxis, mucocutaneous bleeding, easy bruising, and petechiae (Table 2-1). Disorders of platelet adhesion can arise due to several factors, most notably abnormal or absent vWF, defects in GpIb (Bernard–Soulier syndrome), or abnormalities of the subendothelial connective tissues (Ehlers–Danlos syndrome).

von Willebrand disease (vWD) patients have clinical symptoms consistent with a primary hemostatic defect due to vWF's role in platelet adhesion to exposed collagen, but they also display symptoms associated with secondary hemostatic defects due to vWF's role as a carrier protein for the blood coagulation protein **factor VIII** (**fVIII**). Patients with vWD will usually show a normal platelet count, prolonged bleeding time, and an abnormal PFA. Related to vWF's role in secondary hemostasis, vWD patients may also have a prolonged **aPTT** (see table 2-4 and What We Do), although frequently it is normal. Depending on the mutation involved, vWF antigen and fVIII antigen levels may also be decreased. vWD is further classified by subtype, depending on the etiology of the disease.

Secondary Hemostasis

Following vessel wall injury, collagen is exposed initiating primary hemostasis and the membrane-bound receptor protein TF is also exposed. The exposure of TF on subendothelial cell types such as smooth muscle cells and fibroblasts leads to the initiation of **secondary hemostasis**, a process involving the coagulation cascade (**Figures 2-64** and **2-65**).

The coagulation cascade is composed of a series of protein zymogens, identified by Roman numerals with the subscript "a" denoting the active form, whose activation subsequently activates downstream zymogen factors.

The **canonical coagulation cascade** consists of three pathways: the **extrinsic pathway** initiated by the exposure of subendothelial TF, the **intrinsic pathway** or contact pathway, initiated by a complex of HMWK, prekallekrein and fXII, and the **common pathway**, into which both the intrinsic and extrinsic pathways feed (Figure 2-64).

The culmination of the coagulation cascade is the conversion of prothrombin to **thrombin**, an important protease that cleaves fibrinogen to fibrin to form a clot and also feeds back to regulate several important proteins and cofactors involved in the cascade (Figure 2-65).

In the **extrinsic pathway**, exposed TF binds to circulating fVIIa, leading to the formation of the TF–VIIa complex. TF-VIIa complex cleaves fIX to fIXa and also activates fX to fXa directly in the presence of calcium. fXa then feeds into the common pathway and forms the prothrombinase complex with cofactor fVa, calcium, and a phospholipid surface, usually provided by platelets at the site of vessel injury (Figures 2-64 and 2-65). The prothrombinase complex subsequently converts prothrombin to thrombin. This initial burst of thrombin plays a large role in maintaining the activity of the coagulation cascade as it can feed back to activate the cofactors fV and fVIII, leading to increased thrombin generation. Thrombin also cleaves fibrinogen to fibrin, the structural protein that stabilizes the platelet plug formed during primary hemostasis. Finally, thrombin can activate the transglutaminase fXIII to fXIIIa, leading to the stabilization of the clot by cross-linking of the fibrin fibrils.

The intrinsic pathway has a role in maintaining hemostasis in abnormal physiology, such as in hyperlipidemia, or in response to abnormal constituents of the blood, such as bacteria. The initiation of the intrinsic pathway occurs upon the formation

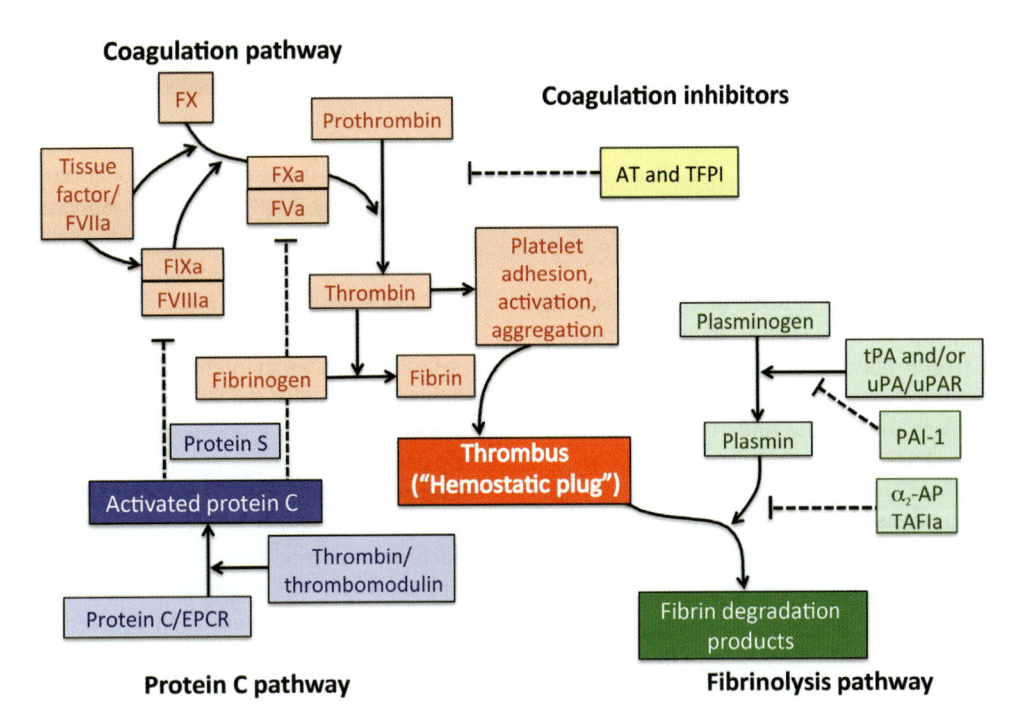

FIGURE 2-65 Hemostasis—overview of pathways.

of a complex of HMWK, prekallekrein, and fXII on a negatively charged surface such as exposed collagen, phospholipids, oxidized LDL, or bacterial cell walls. Activation of this pathway leads to the conversion of fXII to fXIIa by kallikrein, which activates fXI to fXIa (Figure 2-64). Active fXIa subsequently activates fIX to fIXa. The **tenase complex**, consisting of fIXa, fX, the cofactor fVIIIa, and calcium, is formed on a phospholipid surface and leads to the activation of fX to fXa, feeding into the common pathway to produce thrombin and, ultimately, fibrin.

The point at which the extrinsic and intrinsic pathways converge to the **common pathway** is the conversion of fX to fXa (Figures 2-64 and 2-65). The formation of a prothrombinase complex is required for the conversion of prothrombin to thrombin by fXa, and it is usually formed on the phospholipid surface of platelets at the site of injury. The importance of the initial thrombin burst in the activation and maintenance of the coagulation cascade is outlined above, and subsequent increases in thrombin levels lead to the conversion of fibrinogen to fibrin, forming a meshwork that serves to stabilize the initial platelet plug that traps other circulating blood cells. The transglutaminase fXIIIa, which is also activated by thrombin, cross-links the fibrin fibrils of the clot by forming noncovalent bonds between lysine and glutamic acid residues of neighboring fibrils, further stabilizing the fibrin network and platelet plug.

Coagulation Disorders: Vitamin K Deficiency

Vitamin K is a fat-soluble vitamin that is absorbed from the diet in the small intestine and is stored in the liver. It can also be synthesized by endogenous bacterial flora of the small intestine and colon. The three most recognized causes of vitamin K deficiency include inadequate dietary intake, malabsorption in the gut, and impaired uptake and storage by the liver due to hepatic disease. The vitamin K cycle plays a key role in the formation of functional vitamin K-dependent proteins, including prothrombin, VII, fIX, fX, and proteins C and S. These proteins contain post-translationally modified γ-carboxylated glutamic acid (**Gla**) residues. During the vitamin K cycle, vitamin K undergoes a reduction and an oxidation, the oxidation step being critical for the formation of Gla residues via addition of a carboxyl group to specific residues on the coagulation protein. Gla residues play a critical role in the calcium-binding abilities of the vitamin K-dependent coagulation factors, resulting in proper folding as well as proper binding to the phospholipid membrane of platelets.

Vitamin K deficiency causes reduced activity of prothrombin, fVII, fIX, fX, and proteins C and S, leading to prolongation of both the aPTT and the PT since members of the intrinsic, extrinsic, and common pathways are affected. Manifestations of vitamin K deficiency may include easy bruising, mucocutaneous bleeding, and heavy menses in females, and these symptoms can be ameliorated by administration of parenteral vitamin K. Rare mutations in the genes coding for enzymes critical in the vitamin K cycle lead to combined deficiencies of all vitamin K-dependent proteins.

Coagulation Disorders: Disseminated Intravascular Coagulation (DIC)

Acquired disorders of coagulation, which are more common than inherited disorders, frequently involve abnormalities of multiple clotting factors. DIC involves localized focal thrombosis at multiple sites, but paradoxically results in hemorrhage. DIC is characterized by (1) abnormal activation of coagulation, (2) generation of thrombin, (3) consumption of clotting factors leading to hemorrhage, and (4) peripheral destruction of platelets (Table 2-1). DIC is frequently associated with gram-negative sepsis, severe burns, obstetrical disasters, certain leukemias or tumors, shock, and insect or snake venom exposure.

The diagnostic hallmarks of DIC include:

- Prolonged PT (due to consumption of Factor VII)
- Low platelet count
- Low/falling fibrinogen level
- Elevated fibrin degradation products (FDPs)
- Schistocytes (partially fragmented erythrocytes) on peripheral blood smear.

Treatment of DIC requires removal of the underlying cause, followed by supportive measures including platelet transfusions, fresh frozen plasma, or fibrinogen. In patients with thrombotic complications and possibly heparin is often used as an anticoagulant to stop the underlying thrombotic process responsible for DIC.

Coagulation Disorders: Hemophilia A and Hemophilia B

Hemophilia A and B are hereditary, X-linked, recessive traits that affect the production of fVIII and fIX, respectively. Symptomatic hemophilia A or B patients typically produce less than 5% of normal fVIII or fIX levels, with a close clinical correlation between severity of the disease and factor levels. Hemophiliacs usually have a normal PT, normal platelet count, and normal PFA with an abnormal (or prolonged) aPTT (Tables 2-2, 2-3, 2-4 and 2-6). Hemophilia A and B have clinically indistinguishable symptoms, therefore direct measurements of fVIII and fIX activity should be performed to determine which type of hemophilia is present. In addition, mixing studies should be used to distinguish between a factor deficiency and the presence of a factor "inhibitor" (often of immune origin). Several treatment options are available for patients with hemophilia A and B including genetically-engineered recombinant proteins, plasma products enriched in fVIII and fIX, factor concentrates, and possibly in the near future, gene therapy (see Case 2-6).

Fibrinolysis

Although the formation of a clot is of critical importance in maintaining hemostasis, the breakdown of the clot at the proper time and place is equally as important (Figure 2-65). The system of proteins and cofactors responsible for clot degradation is termed the **fibrinolytic pathway**. The major enzyme involved in the breakdown of the fibrin clot is **plasmin**, a serine protease which circulates in its inactive zymogen form, **plasminogen**. Upon vessel injury, the serine protease **tissue plasminogen activator** (**tPA**) is released from the endothelium and cleaves plasminogen into plasmin (Figure 2-65). An additional serine

CASE 2-6

A 4-year-old boy with a history of tonsillitis and Streptococcal infection in the year prior was admitted to the hospital for a tonsillectomy. Routine admission laboratory work demonstrated a normal CBC with a normal platelet count, and the following pre-surgical coagulation studies: PT: 11 sec (normal range values of 10-13 sec); aPTT: 52 sec (normal range values of 29-42 sec); TT: 19 sec (normal range values of 18-25 sec); PFA time: 6 min (normal range values of 3-8 min) (See Table 2-4 and What We Do for details of tests). Due to the prolonged aPTT, surgery was delayed pending. There was no demonstrated family history of bleeding disorders. However, the child had experienced hemorrhagic episodes when playing touch football with his family. The parents noted that such episodes resulted in what was described as "very deep bruises" on his legs, ankles, and knees. The patient's plasma was further investigated using a "mixing" study in which equal volumes of normal pooled plasma were added to the patient's plasma. The aPTT of this "mixed" plasma corrected to within the normal range. Specific factor VIII and IX assay levels were performed using reference plasma as a comparison. The results revealed that coagulation factor VIII was 10% of its expected normal value. After the identification of the deficiency, surgery was successfully performed with the Transfusion Service ready with the appropriate blood products in case of hemorrhage after surgery. The patient and his family were referred to a Comprehensive Hemophilia Center for further counseling about dealing with Hemophilia A.

TABLE 2-2 Coagulation factor deficiencies related to bleeding disorders.

Deficient Coagulation Factor	General Population Incidence	Mode of Inheritance	Chromosome Involved
Fibrinogen	1:1 million	Autosomal recessive	4
Prothrombin	1:2 million	Autosomal recessive	11
Factor V	1:1 million	Autosomal recessive	1
Factor VII	1:500,000	Autosomal recessive	13
Factor VIII	1:10,000	X-linked recessive	X
Factor IX	1:60,000	X-linked recessive	X
Factor X	1:1 million	Autosomal recessive	14
Factor XI	1:1 million	Autosomal recessive	4
Factor XIII	1:1 million	Autosomal recessive	6 and 1 (2 subunits)

TABLE 2-3 Clinical differences between defects in primary and secondary hemostasis.

Clinical Symptom	Clinical Description	Platelet-Vessel Wall Diseases, 1° Hemostasis Defect	Coagulation Factor Diseases, 2° Hemostasis Defect
Mucosal bleeding		Common	Uncommon
Skin cut bleeds		Common	Minimal
Petechiae	Pin-point hemorrhages due to increased vascular permeability or failure of platelets	Common	Rare
Hematoma	Large pool of blood in subcutaneous tissue or muscle, producing localized swelling and deformity	Rare	Characteristic
Hemarthrosis	Hemorrhage into joint	Rare	Common in hemophilia A and B
Sex of patient		Equal	Predominantly male

protease, **urokinase plasminogen activator** (**uPA**), is also capable of cleaving plasminogen to plasmin, typically in the extravasculature. Plasmin recognizes specific arginine and lysine residues of the fibrin fibrils and cleaves the fibrin into smaller fragments, which are released into the bloodstream. These FDPs may include **D-dimers** specifically produced from cross-linked fibrin clots. D-dimer immunoassays are often used as diagnostic tools in suspected thrombotic disease as they indicate the presence of fibrin in the vasculature.

The fibrinolytic system possesses its own set of regulatory proteins that ensure that the clot is being broken down in the correct temporal and spatial locations. These proteins include **PAI-1**, thrombin activatable fibrinolytic inhibitor (**TAFI**), and α2-antiplasmin.

PAI-1 is a member of the **serpin** family of proteins, is released from platelets and synthesized by the endothelium, fibroblasts and smooth muscle cells, and is primarily responsible for the inactivation of tPA and uPA. Inactivation of tPA and uPA inhibits plasmin formation, thus inhibiting the breakdown of the fibrin clot (Figure 2-65). Increased levels of PAI-1 are seen in several diseases, especially those in which an inflammatory state is present, such as metabolic syndrome and cancer. Increased PAI-1 has also been associated with an increased risk of both arterial and venous thrombosis in these patient groups.

TAFI is a member of the carboxypeptidase B family of exopeptidases, whose main targets are C-terminal lysine and arginine peptide bonds. TAFI circulates as a zymogen and is activated by thrombin when thrombin is bound to TM (Figure 2-65). Activated TAFI inhibits fibrinolysis by directly cleaving the amino acids at the C-terminal ends of the fibrin strands that are required for plasmin binding, thus inhibiting the breakdown of the clot by plasmin. TAFI levels in humans have been correlated with several inflammatory biomarkers, including **CRP**, and have been linked to prothrombotic and antifibrinolytic tendencies in patients with systemic inflammation.

α2-antiplasmin is also a member of the serpin family of proteins and binds rapidly to plasmin, forming a stable 1:1 plasmin–antiplasmin complex, which eventually leads to the clearance of the complex from the circulation, essentially decreasing functional plasmin levels (Figure 2-65).

HUNTING FOR ZEBRAS

Although uncommon, genetic defects in the fibrinolytic system are instructive in demonstrating the important role the system plays in the response to injury.

Type I plasminogen deficiency is an inherited disease manifest by low levels of plasminogen and is the cause of a rare fibrotic disease affecting the mucous membranes throughout the body. The lack of plasminogen leads to the deposition of fibrin in several organs including the conjunctiva and genitourinary tract, and also predisposes patients to an increased risk of thrombosis. The effects seen in plasminogen deficiency highlight the role of plasmin in matrix remodeling and fibrosis, in that absence of plasmin leads to aberrant deposition of fibrous matrix proteins as pseudomembranes at mucosal sites, a process often triggered by injury.

α2-antiplasmin deficiency leads to an increased tendency for bleeding due to increased breakdown of the fibrin clot before vessel damage can be repaired. This deficiency is inherited in an autosomal recessive pattern, and only approximately 40 patients with this deficiency have been identified. α2-antiplasmin deficiency patients may present during infancy with umbilical vein bleeding, and subsequent bleeding episodes are usually effectively managed using fibrinolytic inhibitors. Because plasmin also degrades FV and FVIII, individuals lacking this plasmin inhibitor also show bleeding into joint spaces that is similar to that seen in hemophilia.

TABLE 2-4 Clinical tests to diagnose hemorrhagic disorders.

Test	Sample Source	Abnormal Results from?	Associated with?
PFA	Citrated blood	Thrombocytopenia, ITP, TTP, DIC, aspirin, or NSAIDs	Reduced platelet count or loss of platelet function (aspirin, NSAIDs)
PT	Citrated plasma	Deficiency or inhibitor antibody to one or more of the extrinsic/common coagulation factors	DIC, liver disease, warfarin (anticoagulant) therapy
aPTT (or PTT)	Citrated plasma	Deficiency or inhibitor antibody to one or more of intrinsic/common coagulation factors	Hemophilia A, hemophilia B, hemophilia C
TT (or TCT)	Citrated plasma	Deficiency or abnormality of fibrinogen, or by bolus heparin in central line	DIC, liver disease, fibrinogen defect

Role of the Endothelium in the Regulation of Coagulation

The endothelial cell layer provides another level of regulation of coagulation and fibrinolysis and can act as both a procoagulant and anticoagulant surface depending on the circumstances. The endothelium produces several compounds that are important anticoagulants in vivo.

Heparan sulfate is a glycosaminoglycan whose structure allows it to interact with a wide variety of ligands, the most important of which is **antithrombin** (AT). Heparin sulfate is a particularly good anticoagulant molecule in that its binding to AT leads to enhanced activity of AT, and increased inhibition of thrombin and fXa.

- **AT** is a serine protease inhibitor synthesized in the liver and it directly inhibits many of the proteases in coagulation, with decreasing importance for thrombin, fXa, fIXa, fXIIa, and fXIa, respectively.

The endothelium also produces anticoagulant substances that can play a role in the regulation of the primary hemostatic pathway.

- **Prostacyclin** is synthesized by endothelial cells and serves to inhibit platelet aggregation and adhesion to the vessel wall via a cAMP-mediated pathway, and can also inhibit the platelet procoagulant effects mediated by TXA_2.
- **PAF** is also produced by the endothelium and can expose receptors involved in platelet adhesion and activation, such as P-selectin.
- **Tissue factor pathway inhibitor (TFPI)** is a Kunitz-type protease inhibitor that is synthesized by the endothelium and forms a quaternary inhibitory complex with fXa and fVIIa-TF.

WHAT WE DO
Evaluation of Hemostasis

Diagnosis of vascular and hemostatic defects is of utmost importance for identifying underlying abnormalities and for the treatment of disease. There are many individual tests for determining defects of coagulation and platelet production or function, but the use of these tests in concert with one another provides the most useful set of information, allowing a diagnosis to be ruled in or out (see Table 2-4 and Figure 2-64).

- **Bleeding times** are performed by inducing a wound of fixed depth and length and determining the length of time (minutes) until bleeding stops. The test is most sensitive to defects in vWF and platelet function.
- **PFA** is an automated testing system that employs a mesh coated in a platelet agonist. Patient blood samples are applied to the mesh and time to occlusion of the mesh is measured and is indicative of platelet adhesion and activation.
- **PT** is performed by adding exogenous TF to plasma, initiating the extrinsic pathway of coagulation. Prolonged PT times may suggest defects in the factors of the extrinsic or common pathways including coagulation factors II, V, VII or X and fibrinogen.
- **aPTT** is performed by initiation of the intrinsic pathway, usually by kaolin. Prolonged aPTT times usually suggest defects in factors of the intrinsic or common pathways including coagulation factors II, V, VIII, IX, XI, or XII and fibrinogen.
- **Thrombin clot time (TCT or TT)** is performed by adding exogenous thrombin to plasma and detecting the formation of a clot. Prolongation of the TT is indicative of a defect in fibrinogen, and follow-up using a specific fibrinogen assay will confirm this finding.
- **Combined use of PT and aPTT** as a first line screen is of particular importance in determination of hemostatic disorders. Prolongation of only one of these tests suggests that the common pathway is *not* affected, and the defect can be localized to either the intrinsic or extrinsic pathways. If both the PT and aPTT are prolonged, a TT assay is performed to identify if fibrinogen is affected in the common pathway. **Specific functional assays** measuring individual clotting factors can then be employed to specifically identify the deficient or abnormal protein.

The denudation of the endothelium exposes several critical mediators of the coagulant response, including TF and collagen. During normal hemostasis, the endothelial cells provide an anticoagulant surface to keep blood flowing normally through the vessel. Endothelial cells express two important molecules that aid in the anticoagulant properties of the vessel wall: **thrombomodulin** (TM) and **activated protein C** (APC). TM is a membrane-bound protein found on the surface of endothelial cells, which interacts with thrombin in a 1:1 stoichiometric complex. Thrombin bound to TM has no procoagulant activity. The complex of thrombin-TM cleaves circulating **protein C** when it is bound to its **endothelial protein C receptor** (EPCR), to form **APC**. APC proteolytically inactivates fVa and fVIIIa, in the presence of its cofactor **protein S**, by cleaving residues within each of the activated cofactors, thus shutting down the coagulation cascade (Figure 2-65). The importance of the APC anticoagulant system is highlighted by cases in patients who have factor V_{Leiden}, a mutation in factor V that renders it unable to be cleaved by APC. Patients homozygous for factor V_{Leiden} are resistant to APC-mediated inactivation of fVa, and have a harder time shutting down the production of thrombin, leading to an increased risk of thrombosis in the venous circulation.

The APC pathway also plays a role in the inflammatory response. APC itself exhibits anti-inflammatory properties, including protection from sepsis and enhanced inflammatory response to endotoxin, which are thought to arise from the inhibition of thrombin's proinflammatory properties. APC can directly downregulate an inflammatory response by altering several pathways involved in inflammation, including NF-κB and TNF-α, in endothelial cells and monocytes.

AGING: DETERMINATION OF LIFE SPAN

Even with our increasing understanding of disease progression and treatment and with the multiplicity of mechanisms with which our body copes with injury, we all die. We, as do all other species, have a characteristic maximal **life span** that we do not exceed. Why is this so? The physicist might answer entropy, defined as the inevitable thermodynamic tendency toward disorder in systems. In attempting to understand the process of aging, specific factors, some endogenous, the inevitable result of our genetic background and metabolism; others exogenous, environmental and subject to modification, interact to determine our **life expectancy**, the average number of years of life remaining to us at a given age.

Defining Aging

Aging can be thought of as the stochastic (random) accumulation of damage to cells of which we are comprised. This ongoing damage is countered by defense and repair mechanisms that vary in efficiency from individual to individual and which tend to fail with age. It is often said that the best path to a long life is to choose one's parents wisely. There is truth in this as there is about a 30% heritable component to longevity. Attempts to link specific genetic loci to prolonged life remain controversial; however, variation at the FoxO3 locus is associated with longevity in several populations. FoxO proteins are transcription factors involved in the control of a variety of cellular processes likely to be associated with aging including DNA repair, tumor suppression, resistance to oxidative stress, and induction of apoptosis. The aging process is **multifactorial** (having genetic and environmental components) and involves many genes but aging is associated with a common set of phenotypic and cellular changes; a decreasing ability of organ systems to maintain baseline homeostasis that is magnified by stress. Much of this decline is explained by reduced regenerative ability related to tissue stem cell population loss. Characteristic organ-specific changes are associated with aging. Chronic diseases of the cardiovascular system, joints, and pulmonary system occur in 50%, 35%, and 10% of individuals over age 65, respectively. The manifestations of type 2 diabetes occur in about 15% of this population. The multisystem effects of such chronic diseases and the occurrence of cancer are almost inevitably noted on autopsies of the elderly as either the cause of, or major contributing factors to, death.

Cellular Senescence and Telomere Decay

Primary somatic cells can replicate only a limited number of times (the Hayflick limit). The internal "counter" proposed by Hayflick is telomere length. Absent a functional telomere maintenance complex composed of **telomerase transcriptase** (TERT, telomerase reverse transcriptase), a complementary RNA (TERC) and a protein (dyskerin), which binds and stabilizes TERT and TERC; each replicative cell cycle leads to telomerase shortening (because of the problem of semiconservative replication of DNA "ends"). This is best demonstrated in humans in studies of telomere length of white blood cells in relation to donor age (Figure 2-66).

Although telomere length differs greatly between species (and even between inbred mouse strains), there is no obvious absolute relationship between telomere length and species life span. Telomerase is active during embryogenesis but is inactivated in most somatic cells after birth (the major exception being stem cells that normally have stabile telomere length). Telomere shortening beyond some critical length will lead to activation of the DNA damage response followed by cellular senescence and apoptosis via the p53 pathway (Figure 2-67).

In the absence of an active p53 pathway tumorigenesis can occur. Many neoplasms have reactivated telomerase presumably allowing for unlimited replicative potential and selective clonal advantage. Several progeria (premature aging-see below) syndromes have been associated with abnormalities in the telomere maintenance complex, the clearest example being the spectrum of disorders termed **dyskeratosis congenita** (DC). DC is characterized by mucocutaneous abnormalities progressing to epithelial tumors, bone marrow failure, and a variety of changes associated with premature aging including

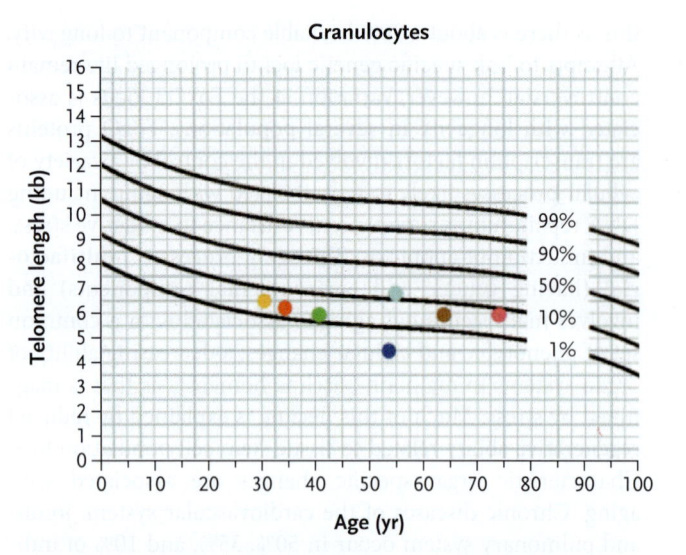

FIGURE 2-66 Telomere length in healthy individuals by age: Solid lines indicate percentile distribution of 400 control subjects. Colored solid points indicate telomere length is seven individuals with mutations in the TERT gene who have marrow failure.

Source: From NEJM, Yamaguchi H. et al, Mutations in TERT, the Gene for Telomerase Reverse Transcriptase, in Aplastic Anemia, Vol. 352, 1419. Copyright © 2005 Massachusetts Medical Society. Reprinted with permission from Massachusetts Medical Society.

gray hair and osteoporosis with death commonly occurring in the second decade. Strikingly, patients have abnormally short telomeres and the five genes known to be associated with DC all code for components of the telomere maintenance complex or are involved in telomere end stabilization (the shelterin complex). The pathogenesis of DC is linked to early failure of essential stem cell pools. For example, early loss of hematopoietic stem cells in DC results in the defects of hematopoiesis that characterize the disease.

Factors in Aging and Their Targets

All cellular constituents are subject to ongoing damage, the majority of which is related to the endogenous products of cellular metabolism, ROS being the prime example. The aqueous cellular environment alone furthers spontaneous hydrolysis of chemical bonds at a significant rate. Since both exogenous and endogenous agents may produce similar damage to biomolecules, the exact source of damage may be difficult to define. Regardless of source, strong evidence suggests that DNA is the primary cellular target for random damage associated with aging. Unlike most cellular biomolecules that can be repeatedly synthesized and, in theory, replaced, the nuclear genome consists of only one diploid copy of DNA that although subject to repair, cannot be replaced de novo. Failure of DNA repair mechanisms is critically associated with accelerated aging (Figure 2-69).

Mechanisms of DNA Damage

The majority of DNA damage detected as mutational events is of endogenous origin. Average rates of base substitution germ line mutations in humans are estimated at about 1.5×10^{-8} per nucleotide per generation with some specific sequences (CpG dinucleotides) having about a ten-fold higher rate. This

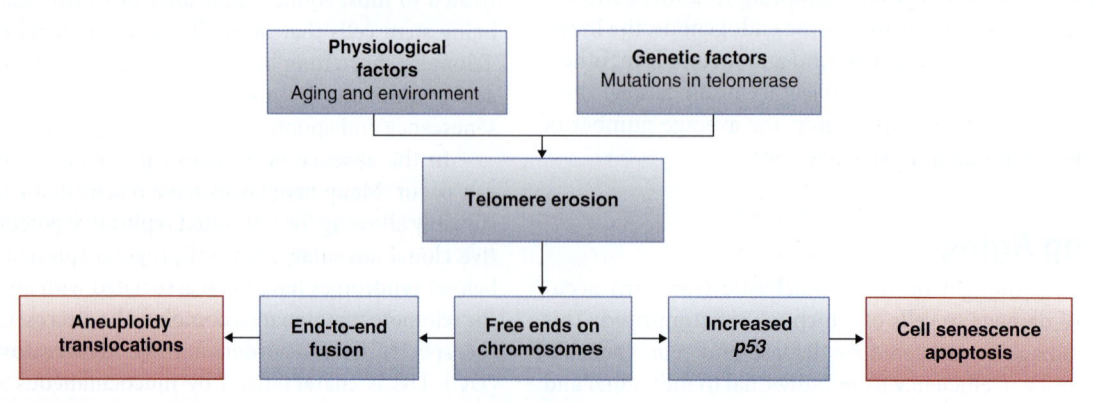

FIGURE 2-67 Telomere erosion and aging: Telomere shortening beyond a critical point leads to uncapped chromosome ends and ultimately cellular senescence or apoptosis.

CASE 2-7

HUNTING FOR ZEBRAS

A 51-year-old female has exhibited a 1-year history of increasing pulmonary distress including increasing exertional dyspnea (shortness of breath), dry cough, and abnormal pulmonary function tests suggestive of reduced functional lung volume. Chest radiographs demonstrated parenchymal infiltrates. A high-resolution CT (HRCT) study showed patchy involvement of the basilar and subpleural regions with moderate spared areas of lung parenchyma. Reticular and linear opacities and honeycomb cysts were noted. Clinical and radiological features were considered to be characteristic of idiopathic pulmonary fibrosis (IPF). A needle biopsy showed alternating areas of normal and abnormal lung with aggregates of proliferating fibroblasts intermixed with areas of interstitial fibrosis (collagen deposition) and honeycomb change. Little inflammation was noted **(Figure 2-68)**.

The histological features were consistent with a diagnosis of usual interstitial pneumonia (UIP). IPF is considered to be the clinically defined synonym for UIP. The patient became increasingly hypoxemic at rest and died while being considered for lung transplantation.

UIP/IPF is an uncommon disease with an incidence rate of about 10 per 100,000 persons per year in a population greater than 50 years of age. The disease is extremely rare in children. The etiology of the disease is unknown, but it is suggested that an endogenous or exogenous agent leads to alveolar cell damage. Activation of the damaged intra-alveolar cells activates mesenchymal interstitial cells leading to fibroblastic proliferation, collagen deposition, and scarring. Support for this hypothetical mechanism of pathogenesis is provided by rare instances of UIP/IPF associated with genetic mutations of serum surfactant protein C thought to result in damage to type II alveolar epithelial cells.

The Zebra: The patient's history suggested a family history of UIP/IPF having reported that her mother died at age 63 of a similar clinical condition. Family studies disclosed that a daughter of the patient died at age 16 of marrow failure following bone marrow transplantation for aplastic anemia. A 14-year-old son was currently under therapy for aplastic anemia. A 12-year-old daughter showed no signs of disease. *The syndrome of familial bone marrow failure and IPF/UIP has recently been associated with autosomal dominant defects in the telomerase maintenance complex (TMC) consisting of the telomerase reverse transcriptase (hTERT), and an RNA component (hTR).* The proband and the surviving affected son both had the identical mutation in hTERT (not found in the unaffected sib) and also had abnormally short telomeres.

Mutations in the TMC show **genetic anticipation** (earlier onset of symptoms) as telomeres become increasingly short in subsequent generations. Thus, the initial generation expressing TMC mutations exhibits UIP/IPF in the fifth decade of life. The next generation develops aplastic anemia/marrow failure in the second decade and perhaps subsequent generations would develop the severe progeric syndrome DC discussed in the text. In all cases, failure of essential stem cell pools is linked to the pathogenesis of the disease, emphasizing the potential role of telomere decay in cellular senescence.

As discussed in the text, DC is a severe progeric syndrome also associated with mutations of the hTERT and hTR genes. IPF/UIP occurred in the absence of other symptoms of DC; however, a common occurrence in DC is marrow failure.

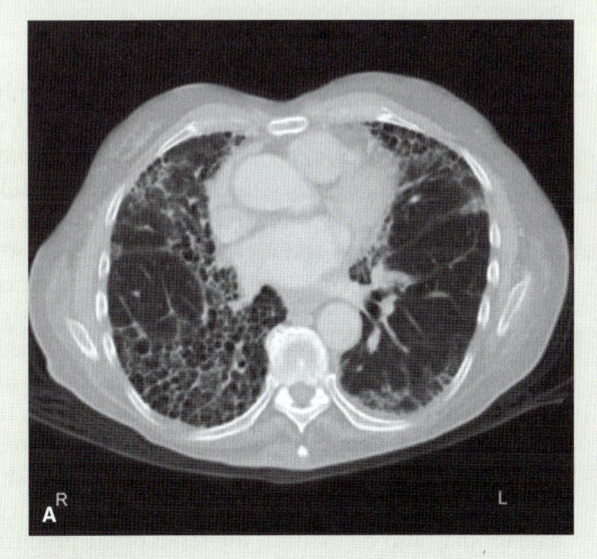

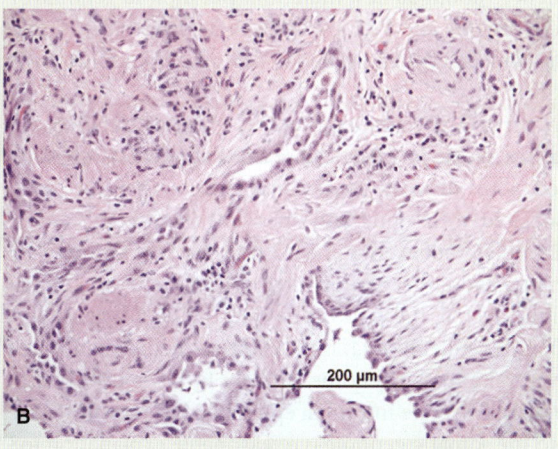

FIGURE 2-68 **(A)** Axial high-resolution CT image of lung base of patient with idiopathic pulmonary fibrosis/usual interstitial pneumonia (IPF/UIP). Right lung (R) shows marked peripheral cystic areas "honeycombing" characteristic of the disease (image courtesy Dr. Karen Birchard). **(B)** Biopsy specimen of patient (H&E stain) demonstrates aggregates of proliferating fibroblasts and acellular interstitial fibrosis (collage deposition).

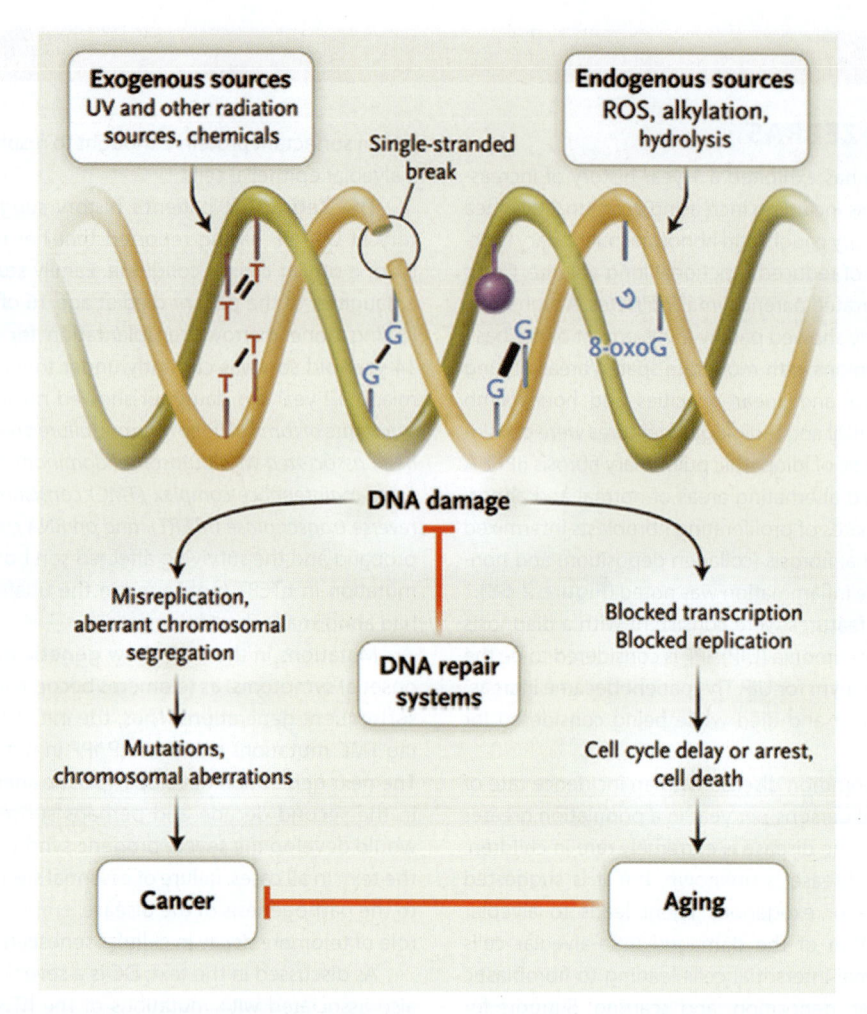

FIGURE 2-69 DNA damage, aging, and cancer: DNA damage in somatic cells may be the result of endogenous or exogenous agents. If unrepaired such damage may lead to cellular senescence, and the process of aging or result in permanent changes to the genome and cancer (modified from indicated reference).
Source: From NEJM, Hoeijmakers J, DNA Damage, Aging, and Cancer, Vol. 361, 1475–1485. Copyright © 2009 Massachusetts Medical Society. Reprinted with permisson from Massachusetts Medical Society.

is equivalent to about 80 new mutations per diploid genome of which between one and four are likely to be deleterious. Small insertions and deletions are about 6% as common as base substitutions.

Such **germ line** mutational events effect population fitness and can result in genetic disease. Pathologists are also concerned with **somatic mutational events** that are critically associated with aging and oncogenesis. Somatic mutations accumulate between 4 and 25 fold faster than those in the germ line and target all nucleated cells. One estimate suggests that by age 60, the cells of the intestinal epithelium will have >10^9 independent mutations. As the individual continues to age every site in the genome is likely to have at least one mutation in at least one intestinal epithelial cell. It is clear that damage to the somatic genome is a reasonable explanation for age-related disease and dysfunction.

Oxidative DNA damage: ROS are an inevitable product of mitochondrial respiration during which several percent of the oxygen is converted into the superoxide anion radical ($O_2^{-\bullet}$). This is rapidly dismutated to hydrogen peroxide that in the presence of iron or copper generates the highly reactive hydroxyl radical (OH•), a potent DNA oxidant. A second important DNA oxidant, peroxynitrite ($ONO2^-$) is produced by the reaction of hydroxyl radical with nitric oxide. The inflammatory reaction, which is critical in host defense and pathogen destruction, also serves as a rich source of potent oxidants capable of damaging DNA and other cellular components (discussed in Molecular mechanisms of necrosis). Oxidative damage to DNA produces a variety of modified bases (for example 8-oxo-guanine (8-oxo-DG)). Because 8-oxo-DG pairs with adenine it produces GC → TA transversions. The base excision repair system (BER) is effective in removing oxidative DNA damage but yields apurinic/apyrimidinic (AP) sites that if not repaired are in themselves mutagenic. Oxidative DNA damage may also be indirect, the result of the production of highly reactive epoxides and aldehydes formed through the oxidation of the polyunsaturated fatty acid residues of phospholipids or by the oxidation of endogenous estrogens.

DNA alkylation: Small molecules from both endogenous and exogenous sources can lead to the methylation of DNA.

The most frequently produced lesions are the generation of 7-methylguanine and 3-methyl adenine. Both altered bases can lead to blocking of replication and the generation of AP as a result of BER. Although *N*-nitroso compounds found in cigarette smoke and dietary products such smoked and nitrate cured meat and fish are the most significant exogenous sources of DNA alkylating agents, endogenous reactants (most notably S-adenosylmethionine) may also produce mutagenic DNA adducts.

Hydrolysis and hydrolytic deamination: The glycosidic linkage between base and deoxyribose is subject to a variety of N-glycosylases important in BER but is also subject to spontaneous hydrolysis yielding predominantly apurinic sites with as many as 10,00 lesions per cell per day being formed. Although such sites are efficiently repaired, a significant steady state level of AP sites occurs. Such sites are mutagenic (AP sites→T preferentially). As noted above CpG sites are preferentially subject to mutation. Such sequences are involved in the silencing of genes via the formation of 5-methylcytosine. This methylated base is spontaneously deaminated to uracil. BER results in a GT mismatch (see above) that ultimately results in a GC→AT transition; a common single site mutation found as the cause of genetic disease.

Endogenous Mutagens and Aging

Endogenous agents are responsible for the majority of human mutations. Most DNA damage produced by such mutagens (ROS for example) is repaired by the base excision repair system (as discussed above). Evidence for the role of endogenous-mediated DNA damage in aging (and aging-related disease) in humans is less clear and relies on differences in the activity of components of the BER in cells taken from young versus elderly donors (and similar work in animal models).

The strongest evidence for the role of DNA damage in aging is provided by the **progerias**, disorders in which the affected individuals demonstrate accelerated aging of multiple body systems. Such syndromes are associated with lesions in pathways involved in DNA repair and maintenance (see below). One progeric syndrome, **Cockayne syndrome group B** (CSB) has, among other defects, impairment of BER of oxidative damage (and in particular, removal of 8-oxo-DG adducts). The role that defective repair of oxidative damage to DNA plays in the generation of the progeric phenotype of CSB is unclear. More dramatic evidence for the role of DNA damage in aging comes from studies of additional defects in DNA repair systems including nucleotide excision repair, double-stranded break repair, DNA cross-link repair, telomere maintenance and also defects in the function of the nuclear lamina.

Progeroid Syndromes

A dramatic tool in the study of the pathogenesis of aging are the progerias, inherited diseases that demonstrate many of the changes associated with the aging process but at a greatly accelerated rate. The genetic lesions responsible for the various progeric syndromes would seem to provide a clear cut etiological target for the pattern of accelerated aging but the link between lesion and phenotype is often speculative. However, defects in the maintenance of genomic stability in somatic cells appear to be a common theme. Although the progerias show many of the characteristic changes accompanying aging they are all, to some extent, **segmental** in that not all tissues in the affected individual demonstrate early aging. Confusingly, the progerias also show lesions not characteristic of the normal aging process or that are atypical in terms of tissue expression. Increased risk of neoplasias of epithelial origin are characteristic of the aging process, however several progeric syndromes (Cockayne syndrome group B, **Hutchison–Guilford Progeria and Werner syndrome**) either show no increase in neoplasia or demonstrate an increase in tumors of mesenchymal origin, This suggests that when DNA damage occurs there may be a tradeoff between processes resulting in cell death and aging or incorporation of the damage in the somatic genome and cancer (Figure 2-69).

Hutchinson–Gilford Progeria (HGP)

HGP is a member of the **laminopathies**, diseases that result from mutation of the **lamin** family of intermediate filament proteins that are found in close association with the inner nuclear member and in the nucleosome of all differentiated cells. HGP results from specific dominant mutations of the *LMNA* gene that codes for lamin A (and also lamin C via alternative splicing). Mutations in other areas of LMNA are responsible for a confusing array of conditions resulting in muscular dystrophies, lipodystrophies and neuropathy. HGP is an uncommon disease (about 1 in 4 million live births) that results from mutations that result in an aberrantly processed isoform of lamin A termed **progerin**. Progerin retains a prenylation site normally cleaved from the mature lamin A protein and is permanently farnesylated (Figure 2-70).

In HGP accelerated aging begins in the second year of life and results in death at a median age of 13, usually from cardiovascular diseases (including stroke, atherosclerosis and congestive heart failure). Patients also demonstrate early loss of hair and subcutaneous fat, aging of the skin and facial features, osteoporosis and lack of joint mobility. Cognitive development is not retarded and remains age appropriate. The presence of the inappropriately processed progerin isoform has been linked to the progeric phenotype in murine models, and the use of inhibitors of farnesylation is under evaluation in the treatment of the human disease. Although the etiology of HGP at the molecular and biochemical level is clear, the pathogenesis of the resulting progeria is not. HGP cells demonstrate many features of cellular senescence including altered nuclear morphology and reduced proliferative capacity. Such cells appear to suffer increased levels of DNA damage and accumulate ROS at a higher than normal rate suggesting that accumulated DNA damage and altered gene expression may contribute to the progeric phenotype.

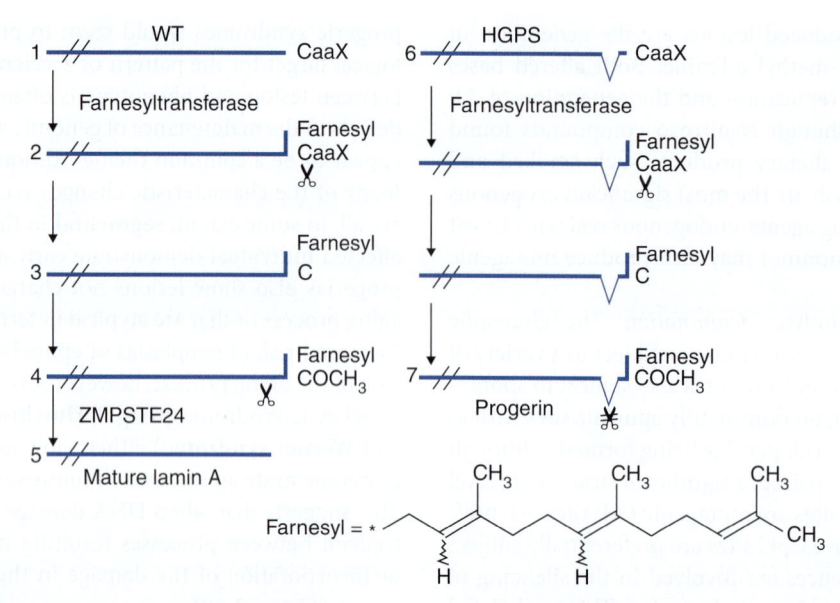

FIGURE 2-70 Processing of prelamin A in Hutchinson–Gilford progeria syndrome: In normal individuals (WT), prelamin A (1) undergoes farnesylation (2), is cleaved by an endoprotease to remove the CaaX motif (3), the terminal farnesyl cysteine is methylated (4), and finally the terminal 15 amino acids are cleaved by a protease (ZMPSTE24), resulting in (5) mature lamin A. In Hutchinson-Gilford progeria (HGPS), alternative splicing deletes 50 amino acids (6) removing the ZMPSTE24 cleavage site. This results in (7) progerin, a mutant form of lamin A that is permanently farnesylated. CaaX cysteine (aliphatic residue) and the farnesylation motif (many possible residues).

Werner Syndrome (WS)

WS is an autosomal recessive progeria that results from mutations in the *WRN* gene encoding a human RecQ helicase that has a major role in DNA replication, cell cycle progression, DNA repair, and telomere maintenance. In Japanese populations the disease is relatively common with a frequency of 1/30,000. WS might be considered an "adult onset progeria" when compared to HGP. Affected individuals show essentially normal development until the third decade although they lack an adolescent growth spurt and consequently have a strikingly short adult stature. Initially skin atrophy and loss and graying of hair are noted. Ultimately age-associated changes including cataracts, hypogonadism, osteoporosis atherosclerosis and diabetes occur with death ensuing in the fifth decade, most commonly from malignancy or myocardial infarction. Although neoplasms are common in WS, their type and distribution is unusual. Mesenchymal cell tumors (sarcomas) are far more common than in non-WS individuals and these may occur in multiple and unexpected primary sites. Which of the protean activities of the WS protein in maintaining genomic integrity are related to the WS phenotype is unclear, although indirect evidence suggests that telomere maintenance may be critical.

Aging and Nutrition

Caloric restriction prolongs life span and suppresses age related degenerative changes in organisms ranging from yeast through rodents and primates. Studies in invertebrates and mammals support the involvement of two interacting cellular signaling pathways in mediating this prolongation; the **insulin-like growth factor1** (IGF1) pathway and the "target of rapamycin" (mTOR) pathway. The mTOR pathway serves as a nutrient sensor, either stimulating protein synthesis and cell growth in the presence of amino acids and carbohydrates or promoting cellular stress response reactions, activation of cell maintenance pathways, autophagy and mitochondrial biogenesis when nutrient starvation occurs. Components of the TOR pathway also interact with the IGF1 signaling pathway by activating the AKT protein kinase. AKT serves to phosphorylate FoxO transcription factors and inhibit their transcriptional activity. FoxO transcription factors regulate a variety of cell processes of presumptive importance in aging including cell death, cell cycle arrest, oxidative stress resistance and DNA repair (Figure 2-71).

Hence, caloric restriction could influence life span by effecting a shift in the pattern of cellular metabolism from a growth to a stress protective pattern consistent with life span extension via downregulation of the IGF-1/insulin and/or TOR pathways acting to activate FoxO transcription factors. FoxO factors can also be activated by oxidative stress or nutrient depletion. The importance of FoxO in aging is well established in invertebrates but less certain in vertebrates. Mouse strains with reduced levels of IGF1 (dwarf mouse strains) and mice treated with TOR inhibitor (rapamycin) have prolonged life span as is reported for humans with certain FoxO3 variants.

A third pathway implicated in the effects of caloric reduction on life span involves **sirtuins**, evolutionarily conserved NAD-dependent deacetylases. In mice SIRT1 expression is necessary for the life prolonging effects of caloric restriction

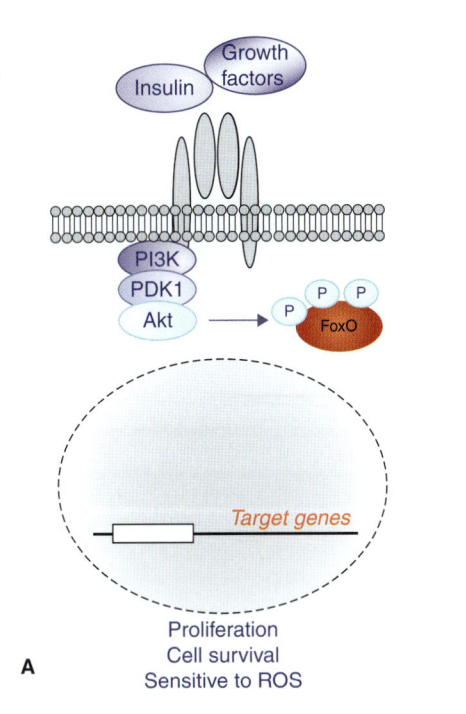

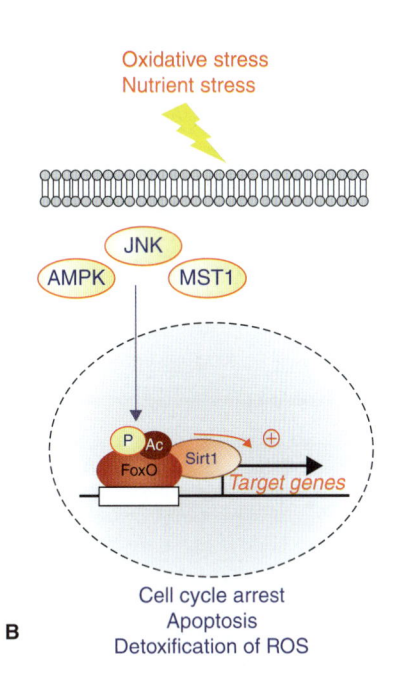

FIGURE 2-71 Negative and positive regulation of FoxO transcription factors: **(A)** In the presence of growth factors, FoxO is phosphorylated and transported from the nucleus inhibiting the transcription of FoxO-dependent genes. Cell survival and proliferation are promoted. **(B)** In the presence of nutrient or oxidative stress, FoxO translocates to the nucleus and furthers the cellular stress response including increased detoxification of reactive oxygen species, cell cycle arrest, and apoptosis. AMPK (AMP-dependent kinase), JNK (Jun-N terminal kinase), MST1 (mammalian Ste20-like kinase), Sirt1 (Sirtuin 1 deacetylase), PI3K (phosphatidylinositol 3-kinase), and PDK1 (3-phosphoinositide-dependent protein kinase-1).

and plays a role in the activation of FoxO transcription factors by serving to bind to and deacetylate them. SIRT1 is implicated as a regulator of cellular pathways important in stress resistance, metabolic status, and mitochondrial biogenesis although which of these roles is important in the response to caloric restriction is unclear. What is clear is that nutritional modification in humans has a profound effect on the prevention and amelioration of chronic disease states associated with aging such as the so-called metabolic syndrome, insulin resistance, and type II diabetes.

CHAPTER 3

Environmental Injury

John Butts, M.D.

INTRODUCTION

External factors, forces, and agents play a significant role in the causation of human disease. The environment in which we live is hardly benign and we are constantly exposed to its potential hazards. These include physical, chemical, thermal, and electrical forces as well as ionizing radiation. Noncommensal microbiological organisms are also external agents. While within the spectrum of human disease there are conditions where external factors have little or no role, such as some inherited disorders of metabolism or the muscular dystrophies, in most human afflictions external factors interact with host factors to produce disease. Certain lung cancers are linked to cigarette smoking and liver disease is a well-documented consequence of heavy alcohol consumption, yet in spite of the clear evidence that links these two agents to these diseases, it is also the case that only a minority of smokers and drinkers respectively develop them. At the other end of the spectrum lie the instances where external forces or agents are essentially the only factors as in trauma from a natural catastrophe like an earthquake or a man-made event such as a motor vehicle crash.

The environmental hazards any one individual is exposed to are determined by a variety of factors including geography, socioeconomic status, and culture. This is true not only for infectious entities such as malaria which depends on an insect vector that itself requires certain climatic conditions for its existence but also for various forms of trauma. Cobra bites are a common problem in India but not in the United States. Motor vehicle-related injuries, gunshot wounds, cutting injuries, and disorders related to contaminated air and water vary from country to country and regionally within countries just as do the incidence of infectious and other diseases.

This chapter will deal with diseases or conditions that are primarily the result of external factors but will not discuss diseases caused by microorganisms except to mention that infections, often from normal flora, are a common complication of trauma and remind readers that many vectors that spread infection require the physical trauma of a bite to inoculate the host. Tetanus caused by a toxin produced by the bacillus, *Clostridium tetani*, usually occurs after the introduction of that soil-dwelling organism into tissues as a consequence of a wound and similarly gas gangrene from *Clostridium perfringens* and other species. In the days before vaccination for tetanus, antiseptic surgery, and antibiotics, these entities were a common often-fatal complication of agricultural, martial, and other trauma and in some areas of the World today remain so.

INJURY

A measure of the burden of injury to the healthcare system in the United States is the fact that one-third of all emergency department (ED) visits in 2008, some 42.8 million, were injury related (Table 3-1). Injury is the leading cause of death for people ages 1–44 years in the United States, and because these deaths are in younger individuals, the years of potential life lost is greater than many conditions that account for a greater number of deaths (Table 3-2).

Acute injuries have immediate consequences for the victim with the potential for subsequent and long-term complications. Recurring trauma, even that which has little apparent immediate consequence, can also lead to disorders. A single episode of heavy ethanol intake may lead to acute intoxication with little or no subsequent complications, while repeated episodes can result in cardiomyopathy and/or cirrhosis of the liver, two of the many potential consequences of chronic alcohol abuse. If the acute ingestion is large enough, however, it may lead to fatal respiratory depression. Moreover, in an inebriated state an individual is at greater risk of additional injury whether by falling, attempting to drive a motor vehicle, leaving a pot on the stove and starting a fire, or becoming involved in an activity that they would not have undertaken in a sober state.

TABLE 3-1 Emergency department visits for selected injury-related causes.

Unintentional	66.9%
Falls	22.8
Motor vehicle traffic	9.3
Poisoning	1.6
Intentional	6%
Assaults	4.3
Self-inflicted	1.6
Adverse effects of medical treatment	4.7%
Alcohol and drug use	4.6%

2008 US ED visits for selected injury-related causes—CDC data.

A driver injured in a motor vehicle crash sustains some degree of immediate impairment, depending on the severity of the crash. The period required for recovery will also vary accordingly. During that period they are at risk of a variety of complications including infection and deep vein thrombosis with pulmonary embolism. In many instances of trauma, recovery is incomplete and the affected individual will thereafter function at a lower level than before the incident, thereby suffering a diminished quality of life. If there is sufficient impairment, such as paralysis or severe brain damage, susceptibility to pressure sores, infection, and other long-term complications may lead to a significantly reduced life span.

Repeated injuries due to chemicals or toxins can lead to disease as is the case for smoking and ethanol. This may also occur after physical and other modes of trauma. Examples include repetitive motion disorders such as carpal tunnel syndrome, osteoarthritis in the limbs of athletes, professional or otherwise, and traumatic encephalopathy. This latter condition, dementia pugilistica, was first noted in boxers following repeated blows to the head, and is now being recognized in football players and other participants in activities where concussions are common. External factors that can lead to injury can be separated into five major categories: physical, chemical, thermal, electrical, and ionizing radiation.

1. **Physical injuries** are those that are related to mechanical interactions and are the most common types of acute injuries from external forces seen in medicine. Motor vehicle wrecks, gunshot wounds, stabbing and cutting injuries, falls, and various mechanical asphyxias fall into this category. We include in this category the effects of pressure and altitude.
2. **Chemical injury** includes exposure to noxious or asphyxiant gases, medications both legal and illegal, and other chemical, metals, and mineral agents.
3. **Thermal injury** results from the exposure to fire and other sources of heat as well as intensely cold surfaces. Environmental exposure to heat or cold may also lead to local injury and/or systemic dysfunction.
4. **Electrical forces** include the natural phenomenon of lightning as well as exposure to man-made electrical currents.
5. **Ionizing radiation** employed as a therapeutic and diagnostic modality in medicine can also lead to unintended injury. Such radiation is also present naturally in our environment and the specter of the consequences of the detonation of a nuclear bomb or a mishap at a nuclear power plant currently "haunt" our society. Solar radiation can potentially lead to both acute and chronic health problems.

TABLE 3-2 Years of potential life lost (YPPL) before age 75.

Cause of Death	YPPL	Total Percentage (%)
All causes	20,486,000	100
Malignancies	4,327,000	21.1
Unintentional injury	3,272,000	16.0
Heart disease	3,054,000	14.9
Perinatal disease	1,093,000	5.3
Suicide	1,009,000	4.9
Homicide	783,000	3.8
Congenital abnormalities	588,000	2.9
All others	6,359,000	31.0

Underlined text are causes of death relating to injury.
All races and both genders included.
Source: CDC/National Center for Health Statistics, National Vital Statistics System 2007 data.

QUICK REVIEW

The same paradigm with which physicians approach the diagnosis of "natural" illnesses is utilized as a first principle in the consideration of injuries from external factors. History, signs and symptoms, supplemented by laboratory tests and imaging studies are used to identify the basic pathological process, the underlying disease, which explains them. Similarly, in the case of trauma, one accepts that injuries caused by a particular injury mechanism will be similar in appearance and character. That is, a sharp object, a bullet or a blow from a blunt instrument will produce distinctive injuries that can be recognized as to their source. Likewise, electrical and thermal forces cause distinctive and recognizable injuries. Drugs or toxins may also produce characteristic signs and symptoms that can be utilized to identify a specific agent. In evaluating physical injuries, this is often referred to as recognizing **patterned injury**. The appearance of an injury reflects the nature of the object and force that caused it and allows the informed observer to infer the cause of an individual injury from its appearance.

A second principle is that particular situations in which injuries occur produce groupings or larger patterns of injury. Thus, the driver of a motor vehicle that collides head-on with an immoveable object will be thrown forward as the vehicle decelerates. If unrestrained, their chest will strike the steering wheel and their head the windshield. This may produce visible external injuries to the head and chest as well as typical internal organ damage. Awareness of the nature of the injury incident in such a case is important to the evaluating physician when the victim arrives at ED as it helps inform what diagnostic and therapeutic steps may need to be taken. Failure to appreciate the underlying causes of injuries may have consequences beyond a failure to adequately provide immediate medical care. If it is not recognized that the injuries a patient presents with are inconsistent with the explanation provided by the patient or their caretaker(s), that patient may be returned to a environment where they are at risk of further injury or even death. This is particularly the case for injuries inflicted in abusive relationships. Infants are unable to speak for themselves, and older children, spouses, partners, and the elderly may be unwilling to reveal the true source of their trauma because of fear or shame. Similarly the failure to recognize that a toxin exposure may have an environmental cause, or that the patients symptoms are due to a toxin, may result in the patient being sent back to be further exposed.

It then follows that in the evaluation of injury from external forces not only must the immediate cause of the injury be identified but also an understanding of how the victim encountered the injurious force must be sought.

It is customary to separate traumatic injuries into three categories based on the circumstances in which they are incurred: unintentional (accidental), self-inflicted, and assaultive, (deliberately caused by another human). The latter two are referred to as "intentional" injuries and assaultive is sometimes also referred to as "violent." *When applied to fatal injuries, this leads to the classification of trauma-related deaths as accident, suicide, or homicide.* These designations are referred to as "manners" of death. An unintentional (accidental) injury is one that is not the consequence of a deliberate human action intended to cause harm, but it is important to appreciate that many injuries deemed unintentional are in fact the consequence of actions intentionally undertaken by the injured or another party, actions that may clearly have put the injured party at significant risk. In fact, the line that delineates intentional from unintentional when the risk of self or other injury is high and clearly apparent to the neutral observer can be difficult to draw and presents a recurring dilemma in medicolegal death investigation and certification as well as in the courts regarding legal culpability. For instance, when a chronic drug abuser dies of an overdose is it the consequence of a miscalculation, carelessness, desire for a better "high," or a calculated intent to end it all? Some "recreational" activities are more dangerous than others, for example, mountain climbing versus vegetable gardening. At what point does the likelihood of injury inherent in a voluntary activity dictate that a resulting injury and death is suicide rather than accident? Most accident insurance policies have exclusions for activities the insurance company considers too dangerous to cover even though a death occurring during that activity would be certified as accidental by a medicolegal authority. Designating an injury or death as "accidental" does not mean either that there can be no criminal or civil culpability on the part of another human agency. Similarly, classifying a death as a homicide does not necessarily mean that someone is criminally liable. Crimes and civil liability are defined by law and manner of death classification is intended primarily for epidemiological purposes as is the similar designation of nonfatal injuries as unintentional, intentional, self-intent, and assault. Strategies to reduce the number of head injuries due to falls are quite different from those due to assaults.

WHAT WE DO
Medicolegal Death Investigation

Forensic pathologists play a major role in the area of medicolegal death investigation. This historically derives from pathologists' involvement with morbid anatomy and autopsies. In fact many of the first autopsies noted in the literature were performed for medicolegal reasons. While the heyday of the autopsy as a tool in our understanding of basic disease processes may have passed, the autopsy still remains an essential diagnostic procedure in determining cause of death and gathering needed information in deaths that occur suddenly and unexpectedly or as a result of trauma. These deaths in most of the world require medicolegal investigation and certification. This is the subspecialty of forensic pathology. In medicolegal death investigation, a medicolegal authority (MLA) assumes jurisdiction and control over certain decedents in order to ascertain why they died. The forensic pathologist may be the MLA, which in the United States is usually a Medical Examiner or Coroner, or may be employed by the MLA. Medical Examiners are appointed officials and ordinarily physicians, although not always forensic pathologists. Coroners are for the most part elected lay officials, though in a few states they must be physicians in order to run for the office. There is no uniformity in the organization of medicolegal death investigation systems within the United States, which are state and/or county based. There is even some variation in which deaths must be reported among the states. With a few exceptions, however, it is the case that all deaths related to acute trauma must be reported to the MLA and the MLA is responsible for certifying them. Deaths due entirely to natural disease are ordinarily certified by the decedent's attending physician.

Medicolegal death investigation systems have an important surveillance function since unexpected and unexplained deaths also come under their jurisdiction. They have played a role in the identification of a number of emerging infectious entities over the years including AIDS, Hantavirus, and Legionnaires disease. Data amassed by Medical Examiner and Coroner's offices are critical in monitoring deaths due to trauma, drugs, and medications. This data provides the epidemiological information necessary to both identify areas where interventions are possible and the basis for determining whether such interventions once implemented have been successful.

As mentioned previously, patients may exhibit signs and symptoms from underlying natural disorders as well as injuries, the consequence of an untoward interaction with the environment. Traumatic injuries may lead to disorders that are not considered external, like pulmonary emboli or infection. It is important, however, to recognize a connection when it is there since to ignore it is akin to treating symptoms of disease without addressing the underlying cause. Pathogenic sequences connect causes and effects. In such sequences, each entity listed is the consequence of the one preceding it. A myocardial infarct results from myocardial ischemia due to diminished or interrupted coronary blood flow that is the consequence of coronary restriction from atherosclerosis. The underlying or proximate condition leading to the infarct is then atherosclerosis. An individual might develop sepsis due to peritonitis that was caused by a bowel injury incurred in a motor vehicle wreck. The wreck is then the underlying or proximate cause of the sepsis. This is particularly important in the process of death certification where the certifier must decide what the underlying disease condition leading to death was. Many deaths are inaccurately certified in regard to their cause when the certifier assigns it to the last process, the one immediately preceding death, and fails to include the underlying cause of that condition. In the case of the last example, attributing death to sepsis due to peritonitis without including the trauma would result in the death being classified as natural rather than unnatural. Failing to link pulmonary fibrosis to asbestos exposure or liver failure to acetaminophen toxicity conceals the contributions of those external factors to human disease.

FACTORS INFLUENCING PHYSICAL INJURY

Physical injury may occur when a moving individual strikes a solid object or surface or a stationary individual is impacted or compressed by a moving object or force. In such interactions, there are several factors that determine the likelihood that significant injury will result.

Quantity of Force Involved: Kinetic Energy

All moving objects or bodies have kinetic energy and as the amount of energy in an interaction increases so does the likelihood of injury. Kinetic energy is the product of the mass of an object times the square of the velocity divided by two. As the mass (weight) increases, there is a direct proportional increase in the amount of energy, while as the velocity increases the energy goes up by the square of the velocity increase. For example, if a baseball and a car were both traveling 30 miles per hour, one could safely catch the baseball, but certainly not the car because the baseball weighs less than half a pound while the car weighs 3000 lb. Similarly a jump from a 3 foot platform to the ground would seldom lead to injury, but the same person jumping from a 32 foot platform would be likely to suffer serious perhaps even fatal injury. The additional velocity imparted by the acceleration of gravity over the 29 foot difference imparts to the moving body sufficient kinetic energy to distort and disrupt internal structures when the individual impacts the ground.

Area over which force is applied: The likelihood of injury is also related to the area over which the particular force is applied. Concentration of the energy of impact over a small area can overcome the resistance of the tissues to deformation and penetration. This can allow entry of an object into the body leading to damage to deeper internal organs. Even in the absence of penetration, there may be sufficient local deformation to cause mechanical disruption of underlying organs and tissues. Bullets, knives, arrows, and other sharp objects have the potential to cause serious injury because they can overcome the resistance of the skin and often underlying bone to reach vital organs and structures, even though the quantities of kinetic energy involved are not large. Similarly a blow from a bat, pipe, or club concentrates the area over which the energy of the impact is dissipated, resulting in more local and/or even deeper injury than would have occurred if the impacting surface was broader. The same applies in reverse when a moving body impacts a stationary surface, for example, stepping on a nail or falling and striking the projecting edge of a piece of furniture.

Time interval during which force is applied: Another factor is the time interval over which the interaction occurs. If it can be lengthened, the likelihood of injury can be lessened. The padding of helmets and dashboards in part does this. It is the principal that allows "bungee" jumping and the different consequences that follow diving into a swimming pool full of water versus one that is empty. In both instances, the energy generated by the fall is safely absorbed and dissipated over distance and time by the elastic cords in the first instance and the yielding water in the second.

Tissue resistance to force: The body's tissues also vary in their resistance to trauma with bone being more resistant that skin. Internal connective tissues are more resistant than muscle that is more resistant than internal organs such as liver and spleen.

Body area(s) affected by force: The significance of any injury to the overall health of an organism is related to the parts affected in addition to the extent of tissue disruption. Injuries that compromise the vital functions of respiration and circulation have the greatest potential to be immediately life threatening, whereas injuries to the extremities or noncritical organs are more potentially survivable, particularly with timely appropriate medical treatment. Many of these factors are not only exploited in the design of weaponry but are also utilized in devising protective strategies. Seat belts, cushioned dashboards, air bags, protective armor, and bicycle helmets all attempt to decrease the likelihood of injury to internal organs in forceful interactions by dissipating the forces of collisions over a larger area extending the interval over which they are dissipated as well as shifting them to tissues of greater resistance.

Fitness of individual: A last factor to be considered is the fitness of the individual injured. Significant preexisting medical conditions as well as the extremes of age may render one individual less likely to survive a given degree of insult than a fitter individual. Older persons are often more fragile and have a diminished capacity for tissue repair. Survival from severe burns, for instance, is inversely proportional not only to the extent and severity of the burns but also to the age of the victim. Injuries of an extent that would easily be survived by younger individuals often prove fatal to the elderly, and a fall leading to a broken hip, rapid decompensation, and death is a common occurrence. Infants and small children have the optimal capacity for repair but are relatively more fragile—an impact that might only bruise an adult can prove fatal to an infant.

HISTOPATHOLOGY OF PHYSICAL TRAUMA

The histopathology of physical trauma is that of inflammation and wound repair and is virtually never employed in the evaluation of nonfatal injuries. In the investigation of fatalities, however, microscopy can aid in the determination of the age

CASE 3-1

A 2-year-old boy is brought to an emergency room (ER) with a complaint of abdominal pain, having collapsed while being bathed at home by a relative. He experiences respiratory arrest, cannot be resuscitated and is pronounced dead at the ER. Autopsy reveals multiple cutaneous bruises including some on the abdomen (Figure 3-1A). Internal examination reveals a mesenteric tear (Figure 3-1B arrow), a laceration of the small bowel and active peritonitis (Figure 3-1C arrow).

Death was deemed due to peritonitis consequent to a blow or blows to the abdomen that ruptured the bowel. Suspicion initially focused on the relative but the degree of inflammation at the site of the rupture (Figure 3-1D) indicated that the fatal injury must have occurred at least a day prior to death implicating a different caregiver.

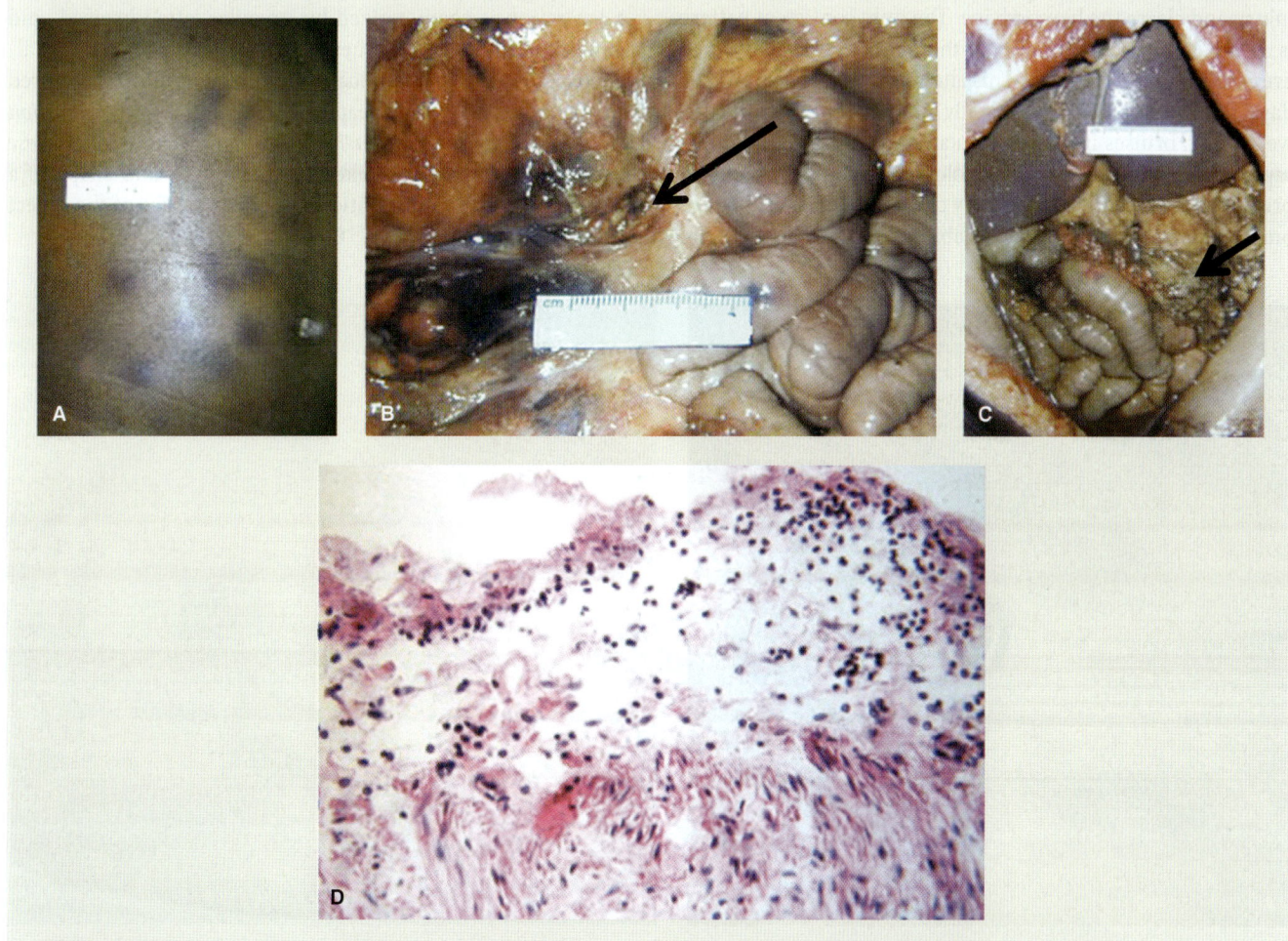

FIGURE 3-1 (A) External examination illustrating multiple abdominal bruises. (B & C) Internal examination showing mesenteric tear (B at arrow) and peritonitis (C at arrow). (D) Microscopic section of bowel wall at site of injury demonstrating acute inflammation.

of bruises, lacerations, and hemorrhages. (Case 3-1) It may also be helpful in confirming the presence of powder residues in close range or contact gunshot wounds.

MECHANISMS OF PHYSICAL TRAUMA

Blunt Injury

Interactions that lead to injury may be characterized as blunt, sharp, or penetrating, although there is overlapping between these categories. Blunt trauma can result from falls and blows from objects with blunt (as opposed to sharp) surfaces as well as collisions with blunt objects or surfaces. The majority of physical injuries encountered in most medical practices will fall into this category. Blunt force interactions can produce the following.

Bruises (contusions): These result from the mechanical disruption of blood vessels. Blood escapes into the surrounding tissues leading to swelling and discoloration. Although cutaneous bruises are the most visible they can also occur within internal organs and tissues. Cutaneous bruises can be visually aged, although not precisely. Fresh bruises are reddish-purple and change color as the body "repairs" the injury and clears the hemorrhage. The only consistent pattern is a change to yellow initially at the periphery of the bruise, eventually fading to brown. This alteration first appears at 1–3 days postinjury. Bruises generally are resorbed within 3–4 weeks with bruises in more vascular areas disappearing more rapidly. In instances where histological examination of the bruise is possible, greater accuracy can sometimes be obtained but there is still considerable variability.

The shape of a bruise reflects the shape and nature of the object that struck the body or the surface that the body struck. This is important for both forensic and clinical reasons. Recognizing that the looped bruises noted on a child's back during an hospital ER visit were the result of its being "disciplined" with a cord or belt rather than by playing with the family dog per the history given by the caretaker could lead to a potentially lifesaving intervention (Figure 3-2).

Abrasions (scrapes, "burns"): These are the consequence of interactions that are tangential to the injured surface and result in damage or loss of the superficial and often deeper layers of skin. Such injuries are common in sports and the ordinary play of children and adults. They can be particularly extensive when high-speed interactions are involved such as a fall from a moving vehicle, such as a motorcycle (Figure 3-3).

Lacerations (tears): These occur when the integrity of the skin or other tissue is disrupted due to crushing or torsional forces. They are more common over bony prominences where skin can be compressed between an impinging object or surface and underlying bone. An identical blow to the head that leads to a scalp laceration may only produce a bruise in a part of the body without underlying bone such as the abdomen. A laceration is characterized by irregular, often bruised, and abraded margins. The tissues at the margins may be devitalized to the extent that clinically debridement may be required before the edges can be reapproximated. *The term laceration should only be used for injuries of this nature and not for those caused by sharp objects.* Like bruises the size and shape of a laceration provide information about the nature of the object or surface that produced it (Figure 3-4).

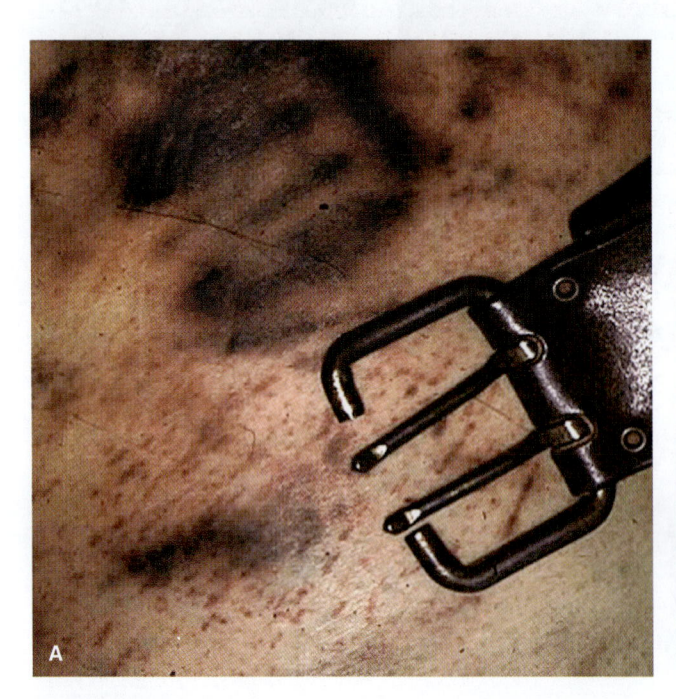

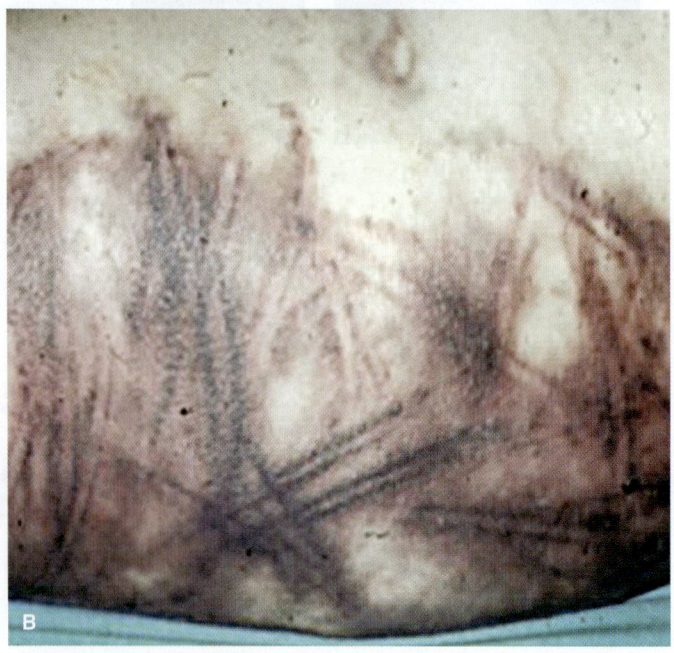

FIGURE 3-2 (A) Bruises may take the shape of the object that caused them—in this case a belt buckle. (B) "Tramline" bruises showing a distinctive parallel pattern result from skin impact with elongated rounded objects that force blood to the margins of the impact. This example shows curving of the bruises produced by a flexible object; an electrical cord.

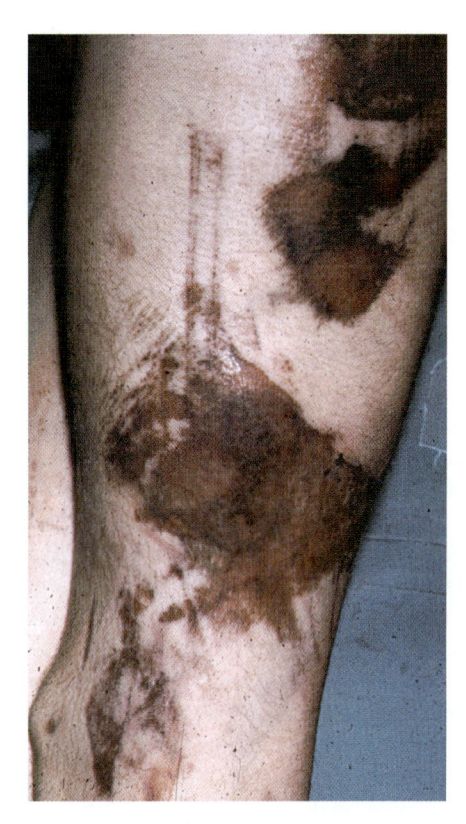

FIGURE 3-3 Thigh abrasions produced by sliding contact with pavement.

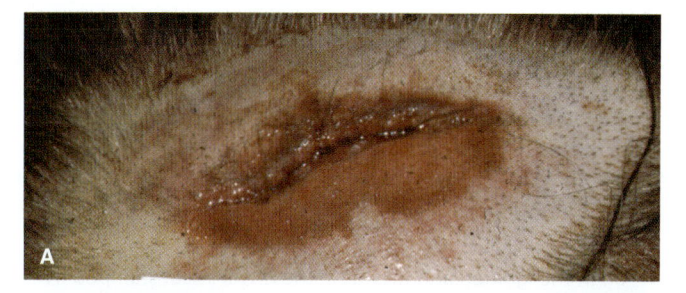

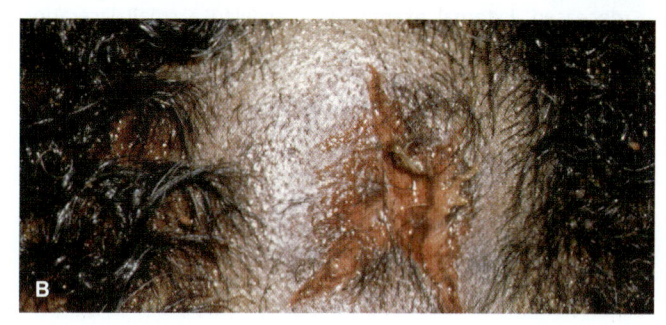

FIGURE 3-4 **(A)** A linear scalp laceration produced by impact with a long blunt-edged object. **(B)** Stellate scalp laceration produced by a hammer blow. The skin has split radially outward from the point of contact. Note **(A)** is upper image.

Avulsions: These are shearing injuries caused by tangential forces. In an avulsion, the skin or tissues are substantially separated from the deeper underlying structures. A common example would be the separation of a fingernail from its bed by catching it on a protruding object. So-called "scalping" injuries where the skin of the scalp is torn and separated from the underlying skull would be another example.

Fractures: Bone may be disrupted by compression, twisting, or bending. Such fractures are described as "incomplete" when the broken parts are not separated, "complete" when they are, "comminuted" when complete and the fracture results in more than two fragments. When the overlying skin is lacerated by broken bone, it is designated as "compound." "Pathologic" fractures are those that occur at sites where bone has been weakened by natural diseases such as tumor or osteoporosis. Such fractures can be the consequence of ordinary weight bearing. There are many specific clinical designations for the fractures of various bones, often eponymic, in part, reflecting the frequency with which such injuries are consistently seen in the clinical setting; for example, Le Fort I, II, and III fractures describe trauma to the maxillae and adjacent bones, resulting from blows or other facial impacts. This reflects the earlier touched upon principle that particular injury situations often result in predictable patterns of injury.

Sharp Injury

Incised wounds (cuts): These are injuries produced by objects with sharp or cutting edges such as knives, scalpels, or broken glass. They should not be described as "lacerations!" Such injuries are characterized by distinct linear margins without bruises or abrasions. The tissues are cleanly separated down into the depths of the wound (Figure 3-6). Most "stab" wounds are caused by sharp implements and are discussed further below.

Chop injury: Instruments with sharp edges that are also very heavy produce injuries with both sharp and blunt force characteristics when they are used as weapons. These include axes, machetes, cleavers, brush hooks, and swords. The resulting skin wounds often have straight clean margins, since these weapons have sharp edges. When firm underlying tissue or bone is struck, it may be cleaved to an extent that would not have been possible with a lighter cutting implement. Impacted bone may show a straight-edged defect identical to the chop mark that results when an axe strikes a piece of wood. The rest of the bone underlying the impact site may also break, resulting in a complete fracture.

Penetrating Injury

Penetrating injury: These injuries can be caused by both blunt and pointed objects and those with sharp edges as well as projectiles and are characterized by the fact that they have passed through the skin and extended deeper into the body. The extent of internal trauma cannot always be appreciated by the external appearance of a wound (Case 3-2). If a wound passes completely through the body, it is described as "perforating." These terms may also be used to describe an injury to an individual organ or body structure.

Stab wounds: Such wounds are usually sharp force injuries caused by knives or knife-like objects but can also result from the thrust into or the impaling of the body onto other pointed objects, for example, screwdriver or ice pick. The depth of the

CASE 3-2

A 27-year-old man got into an argument at a bar and was struck in the head with a pool cue. He was not rendered unconscious, left the premises under his own power and was seen to get into his vehicle and drive away. A few hours later his truck was noted parked on the shoulder of a nearby road. The key was turned off in the ignition and he was in the driver's seat slumped over deceased. External examination revealed a small laceration of the left supraorbital area and a periorbital ecchymosis (Figure 3-5A).

Internal examination demonstrated a partly depressed comminuted fracture of the underlying frontal bone (Figure 3-5B). The fracture line passed through the vascular groove on the inner table of the skull carrying the middle meningeal artery disrupting that vessel causing a large epidural hemorrhage (EDH). This expanding mass had led to left-sided transtentorial brain herniation and his death (Figure 3-5C).

Intracerebral hemorrhage is a common consequence of head trauma and can occur in the epidural, subdural, and/or subarachnoid compartments (EDH, subdural hemorrhage [SDH], and subarachnoid hemorrhage [SAH], respectively). EDH is almost always associated with a skull fracture that tears an imbedded or adherent arterial vessel. Because of the middle meningeal artery's course within a vascular groove in the relatively thin squamous portion of the temporal bone, it is particularly vulnerable. SDHs are usually seen over the cerebral convexities and are felt to be resulted from the tearing of veins bridging the subdural space along the falx. SAH results from disruption of meningeal or other vessels on the surface or base of the brain as may happen with the ruptue of congenital lesions, "berry" aneurysms, of the circle of Willis (see Chapter 21). SAH can also accompany cerebral contusions or from blood dissecting to the surface from deeper intracerebral bleeding.

EDH and SDH become intracranial space occupying lesions and may lead to brain stem herniation. The mechanism whereby "pure" acute SAH causes death is not entirely clear but may involve vascular spasm. In instances of EDH, SDH, and SAH, there may also be accompanying traumatic cerebral parenchymal injury that may be of greater significance than the extracerebral blood. The rapidity with which the bleeding occurs is an important factor. Slow accumulations of blood, particularly in SDHs, are often well tolerated with little or no symptoms, becoming chronic and in some instances eventually being largely organized and resorbed while a similar volume of blood accumulating more rapidly would lead to herniation and death.

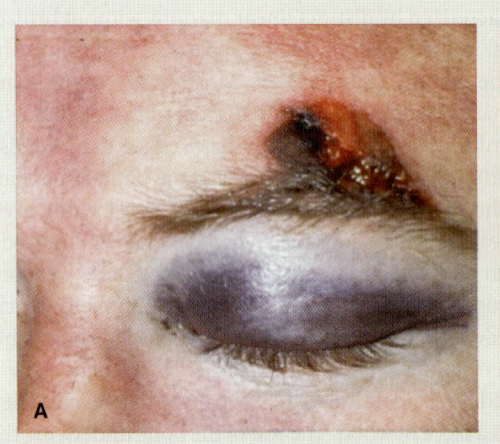

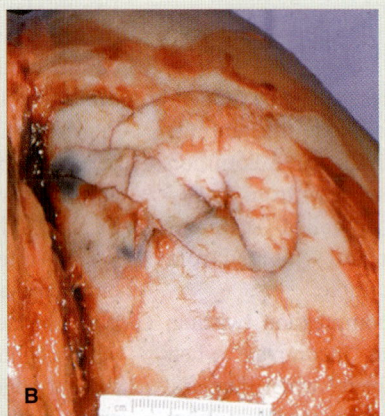

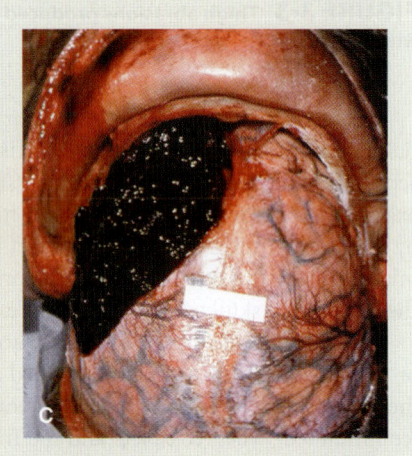

FIGURE 3-5 (A) External examination—note laceration and periorbital ecchymosis (bruising). (B) Internal examination demonstrates a partially depressed fracture of the underlying bone disrupting the middle meningeal artery. (C) Demonstrates the resultant large epidural hemorrhage.

wound cannot be judged by the appearance of the wound in the skin and what appears to be a small cut in the skin may in fact be a potentially lethal wound to deeper internal organs. Since a blade cuts as it passes through the skin, the defect in the skin can be longer than the width of the blade itself, and because the body and tissues are compressible, the depth of the wound may be greater than the length of the stabbing instrument. The depth may also be less since the instrument may not be fully inserted.

Gunshot wounds: These are penetrating injuries produced by rapidly traveling projectiles of small size. It is the high speed of these objects and the small area over which their resultant kinetic energy is applied that causes injury, not their mass (weight). In most firearms, the projectile whether bullet or shot is accelerated down a hollow metal tube, the gun barrel, by an expanding cloud of hot gases generated by the ignition of a quantity of gunpowder, although there are guns that use other sources of gas such as CO_2 or compressed air to propel their missiles. Some of the latter can achieve velocities comparable to gunpowder weapons, though their projectiles are usually much smaller. Nonetheless they can still produce serious and even fatal trauma. The projectiles fired from guns are usually composed of lead because of its density and relatively low melting temperature that allows it to be easily cast into various shapes.

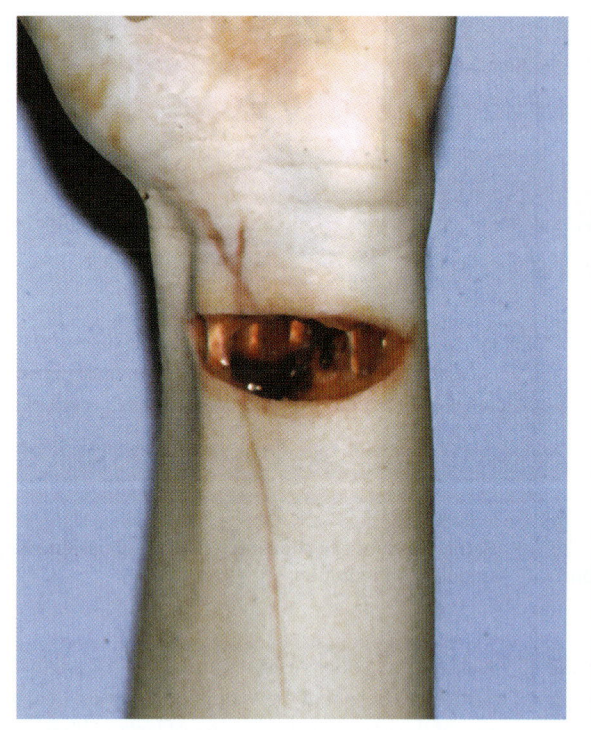

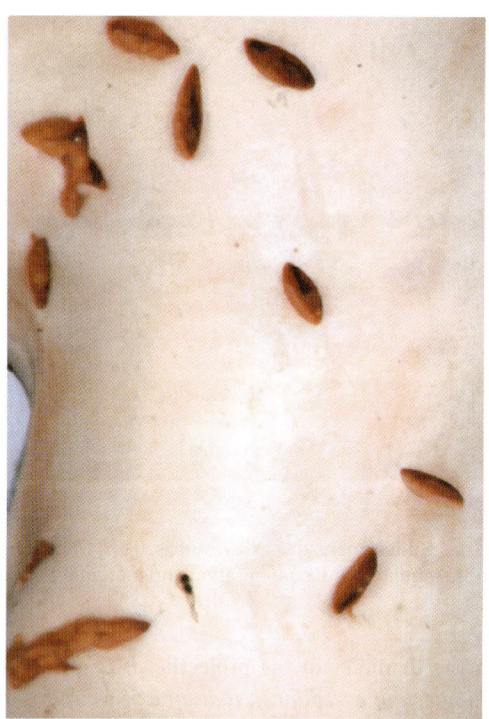

FIGURE 3-6 **Two examples of incised wounds.** (Left) Incised wound of the wrist with suicidal intent. Note presence of tentative or hesitation cuts crossing the wound often characteristic of suicidal injuries. (Right) Homicidal incised wounds that demonstrate "clean" margins and characteristic gaping in the direction of tissue tension.

The projectiles are either cylindrical, generally with a rounded or pointed nose; (bullets), or spherical (shot). The former are used in rifled weapons and the latter in smoothbore weapons (shotguns). Rifled weapons have spiral grooves cut into the bore of the gun barrel that imparts a spin to the bullet as it passes through. This, combined with the elongated shape of the projectile, gives the projectile greater ballistic stability allowing it to travel further and straighter. In a rifled weapon, only one projectile at a time travels down the barrel, although they may be capable of firing many times in rapid succession. Long-barreled rifled weapons are called rifles and short barreled ones handguns. The internal diameter of the gun barrel is its caliber that may be given in inches or millimeters. This determines the diameter of the bullet. Shotguns are smooth bored, have no internal rifling, and are designed to fire multiple projectiles, or "load," at once. This load of shot spreads out after leaving the barrel to produce a cloud of projectiles, the better to strike a small moving target, such as a flying bird. Small shot for hunting birds is called "birdshot" and larger shot or pellets for bigger game is called "buckshot." The diameter or bore of a shotgun is described in terms of its "gauge" (which is, for larger bore guns, the number of lead balls the diameter of the barrel that it takes to make up a pound). Both bullets and shot vary in size, but bullets also show considerable variation in shape while shot is always spherical. Bullets may be composed solely of lead or may be coated with another metal, "jacketed." These variations in shape and covering, in addition to variation in size (caliber), are intended to enhance the performance of the gun and/or the bullet. Lead shot may also be thinly coated with another metal and some shot are made of steel to curb lead poisoning in birds who ingest the spent shot while feeding. Large single projectile rounds, usually referred to as slugs, may be used in shotguns for larger game. Early guns, both long barreled and short, were smooth bored and usually fired single lead balls.

A bullet striking the body may not only penetrate it but may also pass completely through the body. Gunshot wounds are the most common form of perforating injuries. For medicolegal purposes, it is critical to distinguish wound entrances from exits, and it is ordinarily possible to do so in the case of gunshot wounds and often stabs and other perforating trauma.

Entry bullet wounds: When a bullet impacts a surface perpendicularly in a nose first configuration, it produces a defect that is rounded and regular in appearance. On the skin, there is often a thin collar of abrasion at the margins of the defect. Lead or other residue on the bullet may also be deposited at this margin and appear as an encircling fine gray residue or "wipe-off." If the impact is at an acute angle, the defect may be elongated or elliptical in shape. The configuration of the nose of the bullet will to some degree affect the appearance of the defect as well as the presence of intervening clothing. Typically the actual defect is slightly smaller than the diameter of the projectile. Individual shotgun pellet entry wounds will have the same appearance as bullet entry wounds **(Figure 3-7 left)**.

Exit bullet wounds: When a projectile exits the body, it tends to produce an irregular wound as the skin is stretched outward from within. Since the projectile is not impacting the epidermis, there is no abrasion collar. The projectile may have expanded or become distorted during its passage through the body or in the case of a bullet may now be traveling sideways or base forward so that the defect it produces is usually

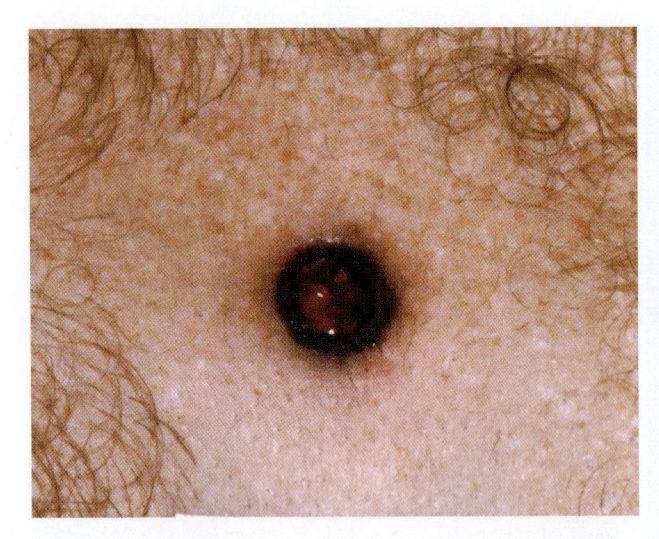

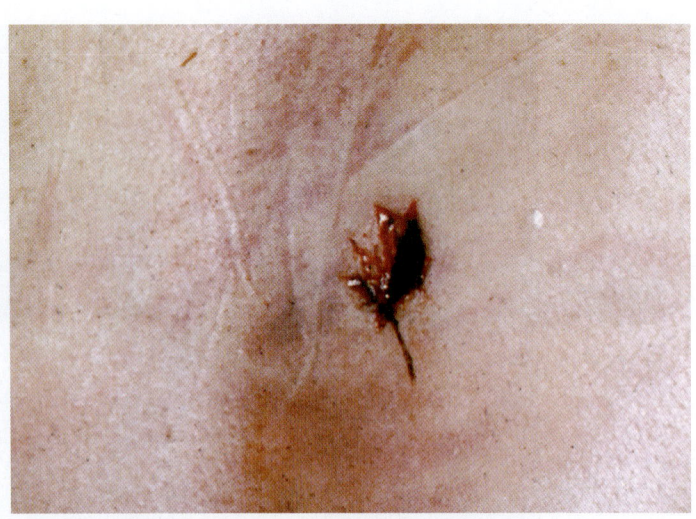

FIGURE 3-7 Bullet entry and exit wounds. (Left) Gunshot entrance—note regular round configuration and marginal abrasion. (Right) Gunshot exit showing lack of marginal abrasion and an irregular configuration.

larger than the diameter of the projectile. *It is generally the case, (with important exceptions), that an exit wound is larger than the corresponding entrance wound* (Figure 3-7 right).

The core of disruption that a projectile produces along its course is related to the size of the projectile and its velocity, that is, its kinetic energy. As bullets become larger and/or move faster, they tend to produce more damage to the organs and tissues that they pass through. As a bullet becomes heavier, it also becomes larger and thus has a greater cross section leading to a larger path of injury. Some bullets are designed to expand as they pass through tissue also increasing their cross-sectional area. Similarly longer bullets tend to tumble or "yaw" as they pass through tissue and the greater exposed surface produces a larger and potentially more destructive wound track. If a bullet fragments and disperses into the tissues, it may produce more damage than a bullet that remains intact and bone struck by projectiles can also fragment and be driven into tissues along the wound track.

The velocity of projectiles varies from around 700–1500 feet/second for handguns up to 3000+ feet/second for high-velocity rifles. The lower velocity weapons tend to produce wound tracks that are approximately the diameter of the bullet, while high-velocity bullets, because of their higher kinetic energy, produce larger wound tracks than low-velocity bullets of the same diameter or caliber.

Range of fire: The distance between the muzzle of the gun and the object struck by the projectile is also an issue in gunshot wounds. It is particularly critical in determining whether a wound could have been self-inflicted and may be of importance in subsequent legal proceedings on other occasions. Range of fire may be characterized as contact, close or distant (Case 3-3).

Contact: The muzzle of the gun is against the body at the time it is discharged which is the typical situation in a suicidal wound. The expanding hot gases from the ignited powder follow the bullet into the tissues and can be visualized within the wound itself as gray sooty residues and intact or partly burned powder particles. There may be visible burning or "searing" of the margins of the entrance. In the case of large caliber weapons, the propellant gases may tear or disrupt the skin at the margins of the entrance, leading to a large irregular often stellate wound. This is most common in wounds of the head where underlying bone inhibits the dispersal of the propellant cases. With high-velocity rifles and shotguns, the head may be massively disrupted with complete or partial exenteration of its contents. If the contact is not tight, gases may escape at the margins leading to wider soot deposition and searing, burning, around the entrance.

Close: Wounds where the weapon is not in contact but close enough that powder residues can be seen on the skin or clothing. This takes the form of soot, the fine particulate smoke produced by the largely complete combustion of the powder and "stippling" or "tattooing", minute lacerations of the skin produced by the impact of unburnt or partly burnt powder particles. As the distance from muzzle to skin increases less of the lighter fine soot reaches the skin and the larger powder particles spread out producing a wider pattern of stippling. Beyond several feet, very little of these powder residues reach the skin.

Distant: No visible residues reach the skin. In the case of most weapon discharges greater than a few feet away, these residues do not reach the skin in sufficient quantity to be visualized with the eye. In the case of shotguns, which discharge multiple projectiles simultaneously, the spread of the pellets can be used to approximate the muzzle to victim distance up to many yards away (Figure 3-8).

Pressure Injury

Injury resulting from pressure phenomena takes several forms.

Blast: An explosion generates a pressure wave that moves at the speed of sound. As it passes through media of different density, the speed of the wave changes. This can lead to

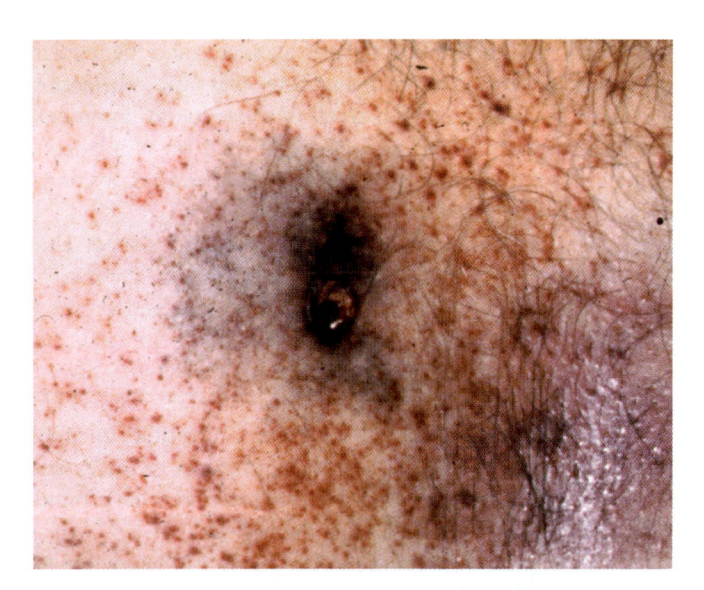

FIGURE 3-8 A close range chest wound showing a pattern of stippling accompanied by deposition of gray soot immediately adjacent to the entry wound.

the disruption of internal organs at air–tissue interfaces as the wave moves through the body. This internal trauma can occur in the absence of visible external injury. A blast may also cause massive direct disruption to the body, depending on its intensity and the proximity of the victim. The explosion may fragment objects in the environment and/or the explosive device itself may fragment, which many bombs, grenades, mines, and other antipersonnel devices are designed to do. These objects and fragments may then produce penetrating projectile injuries in addition to any pressure wave effects. If the explosion generates heat, thermal injury may also occur.

Elevated atmospheric pressure: In circumstances where individuals are exposed to increased barometric/atmospheric pressures, injury may occur upon their return to normal atmospheric pressure. On a too rapid return to lower pressure, gases that have dissolved in the blood (primarily nitrogen from air) come out of solution and form minute bubbles within the blood and tissues where they cause mechanical disruption and interfere with the microcirculation. If severe enough, the bubbles may produce strokes or myocardial ischemic events. First described in workers laboring in underwater pressurized chambers, "caissons," during the construction of tunnels and bridges, it is known as caisson's disease or the "bends." Today, it is mainly a hazard for divers both recreational and professional. Treatment involves placing the affected individual back into an environment of higher pressure, usually in a hyperbaric chamber, to redissolve the offending gases and then slowly decompress them.

Decreased atmospheric pressure: As one ascends from sea level, atmospheric pressure decreases and with it the partial pressure of oxygen. At elevations over 3000 m, the risk of a variety of altitude-related illnesses increases especially for individuals coming from lower altitudes who have not allowed themselves to become acclimated. The most feared

CASE 3-3

A young male calls 911 and states that he was shot during an attempted robbery. He has a wound in his thigh (Figure 3-9). The authorities are suspicious of his story as he states that the assailant was standing several yards away, facing him when the shot was fired. However, the wound track is upward (see arrow upper view) and there is powder residue and soot around the entry wound (see arrow in detail of entry wound). Both wound direction and range of fire are inconsistent with the victims claim and it was concluded that the wound was self-inflicted.

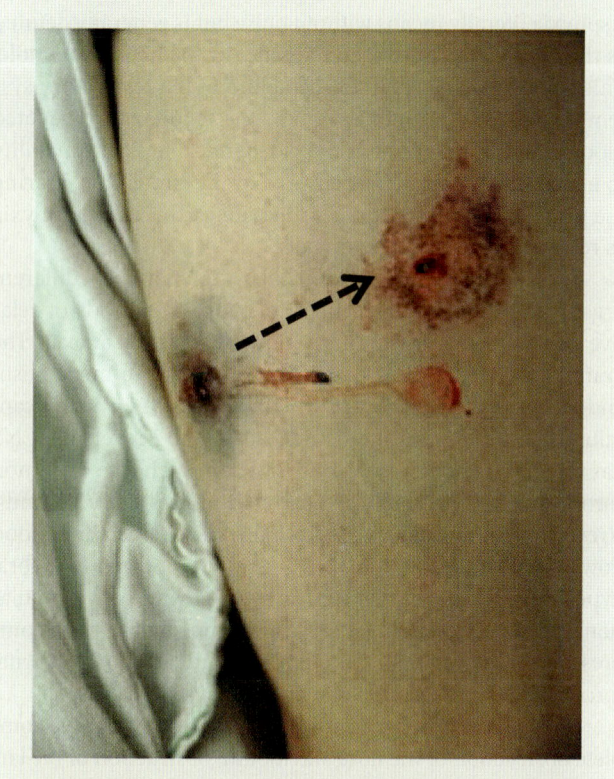

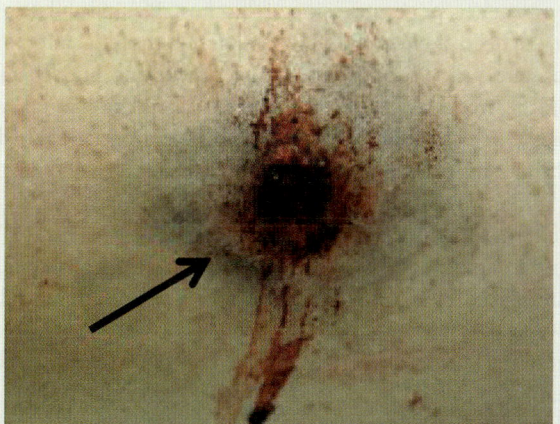

FIGURE 3-9 Upper photo demonstrates upward course of wound track (arrow). Lower photo is the detailed view of entry wound surrounded by abundant sooty powder residue and soot (arrow).

consequence is the development of pulmonary and cerebral edema. This constitutes a medical emergency with return to lower altitude necessary if the individual affected is to survive. Other altitude-related conditions include systemic edema, retinal hemorrhages, general deterioration in physical and mental performance, flatus and acute mountain sickness. The latter is characterized by headache, insomnia, dizziness, fatigue, nausea and/or vomiting, loss of appetite, increased heart rate, and shortness of breath on exertion. There is considerable variability among individuals in their susceptibility to these illnesses.

Asphyxia

Asphyxia literally means without pulse but is generally defined as the deprivation of oxygen to tissues or the body as a whole. This can occur as a result of the failure of the respiratory system to take oxygen into the body, the failure of oxygenated blood to reach tissues or at the biochemical level the inability to utilize the oxygen being delivered by the circulation. During the process of death, all tissues ultimately experience asphyxia as respiration and circulation fails.

Oxygen is essential for cellular function but different organs and tissues vary in their tolerance to periods of relative or complete oxygen deprivation, hypoxia, or anoxia. The brain is the organ most dependent on oxidative metabolism and periods of anoxia that would not result in significant injury to other organs and tissues can lead to irreversible CNS damage. Obstruction of blood flow through the common carotid arteries will lead to loss of consciousness after 6 seconds. Irreversible brain injury will generally result if cerebral blood flow is interrupted for more than 3–4 minutes. Stagnant cerebral hypoxia is not as well tolerated as hypoxia with active circulation, thus the changes in CPR practice emphasizing chest compressions over respiratory, mouth-to-mouth, support. External forces and factors can cause asphyxia in a variety of ways.

Compromise of breathing: This may result from the complete obstruction of the nose and mouth, obstruction of the larynx or trachea, or compression of the chest. Placing a plastic bag over the head, a child choking on a piece of hotdog, and a man whose auto slips off a jack while he is working underneath it are respective examples of these mechanisms. Individuals with some degree of mobility impairment are at a particular risk of such injury. Small infants are susceptible because should they work their way into a position where their breathing is compromised, they are unable to extricate themselves. This is often the case in infant deaths related to unsafe sleeping environments. An infant placed in an adult bed may roll off and become wedged between the mattress and a nearby wall or headboard. Before infant crib standards were established in 1973, there was wide variation in crib sizes, the spaces between the slats on the sides, and the sizes of crib mattresses. These variations created situations where the slats were spaced widely enough for the bodies of small infants to slip between and hang themselves when the larger head would not pass through. Mattresses that did not fit tightly enough created spaces where they met the headboard and sides large enough for infants to slip into. Projecting posts or decorations could catch on articles of clothing and suspend the infant. With the adoption of crib standards and the regular review of fatal incidents involving cribs, playyards, portacribs and other such devices with recall of those found hazardous there has been a significant decrease in such tragic incidents though they are still now seen with old or defective cribs or as noted improvised sleeping arrangements.

Adults impaired by drugs or alcohol are also at risk whether by passing out in a position where their face is covered by an impermeable surface or becoming wedged between furniture or other objects in their environment with resulting chest compression. Elderly demented or otherwise impaired adults, particularly, if restrained, have similar risks. Such restrained individuals may, in an attempt to escape, become wedged under bed rails or twist their restraints to the extent that they suffer chest compression. If the restraints get around the neck, they may, in effect, hang themselves.

Compromise of circulation: Any pressure or restriction to a body part sufficient to interrupt or significantly restrict blood flow distally can lead to ischemic injury, asphyxia, to the parts affected. A simple example is the arm that "falls asleep" when left draped over a chair or bent under us while we sleep. In spite of the unpleasant temporary sensations of woodenness and "pins and needles," this almost never has any long-term consequence. In fact, short-term interruption of the blood supply to an extremity may be employed in surgery to ensure a bloodless field. When pressure is applied to the neck, however, cerebral blood flow can be compromised with potentially rapidly fatal consequences. This is the usual mechanism of death in suicidal hangings. The constricting noose or ligature initially restricts cerebral blood outflow through the internal jugular veins and then arterial flow into the brain through the common carotids. It is almost never the case that there is a bony neck injury. Neck injury is ordinarily only seen if there is a long drop before suspension occurs. Fracture of the cervical spine with high cord damage is the intended mechanism of death in "modern" judicial executions by hanging. Cerebral anoxia also occurs in assaults involving strangulation whether manual, or by ligature. *Damage to rigid internal neck structures like the hyoid bones and thyroid cartilages is rare in suicidal hangings but common in assaults. Also frequently noted in such assaults are facial and conjunctival petechiae. The latter may become confluent.*

Entanglement in ropes or cords is an important cause of unintentional injury in children. Dangling cords for draperies and blinds are a particular hazard to infants and small children. Many infants have been asphyxiated when cords or strings attached to toys dangled into their cribs became twisted around their necks. Cords holding pacifiers and drawstrings in clothing are similarly dangerous. In such cases, visible injury to the body is usually confined to marks caused by the offending string or cord.

Compromise of cellular respiration: A variety of chemicals and toxins interfere with cellular utilization of oxygen. These include cyanide and carbon monoxide that are discussed in another section of this chapter.

Drowning: A number of mechanisms have been proposed as causative factors in drowning; however, the simple fact remains that we cannot breathe underwater. Although there are other physiological events that may occur during a drowning episode, ultimately death results from asphyxia. Survivors of drowning episodes may develop pulmonary complications from aspirating contaminated water in addition to any hypoxic cerebral injury. Many who are initially successfully resuscitated eventually succumb to adult respiratory distress syndrome (ARDS, see Chapter 8), although usually also having sustained significant cerebral damage from hypoxia. Victims of immersion in cold water, particularly children, may be more salvageable than when the event occurs in warm water because of the protective effects of the rapidly induced hypothermia on the central nervous system (or brain).

Oxygen-deficient environments: Some asphyxiations result from a lack of oxygen in the local environment. This may occur if the air is displaced by other gases or fumes even if those gases or fumes are not themselves toxic. Under some conditions oxygen may be depleted in a confined location by biological or chemical processes and of course it is deficient at high altitude. Most of these conditions involve occupational, industrial, or agricultural settings. Tanks utilized to store volatile chemicals may still be filled with fumes after being emptied and unless thoroughly ventilated may be deadly for any workers entering them without an independent source of air. Oxygen-deficient atmospheres can be found in wells and other underground spaces such as sewers. In agricultural settings, silos, grain bins, and manure pits also pose similar risks as well as the possible presence of toxic gases. Individuals may create oxygen-deficient atmospheres during the course of inhalant abuse and inadvertently asphyxiate themselves or do so deliberately as a suicide mechanism. In recent years, helium has become a popular agent for the latter.

Asphyxias may occur when externally supplied air for breathing does not contain sufficient oxygen. There are strict regulations and standards regarding the storage of compressed gases destined for industrial, medical, or other uses in part to ensure that such gases are only used for their intended purposes. In spite of these engineering controls, people still manage to connect incorrect cylinders to gas lines. There have been multiple instances involving hospitals and other care facilities when oxygen lines to patient care units were erroneously connected to other gases with tragic result.

Pathological Findings in Asphyxia

There are no specific pathological findings in asphyxias. Pulmonary congestion and edema are commonly present often accompanied by some degree of intra-alveolar hemorrhage but these are nonspecific changes. The means by which the asphyxiation was effected may result in recognizable injuries such as ligature marks in hangings and ligature strangulations (**Figure 3-10**).

Internal neck trauma is common in assaultive strangulations. Moreover, during the assault other physical injuries may be incurred by the victim (**Figure 3-11**). In mechanical or positional asphyxias pressure marks, bruises and abrasions may be found marking points of contact between the victim and the compressing surfaces. In instances of neck constriction or chest compression fine capillary hemorrhages, petechiae, of the eyes and skin above the constriction/compression

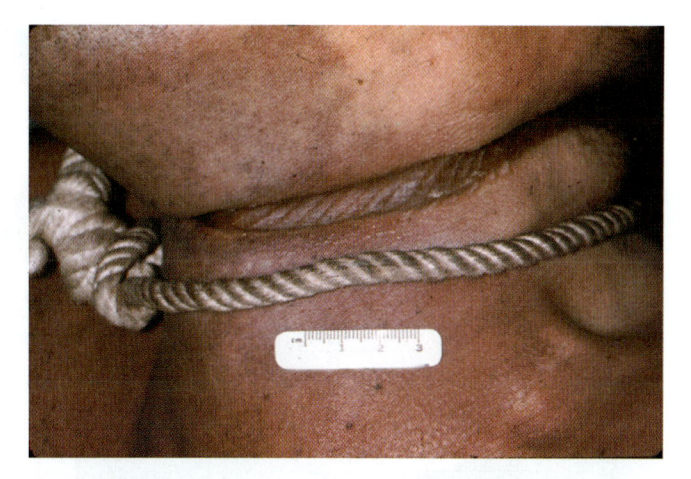

FIGURE 3-10 Ligature marks in a suicidal hanging. The mark reflects the pattern of the rope used (shown below).

may occur. In many instances, however, the identification of asphyxia as the cause of death or injury comes from history and witness accounts. As earlier noted the brain is much more susceptible to anoxic/hypoxic injury than other organs and tissues. This leads to situations where an individual is removed from an asphyxiating environment, e.g. drowning, hanging, in time to preserve all organ functions other then that of the brain. Depending on the severity of the anoxic period varying patterns of cerebral injury may be seen (see Chapter 21).

Complexity of Injuries

Many injury situations produce a complex of different types of injuries. As mentioned, an explosion can produce blunt force, penetrating, and thermal injuries. Similarly, the occupant of a motor vehicle that wrecks could incur blunt force injuries, cuts from broken glass or sharp metal, and thermal trauma should a fire break out. Occupants trapped in collapsed passenger compartments may be mechanically asphyxiated or drowned should the vehicle end up in a body of water.

Occupational Injuries

While occupational injuries will be further addressed in the chemical injury section, in the United States, the majority of acute occupational injuries and certainly the fatal ones are the consequences of physical trauma. In 2010, 87% of such fatalities were due to physical trauma with transportation-related incidents being the most common (**Figure 3-12**).

Fatal workplace injuries occur mostly in men, who while accounting for 56% of the total hours worked constitute 92% of the fatalities. As would be expected certain industries and occupations are inherently more dangerous and have higher rates or injury both fatal and nonfatal (**Figure 3-13**).

Construction had the highest number of fatalities, while agriculture, forestry, fishing, and hunting had the highest rates. Workers employed in fishing and logging followed by aircraft pilots and engineers respectively topped the occupations with high fatality rates (**Figure 3-14**).

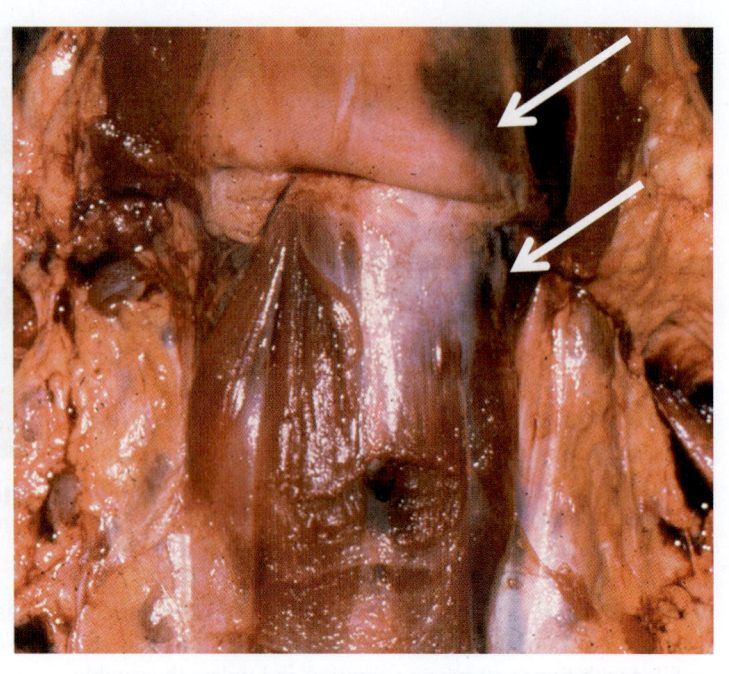

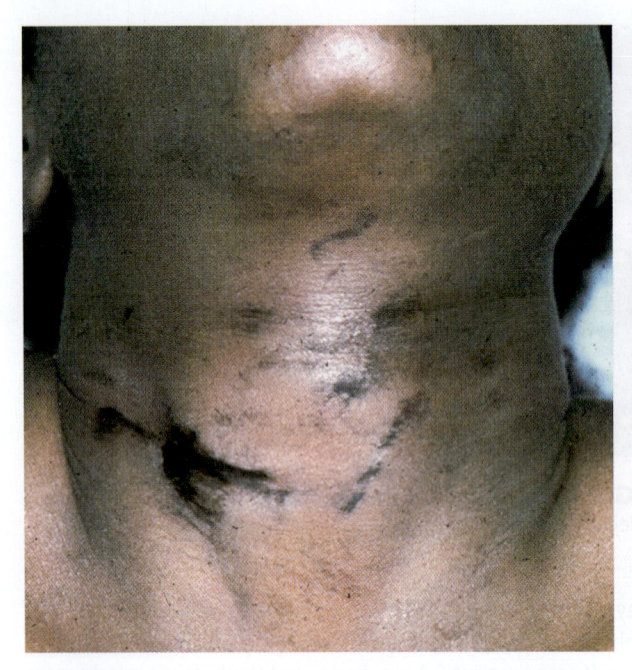

FIGURE 3-11 Manual strangulation. (Left) Abrasions and bruises are visible on external examination. (Right) Internal examination demonstrates hemorrhages (arrows). There was also a fracture of the hyoid bone.

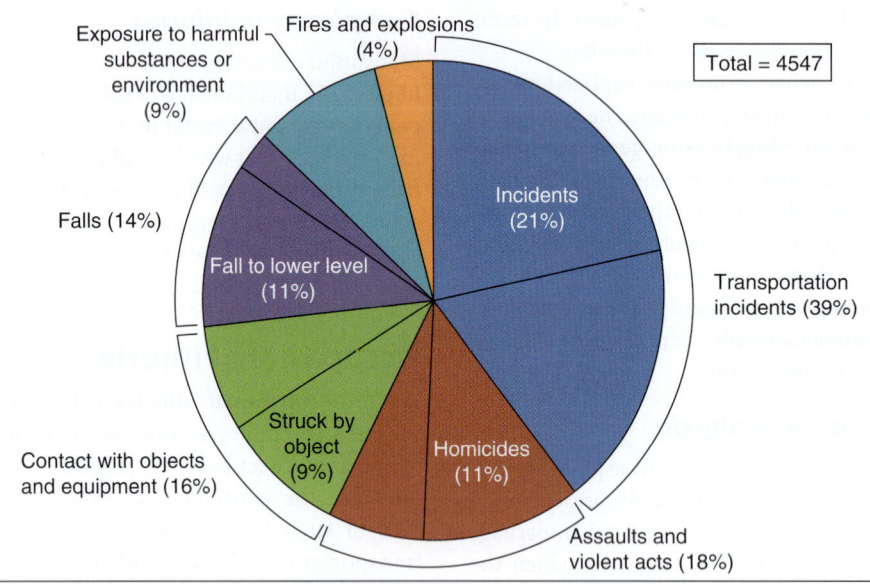

FIGURE 3-12 Manner in which fatal work injuries occurred (2010 data). Data for 2010 are preliminary. Note: Percentages may not add to totals because of rounding. Transportation counts are expected to rise when updated 2010 data are released in Spring 2012 because key source documentation on specific transportation-related incidents has not yet been received. Source: U.S. Bureau of Labor Statistics, U.S. Department of Labor, 2011.

> More fatal work injuries resulted from transportation incidents than from any other event. Highway incidents alone accounted for more than one out of every five fatal work injuries in 2010.

Total = 4547

- Transportation incidents (39%)
  - Incidents (21%)
- Assaults and violent acts (18%)
  - Homicides (11%)
- Contact with objects and equipment (16%)
  - Struck by object (9%)
- Falls (14%)
  - Fall to lower level (11%)
- Exposure to harmful substances or environment (9%)
- Fires and explosions (4%)

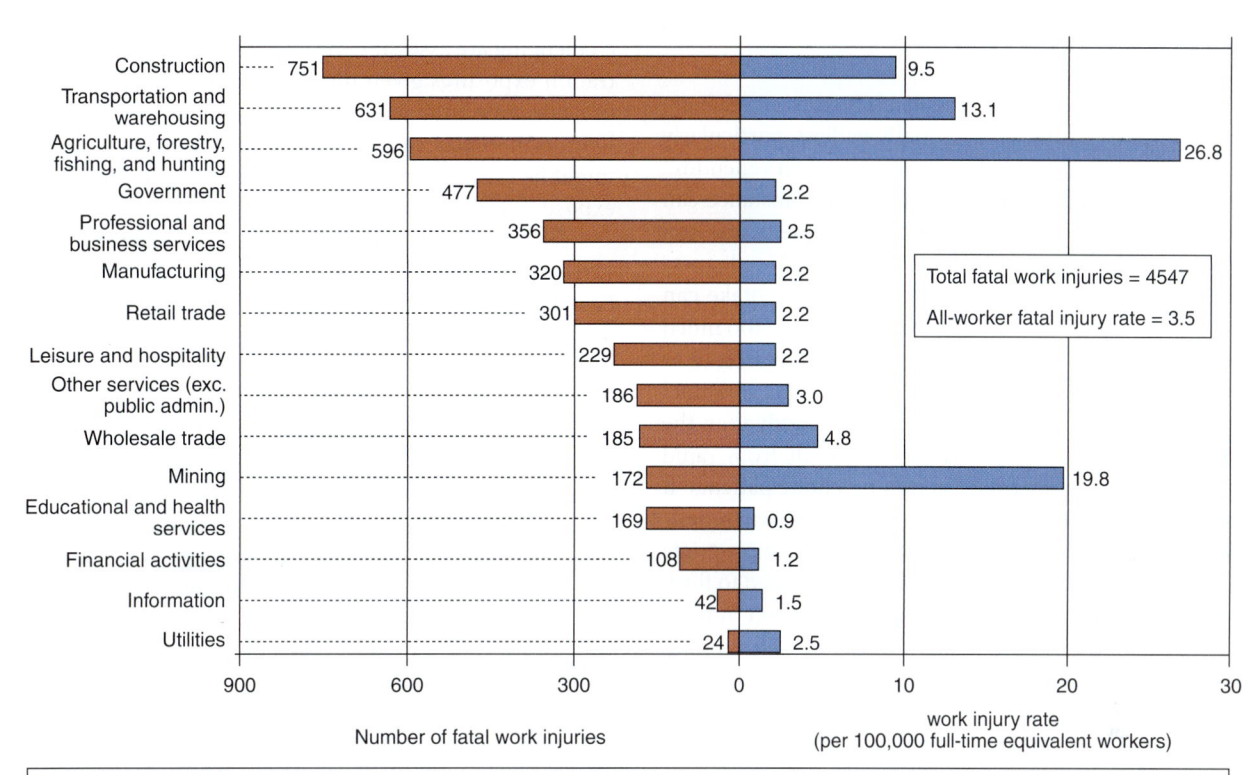

ENVIRONMENTAL INJURY 107

Industry	Number of fatal work injuries	Work injury rate (per 100,000 full-time equivalent workers)
Construction	751	9.5
Transportation and warehousing	631	13.1
Agriculture, forestry, fishing, and hunting	596	26.8
Government	477	2.2
Professional and business services	356	2.5
Manufacturing	320	2.2
Retail trade	301	2.2
Leisure and hospitality	229	2.2
Other services (exc. public admin.)	186	3.0
Wholesale trade	185	4.8
Mining	172	19.8
Educational and health services	169	0.9
Financial activities	108	1.2
Information	42	1.5
Utilities	24	2.5

Total fatal work injuries = 4547
All-worker fatal injury rate = 3.5

Construction had the highest number of fatal injuries in 2010. Agriculture, forestry, fishing, and hunting sector had the highest fatal work injury rate.

FIGURE 3-13 Number and rate of fatal occupational injuries by industry sector (2010 data). Source: U.S. Bureau of Labor Statistics.

Occupation	Number of fatal work injuries	Fatal work injury rate (per 100,000 full-time equivalent workers)
Fishers and related fishing workers	29	116.0
Logging workers	59	91.9
Aircraft pilots and flight engineers	78	70.6
Farmers and ranchers	300	41.4
Mining machine operators	23	38.7
Roofers	57	32.4
Refuse and recyclable material collectors	26	29.8
Driver/sales workers and truck drivers	683	21.8
Industrial machinery installation, repair, and maintenance workers	96	20.3
Police and sheriff's patrol officers	133	18.0

Total fatal work injuries = 4547
All-worker fatal injury rate = 3.5

Fatal work injury rates were highest for fishers, logging workers, and aircraft pilots and flight engineers in 2010.

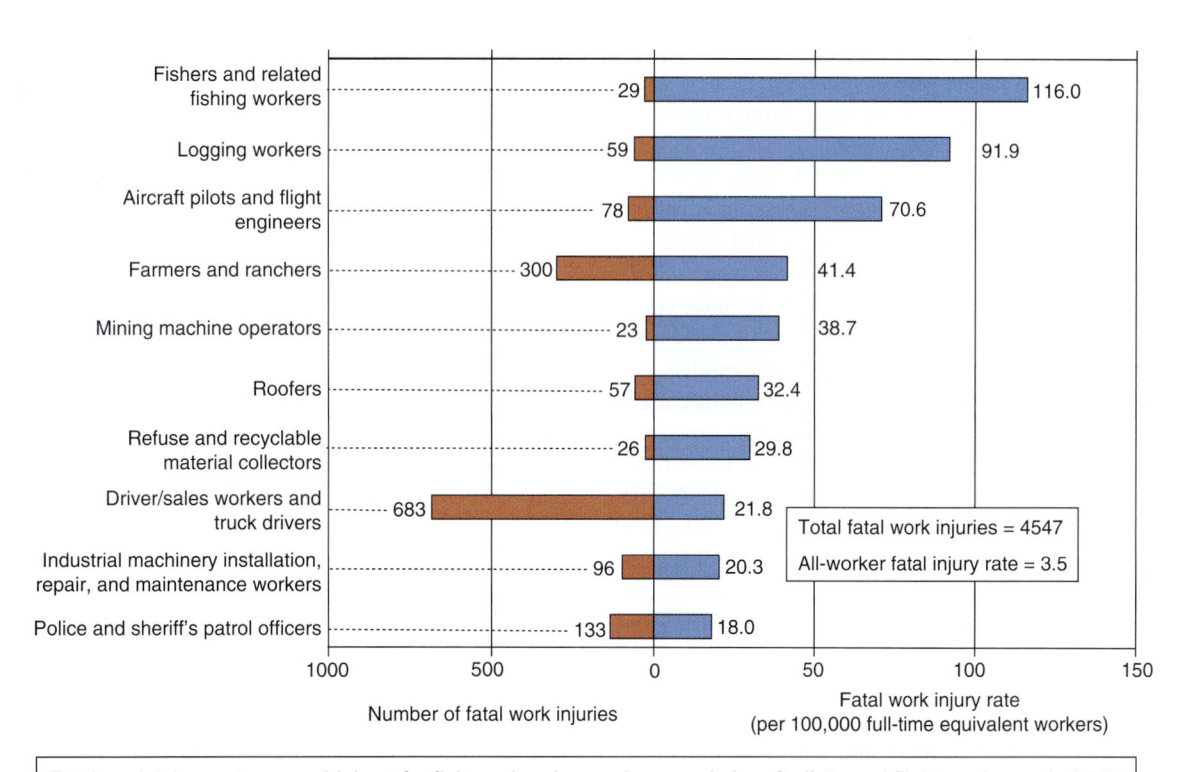

FIGURE 3-14 Occupations with high fatal work injury rates (2010 data). Source: U.S. Bureau of Labor Statistics.

CHEMICAL INJURY

The list of substances, minerals, chemicals, toxins, etc. that are potentially toxic to humans is essentially endless, particularly if we remember Paracelsus' dictum, "sola dosis facit venenum," only the dose makes the poison. Virtually any substance can be toxic if taken in excess, even essential dietary elements. Iron is necessary for the formation of hemoglobin, and inadequate dietary intake leads to anemia but excess dietary intake can lead to hemosiderosis with resulting organ damage. Too much iron in the form of ferrous salts taken at one time can lead to acute poisoning. Is there a substance as innocuous as water? Yet water can be toxic if more is taken into the body than the kidneys can clear. Water intoxication can result from rapid excess ingestion as is sometimes seen in psychotic patients. It can also be an iatrogenic complication of therapy when nonelectrolyte solutions are given to patients with inappropriate antidiuretic hormone secretion or sterile water is used to flush operative sites. Water toxicity also occurs in marathon runners who over hydrate during their run. The excess water dilutes the intravascular volume and the resulting hyponatremia can be fatal.

Toxic chemical exposures, acute or chronic, can occur in the home, workplace, hospital, and the great outdoors. Some of these exposures are natural since numerous toxic substances are already present in the environment such as plant toxins or high arsenic concentrations in some groundwater. Others are man-made, both in regard to the origin of the toxic substance and the circumstances in which they are encountered, such as exposure to solvents in a chemical plant. Man-made substances also escape into the natural environment where they can become hazards as in the case of mercury released from industrial processes into the environment accumulating in the flesh of fish.

The determination that a particular substance is potentially toxic usually begins with the recognition of an apparent association between the use of or exposure to that substance and some malady. The association is confirmed by epidemiologic studies demonstrating that the malady is more common in exposed individuals than unexposed or in those with greater exposure than those with less. Animal models are utilized to support the association and to try to define toxic levels as well as set permissible levels for human exposure. This latter process involves exposing the animals to increasing quantities of the substance and determining the lowest dosage that produces an effect, the threshold dose, which is then used to define a permissible exposure level. Epidemiologic studies are complicated by many factors particularly those involving determining the actual exposure to the substance in questions in the subject groups and identifying an appropriate control group for comparison. Animal studies can be problematic since there are physiological differences between humans and other animals and it may be difficult to approximate conditions in the real world in the experimental setting. Many animal studies utilize exposures many times greater than what humans would experience. Particularly challenging are assessing the effects of long-term low concentration exposures given the long life of humans versus those of laboratory animals. It is in fact difficult to know what the long-term effects to low concentrations of many substances might be raising concerns about our ability to set permissible exposure limits to such substances.

Substances taken into the body are distributed within its various compartments, depending on the chemical properties of the substance. Water-soluble molecules like ethanol are distributed throughout the total body water while others that are more lipophilic move more easily into lipid-rich organs and tissues and are concentrated there. Inhaled particulate materials such as asbestos fibers lodge in the lungs where they do their damage. Most chemicals are metabolized to some degree and both metabolites and residual parent drug are cleared from the body through urine, bile, and/or feces. In some instances, the metabolite of the drug or chemical may be more toxic than the parent substance itself.

Drugs and Medications

The misuse and/or abuse of drugs and medicines is a significant medical and legal problem in much of the world. Even appropriately used medications can have side effects or produce complications more serious than the conditions for which they were prescribed. It is well recognized that iatrogenic injury from medications is a major cause of morbidity and even mortality in both inpatient and outpatient settings.

Medications can cause injury in several ways. If an excess of medication is taken, an overdose can result. Drugs vary in their therapeutic index, essentially the difference between the dosage necessary to produce a therapeutic effect and what will be toxic. Drugs with low therapeutic indexes, like digoxin, have to be carefully monitored to prevent patient injury. Drugs with abuse potential are also likely to result in overdose since users may increase dosage to "improve" the pharmacologic effect they are seeking. Drug interactions can lead to overdoses. If one medication affects the metabolism or clearance of another, it can cause a buildup of the other with a resulting increase in its pharmacologic effects. The anticoagulant, warfarin, is an example of a medication whose effects can be augmented or diminished by numerous other medications as well as dietary substances. The simultaneous intake of multiple medications that have similar potentially toxic side effects sometimes leads to injury even when none of the medications is itself present in a toxic concentration. Sometimes the respiratory depressant effect of ethanol is the additional factor that changes an instance of abuse into a fatality.

Virtually all medications have side effects and some of these can be injurious. There are a variety of hypersensitivity reactions that can occur to medications ranging from minor to disabling or even fatal such as erythema multiforme (see Chapter 20). Erythema multiforme has been associated with a number of medications including barbiturates, penicillins, sulfonamides, and phenytoin. Acute allergic reactions from hives to frank anaphylaxis can occur. These usually involve an initial exposure with sensitization and then a reaction on rechallenge but anaphylaxis may occur without a history of an initial sensitizing exposure. Drugs with greater risk of such allergic reactions include penicillin. Iodinated radiocontrast materials may also cause anaphylaxis, though it is believed to be through a different mechanism as is that seen in individuals allergic to aspirin and other NSAIDs.

When medications are abused, they are often taken by individuals for whom they are not prescribed or, if prescribed, in quantities in excess of that which was prescribed. This may result in an overdose where the pharmacological effects of the drug are paramount. In a situation of abuse, moreover, not only may the quantities of the medication be supratherapeutic but also the route of administration inappropriate. For example, medication in pill form intended for oral ingestion may be ground up and injected intravenously (IV). With street or illicit substances, there are no standards of purity, and in addition to the drug/medication of interest, a variety of other substances may be, and usually are, present. While some may be inert, others are pharmacologically active and potentially toxic. It is also common for abusers to ingest multiple substances/medications at the same time further compounding the problem.

Abusers administering drugs to themselves and/or others put themselves at risk of a variety of diseases and complications beyond those related to the pharmacological effects of the drugs involved. The sharing of syringes and needles by IV drug users has been linked to the spread of infectious agents including hepatitis B and C, HIV, and malaria. Unclean needles and poor injection hygiene can lead to abscesses or cellulitis at injection sites. Right-sided endocarditis is seen in IV drugs abusers. The insoluble components of ground oral medications or materials used to "cut" street drugs become lodged in the microvasculature of the lungs where they induce a striking foreign body granulomatous reaction that can lead to right-sided heart failure, cor pulmonale. Inhalation of powdered cocaine can lead to nasal septal perforation.

Addiction to illicit drugs, legal medications, or alcohol is itself a serious problem with a significant cost to society in addition to the damage it does to the individuals involved and their families. The addict may be unable to function normally in society or support themselves and their families. Some resort to criminal acts and enterprises in order to maintain their habits. Those addicts living marginal existences are at risk of all the medical and nutritional problems associated with such a lifestyle. The production and distribution of illegal drugs is itself a criminal enterprise often associated with violence and users, particularly those that also deal drugs, may become victims. The classes of drugs most abused with the exception of ethanol are the narcotic analgesics, the stimulants, and the anxiolytics.

Narcotic analgesics: These include the medications extracted from the opium poppy, *Papaver somniferum*, mainly morphine and codeine. Heroin, diacetylmorphine, is not utilized clinically but is the main form of street opiate. A variety of synthetic opioids are also available and abused including hydrocodone, oxycodone, hydromorphone, oxymorphone, and others like fentanyl, propoxyphene, and methadone. These substances are respiratory depressants and taken in overdose may cause death via central respiratory depression. There is evidence that methadone and propoxyphene, a related compound, have cardiac effects as well. Generally apart from the serious consequences of addiction noted above and those of acute intoxication, these substances (in and of themselves) have little or no long-term/chronic toxicity.

Stimulants: Cocaine and amphetamines are the major drugs in this group. They are abused for their excitatory effects and their toxicity is felt to be primarily cardiac, with deaths resulting from lethal arrhythmias. They may also precipitate what is termed "excited delirium." This is not an overdose phenomenon but a drug-induced state characterized by bizarre, hyperactive, behavior often culminating in cardiovascular collapse and death. It often becomes particularly problematic when the bizarre behavior leads to law enforcement or bystander intervention and restraint of the victim. Following the collapse concerns are understandably raised that the fatal outcome was the consequence of traumatic asphyxia or physical injuries sustained in the course of the restraint.

Cocaine: It may be taken in the form of the hydrochloride salt, powder, or in a crystalline form, the free base. The latter is often referred to as "crack" because of the cracking noise it makes as it is heated prior to inhaling its vapors. It may be inhaled, snorted—intact, inhaled while it is heated—smoked, or injected. It is not ordinarily ingested except regrettably occasionally in an attempt to hide evidence with often lethal results. Cocaine and amphetamines raise heart rate, cardiac output, and blood pressure. Acute cerebrovascular hemorrhages have also been linked to their use. Cocaine may cause coronary artery spasm, and there is ample evidence linking chronic cocaine use to accelerated coronary atherosclerosis and cardiomyopathy.

Methamphetamine: It is often produced in-house "laboratories" from the over-the-counter precursor drug pseudoephedrine and has become a serious problem in many parts of the United States. This is not only because of its potent addictive potential and its pharmacologic effects but also because its clandestine production involves the use of explosive and corrosive chemicals. These "labs" are often located in homes and trailers where families including children may be living. Chronic methamphetamine users may exhibit evidence of premature aging and striking deterioration of their dentition. The latter has also been noted in cocaine abusers. Methamphetamine may be ingested orally, smoked or injected.

Anxiolytics: There are a large number of medications in this group many of which in addition to their antianxiety properties are utilized as sleep aids and muscle relaxants. The most widely prescribed are the benzodiazepines including alprazolam, diazepam, and chlordiazepoxide among others. They vary considerably in their fatal overdose potential but when, as is often the case, they are taken with in combination with other drugs or ethanol in a situation of abuse they may augment the respiratory depressant effects of the other agents.

Hallucinogens: Hallucinogens such as LSD are dangerous largely due to their mind-altering effects that may lead intoxicated individuals to seek out or unwittingly place themselves in situations where they may be physically harmed.

Inhalants: Another broad group of abused substances is the inhalants. Many of these are low molecular weight hydrocarbons that serve as the propellants in aerosol dispensers. Some inhalants are volatile solvents while others gases with various uses. The propellants include propane, butane, and isobutane as well as fluorinated hydrocarbons. Chlorofluorocarbons (CFCs) were once utilized as propellants but are now banned in most countries because of concerns about their effects on earth's ozone layer. Some CFCs, however, are still used as refrigerants and may be diverted for abuse in that form. When inhaled, "sniffed" or "huffed," for a high, these chemicals have the potential to destabilize the myocardium and consequently precipitate lethal cardiac arrhythmias. Volatile solvents like toluene in glue can have similar effects. Helium, nitrous oxide, and propane may also be sniffed. Asphyxiation may result if a volatile is utilized in a setting where it displaces the air that the abuser is breathing creating an oxygen-deficient atmosphere. This most commonly involves putting a plastic bag over the head to confine the fumes or utilizing a mask.

Acetaminophen: This commonly utilized analgesic and antipyretic deserves inclusion because of its potential for hepatotoxicity in overdose; as such it is the most common cause of acute liver failure in the United States and Great Britain. The drug came into wide usage as a replacement for aspirin in large part because of its much lower incidence of undesirable gastric side effects. Probably because of its availability, ingestion of large quantities in suicide attempts and "gestures" occurs frequently. In overdose, the liver becomes unable to conjugate the drug into the forms in which it is ordinarily excreted from the body in the urine. This leads to the formation of a toxic metabolite and cellular damage. Liver necrosis appears some days after the ingestion that histopathologically is characterized by bland central necrosis. This catastrophe can be averted by the administration of *N*-acetylcysteine within the first 8–10 hours of ingestion. This helps restore liver glutathione stores needed for the conjugation of the parent drug. Chronic alcohol abuse, fasting, and use of some anticonvulsant drugs can increase the potential for acetaminophen to reach toxic levels with heavy but otherwise nontoxic ingestions. Another important factor is the presence of acetaminophen in many different products. Individuals may be unaware of how many of the over-the-counter medications they are taking contain the drug and inadvertently attain toxic concentrations.

Alcohols: There are four alcohols commonly involved in human toxicity: methanol, ethanol, isopropanol, and ethylene glycol.

Methanol, methyl alcohol or wood alcohol, is most commonly used as a solvent. It is at times ingested, usually by alcoholics, as a substitute for ethanol. It is highly toxic and metabolized to formaldehyde and formic acid. It initially produces intoxication, and one of the potential complications of its use is blindness. It is metabolized by alcohol dehydrogenase and thus one of the treatments for methanol poisoning is to administer ethanol which competes with and slows methanol's metabolism.

Isopropanol, isopropyl or rubbing alcohol, is used as a disinfectant and a fuel. It is approximately three times as toxic as ethanol and like methanol is metabolized via the alcohol dehydrogenase pathway. Its major metabolite is acetone, and acetone levels in individuals who ingest isopropanol will approach the same levels that were initially achieved by the parent compound as metabolism proceeds. As with methanol treatment of isopropanol ingestion consists of the administration of ethanol. Like methanol, isopropanol may be utilized as a substitute of ethanol by alcoholics.

Ethanol, ethyl or beverage alcohol, is a widely consumed and equally widely abused drug. Produced via the fermentation of sugars by yeast it is the "active" ingredient in a vast range of alcoholic beverages including beers, wines, and the stronger distilled spirits. Ethanol in beverages is usually described in terms of the percentage of ethanol present per unit of volume. Beers range from 3.2 to 3.5% upward, wines 9% to 13% and distilled spirits 20% to 50%, although there are exceptions. Distilled spirits are sometimes classed by their "proof" which is a number that is equal to twice the ethanol percentage. The highest percentage of ethanol that can be distilled from an aqueous solution is 95 yielding a 190 proof "beverage." Ninety-five percent ethanol has a variety of laboratory and commercial uses including a solvent and disinfectant. Sometimes substances will be added to 95% ethanol to discourage its consumption—this process is called "denaturing" and the resulting product "denatured alcohol."

Ethanol is an anesthetic and in low doses has a disinhibiting effect. At higher concentrations, it affects coordination and in toxic dosages can lead to loss of consciousness, coma, respiratory depression, and death. Extensive studies have demonstrated that slowing of reflexes and loss of coordination begins in the vast majority of individuals at blood ethanol concentrations of 50 mg/dL. Consequently driving while intoxicated/driving under the influence (DWI/DUI) levels in the United States are set at 80 mg/dL, although this is usually phrased as .08%, a concentration of ethanol in the body of .08% by volume. In a "standard" 70 kg male, a quickly ingested standard drink (a drink consisting of a 12 oz beer, 4 oz glass of wine, or mixed drink containing an ounce of ethanol) on an empty stomach will produce a blood ethanol concentration of 15–20 mg/dL. Thus, such an individual would have to consume approximately four "standard drinks" in the space of an hour to be judged as DWI/DUI using the .08% level. Ethanol distributes throughout total body water and concentrations achieved after a particular dose will thus vary, depending on the weight of the individual. There is also data that indicate that women will experience a more rapid increase in blood alcohol after an equivalent ingestion versus a male of the same weight. Food in the stomach blunts the rise after ingestion and may lower the peak ethanol concentration versus intake with an empty one. Ethanol is metabolized in the stomach and liver primarily by the enzyme alcohol dehydrogenase to acetaldehyde that is then metabolized to acetic acid. Ethanol is metabolized or cleared at a rate of approximately 19 mg/dL per hour.

There is some variability among individuals in the intoxicating effects of alcohol, and chronic heavy users develop some degree of tolerance. Naïve drinkers are at risk of respiratory depression and death at concentrations of 350–400 mg/dL. Lower concentrations can prove fatal as well if they lead to loss of consciousness in a position where respiration is mechanically compromised or the inebriate vomits and cannot clear their airway. Acute intoxication can also lead to a variety of injuries through falls, loss of control of moving vehicles, or an innumerable variety of circumstances where the alcohol "altered" senses lead the inebriate into a dangerous situation or prompt him/her into an action they would not have undertaken in a sober state.

While mild regular ethanol consumption, 3–4 standard drinks per day, is not necessarily harmful and may even have beneficial cardiovascular effects, heavy chronic consumption, 10 or more drinks per day, is dangerous. Consequences may include alcoholic liver disease, gastritis, pancreatitis, and dilated cardiomyopathy. See Chapters 9, 10, and 11 for additional details. Alcoholics can suffer from skeletal muscle weakness and alcohol negatively affects the immune system leading to an increased susceptibility to infection. Heavy consumption is also linked to cancers of the oral cavity, larynx, and esophagus. Consumption of alcohol by pregnant women may lead to fetal alcohol syndrome in their infants characterized by microcephaly, facial dysmorphology and malformations of the brain, and cardiovascular and genitourinary systems.

Carbon monoxide: This colorless, odorless gas is the product of the incomplete combustion of carbon containing compounds and oxygen. It has an affinity for hemoglobin that is approximately 240 times greater than that of oxygen, and the resulting carboxyhemoglobin is unable to transport oxygen to the tissues. It also binds to mitochondrial enzymes and interferes with cellular respiration at the molecular level. CO in the body is commonly measured and expressed in terms of the percentage of hemoglobin saturation. CO bonding to hemoglobin is not an irreversible process but the equilibrium greatly favors it over formation of oxyhemoglobin. In individuals unexposed to elevated ambient CO there is only a fraction of a % carboxyhemoglobin in the blood. With CO exposure through cigarette smoking saturations of 5–6% can be seen. Symptoms of headache and nausea can develop at saturations of 20% and saturations over 40 can be fatal in individuals with preexisting medical conditions, while 50–60% is fatal in healthy individuals.

CO from internal combustion engines is a particular hazard to humans, although the addition of catalytic converters to automobile exhaust systems and requirements that those systems be intact have decreased the number of fatalities due to unintentional auto exhaust poisonings. Auto exhaust also contains other asphyxiant gases including CO_2 and nitrous oxides so suicidal "poisonings" via exhaust run into the passenger compartment and closed garages still occur even though blood carbon monoxide saturation levels are not always elevated. Serious intoxications and deaths are seen when other types of internal combustion devices are utilized in enclosed spaces, for example, generators and gasoline powered tools. Motorcycles, lawn mowers, and other garden and home devices if run in a garage, shed, or basement can generate enough CO to produce poisoning and death. CO is also produced in varying quantities by portable heating devices that burn hydrocarbons. CO poisoning should be suspected in individuals presenting with symptoms of weakness, nausea, and headache during the heating season particularly if the symptoms are present in multiple household members. In these cases, the source of the CO is usually a heating system/device that has been improperly installed or when an exhaust vent becomes obstructed. In times of power failures, generators and inadequately vented gas-powered space heaters are often the culprits. Burning charcoal generates a large volume of CO, and when it is used for heat or cooking inside a dwelling can have tragic consequences. It may even be utilized as a means of suicide. CO poisoning is treated with oxygen. Inhalation of 100% oxygen decreases the half life of carboxyhemoglobin in the body from 4–5 hours to a little over 1 hour and under hyperbaric circumstances to less than half an hour.

Tobacco: Tobacco use, mainly in the form of cigarette smoking, constitutes a significant public health hazard in the United States and other countries. Cigarette smoking is felt to cause approximately 400,000 premature deaths yearly in the United States and as such the single greatest potentially preventable cause. Smoking has been linked to cancer, cardiovascular disease, pulmonary disease, and low birth weights in infants born to smokers. Smokers have a decreased life expectancy that is proportional to the number of years smoked. Many of the risks of smoking decrease significantly if the smoker quits.

It is estimated that 85% of cases of lung cancer are smoking related and smokers also are at greater risk of cancers of the oral cavity, larynx, esophagus, kidney, colon, and cervix. Consumers of smokeless tobacco products, chewing tobacco, and snuff are also at risk of oral cancer as well as gum and dental disease.

Coronary atherosclerosis is the primary cardiovascular consequence of smoking, and smokers have a greater incidence of sudden cardiac death. Atherosclerotic disease is not confined to the coronaries but may be noted in the aorta and other vessels. Respiratory complications in addition to neoplasms include bronchitis and chronic obstructive pulmonary disease, mainly in the form of emphysema.

These conditions are not confined solely to the smokers themselves. Nonsmokers who are exposed to cigarette smoke in the workplace or home may also be affected demonstrating an increased risk of lung cancer and coronary atherosclerosis versus the nonexposed. Children growing up in homes where cigarettes are smoked have a higher incidence of respiratory illnesses. Because smoking involves combustion it is an underlying cause in many fire and/or explosion related injuries and deaths.

Cyanide: Sodium and potassium cyanide salts are not commonly present in the home but are readily available in laboratories and utilized in industrial processes. Cyanide is a potent and fast-acting poison that binds to cytochrome c oxidase involved in cellular oxidative processes. It has been famously utilized for suicides and homicides—in the case of the latter particularly in fiction. When the salts are combined with acid, hydrocyanic gas is produced—this was the method utilized in judicial executions involving so-called gas chambers, and hydrogen cyanide gas was infamously employed by the Nazis in their extermination camps. Cyanide containing baits have been utilized to control "undesirable" animals in the wild such as feral pigs, foxes, and coyotes. There were a number of drug tampering incidents in the 1980s where capsules containing acetaminophen were removed from store shelves, refilled with cyanide, and then replaced. In one episode, never solved, seven people were killed. These tragedies led to extensive changes in the packaging of over-the-counter medications including moving away from capsules to solid tablets and tamper resistant packaging. Some plants contain compounds that can produce cyanide on ingestion. A notorious episode involved a quack cancer "cure" called laetrile made from apricot pits that resulted in cases of cyanide poisoning and notably uncured cancers.

Insecticides: Many of these compounds are neurotoxins and highly toxic to humans. Exposure can occur in agricultural situations or tragically in the home or shop when such chemicals are mishandled or improperly stored. The reuse of milk, drink, or other food containers to mix or store such chemicals has led to many unintentional poisonings. This is also the case for other substances in the home from detergents to plant fertilizers. Should containers normally containing food or similar consumables be reused for the storage of other substances, they should be clearly relabeled and never be stored near consumables. Conversely consumables should never be kept near potentially toxic materials.

Heavy metals: Those of primary concern are lead, mercury, and arsenic. These elements have and continue to have numerous industrial and other uses and are common in the environment.

Lead was once a common constituent of paint pigments and while now banned for that purpose in most parts of the world is still found in dangerous concentrations in some older paints. When lead containing paints deteriorate, the dust and flakes may be ingested by young children. Lead is neurotoxic, particularly in the young, and can lead to stunted intellectual development at levels of intake below those required to produce signs of overt intoxication.

Mercury is similarly highly neurotoxic to the developing human. This concern has led to recommendations that pregnant women abstain from or limit their consumption of fish that may contain higher concentrations of mercury because of contamination of the waters in which they grew. Top predatory fish like tuna are also considered potentially dangerous since they accumulate in their flesh the mercury contained in the smaller fish that they feed on.

Arsenic is an element that is naturally present in some areas of the world in sufficient quantity to contaminate water supplies without the assistance of man (Bangladesh being notable). These lower concentrations are associated with higher prevalence of certain cancers in the affected populations. Arsenic was once a common ingredient in insecticides and rodenticides where it caused both unintentional and intentional poisonings. It was a favorite poison in the middle ages and later to the extent that laws were passed to prohibit its inclusion in embalming fluids in order to prevent poisoners from claiming that the arsenic found in their victims was an artifact of the embalming process.

Occupational Chemical and Substance Exposure

Chronic exposure to a variety of chemicals and other substances in occupational or industrial settings has been linked to a variety of specific diseases: benzene to aplastic anemia and leukemia and vinyl chloride to angiosarcoma of the liver. Acute injury from contact with toxic chemicals or substances is a hazard in any occupation where such substances are present. Poisoning from pesticides, for instance, is a particular risk of agricultural workers.

Exposure to dusts among miners, welders, sand blasters, and others causes a group of pulmonary diseases termed the pneumoconioses. These dusts include coal, silica, asbestos, and beryllium as well as some metal salts. While there are differences in their pathogenesis and their histopathology, these conditions all primarily result in pulmonary scarring and can cause significant disability or death. Additionally asbestos has been linked to mesothelioma and cancers of the upper and lower respiratory tract as well as the gastrointestinal (GI) tract. Various industrial or agricultural organic dust exposures have been linked to hypersensitivity pneumonitis and reactive airway disease, asthma.

Air Pollutants

The burning of wood and fossil fuels releases large quantities of combustion product gases and particulate matter into the atmosphere that can cause or contribute to human disease. These gases include nitrogen and sulfur dioxides as well as carbon monoxide and dioxide. Within the atmosphere, the nitrogen and sulfur oxides may be further oxidized to sulfuric and nitric acids. In summer, nitrogen oxides and other hydrocarbons interact with solar radiation to produce ozone, one of the major components of smog. These elements are primarily irritants to the lower respiratory system and are particularly hazardous to children and individuals with pre-existing pulmonary disease, especially reactive airway disease, asthma.

Toxins of Natural Origin

Many toxins of natural origin are present in the environment including the previously mentioned arsenic. These include toxic chemicals within food plants such as oxalic acid in the leaves of rhubarb and cyanogenic glycosides in cassava or manioc, an important staple in many parts of the world.

Inadequate processing of the latter prior to consumption can lead to poisoning. Various mushroom species contain potent hepatotoxins. Most of these plant toxins do not pose a great risk to those buying their food in stores but are a potential risk to those who go out and harvest naturally growing edible plants. Misidentification of plants is the cause of numerous ED visits and some fatalities in the United States. Epidemic poisoning from ergot alkaloids produced by molds growing on rye and other grains was a common affliction during the middle ages and was called Saint Anthony's Fire. Aflatoxin B produced by a fungus that grows on peanuts and corn is one of the most potent carcinogens known and is felt to contribute to the high incidence of liver cancer in some parts of the world. In the United States, aflatoxin levels in milk are monitored because of potential feed-corn contamination. Animal tissues are not immune from risks. Both wild and domesticated animals harbor parasites and bacteria that can lead to human disease if the flesh is inadequately prepared like enterohemorrhagic *Escherichia coli* that causes hemolytic-uremic syndrome. Some fish and shellfish may accumulate toxins from the dinoflagellates that they feed on and their consumption can cause ciguatera poisoning.

Hormones: Hormonally active medications include oral contraceptives (OC), estrogens, somatropin, and others.

OC users have a higher risk of deep venous thromboses and resulting pulmonary emboli, although that risk is decreased with modern formulations. Some studies indicate a slightly increased risk of breast cancer in OC users who started using them at a young age. OC users had a decreased risk of ovarian and endometrial cancer. Benign tumors of the liver, hepatic adenomas are associated with OC use. Estrogen therapy for menopausal symptoms and osteoporosis prevention increases the users risk of endometrial cancer. The addition of progestin, a synthetic progesterone, decreases that risk but may increase the risks of breast cancer and various cardiovascular complications, venous thrombosis and dementia. Diethylstilbestrol (DES) is a synthetic estrogen that was prescribed to pregnant women beginning in the 1940s to prevent premature labor and miscarriages. Women who took DES during their pregnancy were later found to have an increased risk of breast cancer and their daughters a greatly increased risk of a rare vaginal and cervical cancer, clear cell adenocarcinoma, as well as an increased risk of breast cancer.

Somatropin, human growth hormone, used to be obtained from processing donated human pituitary obtained at autopsy. In 1985, several cases of Creutzfeldt–Jakob disease were diagnosed in individuals who had received the hormone and subsequently some 28 cases were identified. Somatropin is now synthesized rather than obtained from human tissues, so this is no longer a risk. This example demonstrates the risks inherent in using materials collected from human sources for therapeutic purposes. When biological source materials are pooled (as was the case for the pituitaries and also for HIV contaminated factor VIII and IX concentrates used to treat hemophilia), there is the possibility that a sample obtained from one infected individual can lead to the infection of many others. The development of screening tests and improved methods of processing such materials have minimized these risks.

Testing for Toxic Agents

Implicating drugs, medications, and toxins as causative agents in human disease can be a complicated matter. In the case of an acute fatal exposure, such as a drug overdose, the appropriate history and symptoms coupled with the finding of the offending agent in the blood and/or tissues of the victim in toxic concentrations usually suffice. This involves both the qualitative and quantitative characterization of the agent since the mere presence of a substance does not necessarily mean that it was the cause of the overdose. For forensic, legal, purposes drug identifications must ordinarily be confirmed by more than one independent methodology. In the clinical setting of a possible drug intoxication, qualitative "screens" are often run on urine. The results are useful in clinical decision making but positive results may be invalid for legal purposes unless confirmed by another methodology because of the possibility of false positives due to cross reacting substances. For some substances, quantitation is important in the clinical setting as it is essential for treatment decisions; for example, acetaminophen concentrations are measured to determine whether *N*-acetylcysteine will be administered.

Postmortem toxicology is further complicated by sample issues. Clean uncontaminated blood or urine can be obtained from living individuals for analysis but in the deceased the samples are often hemolyzed or even decomposed and cannot be analyzed by the same methods employed in the clinical lab. Drugs and medications in the living are distributed, often unevenly, within the various body compartments and this distribution is maintained by the circulation, the integrity of cellular membranes, and other active processes. After death, these substances often redistribute in the body leading to the finding of concentrations in some samples that are different from what they would have been at the moment of death. To avoid misinterpretations, the testing of samples drawn from different sites including tissues is required.

When attempting to implicate environmental factors, testing is required to demonstrate the presence of the substance in question in the air, food, water, etc. that is thought to be the source. Often, however, the substance is not present continuously in the environment or the concern arises years after the period of exposure may have occurred. The offending substance may not be stored in the body of its victims or by the time that the concern is raised may have been cleared. As the sensitivity and capability of testing methodologies improve, it has become possible to detect quantities of substance at levels orders of magnitude lower than previously with the not unexpected finding of chemicals that had not been detected before in environmental samples. The significance of many of these findings in terms of human disease causation is unknown.

> ### HUNTING FOR ZEBRAS
>
> During routine water supply testing, it was discovered that volatile organic chemicals, (VOCs), were present in some of the wells supplying water to a large military base. Initial results identified tetrachloroethylene (PCE) and trichloroethylene (TCE). Benzene was later also detected in one of the systems. The wells had been in existence for some 40 years at the time contaminants were detected, so hundreds of thousands of individuals had potentially been exposed This included the families (and children) of soldiers in who lived in base housing. Not unexpectedly many soldiers and their dependents who had lived or worked on the base have developed illnesses including cancers and many of them and/or their families attribute their illnesses to the chemicals found in the water. An extensive epidemiological study is currently underway to determine if there is an increased incidence of a variety of diseases in this exposed population versus a similar unexposed population.
>
> Even if that study were to show that there was an excess of cases of a particular illness in this group can it be said that any one of those affected individuals developed illness solely due to the exposure? Imagine for illustrative purposes that the incidence of "malignancy X" is 3 cases yearly per 100,000 in the general population, and in the exposed group the incidence was found to be 6. Assuming that this difference was determined to be statistically significant and all other possible contributing factors could be ruled out which 3 of the 6 cases was actually due to the exposure?
>
> This is one of the dilemmas that recurs repeatedly in attempting to attribute causation to environmental agents suspected (or, as is true in this example, known) to cause human disease. While it is often possible to implicate the contribution of an agent to the population burden of an illness, it may not be possible to prove that an individual instance of the illness was caused by the agent unless there is some marker of the condition that links disease occurrence to individual exposure. (For example, with lung disease and asbestos exposure where the co-occurrence of asbestos bodies and lung disease is probative.)
>
> Nonetheless such specific attributions of individual causation are routinely made within the framework of legal and political systems. Individuals with conditions known or sometimes only suspected to have links to environmental factors are awarded damages or compensation for the failure of some agency or entity to prevent or ameliorate that exposure even when the scientific basis for that attribution is felt by many to be weak or totally lacking. This does not argue against the undoubted serious public health burden produced by a variety of environmental contaminants but highlights the scientific, legal, and political difficulties in dealing with the human costs of such damage to the environment. These are issues in which the pathologist may well become involved.

THERMAL INJURY

Burns

Contact with hot surfaces, fluids, gases, flame, and exposure to radiant heat can lead to burns. Cutaneous burns may be separated into three categories, first-, second-, and third-degree based on the depth of injury.

First-degree burns are characterized by redness, erythema, and pain. Sunburn from exposure to excess solar radiation or the lamps of a tanning device are typical examples. These heal without short-term sequelae, except in the more severe instances where subsequent superficial desquamation of the keratin-containing layer of the skin (peeling) occurs. The melanocytes in the skin are also stimulated to produce melanin leading to a tan. Long-term consequences of exposure to such radiant energy include a variety of degenerative actinic changes as well as an increased incidence of basal and squamous cell carcinomas. Malignant melanoma has been linked to episodes of heavy sun exposure with burns at a young age—particularly in lightly pigmented individuals.

Second-degree burns are characterized by the separation of the epidermis from the underlying dermis with blister formation. Because islands of epidermis remain around the dermal adnexal structures, hair shafts, sweat, and other glands, the epidermis can regenerate to cover the denuded areas and such burns generally heal without scarring.

Third-degree burns damage the adnexal structures of the dermis and lack any surviving epidermis. Hence, these burns can only heal by growth inward from the viable margins of the wound. Third-degree burns of any significant size cannot completely close in this fashion and remain as open sores. Such injuries must be treated with grafts of epidermis taken from areas of intact, uninjured skin. Deeper, charring, injuries are sometimes called fourth-degree burns. Some prefer to dispense with this classification and more simply characterize burns as either partial or full thickness. First- and second-degree burns would thus be partial thickness while third- and fourth-degree burns would be full thickness **(Figure 3-15)**.

Direct acute thermal injury leads to denaturation of proteins. Most such injuries will involve the skin but internal "burns" can occur as the result of the ingestion of caustic substances such as strong acids and bases. Although no heat is involved, tissue injuries caused by such substances, whether external or internal, are also referred to as burns. Lasers and electrocautery devices work through the thermal coagulation of tissue. Focal internal thermal damage beyond what was therapeutically intended can be a complication of operative and other therapeutic procedures.

Loss of the protective epidermis of the skin has several consequences including fluid loss through the now exposed dermal and subdermal tissues and providing a route for the entry for microorganisms into the body. Patients with

Scalding

Scalding is a mode of thermal injury that warrants further discussion. While this most commonly occurs when hot water comes into contact with skin, any sufficiently hot liquid can produce the same effect. Scalding can result from splashing, pouring, or immersion and the pattern of burns produced mirrors the mechanism (Case 3-4). As the temperature of a liquid increases above normal body temperature so does its potential to scald. Water at 160°F will burn adult human skin essentially instantaneously while 30 seconds exposure is required at 130° (Figure 3-16).

Since the process involves the transfer of heat energy from the liquid to the skin, the length of time of contact and the volume of liquid may also be factors. Liquids of greater density carry more energy so a droplet of boiling water contains less heat energy than one of cooking oil. Moreover, the oil may be heated to temperatures that greatly exceed that of boiling water.

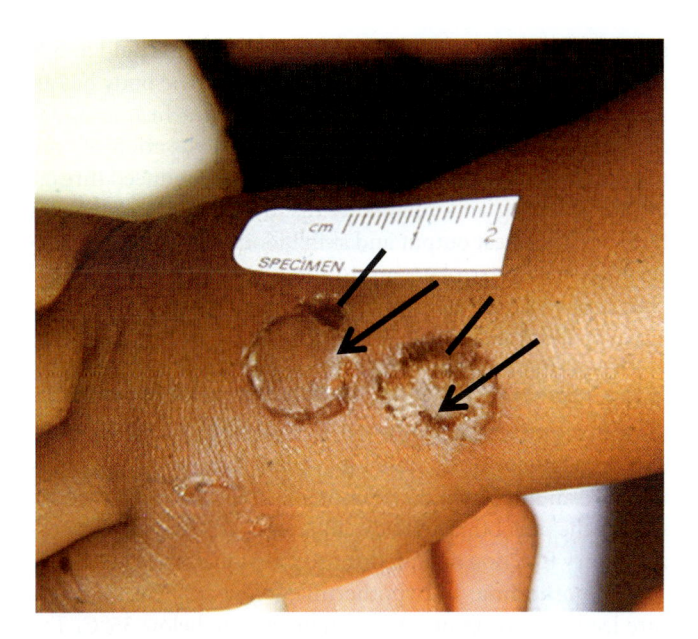

FIGURE 3-15 Burns on the arm of an infant from contact with a butane lighter. Blisters (arrow) are second-degree burn. Depressed areas (line) are third-degree burn and will heal with scarring.

extensive burns have serious problems with fluid balance and require vigorous volume and electrolyte support. They are in a hypermetabolic state and at great risk of infections. Their management is one of the most challenging in medicine and is optimally undertaken in specialized burn centers. Recovery and rehabilitation is a long and daunting process and great efforts must be expended during that process to minimize scarring and preserve the mobility and function of damaged limbs and other mobile structures.

Another potential complication is lower respiratory tract injury from the inhalation of toxic products of combustion as well as particulate matter. This can cause both acute and long-term pulmonary damage. ARDS is a feared complication. Hot or superheated air can cause upper airway damage but will not reach the lower airways. Steam and hot particulate matter, however, can carry thermal energy deep into the airways and lungs.

ENVIRONMENTAL THERMAL INJURY

Environmental exposure to heat and cold represents a threat to organisms whose biochemical processes require maintenance of an optimal internal temperature. When internal temperatures stray significantly above or below that temperature, 37°C in humans, those processes break down with eventually fatal consequences.

Hyperthermia: Hyperthermia occurs when ambient temperatures exceed normal body temperature, and normal cooling mechanisms such as sweating are overwhelmed. It may also occur as a consequence of excessive internal heat generation due to fever or hypermetabolic states.

Heatstroke represents the most severe of several stages of heat stress. In heatstroke, sweating fails and as body temperature rises cardiovascular collapse may ensue. The victim may develop confusion, delirium, headache, chills, and seizures. Their skin is usually hot and dry.

Water Temperature Effects on Adult Skin

Temperature	Time Exposure for Each Type of Burn Injury	
Degree Fahrenheit	Second-Degree Burns	Third-Degree Burns
111	220 Minutes	400 Minutes
113	120 Minutes	180 Minutes
115	30 Minutes	60 Minutes
118	15 Minutes	20 Minutes
120	5 Minutes	10 Minutes
124	2 Minutes	4.2 Minutes
130	18 Seconds	30 Seconds
140	3 Seconds	5 Seconds
150	Instant	<2 Seconds
158	Instant	<1 Second

Second-Degree Burns include blistering and scarring.
Third-Degree Burns cause irreversible damage to epidermis and subdermal tissue.

FIGURE 3-16 **Water temperature effects on human skin.** Time to result in second- and third-degree burn. Data from the American Society of Sanitary Engineers.

CASE 3-4

Emergency medical services was called to an apartment where a 2-year-old child was found unresponsive in a bathtub. The mother stated that she left the child unattended in the tub for only a few minutes. Testing revealed the temperature of the hot water coming from the tap to be 150°F. The child shows diffuse scald burns consistent with immersion as a mechanism of injury (Figure 3-17).

Each year, approximately 3800 injuries and 34 deaths occur in the home due to scalding from excessively hot tap water. The majority of these accidents involve the elderly and children under the age of five. The U.S. Consumer Product Safety Commission (CPSC) urges all users to lower their water heaters to 120°F (Document #5098 US CPSC). Public education campaigns and building code changes to lower residential hot water temperatures have significantly reduced the number of home scalding injuries.

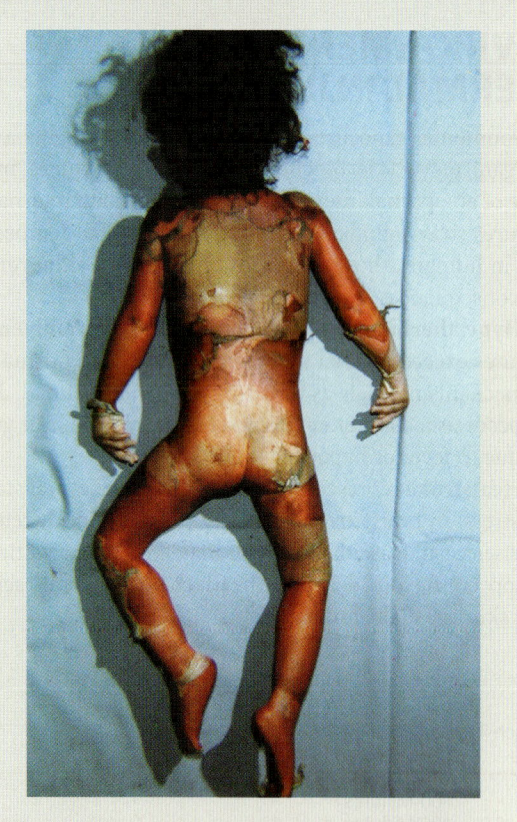

FIGURE 3-17 Photo demonstrates scalding injury.

Heat exhaustion is a milder form with symptoms of weakness and nausea. They are usually sweating with a normal or slightly elevated body temperature and appear pale and clammy with fast shallow breathing. Other milder heat stress-related symptoms can include cramps, syncope, and rash. Heat stress is often seen in the context of vigorous exercise in a warm environment, particularly if the victim is not accustomed to the heat and/or there is inadequate fluid intake to match the losses from sweat and exercise. The body has an adaptive mechanism for hot environments in heat acclimatization. This response to exercise-induced elevation of core temperatures in a hot environment includes a reduced threshold for sweating and cutaneous vasodilatation accompanied by increased sweat output and skin blood flow. Hence, it is no surprise that heatstroke tends to appear in athletes early in the course of rigorous late summer training regimens after they have spent the earlier part of the summer in relative inactivity.

Hyperthermia deaths also increase in the United States during heat waves particularly in large northern cities among the infirm and elderly whose living quarters lack adequate ventilation let alone air conditioning. Preexisting medical conditions are an important contributing factor. Some medications, such as the phenothiazines, can interfere with internal thermoregulatory function and predispose individuals to heatstroke.

Hypothermia: In hypothermia, a low ambient temperature leads to a drop in internal temperature below 35°C. The body initially responds by reducing blood flow to the skin and involuntary shivering follows, the muscular activity generating heat. When at some point these mechanisms fail, blood flow to the skin resumes and the resulting flushing may lead to a perception of overheating and a phenomenon known as "paradoxical undressing" where the victim removes items of clothing in spite of clearly being in an environment where such was needed. As the body cools, metabolic activity slows along with oxygen consumption (allowing induced hypothermia to be utilized as an operative adjunct in cardiac and brain surgery). The danger of hypothermia increases as ambient temperature drops. Adequacy of protective clothing is a factor as well as host fitness. As is the case in hyperthermia, the risk increases with age. Body habitus plays a role with heavier individuals less susceptible than thin ones. Loss of heat is greatly accelerated by convection and moisture. Wet clothing often loses its insulating properties and cold water immersion leads to rapid cooling. Water temperatures that are acceptable as outdoor air temperatures can lead to hypothermia. For example, prolonged exposure to water at a temperature of 26°C (79°F) can lead to hypothermia. A water temperature of 10°C (50°F) often leads to death in 1 hour; water temperatures near freezing can cause death in as little as 15 minutes. Ethanol consumption is a risk factor for hypothermia in two ways. First its behavioral effects can put the individual in an environment where they are at risk, and second its vasodilator effects increase heat loss from the skin.

Hypothermia can also cause local injury, the most familiar of which is frostbite. The lowered temperature leads to a failure of local circulation and resulting ischemic injury to the tissues. Small vessels are damaged and if circulation is restored there is vascular leakage, thrombosis, and ultimately necrosis of the devitalized tissues. Chronic exposure to cold in some individuals can lead to skin ulcers, chilblains, and a severe debilitating condition called "trench foot" often appeared in soldiers forced to spend long periods sitting or standing in wet trenches in the winter.

ELECTRICAL INJURY

Electricity is characterized in units of pressure, electromotive force (EMF) or volts, and volume of flow, amperes. The relationship between these is expressed by Ohm's law, $I = E/R$, where "I" is current flow or amperes, "E" is EMF or volts, and "R" is the resistance of the medium through which the current is passing in ohms. Thus as voltage rises, given a fixed resistance, the flow, amperage, also rises. If resistance increases with constant voltage, current flow decreases. As current passes through a medium, a conductor, it generates heat that is proportional to the volume of current and the resistance of the conductor.

Static Electricity Injury

Electricity has two forms for our concern: static and generated. Static electricity results from the frictional buildup of charges on moving objects or surfaces in the environment. We are all familiar with this phenomenon as it manifests itself in the shock we experience when we touch an object after shuffling across the carpet on a winter day. While the actual voltages involved are high, there is negligible current flow and such discharges are not ordinarily directly harmful to individuals. However, a static discharge can serve as an ignition source in the presence of inflammable fumes or dusts and they also represent a significant hazard to sensitive electronic equipment.

The truly dangerous form of static electricity is lightning. Peak current flow in a discharge can approach 3000 amperes and generate temperatures over 20,000°C. Lightning strikes kill approximately 60 people yearly in the United States and injure several hundred more. Most individuals struck are engaged in outdoor activities. In the United States, the states with the highest number of fatalities are Florida and Colorado, respectively. The mechanism of death is usually cardiac asystole, although burns can also result. Survivors may have neurological sequelae.

Generated Electricity Injury

Generated electrical currents come in two forms: direct and alternating. In direct current, the flow of charge is unidirectional by convention from "positive," high potential to "negative," low potential. In alternating current, the direction of flow reverses or "cycles" a certain number of times per second, commonly 60. Most electronic and battery-powered devices utilize direct current, while virtually all electric transmission is AC since it is a much more efficient means of sending current long distances utilizing high voltages that can be easily stepped down to lower voltages by transformers for end users. AC current is more dangerous to humans because of its potential to induce ventricular fibrillation should a current pass through the heart. High-voltage transmission lines carry current in the hundreds of thousands of volts; neighborhood distribution lines are at approximately 7000 volts that is stepped down to residential electrical service in the United States at 120 and 220 volts. Voltages of greater than 50 are potentially sufficient to overcome skin resistance in humans so even household circuits can produce fatal "shocks." Household service lines are usually insulated, but the distribution lines are not and many electrocutions occur when ladders, antennas, pruning devices, and other conductors inadvertently contact these lines.

Mechanism of Injury

Currents passing through the body can, in addition to affecting cardiac activity, affect other muscles inducing contraction of voluntary muscles. A current flow of 20 mA can cause tetany, 100 mA can cause ventricular fibrillation, while 2 amperes can lead to ventricular standstill. Current passing through the brain can cause seizures. While the internal tissues offer little resistance to electrical current, dry skin has a high resistance. Thus, when a person comes into contact with a sufficient source of current to effect entry, burns may be produced at the point of contact with the electrical source as well as at the point where the current "exits," that is, where the body is grounded to a point of lower electrical potential. Such burns often take a characteristic appearance with a central pale area or blister and a surrounding ring of reddening or erythema. With high current flow, there may be charring at the points of contact (Figure 3-18).

In very high-voltage electrocutions, there may be deep internal injury from the heat generated as the large volume current passes through muscle and other tissues; survivors may require extensive debridement of the damaged areas. Such injuries are a serious risk for lineman and other occupations that work with high-voltage electrical lines.

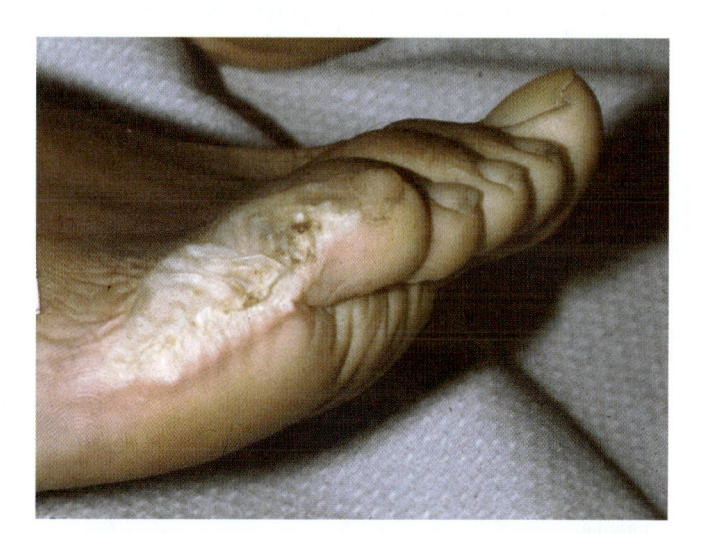

FIGURE 3-18 Electrical burn on the foot of an individual who came into contact with a source of high voltage. There were corresponding burns on the sock and shoe, the point where the individual was grounded. Note the central blistering and surrounding margin of erythema. He had additional burns at the point of contact with the energized wires.

When voltages above 5–700 are involved, actual direct contact with a conductor at high potential is not necessary as the current can jump or "arc" to the point of lower potential.

RADIATION INJURY

Radiation is energy in the form of waves and/or particles traveling through space. It includes electromagnetic energy and particles (alpha and beta particles for example) emitted by radioactive elements and other sources. It can be subdivided into ionizing and nonionizing based on whether the radiation has sufficient energy to remove electrons from atoms or molecules. Ionizing radiation is more likely to cause injury to humans than nonionizing via generation of free radicals and other reactive compounds.

Environmental Radiation

Radiation is ubiquitous in the environment from multiple natural sources primarily cosmic rays from space and naturally occurring radionucleotides. Any individual's exposure to these is determined by geography, for instance, greater at higher altitudes and in areas with more natural radioactive elements in soils, rocks, and water. Stone and brick houses have a higher level of background radiation than wooden ones. Currently about half of the radiation exposure the average person is subject to comes from man-made sources, more than 95% of this from medical procedures. Absent medical sources, the bulk of exposure that the average person is subject to comes from natural sources (especially radon) (Table 3-3).

Radon is an element of particular public health concern because it is present in significant concentrations in rocks in many parts of the world and can accumulate in better-sealed modern structures when it seeps out into soils, air, and water. Radon decay products, radon daughters, are inhaled by the inhabitants of these buildings. *It is believed that radon is the second leading cause of lung cancer behind only cigarette smoking.*

Acute and Chronic Effects of Radiation

Ionizing radiation is measured in terms of the ionization potential—the amount of radiation necessary to create a charge in a volume of matter. Traditionally, this was expressed in roentgens. A more biologically significant measurement is the absorbed dosage or energy deposited. This is expressed in rads or grays (Gy). A Gy is the amount of radiation required to deposit a joule of energy in 1 kg of matter (100 rad = 1 Gy). A rem is the dose of radiation that causes a biological effect equivalent to one rad of x or gamma rays. Another term is the sievert (Sv) that is the absorbed dose in Gy multiplied by a weighting factor to reflect the fact that certain forms of radiation have greater biological effects than others.

High-energy ionizing radiation has the capacity to directly kill cells as well as to produce alterations in DNA by hydrolyzing water creating free radicals. Replicating cells are more sensitive to such damage than those that are not. Thus, many of the manifestations of radiation poisoning appear in the GI tract and hematopoietic systems where normal cellular replication occurs at high rates and whole body radiation is not tolerated as well as localized exposure.

Whole body doses of 200 rem, 2 Sv, can prove fatal from GI and hematopoietic complications over a course of several weeks. Dosages of greater than 1000 rem, 10 Sv, can prove fatal in hours secondary to CNS injury. These conditions are referred to as acute radiation syndrome or radiation sickness (Table 3-4).

The chronic effects of radiation exposure are also dose dependent and primarily involve an increase in the incidence

TABLE 3-3 Sources of radiation exposure in the United States.

Source	Natural Sources (All Radiation) (%)	Man-Made Sources (All Radiation) (%)
Medical procedures		50
Nuclear medicine		12
Consumer products		2
Radon/thoron	37	
Cosmic (space)	5	
Terrestrial (soil)	3	
Internal	5	
Industrial/occupational	0.1	
Total radiation	50 (310 millirem)	50 (310 millirem)

Reprinted with permission of the National Council on Radiation Protection and Measurements, NCRP Report No. 160, http://NCRPpublications.org

TABLE 3-4 Radiation dosage associated with event.

Event	Dose (Millisieverts)
Single dose fatal within weeks	10,000
Single fatal dose exposure at Chernobyl (within 1 month)	6000
Single dose producing nonfatal radiation sickness	1000
Accumulated dosage estimated to cause cancer in 5% of people	1000
Maximum radiation level at Fukushima site (March 2011) per hour	400
Exposure of relocated Chernobyl residents	350
Recommended limit for radiation workers every 5 years	100
Dose in full-body CT scan	10
Mammogram	0.4
Chest X-ray	0.1

WNA, Radiologyinfo.org

of neoplasms. Linked cancers include those of the skin, leukemia, bone, lung, and in children thyroid.

Nonionizing electromagnetic radiation can produce injury mainly through the generation of heat leading to burns. There are concerns about the carcinogenic potential of radio and microwaves but at this time there is no convincing evidence to that effect. The hazards of ultraviolet radiation are well documented and range from the acute agony of sunburn to the changes of premature aging with repeated intense exposures. Basal and squamous cell cancers of the skin are another consequence as well as malignant melanomas. Fair skinned individuals are at much greater risk of these complications than heavily pigmented ones.

Radiation Therapy-Associated Injury

Radiation therapy involves divided, fractionated, doses of up to 80 Gy to localized areas. In addition to the intended target tissue, usually a neoplasm, surrounding normal tissues will be damaged. Vascular injury with thrombosis and resulting ischemic injury leads to fibrosis within the tumor and immediately adjacent tissues. As the beam of ionizing radiation passes through other tissues on its way to the target, those tissues will also incur injury. Radiation-induced pneumonitis, gastritis, proctitis, cystitis, and dermatitis are common complications of radiation therapy when those tissues are in the path of the directed beam or adjacent to implanted radioactive materials, brachytherapy. Delayed complications may be seen as a result of radiation induced fibrosis. Secondary neoplasms can also appear in patients successfully treated with radiation. In the case of Hodgkin disease radiation therapy, an increased risk of neoplasms of the lung, breast, and thyroid has been noted in addition to excess late mortality from cardiac disease. Of note is that younger age at treatment is related to a greater incidence of breast and thyroid cancers in this group reflecting greater organ radiosensitivity in the young.

IATROGENIC INJURY

Iatrogenic injury includes all injuries or illnesses that are caused by medical treatment or diagnostic procedure. By this definition, it encompass some conditions that would not fit within the meaning of trauma and injury that we have used previously in this chapter such as an infection complicating surgery or developing from an indwelling catheter. Considered in a broad perspective, however, iatrogenic injuries are a hazard of a specific "environment" and often do involve external agents in the form of chemicals (therapeutic drugs or solutions), physical manipulations of the patient or radiation. Institute of Medicine reports have identified medication errors as the most common of such events and estimated that tens of thousands of preventable deaths and hundreds of thousands of injuries to patients occur yearly. Regardless of the true numbers incidents of iatrogenic injury are unfortunately not rare and are costly in terms of morbidity and mortality.

Medication errors include administering the wrong drug as well as the right drug in either excessive or inadequate quantity Case 3-5. Drug side effects or reactions that lead to patient injury are not necessarily errors but have similar consequences.

Physical injuries also occur in hospitals, clinics, physician's offices, or other treatment facilities and range from falls to surgical mishaps. All operative and interventional procedures have some degree of inherent risk that must be balanced against their potential benefit to the patient as attested by informed consent documentation. Some errors have occurred so frequently that what seem to be obvious strategies are routinely employed to prevent them. These include placing patient identification bands immediately upon admission to be sure that right person receives the correct medication or goes to the OR. Marking the site of planned procedure to ensure that the right organ or extremity gets operated on is another example. It is a continuing challenge to develop protocols, refine procedures, and implement strategies to ensure that such events do not occur and medicine is actively examining other procedurally oriented disciplines for inspiration.

CASE 3-5

A young child was brought to an ED after a fall leading to a broken arm. The break was realigned and the arm was casted. For pain control, an intramuscular injection of meperidine (Demerol) was administered. A prefilled syringe was employed for the injection. The child was noted to be somnolent at discharge and during the ride home with his parents became unresponsive. He was returned to the ER in cardiorespiratory arrest and could not be resuscitated. The postmortem examination revealed a lethal concentration of hydromorphone (Dilaudid) in his blood. When the medication stocks at the ED were audited, it was found that a 2 mg prefilled syringe of Dilaudid was missing and there was one additional syringe of Demerol present. The medications were stored in alphabetical order by brand name with Demerol next to Dilaudid. Moreover the syringes were of similar size and the labeling also similar in appearance and coloring. Unfortunately, while the meperidine syringe contained a dosage appropriate for a small child, the hydromorphone syringe contained an adult dose.

Errors in medication administration have many causes. In this case, it was a human error that might have been averted if the two medications had not been stored side by side and the syringes in which they were contained had not appeared virtually identical.

Clinical Practice: Anatomic Pathology

CHAPTER 4

William K. Funkhouser, M.D., Ph.D.

THE FIELD OF DIAGNOSTIC ANATOMIC PATHOLOGY

Anatomic pathology is that field of study which describes gross and microscopic anatomic abnormalities in organisms, tissues, and cells, with the goal of diagnosing individual diseases. The field encompasses autopsy pathology, surgical pathology, and cytopathology.

WHAT WE DO

Autopsy pathologists make a set of gross and microscopic diagnoses on a dead patient, and then define the causal relationship between these different diagnoses. For example, if a patient dies in septic shock with renal failure, acute pyelonephritis, lung failure, and mental status changes, then the logical progression of these multiple diseases is "acute pyelonephritis, leading to septic shock and multiorgan (renal, pulmonary, and CNS) failure." The logical ordering of diagnoses requires understanding of the body's normal structure/function, knowledge of the antemortem events, and an ability to integrate these facts with morphologic observations made at the time of autopsy examination. When done correctly, it creates closure for both the family and the treating clinical team, because it coherently explains the disease processes leading to death. TV has made a detective of the autopsy pathologists involved in criminal cases; these **forensic** pathologists do double duty as physicians and expert witnesses when they get drawn into the legal drama of assignment of blame and guilt. Thanks to these portrayals, noncognoscenti in the lay public think that all pathologists are autopsy pathologists. Although the majority of pathologists have had training in the area of autopsy pathology, most of their anatomic pathology effort involves surgical pathology and cytopathology.

WHAT WE DO

Surgical pathologists use the same understanding of the body's normal structure/function, knowledge of concurrent clinical and laboratory abnormalities, and ability to integrate these facts with morphologic observations to make gross and microscopic diagnoses on *living patients who undergo surgical biopsies or resections of abnormal individual organs.* These diagnoses also inform the patient, family, and treating clinical team, and do so at a time when the patient can hopefully be treated to slow or eliminate the disease process.

TV pays no attention to surgical pathologists, even though most pathologists practice surgical pathology. Lawyers, on the other hand, pay close attention to surgical pathologists because of the potentially lucrative monetary awards tied to missed or delayed diagnoses. Surgical pathology is an umbrella field, with specialists for each of the organ systems. Some of these organ systems are sufficiently complex and subtle that they merit case diagnosis by subspecialty-boarded pathologists, for example, **neuropathology**, **hematopathology**, and **dermatopathology**. Hematopathology is a unique subgroup, in that it integrates data from a variety of other sources (flow cytometry, cytogenetics, and molecular pathology) with standard microscopic examination of lymph node, spleen, and marrow.

> **WHAT WE DO**
>
> **Cytopathologists** diagnose diseases based on scant samples that typically show only cellular features, that is, samples lacking elements of tissue architecture. These specimens include **fine needle aspirates** (FNAs), **scrape smears** (think PAP smears), paraffin-embedded **cell blocks**, and **needle cores**.

High-volume fluids, for example, large pleural effusions, can be pelleted by centrifugation, fixed in formalin, embedded in paraffin as cell blocks, then sectioned and stained as are surgical pathology paraffin blocks. Needle cores can be received along with FNA specimens, and do give architectural context to the abnormal cell population. TV pays no attention to cytopathologists, either, even though many pathologists practice cytopathology, but lawyers are interested for the same reasons as above.

SUMMARY

To summarize, anatomic pathology is an umbrella set of diagnostic specialties that includes the following:

- **Autopsy pathology:** The entire deceased person is available for diagnosis.
- **Surgical pathology:** Limited specimens including biopsies and resections from living persons are available for diagnosis.
- **Cytopathology:** Very limited specimens with limited or no architectural context from living persons are available for diagnosis.

CURRENT PRACTICE OF DIAGNOSTIC ANATOMIC PATHOLOGY

Diseases can be distinguished from each other based on differences at the molecular, cellular, tissue, fluid chemistry, and/or individual organism level. One-hundred fifty years of attention to the morphologic and clinical correlates of diseases has led to sets of clinical, radiographic, pathologic, and laboratory diagnostic criteria for the recognized diseases, as well as a reproducible nomenclature for rapid description of the changes associated with newly discovered diseases. The set of genotypic and phenotypic abnormalities in the patient is used to determine the diagnosis, which then infers a predictable natural history, and which can be used to optimize therapy by comparison of outcomes among similarly-afflicted individuals. The disease diagnosis becomes the management variable in clinical medicine, and management of the clinical manifestations of diseases is the basis for day-to-day activities in clinics and hospitals nationwide. The pathologist is responsible for integration of the data obtained at the clinical, radiographic, gross, microscopic, and molecular levels, and for issuing a clear and logical statement of diagnoses in a timely fashion.

Clinically, diseases present to front-line physicians as patients with sets of signs and symptoms. **Symptoms** are the patient's complaints of perceived abnormalities. **Signs** are detected by examination of the patient. The clinical team, including the pathologist, "works up" the patient based on the possible causes of the signs and symptoms (the **"differential diagnosis"**). Depending on the differential diagnosis, the **workup** typically involves history taking, physical examination, radiographic examination, fluid tests (blood, urine, sputum, stool), and possibly tissue biopsy.

Radiographically, abnormalities in abundance, density, or chemical microenvironment of tissues allow distinction from surrounding normal tissues. Traditionally (since Roentgen's discoveries in the late 19th century), imaging technology was based on differential absorption of electromagnetic waves by tissues that led to summation differences in exposure of silver salt photographic films and, now, digital detectors. Tomographic approaches such as CT (described in 1972) and NMR/MRI (described in 1973) complement summation radiology, allowing finely detailed visualization of internal anatomy in any plane of section. In this modern era, ultrasound allows visualization of tissue with acoustic density differences, for example, a developing fetus or gallbladder stones. Most recently, physiology of neoplasms can be screened with **positron emission tomography** PET (described in 1977) for decay of short half-life isotopes such as fluorodeoxyglucose. Neoplasms with high metabolism can be distinguished physiologically from adjacent low-metabolism tissues, and can be localized with respect to normal tissues by pairing PET with standard CT. *The result is an astonishingly useful means of identifying and localizing new space-occupying masses, assigning a risk for malignant behavior and, if malignant, screening for metastases in distant sites.* This technique is revolutionizing the preoperative decision-making of clinical teams, and improves the likelihood that patients undergo resections of new mass lesions only when at risk of morbidity from malignant behavior or interference with normal function.

Pathologically, disease is diagnosed by identifying gross and microscopic abnormalities, then determining whether these morphologic findings match the set of diagnostic criteria previously described for each disease. Multivolume texts are devoted to the epidemiology, clinical presentation, and gross/microscopic diagnostic criteria used for diagnosis, prognosis, and prediction of response to therapy. Pathologists diagnose disease by generating a differential diagnosis, then finding the best fit for the clinical presentation, the radiographic appearance, and the pathologic (both clinical laboratory and morphologic) findings. Logically, this "Venn diagram" of the clinical, radiologic, and pathologic differential diagnoses should overlap. Unexpected features expand the differential diagnosis, and may raise the possibility of previously undescribed diseases. For example, Legionnaire's disease, human immunodeficiency virus (HIV), Hantavirus pneumonia, and severe acute respiratory syndrome (SARS) are examples of newly described diagnoses in the last 40 years.

The mental construct of **etiology** (cause), **pathogenesis** (progression), **natural history** (clinical outcome), and **response to therapy** is the standard approach for pathologists thinking about a disease. The **prognosis** reflects the integration of the expected natural history and the expected response to therapy. A disease may have one or more etiologies (initial causes, e.g., agents, toxins, mutagens, drugs, allergens, trauma, or genetic mutations). A disease is expected to follow a particular series of events in its development (pathogenesis), and to follow a particular clinical course (natural history). Disease can result in a temporary or lasting change in normal function, including patient death. Multiple diseases of different etiologies can affect a single organ, for example, infectious and neoplastic diseases involving the lung. Different diseases can derive from a single etiology, for example, emphysema, chronic bronchitis, and small cell lung carcinoma in long-term smokers. The same disease (e.g., emphysema of the lung) can derive from different etiologies (e.g., emphysema from either alpha-1-antitrypsin deficiency or cigarette smoke).

Modern diagnostic anatomic pathology practice hinges on morphologic diagnosis using the **hematoxylin and eosin (H&E) stain**, supplemented by special stains, immunohistochemical stains, cytogenetics, and clinical laboratory findings, as well as the concurrent clinical and radiographic findings. Sections that meet all of these criteria are diagnostic for the disease. If some, but not all, of the criteria are present that are required to make a definitive diagnosis, the pathologist must either equivocate or make an alternate diagnosis. Thus, a firm grasp of the diagnostic criteria, and the instincts to rapidly create and sort through the differential diagnosis, must be possessed by the diagnostic pathologist.

The pathologic diagnosis has to make sense, not only from the morphologic perspective but also from the clinical and radiographic vantage points as well. It is both legally risky and professionally damaging to make a clinically and pathologically impossible diagnosis. In the recent past, limited computer networking meant numerous phone calls to gather the relevant clinical and radiographic information to make an informed morphologic diagnosis. For example, certain diseases such as squamous and small cell carcinomas of the lung are extremely rare in nonsmokers, such that a small cell carcinoma in the lung of a nonsmoker would merit screening for a non-pulmonary primary site of origin. Fortunately for pathologists, computing and networking technologies now allow us access to pre-op clinical workups, radiographs/reports, clinical lab data, and prior pathology reports. All of these data protect pathologists by providing them with the relevant clinical and radiographic information, and protect patients by improving diagnostic accuracy. *Just as research scientists "ignore the literature at their peril," diagnostic pathologists "ignore the presentation, past history, clinical workup, radiographs, and prior biopsies at their peril."*

Beyond H&E: Techniques in Tissue Analysis

A wealth of information is conveyed to a service pathologist in a tried-and-true H&E section. Analogous to the fact that a plain chest X-ray is the sum total of all densities in the beam path, the morphologic changes in diseased cells and tissues are the morphologic sum total of all of the disequilibria in the abnormal cells. For most neoplastic diseases, morphologic criteria are sufficient to predict the risk of invasion and metastasis (the malignant potential), the pattern of metastases, and the likely clinical outcomes. For example, the etiology and pathogenesis in small cell lung carcinoma can be inferred (cigarette smoking, with carcinogen-induced genetic mutations), and the outcome predicted (early metastasis to regional nodes and distant organs, with high probability of death within 5 years of diagnosis).

However, there are limitations to morphologic diagnosis by H&E stains.

- The lineage of certain classes of neoplasms, for example, "small round blue cell tumors," "clear cell" neoplasms, "spindle cell" neoplasms, and "undifferentiated" malignant neoplasms, is usually clarified by immunohistochemistry, frequently clarified by cytogenetics, and sometimes clarified by transmission electron microscopy (TEM).
- There are limitations inherent in a "snap-shot" biopsy or resection. The etiology and pathogenesis can be obscure or indeterminate, and rates of growth, invasion, or timing of metastasis cannot be inferred.
- Observed morphologic changes may not be specific for the underlying molecular abnormalities, particularly the rate-limiting (therapeutic target) step in the pathogenesis of a neoplasm. For example, *RET* gain of function mutations in a medullary thyroid carcinoma will require DNA level screening to determine germ line involvement, familial risk, and presence or absence of a therapeutic target.
- The morphologic appearance may be identical for two different diseases, each of which would be treated differently. For example, H&E stain of a liver allograft biopsy cannot morphologically distinguish the host lymphoid response to hepatitis C antigens from the host lymphoid response to allo-HLA antigens. This is obviously a major diagnostic challenge if the transplant was done for hepatitis C cirrhosis, knowing that the probability of recurrent hepatitis C virus infection in the liver allograft is high.

Immunohistochemical Techniques

Paraffin section **immunohistochemistry** (using antibodies of known specificity on tissue sections) has proven invaluable in neoplasm diagnosis for clarifying lineage, improving diagnostic accuracy, and guiding customized therapy. If neoplasms are poorly differentiated or undifferentiated, the lineage of the neoplasm may not be clear. For example, sheets of undifferentiated malignant neoplasm with prominent nucleoli could represent undifferentiated carcinoma, large cell or anaplastic lymphoma, or melanoma. To clarify lineage, a panel of immunostains is performed for proteins that are expressed in some of the neoplasms, but not in others. Relative probabilities are then used to lend support ("rule in") or exclude ("rule out") particular diagnoses in the differential diagnosis of these several morphologically similar undifferentiated neoplasms.

Immunohistochemistry can help to make critical distinctions in diagnosis that cannot be accurately made by H&E alone. Examples of this would include demonstration of myoepithelial cell loss in invasive breast carcinoma but not in its mimic, sclerosing adenosis, or the loss of basal cells in invasive prostate carcinoma.

Another role of immunohistochemistry is to identify particular proteins, for example, nuclear estrogen receptor (ER) or the plasma membrane HER2 proteins, both of which can be targeted with inhibitors rather than non-specific systemic chemotherapy. *H&E morphology currently remains the gold standard in this diagnostic process, such that immunohistochemical data support or fail to support the H&E findings, not vice versa.*

Probability and statistics are regular considerations in immunohistochemical interpretation, since very few antigens are tissue- or lineage-specific. Cytokeratin is not only positive in carcinomas but also in synovial and epithelioid sarcomas. Immunohistochemistry results are always put into the context of the morphologic, clinical, and radiographic findings. For example, an undifferentiated CD30(+) neoplasm of the testis supports embryonal carcinoma primary in the testis, whereas a lymph node effaced by sclerotic bands with admixed CD30(+) Reed–Sternberg cells supports nodular sclerosing Hodgkin's disease.

New molecular data for both neoplastic and non-neoplastic diseases will most likely benefit unaffected individuals by estimating disease risk, and will most likely benefit patients by defining the molecular subset for morphologically defined diagnostic entities, thus guiding individualized therapy.

Errors in Pathology Practice

We are human, and all humans make **errors**. Anatomic pathologists have specialty board recognition of expertise in gross and microscopic diagnosis. During their practice careers in service pathology, they will add to their fund of knowledge an appreciation of morphologic subtlety, overlap of sets of diagnostic criteria, probabilities of certain diseases as a function of age/race/sex/location, test performance, and potential pitfalls. *Such hard-won experience sometimes comes by way of making errors.* Errors can be as mundane as a clinic's mislabeling of the specimen (a **clerical error**) before it is accessioned in the pathology department. Such an error is not the pathologist's fault, but it is the pathologist's responsibility to detect and correct it. Ideally, such a **pre-analytical error** would be detected by the accessioning technician, who would resolve the error with the submitting clinic. If the mislabeling error makes it past the accessioning window, then it becomes the responsibility of the gross room personnel (for surgical pathology), cyto prep personnel (for cytopathology), histology technicians (for histology), or the sign-out diagnostic pathologist to detect the problem, based on discrepancies related to history, organ, amount, gross appearance, or microscopic determination of organ of origin. Pathology accessioning, **grossing** (the trimming and dissection of submitted specimens so as to provide samples suitable for histopathological processing and analysis), and cyto prep personnel can make these same mislabeling errors after taking possession of the clinical specimen, and such clerical errors (regardless of source) can be difficult or impossible for the diagnostic pathologist to detect. It is easy to imagine how such a stealth error could make it past the entire pathology team when a bolus of biopsies from eight different heart transplant patients all get accessioned the same morning, and all submitted biopsies have equal numbers of similar-appearing myocardium. Another example would be receipt of a set of 8–12 endoscopic biopsies of colon from a patient, say, Ms. Johnson, who has inflammatory bowel disease (IBD). Common names predispose to clinic mislabeling of specimens with the identifiers of a different, but identically named, person. Pathology's accessioning personnel would never detect such a clerical error, and it may come to our attention months later when we are called by a treating clinician that his Ms. Johnson does not have IBD and did not have biopsies. If a question of specimen misidentification is raised, then molecular methods based on DNA microsatellite length polymorphisms can be used to distinguish tissues from different humans.

Patients depend on us to keep careful track of specimen identity, so practicing pathologists in anatomic pathology, just as in those in clinical labs (e.g., transfusion medicine, hematology, chemistry, and microbiology), are aggressive about recognizing and resolving errors related to specimen misidentification. It goes without saying that in a court of law, there is no defense for a clerical error related to specimen misidentification.

In addition to clerical error, an anatomic pathologist can make a **sampling error**, for example, randomly not sampling the invisible carcinoma in a frozen section specimen (obtained for rapid intra-operative diagnosis), only to find carcinoma the next day in the formalin-fixed permanent specimen derived from the original frozen specimen. In both the frozen section room and in daily sign-out of permanent (formalin-fixed, paraffin-embedded) sections, there is always the possibility of misinterpretation (**cognitive error, interpretive error**). Misinterpretation in the frozen section room can lead to unnecessary or incorrect surgical procedures, and misinterpretation of permanent sections can lead to unnecessary or incorrect medical or surgical therapies. Hence, errors in anatomic pathology can lead to unnecessary procedures, cost, and/or patient morbidity, such that error reduction efforts deserve serious attention.

The worst-case scenario is when the diagnostic sign-out pathologist does not recognize the error, and generates a final diagnostic report that is electronically embedded in the computerized clinical records. Treating clinicians assume that our final reports are accurate; in the case of an incorrectly labeled or misinterpreted specimen, treating clinicians unknowingly read, integrate, and make treatment plans based on an inaccurate diagnosis.

> **WHAT WE DO**
> To minimize the risk of errors, all accessioning, grossing, and histology personnel, as well as all sign-out diagnostic pathologists, are trained to do their jobs on only one case at a time, to have a healthy respect for human errors, to show potential problems to more-experienced colleagues, and to face near-misses and actual errors head-on and quickly. When the sign-out pathologist becomes aware of an error, the error is discussed directly with the treating clinician, reported in a revised report, and discussed candidly in a regular departmental morbidity and mortality (M&M) conference. In this way, recurring errors of a particular type can be used to identify systematic problems that can be resolved.

FUTURE PRACTICE OF DIAGNOSTIC ANATOMIC PATHOLOGY

Diagnostic anatomic pathology will continue to use morphology and complementary data from protein (immunohistochemical) and nucleic acid (cytogenetics, in situ hybridization, DNA sequence, and RNA abundance) screening assays. Data derived from both current and new technologies will be integrated into the diagnostic process in order to reduce the cost and turnaround time while improving diagnostic accuracy and utility. Some of the newer diagnostic technologies of significance to pathologists follow.

Smaller Diagnostic Biopsies with Larger Clinical Significance

Since the advent of flexible endoscopy in the 1980s, CT-guided percutaneous techniques in the 1990s, and PET (metabolic) imaging for localization and staging in the 2000s, the trend has been for surgical pathologists to receive smaller and smaller specimens for initial diagnosis of new neoplasms. For example, a patient with a 15 cm diameter soft tissue mass deep in the thigh may be biopsied by percutaneous needle core using CT guidance, generating a 0.1 cm × 1.5 cm diameter core of the neoplasm. The reader will recognize the challenge of extrapolating from findings on a tiny core to a large heterogeneous mass. However, this is exactly what is required in daily practice: pre-resection ("neoadjuvant") chemotherapy and radiotherapy protocols hinge on these needle core diagnoses, and treatment(s) can markedly distort the morphology of the remaining neoplasm.

Integrated Testing

Breast carcinoma is the prototype for molecular subtyping, with major groups being either ER/PR (+), HER2(+), or triple negative [ER(–), PR (–), and HER2 (–)]. Other solid tumors are now being subdivided into analogous molecular subgroups for trial testing of new therapies based on specific molecular lesions. An example would be non-small cell lung carcinoma, in which epithelial growth factor receptor (EGFR) mutant adenocarcinomas can be treated effectively with tyrosine kinase inhibitors. *To identify this minor subset of non-small cell lung carcinomas, we now reflexively test all non-squamous non-small cell lung carcinomas for EGFR mutations, KRAS mutations, and ALK gene rearrangements at the time of original diagnosis.* This integration of molecular, cytogenetic, and morphologic features gives the treating clinical team a better understanding not only of the parent disease type, but also of the particular molecular subgroup, as they decide on therapy.

Individual Identity Determination

For transplant candidates, major histocompatibility complex [MHC; human leukocyte antigen (HLA) in human] screening is evolving from cellular assays and serology toward sequencing of the alleles of the class I and II HLA loci. Rapid sequencing of these alleles in newborn cord blood allows for databasing of the population's haplotypes, facilitating perfect matches for solid organ and bone marrow transplants. In parallel, PCR amplification of highly polymorphic DNA "microsatellite" repeat sequences can be used to distinguish two humans with certainty. This technology allows accurate measurement of allo-bone marrow engraftment, and can also be used in surgical pathology and cytopathology to resolve questions about possible specimen mis-identification, as noted above.

Rapid Cytogenetics

Current uses of in situ fluorescence and colorimetric hybridization techniques (FISH and CISH) to screen for viruses (e.g., EBV), light chain restriction (in B lymphomas), and copy number variation (e.g., HER2 gene amplification) demonstrate the benefit of in situ nucleic acid hybridization assays. It is possible that interphase FISH/CISH will become rapid enough to be used in the initial diagnostic workup, for example, for neoplasm-specific translocations, ploidy analysis and gene amplification of receptor tyrosine kinase genes.

Rapid Nucleic Acid Sequence and RNA Abundance Screening

Current uses of nucleic acid screening for *BCR-ABL* translocations (see Chapter 14), donor:recipient ratios after bone marrow transplant, microsatellite instability in colon and endometrial carcinomas, quantitative viral load, and single gene mutations demonstrate the benefit of nucleic acid screening in diagnosis

CASE 4-1

ILLUSTRATIVE CASE

A 82-year-old man ex-smoker (40 pack-years, quit 30 years ago) presents with a 1-month history of intermittent memory difficulties and progressive headache. Brain MRI showed a 5.2-cm diameter heterogeneous solid and cystic mass in the left temporal lobe. Chest CT showed a 1-cm diameter right upper lobe nodule. Cell block of the cytology specimen from the cystic mass is shown in **Figure 4-1A**. H&E stain of the biopsy

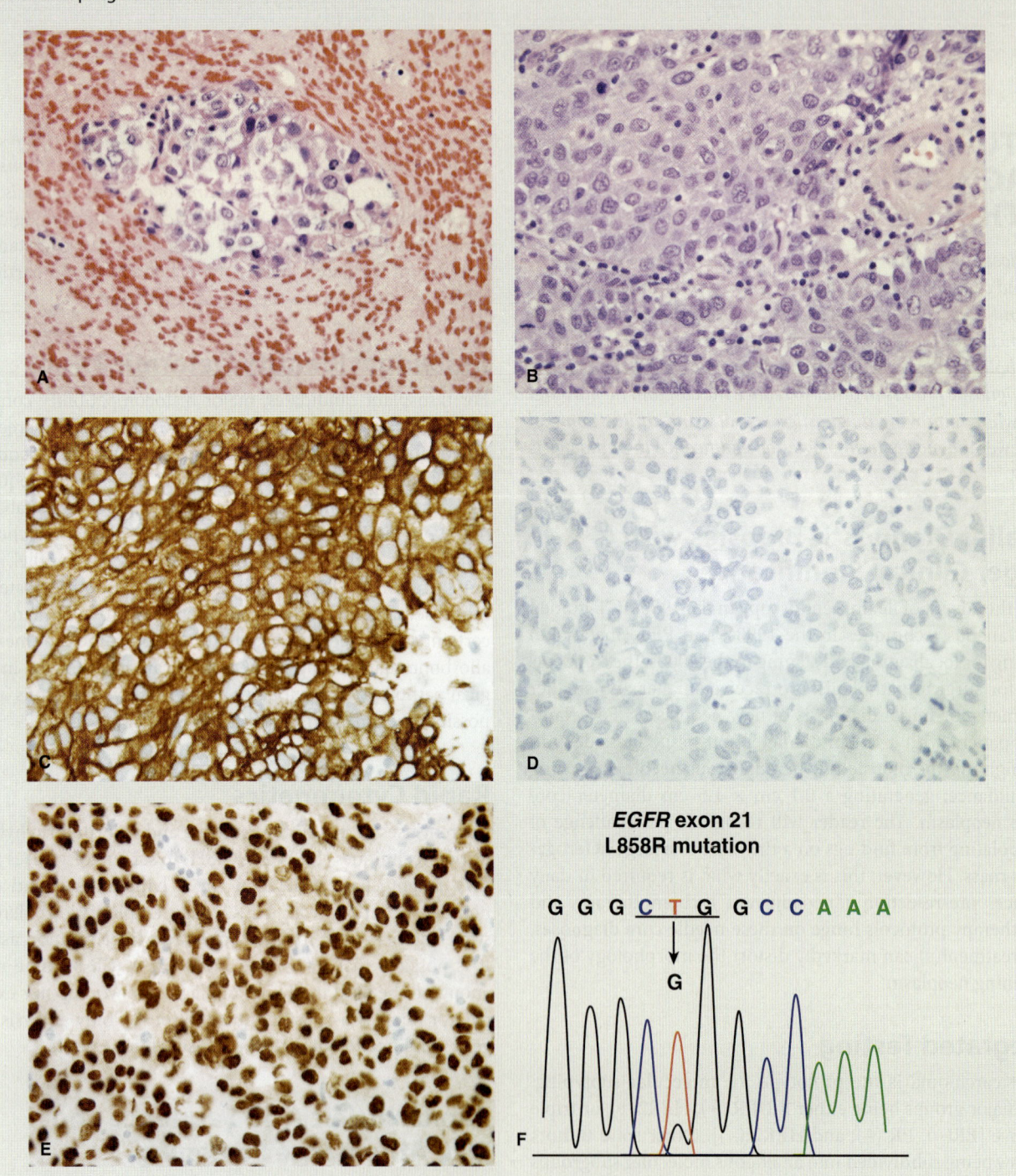

FIGURE 4-1 Description of illustrative case. **(A)** An H&E of the cell block derived from a cytology specimen of the cystic mass. **(B)** A section of the brain biopsy. **(C)** Positive immunostaining for cytokeratin CK7. **(D)** Negative staining for cytokeratin CK20. **(E)** Positive staining for TTF-1. **(F)** A small portion of the Sanger sequence for *EGFR* exon 21, showing one of the two common activating mutations in EGFR-mutant lung adenocarcinomas. The arrow indicates the missense mutation. Source of 1 A-E: W.K. Funkhouser; Source of 1 F: De Oliveira Duarte Achcar R, Nikiforova MN, Yousem SA. Micropapillary Lung Adenocarcinoma, AJCP 2009 131:694-700.

of the brain lesion is shown in Figure 4-1B, with immunostains for CK7, CK20, and TTF-1 shown in panels Figure 4-1C–E. Figure 4-1F shows a portion of the Sanger sequence of *EGFR* exon 21, with an arrow showing the point mutation T ≥ G at position 2573 (c.2573T > G); this coding sequence mutation would result in an amino acid substitution of leucine to arginine (L ≥ R) at EGFR codon 858 (p.L858R)858 (p.L858R).

The immunostaining in this case argues for a metastasis derived from a non-small cell lung carcinoma, specifically an adenocarcinoma. TTF-1 positivity is lineage specific for cells derived from the thyroid and the terminal respiratory unit and is most frequently associated with pulmonary adenocarcinomas. The observation of CK7 positive and CK20 negative staining (as seen in this case) lends additional support to the diagnosis of a metastasis derived from a pulmonary adenocarcinoma. About 20% of such tumors demonstrate mutations of the *EGFR* gene. Patients demonstrating this particular mutation in exon 21 of *EGFR* (L858R) are candidates for first-line treatment with erlotinib, an EGFR inhibitor that has been shown to be effective in prolonging progression-free survival in patients. Hence, this example of integrated testing has revealed an important potential therapeutic option for the patient.

and management. It is possible that each new solid or hematopoietic neoplasm will be promptly defined as to ploidy, translocations, gene copy number differences, DNA mutations, and RNA (both micro and messenger) expression cluster subset, allowing more accurate and rapid diagnosis, individualized therapy, and sensitive residual disease screening. Although neoplasms are likely to be heterogeneous, deep-sequencing techniques may be able to define "driver" mutations that can serve as the starting point for individualized chemotherapy.

Computer-Based Prognosis and Prediction

Current uses of morphology, immunohistochemistry, and molecular pathology demonstrate their benefit through improved diagnostic accuracy. However, diagnosis, extent of disease, and molecular subsets are currently imperfect estimators of prognosis and response to therapy. Relational databases that correlate an individual's demographic data, family history, concurrent diseases, morphologic features, immunophenotype, and molecular subset, and which also integrate disease prevalence by age, sex, and ethnicity using Bayesian probabilities, should improve accuracy of prognosis and prediction of response to therapy. As risk correlates are developed, it is possible that healthy individuals will be screened and given risk estimates for development of different diseases.

Serum Biomarkers

Current clinical use of prostate-specific antigen (PSA) to screen for prostate carcinoma, AFP to screen for yolk sac tumor, hCG to screen for choriocarcinoma, and catecholamines to screen for pheochromocytoma demonstrates the benefit of serum biomarkers in detection of neoplasms and monitoring of their response to treatment. It is likely that high-sensitivity screening of single and clustered serum analytes using proteomic and metabolomic technologies will lead to improved methods for early detection of neoplasms, autoimmune diseases, and infections.

SUMMARY

An anatomic pathologist uses gross and microscopic observations to diagnose diseases. Pathologic description and diagnosis are the *lingua franca* of clinical medicine, and so are foundational elements of medical education. The key concepts of thinking about any disease process are its *etiology* (initial cause), *pathogenesis* (stepwise progression), *natural history* (clinical outcome), *response to therapy*, and *prognosis* (integration of the expected natural history and the expected response to therapy). Ideally, disease diagnosis is reproducible through use of specific diagnostic criteria at the clinical, radiologic, lab, and morphologic levels, such that all members of the clinical team are confident in the diagnosis prior to therapy initiation. Morphologic diagnosis frequently drives therapy, such that anatomic pathologists' diagnostic reports inform the minds, and guide the hands, of the treating clinical teams. Assuming that we can figure out how to analyze scant numbers of cells, the future is bright with the expectation that rapid resequencing and cytogenetic technologies will provide complementary diagnostic, prognostic, and predictive data at the time of initial diagnosis.

Clinical Practice: Molecular Pathology

Margaret L. Gulley

CHAPTER 5

CASE STUDY

A 30-year-old man developed liver cirrhosis and diabetes. Laboratory studies showing high serum ferritin and high transferrin saturation led to the hypothesis that iron toxicity to the liver and pancreas contributed to his cirrhosis and diabetes. A blood specimen was tested for mutation in the *HFE* gene that is responsible, at least in part, for hereditary hemochromatosis. Polymerase chain reaction (PCR) followed by melt curve analysis was performed, and a pathologist interpreted the findings as *HFE* C282Y mutation without wild-type DNA at that locus. Homozygous *HFE* gene mutation with the predicted amino acid substitution predisposes to iron overload by overabsorption of iron from the diet. He was treated with therapeutic phlebotomy until his serum iron levels returned to the normal range. He remains at risk for iron overload, and he should be periodically monitored and managed accordingly. A genetic counselor educated him about the increased risk of iron overload faced by blood relatives if they, too, inherited two mutated alleles of the *HFE* gene.

The practice of molecular pathology capitalizes on analysis of deoxyribonucleic acid (DNA) and ribonucleic acid (RNA) to inform medical decision making. Each nucleated cell in the body contains a complete set of DNA inherited from parents, constituting the person's *genome*. DNA is the blueprint by which cells catalog, express, and transmit genetic information. The human genome is composed of 3 billion pairs of nucleotides divided among 46 chromosomes containing about 25,000 different protein-coding genes plus additional genes encoding RNA that is not translated into protein. There are two copies of every gene—one of paternal and the other of maternal origin. Transcription factors act on gene promoters to regulate gene transcription, as do chromatin modifications such as DNA methylation and histone acetylation.

MOLECULAR TECHNOLOGIES

Molecular assays rely on the ability to find a specific nucleotide sequence in DNA or RNA by using a nucleic acid probe targeting that sequence. A probe is a single-stranded segment of nucleic acid whose nucleotide sequence is complementary to the target sequence of interest. A probe binds to its target through a process called *hybridization*, and then the probe is detected or its effects (e.g., priming DNA synthesis) are evaluated using various detection strategies (see **Figure 5-1**).

> ### QUICK REVIEW
> The molecular technologies most commonly implemented in clinical settings are PCR, *in situ* hybridization, DNA sequencing, Southern blot analysis, and array technology. Benchwork is performed by medical technologists, while pathologists and other clinical laboratory scientists are responsible for interpreting findings and for consulting with health-care providers on the indications of testing and the medical implications of results.

MEDICAL APPLICATIONS OF MOLECULAR TECHNOLOGY

Analysis of nucleic acid sequences in patient samples helps in diagnosis, classification, prognosis, predicting efficacy of therapy, documenting response to therapy, monitoring disease burden, identifying relapse, and screening for disease in high-risk populations. The range of diseases is quite broad and includes heritable disease, cancer, and infectious disease. Heritable disease is, by definition, a disorder resulting from abnormal DNA (chromosomal DNA or mitochondrial DNA). Cancers harbor acquired genetic changes that are responsible for malignant behavior, such as an activated oncogene or an inactivated tumor suppressor gene driving cell proliferation. Finding a tumor-related molecular defect can help confirm a diagnosis of cancer and can further serve as a tumor marker for monitoring disease burden during therapy. For infectious disease diagnosis, each pathogen has its own genome composed of DNA or RNA for which molecular assays may indicate the presence of, amount of, and drug-resistance sequences encoded by a given microbial agent. Drug efficacy or toxicity might be influenced by sequence variants encoding factors important in drug metabolism, distribution, or effectiveness. A pharmacogenetic test can predict which drug

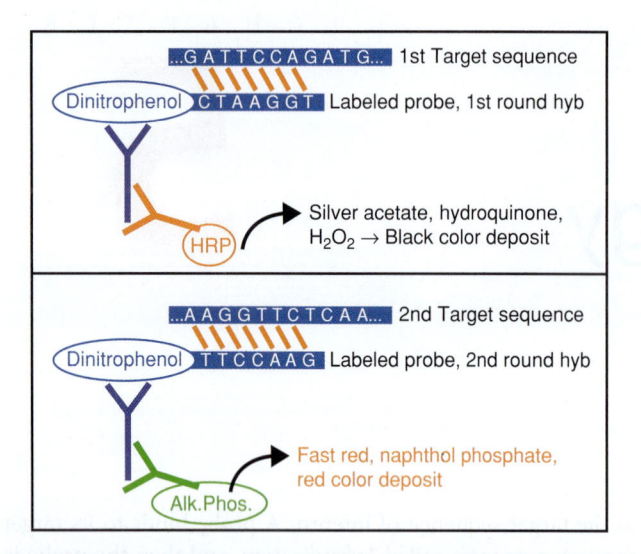

FIGURE 5-1 DNA is composed of complementary strands of nucleotides that are connected by hydrogen bonds between adenine (A) and thymine (T), or between guanine (G) and cytosine (C). In the laboratory, the two strands of DNA may be dissociated from one another by heating them to near boiling (94ºC) or by treating with an alkaline solution (high pH). Single-stranded patient nucleic acid may then hybridize to a complementary probe. In the examples depicted here, labeled probes hybridize to target sequences in patient DNA, and then a detection system deposits black or red chromagen at the locus where the probe is bound.

or dose of drug is most likely to improve outcome in a given patient.

Specimen Preparation

Specimens submitted to a clinical laboratory for genetic testing are collected and handled with care to preserve intact DNA and RNA for downstream analysis. DNA and RNA can be extracted from a wide range of specimens (e.g., blood, marrow and other body fluids, frozen or formalin fixed paraffin embedded tissue, buccal swabs, and needle aspirates) by first using detergent and proteinase enzymes to lyse cellular lipid membranes and degrade proteins. Semiautomated instruments facilitate further purification of DNA or RNA based on preferential binding to a glass or similar surface. DNA and RNA are quantified by spectrophotometry. While DNA is relatively stable, RNA is unstable by virtue of its susceptibility to degradation by ubiquitous enzymes collectively termed *RNase*. Special precautions are required to assure the integrity and quality of nucleic acid from the time of collection through the various hybridization procedures described below. Instructions for collection, transport, and storage of specimens are provided by the testing laboratory.

LABORATORY PROCEDURES

Polymerase Chain Reaction

PCR is a method of replicating a short sequence of DNA, typically about 100 bases in length, so that it may be more easily detected, quantified, or further analyzed for genetic alterations. Although several other technologies have been invented to amplify nucleic acid sequences or probe signals, PCR remains the most commonly used analytic method in molecular testing laboratories (see Figure 5-2).

PCR is the technology of choice among pathologists because of (1) exquisite sensitivity to low numbers of target sequences, (2) small sample size requirement (theoretically only one molecule), and (3) speedy and relatively inexpensive automated test systems. The major disadvantage is the extreme care required to avoid contamination of samples and reagents by extraneous DNA. Abundant amplicons generated from previous reactions are especially concerning, and strategies have been developed to fragment these potential contaminants. Physical separation of pre- and post-amplification work areas is recommended.

Interestingly, the DNA polymerase used in PCR reactions is "thermostable," meaning that it can endure near-boiling temperatures and still remain active. This feature allows the reaction to continue during repeated cycles of heating and cooling without significant loss of enzymatic function. The polymerase is derived from bacteria such as *Thermus aquaticus* (*Taq*) that evolutionarily adapted to live around geysers or hot springs.

Variations on PCR Reactions

In *real-time PCR,* one or two fluorescent internal probes are added to the mixture so that they may mark amplified products to be quantified by a sensor during every amplification cycle. By comparing results to a series of standards, one can extrapolate how much target DNA was present in the original sample. This procedure may also be called *quantitative PCR* (see Figure 5-3).

Reverse transcription PCR (rtPCR) is a common method to detect and measure RNA. First, extracted RNA is converted to complementary DNA (cDNA) by the enzyme reverse transcriptase, and then PCR amplifies a segment of the cDNA. By designing PCR primers to bind in exons flanking a large intron, one can distinguish cDNA from native DNA. Other RNA-based detection methods include nucleic acid sequence-based amplification (NASBA), transcription-mediated amplification (TMA), and array-based technologies such as the Nanostring nCounter system. Any of these methods can be used to measure gene expression, or to detect RNA viruses such as HIV, hepatitis C, or HTLV1.

In *multiplex PCR,* two different target DNAs are amplified in the same reaction. The second reaction is typically a control amplification of an endogenous or spiked DNA that serves to verify that extraction and amplification worked as expected.

In *meltcurve analysis,* a mutation is predicted when an internal probe is shown to melt away from its complementary strand at an abnormal temperature. The probe melting process is accomplished in the same reaction vessel in which the PCR

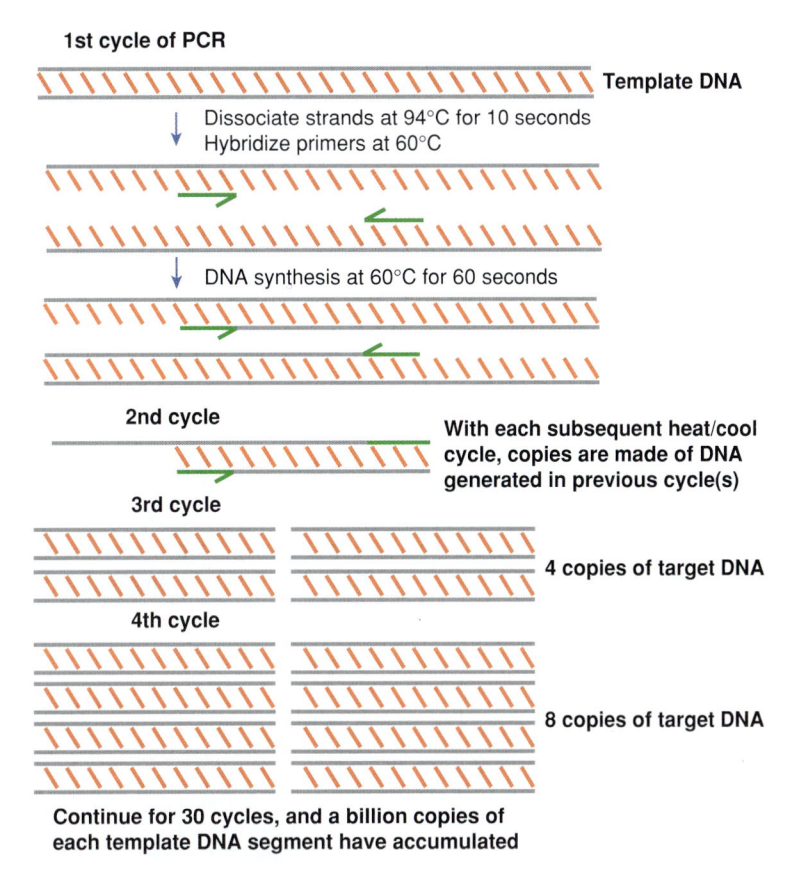

FIGURE 5-2 *PCR is a method of enzymatically amplifying a particular segment of DNA through a process of repeated cycles of heating, cooling, and DNA synthesis in an instrument called a thermocycler.* First, patient DNA is mixed with two short oligonucleotide probes called primers (green half-arrows) that define the segment to be amplified. Also in the mix is an enzyme called DNA polymerase that begins at the 3′ end of the primer and proceeds to incorporate nucleotides to make double-stranded DNA. In each cycle of the reaction, the sample is first heated to dissociate the two strands, then cooled to facilitate primer binding and initiation of enzymatic DNA replication. In each cycle, the products of previous cycles serve as templates, permitting exponential accumulation of replicate DNA copies. After 30 cycles, which takes only a couple of hours, up to 2^{30} (about a billion) copies of the DNA segment have been generated. Depending on the purpose of the test, the PCR products are then detected, quantified, or further analyzed for sequence variants.

was done, thus minimizing the risk of amplicon contamination by containing all amplicons in a sealed vessel (see **Figure 5-4**).

Clinical utility of PCR is well established to (1) diagnose or monitor infectious disease by amplifying the foreign nucleic acid, and detecting sequences associated with antibiotic resistance; (2) detect a particular cancer-associated defect, such as activating *JAK2* point mutation in myeloproliferative disease, or clonal T cell receptor gene rearrangement in T cell lymphoma; (3) measure residual disease post-therapy by amplifying a disease-specific molecular marker, such as *PML–RARA* fusion transcripts in acute promyelocytic leukemia patients; (4) determine pharmacogenetic markers to help select a drug regimen or dose, such as a tyrosine kinase inhibitor drug for leukemia harboring *BCR–ABL1*; (5) detect congenital defects of fetal DNA enriched from maternal blood; (6) perform identity testing for forensic investigations, engraftment assessment of an allogeneic stem cell transplant, or helping match samples to their source.

In Situ Hybridization

In situ hybridization permits localization of particular sequences within cells or tissues immobilized on glass slides. This procedure begins with protease and detergent treatment to permeabilize cell membranes, rendering the target DNA or RNA accessible to a labeled probe that is added in excess. The probe can vary from 20 to over a million bases in length and is complementary to the sequence of interest. After probe hybridization, unbound probe is washed away, and bound probe is then localized using signal detection chemistry. Counterstaining facilitates microscopic visualization of the labeled probe in the context of histologic features and cytologic detail (see **Figure 5-5**). Theoretically, a single copy of target sequence is detectable using brightfield microscopy. Duplexing by simultaneous or sequential hybridization to two different probes, each with a different label, can help colocalize two targets (see Figures 5-1 and **5-6**).

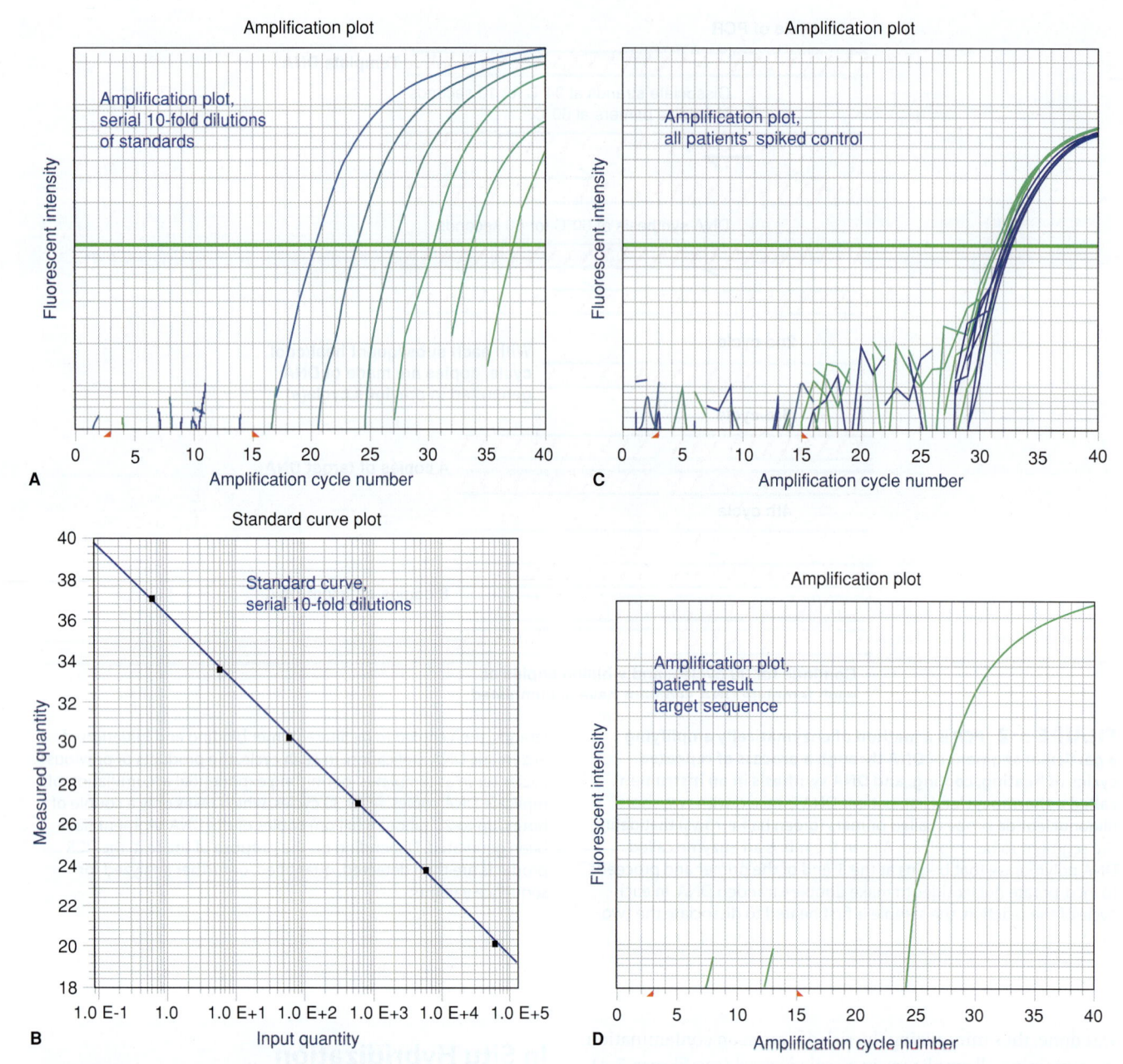

FIGURE 5-3 Real-time PCR is a technology to precisely measure amount of DNA template in a patient sample by monitoring the amount of fluorescence at the end of each amplification cycle in comparison to a series of standards of known DNA level. A sensor detects signal from a fluorochrome-labeled internal probe that hybridizes to PCR products during each cycle, and results are visualized on amplification plots (**A, C, D**) and a standard curve (**B**). The cycle number at which the fluorescence signal crosses the intensity threshold (green line) is inversely related to the initial DNA concentration. Serial dilutions demonstrate assay sensitivity and linearity across five orders of magnitude (**A,B**). A spiked control is recovered in equivalent amounts across all patient specimens in the run (**C**). An individual patient demonstrates a positive result that can be further quantified by extrapolation to the standard curve (**D**).

DNA Sequencing

One can determine the nucleotide sequence of a given gene segment and compare it with that of a reference sequence to find mutation, deletion, insertion, translocation, and other genetic events associated with disease. In the classic Sanger sequencing method, a segment of extracted DNA is first PCR amplified to enrich the sequence of interest using specific primers, DNA polymerase, and deoxyribonucleotides (dNTPs) that are the building blocks for making a cDNA strand (see Figure 5-2). In a subsequent round of replication, a portion of the dNTPs that are added to the reaction cannot sustain chain elongation, so each complementary strand that is being lengthened eventually terminates at a random position. The strands are separated by size using electrophoresis, and the labeled nucleotides marking the terminus of each elongated strand are detected to sequentially order A, T, G, and C incorporation into the copied DNA.

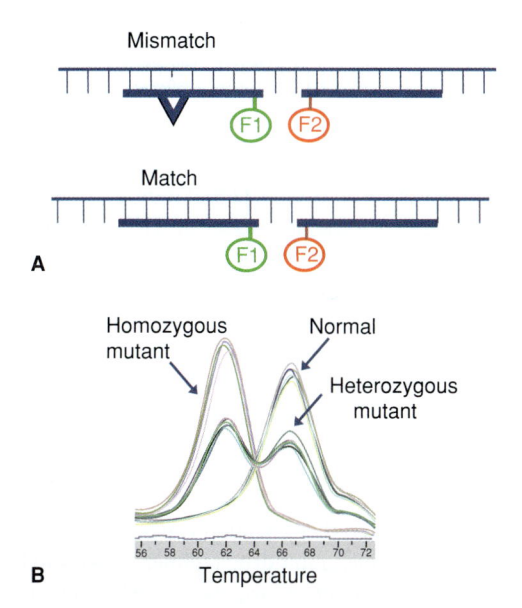

FIGURE 5-4 **Melt curve analysis helps identify sequence variants in PCR products.** **(A)** The products are hybridized to probes labeled with a red or green fluorochrome, and then the reaction is gradually heated until the probes dissociate from their complementary target sequence. As the probe melts off its complementary strand, there is a measurable change in the level of fluorescence resonance energy transfer (FRET) between the two fluorochromes. A probe that is perfectly matched to its target dissociates at a higher temperature compared with a probe that has a mismatch by virtue of a sequence variant. **(B)** In these melt curve graphs, each patient result is classifiable as normal or variant (and heterozygous *versus* homozygous) for the *HFE* C282Y mutation in which adenine substitutes for guanine at nucleotide position 845. In the associated triplet codon, this base substitution suggests a tyrosine (Y) for cysteine (C) substitution at amino acid position 282 in the translated protein that is responsible for regulating iron absorption in the gut.

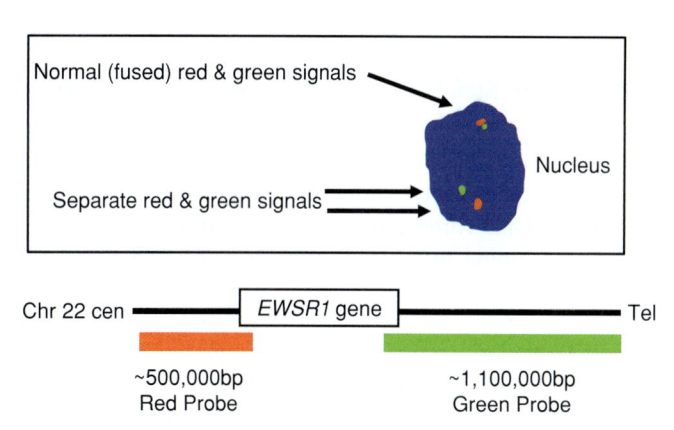

FIGURE 5-6 **FISH analysis helps confirm a diagnosis of Ewing sarcoma by demonstrating a break within the *EWSR1* gene on chromosome 22.** In this break-apart probe strategy, fluoresceinated probes normally flank the *EWSR1* gene. In the nucleus shown here, abnormal (separate) red and green fluorochromes signify disruption of one copy of the *EWSR1* gene. In contrast, the normal allele is intact as evidenced by fused red and green signals indicating that the two probes are juxtaposed as a consequence of binding the same chromosomal locus.

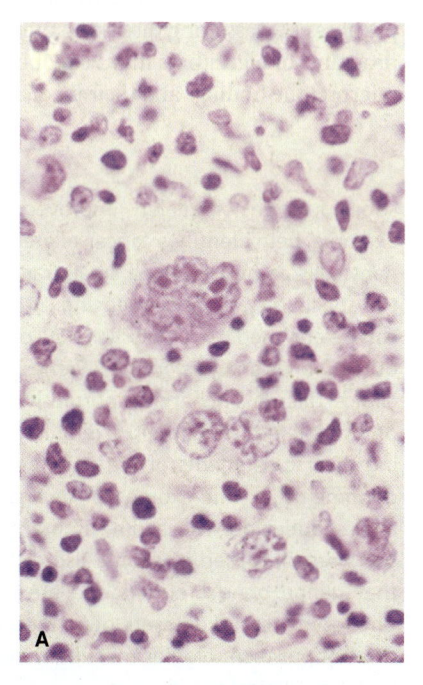

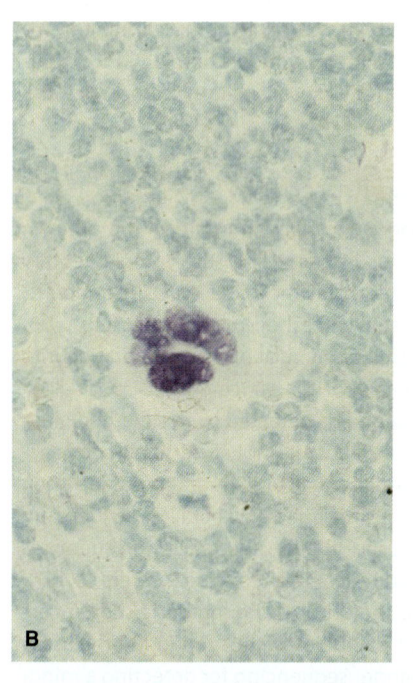

FIGURE 5-5 **In situ hybridization permits visualization of RNA within the context of cytomorphology in tissue sections on a glass slide.** In this example, pathologist interpretation of an **(A)** hematoxylin and eosin (H&E) stain and **(B)** in situ hybridization to *Epstein–Barr virus encoded RNA (EBER)* transcripts reveals that the viral gene product is localized to Reed–Sternberg cells in a case of Hodgkin lymphoma, while surrounding lymphocytes lack this viral RNA.

Variant in Situ Hybridization Procedure Using Fluorochrome Labels

Fluorescence in situ hybridization (FISH) detects and localizes specific DNA sequences in G-banded metaphase or interphase chromosomes using a probe labeled with a fluorochrome that glows brightly when stimulated by light of the appropriate wavelength. Duplex hybridization (e.g., one probe glowing green and another probe glowing red) facilitates interpretation of the number or structure of selected portions of chromosomes (see Figure 5-6). The results can identify or confirm structural alterations that are difficult to discern by standard chromosomal G-banding techniques.

Examples of clinical use of in situ hybridization include (1) identify DiGeorge syndrome characterized by deletion of a small segment of chromosome 22 that is detectable by FISH but may be difficult or impossible to see on a routine karyotype of metaphase chromosomes (2) localize foreign organisms to lesional cells to help diagnose disease involving a pathogen that might also exist as "normal flora," such as Epstein–Barr virus or human papillomavirus, or (3) quantify gene expression by, for example, hybridizing IGK and IGL (kappa and lambda light chain) RNAs as a test for B cell clonality.

Sanger sequencing is considered the gold standard method for characterizing DNA nucleotide sequence. For a disease in which the precise site of mutation varies among affected patients, such as cystic fibrosis for which any of >500 different disease-associated variants might be present in the *CFTR* gene, segments of DNA up to several hundred base pairs can be analyzed in a single sequencing reaction to facilitate identification of disease-causing mutations. DNA sequencing is labor intensive since each result is typically verified by sequencing the opposite strand, and interpretation of the findings requires expert analysis by a pathologist or other laboratory physician to distinguish benign polymorphism from actionable mutation. Mutant DNA must comprise >20% of elongated DNA in the reaction to be detected by this method.

Examples of clinical use of DNA sequencing include (1) detect any of the various mutations of the *HBB* (beta globin) gene responsible for causing beta thalassemia, (2) sequence the tyrosine kinase domain of *BCR–ABL1* to predict drug resistance in leukemia patients treated with a tyrosine kinase inhibitor, (3) sequence genes encoding multiple members of the EGFR signaling pathway in colorectal or lung cancer tissue to predict response or resistance to targeted therapy, and (4) perform HIV genotyping to help predict which multidrug regimen is likely to be effective against the viral sequence variants detectable in that patient.

Microarray Technology for Gene Expression Profiling

Microarray expression profiling involves simultaneous measurement of multiple transcripts to help classify disease and predict outcome in response to therapy. In the most commonly used microarray procedures, a chip has been spotted with many (dozens to millions) of different DNA probes complementary to the genes of interest. Extracted RNA from a patient is reverse transcribed to make labeled cDNA, which in turn is hybridized to the array. A sensor quantifies the hybridization signal at each spot to quantify the amount of each patient RNA species that is targeted. Data is analyzed and the pattern of expression in the patient specimen is matched to a database of known patterns for purposes of classifying disease or predicting outcome. Software programs or algorithms may be required to help the pathologist interpret the findings and their medical significance.

Variant Sequencing Procedures

Like Sanger sequencing, *pyrosequencing* detects the order in which nucleotides are incorporated into the complementary strand that is synthesized from the patient's DNA template. However, the *pyrosequencing* method relies on sensing pyrophosphate that is released upon nucleotide incorporation into the growing strand. Mutant DNA must comprise >5% of elongated DNA in the reaction to be detected by this method.

Clinical laboratories are increasingly using new sequencing methods by which patient DNA is fragmented and then randomly sequenced using massive parallel sequencing reactions. Software is used to align the resulting sequences against a reference sequence. The "coverage" refers to how many times the same region of the genome is sequenced, and typically coverage is >20 times, thus rendering the assay more sensitive than Sanger sequencing for detecting a minor subpopulation of alleles. Improved sensitivity could, for example, help identify a cancer-related change even if malignant cells comprise only a small fraction of cells present in the specimen. Before sequencing, DNA segments of interest can be enriched (e.g., by PCR, rtPCR, or other selection methods) to focus analysis on those genes relevant to solving the clinical dilemma at hand. Importantly, targeted resequencing of multiple genes can help screen for genetic defects involving diverse segments of the genome. If desired, the whole genome or just the exome can be analyzed by massive parallel sequencing. The exome is the estimated 1.5% of the genome composed of exons, also called coding sequences, that define gene products and are more likely to impact phenotype. Large datasets generated by these novel high-throughput technologies must be mined to identify variants and their clinical significance.

Since each class of disease typically has a unique expression profile, microarray analysis is a powerful strategy to gain added value beyond what traditional morphology or immunohistochemical assays can provide. Information gleaned from expression profiling has also led to improved understanding of disease pathogenesis, which in turn helps investigators develop novel therapeutic strategies to overcome the aberrant biochemical pathways operative in the disease. Arrays tend to be relatively insensitive to low level disease, but the array data may point to a disease-specific finding that can then be confirmed by a more sensitive assay (e.g., rtPCR, immunohistochemistry, or flow cytometry) for monitoring minimal residual disease.

Examples of clinical use of array technology include (1) classify the intrinsic subtype of breast cancer and calculate the likelihood of tumor recurrence; (2) predict the histogenesis of a "tumor of unknown origin"; (3) detect any of dozens of respiratory pathogens in a sputum specimen; (4) predict outcome in response to cancer therapy beyond that which is forecast by traditional morphology, immunophenotype, and karyotype; and (5) find congenital defects not visible by karyotype.

THE PATHOLOGIST'S ROLE

Clinical laboratories are required to have a clinical consultant who can advise on indications of testing and on clinical use of test results. Patient-specific findings are typically interpreted by a pathologist who composes a report describing the results and their medical significance. There are two phases of assay

Variant Array Technologies

In clinical trial settings, expression data on all 25,000 genes can be mined to identify a short list of transcripts that is informative for the clinical situation at hand. An assay can then be designed targeting a smaller number of analytes that are measurable using well-established multianalyte array technologies (e.g., rtPCR panels) that are amenable to use on scant specimens or formalin fixed paraffin-embedded tissue (see **Figure 5-7**).

A gene dosage array is a panel of DNA probes that measures copy number of each of dozens to millions of targeted segments of the genome in a patient sample. In healthy cells, each chromosomal gene is present in two copies (one inherited from mother, and the other from father). Certain heritable diseases (e.g., Down syndrome) or certain tumors (e.g., myeloma) have consistent copy number changes conferring diagnostic or prognostic information. Gene dosage arrays have two major technologic variants: *Comparative genomic hybridization* compares gene copy number in the patient with that of a reference genome, and a *single nucleotide polymorphism (SNP) chip* additionally can assess copy neutral loss of heterozygosity (both alleles from the same parent).

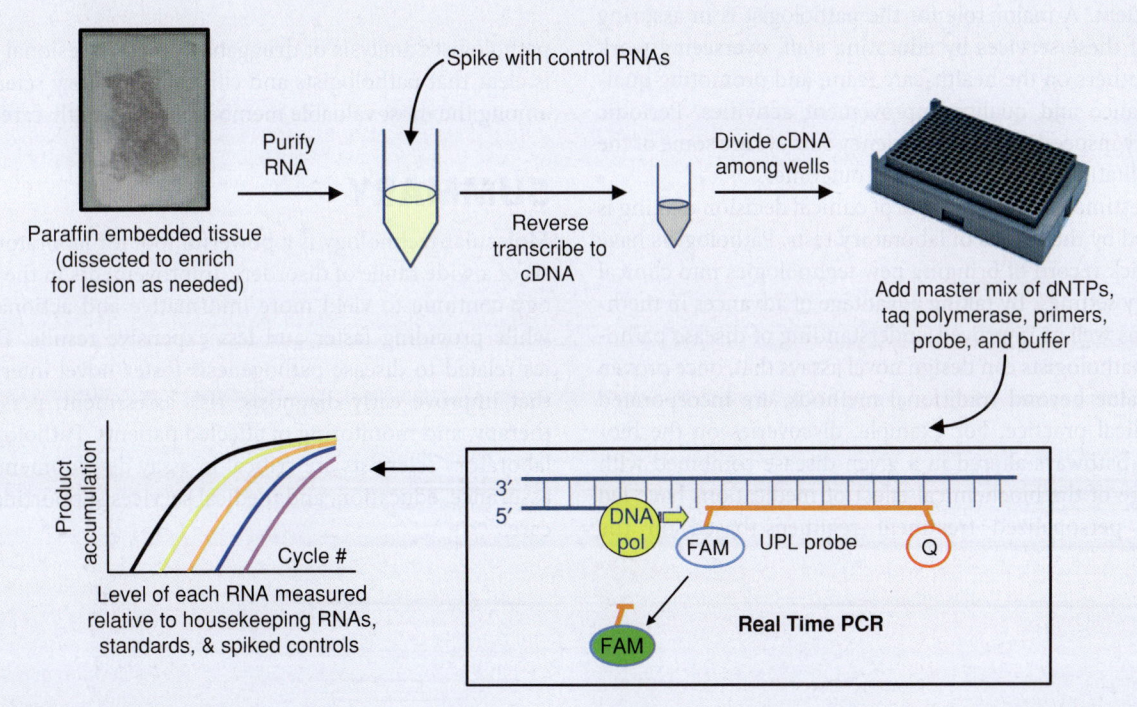

FIGURE 5-7 Array technology permits simultaneous quantification of dozens to millions of analytes. In the array-based rtPCR panel depicted here, RNA is extracted from paraffin-embedded tissue and then spiked with a control sequence before being reverse transcribed to cDNA. The cDNA is divided among wells for real-time rtPCR measuring multiple separate RNAs (e.g., to classify RNA expression profile, or to detect multiple RNA viruses).

interpretation, *analytic* and *clinical*. In analytic interpretation, the pathologist generates a reportable result by first examining the controls to determine if they behaved as expected and then examining the patient data to devise an informed result. In clinical interpretation, the pathologist synthesizes the findings with other clinicopathologic information on that patient or in a relevant population of patients to deduce the medical significance of the result. In some cases, follow-up action is recommended. Pertinent limitations of the test are acknowledged. This interpretive process requires medical judgment based on thorough knowledge of the procedures employed and the clinical factors impacting on and affected by the laboratory findings.

Another role for the pathologist is in selecting the laboratory's test menu, and in conducting validation studies to assess the performance of an assay prior to its implementation. Any change to a test system must also be validated prior to use (e.g., apply the assay to a novel specimen type, new instrument, or protocol improvement). Validation study components are listed in Table 5-1. The laboratory director reviews the validation data and vets the assay as well as the competency of testing personnel prior to initiating the service.

Recent emphasis on preanalytic specimen preparation methods is motivated by recognition that a test result is only as good as the specimen input into the test system. For blood, biopsy, and other cellular specimens, the pathologist is crucial for histopathologic examination and selecting appropriate tissue for testing.

As a physician, the pathologist is responsible for the health-care services provided by their testing laboratory for a given patient. A major role for the pathologist is in assuring quality of these services by educating staff, overseeing work done by others on the health-care team, and promoting quality assurance and quality improvement activities. Periodic laboratory inspections and proficiency surveys are some of the tools facilitating progress and good outcomes.

It is estimated that over 70% of clinical decision making is influenced by the results of laboratory tests. Pathologists have a long track record of bringing new technologies into clinical laboratory settings. By taking advantage of advances in methodology as well as improved understanding of disease pathogenesis, pathologists can design novel assays that, once proven to add value beyond traditional methods, are incorporated into medical practice. For example, discoveries on the biochemical pathways altered in a given disease combined with knowledge of the biochemical effect of medications have led to more personalized treatment regimens based on the pathologist's analysis of druggable targets in lesional tissue. It is clear that pathologists and clinical laboratory scientists are among the most valuable members of the health-care team.

TABLE 5-1 Steps in validating a laboratory test.

- Assess clinical need
- Define anticipated benefits, risks, and minimal performance requirements
- Literature review
- Choose analytic method; develop & pilot test a *standard operating procedure*
- Design a study to assess performance characteristics: *sensitivity, specificity, reproducibility, linearity, analytic measurement range, interfering substances, etc.*
- Assemble reagents, supplies, equipment, software, controls, standard reference materials, and trained personnel
- Perform pilot studies on a reasonable number and representative distribution of specimen types and patients generating the range of results (e.g., normal and mutant and low-to-high values); tweak and retest as needed to improve performance
- Define clinical indications of testing, acceptable specimen types and criteria for rejection, controls, reference materials, interpretation and reporting guidance, troubleshooting tips, critical values, normal range, proficiency testing plan, clinical benefits, and risks of testing
- Calculate costs, develop ordering and billing procedures and reporting mechanism
- Compose "procedure manual," "validation report," and instructions for health-care personnel
- Laboratory director uses medical judgment to vet whether the assay is at least as good as what was previously available to the patient population by comparison to a valid assay and/or to clinicopathologic findings
- Educate laboratorians, clinicians, and relevant health-care providers
- Surveillance and periodic update

SUMMARY

Molecular technology is a powerful tool for laboratory analysis of a wide range of disorders. Improvements in the technology continue to yield more informative and actionable data while providing faster and less expensive results. Discoveries related to disease pathogenesis foster novel interventions that improve early diagnosis, risk assessment, personalized therapy, and monitoring of affected patients. Pathologists and laboratory scientists are critical in assay development, quality assurance, education, and medical services supporting patient care.

Clinical Practice: Laboratory Medicine and Patient Care

CHAPTER 6

Catherine A. Hammett-Stabler, Ph.D., DABCC, FACB

INTRODUCTORY CASES

CASE 6-1

GW is a 23-year-old female who is seen by her family medicine physician following several months of increasing fatigue and generally not feeling well. She reports she has lost 16 lbs over the past 6 months without dieting. She is applying to medical school and thinks this may be stress related.

CASE 6-2

RM is a 52-year-old male who presents to the emergency department with mild chest pain and shortness of breath. He reports that his symptoms began about 3 hours ago just before landing at the local airport after a 18-hour flight from Asia.

LABORATORY MEDICINE

Laboratory medicine will play a critical role in the workup of each of the above patients. The importance of the history and physical must not be understated, but the data often obtained from these activities are subjective or dependent on the patient and the stage of the condition. Furthermore, the signs and symptoms of many diseases are similar, so much so, that patients can be misdiagnosed or mismanaged without additional data. Consider, for example, the number of disorders that can cause the fatigue and weight loss reported by the patient in Case 6-1. Is the shortness of breath and chest pain reported in Case 6-2 due to a cardiac or respiratory problem?

As will be seen, the tests ordered by their respective clinicians and the results reported by the clinical laboratory will make the diagnosis in one patient and will greatly influence additional decisions for the other. These are but two examples in which the judicious use of clinical laboratory testing proves to be one of the most effective and economical ways of acquiring objective data that can clarify many presentations. Today's clinician has several thousand individual tests at his or her disposal.

The goal of this chapter is to introduce you to laboratory medicine and the clinical laboratory thus removing some of the mystery of what happens when you order a laboratory test or take a sample to the laboratory, and to help you understand how to better use and evaluate laboratory tests so that you will be more efficient and effective in ordering tests and interpreting results.

WHAT WE DO

The use of this part of pathology, **laboratory medicine** (Figure 6-1), is so important to patient care that the clinical laboratories in these United States produce more than 7 billion test results each year that are used to derive a diagnosis, determine disease severity, assess risk factors, select and monitor interventions and treatments, formulate prognoses, and to evaluate or avoid potential adverse outcomes.

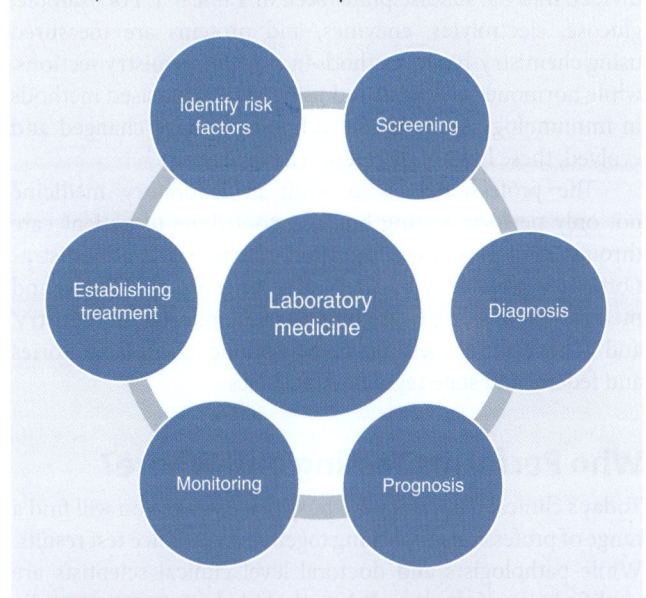

FIGURE 6-1 The role of laboratory medicine in patient care.

TABLE 6-1 Laboratory medicine disciplines.

Discipline or Section	General Role	Examples of Tests
Transfusion medicine (blood bank)	Collection, testing, processing, dispensing of blood and blood products for transfusion	Blood (ABO) typing, cross-matching
Clinical chemistry	Testing for a wide range of analytes from small ionic species and organic molecules to proteins, drugs, and hormones; includes toxicology, endocrinology, blood gases, and metabolic testing	Creatinine, sodium, potassium glucose, troponin, cholesterol, TSH, free thyroxin (free T4), drugs of abuse in urine, blood gases
Cytogenetics	Chromosomal analysis using fluids (blood, amniotic fluid, etc.), tissues and cells, uses techniques such as fluorescence in situ hybridization (FISH)	Karyotype (peripheral blood chromosome analysis), X/Y centromere analysis and subtelomere analysis
Hematology and coagulation	Identification and counting of blood cells	Complete blood count, differential, prothrombin time (PT), activated partial thromboplastin time (APTT, PTT), factor VIII assay, fibrinogen antigen, sickle cell testing, identification of hemoglobinopathies
Immunology and histocompatibility	Testing related to the cellular and humoral immune function, uses techniques such as immunoassay and flow cytometry	Leukemia and lymphoma markers
Medical microscopy and urinalysis	Examination of body fluids other than blood using microscopic, physiochemical, and macroscopic techniques	Urinalysis, specific gravity, pH, crystal identification, ketones
Microbiology	Detection and identification of pathogens and infectious agents includes bacteriology, mycology, parasitology, and virology.	Hepatitis testing, HIV testing
Molecular diagnostics	Performs genetic testing at the gene and protein level	Factor V Leiden DNA, BRCA 1/2 gene mutations, Fragile X syndrome (*FMR1* gene mutation), hemochromatosis, (*HFE* gene), CYP450 polymorphisms

LABORATORY MEDICINE AND THE CLINICAL LABORATORY

Laboratory medicine is the part of pathology typically associated with the provision of laboratory test results. Traditionally, these tests were grouped according to the instruments and techniques used to perform the analyses, and the field is usually divided into the subdisciplines seen in Table 6-1. For example, glucose, electrolytes, enzymes, and proteins are measured using chemistry-based methods in clinical chemistry sections, while hormones are measured using antibody-based methods in immunology sections. As technologies have changed and evolved, these lines of distinction have blurred.

The professionals who work in laboratory medicine not only perform testing but also contribute to patient care through clinical service, education, research, and administration. They practice in a variety of settings from hospitals and medical schools, to private reference laboratories, in industry, and in government settings such as public health laboratories and federal and state regulatory agencies.

Who Performs Testing and Where?

Today's clinical laboratory is a busy place where you will find a range of professionals working together to produce test results. While pathologists and doctoral level clinical scientists are qualified to perform the analytical procedures, most generally do not engage in these activities, but instead provide testing oversight and administration. They work closely with the technical staff to determine what tests will be performed, to select the instrumentation and methods, and to assure appropriate quality practices are in place. These behind the scene roles are absolutely critical to patient care. As part of the clinical services they provide, these individuals guide other clinicians and providers in selecting the best or most appropriate test for the need, in interpreting the result, and in understanding the clinical performance and limitations of the tests. Who physically performs the analysis depends upon the complexity of the test method, a classification determined by the FDA.

A small, but growing portion of testing is performed by other health professionals such as nurses using small, portable devices often in the immediate patient setting. The latter is known as point of care testing (POCT) and even when performed by nonlaboratorians is often managed by the laboratory medicine department. Clinical testing is performed in other locations such as physician offices, free standing ambulatory centers, and in public health laboratories.

Regardless of the setting, any facility in the United States performing testing for patient care is regulated under the Clinical Laboratory Improvement Act of 1988 (CLIA) and its subsequent amendments. This includes all of the aforementioned settings outside of a clinical laboratory including physician offices. These regulations were established to assure accuracy, reliability, and timeliness of the test result used in patient care whether for health assessment or for the diagnosis, prevention, or treatment of disease. The regulations not only establish the various levels of testing based on the complexity of the method and instrumentation but also establish criteria for all levels of

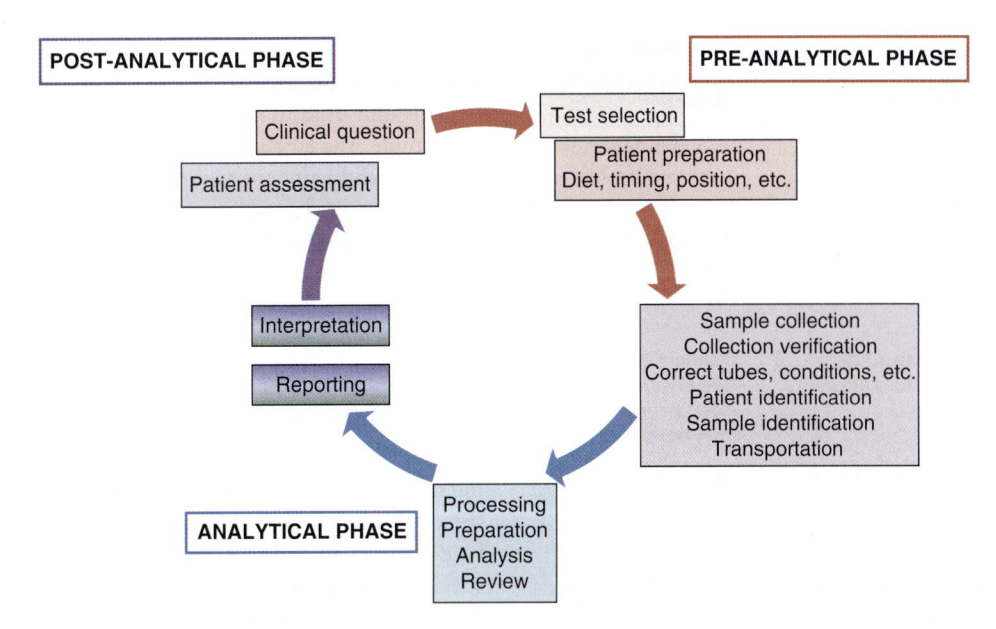

FIGURE 6-2 Total testing process. Testing begins with the evaluation of the patient and the decision to order a test, and is completed when the result is acted on. In this scheme, testing is divided into the preanalytical, analytical, and postanalytical phases with many steps taking place outside the laboratory. As the colors indicate, these steps are interrelated.

personnel, all phases of analytic testing, and quality assurance. The regulations mandated by this federal law are monitored by a variety of agencies such as the Joint Commission on Accreditation of Healthcare Organizations (the Joint Commission), College of American Pathologists (CAP), American Association of Blood Banks (AABB), among others.

THE TOTAL TESTING PROCESS

Laboratory medicine uses a systems-based approach known as the total testing process. In this, testing begins with the clinical decision to order a test and ends when the result is acted on. By approaching testing from this perspective, pathologists and laboratory scientists are able to monitor and assess all of the activities and processes that impact a test result and therefore the care of the patient. The following sections will provide a broad overview of the total testing process (**Figure 6-2**) with brief descriptions of key operations and concepts to prepare you to understand and use the laboratory more effectively.

> ### QUICK REVIEW
> The testing process is divided into the preanalytical, analytical, and postanalytical phases with each phase consisting of multiple steps many of which take place outside of the laboratory (Figure 6-2).

The Preanalytical Phase of Testing

The testing process begins with an interaction between the clinician and the patient, perhaps in the form of a physical examination or a history of current symptoms. Studies of laboratory-related medical errors in diagnosis find that about half are due to failure to use the correct test indicated for the disorder in question. Admittedly, this part of the process is complicated by the fact that testing has changed rapidly over recent years both in terms of new analytes and technologies. Laboratory medicine professionals are challenged to stay abreast of these changes and it is more so for those outside.

There are several approaches used in deciding what tests to order. Some take the "shot-gun" approach, in which as many tests as possible are ordered, to cover all aspects of the differential. Such an approach is not time or cost-effective for anyone—physician, patient, or laboratory. Testing schemes will differ depending on the use, that is, the question(s) you are asking and the setting. For example, one test may be appropriate when screening an apparently healthy newborn for thyroid disease but additional tests will be needed when evaluating a 42-year-old woman who has clinical symptoms of thyroid disease.

To help put this in perspective, consider the patient presented in Case 6-1: The differential diagnosis of weight loss includes malignancy, chronic illness, gastrointestinal disease, malabsorption, drug use, diabetes, hyperthyroidism, and pheochromocytoma. The shotgun approach could include several tumor markers, C-reactive protein, complete blood count (CBC) including differential, electrolytes, albumin, total protein, glucose, thyroid stimulating hormone (TSH), thyroxine, urine drug screens, and urinary metanephrines and catecholamines. In the history, you determine that the patient has had several occurrences of vaginal yeast infections the past year, and has experienced an increase in thirst and urination. Her vital signs include a blood pressure of 119/78 mmHg and pulse of 80 bpm. She admits to being stressed during the examination because she is worried. Armed with this information, some of the disorders associated with weight loss move up in terms of likelihood and one might consider if the patient has

TABLE 6-2 Examples of specimen types and use.

Specimen Type	Examples of Tests	Collection
Serum	Troponin, glucose, creatinine, drugs, metals	Red, gold, brown, royal blue top tubes
Plasma EDTA Heparin Citrate	Hematology testing Chemistry testing Coagulation testing	Lavender tube Green top tube Blue top tube
Urine	Sodium, protein, infectious organisms, drugs	Random, timed, preservatives, and special containers may be needed
Cerebral spinal fluid	Protein, infectious organisms, glucose	Sterile plastic vials

diabetes or hyperthyroidism. One might still decide to include some basic tests to assess general health such as total protein, renal function, and a CBC, but emphasis will be placed on the glucose and TSH results.

Having considered which tests are appropriate to order, there are preparations that still need to take place before any samples are collected: some tests require the patient be fasting or have followed a specific diet for several days, others should be collected at specific times of the day, while others should be collected just before a medication is given. Some of these variables will be discussed below in the section on **biological variation**. In addition one must think about the type of specimen needed for testing (Table 6-2). Serum, the most common sample type, requires blood be collected into a phlebotomy tube that does not contain an anticoagulant. Plasma, whole blood, urine, feces, other body fluids, and even tissues are also used. Today, most laboratories have patient preparation and collection information readily available online, but when in doubt, talk to the laboratory performing the testing as requirements for some tests will vary between laboratories because of differences in methods used. Recognize that phlebotomy takes practice and skill—aspects that potentially impact the result include the patient's position, stasis from the placement of the tourniquet, clenching of the fist, even order of tube collection.

> ### QUICK REVIEW
> Most errors related to testing take place in the preanalytical phase:
> - Test—incorrect test is ordered
> - Patient—not prepared
> - Samples—improperly identified, collected, or handled

Each sample must be annotated with sufficient information to assure it can be tracked to the patient from whom it originated. At a minimum, this includes the patient's name and medical record number along with the date and time of collection. Failure to comply with this requirement results in samples being rejected for analysis. Many hospitals have implemented the use of devices that are carried to the patient's bedside and used to scan the armband to generate a label for the sample. The labels display the patient's identification information both in alphanumeric form and as a barcode.

The importance of the preanalytical phase cannot be overemphasized. Neither staff nor technology can correct for an improperly collected, incorrect, or invalid sample. Of the total process, this is the phase during which most errors occur—up to 75% of all errors take place before the sample reaches the laboratory.

The Analytic Phase

Clinical laboratories are typically divided into sections based on the subspecialties described earlier. The technologists and staff in these areas follow well-defined procedures to perform the analytic phase of testing that leads to a result. This phase includes specimen processing and preparation, the actual testing of the specimen, review and verification of results, and quality control.

When the sample is received into the laboratory, it and the accompanying orders (paper or electronic requests for testing) are reviewed to verify identification and that the correct specimen types have been collected. It is not unusual for a patient to have 5–15 tests ordered that may necessitate multiple sample types to be collected. During processing, the sample is triaged based on the degree of urgency with stat or urgent samples being given priority. Additional handling or processing may be necessary, such as centrifugation, before the sample is ready for testing.

Testing may need to be repeated or verified before the result is released, and issues may arise at various steps of the process that cause a sample to be declared unsuitable and rejected, or resulted with a cautionary comment. Discovering that a sample is hemolyzed is the most common example of such an event.

> ### IN TRANSLATION
> Hemolysis occurs when erythrocytes are damaged allowing their contents to be released. This occasionally occurs in vivo due to several pathological conditions, but its occurrence during phlebotomy or sample processing renders samples unsuitable for testing for several reasons. First, erythrocytes contain many chemicals in addition to hemoglobin: potassium, magnesium, iron, lactate dehydrogenase, and aspartate aminotransferase, to name a few. The amounts of these compounds can be considerable—the amount of potassium within erythrocytes is 30-fold above that found in plasma; the amount of lactate dehydrogenase is 150-fold. Obviously, release of these intracellular constituents falsely raises the serum or plasma concentrations. Less obvious is the fact that the release of erythrocyte contents into the plasma dilutes the extracellular constituents, such as sodium, and the result would be falsely decreased. In addition, one or more of the chemicals released into the sample may interfere with an analytical method.

Throughout the analytical process, quality assurance tools are used to reduce and identify errors and to determine if methods or instruments are performing to specifications. All of these steps are done to produce the most accurate test possible. CLIA and other regulations require laboratories monitor each method as long as it is used for patient care. Performance parameters of clinical importance include precision (imprecision), accuracy, analytical sensitivity, and analytical specificity.

> **QUICK REVIEW**
>
> Analytical performance characteristics that are clinically important include the method's:
>
> - Precision—describes repeatability of measurements from one to another
> - Accuracy—describes trueness of measurements
> - Analytical sensitivity—defines the lowest concentration accurately measured
> - Analytical specificity—defines ability of method to accurately detect and measure the analyte

> **QUICK REVIEW**
>
> Precision is the closeness of agreement between replicate measurements of a single sample for a given test, while accuracy refers to the closeness of a measurement to the true value. Laboratories quantify these parameters using measures of imprecision and bias, respectively. Imprecision is the measure of the random error between measurements expressed as the standard deviation (SD) or coefficient of variation (CV). The % CV is calculated by dividing the SD by the mean of the series of measurements multiplied by 100%.

Imprecision increases over time as instruments and reagents age. It is important for patient care because of how test results are reviewed and interpreted. The first thing the physician does is to compare the result with the reference range. How reference ranges are derived will be described shortly but for now just realize these represent the range of values expected for a nondiseased individual. Next, the results are often compared with previously obtained test results to look for a change. Neither of these would be possible if the testing methods differed significantly from testing to testing.

Accuracy is assessed by testing samples or other materials with known concentrations. It is entirely possible, though clearly problematic, that a method could be extremely precise but very inaccurate. Such issues arise when the standard to which a method is calibrated is flawed—perhaps it was made improperly, has degraded or become contaminated.

The analytical sensitivity of a method is, by definition, the lowest concentration of the analyte reliably measured. Analytical sensitivity is important for those tests where very low concentrations have clinical significance or where this characteristic is used to establish clinical decision points. An example of a test where very low concentrations have clinical consequences is troponin because any detectable troponin is considered indicative of myocardial cell injury.

The analytical specificity of a method reflects its ability to measure the analyte being tested in the presence of potentially interfering substances. Interfering substances include hemolysis and lipemia—the most common interferences encountered—as well as, structurally similar compounds (e.g., other glucocorticoids when testing for cortisol) and unexpected, totally unrelated materials (e.g., supposedly inert ingredients in phlebotomy blood collection tubes). This parameter is often assessed by conducting cross-reactivity studies in which increasing amounts of the suspected material or chemical are added to samples, testing the samples, and then calculating the percentage of cross-reactivity. A complete assessment for every potential interfering substance would be impossible to perform, hence the best resource for detecting interferences in a laboratory test is often the clinician who communicates with the laboratory and relates that the results do not fit the expected picture Similarly, clinicians find their best resource for information regarding potential interferences to be the testing laboratory performing the testing. Because of the different methods in use, one must be certain that reference information applies to the local test.

The Postanalytical Phase

Once the analysis is complete, the results are reported. Note the report begins with the identification information that was provided. The report also notes the date and time of collection. Each test is identified by name followed by the result with units. Each result is accompanied by a reference range. Results that exceed the reference range are usually flagged so as to draw attention to them. The report may also include an interpretation and, when appropriate, additional recommendations for testing. Additional comments that may be found include identification of tests sent from the reporting laboratory to outside laboratories for testing and issues affecting the quality of the result, for example, the presence of hemolysis.

Interpretation may be performed by the pathologist or doctoral-level clinical scientist in the laboratory but is usually the responsibility of the ordering clinician, who must also determine the appropriate treatment and follow-up. Only when the result is acted on is the test complete in the view of laboratory medicine and the philosophy of the total testing process. *Unfortunately, 32% of laboratory-related medical errors were due to failure on the part of the ordering clinician to act on the results in a timely manner.*

UNDERSTANDING AND INTERPRETING TEST RESULTS

Reference Ranges

Test results cannot be interpreted without knowledge of the results one would expect to see in a healthy individual. These values are usually referred to as the reference range—other terms you may hear include normal range, normal value,

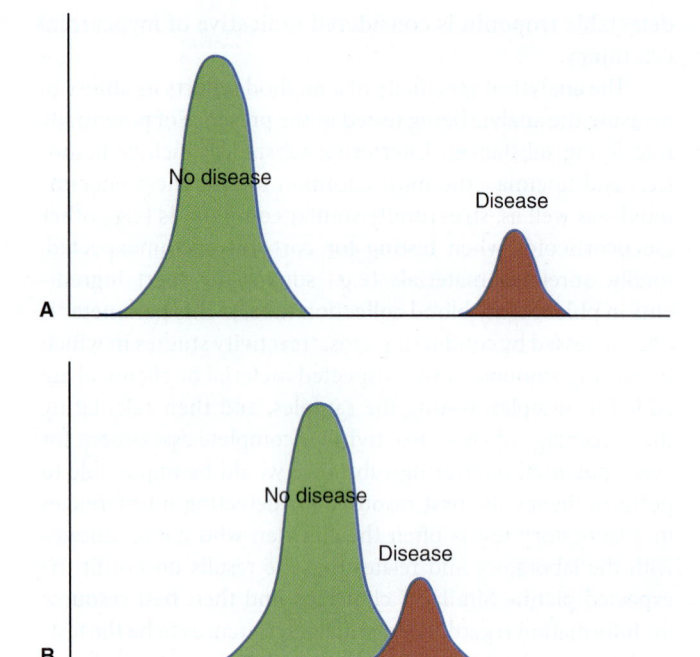

FIGURE 6-3 Distribution of results in healthy or nondiseased and diseased individuals. **(A)** Example in which results between the two populations are clearly separated. **(B)** Example in which results overlap.

reference interval, and expected range. There are some tests for which clinical decision limits are used instead of reference ranges and these will be discussed below.

Laboratories are required to verify or establish reference ranges for each method they perform and to publish these ranges with each result. Briefly, this process includes the identification of inclusion and exclusion criteria, selection of apparently healthy subjects who meet these criteria, procurement of samples under controlled conditions, testing, and data analysis. Inclusion and exclusion criteria include factors such as exercise, time of day, foods, or prescribed drugs that are known to impact the result, and so on. Ranges may also vary with gender and age.

> **IN TRANSLATION**
>
> The enzyme alkaline phosphatase serves as an excellent example of an analyte where the reference ranges depend on age and gender. In our laboratory, the range for adults (>age 20 years) is 38–126 U/L. Since a significant portion of alkaline phosphatase found in the circulation is derived from the bone isoenzyme, growing children are expected to have higher alkaline phosphatase activity due to its expression in bone growth and development. Thus, it is appropriate for the alkaline phosphatase of a growing 5 years old to fall between 150 and 380 U/L. Even higher levels are appropriate for a 15-year-old (up to 525 U/L for a male but only 230 for a female). Such levels of activity in a sample from an adult would suggest pathology.

Ideally, the reference range is clearly separated from the values seen in patients who have disease (Figure 6-3A). For many tests, the results seen across the healthy population are distributed in a Gaussian or bell-shaped distribution pattern, but the distribution may be skewed to one side or nonparametric. Complicating matters, some overlap typically occurs between the healthy and diseased populations so that some healthy individuals will have "abnormal" results and some patients with the disease will have test results that fall within the reference interval (e.g., when a patient presents early in the disease or has a mild form). Understanding the clinical sensitivity and specificity of the test helps in these cases.

For many tests, reference ranges are standardized across laboratory methods; that is, the ranges change very little regardless of the laboratory or the method. Several examples of such tests include sodium and potassium. However, the reference ranges for many enzymes vary considerably with the method used. Lactate dehydrogenase (LD) is a good example as methods are based either on the enzyme's ability to convert lactate (L) to pyruvate (P) or the reverse (P → L). Not only does the reaction used make a difference but the temperature at which the test is performed also impacts the reference range. The adult reference range for a L → P method at 30°C is 35–100 U/L, but is typically 100–190 U/L at 37°C. When the laboratory uses a P → L-based method, the range is 140–280 U/L at 30°C but 208–378 U/L at 37°C. The take home lesson here is to double check reference ranges and to not assume that what you read in one text or used in the hospital in which you trained is applicable. While there are several efforts underway to harmonize reference ranges, this will take several years to accomplish.

Clinical Decision Limits

In some instances, it is more appropriate to use **clinical decision limits** (also called medical decision limits) in place of population-based reference ranges. These criteria are based on data derived from outcome studies or on the diagnostic performance of the test.

The various lipids used in the diagnosis of hyperlipidemia and the assessment of a patient's risk of cardiovascular disease are among the best examples of tests for which outcome-based clinical decision limits are now used instead of reference ranges. Prior to the early 1980s population-based ranges were used for lipids; and in fact, 150–300 mg/dL is listed as the reference range for cholesterol in a ca 1984 text. But a number of investigators, such as those who conducted the Framingham Study, had shown many individuals whose cholesterol levels exceeded 200 mg/dL developed coronary artery disease. Thus, in 1984, the National Cholesterol Education Program recommended the adoption of clinical decision-based limits for these tests. The current recommendations classify cholesterol levels not only by the absolute concentration but also with the patient's other risk factors in mind (family history, smoking history, etc.). These will be discussed in greater detail in the cardiovascular chapter.

CLINICAL PERFORMANCE OF TESTS

Sensitivity, Specificity, Predictive Value, and Analytical Versus Biological Variation

Clearly, laboratories strive to use sound and robust methods. But the question must be asked, do these "analytically sound" results translate into clinically useful results? Hence, it is important to define the expectation that a true positive result is associated with the disease or process of concern (e.g., the finding of a protein at or above a specific concentration indicates cancer), while a true negative result indicates the lack of pathology or the process of concern.

> **QUICK REVIEW**
> The clinical sensitivity of a test describes the probability that the test will be positive in the presence of a disease, while specificity describes the probability that the test will be negative in the absence of disease. These can be calculated by the following equations:
>
> $$\text{Sensitivity} = \frac{\text{True positive}}{\text{True positive} + \text{false negatives}} \times 100\%$$
>
> $$\text{Specificity} = \frac{\text{True negative}}{\text{True negatives} + \text{false positives}} \times 100\%$$

False negatives are those patients who have disease but whose test result indicates otherwise. Similarly, false positives are those patients whose test result indicates that they have disease but in reality do not. Sensitivity and specificity of tests are inversely related.

As noted earlier, the distribution of test results obtained for nondiseased individuals very often overlaps with the range of results obtained for patients with the disease in question. Thus as seen in Figure 6-3B, where one sets the cutoff or clinical decision point separating nondisease from disease impacts the sensitivity and specificity. If the decision point is moved so that sensitivity is improved, specificity will decrease.

These data can be used to determine how well a given test meets specific uses. For example, a test used to screen for disease in the general population should have good sensitivity, that is, it should produce as few false negatives as possible because the goal of screening is to detect anyone who might have the disease but be asymptomatic. Good sensitivity is also needed for tests used to diagnose diseases that should not be missed. Furthermore, tests used to diagnose treatable diseases where false-positive results could cause serious trauma (physical, psychological, or economic) should also have high sensitivity.

However, tests used to confirm the presence of disease should have few false positives in order to establish that a disease is present, and for this reason confirmatory tests should have good specificity. High specificity is also required for those tests used to identify diseases for which there is no treatment or cure, for those used to diagnose diseases for which knowledge that the disease is absent has psychological or public health value, and where false-positive results can lead to serious trauma to the patient.

The predictive value of a test depends on sensitivity, specificity, and the prevalence of a disease in the population tested. Prevalence is the number of cases of a disease in the population being tested at a given time. Incidence refers to the number of cases observed over a period of time.

> **QUICK REVIEW**
> The positive predictive value describes the probability that a positive test result will accurately reflect the true presence of disease:
>
> $$\text{Positive predictive value} = \frac{\text{True positives}}{\text{True positive} + \text{false positives}} \times 100\%$$
>
> In other words, it asks the question: if the patient has a positive result, what is the likelihood that the patient has the disease?
>
> The ability of a negative test result to predict the absence of disease is calculated by
>
> $$\text{Negatives predictive value} = \frac{\text{True negatives}}{\text{True negatives} + \text{false negatives}} \times 100\%$$
>
> It asks the question, if a patient has a negative test result, then what is the probability that the patient is disease free? A test's negative predictive value is clinically useful because it gives one a sense of the correctness of a negative result for a given patient and indicates its utility in ruling out disease.

Clinical decision limits can also be based on the diagnostic performance of a test, that is, the test's sensitivity, specificity, and predictive value. An example of the use of test performance to establish limits is seen in Case 6-2; a 52-year-old man who presents to the emergency department with mild chest pain and shortness of breath that began at the end of a long-duration flight. This history raises the possibility that his symptoms are indicative of a thrombotic event, such as a pulmonary embolism (PE). Unfortunately, there is no test specific for PE or thrombosis, but we know that an increase in coagulation correlates with increased fibrinolysis, and that fibrin degradation leads to an increase in fibrin fragments known as D-dimers. These fragments increase with deep vein thrombosis, pulmonary emboli, streptococcal infections, thrombocytopenia, and several other conditions, so the test is not specific for any of these conditions. In other words, a result above a defined concentration indicates increased fibrinolysis, but does not specifically rule-in any of the conditions. The test's greatest value is being used to eliminate or "rule-out" these conditions, if the result is less than the clinical decision point. If the test result is above the clinical decision point, then the patient can be triaged to the appropriate confirmatory testing. In this particular case, the D-dimer was below the decision point and so the patient did not undergo a CT scan or ultrasonography appropriate to aid in the diagnosis of a PE. Another laboratory test, troponin I, performed at the same time, however, was significantly elevated above the clinical decision point and cardiac catheterization indicated a blocked coronary.

Biological Variation

The body is not static. For example, changes occur every day due to stressors, growth, and cell cycling. In response, analytes change throughout the day, from day to day, and over longer time intervals—that is, they show **biological variation**. Many hormones respond to sleep-wake or light-dark cycles to give distinct patterns of increasing and decreasing concentrations over the 24-hour period (these are known as circadian or diurnal patterns). These same hormones may also respond to stress, to temperature, to exercise, to food, which cause random changes in concentrations. The highest concentrations of cortisol and ACTH, for example, are seen in the morning about 0800 hours. Concentrations decline gradually afterward and throughout the day until they reach the lowest point about 2000 hours. Episodic release of the two will be encountered throughout the day in response to stress or other events. Other hormones exhibiting a circadian pattern include TSH and growth hormone.

Circadian patterns differ. For example, the circadian pattern observed for TSH reaches highest concentrations around 2400 hours then declining to its nadir between noon and mid-afternoon. Like cortisol and ACTH, this hormone will also be released in pulses throughout the day. Circadian patterns are not exhibited by only hormones; nonhormones with such patterns include potassium, creatinine, and iron. One must therefore need to consider a patient's sleep–wake cycle when interpreting results of these analytes.

The methods and instruments in use today have good analytical precision so that when analytes are followed closely, for example, by repeat testing over several days or weeks, much of the difference seen between the measurements may be due to biological variation. Thus, it is helpful to consider both analytical precision and biological variation when using a test to follow the course of a disease or the response to treatment. Since it is not practical to determine every patient's personal biological variation, you will find it useful to turn to studies in which these have been estimated in healthy populations. For example, sodium, albumin, and calcium change little from day to day in a healthy individual, while others such as triglycerides, iron, and TSH vary quite a bit.

QUICK REVIEW

So how does one handle the variability in a series of test results? How can one distinguish the impact of analytical and biological variations from pathological changes? Total intraindividual variation represents the combined influence of analytical and biological variation and can be estimated by the formula

$$CV_i = \sqrt{CV^2_{bi} + CV^2_a}$$

where CV_i is the total coefficient of variation for the intraindividaul variation, CV^2_{bi} is the biological intraindividual coefficient of variation, and CV^2_a is the analytical coefficient of variation. By multiplying the CV_i by 2.77, one can determine the least significant change. Two results should differ by this amount to be considered statistically significant.

DEALING WITH UNEXPECTED RESULTS

The natural response of many clinicians on receiving an unexpected result is to wonder what the laboratory has done incorrectly. Errors certainly do occur within the clinical laboratory or testing setting. Given the volume of testing and the fact that instruments are human inventions, such error is inevitable. However, most of the instruments and methods in use are extremely robust. Repeat testing of the sample verifies or confirms the result >99% of the time in one major clinical laboratory. That does not suggest that the results are always clinically correct. A result may repeat yet be incorrect due to interference from hemolysis, an unreported contaminant in the phlebotomy tube or from an over-the-counter medication the patient did not admit to taking. Other nonanalytical causes of unexpected results include unanticipated or detected pathology, unrecognized changes in physiology, pharmaceutical interactions or effects, improper patient preparation, or incorrect specimen collection or handling. Talk to the laboratory before ordering repeat testing. *Laboratories consider the clinician who is using the result in the care of the patient from whom the sample was derived as the best quality assurance indicator.*

SUMMARY

The Value of Laboratory Testing

For many years, it has been stated that about 70% of medical decisions are based on laboratory test results. Unfortunately, these claims were derived originally from loosely acquired data using physician surveys and chart reviews. Medical economists found it challenging to firmly determine the value of testing in this country because of its ready availability. However, a careful recent study demonstrated that testing narrowed the differential diagnosis in 93% of the cases, changed disposition in 43% of the cases in which it was performed, and substantially changed treatment in 75% of the cases.

Economically, laboratory testing is one of the greatest values in patient care. Yes, the billions of tests performed do contribute to the overall health-care budget, but laboratory testing represents only 2.3% of US health-care expenditures. When used wisely, it is an effective and efficient tool. Because laboratory testing impacts the care of so many patients, it is clear why laboratory medicine, the part of pathology that provides this service, is considered one of the most important contributors to patient care. It is essential to the health-care system and key to many clinical decisions.

CHAPTER 7

The Vascular System

Karen L. Kelly, M.D.

INTRODUCTION

Blood moves through the vascular system secondary to pressure and osmotic gradients similar to a plumbing system, but, unlike our household pipes, the system of blood vessels is not made up of static and inflexible structures. The vascular system is dynamic and always changing to regulate blood flow to the body and its essential organs. The system of blood vessels with the heart at its center is critical for delivering oxygenated blood and essential nutrients to organs and tissues and removing and transporting waste products.

This chapter will cover the normal circulatory system and its structures and congenital and acquired diseases including atherosclerosis, trauma, and inflammatory and infectious processes. The pulmonary vascular system and its diseases will also be discussed.

EMBRYOLOGY OF BLOOD VESSELS

The cardiovascular system develops very early in gestation (as early as 15–16 days) due to the limited energy sources available from the egg and yolk sac. The cardiovascular system delivers nutrients to the increasingly actively dividing cells and disposes of waste products through its connections with the maternal vasculature of the placenta. The heart and blood vessels are created from the mesoderm that forms blood islands (isolated cell masses) around which the endothelial tubes are formed. Vascular smooth muscle cells and connective tissue derived from the local mesoderm then surround the endothelial tubes. The heart begins to beat and blood begins to circulate throughout the blood vessel network around the 4th week of gestation (Figure 7-1).

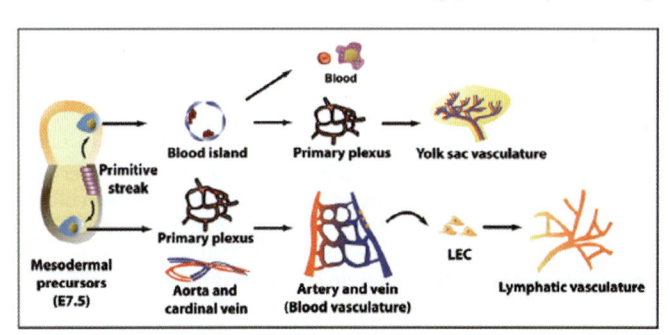

FIGURE 7-1 Embryological development of blood vessels. In the extraembryonic yolk sac, mesodermal precursor cells aggregate to form blood islands, the sites of development of endothelial and primitive blood cells. Within the blood islands, centrally-located cells become primitive blood cells, whereas outer cells give rise to endothelial cells (ECs). ECs then form the vascular primary plexus which is subsequently remodeled to form the yolk sac vasculature. In the embryo proper, mesodermal precursor cells differentiate into the vascular primary plexus and major vessels, aorta, and cardinal vein. After arterial and venous ECs are specified, the complex blood vasculature is formed via extensive remodeling. At embryonic day (E) 9.5, a subset of ECs of the cardinal vein acquires a lymphatic endothelial cell (LEC) fate and develops into lymphatic vessels.
From Park C, Kim TM, Malik AB. Transcriptional regulation of endothelial cell and vascular development. *Circ Res*. 2013;112:1380–1400.

QUICK REVIEW
Normal Anatomy of Blood Vessels
Blood vessels consist of arteries, veins, and capillaries that are categorized according to their structure, size, and function. The arterial system carries oxygenated blood away from the heart to the organs and periphery providing oxygen and nutrients to the cells at a distance. The capillary system is responsible for the exchange of new supplies and the waste products. The venous system carries the deoxygenated blood with its waste products back to the heart for transport to the lungs for replenishment of oxygen. Lymphatics are a back-up system that operates to assist the vascular system.

Arteries are made up of three layers: the intima, media, and adventitia. The intima is composed of a confluent, single-cell layer of endothelium lining the blood vessel lumen, a basement membrane, and subendothelial connective tissue along the luminal side of the internal elastic lamina.

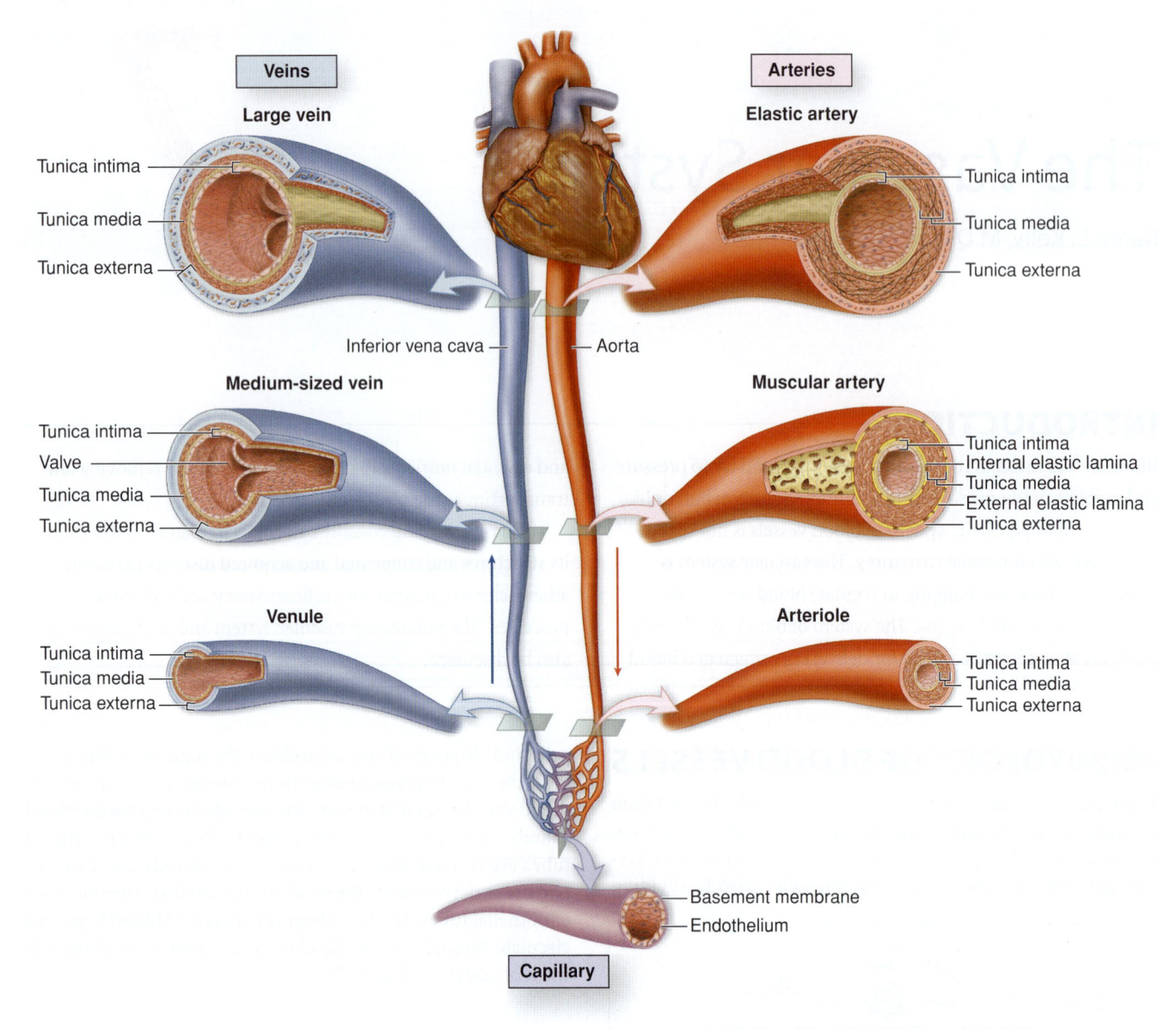

FIGURE 7-2 Vessels of the blood circulatory system. The heart is the principal organ of the blood circulatory system, pumping blood throughout the body and providing one of the forces by which nutrients leave the capillaries and enter tissues. Large elastic arteries leave the heart and branch to form muscular arteries. These arteries branch further and enter organs, where they branch further to form arterioles. These arterioles branch into the smallest vessels, the capillaries, composed by a single cell layer allowing exchange of nutrients and waste products between blood and surrounding tissue. Capillaries then merge to form venules, which merge further into small- and later medium-sized veins. These veins leave organs and form larger veins that eventually bring blood back to the heart. From Mescher AL. *Junqueira's Basic Histology Text & Atlas*. 12th ed. New York, NY: McGraw-Hill Lange; 2010. Figure 11-1, page 186.

The cells of the intima derive their nutrients and oxygen directly from the luminal contents. The media is the middle and thickest layer of the artery bounded by the internal and external elastic laminae. Its components include smooth muscle fibers and collagen. Additional components (elastic fibers) vary depending on the size and function of the artery. Changes in the arterial media are due to local adaptations for mechanical or metabolic needs of the organ or tissue. These adaptive structural changes are primarily seen in the media and external elastic lamina. The outermost layer, the adventitia, is composed of the external elastic lamina, connective tissue, nerves, and small blood vessels (vasa vasorum). The vasa vasorum are the "artery's artery" and are the source of nutrients and oxygen for the arterial media.

The arterial system, responsible for conducting the blood to the periphery and for creating peripheral resistance, is divided into three types based on size, structural features, and function. The three arterial types are divided by their medial components and include elastic arteries, muscular arteries, and small arteries and arterioles.

Elastic arteries are the large-diameter, low-resistance arteries of the body and include the aorta (the largest blood vessel in the body), aortic branches (the brachiocephalic, subclavian, common carotids, and iliac arteries), and the pulmonary arteries. The media of the elastic arteries is rich in elastic fibers arranged in compact layers that alternate with smooth muscle cells. The elastic component allows for expansion of the artery during cardiac systole (contraction of the heart), creating kinetic energy for elastic recoil and propulsion of blood to the periphery during cardiac diastole (relaxation of the heart). The media of the elastic arteries is supplied with oxygenated blood and nutrients through the small arteries throughout the adventitia.

The muscular, **medium-sized arteries** are considered the distribution system and conduct the blood to the organs and periphery. The major muscular arteries to be discussed include the coronary, renal, and femoral arteries. The media of these arteries is composed of a circular to spiral arrangement of smooth muscle cells without elastic fibers. The lack of elastic fibers allows more efficient contraction of the artery in response to appropriate stimulation. The internal and external elastic laminae are the only elastic elements of the muscular arteries. As the muscular arteries branch, the media thins, the internal elastic lamina disappears, and the intima is a single layer of endothelial cells (ECs).

Small arteries and arterioles are differentiated by size: small arteries are <2 mm and arterioles are 20 to 100 μm in diameter. They are made up of a single-cell layer of endothelium, a few layers of smooth muscle cells, and adventitia. Small arteries and arterioles are critically important as they regulate regional blood flow and systemic blood pressure by changes in the caliber of the lumen.

The small arteries and arterioles lead to the **capillary system** where exchange of nutrients, oxygen, and waste products actually occurs through the smallest (diameter of a red blood cell), thin-walled (single endothelial layer supported by scattered smooth muscle cells) vessels. The capillary system has a markedly increased surface area and decreased flow velocity to maximize the exchange between the blood and tissues. The highest density capillary systems are found in organs and tissues with a high metabolic rate (myocardium). ECs are semipermeable allowing for exchange controlled by molecular size and charge of the substrate. Like other portions of the vascular system, capillaries are modified according to the tissue or organ they supply by alterations of their ECs creating changes in permeability and their ability to transport substances across cell membranes (pinocytosis). For example, fenestrated capillaries in renal glomeruli are specifically adapted to allow filtration of plasma.

From the capillary system, the blood begins its return to the heart through postcapillary venules (small veins), to collecting venules, to small veins, medium veins, and large veins. Veins are thin-walled, large–volume, and large-diameter vessels with less-organized walls. They are also surrounded by less support allowing for irregular dilatation, compression, and penetration by tumor and inflammatory cells. Collectively, the venous system contains approximately two-thirds of our blood volume at one time. Reverse flow is prevented by venous valves.

Lymphatics are thin-walled, endothelial-lined channels that serve as a back-up for the vascular system by collecting interstitial fluids and returning them to the vascular system via the thoracic duct. Of note, lymphatics are very important as they are easily accessed by tumor cells and microorganisms leading to dissemination of disease.

The **pulmonary vasculature** is a crucial part of the cardiovascular system as it carries deoxygenated blood from the right side of the heart to the lungs. If this pathway is disrupted or interrupted, the blood can no longer reach the lungs for oxygenation leading to death.

Embryologically, the aorta and main pulmonary artery are formed from the truncus arteriosus (the single blood vessel arising from the heart) by septation. Therefore, prior to birth, the main pulmonary artery is a large elastic artery similar to the aorta. After birth, its elastic fibers become less organized (**Figures 7-2** and **7-3**).

DISEASES OF THE VASCULAR SYSTEM

Congenital Vascular Anomalies

Congenital vascular anomalies are most commonly vascular structures with abnormal branching and anastomotic connections that are developed in utero. However, such congenital abnormalities are not necessarily genetically transmitted. Two important congenital vascular anomalies include the **berry aneurysm** and the **arteriovenous malformation (AVM)**.

Berry Aneurysm

The berry aneurysm is a **saccular aneurysm** (a dilated outpouching of a blood vessel that forms a sac-like structure with its artery at its base) found in approximately 2% of autopsies and in 3% to 6% of the general population. The abnormality is most commonly found intracranially. At birth, the arterial medial layer is abnormal creating a focal weakness in the arterial wall. The dilated outpouching is not present at birth, but forms over time with increased vascular pressure and various risk factors including cocaine use and cigarette smoking. The majority (90%) of berry aneurysms are found in the anterior cerebral circulation of the circle of Willis at its major branch points (internal carotid arteries, anterior communicating arteries, etc.), where there is significant turbulence and shear forces. Multiple aneurysms in a single person are seen in 20% to 30% of cases. Annual rupture rates in one large study showed that aneurysms <10 mm had a rupture rate of 0.05%. Rates of rupture were higher (~1%) for aneurysms >10 mm in diameter, those that were symptomatic, or those located in the posterior circulation.

Most aneurysms are clinically silent and asymptomatic, remaining undetected until rupture. Clinical presentation of a ruptured berry aneurysm (the first presentation in over 50% of cases) is most commonly "the worst headache of my life"

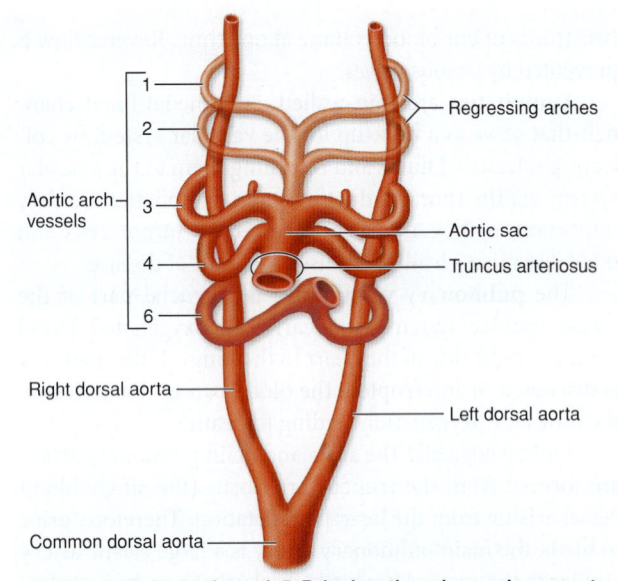

Aortic Arch Vessel	Postnatal Structure Formed by Vessels
1	Small part of maxillary arteries
2	Small part of stapedial arteries
3	Left and right common carotid arteries
4	Right vessel: proximal part of right subclavian artery Left vessel: aortic arch (connects to the left dorsal aorta)
6	Right vessel: right pulmonary artery Left vessel: left pulmonary artery and ductus arteriosus

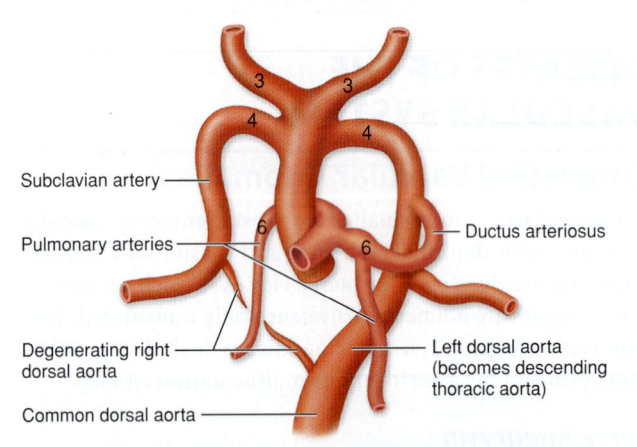

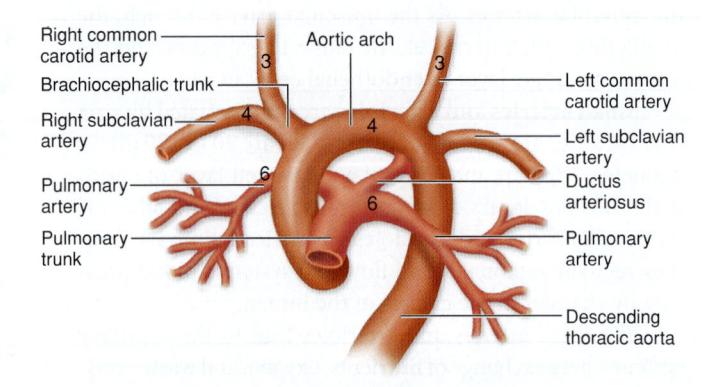

FIGURE 7-3 Thoracic artery development. Aortic arch vessels form most of the major thoracic and head and neck arteries. From McKinley M, O'Loughlin VD. *Human Anatomy*. 2nd ed. New York, NY: McGraw-Hill; 2008. Figure 23.24, page 714.

with nausea and vomiting. There may be a loss of consciousness. The ruptured aneurysm leads to a **diffuse subarachnoid hemorrhage** (blood over the surface of the brain below the arachnoid) **(Figure 7-4A)**. The hemorrhage leads to contraction of cerebral vasculature (vasospasm) and decreased blood flow, which leads in turn to decreased oxygenation of the brain or cerebral ischemia. Rupture of a cerebral aneurysm is a medical emergency due to the significant morbidity and mortality. With the first rupture, 25% to 50% of patients will die. Some patients may regain consciousness while others will not.

Gross pathology of the aneurysm is a sac-like structure protruding from its artery. Histologically, the aneurysm wall is made up of a thickened, hyalinized intimal layer and adventitia. The media in the area of the aneurysm is absent (Figure 7-4B). The frequency of berry aneurysms varies by anatomic location **(Figure 7-5)**.

While the majority of berry aneurysms are sporadic and not genetically transmitted, they may be associated with polycystic kidney disease (autosomal dominant polycystic kidney [ADPK] disease), Ehlers–Danlos and Marfan syndromes, neurofibromatosis type I, fibromuscular dysplasia, and coarctation of the aorta.

Arteriovenous Malformation

AVMs (also known as arteriovenous fistula) are abnormal direct communication between arterial and venous vessels without the interposed, normal capillary system leading to a short circuit of blood flow. These abnormalities are more commonly found in men (2:1) and are most likely to be clinically recognized between 10 and 30 years of age. They may present as a new-onset seizure disorder with stroke-like symptoms or rupture.

CASE 7-1

A previously healthy, 30-year-old woman complained of the "worst headache" of her life before collapsing at an aerobics class. She was rushed to the local emergency department where it was found on CT scan that she had diffuse subarachnoid hemorrhage. An autopsy showed a ruptured cerebral berry aneurysm (Figure 7-4)

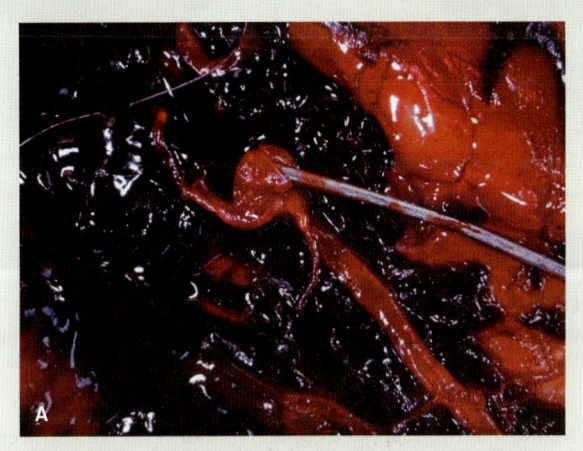

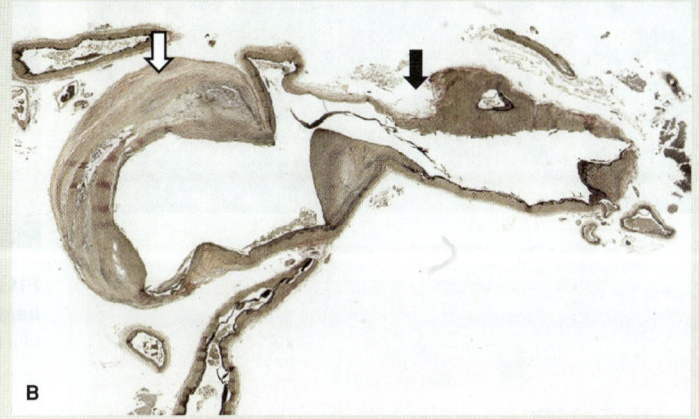

FIGURE 7-4 (A) Acute subarachnoid hemorrhage secondary to ruptured berry aneurysm: probe indicates ruptured saccular aneurysm of middle cerebral artery. Note the large thrombus on the left of image. From Department of Pathology and Laboratory Medicine, University of North Carolina at Chapel Hill. **(B) Berry aneurysm (elastic tissue stain).** Area of rupture is shown by a black arrow. Area of dilatation and disorganization of elastic tissue is shown by a hollow arrow. From Department of Pathology and Laboratory Medicine, University of North Carolina at Chapel Hill.

Grossly, the AVM appears as worm-like channels. Histologically, the enlarged blood vessels show abnormal arteries and veins (Figure 7-6).

Capillary Hemangioma

An abnormal, localized, usually superficial collection of capillaries commonly seen in infancy or childhood (with a frequency of 1:200) is termed a **capillary hemangioma** (Figure 7-7A). A number of these collections are present at birth (30%) and may enlarge with a child's growth. They are most often seen on the head or neck, but up to one-third can be found in the liver, spleen, or kidneys. These collections do not undergo malignant transformation. Most (75%–90%) will regress by 7 years of age.

The usual "**strawberry**" **hemangioma** (birth mark) seen in infants and children may show rapid growth initially and may be multiple. Grossly, they are bright red to blue in color, are level with the skin surface, and have an intact epithelial surface. Histology shows an unencapsulated aggregate of closely spaced, thin-walled, blood-filled, endothelial-lined capillaries.

Another type of vascular "tumor" is a **cavernous hemangioma**, a similar collection of larger-caliber vessels usually situated more deeply in tissues or organs (Figure 7-7B).

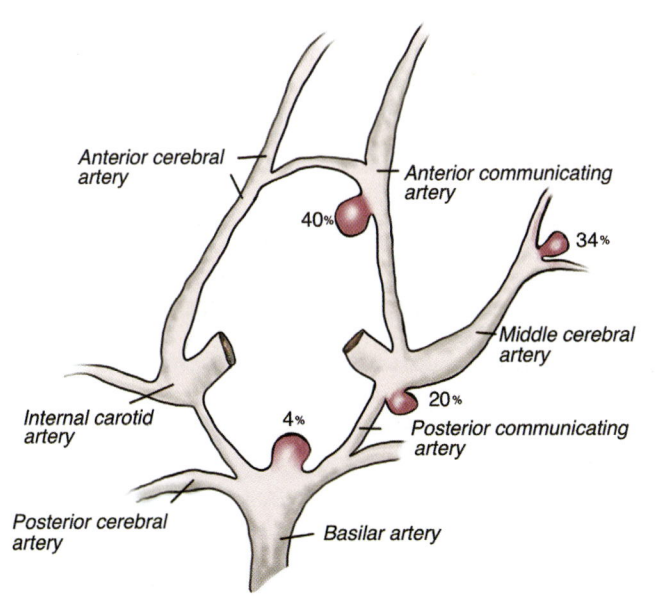

Vascular Ectasias

Vascular ectasias are localized dilatations of preexisting blood vessels usually seen in the skin or mucous membranes that create a focal red lesion.

The **nevus flammeus**, also known as the "port-wine stain," is most commonly seen over the face and neck in the distribution of the trigeminal nerve. It may be associated with **Sturge–Weber syndrome** that includes port-wine stain of the face and venous angiomas of the leptomeninges (covering of the brain) and may cause mental retardation, seizures, and strokes. In patients with nevus flammeus, it is necessary to determine whether there are associated cerebral vascular abnormalities.

FIGURE 7-5 Most common sites of intracranial aneurysms (**berry aneurysms**). From Department of Pathology and Laboratory Medicine, University of North Carolina at Chapel Hill.

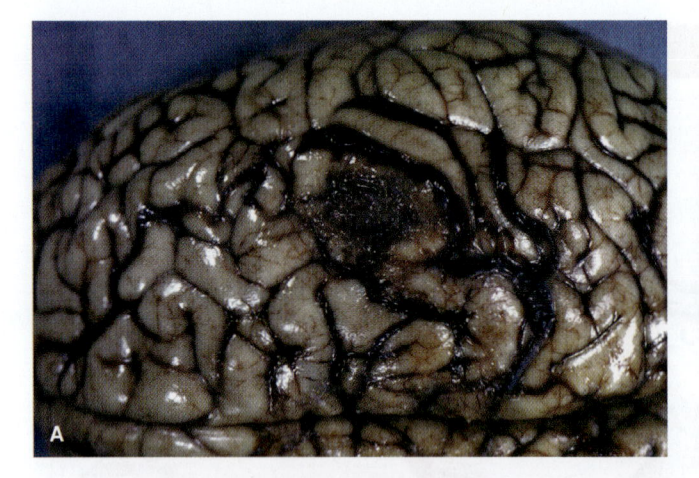

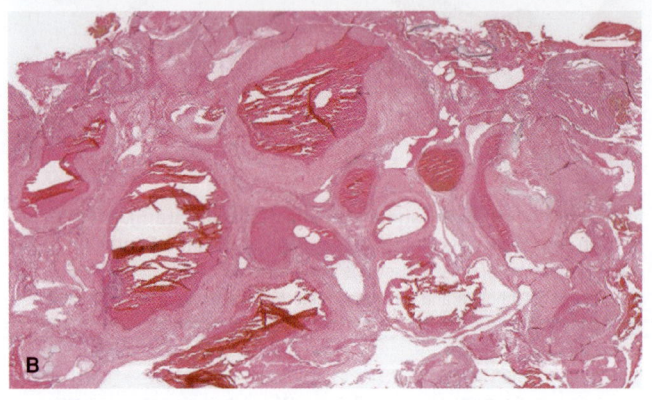

FIGURE 7-6 Arteriovenous malformation of the brain. **(A)** Gross fixed tissue, external cortical view. From Peter Anderson D.V.M., Ph.D., PEIR Digital Library Image 9386. **(B)** Microscopic view (low power). From Department of Pathology and Laboratory Medicine, University of North Carolina at Chapel Hill.

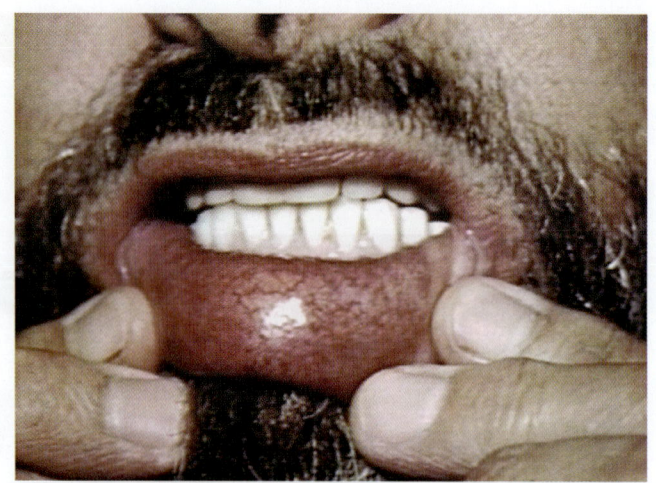

FIGURE 7-8 Osler Weber Rendu disease (hereditary hemorrhagic telangiectasia). Characteristic telangiectasias on the lip of a patient. From Peter Anderson D.V.M., Ph.D., PEIR Digital Library Image 212369.

Malformations of dilated capillaries and veins are also seen in autosomal dominant inherited **Osler–Weber–Rendu disease**. These patients may have these dilated collections of vessels involving their oral cavity, lips, lungs, gastrointestinal tract, or urinary system. As these vascular collections are structurally abnormal, they are at risk for rupture or bleeding (Figure 7-8).

Nonatherosclerotic Diseases

Aortic Dissection

Aortic dissection (also called "dissecting aortic aneurysm") is a rare but frequently fatal process caused by an intimal–medial tear that allows passage of aortic blood from the true aortic lumen into the medial layer of the aorta creating a **false lumen**. Aortic dissection has an incidence of 5 to 30 cases per 1 million per year (approximately 2000 cases per year) with a male predominance (2:1) and a peak occurrence in 60- to 70-year-olds. The most common risk factor for an acute aortic dissection in those without an inherited connective tissue

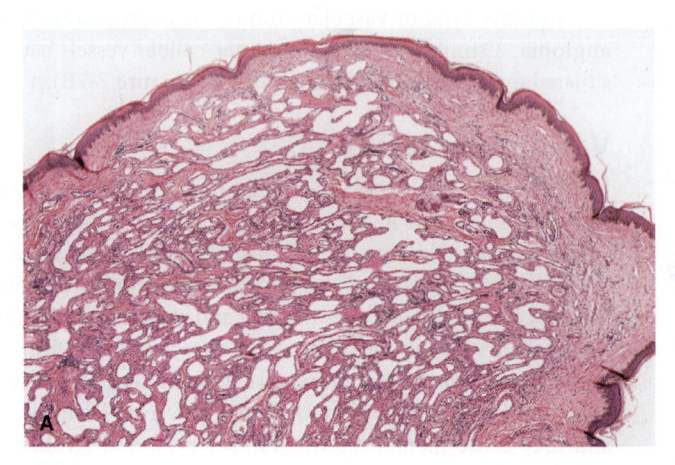

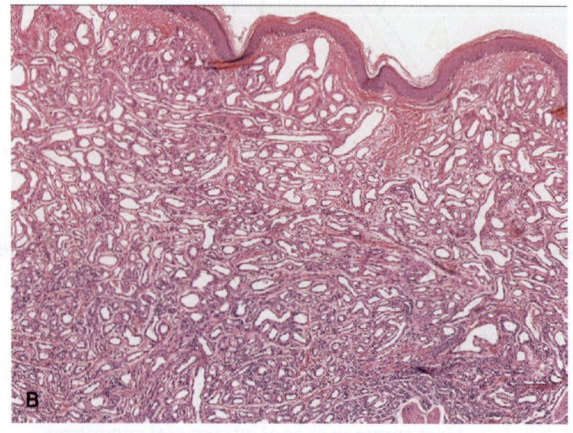

A **spider telangiectasia** is a radial, often pulsatile array of dilated subcutaneous small arterioles usually seen on the face, neck, and chest. They appear to be related to increased systemic estrogen and are often seen in pregnant women and alcoholics with hepatic cirrhosis.

FIGURE 7-7 Hemangiomas (microscopic views). **(A)** Hyperplastic capillary hemangioma of the skin. **(B)** Cavernous hemangioma of the liver. From Department of Pathology and Laboratory Medicine, University of North Carolina at Chapel Hill.

CASE 7-2

A 67-year-old man, with a history of treated systemic hypertension, suddenly grasped his chest and collapsed while at a local grocery store. Emergency medical services found him unresponsive with a weak pulse. He was rushed to the emergency department where he could not be resuscitated. Autopsy showed a large **hemopericardium** (blood in the pericardial sac) and an aortic dissection with rupture of the ascending aorta (**Figure 7-9**).

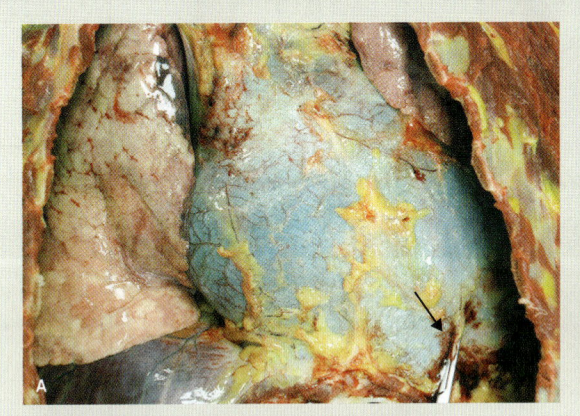

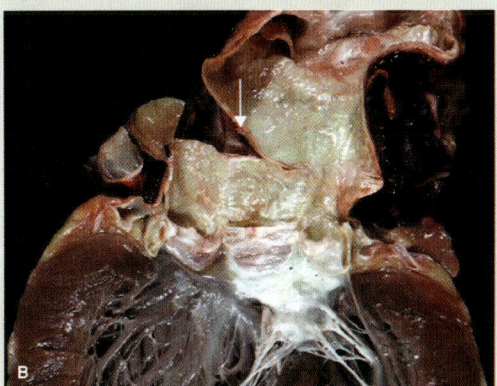

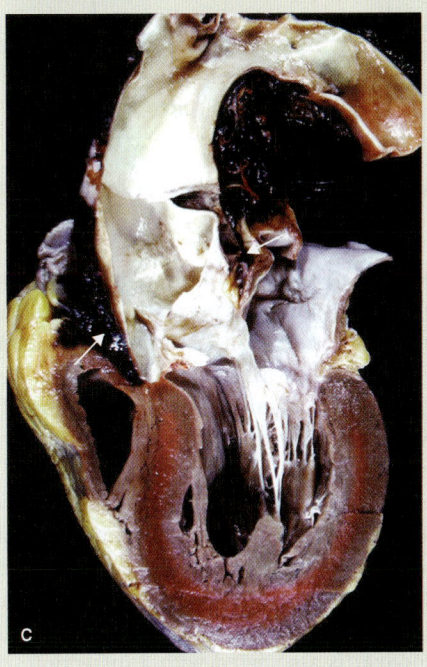

FIGURE 7-9 Aortic dissection. **(A)** View of the chest demonstrating hemopericardium. Note extravasated blood at the point of disruption of the pericardium (arrow). From Vincent J. Moylan, Jr., M.S., P.A. (ASCP), Department of Pathology and Laboratory Medicine, University of North Carolina at Chapel Hill. **(B)** Heart with aorta opened to show the origin of the intimal-medial tear leading to the dissection above the aortic valve (arrow; DeBakey type I; see Figure 7-10). **(C)** Aorta in cross-section to show blood between the layers of the media (false lumen) (arrow). Figures 7-9b and 7-9c: From Department of Pathology and Laboratory Medicine, University of North Carolina at Chapel Hill.

disorder (see below) is systemic hypertension (70%–80% of patients). Other risk factors include prior traumatic injury, including iatrogenic, procedure-related injury, aortitis, and medial dysplasia. Cocaine use, which causes a rapid and acute elevation of blood pressure, is also a risk factor and can lead to aortic dissection in younger patients.

Aortic dissections are classified according to their anatomic location and duration of symptoms. The two most frequently used classification schemes are the DeBakey and the Sanford classifications. The Sanford classification is simplest to understand and is based on the site of the dissection. Sanford type A denotes involvement of the ascending thoracic aorta, regardless of its site of origin. Sanford type B indicates that the ascending aorta is not involved. The DeBakey classification is more complicated, but is most commonly used clinically by surgeons. The most common aortic dissection seen in approximately 54% of cases, the DeBakey type I dissection, indicates that the intimal-medial tear is in the ascending thoracic aorta with the dissection extending distally to the descending thoracic aorta. In DeBakey type II dissections, the intimal-medial tear again is in the ascending thoracic aorta, and the dissection is limited to this region of the aorta. DeBakey type II dissections occur in approximately 20% of patients. In DeBakey type III dissections, the intimal-medial tear is located distally, usually in the distal aortic arch or the proximal descending thoracic aorta. Type III is divided into two subtypes: type IIIa indicates that

Classification of aortic dissection

60%	10%–15%	25%–30%
DeBakey I	Debakey II	Debakey III

FIGURE 7-10 **DeBakey dissection Scheme.** From Department of Pathology and Laboratory Medicine, University of North Carolina at Chapel Hill.

the dissection, by retrograde extension, involves the ascending thoracic aorta; type IIIb indicates that the dissection is limited to the distal aorta without involvement of the ascending region (Figure 7-10). The determination of the origin of the dissection is crucial for the surgeon who must know where to enter the chest for the aortic repair.

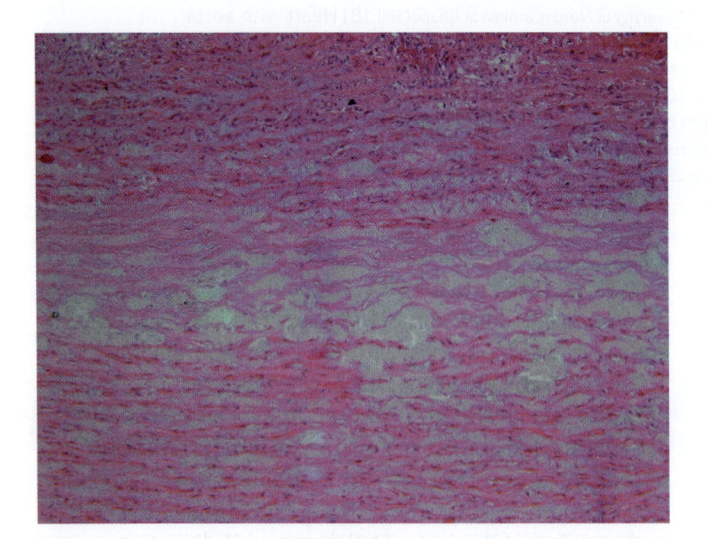

FIGURE 7-11 **Cystic medial necrosis.** The acellular myxoid material (blue) divides and disrupts the elastic fibers of the media. These changes predispose the individual to developing an aortic dissection. From Kemp WL, Burns DK, Brown T. *The Big Picture Pathology.* New York, NY: McGraw-Hill Lange; 2008. Figure 9-8, page 100.

The mechanism of the intimal–medial tear that leads to an acute aortic dissection is presently unknown, although theories abound. The common factor in those with an aortic dissection is acquired or inherited aortic medial weakness (also known as "**cystic medial necrosis**"). Aortic medial weakness occurs with disruption and interruption of elastic fibers and is a microscopic diagnosis (see below) (Figure 7-11).

The pathology of the gross specimen shows a usually horizontal to hockey-stick-shaped intimal-medial tear of the proximal ascending aorta approximately 1 to 3 cm above the aortic valve. Separation between the layers of the aorta with blood clot between the inner and outer medial layers will be seen if the tear is associated with a dissection. Multiple intimal tears and evidence of healing or healed dissections may be seen along the descending thoracic and abdominal aorta as these are most commonly asymptomatic.

Histology of an acute aortic dissection shows separation between the intima-inner two-thirds of the media and the outer one-third of the media–adventitia with hemorrhage between these layers. In elderly hypertensive patients, the aortic media is usually histologically normal without obvious changes of medial weakness (Figure 7-12).

Clinical symptoms are most commonly an abrupt onset of severe chest pain. The location of the pain is usually associated with the location of the dissection: anterior chest pain is associated with dissection involving the ascending aorta (DeBakey type II) and back or interscapular pain is associated with dissection of the distal aortic arch or descending thoracic aorta

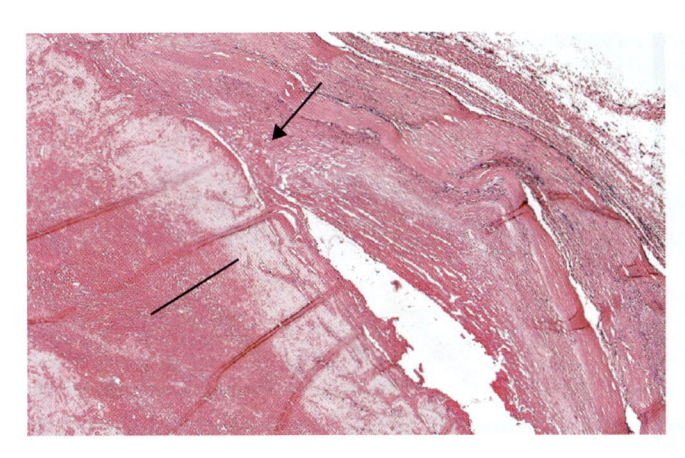

FIGURE 7-12 **Histology of an aortic dissection.** An area of medial disruption in the aorta is shown (arrow). The dissecting blood (thrombus) occupies the lower portion of the image (line). (See also Figure 7-9C.) From Department of Pathology and Laboratory Medicine, University of North Carolina at Chapel Hill.

(DeBakey types I and III). Additional symptoms include syncope, stroke, paraplegia, and sudden death. Often symptoms will vary according to areas of the aorta affected. Patients may present with cough or dysphagia due to compression of the trachea or esophagus by the enlarged, dissected aorta. Other symptoms can result from vascular ischemia, as small arteries are no longer supplied with oxygenated blood from the true lumen.

This disease is important because it is a difficult diagnosis to make. Most commonly diagnosed as an acute myocardial infarct, patients are often sent home when their EKGs and cardiac enzymes are normal. These patients go home and have an increased risk of sudden death due to the significant complications of dissection. There is a high mortality rate if the diagnosis is missed.

The most significant complications include rupture of the false lumen and compression of the true lumen and its arterial branches. Rupture of the false lumen that occurs into the pericardium leads to **pericardial tamponade** in approximately 90% of proximal dissections. Continued compression of the true lumen and the aortic branches leads to ischemia of the organs deprived of oxygenation. For example, if the carotid artery branches are involved, the brain may be deprived of oxygen leading to cerebral ischemia and stroke (Figure 7-9A).

Disease processes that are associated with aortic dissection include Marfan and Ehlers–Danlos syndromes, congenitally bicuspid aortic valve, aortic coarctation, Turner syndrome, and aortitis. **Marfan syndrome**, an inherited connective tissue disease, leads to significant aortic medial weakness with large pools of basophilic glycosaminoglycans with significant interruption and disruption of elastic fibers. Patients with Marfan syndrome account for approximately 5% to 10% of all aortic dissections. Approximately one-third of patients with Marfan syndrome develop aortic dissections and must be carefully monitored. **Congenitally abnormal aortic valve disease** is also associated with a significantly increased risk of aortic dissection. Bicuspid disease has a nine times greater risk of aortic dissection than patients with a normal, tricuspid aortic valve. Patients with a unicuspid aortic valve have a nearly 20-fold increased risk. As awareness has increased over time, this process has been dubbed Bicuspid Aortic Disease (BAD).

Surgical treatment of aortic dissections involves placement of an interposition tube graft at the site of the intimal tear that redirects the blood into the true lumen.

Aortitis

Noninfectious Aortitis

The most significant noninfectious inflammatory diseases of the aorta (**aortitis**) include **Takayasu disease** and **giant cell aortitis**. Multiple systemic connective tissues diseases can also involve the aorta and may have disease-specific features. For example, patients with rheumatoid arthritis (RA) may have rheumatoid nodules in the media of the aorta. Regardless of the underlying etiology, the aorta has limited means of reaction to injury and demonstrates the same gross features of acute and chronic phases regardless of the disease process. The gross features of the acute phase show edema and irregularity of the intimal layer. The gross features of the chronic phase of any aortitis shows marked intimal and adventitial thickening of the vessels with interruption and disruption of the medial elastic fibers and replacement fibrosis. The irregular intimal thickening and the contraction of the scarred media leads to wrinkling of the intima and the classic "tree-bark"-like appearance (Figure 7-13). Like the gross appearance, the histologic appearance of aortitis is not specific; the same type of inflammation, including giant cells, can be seen in noninfectious and infectious aortitis. The incidence, patient features, symptoms, and histology all help differentiate the specific type of aortitis in each case. Also, in the chronic phase, aortitis can lead to aneurysm formation anywhere along the aorta. These aneurysms have an increased risk for rupture.

Takayasu Disease

Takayasu disease is a granulomatous inflammation of large- and medium-sized arteries. Multiple synonyms for the disease include pulseless disease, occlusive thromboaortopathy, and young female arteritis. The majority of cases have been seen in Asia and Africa, but cases have been identified worldwide.

Takayasu disease affects women more frequently than men (8:1) most often between 20 and 30 years of age. Approximately two cases per million patients per year are diagnosed in North America and Europe. The disease affects the aorta and the proximal portions of its large branch arteries. Symptoms of the acute phase are similar to all vasculitides and can range from absence of symptoms to fever, weakness, malaise, myalgias, arthralgias, and anorexia. The acute phase can precede the chronic (or occlusive) phase by weeks, months, or years. In the chronic phase, patients may be asymptomatic or may suffer severe systemic complications including stroke, renal artery stenosis, or blindness. Often the patients present with absence of peripheral pulses (96%), bruits (94%), hypertension (74%), and heart failure (28%). The subclavian arteries are involved in approximately 90%, the carotid arteries in 45%, the vertebral

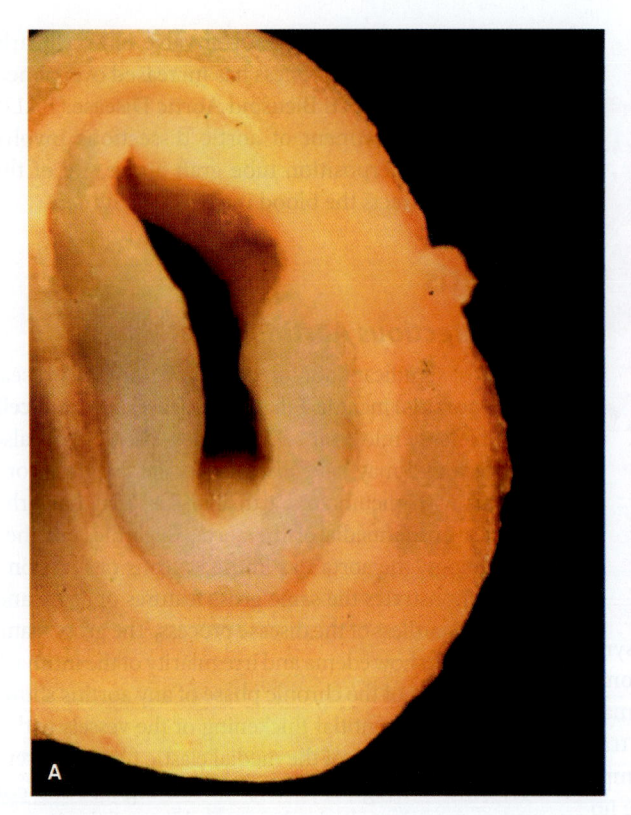

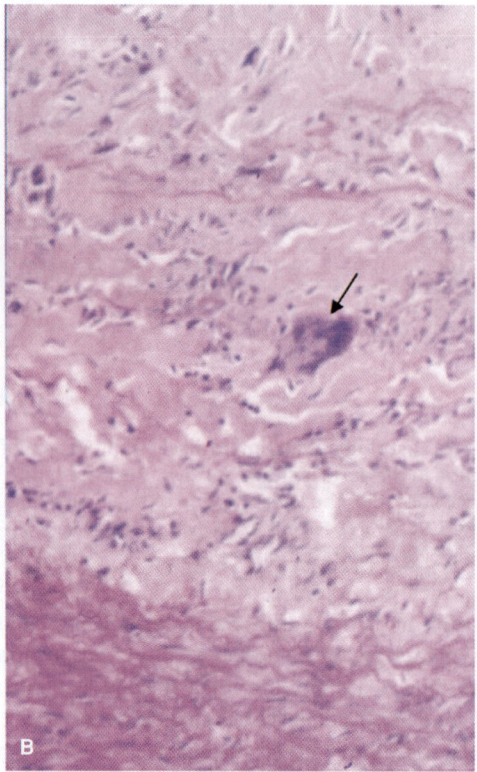

FIGURE 7-13 Takayasu aortitis. Innominate artery of a 27-year-old woman with Takayasu arteritis with arch vessel involvement. **(A)** Extensive intimal thickening is seen with attenuation of the media and adventitial fibrosis. **(B)** Histology revealed degeneration of the media with a dense inflammatory infiltrate, including giant cells (arrow). Image courtesy of Dr. Richard N. Mitchell, Department of Pathology, Brigham and Women's Hospital. From Gornik HL, Creager MA. Aortic diseases. Aortitis Circ. 2008;117:3039–3051.

arteries in 25%, and the renal arteries in 20%. Coronary arteries are involved in 15% of cases and can lead to myocardial infarct and sudden death.

Multisegmental lesions interrupted by normal artery are changes typical of this disease. Cross-section of occluded arteries has a pale, gray, myxoid gross appearance. In order to make the diagnosis, histology, which must be performed, shows chronic inflammation with perivascular cuffing and medial giant cells and patchy medial necrosis in the acute phase. Histology of the late-stage disease shows scattered smooth muscle cells with rare fibroblasts in the markedly thickened and fibrotic intima and large medial areas with loss of elastic fibers replaced by fibrosis (Figure 7-13).

The exact etiology of the disease is currently unknown. Much research has focused on possible autoimmune mechanisms with identification of susceptibility genes and human leukocyte antigen (HLA) alleles. Familial cases of Takayasu disease do occur.

Infectious Aortitis

Syphilitic Aortitis

Syphilitic aortitis is an infectious aortitis, once quite common, accounting for 5% to 10% of all cardiovascular deaths. While it is now less frequent, it is often seen in developing countries and is once again making a come-back in developed countries. Syphilis is caused by infection with the spirochete *Treponema pallidum*. Syphilitic aortitis shows marked lymphoplasmacytic inflammation involving the vasa vasorum (blood vessels in the adventitia that feed the aortic media). The adventitial vessels are attacked by this inflammatory reaction to the bacteria, causing necrosis of the small arteries leading to fibrosis and scarring with eventual occlusion of the arterioles. The medial layer of the aorta suffers ischemia due to the lack of blood flow from the adventitial vessels, leading to acute necrosis and destruction of elastic fibers with eventual fibrosis and scarring **(Figure 7-14)**.

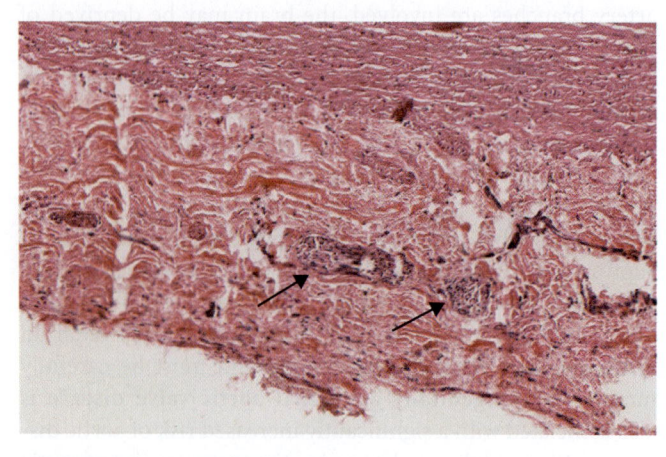

FIGURE 7-14 Syphilitic aortitis. Lymphocytic inflammation of the vasa vasorum is present (arrows). From Department of Pathology and Laboratory Medicine, University of North Carolina at Chapel Hill.

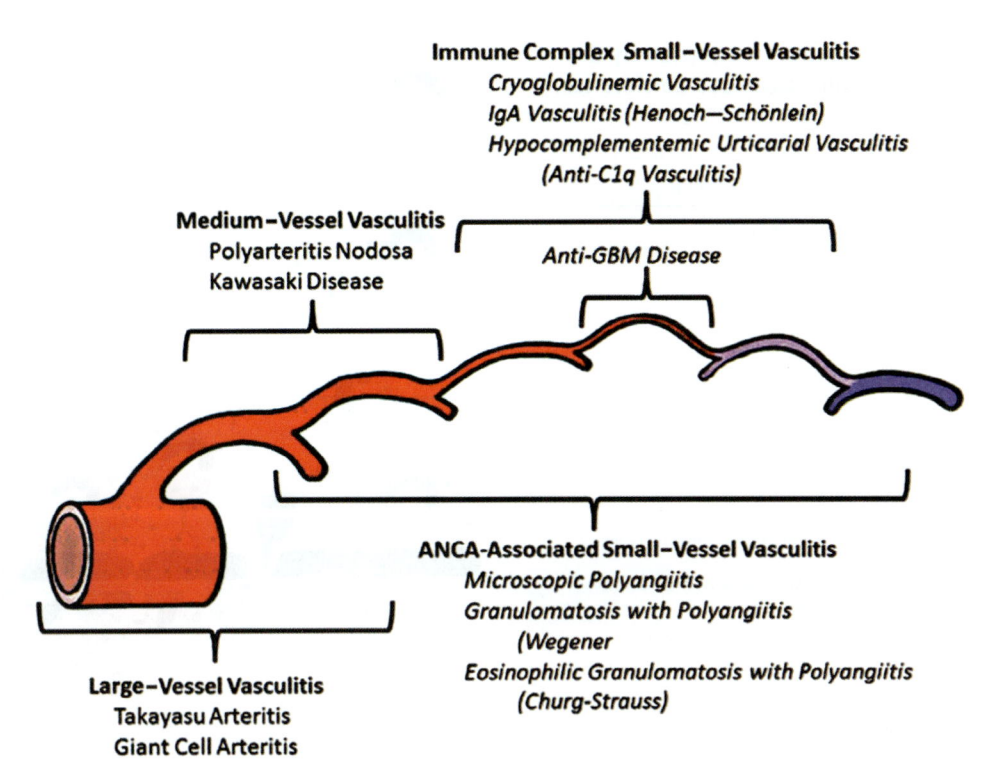

FIGURE 7-15 Vasculitis versus vessel caliber. Distribution of vessel involvement by large-vessel vasculitis, medium-vessel vasculitis, and small-vessel vasculitis. Note that there is substantial overlap with respect to arterial involvement, and an important concept is that all three major categories of vasculitis can affect any size artery. Small-vessel vasculitis predominantly affects small vessels, but medium arteries and veins may be affected, although immune complex small-vessel vasculitis rarely affects arteries. The diagram depicts (from left to right) aorta, large artery, medium artery, small artery/arteriole, capillary, venule, and vein. Anti-GBM, antiglomerular basement membrane; ANCA, antineutrophil cytoplasmic antibody. From Jennette JC, Falk RJ, Bacon PA, et al. 2012 Revised International Chapel Hill Consensus Conference Nomenclature of Vasculitides. *Arthritis Rheum*. 2013;65(1):1–11 (Figure 17).

As discussed earlier, the gross and histologic features of syphilitic aortitis are not specific. Therefore, it is necessary to know the patient's history and serologic status. A patient's serologic status must be positive in order to diagnose syphilitic aortitis.

Vasculitides

Vasculitis is a heterogeneous group of inflammatory processes involving blood vessels of any size in any organ and can give rise to diffuse, nonspecific, constitutional symptoms in patients of all ages. Vasculitides may be classified based on various criteria including infectious versus noninfectious etiology, by size and type of blood vessel involved and specific organ involvement (Figure 7-15).

Noninfectious vasculitis is thought to be initiated by immunologic mechanisms including deposition of immune complexes, cell-mediated immune reactions, or direct antibody attack by circulating antibodies. Infectious vasculitis is caused by direct infection by infectious agents and the body's natural inflammatory reaction to the infection. Inciting agents are largely unknown; however, some types of vasculitis may be associated with viral infections (see **Polyarteritis Nodosa** section). A distinctive mechanism of immune damage, antineutrophil cytoplasmic antibody (ANCA)-associated vasculitis, a form of nonnecrotizing vasculitis with little or no deposition of immune complexes, is predominantly associated with small-vessel disease (small-vessel vasculitis [SSV]; Table 7-1). Figure 7-16 provides an overview of the proposed mechanism of parenchymal necrosis and vasculitis in ANCA-mediated vessel damage.

Diagnosis of vasculitis can be quite difficult as the symptoms are nonspecific and often constitutional. Patients may exhibit weakness, fatigue, weight loss, muscle aches (myalgias), and joint pain (arthralgias) during the acute phase. Some of these processes can cause chronic disease with systemic complications. The diagnosis of a specific type of vasculitis is extremely difficult as the symptoms are similar for each type.

Multiple systems of classification of vasculitides have been proposed, but none encompasses both immunopathologic mechanisms and clinicopathologic entities. The recently proposed 2012 International Chapel Hill Consensus Conference system of nomenclature (Table 7-1) has the advantage in linking the names of vasculitides with the caliber of the vessel affected, although other systems remain in use by diagnosticians.

Giant Cell (Temporal) Arteritis

Giant-cell arteritis, a vasculitis that affects all sizes of arteries, is the most common form of systemic vasculitis in adults. It most commonly affects the temporal artery (therefore, is often called **temporal arteritis**), but may involve any of the cranial arteries and the aorta and its branches. It is rare to make the diagnosis in persons less than 50 years of age (70 years is the average age), with women more commonly affected than men. The incidence increases with age, reaching nearly 1% by

TABLE 7-1 Names for vasculitides adopted by the 2012 International Chapel Hill Consensus Conference.

Vasculitides Nomenclature	
Groups	**Diseases Included in Group**
Large-vessel vasculitis (LVV)	Takayasu arteritis (TAK)
	Giant cell arteritis (GCA)
Medium-vessel vasculitis (MVV)	Polyarteritis nodosa (PAN)
	Kawasaki disease (KD)
Small-vessel vasculitis (SVV)	Antineutrophil cytoplasmic antibody (ANCA)-associated vasculitis (AVV)
	Microscopic polyangiitis (MPA)
	Granulomatosis with polyangiitis (Wegener) (GPA)
	Eosinophilic granulomatosis with polyangiitis (Churg–Strauss syndrome) (EGPA)
SVV/immune complex SVV	Antiglomerular basement membrane (anti-GBMD) disease
	Cryoglobulinemic vasculitis (CV)
	IgA vasculitis (Henoch–Schönlein) (IgAV)
	Hypocomplementemic urticarial vasculitis (HUV) (anti-C1q vasculitis)
Variable vessel vasculitis (VVV)	Behcet disease (BD)
	Cogan syndrome (CS)
Single-organ vasculitis (SOV)	Cutaneous leukocytoclastic angiitis
	Cutaneous arteritis
	Primary central nervous system vasculitis
	Isolated aortitis
	Others
Vasculitis associated with systemic disease	Lupus vasculitis
	Rheumatoid vasculitis
	Sarcoid vasculitis
	Others
Vasculitis associated with probably etiology	Hepatitis C virus-associated cryoglobulinemic vasculitis
	Hepatitis B virus-associated vasculitis
	Syphilis-associated aortitis
	Drug-associated immune complex vasculitis
	Drug-associated, ANCA-associated vasculitis
	Cancer-associated vasculitis
	Others

Source: Jennette JC, Falk RJ, Bacon PA, et al. 2012 Revised International Chapel Hill Consensus Conference Nomenclature of Vasculitides. *Arthritis Rheum.* 2013;65(1).

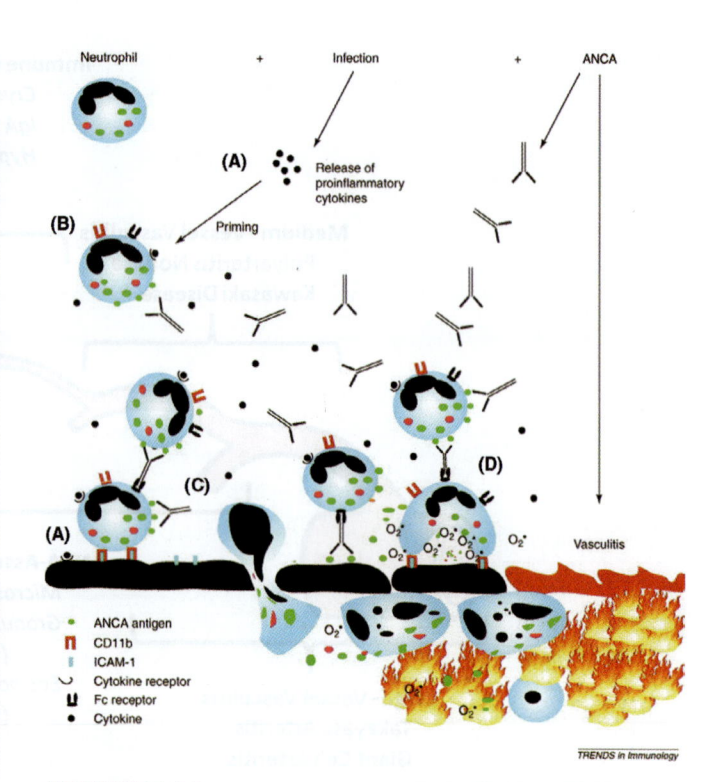

FIGURE 7-16 Proposed mechanism of ANCA-mediated neutrophil responses involved in the pathogenesis of ANCA-associated small-vessel vasculitis. **(A)** Proinflammatory cytokines and chemokines (e.g., tumor necrosis factor α) released as a result of local or systemic infection cause upregulation of endothelial adhesion molecules (e.g., selectins, ICAM-1, and VCAM) and prime the neutrophils. **(B)** Neutrophil priming causes upregulation of neutrophil adhesion molecules (CD11b) and translocation of the ANCA antigens from their lysosomal compartments to the cell surface. **(C)** Engagement of the F(ab')$_2$ portion of ANCA with ANCA antigens on the cell surface and interaction of the Fc part of the antibody with Fc receptors activates the neutrophil, causing increased neutrophil–vessel wall adherence and transmigration. **(D)** ANCA-mediated neutrophil activation also triggers reactive oxygen radical production and possibly causes neutrophil degranulation, with consequent release of proteolytic enzymes, leading to vasculitis. From Heeringa P, Huugen D, Tervaert JWC. Anti-neutrophil cytoplasmic autoantibodies and leukocyte–endothelial interactions: a sticky connection? *Trends Immunol.* 2005;26:561–564.

80 years. The age of onset helps differentiate giant cell (temporal) arteritis from vasculitides that can affect the same arteries in younger patients. The self-limited disease is usually benign clinically with symptoms resolving in 6 to 12 months.

Patients most commonly present with throbbing temporal pain, jaw pain, and headaches. The skin over the temporal artery may be swollen, tender, and red. The affected temporal artery may feel cord-like with areas of nodular thickening. Constitutional symptoms may be present including malaise, fever, weight loss, and generalized muscular aches and stiffness of the shoulders and hips (**polymyalgia rheumatica**). Approximately 50% of patients have visual symptoms, which may progress from transient to permanent blindness in one or both eyes. *As the visual symptoms may progress rapidly, they are considered a medical emergency.* The disease may also affect the heart, brain, or gastrointestinal system leading to, possibly lethal, specific organ infarction. The diagnosis is made through a 2- to 3-cm biopsy of the temporal artery. Patients' response to corticosteroids is usually dramatic with symptoms resolving in days.

The disease is segmental, focal, and chronic with granulomatous inflammation that attacks the internal elastic membrane of the artery. The arterial lumen may be reduced to a slit or may be obliterated by thrombosis. As the disease is focal and segmental, multiple levels of the artery are examined microscopically. In a positive biopsy, aggregates of macrophages, lymphocytes, and plasma cells are admixed with variable

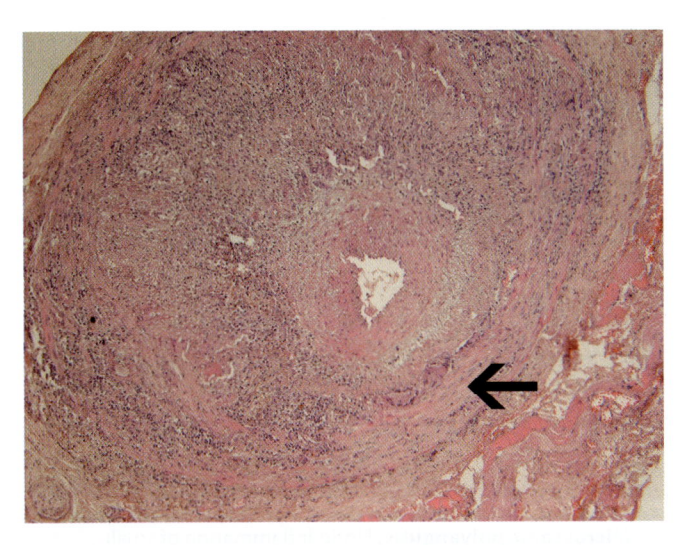

FIGURE 7–17 Giant cell (temporal) arteritis of a cerebral artery. The temporal artery has a wall that contains a striking inflammatory infiltrate including giant cell formation (arrow). From Kemp WL, Burns DK, Brown T. *The Big Picture Pathology.* New York, NY: McGraw-Hill Lange; 2008. Figure 9-11, page 103.

numbers of eosinophils and neutrophils throughout the media and intima. Giant cells tend to be distributed along the internal elastic lamina, but can vary widely in numbers. Both foreign-body giant cells and Langerhans giant cells are seen. The internal elastic lamina can appear swollen, irregular, and fragmented with foci of necrosis (Figure 7-17). Fragments of the elastica can appear in the cytoplasm of the giant cells. The intima is thickened and the media is fibrotic in later stages. Organized thrombi frequently occlude the arterial lumen, and recanalization can occur. Of note, since the disease is focal and segmental, as many as 50% of biopsies may be negative in patients with otherwise classic symptoms. A negative biopsy does NOT mean that the patient does not have temporal arteritis. If the biopsy is positive, the diagnosis is made definitively.

ANCA is negative in giant-cell arteritis. The specific etiology of the disease is unclear, but an association with HLA-DR4 and its occurrence in first-degree relatives support a potential genetic component to its pathogenesis. Morphologic alterations and cellular elements are suggestive of an immunologic reaction. Data suggest that this is a T-cell-dependent disease with activated CD4 T-helper cells. B-cells are absent. Persistent macrophage activation and cytokine production are important features.

Polyarteritis Nodosa

Classic polyarteritis nodosa (PAN) is an acute necrotizing vasculitis of medium and small vessels. Like other vasculitides, PAN affects multiple organ systems leading to variable symptoms, although it most commonly affects the skin, joints, peripheral nerves, gastrointestinal tract, and kidney. Of interest, PAN was a rare disease until the 1940s, when there was a marked rise in its incidence. The widespread use of bacterial antisera, animal toxins, and sulfonamides may have been associated with this increase. The diagnosis of PAN currently appears to be decreasing with a current incidence of approximately 3 to 4.5 cases per 100,000 population per year. PAN affects men more frequently than women (1.6–2:1). Typical presentations include fever, night sweats, weight loss, skin ulcerations or tender nodules, and severe muscle and joint pains that develop over weeks to months. It is important to note that the specific patient symptoms will depend on the arterial system involved, resulting in organ dysfunction.

QUICK REVIEW

The American College of Rheumatology has established criteria to help differentiate PAN from other vasculitides. This committee selected 10 disease features associated with PAN; in order to make the diagnosis, at least 3 of the 10 criteria should be present when the diagnosis is made by radiographic or pathologic means. The 10 criteria include:

- Weight loss of 4 kg or more
- Livedo reticularis (lace-like, purple skin discoloration)
- Testicular pain/tenderness
- Myalgia or leg weakness/tenderness
- Mononeuropathy or polyneuropathy
- Diastolic blood pressure >90 mm Hg
- Elevated blood urea nitrogen (BUN) or creatinine level unrelated to dehydration or obstruction
- Presence of hepatitis B surface antigen or antibody in serum
- Arteriogram demonstrating aneurysms or occlusions of visceral arteries
- Biopsy of small- or medium-sized artery containing neutrophils

Characteristic lesions of PAN in small- and medium-sized muscular arteries are found in a patchy distribution and may extend into larger arteries. The lesions are usually 1 mm in length and may involve a portion or the entire circumference of the vessel and may present as palpable nodules along the course of medium-sized arteries during autopsy. The lesions affecting medium-sized arteries usually occur at bifurcations or branch points. The histologic appearance depends on the stage of the inflammatory process. Lesions of the acute phase demonstrate fibrinoid necrosis with loss of the muscular media and adjacent tissues with deposition of eosinophilic fibrin material. The fulminant acute inflammatory response is composed of neutrophils, lymphocytes, and plasma cells that vary in their proportions. Eosinophils are often numerous. Lesions in the same artery may vary in age and is a characteristic finding. Due to the vascular injury, luminal thrombosis may occur in the involved segment, leading to ischemia and infarct of the distal organ. Due to the vascular injury and weakening of the vessel wall, aneurysms may occur leading to risk of rupture and significant hemorrhage. Chronic, healed lesions show fibrous proliferation of the intima that may result in significant narrowing of the arterial lumen, again leading to tissue ischemia and potential infarcts (Figure 7-18A).

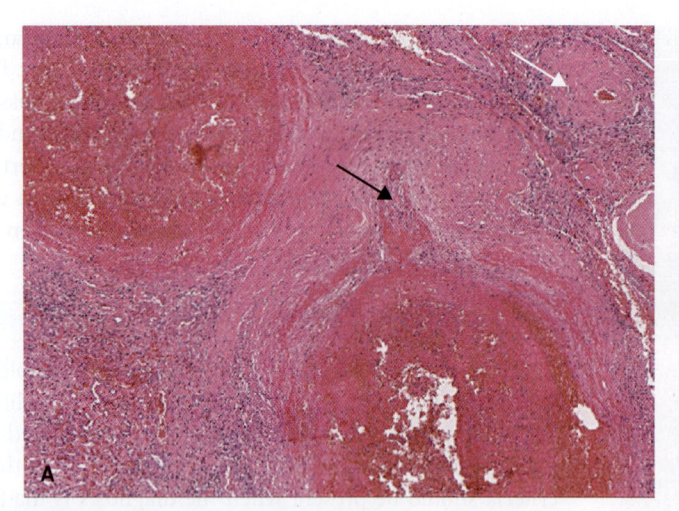

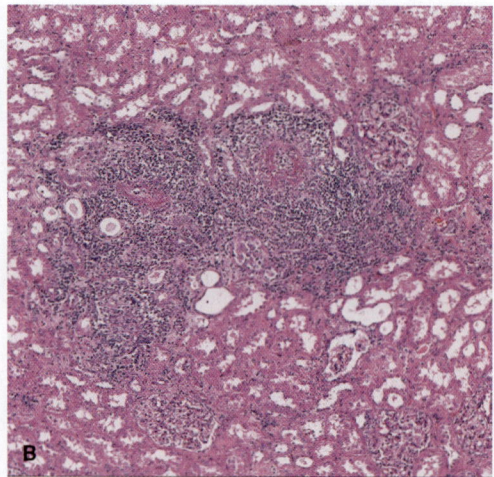

FIGURE 7–18 **(A) Polyarteritis nodosa (PAN).** A large nodular lesion demonstrating an aneurysmal outpouching (black arrow) and fibrinoid necrosis. A chronic healed lesion (white arrow) shows intimal proliferation and narrowing of the vessel lumen.

(B) Microscopic polyangiitis. Florid inflammation of small arteries/arterioles is present. From Department of Pathology and Laboratory Medicine, University of North Carolina at Chapel Hill.

The exact etiology of PAN is unknown and no animal model is available for study. Interestingly, viral infections including human immunodeficiency virus (HIV), hepatitis C virus (HCV), and hepatitis B virus (HBV) infections have been associated with PAN. A strong association between HBV infection and PAN has been related to immune complex-mediated disease and was once the cause of up to 30% of PAN cases. It is believed that viral replication directly injures the vascular wall causing endothelial dysfunction and production of inflammatory cytokines and adhesion molecules. HBV-associated vasculitis always takes the form of PAN and may occur at any time during the course of the disease. Most commonly it occurs within 6 months of the infection. The widespread use of hepatitis B vaccine has significantly decreased the number of HBV-related PAN that now accounts for approximately 8% of all PAN cases.

Additional associated diseases include other infectious diseases, systemic syndromes, and hematologic malignancies.

Left untreated, the 5-year survival rate of patients suffering from PAN is 13%. Approximately 50% of patients die within the first 3 months of onset. Patients with acute abdominal symptoms have a markedly worse prognosis due to extensive bowel involvement. Their usual postoperative course is complicated by infections and delayed healing. Central nervous system involvement has a worse prognosis than does peripheral nerve involvement. Patients with cutaneous PAN without systemic involvement have a benign prognosis, although the disease tends to relapse. Death is most commonly due to uncontrolled vasculitis, infectious complications due to immunosuppression, and vascular complications including myocardial infarction (MI) and stroke. Corticosteroid therapy improves the 5-year survival rate to nearly 50% to 60% to greater than 80% when combined with other *immunosuppressants.*

Microscopic polyangiitis (MPA; formerly known as microscopic polyarteritis) is an ANCA-associated systemic vasculitis with some features similar to PAN with involvement of small arteries and arterioles and the microcirculation (renal glomeruli and pulmonary capillaries) (Figure 7-18B).

Kawasaki Disease

Kawasaki disease (KD), also known as mucocutaneous lymph node syndrome, is a pediatric inflammatory illness of unknown etiology. This disease process is the leading cause of acquired heart disease in childhood in North America and Japan. The

CASE 7-3

A previously healthy, 17-year-old was playing basketball with his friends. He told them he needed a break and went into the house. He didn't return and his friends found him dead on the floor of the kitchen.

Pathology: At autopsy, his heart was markedly enlarged with dilated, aneurysmal coronary arteries. Cross sections showed the coronary arteries (**Figure 7-19 top**) had a thickened wall with intimal fibrosis and thrombotic occlusion of the anterior descending and right coronary arteries. Histology showed a healed arteritis of the aneurysmal coronary arteries. Both histology and gross examination (**Figure 7-19 bottom**) revealed evidence of ongoing ischemic injury and scarring of the myocardium.

This young man's cause of death: sudden cardiac death due to myocardial ischemia following occlusion of giant coronary artery aneurysms due to healed Kawasaki disease.

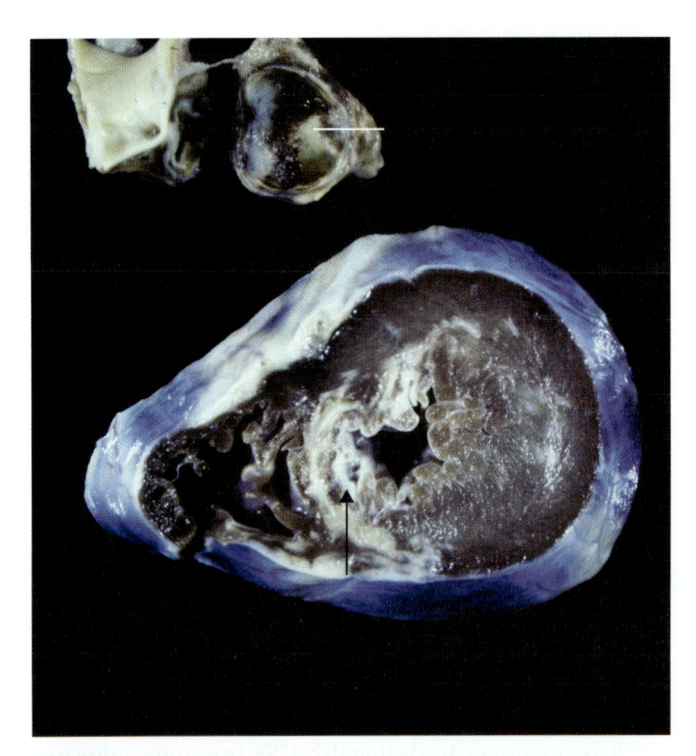

FIGURE 7-19 Kawasaki disease (radiograph). A thrombosed large aneurysm of the left descending coronary artery (line) led to the sudden death of this 15-year-old individual. Marked fibrosis of the left ventricular septum (arrow) and wall is related to long-standing myocardial ischemia associated with the vasculitis. From Department of Pathology and Laboratory Medicine, University of North Carolina at Chapel Hill.

disease is endemic in Japan with an incidence of 20 to 100 cases/100,000 population <5 years of age. In North America, the incidence is 4 to 15 cases/100,000 population. The disease most commonly affects (in order of frequency) Asians, African-Americans, Whites, and Native Americans with a slight male predominance (1.5:1). Eighty percent of affected children are less than 4 years of age. Clinical symptoms include an abrupt high fever that lasts longer than 5 days, conjunctival and oral erythema with erosions ("strawberry" tongue), edema of the hands and feet, erythema of the palms of the hands and soles of the feet, a diffuse skin rash with desquamation, and enlargement of cervical lymph nodes. The disease, similar to other pediatric viral illnesses, is usually self-limited, even without treatment. Although it appears similar to other viral illnesses, no specific infectious cause has been identified. Infections with parvovirus B 19 or with New Haven coronavirus have been implicated in some cases. Various bacterial infections (including *Staphylococcus*, *Streptococcus*, and *Chlamydia*) have been implicated in occasional cases. The common theme in such cases appears to be production of super-antigens that bind to major T-cell receptors resulting in massively activated immune responses in an antigen-nonspecific manner. Autoantibodies to endothelial and smooth muscle cells have been identified in other patients.

The acute phase of the disease causes an acute necrotizing vasculitis similar to PAN that specifically affects the epicardial coronary arteries. Approximately 70% of patients have coronary artery involvement resulting in death in 1% to 2%.

The most important cardiovascular sequelae occur in approximately 20% of patients, ranging from asymptomatic vasculitis to giant coronary artery aneurysms (Figure 7-19). Giant coronary artery aneurysms (7–8 mm) occur in 25% of children and are usually multiple. Significantly, the aneurysms may thrombose leading to myocardial ischemia and infarction.

During the acute phase, the histology is similar to that of PAN, with patchy vascular fibrinoid necrosis with varying collections of neutrophils, lymphocytes, plasma cells, and eosinophils. Of note, the disease is associated with activation of T-cell lymphocytes and macrophages that results in elevated levels of inflammatory cytokines. The resultant, healed aneurysms show destruction and absence of the elastic laminae, medial thinning, and fibrointimal proliferation and organized mural thrombi.

Persistence rate of aneurysms is 72% at 1 year and 40% at 5 years after disease occurrence. Approximately 55% of patients show regression of aneurysms over a significant period (14 years). Regression is inversely related to severity of the initial aneurysm and male gender. Treatment with high-dose aspirin and intravenous gamma-globulin is positively related to aneurysm regression.

After treatment, the long-term rate of an acute myocardial infarct is approximately 1% with a mortality rate of 1%. Patients dying of ischemic sequelae of KD show occlusion of one or more coronary arteries in 75% of cases.

Granulomatosis with Polyangiitis

Granulomatosis with polyangiitis (previously known as Wegener granulomatosis) is a systemic necrotizing vasculitis of unknown etiology that manifests as granulomatous lesions of the respiratory tract including the nose, sinuses, and lungs and as a renal glomerular disease. Men are more commonly affected in their fifth and sixth decades. Studies have demonstrated ANCAs in the blood of approximately 90% of patients; 75% of these are positive for cytoplasmic-ANCA (c-ANCA more currently identified as proteinase-3 (PRTN-3)). It has been suggested that c-ANCAs may activate circulating neutrophils to attack the blood vessels.

Patients usually present with respiratory symptoms including pneumonitis and sinusitis. Chronic sinusitis and nasopharyngeal mucosal ulcers are frequent. The lung is ultimately involved in over 90% of patients. Radiologically, multiple pulmonary infiltrates are prominent and may be cavitary. Hematuria and proteinuria are common due to focal necrotizing glomerulonephritis. Progression to crescentic glomerulonephritis can lead to renal failure. Rash, muscular pains, joint involvement, and neurologic symptoms can occur. Untreated, the disease leads to an 80% mortality rate within 1 year with a mean survival of 5 to 6 months.

Gross pathologic lesions of polyangiitis with granulomatosis show parenchymal necrosis with a geographic pattern and individual lung lesions as large as 5 cm in diameter which may cavitate, giving an appearance similar to those seen in tuberculosis. The vasculitis involves small arteries and veins most frequently in the lung, kidney, and spleen. Histologically, the

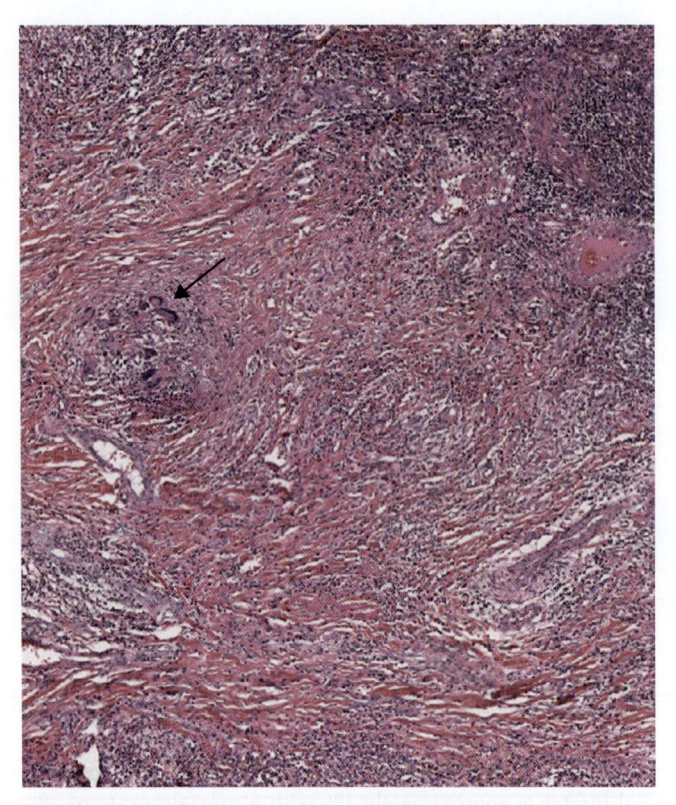

FIGURE 7-20 Granulomatosis with polyangiitis (Wegener granulomatosis). Disease in lung with granulomatous inflammation indicated by an arrow. There is extensive parenchymal necrosis and vasculitis throughout the image. From Department of Pathology and Laboratory Medicine, University of North Carolina at Chapel Hill.

vasculitis is often characterized primarily by chronic inflammation, but acute inflammation, necrotizing and non-necrotizing granulomatous inflammation, and fibrinoid necrosis are often present. Later in the disease, medial thickening and intimal proliferation are common and can lead to narrowing or obliteration of the vessel lumen (Figure 7-20) resulting in tissue ischemia.

Treatment with cyclophosphamide produces complete disease remission and substantial disease-free intervals in most patients. Of note, antimicrobial sulfa drugs significantly reduce the incidence of relapses.

Eosinophilic Granulomatosis with Polyangiitis (Churg–Strauss Syndrome)

Eosinophilic granulomatosis with polyangiitis is a systemic vasculitis with prominent eosinophilic inflammation that affects young persons with asthma or allergies. Churg–Strauss syndrome (CSS) is a rare disease. There is no gender predilection. Several exogenous trigger factors for disease onset or flares have been suspected in some studies and include vaccinations, desensitizations, and medications

Its most typical presentation consists of the appearance of vasculitis manifestations including fever, rash, and central nervous system symptoms in a patient with known allergic rhinitis, nasal and sinus polyposis, and asthma. The combination of blood eosinophilia and inflammatory symptoms is highly suggestive of the diagnosis. Thirty to forty percent of patients with CSS are positive for perinuclear-ANCA with anti-myeloperoxidase specificity.

In addition to the asthma with airflow obstruction, patchy and transient alveolar infiltrates with pleural inflammation can occur. Allergic rhinitis, sinusitis, and/or nasal polyps can be seen in as many as 60% to 80% of patients. Skin lesions including purpura, nodules, and hives occur in approximately 50% of patients. Peripheral neuropathy affects about 50% to 80% of patients and can be severe. Renal manifestations occur in up to 25% of cases and range from isolated urinary abnormalities to rapidly progressive renal failure. *Patients with CSS must be evaluated for cardiac involvement, as such carries a poor prognosis.*

Pathology shows widespread necrotizing lesions of medium- and small-sized arteries, arterioles, and veins primarily of the lungs, kidney, spleen, heart, liver, and central nervous system. The lesions are granulomatous with a prominent eosinophilic infiltrate in and around the vessels, resulting in fibrinoid necrosis, thrombosis, and aneurysm formation similar to PAN. The resultant occluded vessels lead to distal organ ischemia and possible infarct (Figure 7-21).

It is important to distinguish CSS from other diseases with eosinophilia including parasitic and fungal infections, granulomatosis with polyangiitis, eosinophilic pneumonia, and hypersensitivity vasculitis.

Untreated patients have a poor prognosis. Corticosteroid therapy is almost always successful in leading to remission.

Hypersensitivity Vasculitis

Hypersensitivity vasculitis refers to a broad group of inflammatory vascular lesions thought to represent a reaction to foreign

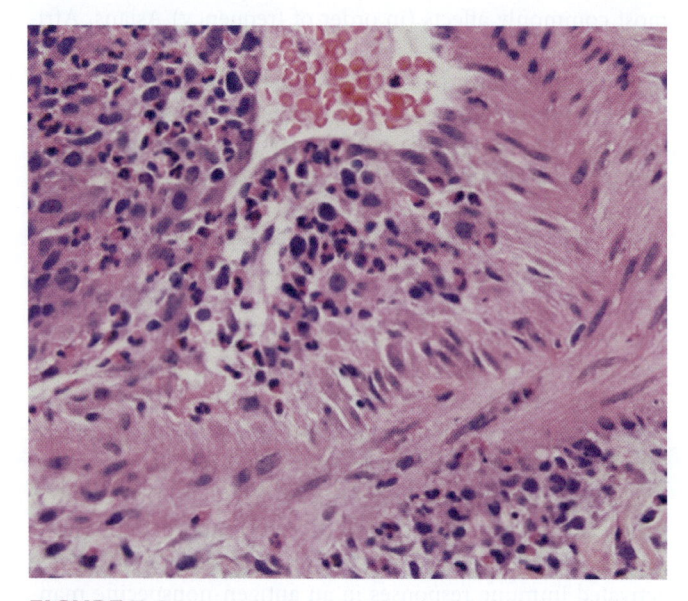

FIGURE 7-21 Eosinophilic granulomatosis with polyangiitis (Churg–Strauss syndrome). The image demonstrates an area of eosinophil rich in small-vessel vasculitis. From Charles Jennette M.D., Department of Pathology and Laboratory Medicine, University of North Carolina at Chapel Hill.

CASE 7-4

A six-year-old boy was brought to his pediatrician with symptoms consistent with group A beta-hemolytic streptococcal pharyngitis and was prescribed a course of amoxicillin. After several days of treatment, the boy complained of severe itching on both forearms, and an extensive rash was noted by his mother. The mother thought the rash was due to "hives" but the boy became increasingly uncomfortable and was returned to the pediatrician. On examination, the pediatrician noted a palpable purpuric rash consisting of multiple 2-mm lesions on his forearms and thighs. He complained of joint pain. A urinalysis was normal. The rash persisted. Concerned over the possibility of severe disease, the pediatrician performed a skin biopsy in an affected region.

The skin biopsy (Figure 7-22) was interpreted as hypersensitivity vasculitis likely related to drug sensitivity. Antibiotics had been discontinued and the rash resolved spontaneously.

Pathology: The lesion was described as demonstrating vascular and perivascular infiltrates predominantly of neutrophils with leukocytoclasia.

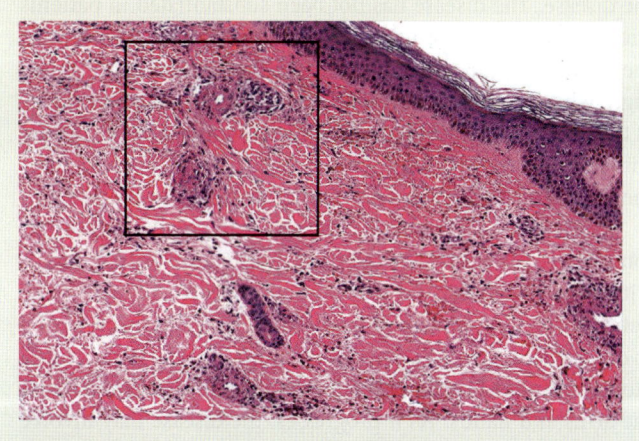

FIGURE 7-22 **Hypersensitivity vasculitis.** Vessels show a predominantly neutrophilic infiltrate with leukocytoclasia (box). From John Woosley, M.D., Ph.D., Department of Pathology and Laboratory Medicine, University of North Carolina at Chapel Hill.

materials. The skin is the most commonly affected organ in primary hypersensitivity reactions, although any organ may be involved. In the case of lesions confined predominantly to the skin, a definitive diagnosis rests on histopathologic examination of the affected tissues. A tissue diagnosis is easily accomplished with cutaneous involvement. Cutaneous vasculitis may occur following administration of many drugs, various bacterial infections (streptococcal and staphylococcal), viral hepatitis, tuberculosis, and bacterial endocarditis. The disease typically presents as palpable purpura, predominately on the lower extremities. Cutaneous vasculitis is usually self-limited, even without treatment.

The most common histologic pattern is a neutrophilic infiltrate of postcapillary venules associated with leukocytoclasia (destruction of white blood cells with karyorrhexis) and evidence of vascular damage including EC swelling, fibrinoid necrosis, and red blood cell extravasation. The vascular lesions of hypersensitivity vasculitis are all at the same stage of development at any given time (Figure 7-22).

Systemic hypersensitivity angiitis may be an isolated entity or may be a feature of other disease processes including collagen vascular diseases and a variety of malignancies. Patients with systemic hypersensitivity angiitis may also have skin manifestations. Small-vessel angiitis may cause microinfarcts of internal organs, which do not usually cause major organ dysfunction.

Subtypes of hypersensitivity vasculitis are all characterized by an immunologically mediated, small-vessel angiitis. They may be distinguished by differing clinical presentations, specific laboratory findings, and/or the presence of an underlying systemic disorder.

- **Serum sickness** is a clinical syndrome resulting from injection of heterologous serum or serum proteins. Classic serum sickness is infrequent today, as heterologous serum is rarely used. However, reactions to nonprotein-containing drugs are common.
- **Henoch–Schönlein purpura**, also known as anaphylactoid purpura, is a systemic small-vessel vasculitis. It appears clinically as a syndrome of nonthrombocytopenic purpura, arthritis, gastrointestinal bleeding, and renal disease. This disease is caused by deposition of immune complexes due to viral or streptococcal infections, medication administration, and ingestion of certain foods. Unlike hypersensitivity vasculitis, IgA is principally detected as part of the circulating immune complex and/or immune deposits within vessels and renal glomeruli (see Chapter 12).
- **Vasculitis associated with mixed cryoglobulinemia**. Diagnosis of this condition is made by the demonstration of a cryoglobulinemia and a small-vessel vasculitis.
- **Vasculitis associated with other systemic diseases**. Necrotizing small-vessel vasculitis has been associated with a number of collagen vascular diseases including systemic lupus erythematosus (SLE), RA, systemic sclerosis, and Sjögren syndrome. Similar small-vessel vasculitides have also been associated with various neoplastic conditions including myeloproliferative disorders, hairy cell leukemia, lymphoproliferative disorders, multiple myeloma, and a variety of carcinomas.

Thromboangiitis Obliterans (Buerger Disease)

As its name suggests, **thromboangiitis obliterans** *(TAO) is an occlusive disease of arteries in the arms and legs almost exclusively seen in young and middle-aged men who smoke heavily.* Previously, the disease was thought to only occur in men; however, increasing numbers of affected women are being reported. While most patients are heavy smokers, the disease has also been reported in cigar smokers and users of smokeless tobacco, demonstrating the significant association between tobacco and the disease. The disease has not been substantiated in patients without some form of tobacco use. TAO is more common in the Mediterranean areas, the Middle East, and Asia. Interestingly, while tobacco is central to the initiation and continuance of the disease, EC dysfunction has been found in arteries not yet clinically involved with the disease. Elevated levels of antiendothelial cell antibodies have also been found in these patients.

Typically, TAO occurs in smokers with the onset of symptoms before the age of 40 to 45 years. The disease usually begins with involvement of the distal small arteries and veins. The patients usually complain of claudication (literally, to limp; used to describe a cramp-like pain most commonly due to decreased blood flow or ischemia) of the feet and legs and occasionally of the arms and hands. As it progresses, the disease may involve more proximal vessels with development of ischemic ulcerations of the distal portions of the toes or fingers. Seventy-six percent of patients had ischemic ulcerations at the time of presentation. Two or more limbs are usually involved in the disease process. No specific laboratory tests are diagnostic of Buerger disease. However, it is important to exclude other diseases that might mimic TAO such as hypercoagulable states, other systemic diseases and illicit drug use. Cocaine and amphetamines ingestion can mimic TAO and show nearly identical arteriographic findings. Therefore, in patients with manifestations of Buerger disease who do not use tobacco, a toxicology screen can be helpful. Angiographic features show multiple segmental occlusions of small- and medium-sized vessels with collateralization around the obstructions (corkscrew collaterals).

The histopathology of the acute phase of the disease is the most diagnostic feature of the disease (Figure 7-23). Biopsy of an acute superficial thrombophlebitis is most likely to show the characteristic lesion of the acute phase. Acute inflammation involves all layers of the vessel wall and is associated with an occlusive, cellular thrombosis. Degenerating neutrophils are at the periphery of the thrombus, and multinucleated giant cells may be seen. The subacute lesion shows organization of the occlusive thrombus. Decreased numbers of inflammatory cells are seen in the vessel wall in the subacute phase. The chronic phase (or end stage) shows the vessel lumen occluded by an organized thrombus. Recanalization of the thrombus may be prominent. Of note, the normal architecture and the elastic laminae of the vessel wall remain intact and allow differentiation from other vasculitides.

Therapy consists of the complete discontinuation of cigarette smoking and the use of any form of tobacco. Complete abstinence is the only way to halt the progression of TAO and to avoid future complications, including amputations. All other forms of treatment are palliative. The risk of amputation in previous smokers is eliminated 8 years after smoking cessation.

Behçet Disease (Adamantiades-Behçet Disease)

Behçet disease is a chronic and multisystem inflammatory disorder with a remarkable ability to involve blood vessels of nearly all types and sizes and involving both veins and arteries. Manifestations may occur at many sites throughout the body because of the diversity of the blood vessels affected, although the disease has a predilection for certain organs and tissues including the eye, mouth, skin, lungs, joints, brain, gastrointestinal tract, and genitals. The disease is most commonly seen in populations from Japan and China to the Mediterranean Sea and develops in persons aged 20 to 30 years.

Patients may develop anterior and/or posterior uveitis (inflammation of the middle, pigmented vascular structures of the eye including the iris, ciliary body and choroid) of the eye. Anterior uveitis causes blurry vision, pain, light sensitivity, tearing, and redness of the eye. Posterior uveitis can be more dangerous with few physical symptoms and can lead to blindness due to damage to the retina.

Painful aphthous ulcers of the mouth are similar to mouth ulcers in the general population; however, they are more numerous, more frequent, larger, and more painful in Behçet disease. These ulcers can be found on the lips, tongue, and the inside of the cheeks and may be single or appear in clusters.

Genital ulcers develop on the scrotum or vulva and are similar to the mouth ulcers, but frequently involve deeper tissues.

Involvement of the central nervous system is one of the most dangerous manifestations of Behçet disease. The disease tends to involve the white matter of the cerebrum and brainstem. Symptoms may include headache, confusion, strokes, personality changes, and dementia. It may also present as "aseptic" meningitis.

Pustular skin lesions can occur anywhere on the skin. Red, tender nodules that occur on the legs and ankles (erythema nodosa) may also appear on the face, neck, or arms. Unlike erythema nodosa associated with other diseases, the skin lesions associated with Behçet disease tend to ulcerate. Aneurysms in the lung may rupture leading to massive lung hemorrhage.

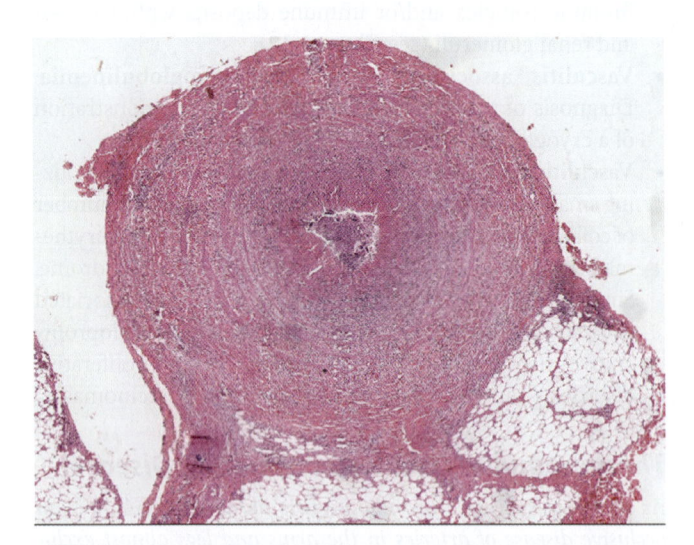

FIGURE 7-23 Thromboangiitis obliterans (Buerger disease). Biopsy of an area of acute superficial thrombophlebitis demonstrates multilayer inflammation of the vessel wall and an occlusive cellular thrombus surrounded by cellular debris. From Department of Pathology and Laboratory Medicine, University of North Carolina at Chapel Hill.

Joints may develop arthritis. Ulcerations may occur anywhere in the gastrointestinal tract from the mouth to the anus, most commonly in the terminal ileum and cecum.

Behçet disease is one of the only forms of vasculitis that has a genetic predisposition. The presence of HLA-B51 is a risk factor for the disease; however, only approximately 5% of cases are familial. Therefore, it is believed that other factors play a role in developing the disease in the presence of HLA-B51. Possibilities include infections (*Streptococci*) and environmental exposures.

The underlying pathologic lesion is a small-vessel vasculitis that predominately affects venules. Biopsies of mucocutaneous lesions show a perivascular infiltration of lymphocytes, plasma cells, and monocytes affecting arterioles and venules. Frank necrosis of small vessels is unusual. Cutaneous vasculitis appears mainly as a venulitis or phlebitis.

Treatment for disease confined to mucocutaneous regions is topical steroids and medications such as colchicine. Corticosteroids may be required for disease exacerbations with some patients requiring low-dose steroids to keep the disease under control. Serious disease with end-organ involvement requires high-dose corticosteroids and other immunosuppressive agents.

Radiation Vasculitis

Acute radiation vasculitis injury shows EC damage, ballooning degeneration of the intimal cells, and necrosis of medial smooth muscle with or without thrombosis of the small arteries and arterioles. The chronic phase shows fibrous intimal proliferation that may lead to significant luminal narrowing. Radiation can lead to significant luminal narrowing of the coronary arteries with resultant myocardial ischemia after chest radiation.

HYPERTENSIVE VASCULAR DISEASE

Systemic hypertension is one of the most important modifiable risk factors for atherosclerotic coronary heart disease, stroke, congestive heart failure, and end-stage kidney disease. Prevention and treatment of hypertension can lead to a significant decrease in morbidity and mortality from the leading causes of death in North America. The effects on end organs increase as the blood pressure increases.

Specific numbers for the systolic and diastolic blood pressure levels are based on epidemiologic studies that relate blood pressure levels to risks for adverse outcomes and on evidence from clinical trials that show a reduced risk of adverse outcomes when hypertension is controlled. The question of what is adequate control has, until recently, been based on the recommendations from the Seventh Report of the Joint National Commission of Prevention, Detection, Evaluation and Treatment of High Blood Pressure (JNC VII) released in 2003 which classify blood pressure for adults 18 years or older:

- Normal—Systolic <120 mm Hg, diastolic <80 mm Hg
- Prehypertension—Systolic 120 to 139 mm Hg, diastolic 80 to 90 mm Hg
- Stage I—Systolic 140 to 159 mm Hg, diastolic 90 to 99 mm Hg
- Stage II—Systolic ≥160 mm Hg, diastolic ≥100 mm Hg

These blood pressure classifications are based on an average of 2 or more readings taken at each of two or more visits after an initial screening. Prehypertension is a new category designated in the JNC VII and is important as it emphasizes that these patients are at risk to progress to hypertension.

These recommendations have been recently reevaluated in the 2014 Evidence-Based Guideline for the Management of High Blood Pressure in Adults Report From the Panel Members Appointed to the Eighth Joint National Committee (JNC 8) (Table 7-2). These guidelines establish thresholds for pharmacologic management of persons based on age and clinical status rather than establishing categories of hypertension. For example, treatment thresholds for nondiabetic, nonrenal disease patients have been defined as greater than systolic 140, diastolic 90 for persons between 18 but less than 60 years of age and systolic 150, diastolic 90 for persons of 60 years old.

Blood pressure is determined by cardiac output and blood volume (pressure = flow × resistance). Blood volume is dependent on sodium and water balance. Blood vessel resistance, regulated primarily at the level of the arterioles, is dependent on hormonal and neural systems. Hormonal components such as the renin–angiotensin, kinin, and prostaglandin systems play important roles in vascular tone. Other factors, including hypoxia and acidosis, can cause significant alterations in vascular resistance.

Clinically, systemic hypertension is divided into two categories: essential (idiopathic) or secondary. Essential hypertension accounts for about 95% of the 50 million Americans with hypertension. Secondary hypertension related to a definable

TABLE 7-2 Evidence-Based Guideline for Hypertension Management (JNC 8).

All adults aged ≥ 18 years with hypertension		
Implement lifestyle intervention		
Set blood pressure goals Initiate blood pressure lowering medication		
Age ≥ 60 yr with no diabetes or CKD Blood pressure goal SBP < 150 mm Hg DBP < 90 mm Hg	Age < 60 yr or all ages with diabetes but no CKD Blood pressure goal SBP < 140 mm Hg DBP < 90 mm Hg	All ages with CKD with/without diabetes Blood pressure goal SBP < 140 mm Hg DBP < 90 mm Hg
Non-Black: Initiate thiazide-type diuretic or ACEI or ARB or CCB alone or in combination Black: Initiate thiazide-type diuretic or CCB alone or in combination		All races: Initiate ACEI or ARB, alone or in combination with another drug class

This table is an abbreviated version of the guidelines published in 2014 Evidence-Based Guideline for the Management of High Blood Pressure in Adults: Report From the Panel Members Appointed to the Eighth Joint National Committee (JNC 8). *JAMA* 2014;311(5):507–520. Refer to the source for complete therapeutic guidelines. DBP, diastolic blood pressure SBP, systolic blood pressure; ACEI, angiotensin-converting enzyme inhibitor; ARB, angiotensin receptor blocker; CCB, calcium channel blocker.

clinical cause makes up less than 5% of cases. Patients presenting with new-onset hypertension should undergo a complete work-up for causes of secondary hypertension, as some of these causes are immediately treatable. Secondary hypertension can be caused by renovascular hypertension (renal artery stenosis, fibromuscular dysplasia), endocrine diseases (including pheochromocytoma, exogenous steroid administration), neurogenic causes, drugs, and toxins.

Etiology of Essential Hypertension

After ruling out causes of secondary hypertension, the remaining 95% of hypertensive cases are considered essential or idiopathic. The pathogenesis of the disease is multifactorial and its etiology has been difficult to completely determine due to the many factors involved in blood pressure modulation, including the vasculature, the central and sympathetic nervous systems, the kidney and many hormone regulators involved, and the effects of diet and medications. Currently, it is believed that multiple factors contribute to the development of hypertension, including an inherited predisposition, excessive dietary salt intake, and increased adrenergic tone.

While epidemiologic and family aggregation studies have definitely established that there is a significant inheritable component for blood pressure, how genetics plays a role has not yet been determined. While the study of rare genetic disorders affecting blood pressure has led to the identification of uncommon causes of hypertension, these have not contributed to the determination of specific genes that may be responsible for hypertension in the general population. Environmental factors are believed to alter the genetic components in many familial cases. The heavy intake of salt has been one factor that has been shown to significantly increase the risk of developing hypertension in genetically predisposed individuals.

The kidney has a central role in maintenance of blood pressure by its ability to regulate sodium and water. Many researchers have shown that the kidney also plays a major role in the development of high blood pressure. The development of hypertension has been demonstrated in the kidney through loss of sodium excretory pathways leading to increased intra-arterial pressures, cross-transplantation studies where the hypertension was transmitted to the recipient by the donor kidney and the major role played by the renin-angiotensin system. One study demonstrated the importance of the nervous system in hypertension by their ability to lower blood pressure in patients with refractory hypertension by denervation of the kidney.

Other studies have revealed the importance of changes in vascular tone as a crucial component of hypertension. The elevated peripheral resistance demonstrated by hypertensive patients, mediated by hormonal regulators, may be altered by targeting specific genes and their signaling pathways. The possibility of hypertension being an autoimmune disease process has also been proposed. Of interest, using this theory, some researchers are attempting to develop a vaccine for hypertension.

Pathologic Changes of the Vasculature in Hypertension

Systemic hypertension, associated with increased atherogenesis, also causes degenerative changes in large- and medium-sized blood vessels. These degenerative changes cause weakness of the vascular wall that can be responsible for rupture of the aorta (aortic dissection) or cerebral vasculature (intracerebral hemorrhage [see above]). Small arteries show hyaline arteriolosclerosis, a pink, homogeneous, hyaline-like thickening of the arterial wall. The arteriolar lumen is most commonly narrowed, leading to decreased flow of oxygenated blood to distal organ structures. The hyalinized appearance of the arterioles is due to leakage of plasma components across the vascular endothelium (due to damage by the increased systemic pressures) and increased production of extracellular matrix by smooth muscle cells. Hyaline arteriolosclerosis is one of the major components of benign nephrosclerosis (see Hypertensive Arterionephrosclerosis section in Chapter 12).

Systemic Effects of Hypertension

Cerebral Hypertension and Intracerebral Hemorrhage

Like the heart lung and kidneys, systemic hypertension causes significant structural changes in the vasculature of the brain. Both systolic and diastolic pressures are important predictors for primary and recurrent stokes. The specific pathological changes are described as both lipohyalinosis (deposition of lipid and hyaline material into the arterial wall) and/or fibrinoid necrosis. The chronic changes result in thickening of the arterioles with deposition of type IV collagen into the arteriolar wall, leading to loss of normal contractile function. Cerebral hypertension may result in spontaneous intracerebral hemorrhage. Aneurysm-like lesions found at sites of the rupture are a likely precursor lesion leading to the acute intraparenchymal hemorrhages. These miliary aneurysm-like lesions are more commonly detected in hypertensive individuals.

Intracerebral hemorrhage in hypertensive patients is a life-threatening disease that carries significant morbidity and mortality. In these patients, the alterations in the arterioles allow blood to extravasate into surrounding brain parenchyma causing destruction of adjacent tissues and possible rupture of the hemorrhage into ventricles or the subarachnoid and subdural spaces (see Case XXX and Chapter 21 "Brain Hemorrhage").

Hypertension and the Eye

Both acute and chronic hypertensive changes may manifest in the eye and range from acute changes of malignant hypertension (see below) to chronic changes from long-term hypertension. As is the case with the cerebral vasculature, retinal vasculature becomes thickened in the setting of chronic hypertension. The normal light reflex of the retinal arterial system is formed by the reflection from the interface between the column of blood and the vessel wall. In hypertension, the

CASE 7-5

A 63-year-old woman with a history of poorly controlled hypertension was brought to the emergency department after collapsing at home. She had been complaining of severe headaches for 2 days. A CT of the head showed a large acute intracerebral hemorrhage with extension into the ventricles (Figure 7-24a). Her neurologic status continued to decline and she was declared brain dead. At autopsy, her heart and kidneys showed chronic hypertensive changes. Examination of the brain showed diffuse brain swelling with massive intracerebral hemorrhage involving the left thalamus and basal ganglia (Figure 7-24b) with extension of the hemorrhage into the ventricular system. Microscopic examination showed widespread acute intraparenchymal hemorrhage. Surrounding brain tissue showed thickened, sclerotic small arteries with perivascular hemosiderin-laden macrophages (Figure 7-24c). (Case provided courtesy of Drs. Diane Armao and Thomas Bouldin Department of Pathology and Laboratory Medicine, University of North Carolina at Chapel Hill.)

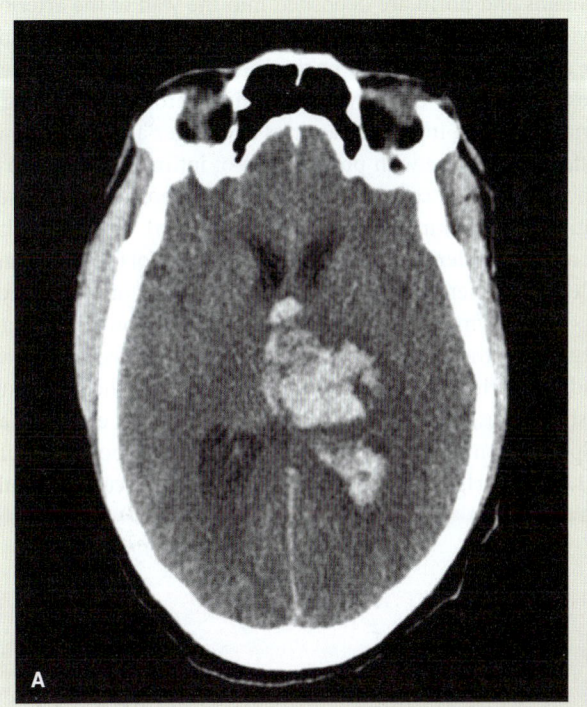

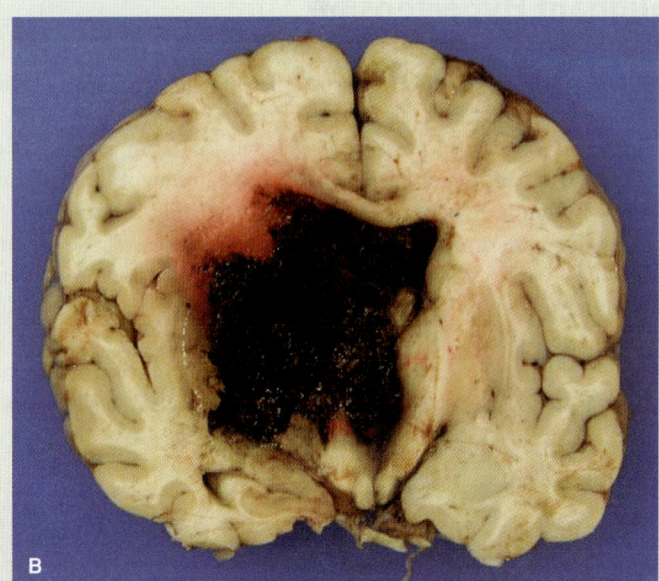

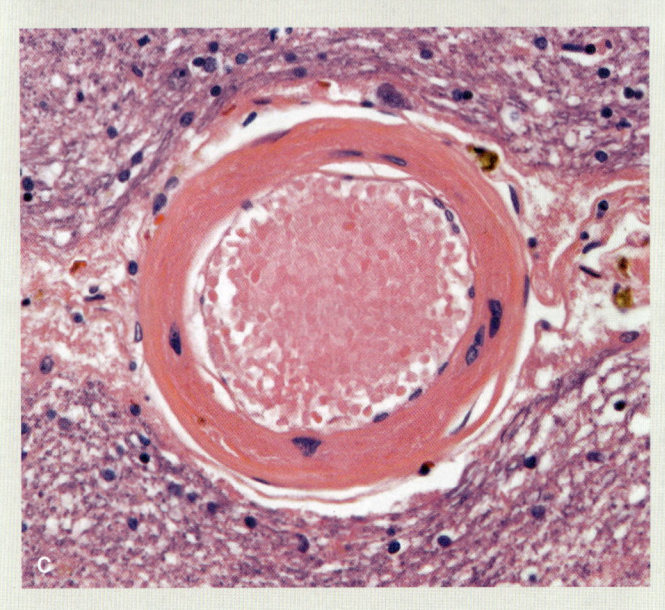

FIGURE 7-24 **(A) CT demonstrating intracerebral hemorrhage. (B)** Autopsy examination of brain with hemorrhage. **(C)** Histopathology of brain tissue. Note hemosiderin –laden macrophages. From Bouldin T, Armao D. Department of Pathology and Laboratory Medicine, University of North Carolina at Chapel Hill.

progression of hyalinization and thickening causes the light reflex to become more diffuse and the retinal arterioles appear red-brown (**copper wire**). As the sclerosis advances, the increased density of the retinal arterioles seen on ophthalmoscopy is referred to as sheathing of the vessels. When the sheathing encircles the entire wall, it produces an appearance of a **silver wire**. Focal narrowing of arterioles due to arteriolosclerosis can impede forward circulation resulting in dilated veins peripheral to the arteriolar/venous crossing. This is known **as arteriovenous nicking** (Gunn sign). Additional retinal changes associated with chronic hypertension include retinal hemorrhages, loss of nerve fiber layers, increased vascular tortuosity, and vascular remodeling due to capillary nonperfusion (microaneurysms and shunt vessels).

Malignant Hypertension

Malignant hypertension, a medical emergency, is the rapid and severe elevation of blood pressure that may lead to end-organ damage of the heart, kidneys, and/or brain. Most commonly, the systolic blood pressure is elevated to 180 mm Hg or higher. Malignant hypertension is much less frequent than idiopathic systemic hypertension, occurring in only a small percentage of patients with elevated blood pressures. Those found to be at risk of developing malignant hypertension are African-American men or someone of a lower socioeconomic status. Poor access to health care also increases the risk. Malignant hypertension may develop spontaneously in a previously healthy individual or as a complication in approximately 1% of previously hypertensive patients. Other causes include any form of secondary hypertension, pregnancy, cocaine, monoamine oxidase inhibitors (MAOIs), oral contraceptives, withdrawal of alcohol, β-blockers, or α-stimulants.

The precise etiology of malignant hypertension is unclear, but the initial event appears to be vascular damage to the kidneys. In the setting of chronic hypertension, it may result from end-stage changes to the arterioles or may be in the setting of arteritis. Injury to the arterioles leads to increased permeability of the small vessels to plasma proteins (including fibrinogen), platelet deposition, and endothelial cell injury. The plasma proteins and fibrin are deposited into the wall of the arteriole, giving the vessels an eosinophilic, homogeneous, and granular appearance (**fibrinoid necrosis,** Figure 7-25a). The arterioles may develop occlusive intraluminal thrombosis leading to renal ischemia. Interlobar arteries and larger arterioles show a different response with proliferation of intimal (believed to be smooth muscle) cells that produce a concentric arrangement with an onion-skin appearance (Figure 7-25b). This **hyperplastic arteriolosclerosis** causes severe narrowing of the arterial and arteriolar lumens and further ischemic changes of the kidneys.

Early symptoms of malignant hypertension depend primarily on the organ system most severely affected initially and can include chest pain, heart failure, headache, and visual disturbances. The most severe symptomatology of malignant hypertension is characterized by diastolic blood pressures >120 mm Hg, papilledema, encephalopathy cardiovascular

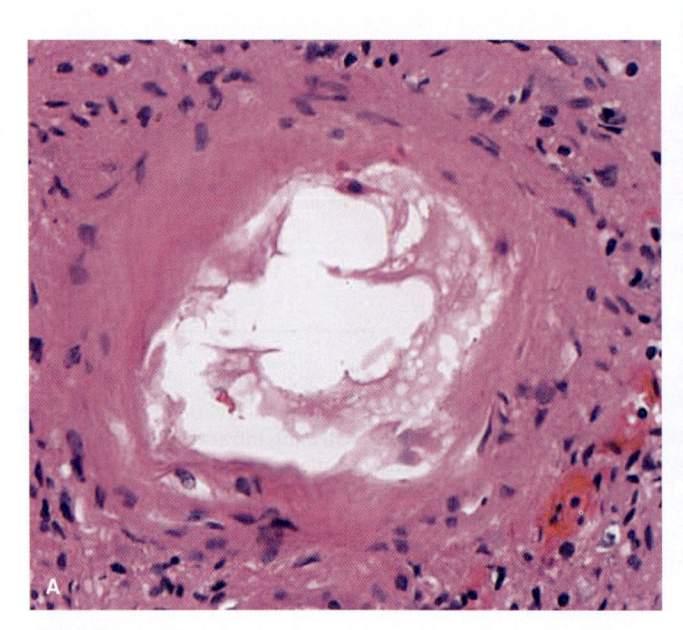

FIGURE 7-25 Malignant Hypertension in Renal Vasculature.
(A) Fibrinoid necrosis N deposited amorphous eosinophilic material in vessel wall. **(B)** "Onion-skin" changes demonstrating proliferation of intimal (smooth muscle) cells. From Department of Pathology and Laboratory Medicine, University of North Carolina at Chapel Hill.

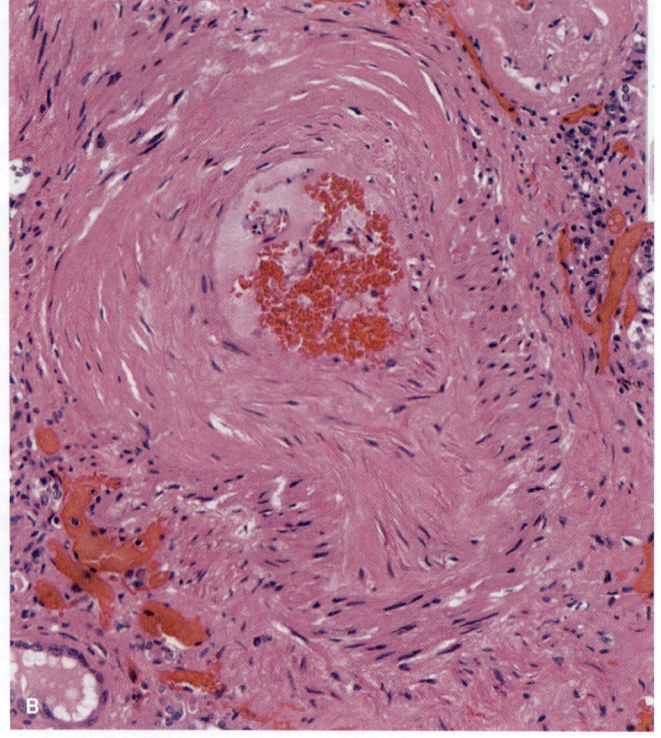

abnormalities, and renal failure. If untreated, malignant hypertension causes significant morbidity and mortality. Often fatal complications include aortic dissection, myocardial ischemia, heart failure, intracerebral hemorrhage, and acute renal failure.

Therapy is to initially reduce the mean arterial blood pressure by approximately 25% over the first 24–48 hours as a rapid reduction may lead to organ hypoperfusion and organ ischemia. Prior to the time of effective treatment, the life expectancy of patients with malignant hypertension was less than 2 years. With current therapy and renal dialysis as a bridge to returning renal function, the survival rate at 1 year is >90% and at 5 years is approximately 80%.

Pulmonary Hypertension

The pulmonary vascular system is one of low resistance with normal arterial pressures approximately one-tenth of systemic (at rest <20 mm Hg). Pulmonary hypertension, defined as mean pulmonary arterial pressures ≥25 mm Hg, presents equally in men and women of all age groups. The mean age at diagnosis is in the 3rd and 4th decades. The current WHO classification system divides pulmonary hypertension (PH) into 5 groups based on the etiology of the condition:

Group 1: Patients with pulmonary arterial hypertension including idiopathic pulmonary arterial hypertension, heritable idiopathic pulmonary arterial hypertension, and PH that is localized to small pulmonary muscular arteries including connective tissue diseases, congenital heart disease, pulmonary venoocclusive disease, HIV infection, persistent pulmonary hypertension of the newborn, and parasitic infections.

Group 2: Pulmonary hypertension due to left heart failure, including systolic or diastolic dysfunction or valvular heart disease.

Group 3: Pulmonary hypertension due to lung disease or hypoxemia including chronic obstructive disease, interstitial lung disease, obstructive sleep apnea, and hypoventilation syndrome.

Group 4: Chronic thromboembolic pulmonary hypertension. These patients have pulmonary hypertension due to vascular obstruction by recurrent thromboemboli.

Group 5: Pulmonary hypertension due to unknown or multifactorial mechanisms.

Pathology: The underlying pathology of pulmonary artery hypertension is dependent on its etiology. In chronic thrombotic/embolic disease, pulmonary arteries and arterioles will show eccentric mounds of acute, organizing and organized thrombus along intimal surfaces. In patients with left heart failure, the major changes of intimal fibrosis will be identified in pulmonary veins.

The morphology of PAH seen in patients with unoperated congenital heart disease includes six grades of structural changes in the pulmonary arteries. Grades 1–3 show progressive medial thickening with adventitial fibrosis in pulmonary arterioles and muscular pulmonary arteries. Grade 3 shows progressive intimal proliferation and fibrosis in smaller pulmonary arteries and arterioles with extension into medium-sized arteries. The characteristic feature of grade 3 pulmonary vascular disease is the widespread occlusion of muscular pulmonary arteries and arterioles by acellular fibrous tissue admixed with fine elastic fibrils. Grades 4, 5, and 6 include plexiform lesions, vein-like branches of hypertrophied, usually occluded, muscular pulmonary arteries, angiomatoid lesions, and cavernous lesions (Figure 7-26). Plexiform lesions are the hallmark of grade 4 pulmonary hypertension and are formed by distention of arteries with formation of sacs with endothelial proliferation and thrombosis. Grade 6 is characterized by necrotizing arteritis with fibrinoid changes of the media with an intimal inflammatory reaction. Lesions of grades 1 and 2 and sometimes grade 3 are reversible (given surgical repair of the inciting cardiac defect). Changes found in grades 4–6 are irreversible.

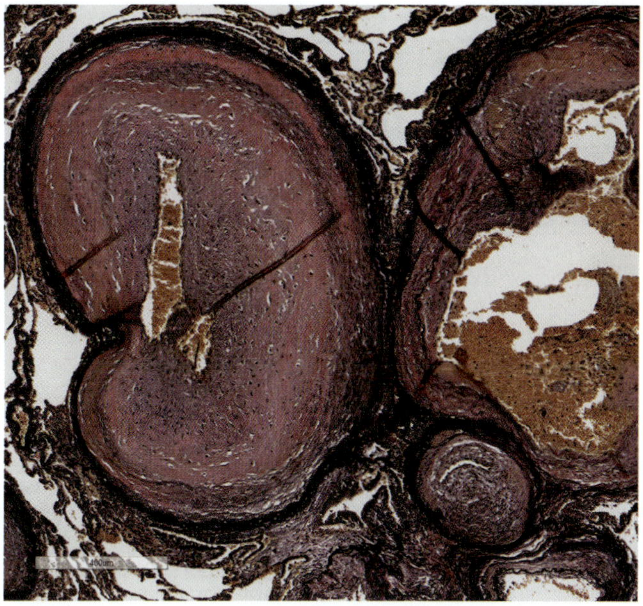

FIGURE 7-26 Vascular Changes in Pulmonary Arterial Hypertension. Pulmonary arterioles/arteries from an individual with uncorrected congenital heart disease. Elastic tissue stain demonstrates adventitial fibrosis. There is also marked medial thickening and occlusion of arteriole. (grade 3 lesion). From Department of Pathology and Laboratory Medicine, University of North Carolina at Chapel Hill.

Pulmonary lung biopsies are now infrequent for grading of pulmonary arterial changes. Clinical studies, including echocardiogram and arteriogram, can provide the necessary information of pulmonary artery pressures and the possible prognosis. Additional aspects of pulmonary vascular disease are discussed in Chapter 8.

ARTERIOSCLEROSIS

Based on Greek words meaning "arteries" (arterio-) and "hardening" (sclerosis), **arteriosclerosis** *is a pathologic process caused by thickening and loss of elasticity of the arterial walls.* The three types of arteriosclerosis include

- Mönckeberg medial calcific stenosis
- Arteriolosclerosis (see above)
- Atherosclerosis

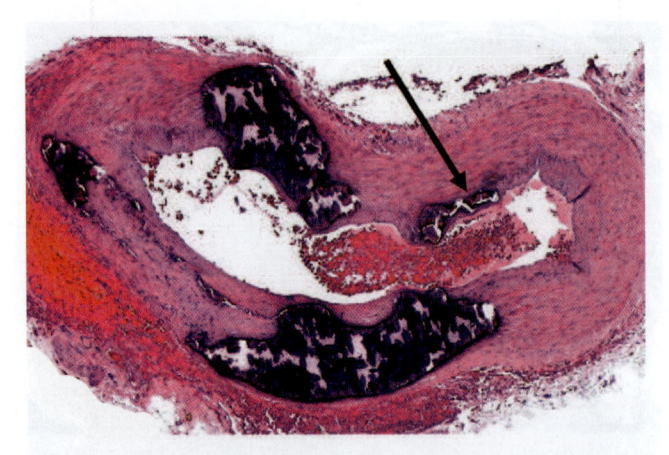

FIGURE 7-27 **Mönckeberg medial calcific stenosis.** Typical appearance of an artery demonstrating medial calcification. An area of calcification of the internal elastica is shown by the arrow. Reprinted from Micheletti RG1, Fishbein GA, Currier JS, Fishbein MC. Mönckeberg sclerosis revisited: a clarification of the histologic definition of Mönckeberg sclerosis. *Arch Pathol Lab Med*. 2008 Jan;132(1):43-7 with permission from Archives of Pathology & Laboratory Medicine. Copyright 2008. College of American Pathologists..

Mönckeberg medial calcific stenosis is the calcification of the muscular media in elderly patients leading to decreased elasticity. This medial calcification does not lead to luminal narrowing or decreased blood flow. It does, however, lead to the decreased ability of muscular arteries to respond to stimuli inducing changes in resistance (**Figure 7-27**).

Atherosclerosis *is the most common type of arteriosclerosis primarily involving end-organ arterial systems including large elastic (aorta, carotids, iliacs) and medium-sized muscular arteries (coronary arteries, femoral, popliteals).* The term reflects the appearance of the atherosclerotic plaque due to accumulation of lipid, smooth muscle cells, inflammation, and connective tissue within the intima. These intimal lesions, called **atheromas** or atherosclerotic plaques, lead to significant morbidity and mortality, therefore, making it important to understand its etiology and pathogenesis.

The **response-to-injury theory**, also now known as *atherothrombosis*, was proposed by Ross and Fuster in the 1990s. This theory with some modification is the current, best accepted hypothesis explaining the pathophysiology of atherosclerosis. It is postulated that atherosclerosis begins with injury of the endothelium, subsequently leading to thrombosis and lipid deposition. In this theory, the interaction between the vascular wall and various physical forces regulate formation of the atherosclerotic plaque by a fibroproliferative and inflammatory response. The typical atherosclerotic plaque (atheroma) is a progressive accumulation of inflammatory cells, smooth muscle cells, lipid, and connective tissue within the intima.

The endothelium is an active and dynamic tissue that produces multiple cytokines, proteins, and tissue factors that allow normal function of the vascular system. ECs prevent thrombosis by production of a layer of heparin sulfate along the luminal surfaces. **Prostacyclin** also prevents thrombosis by preventing platelet aggregation (see Chapter 2). Production of endothelium-derived relaxing factor (EDRF, nitric oxide), a potent vasodilator, and potent vasoconstrictors (endothelin, serotonin, platelet-derived growth factor) allows the endothelium to maintain appropriate vascular tone. Lysis of fibrin is crucial for maintenance of blood flow and is promoted by endothelial production of plasminogen. Selective permeability of various blood components, including lipids, is also an important role of ECs.

Acute or chronic injury of the endothelium causes endothelial dysfunction. Secretion of cytokines and growth, migration, and adhesion factors occurs in the **initiation and formation phase** of the atherosclerotic plaque due to endothelial injury. Multiple growth factors (platelet-derived growth factor, insulin-like growth factor, α- and β- transforming growth factors, fibroblastic growth factor, and angiotensin II) are mitogens produced by activated platelets, macrophages, and dysfunctional ECs.

These mitogenic factors cause alteration of medial smooth muscle cells, important components of the atherosclerotic plaque. The local factors produced by the dysfunctional ECs cause medial smooth muscle cells to lose their contractile elements and thus function. The dedifferentiation also allows increased protein synthesis leading to proliferation and subsequent migration of smooth muscle cells to the intima where they produce and deposit extracellular matrix material, forming a "neointima."

EC injury also alters the selective permeability of normal endothelium, allowing lipid accumulation. The accumulated lipid materials cause further cell dysfunction and injury resulting in increased production of inflammatory cytokines and macrophage and lymphocyte accumulation in response. Mononuclear macrophages participate in further lipid accumulation and release additional factors responsible for continued smooth muscle cell proliferation and production and deposition of matrix proteins. The macrophage component also produces factors that inhibit the growth of reparative ECs. Other factors produced by macrophages lead to endothelial-cell production of platelet-activating factor, tissue factor, and plasminogen-activating inhibitor creating a procoagulative state. In this state, the thrombus that forms along the intimal surface undergoes organization and incorporation into the plaque and further production of factors responsible for smooth muscle cell alterations.

Causes of endothelial cell injury encompass a variety of insults and are thought to include hypercholesterolemia, hemodynamic factors, microorganisms, and exposure to toxic chemicals in the blood (importantly, some derived from cigarette smoking). How each affects the EC is unclear but leads to EC phenotypic alteration by modulation of genetic expression and regulation of production of specific proteins.

Atherosclerotic plaques do not occur randomly, but are characteristically located at branch points and in areas of irregular or turbulent flow stress in arteries. Shear stress and turbulence promote atherosclerotic plaque production at these sites within coronary arteries, the major branches of the aorta, and the large arteries of the upper and lower extremities.

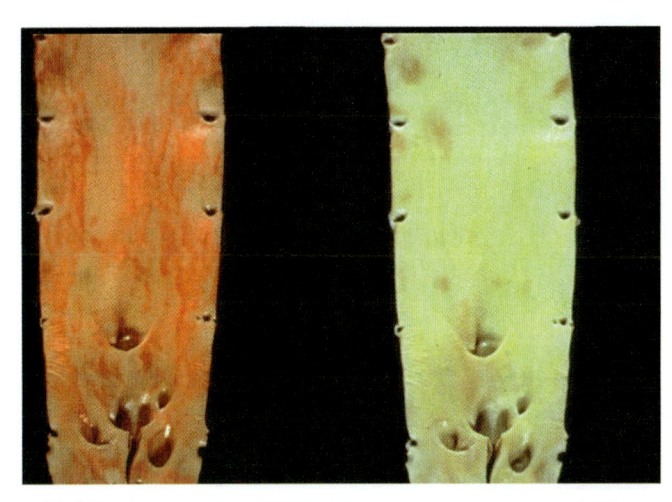

FIGURE 7-28 **Fatty streak lesions of the aorta.** Intimal surface of the aorta. Left image is stained with Oil Red O (a lipophilic stain) to highlight fatty streak lesions. From Department of Pathology and Laboratory Medicine, University of North Carolina at Chapel Hill.

Atherosclerotic (or Atherothrombotic) Lesions

Many autopsy series have shown specific intimal lesions, *fatty streaks,* and intimal thickening, to be present along the aortic intima in all children more than 10 years of age. It is uncertain if these areas of lipid deposition represent precursor lesions of atherosclerosis, as in many populations that do not develop atherosclerosis in later life, fatty streaks may regress with age.

Fatty streaks are flat or minimally elevated, 3- to 5-mm, yellow foci along the intimal aortic surface. Microscopically, islands of intracellular and extracellular lipid accumulation are seen in the intima. The cells within the intima, derived from smooth muscle cells and macrophages, are filled with lipid droplets, creating "foam cells." These foci stain strongly with Oil Red O (a lipophilic stain). There is no collagen deposition in these lesions (Figure 7-28).

Fibrointimal thickening at sites of predilection for atherosclerotic plaques have been shown to also be present in childhood with progression throughout life. Smooth muscle cells have been identified in these thickenings and it has been suggested that these areas of intimal fibrous thickening are precursors to atherosclerosis.

Characteristic atherosclerotic lesions are similar in all populations studied. Grossly, the simple atherosclerotic lesion is an elevated, white-yellow, smooth, irregular, focal lesion with definite borders. The plaques along the intimal surface of the aorta are mostly oval and are oriented along the direction of blood flow. Smaller arteries (carotids, coronary arteries) usually have eccentric lesions. As the lesions progress, the arterial lumen is narrowed further (Figure 7-29). During growth of the plaque, the artery undergoes adaptive changes with remodeling alterations in an attempt to maintain flow. Once the plaque encroaches on 50% of the lumen, the

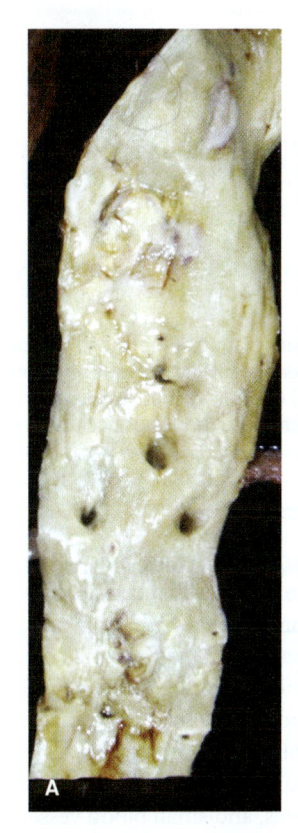

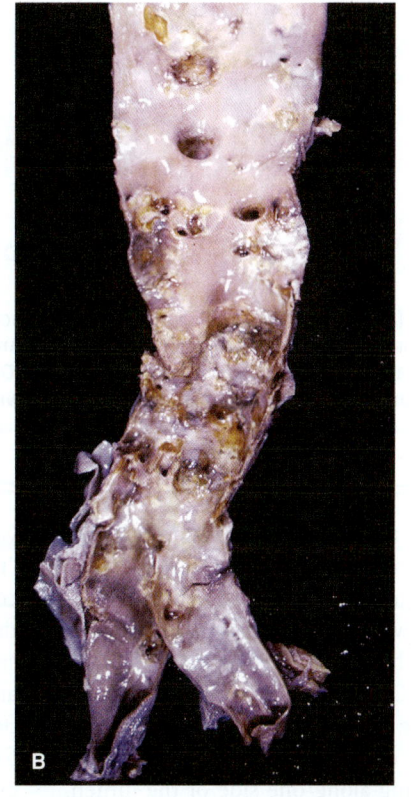

FIGURE 7-29 **Atherosclerotic lesions of the aorta (gross).** **(A)** Fibrofatty plaque. **(B)** Complex lesion. From Department of Pathology and Laboratory Medicine, University of North Carolina at Chapel Hill.

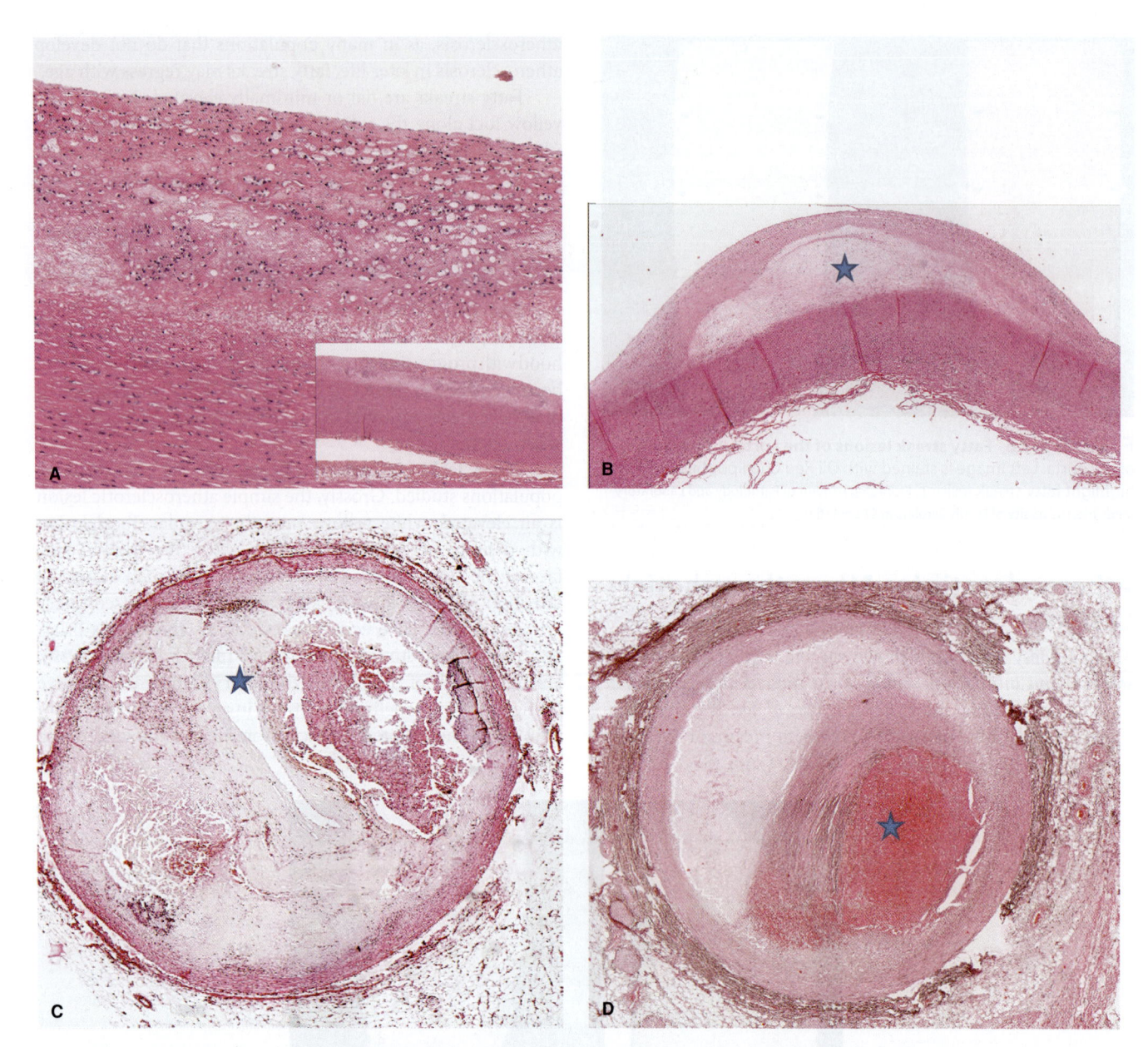

FIGURE 7-30 Atheromas. (A) Simple atheroma. Low-power view (inset) demonstrates fibrointimal thickening. High-power view shows intact endothelial lining and extensive presence of foam cells (lipid-filled macrophages shown with clear cytoplasm) (arrow). **(B)** More mature/advanced (atheroma demonstrating fibrous cap (arrow) and grumous core (star). **(C)** Complicated atheroma with acute plaque hemorrhage compressing the arterial lumen (star). Areas of calcified plaque and lipid debris are present (arrows). **(D)** Complicated atheroma with extensive grumous core (arrow) with acute thrombus occluding the lumen (star). From Department of Pathology and Laboratory Medicine, University of North Carolina at Chapel Hill.

compensatory remodeling is no longer effective and the artery becomes physiologically narrowed.

The atherosclerotic plaque is a complex lesion that is composed of multiple cell types with lipid, matrix material, serum proteins, platelets and white blood cells, necrotic debris, small blood vessels, and crystals. Classifications of atheromas have been proposed based on the descriptive histologic morphology of the plaque. Histology of the **simple atheroma** demonstrates fibrointimal thickening along one side of the lumen. The intimal fibrous mound is covered by endothelium. As the lesion grows, histologic features vary between plaques and can vary from area to area of the same artery (Figure 7-30A). The **"mature"/advanced plaque** is composed of three principle components including cells, matrix, and lipid material. The tissue over the necrotic core, the **fibrous cap**, is composed of smooth muscle cells, macrophages, foam cells, lymphocytes, and connective tissue materials. The histology of the central portion (core) of the lesion demonstrates necrotic debris, foam cells, lipid crystals, foreign-body giant cells, lymphocytes, and small blood vessels. The necrotic debris has a gross, gruel-like appearance, hence the descriptive name "grumous" (Figure 7-30B). *In Greek "athero" means "gruel."*

In the clinical phase of the disease, advanced atherosclerotic lesions are at risk for complications leading to clinical signs and symptoms. Plaques that undergo such complications are known as **complicated plaques.** These complicated plaques have been shown to contain activated mast cells and variable amounts of inflammatory activity, elements that may play a significant role in the potential complications. Some studies have demonstrated the increased presence of matrix metalloproteinases in some plaques leading to increased vulnerability for plaque alterations. Shear stress may also be a component leading to complications of the atheroma.

Complicated plaques can undergo erosion, ulceration, or rupture of the fibrous cap, hemorrhage into the plaque, mural thrombus, calcification, and aneurysm formation. Erosion, ulceration, or rupture of the fibrous cap can lead to release of thrombogenic material from the necrotic core leading to an acute luminal thrombosis. With acute occlusion, the arterial flow is interrupted resulting in organ injury due to lack of oxygen. If the obstruction continues, the end organ will undergo ischemic necrosis manifested by organ-dependent clinical signs and symptoms (Figure 7-30 C and D).

Epidemiology and Risk Factors of Atherosclerosis

Atherosclerosis, a disease of developed countries, causes significant morbidity and mortality in the Western world leading to myocardial injury that is responsible for 20% to 25% of all deaths in the United States. Other countries do not have the same prevalence of atherosclerosis. For example, atherosclerotic disease is significantly less in populations of Central and South America, Africa, and Asia. The mortality rate of ischemic heart disease in the United States is six times that of Japan. What is fascinating is that low-risk populations that emigrate to countries with a higher prevalence of atherosclerosis will acquire the same predisposition as the native population.

The Framingham Study

During the 1940s and 1950s, public health officials became aware of a mounting epidemic of cardiovascular disease. By 1950, one of every three men in the United States developed cardiovascular disease before the age of 60 years. Cardiovascular disease had become the leading cause of death, with life expectancy estimates of 45 years of age. With little knowledge of how to uncover the risk factors, treatment options and means to decrease these deaths, an epidemiologic study was begun. This study attempted to determine the natural history of cardiovascular disease, explore its behavior, and identify any factors that might relate to its development. The initial studies of arteriosclerosis and hypertensive cardiovascular disease became a longitudinal cohort study (the Framingham study) that allowed researchers to determine significant findings regarding the development of arteriosclerosis including:

- 1960—Cigarette smoking increases the risk of heart disease
- 1961—Cholesterol level, blood pressure, and electrocardiographic abnormalities increased the risk of heart disease
- 1967—Physical activity reduced the risk of heart disease
- 1967—Obesity increased the risk of heart disease
- 1967—Menopause increased the risk of heart disease in women

The research results from this study continue to affect current conventional wisdom and treatment recommendations. Recently, the Framingham Heart Study contributed to the discovery of multiple genes that underlie heart disease risk factors.

A second crucial study that significantly contributed to our knowledge of cardiovascular disease was the Multiple Risk Factor Intervention Trial (MRFIT) that began in 1971. This trial attempted to determine whether lowering serum cholesterol and diastolic blood pressures and ceasing cigarette smoking would lower mortality from coronary heart disease. This trial was important in that it demonstrated a significant, graded, and continuous relationship between elevated cholesterol and coronary heart disease.

Two types of **risk factors** *were found to play a role in the development of atherosclerosis. The* **constitutional, nonalterable factors** *include increasing age, male gender, and family history.* The risk of developing atherosclerosis increases with each decade of life **(Figure 7-31)**. As age increases between 40 and 60 years, the incidence of developing acute myocardial injury (a myocardial infarct) increases fivefold. Male gender is a second nonalterable risk factor of atherosclerosis. Men are at an increased risk for developing atherosclerosis and its complications compared to premenopausal women who do not have additional risk factors. As the risk of atherosclerosis increases in postmenopausal women as in men, a protective role of estrogen had been hypothesized. Much research into the cardioprotective effects of estrogen has shown that estrogen binds to receptors on ECs causing increased genetic expression of prostacyclin and nitric oxide synthase, rapid re-endothelialization after injury, and inhibition of smooth muscle cell proliferation.

A positive family history is a well-established predisposition for atherosclerosis and ischemic heart disease. In many instances, it is the familial risk for hypertension, diabetes, or familial hypercholesterolemia that increases the risk for atherosclerosis. Even in families that do not have these additional risk factors, there may be a genetic predisposition leading to the increased risk for atherosclerosis. Since no single gene has been isolated, the genetic risk is most likely polygenetic. A middle-aged man who has a family history of a father with atherosclerotic heart disease before the age of 40 years is at a significant risk for a similar outcome.

Other risk factors were discovered that are potentially **alterable** *in an individual including systemic hypertension, hyperlipidemia, diabetes mellitus, and cigarette smoking. Systemic hypertension* is a major risk factor for developing atherosclerosis at all ages. While the exact mechanism of its effects is currently unknown, it has been established that those with untreated hypertensive blood pressures are at a significantly increased (more than fivefold) risk for ischemic heart disease. Both systolic and diastolic hypertension are known to increase

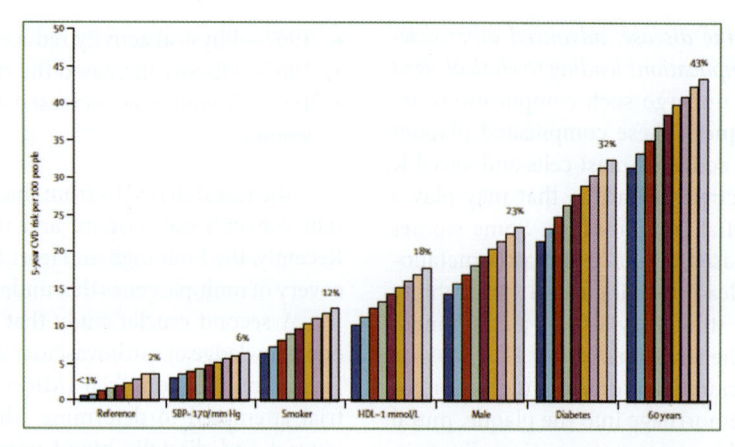

FIGURE 7–31 Risk factors in cardiovascular disease. Absolute risk of cardiovascular disease over 5 years in patients by total blood cholesterol at specified levels of other risk factors (x-axis). Colored bars represent cholesterol concentrations of 4.0 to 8.0 mmol/L at intervals of 0.5 mmol. In each category on the x-axis, additional risk factors are sequentially added. (Reference is a 50-year-old, nonsmoking, nondiabetic woman who is normotensive.) From Jackson R, Lawes CM, Bennett DA, et al. Treatment with drugs to lower blood pressure and blood cholesterol based on an individual's absolute cardiovascular risk. *Lancet* 2005; 365:436.

the risk. Adequate treatment can reduce the incidence of morbidity and mortality due to strokes and ischemic heart disease.

Hyperlipidemia, primarily hypercholesterolemia, is a second potentially alterable risk factor for the development of atherosclerosis. The major implicated component of the total serum cholesterol associated with this increased risk is the low-density lipoprotein (LDL) component that makes up much of the circulating cholesterol and has been positively related to coronary disease. Familial hypercholesterolemia has provided medicine with a natural research project showing that the higher levels of cholesterol are related to higher incidence of coronary disease. Patients with **homozygous hypercholesterolemia** have absent or defective receptors for LDL, resulting in markedly increased serum cholesterol levels and severe complicated atherosclerosis in their early lives (10–20 years of age). Patients with heterozygous genetic defects have 50% abnormal receptor activity and less severe cholesterol levels and demonstrate atherosclerosis later in life than homozygotes.

Conversely, high-density lipoproteins (HDLs) play a protective role with levels inversely related to cardiovascular disease risk. HDLs function to transport cholesterol to the liver for excretion in the bile. HDL levels increase with exercise and weight loss. Postmenopausal estrogen use has been shown to result in higher HDL levels. Moderate alcohol consumption, one to two glasses of red wine per day, also increases HDLs.

Recall that the various blood lipids are transported as lipoproteins complexed to various apoproteins. Lipoprotein a (Lp(a)) is an altered form of LDL containing the apolipoprotein B-100 portion of the LDL linked to apolipoprotein A (apo A). Various epidemiologic studies have suggested a correlation between increased blood levels of Lp(a) and cerebrovascular and coronary artery disease (CAD). This risk is independent of the total cholesterol or LDL blood levels.

Whether increased levels of triglycerides play a significant role in atherogenesis has been recently challenged. Hypertriglyceridemia is usually accompanied by decreased levels of HDL cholesterol, a known risk factor for atherosclerosis. Therefore, increased blood levels of triglycerides may play an important role as a biomarker of atherogenesis. Patients with type 2 diabetes mellitus and/or metabolic syndrome are at a particularly high risk for this dyslipidemia.

Diabetes mellitus, a third potentially alterable risk factor established by the Framingham and other studies, leads to significantly increased vascular complications relative to nondiabetics. In type 2 diabetes mellitus, hyperglycemia leads to insulin resistance, endothelial dysfunction and incorporation of extracellular materials, cholesterol, and proteoglycans leading to a significantly increased risk of atherothrombosis. The incidence of myocardial infarct in patients with diabetes mellitus is twice that of the nondiabetic population. The risk of strokes is also significantly increased. The risk of atherothrombotic-induced gangrene of the lower extremities is as much as 100 times nondiabetics.

Like type 2 diabetes mellitus, type 1 diabetes mellitus (T1D) with hyperglycemia causes endothelial dysfunction, increased circulating free fatty acids, and inflammation. This proinflammatory environment again leads to an increased risk of atherothrombosis. Although childhood deaths from cardiovascular disease are rare, autopsy studies have suggested that subclinical disease may present in early adolescence. The mortality rate from CAD in patients with T1D is 35% by the age of 55 years compared with 4% to 8% in those without diabetes. In the third decade after T1D diagnosis, cardiovascular disease accounts for 67% of deaths. One study showed that intensive glycemic control in T1D patients decreased the risk of cardiovascular events by 57%. Of note, the increasing numbers of obese children are at risk for the early development of metabolic syndrome and type 2 diabetes (T2D).

Cigarette smoking is the fourth potentially alterable risk factor from the Framingham study. Smoking cigarettes releases a complex mixture of at least 4000 constituents. Some of these constituents enter the bloodstream via "mainstream smoke," categorized as the material leaving the mouth end of the cigarette, composed of four major components including carbon monoxide, other gas-phase materials, nicotine, and particulate matter. It is uncertain which components of the cigarette smoke contribute to the pathogenesis of atherothrombosis. However, these various components are responsible for endothelial dysfunction, creation of proinflammatory and procoagulative environments, increased oxidative stress, and alterations in lipid metabolism, all factors known to lead to atherosclerotic changes in blood vessels. Of interest, impaired arterial endothelium-dependent vasomotion has been documented after smoking a **single cigarette**. It has been well documented in men that cigarette smoking is related to increased atherosclerosis in peripheral, cerebral, and coronary vascular beds. The significant increase in numbers of women with cardiovascular disease appears to be related to the increased numbers of women who smoke. The risk of cardiovascular disease is dose-dependent in smokers. Those who stop smoking are able to decrease their risk substantially.

Several additional factors may be possible markers of patients at an increased risk for atherothrombotic events (myocardial infarct, strokes), including plasminogen activator inhibitor 1 and C-reactive protein. Patients with high circulating blood levels of homocysteine (hyperhomocysteinemia) have premature vascular disease, as demonstrated by rare cases of inborn metabolic syndromes leading to homocystinuria. Epidemiologic and clinical studies have shown that individuals without the genetic condition, but with elevated blood levels of homocysteine, show premature atherosclerosis.

Other factors that have been less well demonstrated to be associated with atherothrombosis (referred to as the "soft" risk factors) include lack of exercise, stressful life style (type A personality), and unrestrained weight gain.

It is important to note that risk factors accelerate the progression of the disease. Multiple risk factors have a MULTIPLICATIVE effect on the progression. Two risk factors increase the risk approximately four times. If a patient has three risk factors (hypertension, smoking, and hyperlipidemia), the risk of myocardial infarct is increased seven times (Figure 7-31).

With the results of the Framingham Study and Multiple Risk Factor Intervention Trial (MRFIT) in hand, public health officials began an aggressive campaign to fight the development of cardiovascular disease. Since that time, there has been a 50% decrease in the death rate from ischemic heart disease. From 1963 to 2000, there was a 70% decrease in the death rate from strokes. While the morbidity and mortality rates associated with atherosclerosis have decreased significantly, currently it remains the primary cause of death in both men and women in North America and Europe.

Metabolic Syndrome

Metabolic syndrome is a recent condition that was defined less than 20 years ago. It is widespread and about 47 million Americans (1 in every 6 people) suffer from it according to the American Heart Association. It is not a disease itself, but consists of a group of risk factors that are associated with insulin resistance accompanied by abnormal fat deposition and function. Metabolic syndrome has a high prevalence in African-Americans in the United States, especially affecting African-American women. The higher prevalence of obesity, hypertension, and diabetes in this population puts them at an increased risk of the syndrome. Metabolic syndrome is considered to be an emerging global epidemic with approximately 25% of all European and Latin American adults showing its features. Although metabolic syndrome is a clinical diagnosis and not specifically a 'pathological' disease process, it leads to increased risks of cardiovascular, renal, and cerebrovascular diseases. Understanding the process of diagnosis and the pathogenesis of metabolic syndrome can further help us to understand how it affects these organs and the development of disease.

The American Heart Association and National Heart, Lung and Blood Institute have established guidelines for the diagnosis of metabolic syndrome. Patients who have at least three of the following five conditions can be diagnosed with metabolic syndrome:

- Fasting blood glucose ≥ 100 mg/dL (or receiving drug therapy for hyperglycemia).
- Blood pressure ≥ 130/85 mm Hg (or receiving drug therapy for hypertension).
- Triglycerides ≥ 150 mg/dL (or receiving drug therapy for hypertriglyceridemia).
- HDL-C < 40 mg/dL in men or < 50 mg/dL in women (or receiving drug therapy for reduced HDL-C).
- Waist circumference ≥ 102 cm (40 in) in men or ≥ 88 cm (35 in) in women.

Patients meeting the diagnosis of metabolic syndrome have been shown to have twice the risk of developing clinically significant atherosclerotic coronary artery disease. It also increases the risk of developing diabetes mellitus by five times. A correlation between metabolic syndrome and stroke has recently been suggested. Risk factors for developing the clinical diagnosis of metabolic syndrome in patients include family history, poor diet, and lack of/or inadequate exercise.

The etiology of metabolic syndrome is thought to be caused primarily by insulin resistance and adipocyte dysfunction. In caloric excess, increased energy is stored in adipose tissues, the main lipid storage depot. However, in obesity, lipid excess results in hypertrophy (increase in size) of adipocytes. When the adipocyte is no longer able to process the excess, free fatty acids are released into the circulation, causing triglycerides to deposit in skeletal muscle, the liver, and pancreas. In addition, the adipocyte becomes less sensitive to insulin and begins to produce excess proinflammatory cytokines leading to a chronic inflammatory state. This chronic inflammatory state and ectopic lipid deposition lead to insulin resistance in the liver, skeletal muscle, the pancreas, and endothelial cells.

The resultant insulin resistance in the liver leads to increased glucose output (fasting hyperglycemia) and dyslipidemia with increased plasma levels of fatty acids and triglycerides. In response to the hyperglycemia, insulin secretion

CASE 7-6

A 63-year-old man complains of severe abdominal pain. You are told by your senior resident to examine this man. He tells you to be careful when you palpate his abdomen.

While taking the patient's history, he states that his father died of a ruptured abdominal aortic aneurysm. When you see the patient, he has a large, pulsatile mass in his abdomen. He is sent emergently to surgery and does well (Figure 7-32).

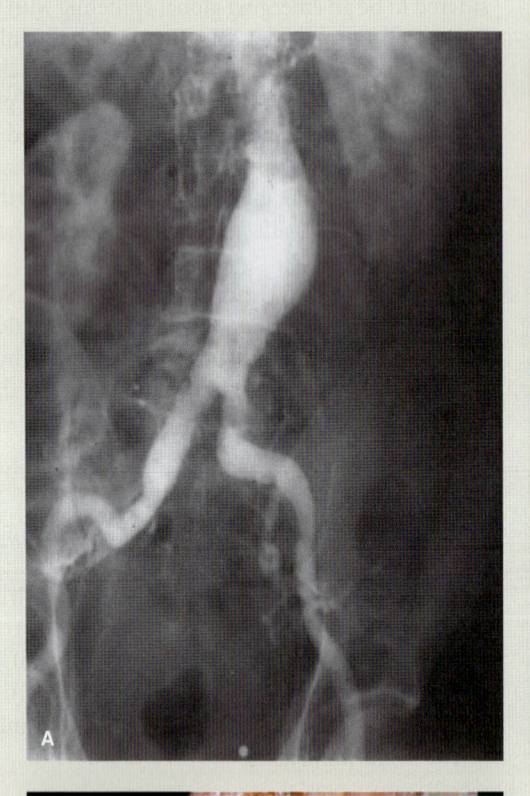

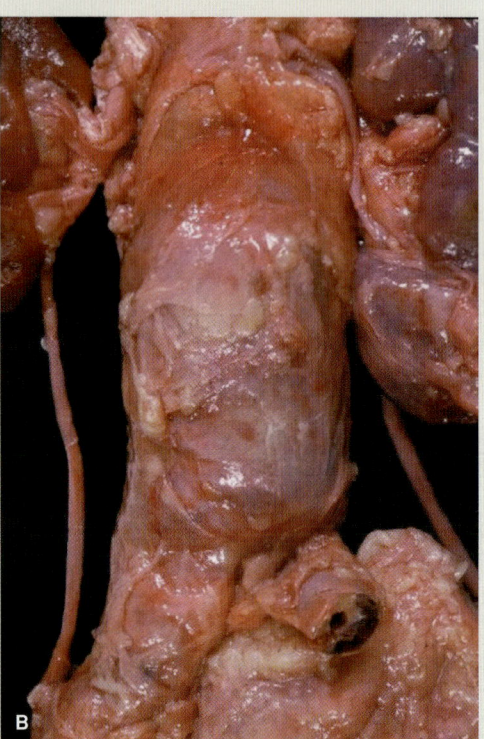

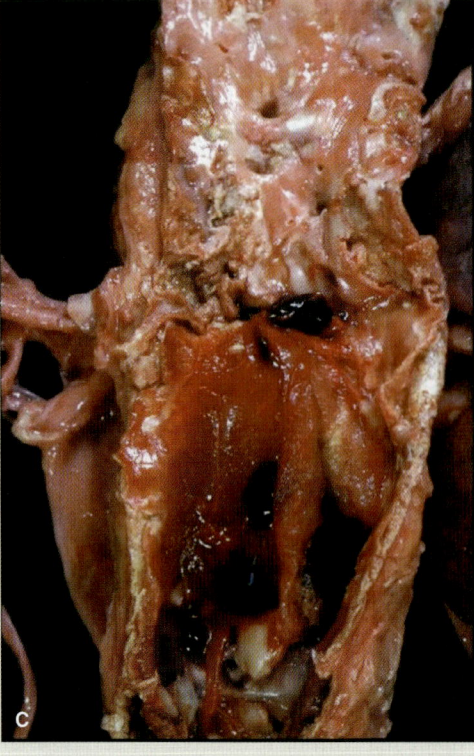

FIGURE 7-32 Abdominal aortic aneurysm (AAA or "triple A"). (A) Frontal view of typical infrarenal AAA seen on radiograph after filling with contrast material. Note large fusiform distal abdominal aneurysm with focal saccular enlargement; also note tortuosity of iliacs affected by atherosclerotic disease. **(B)** Gross view of infrarenal AAA. **(C)** Aneurysm opened. Note extensive atheroma formation on aortic surface and adherent thrombotic material within the lumen of the aneurysm. From Department of Pathology and Laboratory Medicine, University of North Carolina at Chapel Hill.

and β-cell mass is upregulated in the pancreas in an attempt to overcome these changes caused by the insulin resistance. The inability of the pancreas to produce insulin levels high enough to overcome the insulin resistance and limit the hyperglycemia will lead to diabetes.

Insulin activity has a role in controlling the sympathetic nervous system. Increased sympathetic activity occurs in response to increased insulin levels and decreases with fasting. In obese individuals, the sympathetic nervous system activity is increased leading to vasoconstriction of resistance vessels and hypertension. *Thus, insulin resistance is an important process in the development of the features of the metabolic syndrome, including hypertension, hyperglycemia, and triglyceridemia.*

Complications of Atherosclerosis

Abdominal Aortic Aneurysm

Atherosclerosis is the most common cause of **abdominal aortic (and other arterial) aneurysms**. *The overlying atherosclerotic plaque causes compression and erosion of and destruction of the arterial media, leading to significant thinning of the vascular wall.* As the blood travels down the aorta, the systolic pressure causes the aorta to expand. During diastole, the elastic properties of the normal aorta allow it to contract to its original size. In the setting of atherosclerosis and the loss of its medial elastic components, the atherosclerotic abdominal aorta widens during systole and is unable to return to its normal size. Over time, the abdominal aorta will become dilated creating an aortic aneurysm. The abdominal aorta is the most common site of the atherosclerotic aneurysm. However, the aortic arch, descending thoracic aorta, and common iliac arteries may also form atherosclerotic aneurysms.

Abdominal aortic aneurysms (AAAs) are most commonly found below the renal arteries (**infrarenal**) and above the aortic bifurcation. The aneurysms can be **saccular** or **fusiform** and can reach quite large sizes. The aneurysms shows marked, confluent atherosclerosis with severe thinning of the aortic media. The lumen of the aneurysm is filled by bland, laminated, unorganized fibrin thrombus material. Not uncommonly, abdominal aortic atherosclerotic aneurysms are associated with atherosclerotic aneurysms of the common iliac arteries. Histology of the AAA demonstrates the marked thinning of the aortic wall, the severity of the atherosclerosis, loss of the elastic media, and normal adventitia (Figure 7-32).

Atherosclerotic AAAs rarely develop before the age of 50 years and more commonly affect men (6:1). Risk factors for an abdominal atherosclerotic aneurysm include advanced age, male gender, cigarette smoking, family history, obesity, and coexisting coronary or cerebrovascular arterial disease. Of interest, cigarette smoking is the most significant risk factor with smokers having a sevenfold increased risk for AAA. This association with cigarette smoking is similar to the association of cigarette smoking with lung cancer. Ninety percent of AAA patients have been regular cigarette smokers at one time in their lives. Obesity, with its associated proinflammatory properties, has been independently associated with AAA. Genetics also play a role in the increased risk of some patients. Several studies have shown a familial connection of AAA, with an eightfold increase for a first-degree relative. Genetic studies have examined genes involved with extracellular matrix production, the cardiovascular system, the immune system, and signaling pathways. Two single nucleotide polymorphisms on chromosomes 9p21 and 9q33 have disclosed genetic sites that may possibly be associated with the development of AAA. Hypertension and hypercholesterolemia have a weaker positive risk. Female gender, African-American race, regular aerobic exercise, and diabetes mellitus have been shown to be **protective** against AAA.

Approximately 9% to 15% of patients with atherosclerotic abdominal aortas will develop atherosclerotic AAAs. The clinical course of AAAs is continued dilatation over time. An atherosclerotic AAA is defined as aortic dilatation ≥3 cm in diameter. The significance of the aneurysm changes as the aneurysm enlarges. The aneurysm diameter remains the principle clinical determinant of disease progression and risk of complications including death due to rupture of the aneurysm. The risk of rupture of the AAA increases with the relative size of the aneurysm. If the aneurysm ruptures, blood will fill the retroperitoneum and then the peritoneal cavity. Often, the abdominal cavity can contain 1 to 2 L of blood from a ruptured AAA. Clinically, a patient may experience severe abdominal or back pain with the rupture of an AAA. As the blood is leaving the aortic site of rupture at systolic pressures, the patient may collapse shortly after complaining of the pain. The most important factor determining enlargement of the aneurysm is hypertension.

Surgical treatment is the only effective intervention in preventing deaths due to AAA rupture. Patients undergoing emergent surgical repair for a ruptured AAA have a >50% mortality rate. In contrast, patients undergoing an elective repair for an unruptured AAA have a <5% mortality rate. Therefore, current management of AAA involves serial imaging and clinical surveillance of the early stages of the aneurysm (4.0–5.5 cm). As the aneurysm reaches 5 cm, intervention is indicated. Rapid aneurysm enlargement is also a critical indication that intervention is imminent. Approximately 70% of aneurysms will require surgical intervention within 10 years of diagnosis. Endovascular aneurysm repair (EVAR) has been used increasingly as a means of intervention and has been accompanied by decreasing numbers of procedure-related morbidity and mortality. The endovascular graft is deployed via an intravascular catheter system and attaches to the proximal and distal ends of the aneurysm by metal hooks.

Coronary Artery Atherosclerosis

See Case 2-1 in Chapter 2 for a pertinent case.

Coronary arteries are end arteries, meaning that they are the only, major and final arteries to the heart. Therefore, if the blood flow through the end arteries is interrupted, the tissue distal to the obstruction will not be perfused, leading to **ischemic** injury. Ischemia is the state of inadequate oxygen supply to the tissues. It is usually created by an imbalance between the supply (perfusion) and demand of a tissue for oxygen. In addition to decreased oxygen supply, nutrients are not delivered to the tissues and waste products cannot be not removed. Tissues vary greatly in the amount of time they can tolerate this change in oxygen supply, as some tissues are able use anaerobic metabolism to maintain function in the setting of decreased oxygen.

Atherosclerosis affects the coronary arteries and can lead to significant complications including death. In the heart, decreased perfusion leads to loss of aerobic glycolysis and initiation of anaerobic glycolysis. The loss of the major energy supply of the heart (adenosine triphosphate or ATP) and increased amounts of intracellular noxious metabolites lead to decreased myocardial contractility within 2 minutes. The ischemic changes are reversible for a 20-minute period. After 20–40 minutes, these ischemic changes are no longer reversible and cell death and necrosis ensue.

Ischemic heart disease *is a generic, nonspecific term used to describe multiple, related syndromes resulting from myocardial ischemia.* Other terms that are used to describe the vascular deficiency include coronary artery disease (CAD), atherosclerotic CAD (ASCAD), atherosclerotic coronary heart disease (ASCHD) and atherosclerotic cardiovascular disease (ASCVD). More than 90% of cases of myocardial ischemia are caused by decreased blood flow due to coronary artery narrowing by atherosclerotic obstruction.

The pathogenesis of myocardial ischemia results from decreased coronary perfusion with an increase in myocardial demand. Decrease in available blood supply can occur by multiple mechanisms including low blood pressure (hypotension), fixed coronary artery obstruction, and increased heart rate (tachycardia). Increased heart rate decreases the time the heart is in diastole, therefore decreasing the coronary artery filling time. Increased cardiac demand can be caused by increased heart rate and myocardial hypertrophy (increased heart wall thickness) (Chapter 2, Figure 2-3).

Clinical symptoms develop when there is progressive narrowing of the arterial lumen (**chronic obstruction phase**) with a superimposed acute plaque alteration leading to thrombosis and occlusion of the arterial lumen (**the sudden and dynamic phase**). In patients with a fixed atherosclerotic obstruction <75%, the artery remains able to dilate and increase myocardial perfusion to meet increased demand. Coronary arteries with >75% narrowing are no longer able to modulate the need for increased flow. Therefore, patients with atherosclerotic coronary artery obstruction >75% will become symptomatic with an increased need (usually during exercise, stress, etc.). Patients with 90% luminal narrowing may show symptoms at rest. Atherosclerotic narrowing develops over years. With ongoing decreased oxygenation, the heart responds by developing collateral vasculature to provide additional blood flow to the myocardium. Collaterals can be a significant benefit to the patient when an acute plaque event occurs.

Atherosclerotic plaques are dynamic, and their structure is influenced by both intrinsic and extrinsic factors that can lead to life-altering events. Intrinsic influences primarily include the basic plaque structure and its components. Plaque composition contributes to its likelihood of disruption. **Vulnerable plaques** (those at the highest risk for alteration) were first described in the literature as a means to identify patients with an increased risk of subsequent myocardial events. It was proposed that plaque alterations occurred causing the resultant luminal occlusive thrombosis that led to myocardial ischemia. Autopsy studies showed three histologic features thought to be significant in atherosclerotic plaques responsible for acute myocardial events. These features included plaques with increased numbers of foam cells and extracellular lipid (>40% of the total lesion area), plaques with a thinner fibrous cap (<65 μ), and plaques with increased numbers of inflammatory cells. Production of matrix metalloproteinases by macrophages is thought to lead to disruption of the fibrous cap.

Extrinsic influences of plaque behavior identified in these studies included blood pressure, vasospasm, vasoconstriction, increased platelet activity, and emotional stress. Interestingly, angiography studies have shown that the "culprit" lesion does not usually develop from the most severely narrowed atherosclerotic lesion, but is more often a mild to moderately narrowed artery.

Changes in plaques that can lead to acute myocardial events include plaque rupture, intraplaque hemorrhage, or erosion of the fibrous cap. Intraplaque hemorrhage is thought to occur due to disruption of the thin-walled capillaries within the plaque. These plaque alterations are thought to lead to exposure of the grumous plaque debris to the arterial blood leading to thrombus formation and arterial occlusion. Autopsy and angiographic studies have frequently shown that luminal thrombosis is present in patients with acute coronary events **(Figure 7-33)**.

Acute Coronary Syndrome

Acute coronary syndrome is an umbrella term for a group of symptoms and clinical presentations caused by sudden occlusion of the coronary arteries. The clinical symptoms of the acute coronary syndrome include angina pectoris, myocardial infarct, and sudden cardiac death (SCD).

Angina pectoris is intermittent and usually recurrent chest pain due to transient myocardial ischemia. Three types of angina are recognized and include stable ("typical") angina, Prinzmetal (variant) angina, and unstable ("crescendo") angina. **Stable or typical angina** is the most commonly recognized form, which generally occurs during exercise or stress. The pain is most often described as crushing, squeezing, and substernal which may radiate into the left arm or jaw. The pain is relieved by rest or nitroglycerin (which causes venous dilation and decreases venous return to the heart, hence decreased cardiac work). Patients describe the pain as "always the same" when it occurs. Stable angina is due to a fixed atherosclerotic obstruction (usually 75% or more) of one or more coronary arteries. At rest, the artery is able to deliver adequate flow to the myocardium, but with increased demand associated with exercise or stress, the artery is no longer able to maintain adequate flow

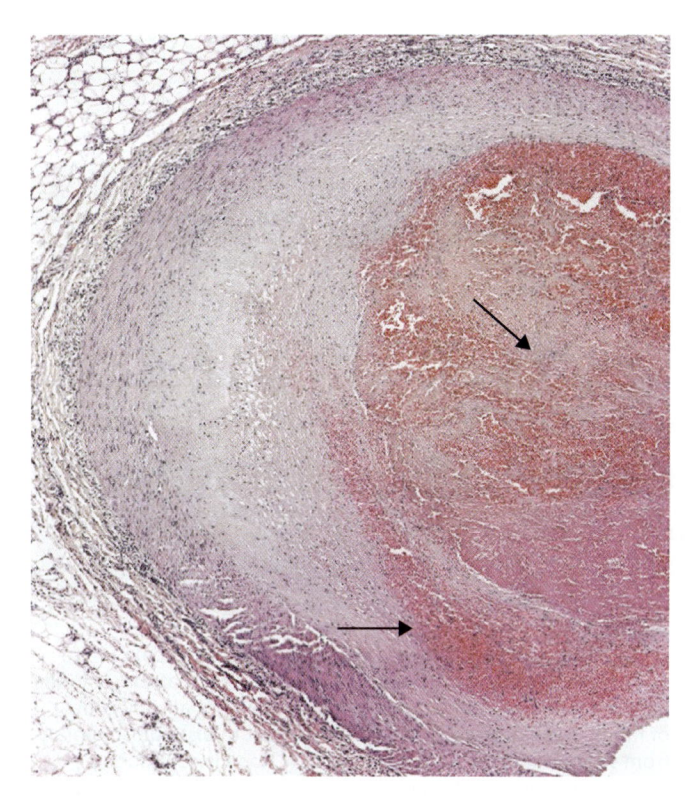

FIGURE 7-33 Hemorrhage into plaque. An area of hemorrhage into an atheroma in a coronary vessel (arrow) was associated with a myocardial infarct. Note the acute occlusive luminal thrombus in reaction to the plaque hemorrhage. From Department of Pathology and Laboratory Medicine, University of North Carolina at Chapel Hill.

leading to ischemia. The ischemia causes the substernal sensation of pain.

Prinzmetal or variant angina occurs at rest and may awaken a patient from sleep. Prinzmetal angina is caused by vasospasm usually near an atherosclerotic plaque and, occasionally, in a normal artery. The exact mechanism of the spasms is not understood. The spasm does respond to administration of vasodilators (nitroglycerin).

Unstable or "crescendo" angina occurs with increasing frequency and is precipitated with less effort each time. Unlike episodes of stable angina, these events last longer, are more intense, and are not relieved by rest or nitroglycerin. Unstable angina is a prodrome of more serious, potentially irreversible myocardial ischemia and has been referred to as **"preinfarction angina."** This pain is caused by an acute plaque change with superimposed luminal thrombus in most patients.

Myocardial ischemia is the leading cause of death in the United States with nearly 500,000 deaths each year. The number of deaths due to ischemic heart disease peaked in 1963. Widespread public information campaigns and education regarding prevention, increase in diabetic control, control of obesity, and aspirin prophylaxis, and advances in diagnosis and therapy have led to a 50% decrease in overall ischemia-related deaths. Although clinical manifestations of coronary artery atherosclerosis may occur at any age, it is most commonly seen in men approximately 60 years of age and in women approximately 70 years of age. Men are more affected by this disease than women until the ninth decade, when the incidence is similar in both genders. Factors that lead to ischemic heart disease are similar to those responsible for the development of atherosclerosis and include systemic hypertension, cigarette smoking, diabetes mellitus, and high blood concentrations of low-density lipoprotein (LDL) cholesterol. As with atherosclerosis, genetic factors and family history play a significant role. Similarly, exercise and moderate consumption of red wine are factors that can potentially decrease the risk of coronary atherosclerosis.

QUICK REVIEW
Normal Heart

The heart is a muscular organ that contracts rhythmically, pumping the blood through the circulatory system. The normal heart weight varies greatly based on the individual's height, weight, and skeletal structure from 300 to 350 g for adult men and 250 to 300 g for adult women. The function of the normal heart is similar to a pump with four chambers forming the mechanic components of the pump, cardiac valves control the direction of the flow, the conduction system determines the rhythm, and coronary arteries provide oxygenation for production of energy.

The walls of atria and ventricles consist of three major layers the **endocardium**, **myocardium**, and **epicardium**. The endocardium consists of a single cell layer of ECs on a thin layer of loose connective tissue containing elastic and collagen fibers. Connecting this endothelial layer to the myocardium is additional connective tissue (often called the subendocardial layer) containing veins, nerves, and branches of the conduction system of the heart **(Figure 7-34)**.

The myocardium, the thickest of the layers, consists of cardiac muscle cells arranged in layers that surround the heart chambers in a complex spiral. The myocardium is much thicker in the ventricles than in the atria. Due to its function as the systemic ventricle, the left ventricle is normally thicker than the right. Cardiac myocytes are connected by a unique intercellular junction called the intercalated disc, which allows mechanical and electrical coupling of individual myocytes.

The heart is covered externally by mesothelium supported by a thin layer of connective tissue that constitutes the epicardium. The epicardium corresponds to the visceral layer of the pericardium, the serous membrane which surrounds the heart. The pericardial cavity between the epicardium and pericardium contains a small amount of lubricant fluid that facilitates the heart's movements.

The oxygen-depleted blood from the systemic circulation enters the heart through the right atrium to the right ventricle, and then is pumped into the lungs via the pulmonary arteries. Within the lungs, the blood is oxygenated and returns to the left atrium through the pulmonary veins.

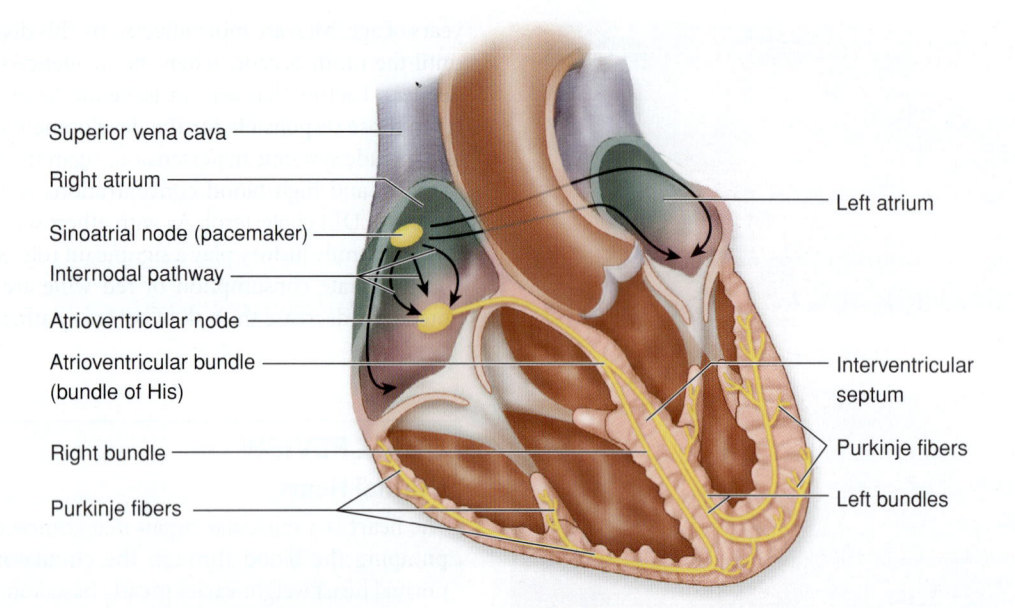

FIGURE 7-34 Major histologic features of the heart. Longitudinal view of the human heart showing the atria and ventricles. The ventricular walls are thicker than those of the atria, principally because of the much thicker myocardium. The **valves** are basically flaps of connective tissue anchored in the heart's dense **fibrous skeleton** region, shown in white. Other parts of the fibrous skeleton are the chordae tendineae. These chords of dense connective tissue attach to the free edge of the atrioventricular valve leaflets and to papillary muscles to help prevent valves from turning inside-out during ventricular contraction. Shown in yellow are parts of the cardiac **conduction system**, which initiates the electrical impulse for the heart's contraction (heartbeat) and spreads throughout the ventricular myocardium. Both the sinoatrial (SA) node (pacemaker), in the posterior wall of the right atrium, and the atrioventricular (AV) node, in the floor of the right atrium, consist of modified myocardial tissue that is difficult to distinguish grossly from surrounding cardiac muscle. The AV node is continuous with specialized bundles of cardiac muscle fibers, the **AV bundle** (of His) which run along the interventricular septum where they branch further as **conducting (Purkinje) fibers** extending into the myocardium of both ventricles. From Mescher AL. *Junqueira's Basic Histology Text & Atlas*. 12th ed. New York, NY: McGraw-Hill Lange; 2010. Figure 11-3, page 187.

The oxygenated blood then reaches the left ventricle and is pumped through the aorta to the rest of the body. This unidirectional blood flow is maintained by two **atrioventricular** valves (the right-sided tricuspid valve and the left-sided mitral valve) and **semilunar valves** (the right-sided pulmonary and the left-sided aortic valves). The leaflets (in the tricuspid and mitral valves) or cusps (in the aortic and pulmonary valves) are composed of three layers. The atrial surface is lined by a single endothelial cell layer. The middle layer (the spongiosa) is composed of elastic fibers and collections of glycosaminoglycans that provide the valves with flexibility. The ventricular layer is composed of dense fibrous tissue and elastic fibers that provide structure to the valve. The valves are attached to strong fibrous rings that are part of the central fibrous skeleton. This dense, fibrous region anchors the base of the valves and is the site of origin and insertion of the cardiac muscle fibers **(Figure 7-35)**.

Different from the semilunar valves, the mitral and tricuspid valves are connected to papillary muscles through cord-like tendons called chordae tendineae. As ventricular pressures rise during systole, the leaflets of the atrioventricular valves are brought together. The papillary muscles with their chordal attachments prevent prolapse of the leaflets.

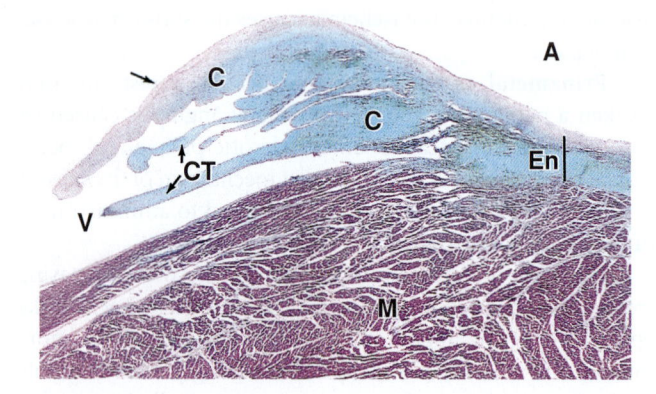

FIGURE 7-35 Valve leaflet and fibrous skeleton. The fibrous skeleton of the heart consists of masses of dense connective tissue in the endocardium which anchor the valves and surround the two atrioventricular canals, maintaining their proper shape. Section through a leaflet of the left atrioventricular valve (arrows) shows that valves are largely connective tissue (C) covered with a thin layer of endothelium. The collagen-rich connective tissue of the valves is stained pale green here and is continuous with the fibrous ring of connective tissue at the base of the valve, which fills the endocardium (En) of this area between the atrium (A) and ventricle (V). The **chordae tendineae** (CT), strands of connective tissue which bind the free edge of valve leaflets, can also be seen here. The interwoven nature of the cardiac muscle fibers, with many small fascicles, in the myocardium (M) is also shown (×20; Masson trichrome). From Mescher AL. *Junqueira's Basic Histology Text & Atlas*. 12th ed. New York, NY: McGraw-Hill Lange; 2010. Figure 11-6, page 189.

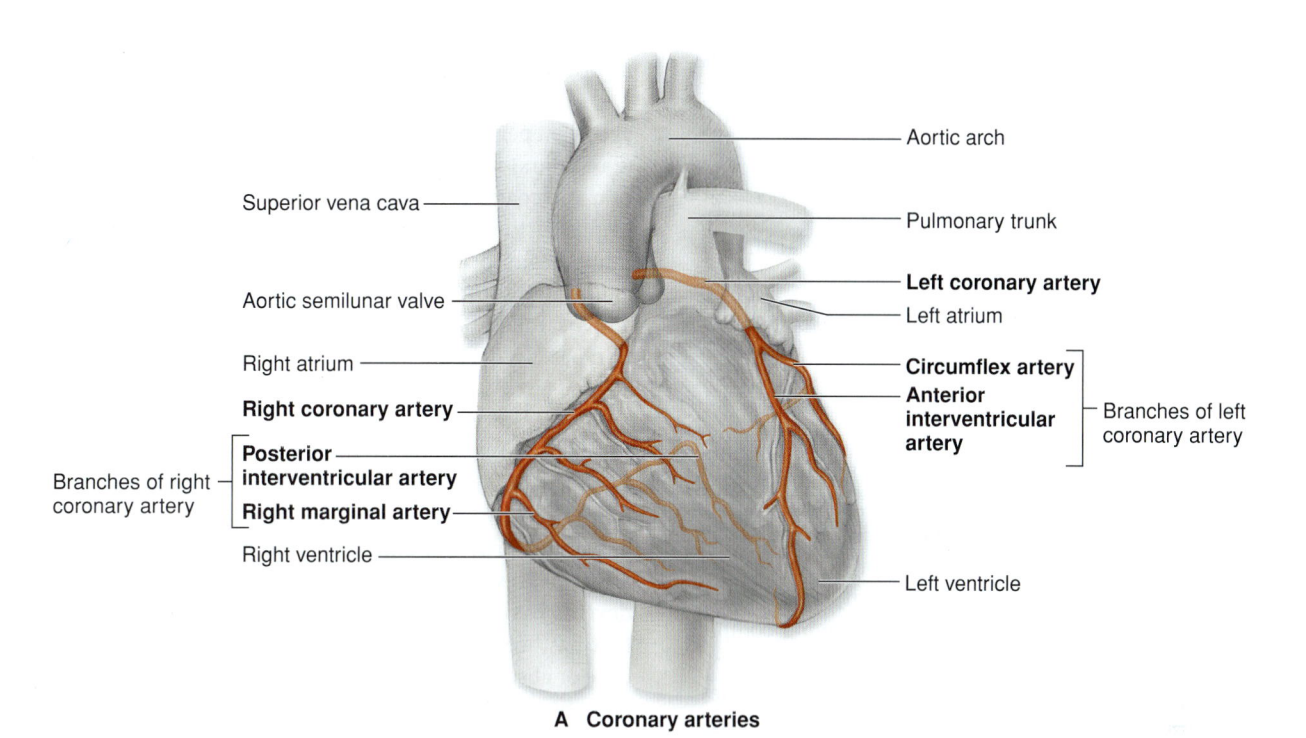

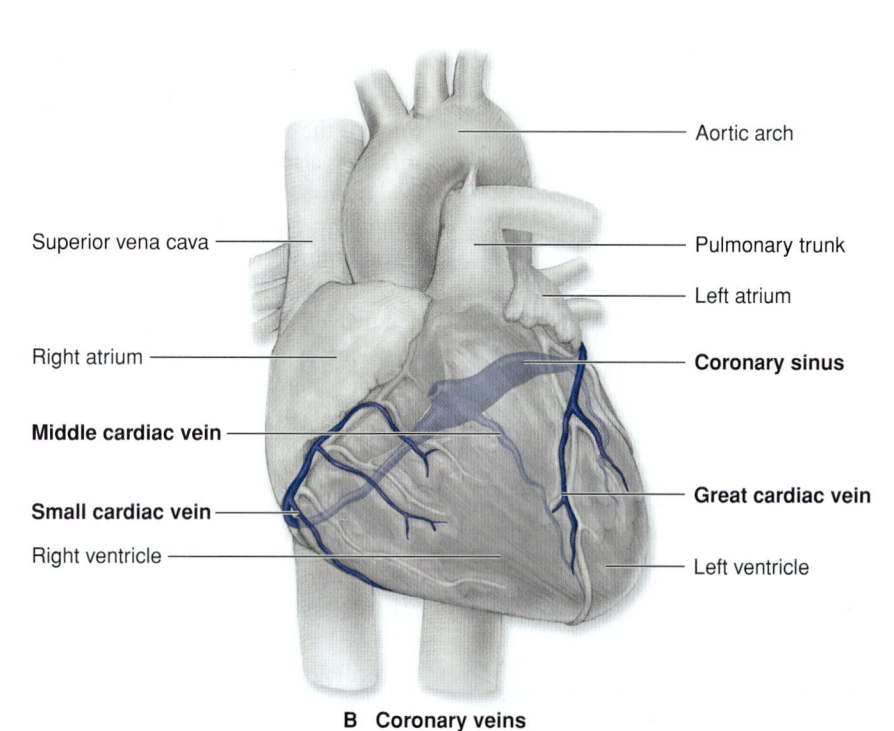

FIGURE 7-36 Coronary circulation. Anterior view of (**A**) coronary arteries and (**B**) coronary veins. From McKinley M, O'Loughlin VD. *Human anatomy.* 2nd ed. New York, NY: McGraw-Hill; 2008. Figure 22-9, page 665.

The heart has a specialized electrical system that generates a rhythmic stimulus for contraction. This system consists of two nodes where the electrical impulse is generated. The first is the sinoatrial node (SA node) located at the junction of the right atrium and the superior vena cava. It is composed of a small mass of modified cardiac fibers that are fusiform, smaller and with fewer myofibrils than neighboring myocytes. It generates electrical impulses of about 60 to 100 beats/minute under resting conditions. Impulses generated from the SA node are transmitted to the second or atrioventricular node (AV node). The AV node is located in the triangle formed by the septal annulus of the tricuspid valve, the mouth of the coronary sinus and the tendon of Todaro and has cells similar to those of the SA node. Specialized fibers from the AV node form the bundle of His, then passes along the top of the interventricular septum and splits into left and right bundles, and then branches further to both ventricles. The cells/fibers of the electrical conduction system are modified cardiac muscle cells functionally integrated by gap junctions (Figure 7-34).

Distally, fibers of the AV bundle appear larger than ordinary cardiac muscle fibers and acquire a distinctive appearance. These conducting myofibers or Purkinje fibers have one or two central nuclei, and their cytoplasm is rich in mitochondria and glycogen. Myofibrils are sparse and restricted to the periphery of the cytoplasm. After forming the subendocardial conducting network, these fibers penetrate the myocardial layer of both ventricles, an important arrangement that allows the stimulus for contraction to reach the innermost layers of the ventricular musculature.

Both parasympathetic and sympathetic neural components innervate the heart. Ganglionic nerve cells and nerve fibers are present in the regions close to the SA and AV nodes, where they affect heart rate and rhythm, such as during physical exercise and emotional stress. Stimulation of the parasympathetic division (vagus nerve) slows the heartbeat, whereas stimulation of the sympathetic nerve accelerates the rhythm of the pacemaker. Afferent nerve fibers between muscle fibers of the myocardium are related to sensibility and pain.

Finally, the heart depends on the coronary arteries for a constant supply of nutrients and oxygen. The two main coronary arteries, the left main and right coronary arteries, arise within the sinuses posterior to the right and left aortic valve cusps. The distribution of coronary arteries can be quite individual. In the most common variant, the right-dominant system, the **right coronary** artery branches into the **right marginal** and **posterior descending** arteries that supply the right and posterior side of both ventricles and the posterior 1/3 of the ventricular septum. The **left main coronary artery** gives rise to **the left anterior descending** and **circumflex** arteries. The anterior descending coronary artery supplies the anterior wall of the left ventricle and the anterior 2/3 of the ventricular septum. The circumflex coronary artery supplies the lateral wall of the left ventricle. (Figure 7-36).

The coronary arteries running across the surface of the heart in the **epicardium**. As they branch, they penetrate into the myocardium, becoming **intramural** arteries. This pattern of blood supply makes the endocardium more susceptible for ischemic injuries due to its distance from the origin of the supply. The coronary arteries fill during ventricular diastole.

MYOCARDIAL INFARCTIONS

MI (heart attack) is the most important form of ischemic heart disease. Of the 1.5 million people in the United States who suffer from an acute MI annually, up to 33% will die; 250,000 die before they reach the hospital each year. The risk of an acute myocardial infarct increases progressively with age.

The classic myocardial infarct is caused by hypoxic damage when perfusion is decreased for an extended period of time (2–4 hours) resulting in a permanent loss of myocardial function and coagulative necrosis of myocardial cells. The ischemia begins furthest from the blood supply or at the myocardium immediately below the endocardium (the subendocardium) and moves through the entire wall thickness. The **location** of a myocardial infarct is usually in a specific anatomic distribution pattern dependent on the anatomy of epicardial coronary arterial circulation. The overall **outcome** of the infarct depends upon the rate and duration of the occlusion and the size of the vascular bed supplied by the artery. An acute occlusion due to an abrupt interruption of blood flow to the myocardium is more likely to result in a severe, larger infarct. If a significant, but nonobstructive, atherosclerotic narrowing of a coronary artery is present for a long period of time, the heart is able to develop a collateral vascular system to supply the myocardium that has been chronically undersupplied. Therefore, the presence or absence of collateral vessels can also factor into the size and severity of the acute infarct. The frequency of occlusion of specific coronary arteries and the distribution of their associated infarcts are shown Table 7-3, Page 189.

Most commonly, infarcts are classified as **subendocardial** or **transmural**. In a subendocardial infarct, the inner one-third of the ventricular wall is involved. The **subendocardial infarct** is also known as a non-ST elevation myocardial infarction (non-STEMI) and as a non-Q wave infarct by electrocardiography. Subendocardial infarcts may be caused by partial thrombotic occlusion of a coronary artery; however, it is more likely that these infarcts are due to transient decreases in oxygen delivery in the setting of severe, fixed ASCAD. Causes of transient hypoxia include decreased oxygen delivery (hypotension, anemia, sepsis) or increased demand (hypertension, tachycardia).

Transmural infarcts involve the entire thickness of the wall, usually in a single-coronary artery distribution. As discussed earlier, the transmural infarct is most commonly caused by acute thrombotic occlusion of a coronary artery associated with atherosclerotic plaque alteration. Clinically, transmural infarcts are known as ST-elevation myocardial infarcts (STEMI) as they cause elevation of the ST segment on electrocardiogram. Transmural infarcts that involve the posterior/inferior left ventricle extend to involve the right ventricle in approximately 15% to 20% of cases. Isolated right ventricular infarcts are exceedingly rare (<1%–3% of cases).

Morphology

The gross and microscopic appearance of myocardial infarcts depends on the length of time the patient survives after the insult. A well-defined progressive sequence of events including necrosis, inflammatory reaction, healing, and repair allows pathologists to accurately age myocardial infarcts for the first several weeks.

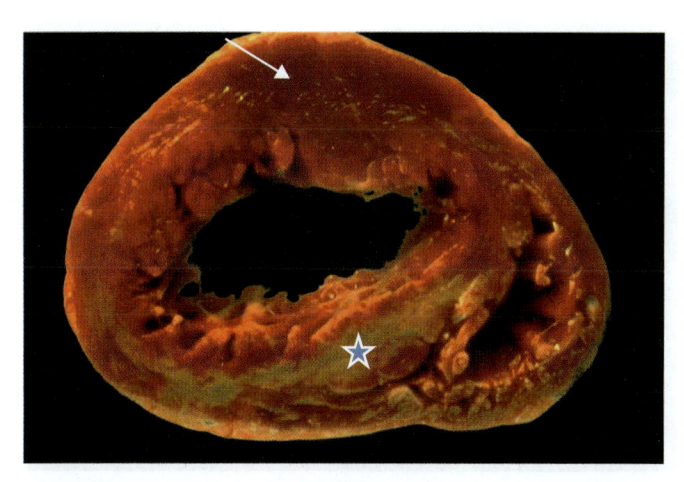

FIGURE 7-37 **Transverse sections of heart postmyocardial infarctions of about 10-hour duration.** Unstained section shows some darkening in the area of infarct (arrow). An area of scar resulting from a prior infarct is also present (star). From Department of Pathology and Laboratory Medicine, University of North Carolina at Chapel Hill.

Gross identification of a very acute myocardial infarct is difficult, as no specific gross features are seen for the first 12 hours after the hypoxic insult. Special "vital" stains may be used to demonstrate these acute infarcts that are not grossly demonstrable. The "vital" stains most commonly used include nitroblue tetrazolium chloride (NBT) and triphenyltetrazolium chloride (TTC). The stains are converted to blue (NBT) and red (TTC) by the enzymes in the viable myocardium. The non-viable myocytes undergo necrosis and loss of the intracellular enzymes. As the necrotic myocardium is unable to convert the stains to the typical color, the necrotic myocardium does NOT stain; the viable myocardium stains (therefore a "vital" stain) **(Figure 7-37)**.

At approximately 12 to 24 hours, the myocardium may grossly appear pale. At 24 hours, the infarct appears pale with a circumferential red rim caused by vascular congestion. The infarct develops a central green color with a peripheral red rim at 2 to 3 days. From 10 to 14 days, the infarct has a depressed, ground-glass appearance at the periphery caused by infiltration of granulation tissue. The infarct is progressively infiltrated by fibrosis until it is a dense, fibrous scar at approximately ≥6 weeks **(Figure 7-38)**.

Like the gross appearance, the microscopic appearance of myocardial infarcts follow a typical healing pattern that can aid in aging the injury. From 6 to 12 hours, ischemic myocytes show changes of coagulative necrosis with contraction bands and cytoplasmic clumping. Acute inflammation (neutrophils) is the first response to the acute myocardial injury.

- Neutrophils first begin to infiltrate interstitial areas (between the myocytes) at approximately 24 hours.
- The number of neutrophils increases dramatically and reaches its peak at approximately 3 days (72 hours). The neutrophils begin to destroy the necrotic myocytes leading to production of cytokines and chemotactic substances that call macrophages to the scene.
- Macrophages engulf and remove the necrotic tissue from days 5 through 7.
- Fibroblasts, chronic inflammation, and granulation tissue begin to enter the area from day 7 through day 10.
- Fibroblasts continue to produce a collagenous scar from approximately 2 to 4 weeks.
- The well-formed scar is complete by 4 to 6 weeks after the injury. Once the scar is formed, it is impossible to age, other than to say it is healed.

Another histologic feature that can be seen in chronically ischemic myocardium is vacuolated myocytes within the subendocardium (myocytolysis). These cells, having been chronically oxygen-deprived, have undergone alterations similar to hibernation. Histologically, the cells appear vacuolated. If adequate perfusion is supplied, these cells will regain normal function (see Chapter 2, Figure 2-4).

Early Complications of Myocardial Infarction

The technologic advances in health-care have led to decreasing patient deaths after an acute myocardial infarction (AMI). In-hospital deaths due to complications from AMI have been reduced from 30% to 7%–10%. While the in-hospital death rate has been significantly reduced, out-of-hospital deaths still claim **up to 50%** *of patients within 1 hour of onset of their symptoms. These patients usually succumb to fatal ventricular arrhythmias prior to receiving any medical attention.*

The risk of complications and overall prognosis of patients who survive the initial period after their acute MI is dependent on infarct size and location and the amount of myocardium involved. Nearly 75% of patients who do survive the initial period will suffer from one or more complications including pump dysfunction, cardiac dysrhythmias, myocardial rupture, pericarditis, or mural thrombus.

Pump Dysfunction

The left ventricle is responsible for generating adequate cardiac output to supply the body. Its pump function is directly affected by the amount of myocardium damaged by an AMI. Most patients will experience some loss of ventricular function as diagnosed by decreased ejection fraction. In approximately 10% to 15% patients, pump failure or **cardiogenic shock** will occur. These are patients who have experienced loss of ≥40% of the left ventricle associated with AMI. Cardiogenic shock has an associated 70% mortality rate. These patients may need insertion of a left ventricular assist device to maintain adequate cardiac function and may require a cardiac transplant.

Cardiac Dysrhythmias

Due to the significant intracellular changes created by ischemia associated with AMI, infarcted myocardium becomes "irritable" leading to an increased risk of abnormal electrical conduction and dysrhythmia. Ninety percent of patients will

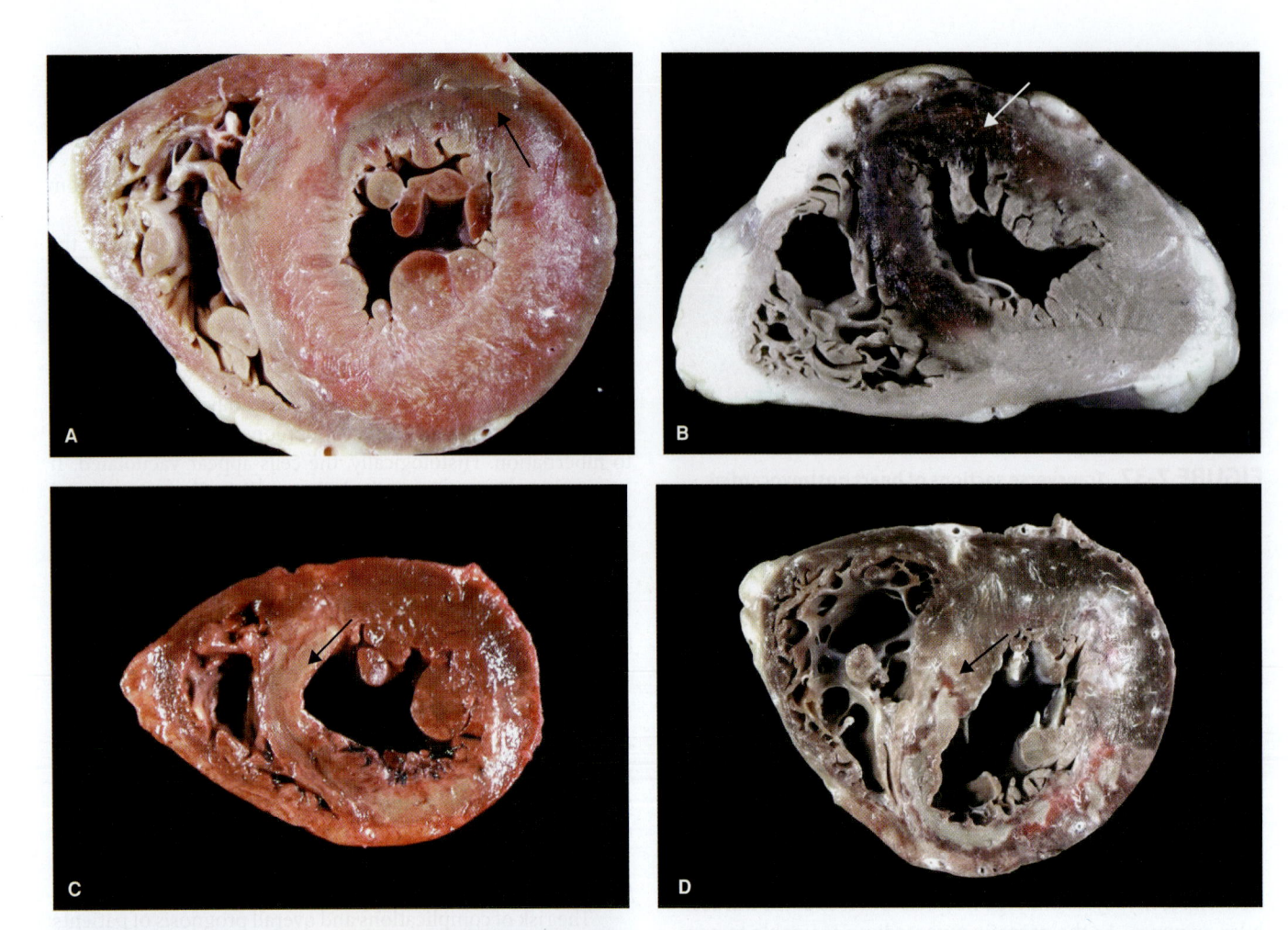

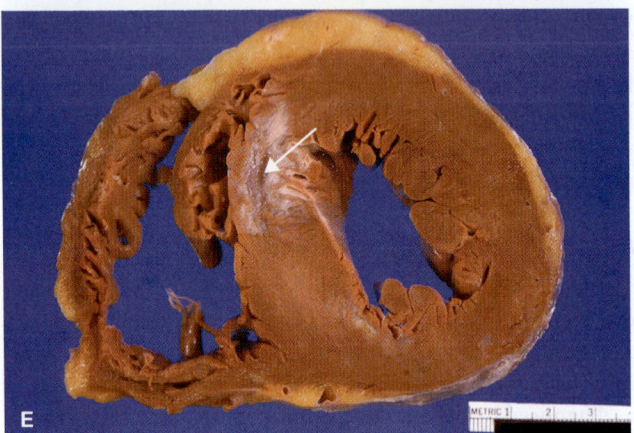

FIGURE 7-38 Sections of heart postmyocardial infarction. **(A)** Acute myocardial infarct resulting 24-hour duration. Note the pale area surrounded by zones of hyperemia (arrow). From Howard Reisner, Ph.D. Department of Pathology and Laboratory Medicine University of North Carolina at Chapel Hill. **(B)** Acute myocardial infarct resulting from thrombosis of the LAD. Forty-eight-hour duration with some degree of reperfusion. The area of infarction (arrow) shows a pale center surrounded by a dark area of vascular congestion and hemorrhage. (For details related to reperfusion injury, see Chapter 2.) **(C)** Acute myocardial infarct resulting from thrombosis of the LAD. Four-day duration. The areas of infarction (arrow) show a greenish central color. **(D)** Acute myocardial infarct resulting from thrombosis of the LAD. Fourteen-day duration. The areas of infarction (arrow) show a glassy appearance and are depressed. From Department of Pathology and Laboratory Medicine University of North Carolina at Chapel Hill. **(E)** Chronic myocardial infarction of greater than 2-month duration. The areas of infarction (arrow) appear as dense fibrous scar. From Peter Anderson, D.V.M., Ph.D., PEIR Digital Library Digital Library Image 16907.

experience some form of abnormal rhythm after an AMI. The patients with a transmural (or STEMI) infarct are at greater risk than those involving the subendocardium (non-STEMI). The highest risk for the most severe ventricular dysrhythmia (ventricular tachycardia/fibrillation) is in the first hour after symptom onset. The risk of a serious dysrhythmia decreases after that first hour. The infarct location can also affect the likelihood of conduction complications. The types of dysrhythmia vary greatly (bradyarrhythmias, tachyarrhythmias) and can include complete heart block if the AMI has involved the conduction system. Significant heart block is more likely in patients with posterior/inferior infarcts.

Myocardial Rupture

Rupture of the myocardium is due to mechanical weakness of the necrotic tissues and most commonly occurs after the dead muscle has been removed from the infarcted area and little collagen has been deposited. Histologically, we know that

CASE 7-7

A 75-year-old woman with a prior history of systemic hypertension is hospitalized with her first acute MI of the anterior left ventricle. She is treated medically and doing well. While walking down the hall with her family, she suddenly collapsed and cannot be resuscitated (Figure 7-39).

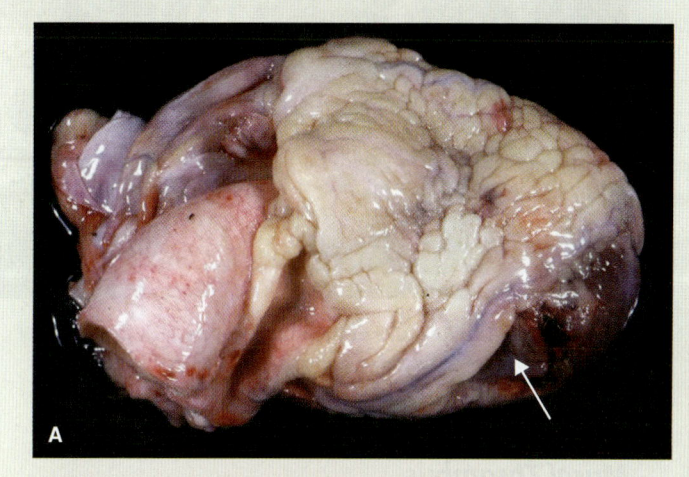

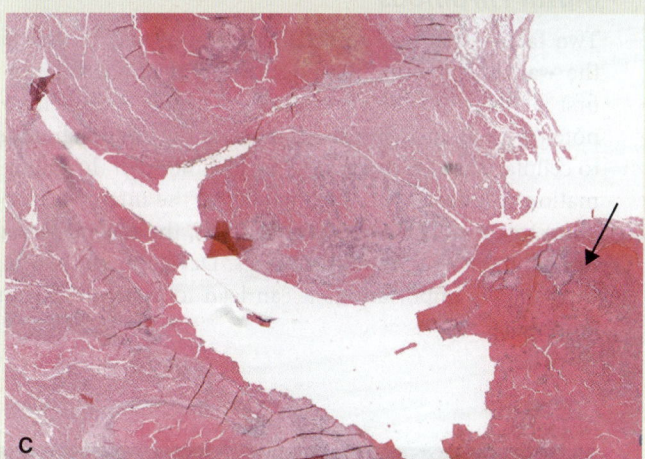

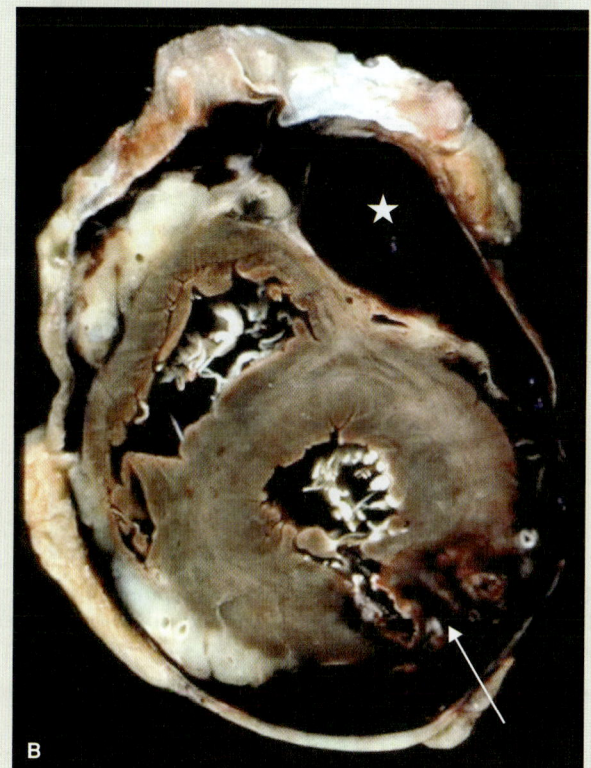

FIGURE 7-39 Myocardial rupture. **(A)** Gross view of the ventricular rupture (arrow). From , Department of Pathology and Laboratory Medicine, University of North Carolina at Chapel Hill. **(B)** Transected heart showing ventricular rupture. Arrow indicates the site of rupture and star the hemopericardium. From Group for Research in Pathology (GRIPE) Image 1771 **(C)** Microscopic view of the site of rupture (arrow). From Department of Pathology and Laboratory Medicine, University of North Carolina at Chapel Hill.

these changes occur at approximately 5 to 7 days postinjury, the time when the largest number of ruptures occurs. However, approximately 25% of ruptures can occur as early as 24 hours postinjury. A third peak of ruptures occurs at approximately 10 days (~10%). Three significant sites of rupture routinely occur and include the free wall of the left ventricle, the ventricular septum, and the papillary muscle.

Rupture of the **left ventricular free wall** can lead to blood rapidly filling the pericardial sac (**hemopericardium**) resulting in **cardiac tamponade** and rapid death. The blood from the heart escapes the left ventricle at systemic pressures leading to rapid filling of the pericardial sac. The pressures from the surrounding blood prevent the heart from relaxing to fill with venous blood. The blood in the pericardium also compresses the veins entering the heart, also decreasing filling. Therefore, the heart is basically empty and compressed leading to absence of blood supplied to the body (especially the brain) and sudden collapse. If circulation is not restored, this can lead to death. Identified risk factors for free-wall rupture include a first myocardial infarct, older age (>60 years of age), female gender, and a medical history of systemic hypertension. Infarcts of the anterior left ventricle are more likely to rupture. The patient described in the case above suffered from rupture of her anterior left ventricle and cardiac tamponade (Figure 7-39B).

Rupture of the **ventricular septum** leads to a ventricular septal defect (VSD) and a left-to-right shunt (blood is shunted

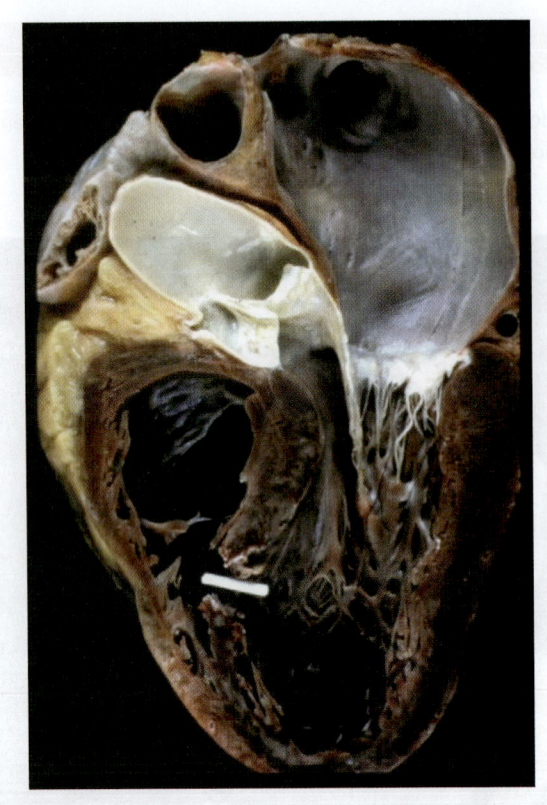

FIGURE 7-40 Rupture of the ventricular septum. Line indicates the point of rupture. From Group for Research in Pathology (GRIPE) Image 1766.

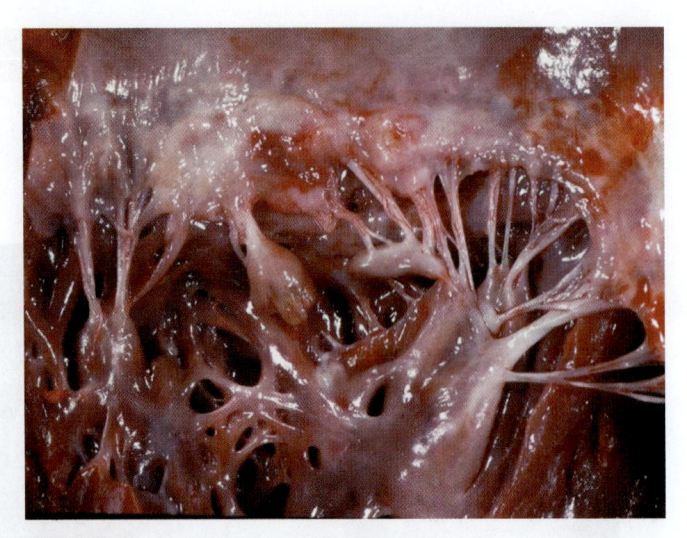

FIGURE 7-41 Rupture of papillary muscle. From Department of Pathology and Laboratory Medicine, University of North Carolina at Chapel Hill.

from high pressure to low pressure). The sudden occurrence of increased blood in the right heart can cause acute right heart failure. Clinically, these patients will have a systolic murmur not heard on previous physical examinations (Figure 7-40).

Rupture of a **papillary muscle** can lead to acute mitral valve insufficiency and acute heart failure. As the papillary muscle no longer serves as an anchor for the valve, increased amounts of blood are sent backward into the left atrium causing back pressure into the lungs. These patients will have sudden onset of shortness of breath and murmurs (both systolic and diastolic) on physical examination (Figure 7-41).

Pericarditis

Transmural myocardial infarcts can elicit an epicardial and pericardial reaction due to the associated inflammatory process resulting in a fibrinous pericarditis. The fibrin and acute inflammatory cells are layered over the epicardium and along the visceral surface of the pericardium. Typically, the pericarditis occurs 2 to 3 days after the infarct causing chest pain that is relieved by alteration in position (sitting forward). Physical examination may reveal a friction rub. Pericarditis usually resolves in several days. A more severe pericardial reaction can lead to a pericardial effusion (fluid collection in the pericardium) or dense adhesions between the heart and the epicardium.

Mural Thrombus

Two factors can lead to the formation of a thrombus along the wall of the left ventricle in the area of the infarct. The first factor is the damage to the ventricular endothelium. As noted with atherosclerosis, damage to the endothelium leads to cellular changes increasing the likelihood of thrombus formation (Figure 7-42). The inability of the infarcted myocardium to contract causes areas of stasis, the second factor for development of a mural thrombus. Development of a mural thrombus is important as it can lead to systemic **thromboembolism**.

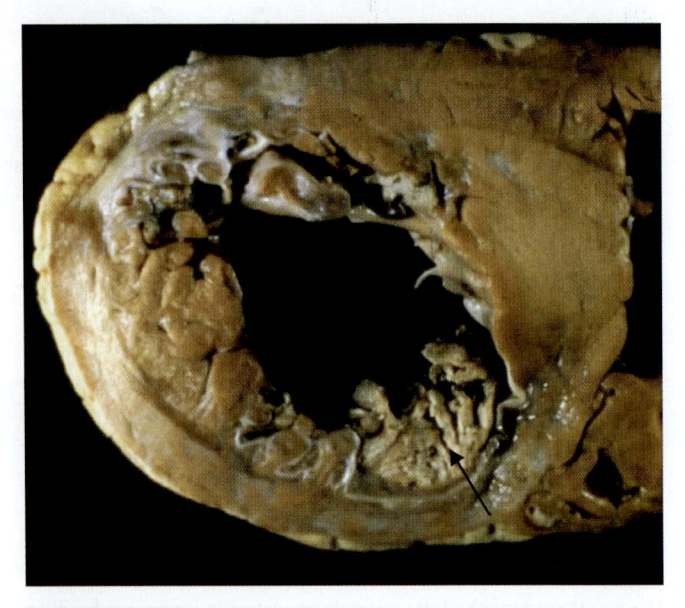

FIGURE 7-42 Mural thrombus. Thrombus is located over a healed infarct (arrow). From Group for Resaerch in Pathology (GRIPE) Image 1762.

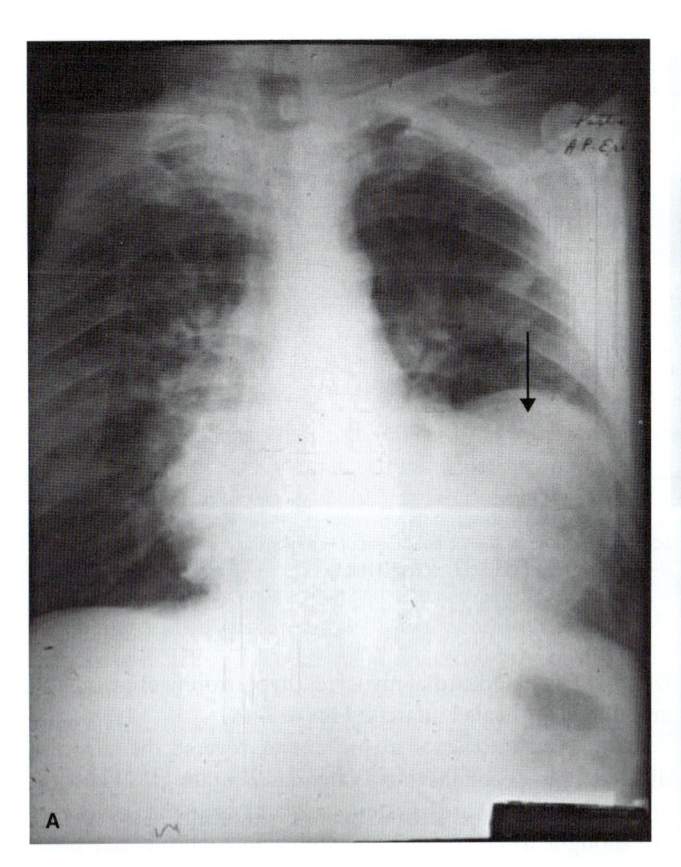

FIGURE 7-43 Ventricular aneurysm. **(A)** Radiograph with large ventricular aneurysm (arrow). **(B)** Gross view of ventricular aneurysm with adherent plicated thrombus (arrow). From Department of Pathology and Laboratory Medicine, University of North Carolina at Chapel Hill.

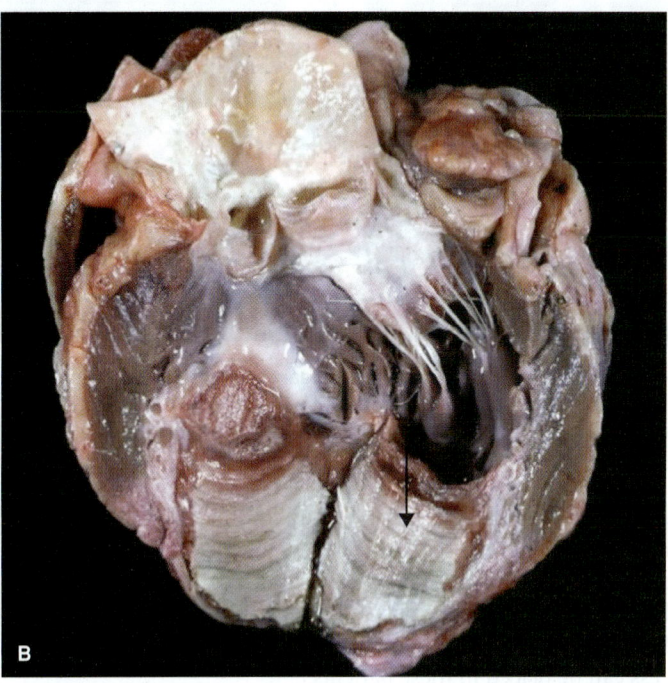

Late Complications of Myocardial Infarct

Ventricular aneurysm is a not uncommon late complication of an anterior or anteroseptal myocardial infarct. These aneurysms are formed from a large, anterior-anteroseptal, transmural infarct that heals with a thinned, dilated wall of scar tissue. Unlike aneurysms of blood vessels, left ventricular aneurysms do not rupture as their wall is composed of dense scar tissue. The dilated aneurysm can lead to significant complications, however, including the formation of mural thrombi and dysrhythmias (Figure 7-43). Anterior wall aneurysms can also lead to congestive heart failure. During systole, the blood in the left ventricle will preferentially enter the ventricular aneurysm rather than being ejected through the aortic valve due to the low resistance of the aneurysm. Blood collecting in the aneurysm will lead to an increase in the blood remaining in the left ventricle at the end of systole (increased end systolic volume). Over time, the increased volume with back up into the left atrium and the pulmonary veins leading to increased pulmonary venous hypertension and eventual heart failure.

The long-term prognosis of patients after an MI depends on the quality of the left ventricular function and the severity of their underlying atherosclerotic coronary disease and the ability to perfuse the remaining viable myocardium. The overall mortality is 30% in the first year after an MI, including those deaths that occur prior to medical treatment. There is a 3% to 4% mortality rate per year after the first year.

After myocardial infarction, the remaining ventricular myocardium attempts to compensate for the loss of viable contractile muscle. During **ventricular remodeling**, the viable myocardium hypertrophies and dilates while the infarcted area scars and thins. Initially, the hypertrophy may be able to compensate for the lost function. With time, however, this adaptation is exhausted leading to ineffective left ventricular function.

Treatment of Acute Myocardial Infarct

The type of clinical treatment of AMI is dependent on the timing of the patient's symptoms, their clinical history, and left ventricular function. Early treatment can include lysis of the coronary artery thrombosis, most commonly using tissue-type plasminogen activator (t-PA) which activates the fibrinolytic system. Other treatments include primary percutaneous coronary intervention (PPCI) or coronary artery bypass surgery.

PPCI involves intravascular introduction of a balloon catheter into the coronary artery lumen and mechanical disruption of the thrombus and atherosclerotic plaque with expansion of the balloon. Depending on the situation, a metallic stent may or may not be placed into the coronary artery lumen as structural support to maintain patency. Long-term

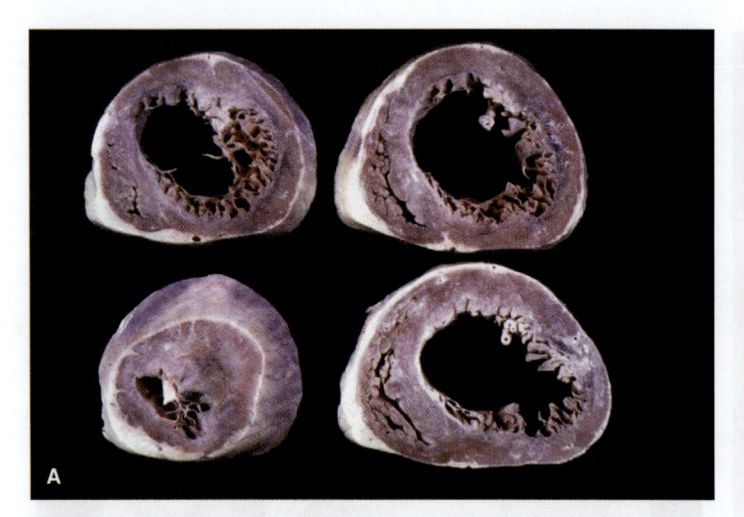

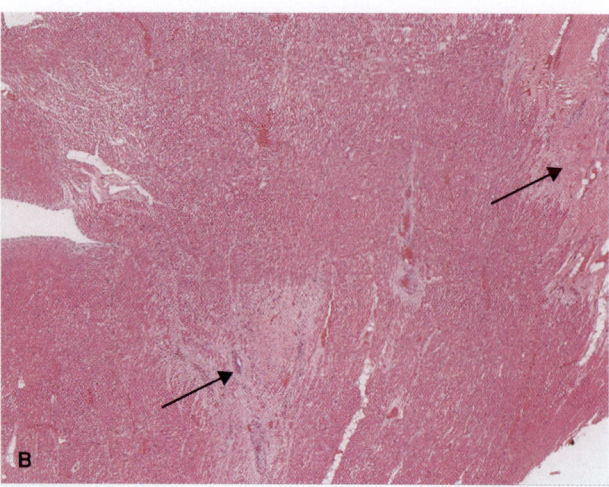

FIGURE 7-44 Chronic ischemic heart disease. **(A)** Multiple sections of the transected ventricle showing extensive scarring in the wall. **(B)** Microscopic view demonstrating multiple areas of scarring (arrows). From Department of Pathology and Laboratory Medicine, University of North Carolina at Chapel Hill.

effects of this treatment depend on the patients and their body's healing processes. Some patient have a rapid and proliferative endothelial healing reaction after angioplasty that can lead to coronary artery obstruction by intimal proliferation. Drug-eluting stents preventing this proliferative healing process can be placed in these patients.

Patients with severe, multivessel atherosclerotic disease may undergo coronary artery bypass grafting (CABG), a more invasive treatment procedure. The surgeon will determine the best possible vessels used to bypass the area of coronary artery obstruction. The left internal mammary artery (LIMA), radial artery, and saphenous veins are the most common vessels used in these surgeries. Saphenous vein grafts most commonly remain patent for approximately 10 years. LIMA grafts, usually grafted to the anterior descending coronary artery, can remain patent for more than 15 to 20 years.

CHRONIC ISCHEMIC HEART DISEASE

Chronic ischemic heart disease (clinically often called *"ischemic cardiomyopathy"*) describes progressive left ventricular failure due to ongoing ischemic myocardial damage or exhaustion of the compensatory mechanisms of the remaining myocardium. Most patients with chronic ischemic heart failure have a history of a prior infarct. Many of these patients continue to experience myocardial ischemia with or without frank infarction. Clinically, these patients have progressive heart failure with increasing shortness of breath, orthopnea, and paroxysmal dyspnea. Mortality is usually due to dysrhythmia.

The wall of the left ventricle of these patients is thickened (hypertrophic) with an enlarged, dilated ventricular chamber. There is often endocardial thickening, and mural thrombi may be present overlying areas of infarct or aneurysm. Dense, gray fibrous scar is in the areas of prior infarcts. Histology of chronic ischemic heart disease shows endocardial thickening, vacuolization of subendocardial myocytes, hypertrophy of myocytes, and fibrosis of healed infarcts (Figure 7-44).

Research into ways to prevent or reverse the myocardial changes secondary to ischemia includes the isolation and infusion of cardiac stem cells. In humans, myocytes are thought to be without the ability to replicate, but bone marrow-derived, pluripotent cells may be able to repopulate mammalian hearts. Present in extremely small numbers, the results of infusion or direct injection of these cells has been disappointing. The cells show myocyte differentiation, but they did not significantly contribute to restoration of function in infarcted areas. In addition, these cells can lead to isolated areas of dysrhythmias.

Other areas of research include identification of micro-RNAs that are associated with myocardial injury and congestive heart failure. Inhibition of specific micro-RNA families can lead to salvage of ischemic myocardium.

SUDDEN CARDIAC DEATH (SCD)

Sudden death is defined as an unexpected death that occurs within 1 to 24 hours of onset of symptoms. Sudden death can be caused by multiple mechanisms including large, saddle pulmonary thromboemboli, subarachnoid hemorrhage due to a ruptured berry aneurysm, and obstruction of the brain's third ventricle by a colloid cyst. While these processes can cause an unexpected death, the majority of sudden deaths are due to cardiac causes. The incidence of SCD varies greatly depending on the group studied; however, it occurs in approximately 0.1% to 0.2% of the general population (or approximately 250,000 to 400,000 deaths) in the United States each year. As was discussed in the previous section, some form of atherosclerotic coronary disease is responsible for approximately 80% to 90% of SCD in those over 35 years of age. In nearly 25% to 30% of patients, SCD can be the first symptom of ischemic heart disease.

In young (<35 years of age) patients, a variety of non-atherosclerotic cardiac abnormalities are responsible for SCD including:

- **Congenital heart disease (CHD)** including coronary artery abnormalities.
- Various forms of **myocardial inflammation or infiltrative process** (myocarditis, sarcoidosis, amyloidosis).
- **Mitral valve prolapse** with its associated intramyocardial dysplasia.
- **Inherited conduction system defects or channelopathies** (long QT syndrome, short QT syndrome, Brugada syndrome) and acquired conduction abnormalities.
- **Cardiomyopathic processes** (hypertrophic cardiomyopathy [HCM], dilated cardiomyopathy [DCM]) including hypertensive heart disease. Left ventricular hypertrophy (LVH) itself, regardless of cause, is an independent risk factor for SCD.

Sudden death in athletes, while seemingly more common due to the wide spread media coverage, is actually a relatively uncommon occurrence. Multiple studies have shown 0.4 to 2.3 deaths per 100,000 athletes per year confirming that sudden death of a young athlete is relatively rare. Most commonly, sudden death occurs during the exertion of exercise or shortly after completion. Cardiac abnormalities are frequently unknown in these athletes prior to their death.

The terminal mechanism in SCD of all types is believed to be a severe, lethal dysrhythmia of ventricular tachycardia, ventricular fibrillation or asystole.

CONGENITAL HEART DISEASE (CHD)

CHDs are abnormalities of the heart and/or great arteries that are present from birth. Most of these abnormalities occur during the formation of the major cardiovascular structures during the 3rd through 8th weeks of gestation. Heart defects occur in approximately 6 to 8 per 1000 liveborn infants, making it the most common birth defect. The incidence of CHD is higher in premature births and stillborns. Approximately 35,000 to 40,000 neonates are born with CHD each year in the United States.

The abnormalities can range from simple, single defects (**atrial septal defect [ASD]**) to more severe forms (**hypoplastic left heart syndrome**). The majority of the abnormalities arise from arrested development of a normal structure or malalignment of structures. Approximately 12 entities make up nearly 85% of congenital heart defects (see Table 7-4).

Although the cause of >90% of CHD is unknown, the remaining 10% have well-defined environmental or genetic influences. Environmental factors that have been well documented include viral infections (including rubella), maternal diseases (diabetes mellitus), and various teratogens (lead exposure, alcohol, drugs). As there is an increased risk of CHD in the offspring or siblings of a patient with CHD, a genetic component to the development of CHD is hypothesized. In addition, multiple chromosomal abnormalities have associated CHD including DiGeorge syndrome; trisomies 13, 15, 18, and 21, and Turner syndrome, further suggesting a genetic influence in CHD.

The embryonic development of the heart is complex. Multiple genes are responsible for a complex series of events that are tightly regulated to create a normal heart. Mutations in genes encoding necessary basic cardiac transcription factors have emerged as major contributors to many forms of CHD. As researchers study the transcriptional factors that control normal heart development, the number of associated factors has grown. Three transcription factors and their genetic and protein associations play a major role in cardiac development: Nkx2-5, GATA4, and Tbx5.

Cardiac septation defects (ASDs, VSDs, and atrioventricular septal defects) make up approximately 50% of all congenital heart defects and comprise the highest number of isolated defects not associated with other genetic syndromes. The genes associated

TABLE 7-3 The frequency of occlusion of specific coronary arteries and the distribution of their associated infarcts.

Anterior descending coronary artery	40%–50%	Anterior and apical left ventricle; anterior two-thirds of the ventricular septum
Right coronary artery	30%–40%	Right ventricle, posterior/inferior left ventricle, and posterior one-third of the ventricular septum (in a right "dominant" coronary circulation)
Circumflex coronary artery	15%–20%	Lateral left ventricle; may also involve the posterior left ventricle and posterior septum in a left "dominant" coronary circulation

TABLE 7-4 Frequency of congenital malformations of heart and great vessels.

Malformation	Congenital Heart Disease (%)
Ventricular septal defect	30–40
Patent ductus arteriosus	10
Atrial septal defect	10
Atrioventricular septal defect	4–7
Pulmonary stenosis	7–8
Coarctation of the aorta	5–7
Aortic stenosis	4–6
Tetralogy of fallot	4–9
Transposition of the great arteries	4–10
Truncus arteriosus	2
Tricuspid atresia	1

with the cardiac septal defects include Nkx2.5, GATA4, and Tbx5. Deletion of the homeobox gene Nkx2.5 in *Drosophila* can prevent heart formation completely. In humans, deletion of the Tinman (named for the heartless character in the Wizard of Oz) gene causes abnormal morphogenesis including atrial, ventricular, and atrioventricular septal defects, tetralogy of Fallot (TOF), and much more complex defects. Conotruncal and outflow tract defects including aortic arch abnormalities comprise approximately 20% to 30% of congenital heart defects. DiGeorge, velocardiofacial, and conotruncal-face syndromes are associated with the deletion of chromosome 22q11. Patients with TOF have a significantly higher incidence of 22q11.2 deletion (See below). Children with CHD are now living into adulthood due to the advancement in understanding of the disease processes and medical therapies.

Terminology and Concepts Associated with CHD

The study of CHD requires the understanding of multiple new terms and concepts. A **shunt** is an abnormal communication between heart chambers or vessels seen in patients with cardiac septation defects. The direction of flow through a shunt depends on basic hemodynamic factors including resistance through the defect and pressures on both sides of the defect. Clinically, shunts are described by their direction of flow. For example, with a left-to-right shunt the blood is flowing from left to right. Right-to-left shunts also occur and will be discussed.

Another important term used when discussing CHD is **cyanosis** (cyan = blue). Deoxygenated blood is darker in color and appears blue relative to the appearance of oxygenated (red) blood. Patients who are poorly oxygenated will appear cyanotic or have a blue appearance around their mouth and fingertips.

CHD can be classified into defects that cause or do not cause cyanosis. The **cyanotic group** of CHD includes the defects that cause a right-to-left shunt. In these patients, the pressures on the right side of the heart are higher than those on the left side causing the blood to flow from right to left. With this alteration in flow, deoxygenated blood from the right heart bypasses the lungs and is sent to the left side of the heart and into the systemic circulation. Depending on the size of the defect and the amount of deoxygenated blood flowing across the defect, the patients may appear blue.

Left-to-right shunts are *initially* **noncyanotic** as oxygenated blood leaves the left heart at systemic pressure and goes into the right heart and the lungs. This shunt significantly increases the blood flow volume and pressures into the lungs. *Recall that increasing blood volume does not provide any benefit to an organ resulting in the arterial vasoconstriction to prevent organ damage due to the increased blood volume and pressure.* Over time, the pulmonary arteries constrict causing increasing vascular resistance to flow or pulmonary hypertension. As the right heart works against increased resistance over time, the right heart becomes hypertrophic and the right heart pressures become the same or higher than the left heart causing reversal of the shunt (right to left). As the shunt reverses, the patients will become cyanotic. This phenomenon of shunt reversal over time is known as *Eisenmenger syndrome*.

Acyanotic CHD is caused by obstructive lesions without the presence of a shunt. Obstructive lesions in CHD are due to abnormally formed valvular structures that are narrowed (**stenotic**) or absence of an opening through a valve (**atresia**). These defects cause alterations in the associated chambers and arteries due to decreased flow.

Noncyanotic Congenital Heart Disease

Noncyanotic CHDs are the most common encountered cardiac malformation. These defects include the cardiac septation defects (ASDs, VSDs, atrioventricular septal defects) and patent ductus arteriosus.

Ventricular Septal Defect

Ventricular septal defects (VSDs) are the most common noncyanotic congenital heart lesion caused by abnormal septal formation during the 5th week of gestation. VSDs are commonly associated with trisomies 21, 13, and 18. The size and position of VSDs are variable ranging from small to large defects involving the entire ventricular septum. The size of the VSD is the primary variable that determines the extent of the patient's symptoms. A patient with a small VSD may not exhibit any symptoms, while a large defect can cause severe symptoms in a newborn.

The ventricular septum forms from the growth of a muscular ridge at the apex of the heart that grows toward the heart base. VSDs can occur anywhere along the septum and are classified according to their location: perimembranous, muscular, and outlet defects (Figure 7-45).

- The **membranous septum** is the most common (90%) location of a VSD. As the defect also involves tissue around the membranous septum, these defects are also known as **perimembranous** VSDs.
- Defects of the muscular septum (**muscular** VSDs) comprise 5% to 20% of VSDs and more commonly occur at the apex of the septum. These muscular defects are often multiple.
- **Outlet VSDs** (5%–7% of defects) occur immediately below the pulmonary valve and above a muscle bundle in the right ventricular outflow tract known as the crista supraventricularis. Thus, outlet VSDs are also known as "supracristal" VSDs.

Clinical features: The size of the VSD is the primary variable relating to the development of patient symptoms. Approximately 50% of small VSDs will close without intervention by 3 years of age. Large defects across the ventricular septal are associated with a left-to-right shunt resulting in increased pulmonary blood flow and transmission of increased pressure to the pulmonary arteries. Infants with a large VSD may show symptoms such as shortness of breath (due to increased pulmonary flow), sweating with exertion (feeding), "fussiness," and fatigue. Auscultation will show a holosystolic murmur created as the blood flows across the defect into the right heart.

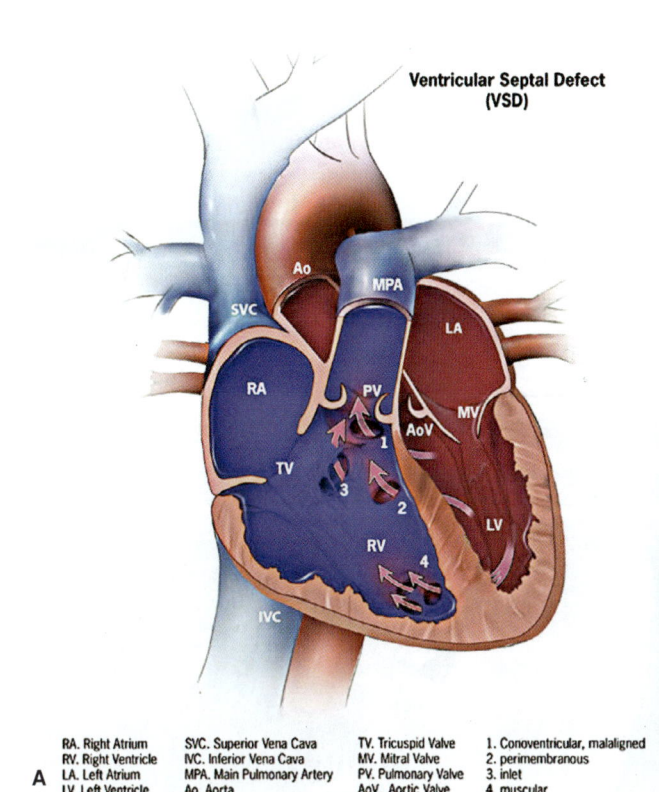

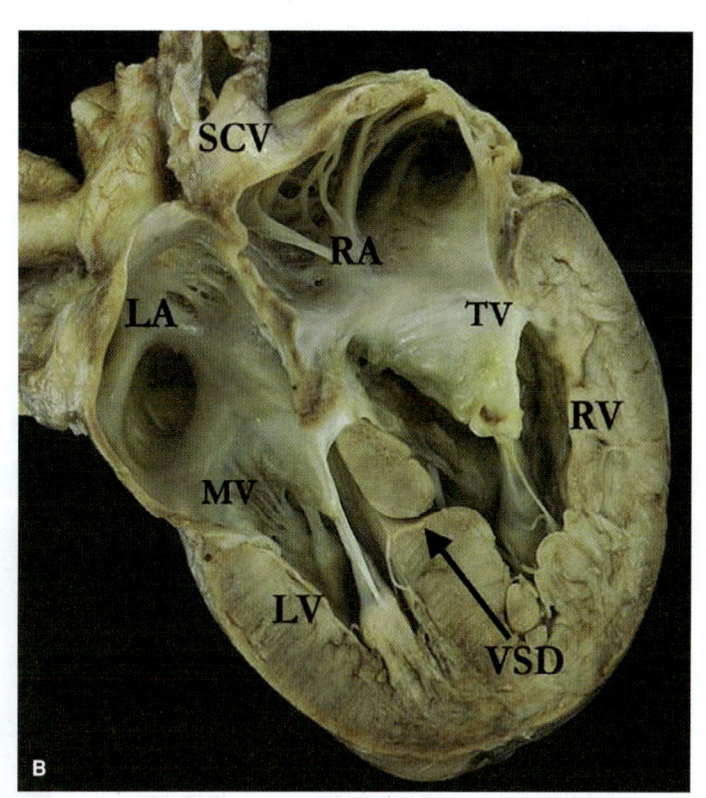

FIGURE 7-45 Ventricular septal defect. **(A)** Diagrammatic representation. From http://www.cdc.gov/ncbddd/heartdefects/vsd_simple-graphic.html (public domain). **(B)** Grossly, the four chamber view of this heart demonstrates a mid septal, restrictive, muscular septal defect (VSD). The atrial septum is intact and there is biventricular hypertrophy. From the Web Portal of the Archiving Working Group of the International Society for Nomenclature of Paediatric and Congenital Heart Disease (ISNPCHD) (http://ipccc-awg.net) and courtesy of Diane E. Spicer BS, PA (ASCP) (The Congenital Heart Institute of Florida [CHIF] and the University of Florida, Department of Pediatric Cardiology). SCV, superior caval vein; RA, right atrium; LA, left atrium; RV, right ventricle; LV, left ventricle.

A split S2 will also be heard due to the increased flow across the pulmonary valve.

Treatment: Small VSDs will usually close without intervention. Infants with large VSDs usually require some type of intervention. Intravenous intervention may be employed to deploy an occluder device into the defect. If a less invasive means cannot be used to close the defect, surgical closure by a patch graft can be done. Once the defect is closed, the infant's lifespan is normal.

If the defect remains unrepaired over the lifetime of the patient, the increased blood flow and increased pressure transmitted to the lungs will result in **pulmonary hypertension**, right ventricular hypertrophy, and reversal of the shunt (**Eisenmenger syndrome**). It is important to note that once significant pulmonary hypertension exists or the shunt has reversed, the defect cannot be repaired. If the defect is closed after shunt reversal, the right heart will rapidly fail without a means to release the significant pressures generated to maintain pulmonary flow.

Atrial Septal Defect and Patent Foramen Ovale

During fetal development, the atrial septum remains widely patent through the formation of multiple defects (ostium primum and ostium secundum) in the septum. These are crucial during fetal life to maintain adequate blood flow to the heart and lungs. Later, the atrial septum undergoes septation (septum primum and septum secundum) to separate the atria. In 80% of patients, these septae fuse and completely seal the atrial septum. In approximately 20% of people, the septae fuse incompletely and allow a small defect at the anterior edge of the fossa ovalis called a **patent foramen ovale (PFO)** (Figure 7-46). Since the left atrial pressures are higher than the right, the flap of the patent foramen remains closed. The presence of a PFO is considered a variant of normal. However, when the right-sided pressures are higher than the left (during sneezing, Valsalva maneuver, coughing), blood can flow into the left atrium from the right. In the majority of patients, this is not significant. However, rarely a venous thrombus may enter the right atrium from the venous system and can cross the PFO into the systemic circulation while the right atrial pressures are increased. This is known as a **paradoxical embolism** and can lead to transient ischemic attacks, cerebral vascular accidents, or other systemic complications. Atrial septal defects occur when the septae do not completely reach the anterior edge of the fossa ovalis.

Morphology: ASDs comprise 10% of CHD and are abnormal, fixed openings in the atrial septum. ASDs are usually isolated defects. The defects are classified according to their location: ostium secundum, ostium primum, and caval defects.

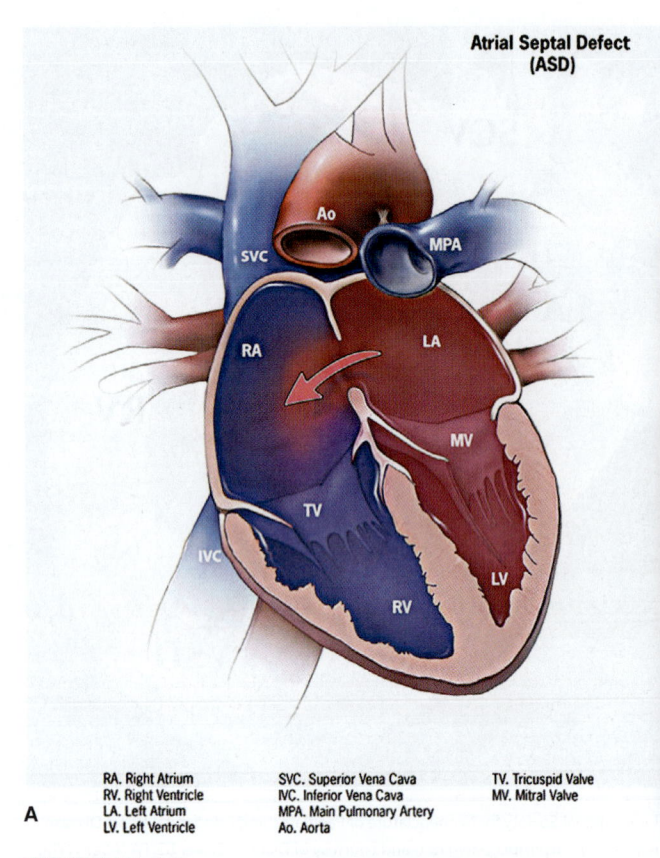

FIGURE 7-46 Atrial septal defect. **(A)** Diagrammatic representation. From http://www.cdc.gov/ncbddd/heartdefects/AtrialSeptalDefect-graphic2.html (public domain). **(B)** The anterior wall of the morphologic right atrium has been dissected away allowing for an anatomic view of the atrial septum (gross). The superior caval vein (SCV) and inferior caval vein (ICV) enter the right atrium in the usual fashion and the coronary sinus (CS) is in its usual position. The septum secundum, or the floor of the fossa ovalis, is fenestrated, giving rise to several small atrial septal defects. The tricuspid valve (TV) guards the inlet to the right ventricle. From the Web Portal of the Archiving Working Group of the International Society for Nomenclature of Paediatric and Congenital Heart Disease (ISNPCHD) (http://ipccc-awg.net) and courtesy of Diane E. Spicer BS, PA (ASCP) (The Congenital Heart Institute of Florida [CHIF] and the University of Florida, Department of Pediatric Cardiology).

- **Ostium secundum** ASDs (90% of ASDs) are usually smooth-walled defects of the septum secundum. The defects can vary in size and can be multiple with a fenestrated appearance.
- Approximately 5% are **ostium primum** defects located in the lowest part of the atrial septum at the level of the tricuspid valve annulus. A cleft in the anterior mitral valve leaflet is associated with this defect. Together these defects are considered a **partial atrioventricular canal defect**.
- **Caval** ASDs (5% of ASDs) are located adjacent to the mouth of the coronary sinus adjacent to the inferior vena cava. **Sinus venosus** ASDs are located high in the atrial septum adjacent to the superior vena cava. This defect is associated with anomalous pulmonary venous drainage into the superior vena cava or the right atrium.

Clinical features: ASDs are usually asymptomatic during early life and are not usually diagnosed until adulthood. The age at presentation is variable, but most are not diagnosed until the third decade, making them the most commonly diagnosed congenital heart defect in adulthood. ASDs are often diagnosed during pregnancy. The increased systemic blood volume of the mother increases the flow across the defect that is then more easily heard by auscultation.

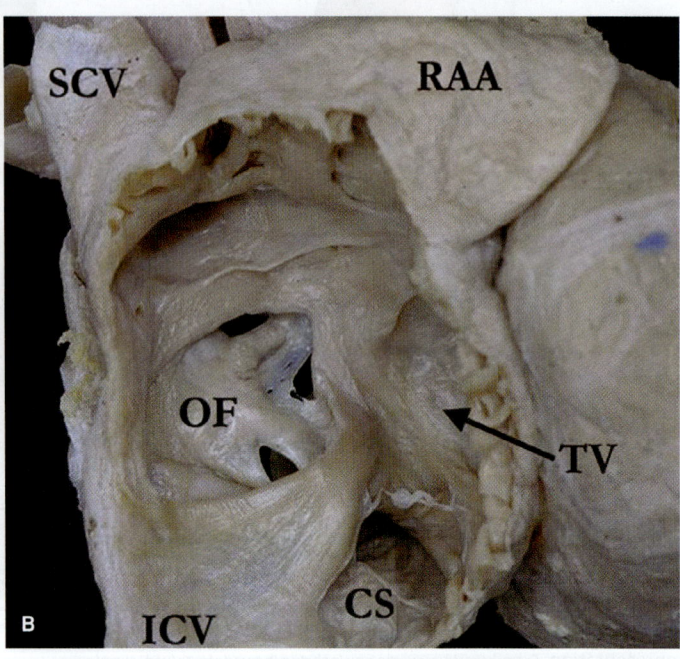

Initially, a left-to-right shunt exists through the defect with increased blood flow (anywhere from two to four times normal) to the pulmonary vasculature. As atrial pressures are low (relative to left atrial pressure) the increased volume is solely responsible for development of pulmonary hypertension in <10% of patients with an isolated ASD. Paradoxical emboli are a risk with an ASD.

Treatment: The rule with ASDs: *Find it, fix it*. Most ASDs are closed using an occluder device placed through the vascular system. This intervention has a low morbidity and mortality risk. Closure of the defect prevents paradoxical emboli and late right heart failure that may occur in a small number patients.

Patent Ductus Arteriosus

The ductus arteriosus is a structure that arises from the proximal left pulmonary artery and connects with the proximal descending thoracic aorta during fetal development. This structure allows the majority of the fetal blood to bypass the lungs and flow through the right heart to the aorta. After birth, the lungs expand and blood begins to flow through the right heart into the pulmonary arterial system due to decreased pulmonary resistance. The ductus arteriosus constricts after birth due to decreased flow and the body's prostaglandin E_2 levels. The lumen becomes occluded by thrombosis, allowing functional closure in the first several days after birth. The ductus arteriosus becomes a fibrotic cord (the **ligamentum arteriosum**) during the first month after birth (Figure 7-47 A and B)

Morphology: A well-formed arterial ostium arises from the proximal left pulmonary artery at the bifurcation with the right pulmonary artery, leading to a short, thick-walled artery into the aorta. The aortic side of the patent ductus arteriosus is usually at the underside of the aortic arch where it becomes the descending thoracic aorta.

Clinical features: In approximately 90% of cases, patent ductus arteriosus is an isolated defect. In 10% of patients, the patent ductus arteriosus (PDA) is associated with a ventricular septal defect or coarctation of the aorta (see later). Females more commonly suffer from patent ductus arteriosus than males.

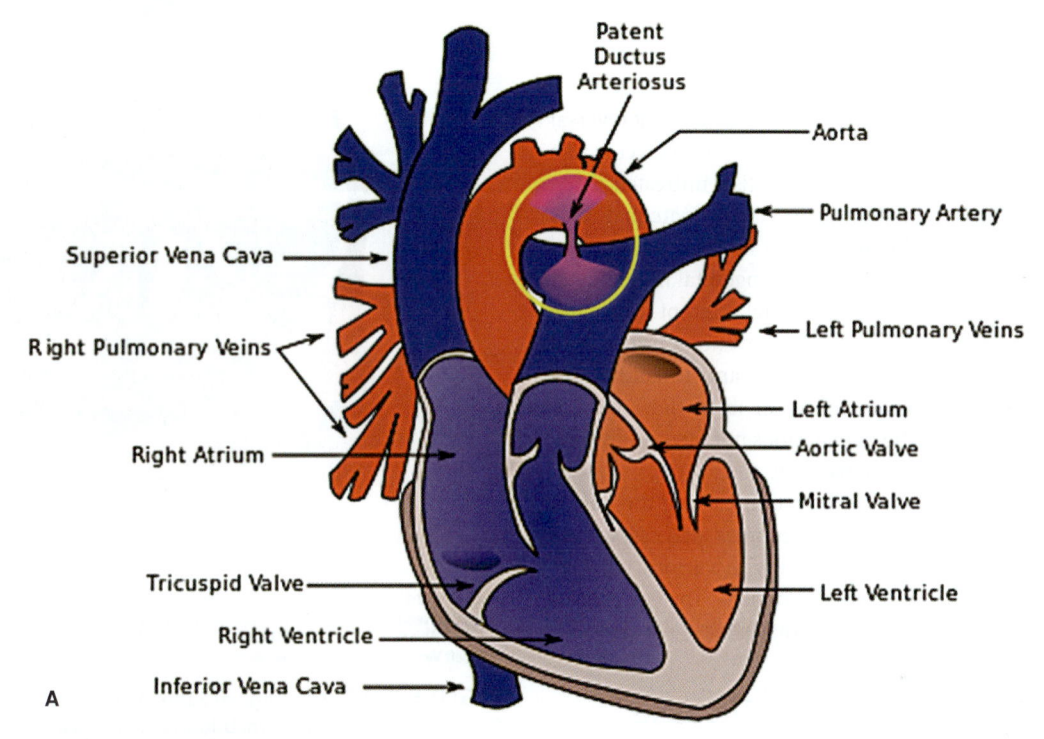

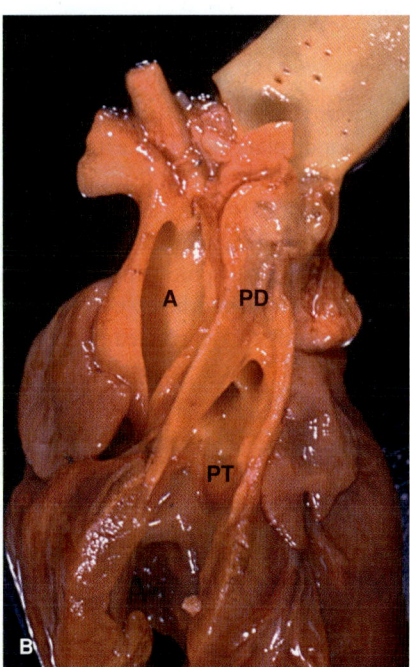

FIGURE 7-47 Patent Ductus Arteriosus (A) Diagrammatic representation. (b) Gross view of patent ductus arteriosus in an infant. A = opened aorta; PD = Patent ductus; PT = Pulmonary trunk.

From http://www.nhlbi.nih.gov/health/health-topics/images/ (public domain) Source: b From Department of Pathology and Laboratory Medicine University of North Carolina at Chapel Hill.

Initially at birth and during childhood, a patent ductus arteriosus is usually asymptomatic. On physical examination, a harsh, machinery-like murmur is heard with auscultation. The murmur is heard in both systole and diastole as blood flows across the patent ductus arteriosus during both cycles. As with a VSD, a patent ductus arteriosus creates a left-to-right shunt, increasing blood flow and systemic pressure to the right heart and pulmonary arterial system. The size of a patent ductus arteriosus, like the VSD, is important, as a large ductus allows transmission of more blood volume and high pressure into the lungs than does a small defect. Clinical symptoms are dependent on the size of the defect and are similar to those seen with a large VSD. If untreated, a patent ductus arteriosus can lead to shunt reversal resulting in Eisenmenger syndrome/complex. This defect is also known to predispose to infective endocarditis if untreated.

Treatment: Clinical wisdom is to close a patent ductus arteriosus as soon as possible unless it is necessary to sustain the infant's life due to a separate, lethal congenital heart defect (see below). Medical therapy is the initial attempt at closure in the first 10–14 days of life using intravenous infusion of prostaglandin inhibitors (nonsteroidal anti-inflammatory drugs (NSAID) such as indomethacin or ibuprofen), once it has been determined that the patient does not have additional cardiac defects requiring ductal patency.

If NSAIDs infusion is not effective in closing the patent ductus arteriosus, a more invasive becomes necessary. Percutaneous methods are routinely used with various types of occluders can be introduced intravenously. The success of catheter occlusion is quite high, but not 100%.

Cyanotic Congenital Heart Disease

In early cyanotic heart diseases, blood is shunted from the right heart into the left heart and cyanosis is evident from birth. The specific defects cause deoxygenated blood (blue) to bypass the lungs and mix with oxygenated blood. The deoxygenated blood decreases the amount of oxygenated blood sent to the body. These infants and children have a slight blue appearance to their lips and skin. The right-to-left shunt can lead to serious systemic complications including polycythemia (increased numbers of red blood cells) and the possibility of paradoxical embolism.

Tetralogy of Fallot (TOF)

TOF, the most common form of cyanotic heart disease, makes up 4–9% of all congenital cardiac abnormalities or approximately 4 per 1000 live births in the United States. TOF is also commonly associated with trisomy 21. The specific collection of abnormalities are named after a French physician, Étienne-Louis Fallot, who first described this CHD in 1888 as "la maladie bleu" (or the blue illness). The four (tetra-) components required to make the diagnosis include:

1. The presence of a ventricular septal defect.
2. "Overriding" of the VSD by the aorta.
3. Obstruction of the pulmonary outflow tract.
4. Right ventricular hypertrophy.

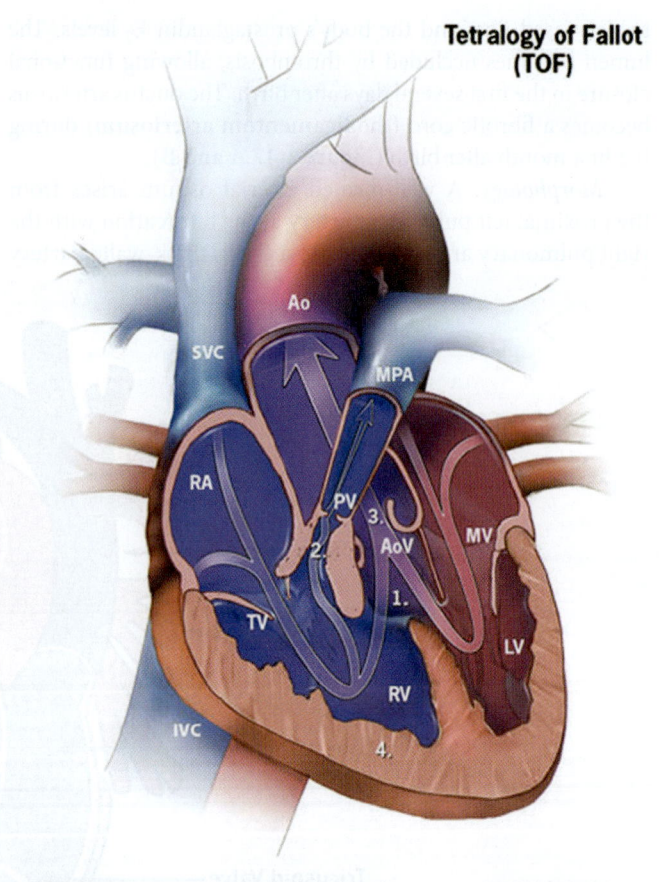

FIGURE 7-48 Tetralogy of Fallot. Diagramatic representation. From http://www.cdc.gov/ncbddd/heartdefects/TetralogyOfFallot-graphic.html

These four characteristics of the disease are the result of anterosuperior displacement of the infundibular septum of the right ventricular outflow tract leading to abnormal septation between the pulmonary trunk and aortic root (**Figure 7-48**).

Morphology: When viewed externally, the right ventricle is markedly hypertrophic (thickened) and makes up the majority of a boot-shaped heart mass (coeur en sabot). The right ventricle leads to a narrowed outflow tract causing pulmonary stenosis. The right ventricular hypertrophy is a result of the obstruction of the outflow tract. The stenosis is most commonly below the pulmonary valve (subvalvular) at the level of the muscle of the infundibulum. The stenosis may also be at the level of pulmonary valve (valvar) or above the valve (supravalvular). The pulmonary valve may also be atretic (no opening) leading to a small main pulmonary artery and pulmonary artery branches that do not form due to lack of flow during development. In cases of pulmonary atresia, the patent ductus arteriosus is the only supply of blood to the lungs.

The usually large VSD is high in the ventricular septum near the area of the membranous septum and the aortic valve can be seen through the VSD when viewed from below (**overriding** aorta). The VSD serves as the major point of outflow for both ventricles. Other abnormalities associated with TOF include a right aortic arch in up to 25%, abnormal coronary artery anatomy (5%), and atrial septal defect (pentalogy of Fallot).

Hemodynamics of TOF show increased right ventricular pressures, right-to-left shunt, decreased pulmonary blood flow, and increased blood flow into the aorta. The single most important morphological variable in patients' clinical severity of symptoms is the degree of **pulmonary obstruction**. Therefore, the more severe the outflow obstruction, the more deoxygenated blood from the right ventricle is shunted through the VSD into the aorta where it mixes with the oxygenated blood from the left ventricle. Patients with mild pulmonary obstruction may present with symptoms similar to an isolated VSD.

Clinical features: Patients with TOF may be cyanotic and symptomatic from birth with most presenting by 6 months of age. Patients with moderate pulmonary stenosis usually present with parental descriptions of the baby "turning blue" and being short of breath with feeding or crying. The infant may also show poor growth (failure to thrive). They may also describe events when the child turns dark blue and squats.

"Tet spells" are a classic symptom of TOF that occur most commonly during stress or strenuous play in young infants of 2–4 months. Events provoking a spell are usually those that decrease oxygen saturation (crying) or decrease systemic peripheral resistance (playing). The child has a sudden and profound cyanotic episode with rapid and deep respirations (hyperpnea), irritability, and prolonged crying. During these episodes, it is obvious that there is a significant increase in the right-to-left shunt with increased amounts of deoxygenated blood entering the systemic circulation through the VSD. The mechanism of the Tet spell is believed to involve an increase in circulating epinephrine during play or stress. Epinephrine has been shown to increase muscle tone of the right ventricular outflow tract, thereby significantly increasing the obstruction to the right ventricular out flow. This then increases the right-to-left shunt through the VSD.

Chest X-ray will show a boot-shaped heart due to right ventricular hypertrophy and decreased pulmonary vascular markings due to decreased blood flow to the lungs. Cardiac auscultation will commonly disclose a harsh, systolic murmur at the left mid- and upper sternal borders with a single S_2 heart sound. The systolic murmur is always due to the pulmonary stenosis. The VSD is silent as the pressures of the right and left ventricle are the same (no pressure gradient). The second heart sound is single as the pulmonary component is markedly reduced. A right ventricular impulse and systolic thrill may be present in some patients.

Treatment: For infants with TOF with pulmonary atresia, the ductus arteriosus must be kept open by infusion of prostaglandin E_1. In young children with severe Tet spells, positioning, calming, oxygen, and medications can relieve the spell. Most older children instinctively know to squat to prevent and interrupt the spells. Surgery is the definitive treatment of choice. Surgery is usually done electively at 3–6 months of age or at any time if severe symptoms are present. The perioperative mortality for complete surgical repair is <5% for uncomplicated TOF. Many patients survive into adulthood after surgical repair. However, if left untreated, survival rates are 55% at 5 years and 30% at 10 years.

Transposition of the Great Vessels (TGA)

Transposition of the great arteries accounts for approximately 4–10% of congenital heart disease abnormalities. TGA is the most common cyanotic congenital heart disease diagnosed in neonates and is more common in infants of diabetic mothers. In 90%, the defect is isolated and is not associated with extracardiac abnormalities. Untreated, the mortality rate of TGA is 30% in the first week of life, 50% in the first month and 90% by the end of the first year. TGA has a male predominance (1.5–3.2:1).

TGA results from discordant connections between the ventricles and their respective great arteries due to abnormal rotation of the conotruncal septum. Due to this abnormal rotation, the right ventricle leads directly to the aorta and the left ventricle leads to the main pulmonary artery to the lungs. Hence, this situation leads to separate, parallel pulmonary and systemic circulations. After returning to the right heart, the deoxygenated blood is returned to the systemic circulation without oxygenation by the lungs. Likewise, the oxygenated blood from the left ventricle is again sent to the lungs. The anomaly is NOT compatible with life. However, in the neonate, the patent ductus arteriosus and patent foramen ovale allow mixing of the blood initially (Figure 7-49).

Morphology: In patients with TGA, the aorta is anterior to the right of the pulmonary artery. Approximately 30–40% of patients have a ventricular septal defect that provides a stable shunt for mixture of blood. Sixty-five percent (65%) of patients have a patent ductus arteriosus or patent foramen ovale (unstable shunt). Of note, approximately 30% of patients with TGA have abnormal coronary artery anatomy. The right ventricle is markedly hypertrophic as it is serving as the systemic ventricle. The left ventricle is thin since it pumps blood into the low-resistance pulmonary circulation.

Clinical features: Severe cyanosis occurs within hours of birth, especially in patients with an intact ventricular septum. These infants rapidly develop metabolic acidosis due to poor tissue oxygenation as the ductus arteriosus begins to close and separate the two abnormal circulatory pathways. The diagnosis in these infants is usually suspected clinically due to the severity of the cyanosis that increases with time. No significant heart murmurs are present with an intact ventricular septum. Chest X-ray can also provide a significant clue to the diagnosis ("egg-on-a-string" appearance) due to the narrowed upper mediastinum. Echocardiogram is diagnostic.

Patients having a ventricular septal defect are less cyanotic. A systolic murmur will be heard as blood travels across the VSD. However, these patients can develop signs of congestive heart failure (shortness of breath, fast breathing, sweating, fast heart rate) in the first 3–6 weeks of life. The exact mechanism of the development of CHF is unknown.

Treatment: As discussed above, infusion of prostaglandin E_1 should begin immediately to maintain ductal patency in a neonate with TGA unless oxygen saturations are only

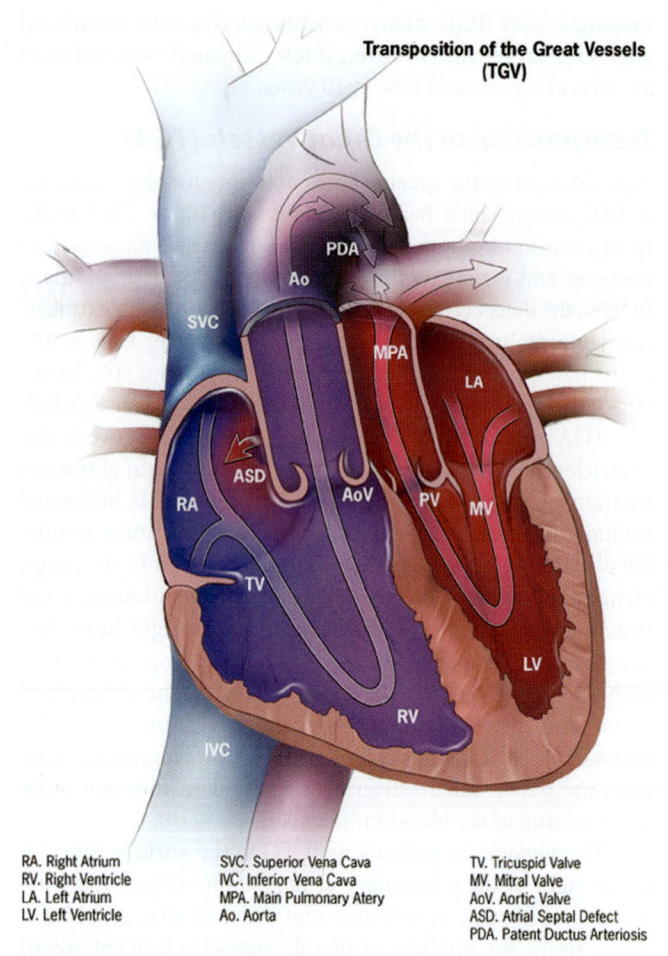

FIGURE 7-49 **Transposition of Great Vessels.** Diagramatic representation. From ww.cdc.gov/ncbddd/heartdefects/d-TGA-graphic.html

mildly decreased and the atrial communication is adequate. For severely hypoxic neonates not responding to prostaglandin infusion, a balloon atrial septectomy (uninflated balloon crosses into left atrium, is inflated and pulled across the atrial septum) to create an iatrogenic atrial septal defect allows mixing of blood and systemic arterial oxygenation.

The current method of definitive repair is an arterial switch operation, typically done during the first week of life. The proximal portions of the great arteries are transected, the coronary arteries are transplanted to the native pulmonary artery root (the neoaorta), and the arteries are switched to their "correct" ventricles. If an associated VSD is present, it is closed using a patch graft during the procedure. After surgery, survival rate into adulthood is >90%.

Truncus Arteriosus

Truncus arteriosus is an uncommon form of CHD comprising about 1% to 2% of congenital heart defects (5–15 of 100,000 live births). Like transposition of the great arteries, there is an increased incidence of truncus arteriosus in newborns of diabetic mothers. While seen infrequently in live births, truncus arteriosus is seen in a large number (5%) of spontaneous abortions and stillborn fetuses. As with other congenital heart defects of the conotruncal region, truncus arteriosus is associated with a microdeletion in the chromosome band 22q11.2 in 30% to 40% of cases.

Morphology: Embryologically, the defect arises from incomplete or failed septation of the truncus (the single artery arising from the heart during development) by the aortopulmonary septum resulting in a single arterial trunk that arises from both normally formed ventricles. A single semilunar valve (the truncal valve) usually sits directly over a VSD that receives blood from both ventricles. The pulmonary arteries arise from the common trunk above the coronary arteries and below the aortic arch. The abnormality has been organized into anatomical classifications primarily based on the location of the origin of the pulmonary arteries. As with transposition of the great arteries, a right-to-left shunt exists with deoxygenated blood mixing with oxygenated blood through the VSD. The degree of cyanosis and hypoxia depends on the ratio of resistances to flow in the pulmonary and systemic vascular beds (Figure 7-50). Multiple additional cardiac abnormalities are associated with truncus arteriosus including abnormal coronary artery origins, interruption of the aortic arch, right aortic arch, and ASD. The abnormal truncal valve can lead to significant valve regurgitation.

Clinical features: Truncus arteriosus can be diagnosed using prenatal ultrasonography in some patients. Most neonates with truncus arteriosus are diagnosed within the first few days of life.

Patients' parents may describe clinical symptoms similar to other cyanotic CHD, including fatigue, failure to thrive, shortness of breath, and sweating with feeding. Cyanosis is often recognized. Patients with significant truncal valve insufficiency may present earlier with profound symptoms of congestive heart failure.

DiGeorge or velocardiofacial syndrome is present in approximately 30% to 35% of patients with truncus arteriosus. Most of these patients have deletions of chromosome band 22q11. In addition to the cardiac abnormalities, the most common noncardiac abnormalities define the CATCH 22 syndrome (**c**ardiac abnormalities, **a**bnormal facies, **t**hymic hyperplasia, **c**left palate, and **h**ypercalcemia related to parathyroid dysfunction). In addition, renal, gastrointestinal, and skeletal abnormalities may occur.

Physical examination will demonstrate a significant cardiac murmur. Chest X-ray will commonly show cardiomegaly and increased pulmonary vascular markings. Echocardiography can definitively diagnose truncus arteriosus and define the exact anatomical features.

Treatment: Primary complete repair of the disease is now the standard of care at most large centers with survival rates of 90% to 95%.

Obstructive Congenital Anomalies

Obstructive lesions in CHD can occur below, at the level of or above the heart valves or along a great artery. An obstructive

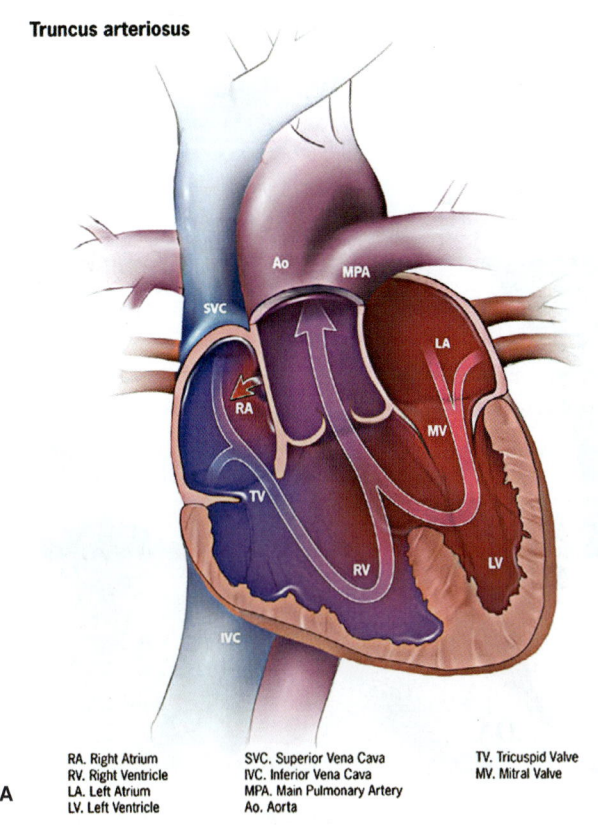

FIGURE 7-50 **Truncus arteriosus.** **(A)** Diagrammatic representation. From http://www.cdc.gov/ncbddd/heartdefects/TruncusArteriosus-graphic.html (public domain). **(B)** Anterior, close-up view of the common arterial trunk (CAT). The right pulmonary artery (RPA) and the left pulmonary artery (LPA) have separate origins from the posterior aspect of the common trunk. The left coronary orifice (LCO) lies between the truncal valve and the right pulmonary artery. The truncal valve is tricuspid and is not thickened. From the Web Portal of the Archiving Working Group of the International Society for Nomenclature of Paediatric and Congenital Heart Disease (ISNPCHD) (http://ipccc-awg.net) and courtesy of Diane E. Spicer BS, PA (ASCP) (The Congenital Heart Institute of Florida [CHIF] and the University of Florida, Dept. of Pediatric Cardiology). SCV, superior caval vein; RAA, right atrial appendage; LAA, left atrial appendage.

lesion prevents flow from reaching developing areas of the heart distal to the obstruction. Without adequate flow during development, these areas are referred to as "hypoplastic" (normally formed but small). Examples of obstructive lesions include coarctation of the aorta, congenital aortic stenosis, mitral and/or aortic valve atresia (also known as hypoplastic left heart syndrome), and tricuspid valve atresia.

Coarctation of the Aorta

Coarctation of the aorta is a localized narrowing of the aortic lumen causing impairment of flow distal to the obstruction. Coarctation represents 5% to 7% of CHD. Males have a higher predominance of the abnormality than females (2:1). Ten to twenty percent of patients with Turner syndrome have coarctation of the aorta. Age at presentation is dependent on the severity of the narrowing.

Morphology: Coarctation of the aorta most commonly occurs at the proximal descending thoracic aorta immediately distal to the aortic ostium of the left subclavian artery. Coarctation can occur as an isolated anomaly or associated with other congenital heart abnormalities including bicuspid aortic valve, VSD, aortic stenosis, and mitral valve disorders. Fifty percent (50%) of patients with coarctation have a congenitally bicuspid aortic valve (Figure 7-51).

The coarctation is formed by a localized medial thickening with infolding of the media and superimposed intimal fibrosis usually forming a shelf-like structure with an eccentric opening or a membranous curtain-like structure with a central or eccentric opening. Most commonly, the narrowing is discrete and localized, but may involve a long segment.

Coarctation has often been divided into two types: (1) infantile (preductal) and (2) adult (postductal). This classification is based on the location of the coarctation relative to the ductus arteriosus. Some authors have questioned the usefulness of this division noting that all coarctations are juxtaductal.

Classically, the coarctation is located immediately distal to the aortic ostium of the left subclavian artery at the proximal descending thoracic aorta. When the aorta is opened, the coarctation forms the shelf-like or curtain-like intrusion into the lumen allowing a small, usually eccentric opening to the distal aorta. Variable degrees of hypoplasia of the isthmus (the aorta between the left subclavian artery and the ductus arteriosus)

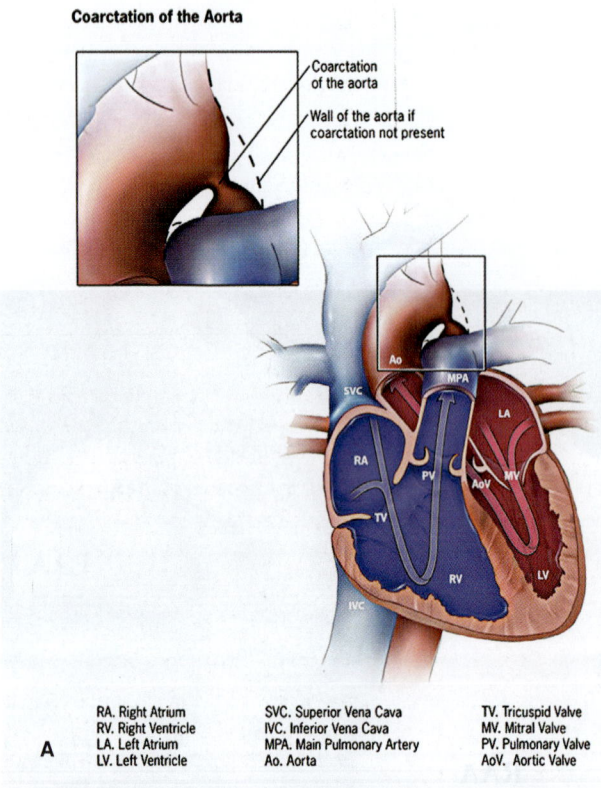

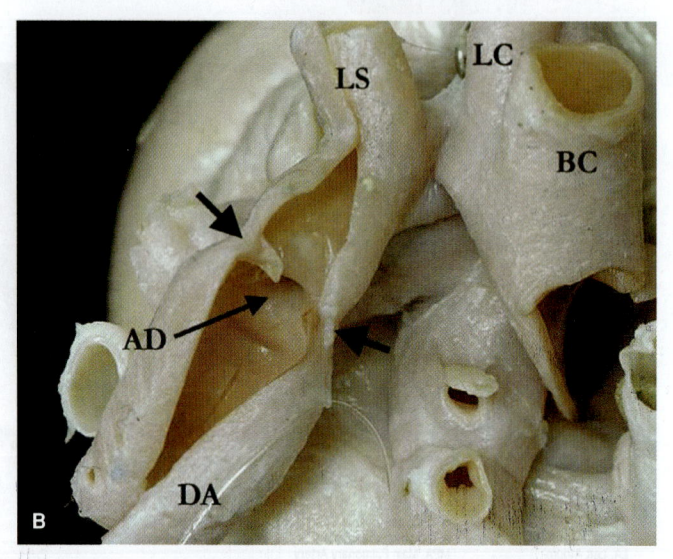

FIGURE 7-51 Coarctation of the aorta. (A) Diagrammatic representation. From http://www.cdc.gov/ncbddd/heartdefects/CoarctationOfAorta-graphic.html (public domain). **(B)** The great arteries exit the ventricular mass in the normal fashion in this anatomic view of the base of the heart (gross). The brachiocephalic vessels branch from the aortic arch in the usual fashion; the ascending aorta and the aortic arch smaller than normal. Just distal to the left subclavian artery (LS) and proximal to where the arterial duct (AD) joins the descending aorta (DA), there is a coarctation (black arrows). From the Web Portal of the Archiving Working Group of the International Society for Nomenclature of Paediatric and Congenital Heart Disease (ISNPCHD) (http://ipccc-awg.net) and courtesy of Diane E. Spicer BS, PA (ASCP) (The Congenital Heart Institute of Florida [CHIF] and the University of Florida, Department of Pediatric Cardiology). SCV, superior caval vein; RAA, right atrial appendage; LAA, left atrial appendage; PT, pulmonary trunk; LPA, left pulmonary artery; BC, brachiocephalic trunk; LC, left carotid artery. (Van Mierop Archive—University of Florida.)

may be present. Dilatation of the aorta immediately distal to the obstruction is common. A jet lesion may be present on the aortic wall directly opposite of the eccentric opening.

The most commonly associated, clinically significant defects include patent ductus arteriosus, VSD, and aortic stenosis. In infants with coarctation of the aorta, nearly 60% have a congenitally bicuspid aortic valve. When coarctation presents in children or in adults, only 30% have an associated bicuspid aortic valve. All patients with coarctation of the aorta will have left ventricular hypertrophy, the extent of which is dependent on the severity of the obstruction.

The current theory of coarctation development is associated with abnormal hemodynamics in the area of the ductus arteriosus.

Histology of the coarctated segment shows smooth muscle and elastic fibers continuous with the aortic media.

Clinical features: Clinical symptoms depend on the severity and location of the obstruction. The diagnosis can present early in infants with congestive heart failure. These patients may present acutely due to closure of the ductus causing a sudden increase in left ventricular afterload.

Older children may present with systemic hypertension of unknown etiology. In these patients, their upper extremities show hypertensive blood pressures. Their lower extremities show decreased blood pressure (due to decreased blood flow and pressure passing through the coarctation). It is necessary to document lower extremity blood pressures in children presenting with hypertension. These children will also develop collateral arterial systems through the intercostal and internal mammary arteries to increase flow to the lower body receiving inadequate flow. Most patients will have a holosystolic murmur on physical examination and may have a palpable thrill.

Treatment: Past studies (mostly autopsy) revealed that the mortality rate of untreated patients with coarctation was 90% by age 50 years, with a mean age of 35 years. Death was often due to complications of hypertension including rupture of intracranial aneurysms and aortic dissection with rupture. Bacterial endocarditis or congestive heart failure also led to death.

Treatment today most often includes percutaneous balloon angioplasty resulting in dilatation of the narrowing. Initial success rate after balloon angioplasty is 80% to 90%. As the child grows, recatheterization may be necessary. Surgical methods or repair include graft widening of the aorta (aortoplasty), subclavian flap repair or resection of the coarctation with end-to-end anastomosis.

Of note, it has been shown that these patients have a very high late morbidity and mortality even after coarctation repair.

Congenital Aortic Stenosis

Congenital aortic stenosis comprises approximately 4% to 6% of congenital heart defects. Obstruction to blood flow through the left ventricular outflow tract can occur at various levels similar to that seen in pulmonary stenosis including subvalvar, valvar, or supravalvar.

The three types of obstruction create similar symptoms and presentations.

Subvalvar obstruction, also known as subaortic stenosis (SAS), is a fixed obstruction to the flow of blood through the left ventricular outflow tract. SAS makes up 15% of cases of congenital aortic stenosis and is associated with additional congenital defects in 25–50% of patients. The most commonly associated anomalies include VSD, patent ductus arteriosus, coarctation of the aorta, bicuspid aortic valve, and several more complex defects. Male to female ratio of occurrence is 2 to 3:1.

The obstruction is caused by a thin, discrete membrane or a fibromuscular ridge located 0.5 to 1.0 centimeter below the aortic valve in 70–80% of patients. The majority of SAS patients become symptomatic during childhood, adolescence, and young adulthood (ages from 10 to 21 years).

Congenital aortic valve stenosis (CAVS) is due to obstruction caused by variable degrees of abnormal valve formation. Approximately 10% to 15% of patients with aortic valve stenosis present in infancy (<1 year of age). Aortic valve stenosis has a strong male incidence of 4:1. As many as 20% of patients with aortic valve stenosis have associated congenital heart defects including patent ductus arteriosus, aortic coarctation, VSD, and more complicated heart abnormalities.

In patients presenting in infancy, the aortic valve is most abnormal and is usually unicuspid. During embryogenesis, the valve cusps fail to separate forming a nearly plate-like, domed membrane with a small valve orifice. Presentation and symptoms are variable and depend on the degree of stenosis. Congenitally bicuspid valves are quite common and are seen in up to 2% of the population. Unlike the congenitally unicuspid aortic valve, patients with a congenitally bicuspid valve do not present with symptoms until later in life (see below and **Figure 7-52**).

Supravalvar aortic stenosis (SVAS), a localized or diffuse narrowing of the ascending aorta above the superior edge of the aortic sinuses, makes up approximately 7% of cases of congenital aortic stenosis. Morphologically, an hour-glass-shaped narrowing above the level of the coronary arteries occurs in 50–75% of cases. Sporadic occurrence of SVAS in 50% of cases is associated with an arterial abnormality or in association with Williams syndrome, an autosomal dominant genetic disorder associated with idiopathic familial hypercalcemia. A familial form also exists that is not associated with Williams syndrome. The exact cause of SVAS is uncertain; however, its association with Williams syndrome suggests an abnormality in an elastin gene. Williams syndrome is caused by an alteration of an elastin gene at band 7q11.

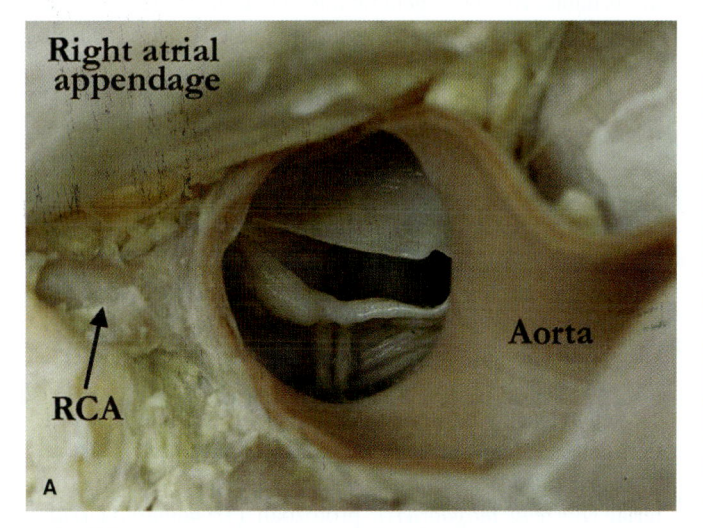

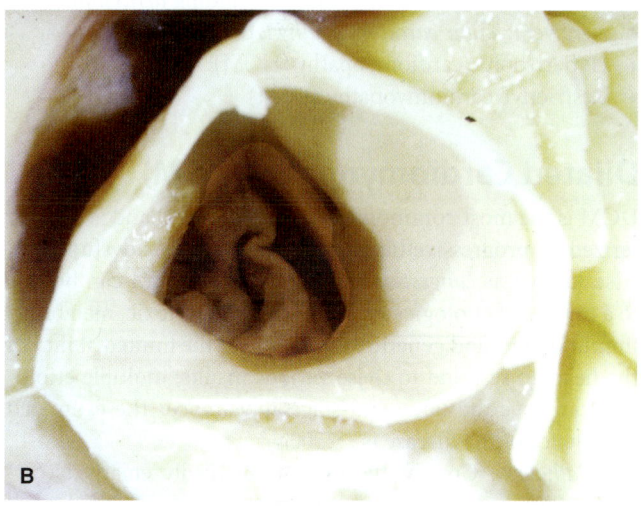

FIGURE 7-52 Bicuspid aortic valve. (A) This arterial view of the aortic valve demonstrates a bicuspid aortic valve. The right and left coronary cusps are fused with a prominent raphe demonstrating the line of nonseparation between the conjoined cusps. The edge of the conjoined cusps is thickened, indicating chronic insufficiency. The noncoronary cusp is of normal thickness. RCA, right coronary artery. (Van Mierop Archive—University of Florida). From the Web Portal of the Archiving Working Group of the International Society for Nomenclature of Paediatric and Congenital Heart Disease (ISNPCHD) (http://ipccc-awg.net) and courtesy of Diane E. Spicer BS, PA (ASCP) (The Congenital Heart Institute of Florida [CHIF] and the University of Florida, Department of Pediatric Cardiology). **(B)** Calcified congenitally bicuspid aortic valve from above. From Department of Pathology and Laboratory Medicine, University of North Carolina at Chapel Hill.

The survival rate following repair of SVAS is approximately 85% at 15 years. Prognosis is dependent on associated congenital anomalies and coronary artery lesions. As coronary artery anomalies are associated with SVAS, patients with SVAS, even after repair, have a higher risk of sudden death.

Clinical features: All patients with left ventricular outflow tract obstruction will show similar symptoms. Most often the asymptomatic patients present for work-up of a cardiac murmur. Patients can present with shortness of breath, angina, and syncope. Initially, these symptoms are most noted during exertion. Angina can occur in as many as 25% of patients with left ventricular outflow obstruction.

Treatment: Timing of treatment of congenital aortic stenosis is similar for all types and is dependent on the severity of the gradient across the valve. Surgical intervention is indicated dependent on severity of symptoms.

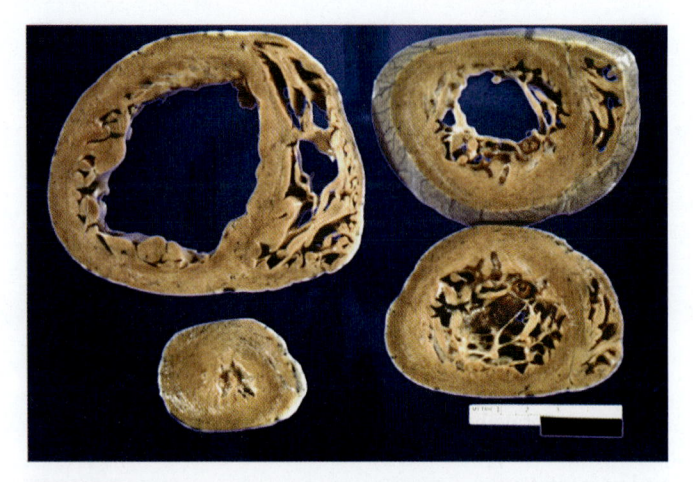

FIGURE 7-53 Dilated familial cardiomyopathy. Gross view of transverse sections of the heart. Note dilation of all chambers. From Peter Anderson DVM, Ph.D. PEIR Digital Library Image 8572.

CARDIOMYOPATHIES

Cardiomyopathy is a primary disease process of the heart muscle. The majority of heart muscle disease processes are secondary to a primary process such as CAD, hypertension, or other. In the case of a cardiomyopathy, the disease is primarily an abnormality of the heart muscle and is confined to the myocardium. The causes of cardiomyopathic processes are extremely diverse and include inflammatory, immunologic, systemic metabolic disorders, muscular dystrophies, and genetic abnormalities of the myocyte. Occasionally, the cause of the cardiomyopathy cannot be determined. These cases are called an idiopathic cardiomyopathy.

Cardiomyopathies are classically divided into three categories:

- Dilated cardiomyopathy (DCM) including *arrhythmogenic right ventricular cardiomyopathy (ARVC)*
- Hypertrophic cardiomyopathy (HCM)
- Restrictive cardiomyopathy (RCM)

Dilated Cardiomyopathy (DCM)

DCM is the most common form (90% of cases) and is characterized by progressive heart dilation and *systolic* dysfunction. Also known as *congestive* cardiomyopathy, DCM can be due to a myriad of etiologies including infectious, toxic, metabolic, immunologic, and genetic causes. Due to the limited ability of the heart to respond to these various insults, multiple etiologies can have the same end-stage appearance. The estimated prevalence of the disease is 1:2500.

Pathology: Grossly, the heart is markedly enlarged (cardiomegaly), heavy (often two to three times the normal heart weight) and "flabby" with enlargement of all chambers. The thickness of the left ventricle may vary. Due to the significant dilatation of the chambers and stagnation of blood, mural thrombi are common and may be the source of distant thromboembolic complications. The normal valves are unable to close completely due to the geometric alterations of the ventricle leading to valve insufficiency. The papillary muscles are moved further apart and the arterial roots dilate leading to valve dysfunction. By definition, the valves, coronary arteries, and other potential vascular etiologies for the dilation are normal. The myocardium is normal in gross appearance (Figure 7-53).

The histology of the heart is nonspecific and does not reflect the underlying etiology. The histologic appearance also does not reflect the severity of cardiac dysfunction. Microscopically, myocytes are hypertrophic with enlarged nuclei. Patchy fibrosis in interstitial and endocardial areas is scattered with chronic inflammatory cells. Some replacement fibrosis may be seen due to ischemic imbalance.

Pathogenesis: At presentation of DCM in the end-stage state, the cause of the original disease process is not easily discernable. However, genetic and research studies have provided insight into a number of definable etiologies including infectious, toxic, and genetic.

Infectious etiologies: Using current technologies, viral RNA from adenoviruses, cytomegaloviruses, and enteroviruses has been identified in some patients with end-stage DCM, providing circumstantial evidence that many cases of DCM can be attributed to infectious etiologies. Enteroviruses including Coxsackie B virus have been studied in depth to determine how the infection leads to the end-stage, dilated state.

Introduction of viral genetic material into myocyte DNA leads to the production of intracellular enterovirus protease 2A that has been shown to directly cleave dystrophin (the defective protein in Duchenne and Becker muscular dystrophy). Destruction of this support protein is thought to lead to cell injury and cytoskeleton disruption. Other infectious causes include bacterial (*Borrelia burgdorferi*), protozoan (*Trypanosoma cruzi*), and rickettsial infections. Autoimmune mechanisms incited by cross-reacting viral proteins may also lead to DCM.

Toxic etiologies: Alcohol abuse is the most common toxic etiology known to cause DCM. Alcohol and its metabolites (acetaldehyde) have a direct toxic effect on the myocardium. In chronic alcoholism, associated deficiencies including thiamine deficiency can lead to beriberi heart disease. Other well-known toxins include doxorubicin (Adriamycin) and cobalt. Adriamycin is a chemotherapeutic agent that causes a dose-related DCM. In 1966, cobalt had been used in Canada to stabilize beer foam and led to DCM, known as beer drinker's cardiomyopathy.

Genetic etiologies: Inherited genetic abnormalities are associated with DCM in 20% to 30% of cases causing familial dilated cardiomyopathy. Cytoskeletal protein abnormalities such as that resulting from mutations in the dystrophin gene seen in Duchenne and Becker muscular dystrophy, mutations in the alpha cardiac actin gene, and mitochondrial enzyme defects are associated with DCM.

A unique DCM is associated with pregnancy and is termed peripartum cardiomyopathy (PPCM). The estimated incidence of PPCM is from 1 case per 15,000 live births to 1 case per 1,300 live births. PPCM has been documented across all ages and races, but is most common in multiparous women. African-American women have a 15.7-fold higher relative risk for PPCM than others. Patients present with symptoms of CHF late in their pregnancy to several weeks postpartum. Approximately 50% of the affected patients recover spontaneously without sequelae. The cause is unknown.

Clinical features: DCM may occur at any age, but most commonly affects patients aged 20 to 50 years of age. Patients present with slowly progressive shortness of breath, fatigue, paroxysmal nocturnal dyspnea, and other signs of congestive heart failure. Upon presentation, the patients' ejection fraction is usually quite low (15%–25% at end stage). As many as 50% of patients die within 2 years of the onset of the disease. Only 25% of patients survive more than 5 years. Most patients die due to progression of the heart failure or dysrhythmias.

Treatment: Treatment is symptomatic ultimately leading to cardiac transplant.

Arrhythmogenic Right Ventricular Cardiomyopathy (ARVC)

Some classifications place ARVC into the dilated cardiomyopathies due to the dilatation of the right ventricle that occurs with the disease. ARVC is transmitted in an autosomal dominant pattern with variable penetrance in familial forms which account for 30% of cases. Patients can present with right ventricular dilatation and failure. Others have significant rhythm disturbances and die suddenly and unexpectedly. The prevalence of ARVC in the general population is estimated to be 1 in 2000 to 1 in 5000. ARVC is the cause of SCD in 11% of cases overall and 22% of athletes in Italy. Patients present between the ages of 10 and 50 years with a mean age of 30 years of age.

Pathology: Grossly, the right ventricle is thin walled and often significantly dilated. The right ventricular myocardium shows focal, often transmural replacement by mature fat with areas of fibrosis. Histology shows replacement of the myocardium with mature fat, increased interstitial and replacement fibrosis and scattered chronic inflammatory cells (usually lymphocytes). Left ventricular involvement may be seen with significant right ventricular involvement (classic pattern), with relatively mild right-sided involvement (left dominant pattern) or parallel involvement of both ventricles (biventricular pattern)

Etiology: ARVC is a disease process related to the **desmosome**. The desmosome, also known as the macula adherens, is responsible for cell-to-cell adhesion and myocyte mechanical coupling for transmission of contractile forces. Diseases associated with desmosomal disruption have shown progressive cell separation, cell death, and replacement by fat and fibrosis. Genetic mutations in five genes related to desmosomal proteins have been found in approximately 50% of clinically diagnosed cases of ARVC. Genes for the protein *plakophilin-2* are the most commonly mutated in 43% of cases (70% of familial cases).

Clinical features: Primary symptoms include dizziness, palpitation, syncope, and shortness of breath in 60% of patients. The remaining 40% may be totally asymptomatic when diagnosed with ARVC at screening examination for affected family members. Patients may be suspected of having ARVC due to nonspecific electrocardiographic or echocardiographic changes or the presence of ventricular dysrhythmias on Holter monitoring. A second possible presentation of patients can be SCD with the diagnosis being made at autopsy. ARVC may be associated with 10% of otherwise unexplained SCD.

The diagnosis is difficult to make, and criteria including electrocardiographic abnormalities, structural or functional abnormalities, tissue characterization, the presence of arrhythmias, and family history must be relied on

Treatment: As the most significant and major goal of treatment in ARVC is the prevention of sudden death, implantation of an internal cardiac defibrillator is recommended in patients with significant, sustained ventricular dysrhythmias.

Hypertrophic Cardiomyopathy (HCM)

HCM, a disease with many names and acronyms, is characterized by LVH of variable morphologies with a wide variety of clinical and hemodynamic abnormalities. Depending on the site of hypertrophy, patients may exhibit diastolic dysfunction, mitral valve regurgitation, left ventricular outflow tract obstruction (30% of cases), and myocardial ischemia. The enlarged, thick-walled left ventricle has a small ventricular chamber and poor myocardial compliance leading to decreased diastolic filling and decreased cardiac output. HCM must be distinguished from hypertensive heart disease, amyloid heart disease, and age-related subaortic septal hypertrophy.

The prevalence of HCM is approximately 1 out of every 500 adults (or 0.2%) as determined by echocardiographic studies in the United States, Japan, and China. The disease is genetically inherited by autosomal dominant transmission, with variable penetrance.

Pathology: Grossly, the heart is markedly enlarged with a thickened left ventricular wall **(Figure 7-54A)**. The left ventricular chamber is small without dilatation. The "classic" form shows disproportionate thickening of the ventricular septum below the aortic valve compared to the left ventricular free wall (ratio of 2.5–3:1). The classic form, also known as idiopathic

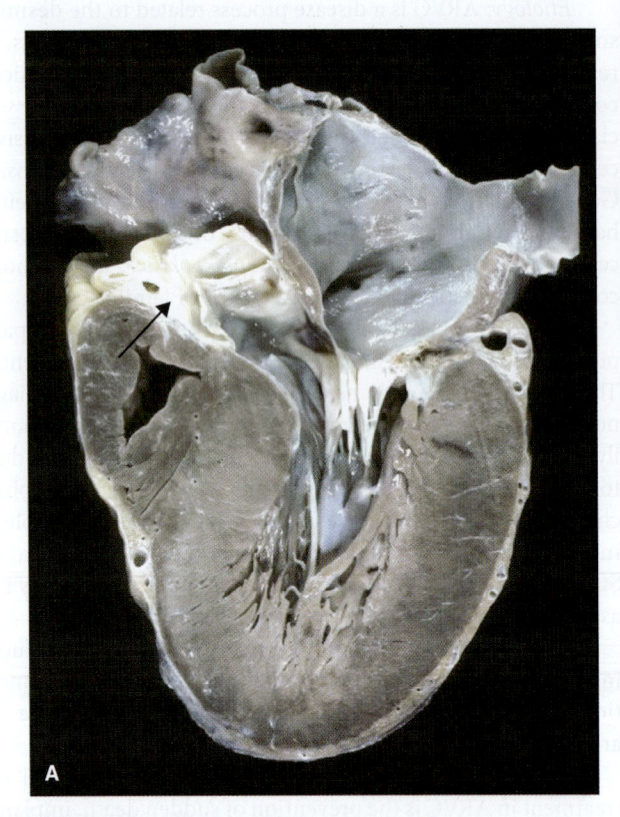

FIGURE 7-54 **Hypertrophic cardiomyopathy. (A)** Gross view. The left ventricular chamber is small with a thickened wall and subaortic endocardial friction patch (arrow). Department of Pathology and Laboratory Medicine, University of North Carolina at Chapel Hill. **(B)** There is a disproportionate thickening of the ventricular septum below the aortic valve (idiopathic subaortic stenosis) (arrow). From Peter Anderson DVM, Ph.D. PEIR Digital Library Image 0453. **(C)** Microscopic view demonstrates myocyte hypertrophy and, notably, disarray of individual myocytes. From Department of Pathology and Laboratory Medicine, University of North Carolina at Chapel Hill.

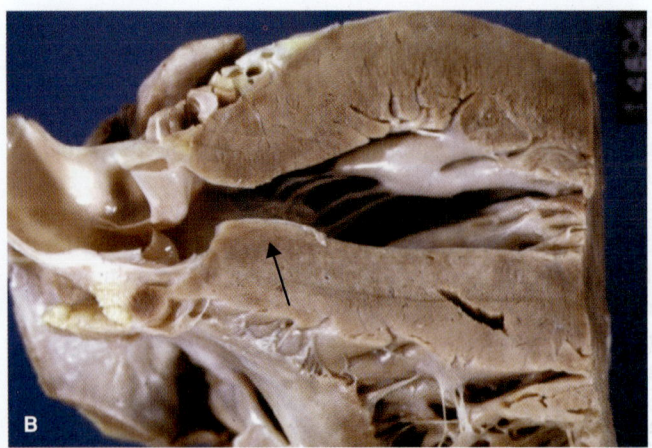

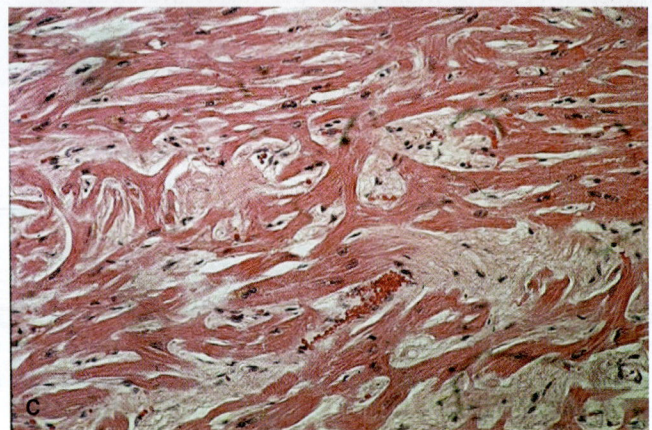

hypertrophic subaortic stenosis and asymmetric septal hypertrophy, is now called hypertrophic obstructive cardiomyopathy (HCM). The significant thickness of the ventricular septum below the aortic valve creates a projection into the left ventricular outflow leading to obstruction of outflow (Figure 7-54B). Due to the physics of flow through the obstruction, the mitral valve is positioned within the outflow tract causing systolic anterior motion (SAM). The irritation of the mitral valve fluttering over the endocardium of the obstruction causes an endocardial friction patch below the aortic valve. As a consequence of SAM, the mitral valve may be thickened or myxomatous. Approximately 10% of cases of HCM show concentric (involvement of all walls) hypertrophy without obstruction.

Histologic features of HCM are necessary for the pathologic diagnosis of the disease. The diagnostic histology shows massive myocyte hypertrophy (diameter >40 μm) and haphazard arrangement of myofiber bundles and/or individual myocytes (**disarray**) (Figure 7-54C). Additional associated histologic features include patchy interstitial and replacement fibrosis and significantly thick-walled intramyocardial arterioles.

Pathogenesis: HCM is a genetically determined disease of the heart muscle that is caused by mutations in genes that encode for sarcomeric proteins of the contractile apparatus. Identified mutations are responsible for about 50% of cases. The most common mutation found is in cardiac myosin binding protein-C. Mutations in cardiac β-myosin heavy chain are the second most common. The consequences of these mutations in contractile protein genes appear to directly affect sarcomeric function. Significant upregulation of other genes (including those responsible for secondary hypertrophy) in response to the mutation also occurs.

Clinical features: The majority of patients with HCM have no or minor symptoms. Many are diagnosed during family screening, on detection of a heart murmur, or due to abnormalities on electrocardiogram. These patients have a better prognosis than those with more severe symptoms. Presentation can occur at any age, but most commonly appears during the pubertal growth spurt. Symptoms include shortness of breath (in 90% of symptomatic patients), angina (in 25% to 30%), syncope (15% to 20% of patients report at least one episode), fatigue, and palpitations. Clinical symptoms *are not directly* related to the presence or severity of the left ventricular outflow tract obstruction.

Patients with HCM are at risk for multiple complications including mural thrombi associated with atrial fibrillation, infective endocarditis, progressive heart failure, and sudden death due to ventricular dysrhythmias. Recent large epidemiologic studies have shown an annual mortality rate of approximately 1% per year with those diagnosed in childhood (unlike those diagnosed as adults) having a significantly higher risk of death. HCM is the most common cause of sudden death in young (<35 years old) athletes (36% of cases in one study). These athletes collapse suddenly during or immediately after exertion. This disease has been found in a disproportionate number of African-American athletes with the majority of these patients not diagnosed prior to their death.

Treatment: Medical treatment involves negative inotropic agents that slow the heart rate prolonging diastole and ventricular filling and decrease outflow obstruction. Additional treatments can include surgical septal myectomy of the obstruction or septal ablation.

Restrictive Cardiomyopathy (RCM)

RCM is the least common form of the cardiomyopathic processes and accounts for approximately 5% of all cases of primary heart muscle disease. RCM is defined as a myocardial disease characterized by restrictive filling and reduced diastolic volume of either or both ventricles with normal or near-normal systolic function and wall thickness. RCM can present similarly to HCM or constrictive pericarditis. The possibility of constrictive pericarditis must be ruled out clinically, as it is a process that can be relatively easily treated with surgery.

RCM is divided into the following types:

- Idiopathic
- Infiltrative
- Treatment-induced
- Others

Idiopathic RCM is a rare subset of patients that present with symptoms of diastolic dysfunction, heart failure, and restrictive hemodynamics with no significant ventricular hypertrophy, endocardial thickening or fibrosis, hypereosinophilia, or other distinct clinical findings. Rarely, a familial pattern has been documented. The disease process may be a form of HCM with a different clinical expression.

Infiltrative RCM is most commonly associated with systemic diseases that also involve the heart such as amyloidosis, sarcoidosis, metabolic storage diseases, scleroderma, and hemochromatosis **(Figure 7-55)**.

Amyloid infiltration of the heart can occur with systemic involvement or may be localized to the heart in the elderly (senile cardiac amyloidosis). Small, raised, yellow nodules may be identified in the atrial endocardium of RCM due to amyloidosis. Amyloidosis is caused by the deposition of fibrils composed of subunits of serum proteins that form insoluble β-pleated sheets. This intercellular deposition accumulates in amounts sufficient to impair organ function.

Treatment-induced RCM can be due to radiation or chemotherapeutic agents. Radiation cardiotoxicity is thought to be due to injury to arterioles within the heart. The injury is thought to be due to reactive oxygen species that disrupt DNA strands. Secondary inflammatory response then leads to fibrosis. The diffusely increased interstitial fibrosis in the heart leads to the restrictive hemodynamics several years after treatment.

Other types of RCM include endomyocardial fibrosis (EMF) and Loeffler endomyocarditis. EMF is a characteristic syndrome with specific epidemiologic features. It is a disease of children and young adults in Africa and other tropical countries characterized by diffuse fibrosis of the apical endocardium of the right ventricle, left ventricle, or both **(Figure 7-56)**. In Uganda, a bimodal peak occurs at ages 10 and 30 years. While the true incidence is unknown, EMF is believed to be the most common form of RCM worldwide. The exact etiology of EMF is unknown, although multiple theories exist. As there are significant regional differences of EMF cases and the lack of a unifying infectious etiology, one thought is a geochemical basis for the etiology. Cerium, a rare element, has been postulated to play a role in the development of EMF. Abundant cerium levels have been shown to occur in areas endemic for EMF. In addition, children have elevated serum levels of cerium in these areas. In areas where the previously abundant cerium presence has decreased, the occurrence of EMF has also fallen.

Loeffler endomyocarditis is due to hypereosinophilic syndrome (HES), a group of disorders marked by a prolonged overproduction of eosinophils, in which infiltration of eosinophils and its mediators causes damage to multiple organs. The third or healed phase of HES with diffuse fibrosis and scarring of the endocardium and myocardium leads to the RCM.

Pathology: The gross appearance of the heart in the various types of RCM is similar. The ventricles are of relatively normal thickness or only slightly thickened, but the heart is heavy by weight. The ventricular chambers are not dilated. The myocardium is rubbery to firm, without specific localized lesions. The atria are commonly dilated due to poor ventricular filling and pressure overload.

Microscopy shows variable degrees of fibrosis. It may also reveal the underlying etiology of the disease. Endomyocardial biopsy may assist in making the diagnosis of a specific etiologic disorder.

VALVULAR HEART DISEASE

The endocardium lining the ventricles is lifted from the surface of the ventricle during embryogenesis to create the valves which are responsible for unidirectional blood flow. The valves are subjected to repetitive mechanical stresses and high pressure gradients over a long period of time (>40 million cycles each year). These factors can lead cumulative damage that can lead clinically to significant heart disease. The normal valves are composed of thin, flexible tissues that also are sturdy to prevent flow reversal and transmission of the significant gradient differences across the valve.

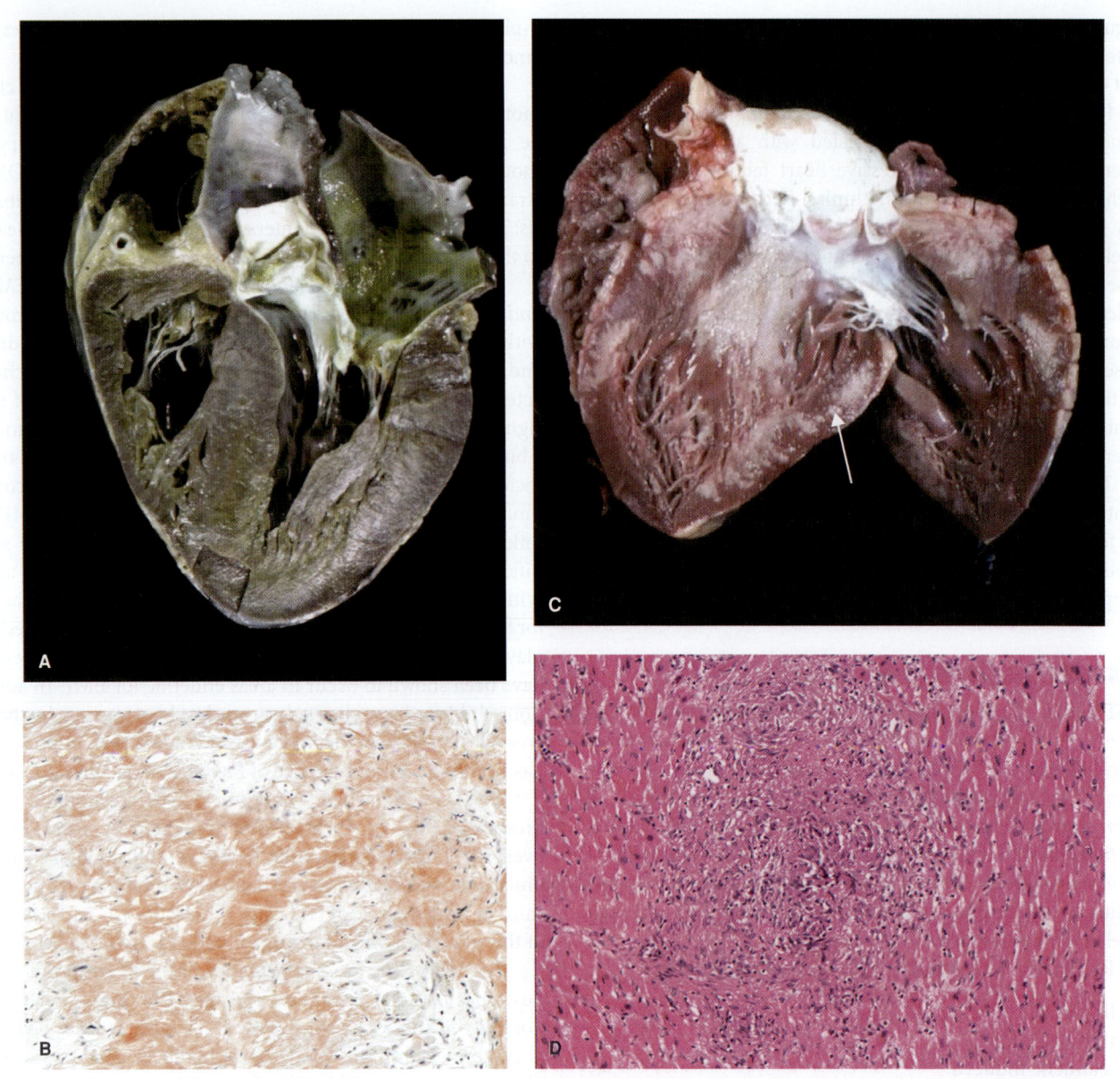

FIGURE 7-55 Restrictive cardiomyopathy. (A) Cardiac amyloid. Note thickened ventricular walls due to amyloid deposition (color cast is artifactual). Note yellow discoloration of atrial endocardium due to amyloid deposition. **(B)** Cardiac amyloid microscopic (Congo red stain). Cardiac myocytes are faintly visible (unstained). **(C)** Cardiac sarcoidosis. Infiltrative process in ventricular wall is visible (arrow). **(D)** Cardiac sarcoidosis. Granulomas are present at the center of the field. From Department of Pathology and Laboratory Medicine, University of North Carolina at Chapel Hill.

Terminology: When discussing valvular heart disease, it is necessary to understand terminology related to valve dysfunction. *Stenosis* indicates that the valve has a narrowed opening. The valve fails to open completely impeding forward flow and causing obstruction. Stenosis is ALWAYS a **primary, chronic** process involving valves. In valve *insufficiency (regurgitation)*, the valve does not close completely allowing reversal of blood flow. The process of insufficiency may be due to a **primary, intrinsic abnormality of the valve** or due to **damage to or alteration of the geometry of the support structures** (papillary muscles, chordae tendineae). Alteration of the valve's support system is classified as secondary or **functional insufficiency**. In the setting of DCM, the geometry of the valve's support structures (especially the papillary muscles) is altered such that the valve leaflets cannot co-apt allowing blood flow reversal during systole. The majority of dysfunctional valves exhibit a mixed picture of stenosis and regurgitation, but one or the other may predominate. The valve disease may also be *isolated* (involving only one valve) or *combined* (involving more than one valve).

The patient's clinical symptoms will be dependent on multiple factors including

- Which valve is involved.
- The degree of valve impairment.

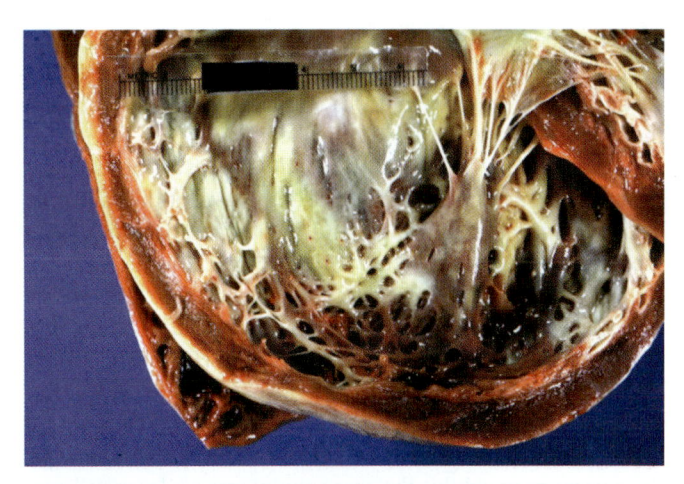

FIGURE 7-56 **Endomyocardial fibrosis.** From Department of Pathology and Laboratory Medicine, University of North Carolina at Chapel Hill.

- The rate of development of the impairment (acute or chronic).
- The rate and ability of the heart to compensate for the impairment.

Valve dysfunction may also be due to a congenital anomaly or acquired impairment. A patient with a congenitally abnormal valve is at risk for later development of superimposed acquired changes. Acquired changes are those that develop over time. **Acquired stenosis** of the aortic and mitral valves comprises two-thirds of **ALL** valve diseases.

The major causes of acquired valve stenosis include aortic valve stenosis (including "senile" calcific aortic stenosis, calcification of a congenitally abnormal aortic valve, and postinflammatory processes [sequelae of rheumatic fever]). The one and **only** cause of mitral stenosis is the postinflammatory process (most commonly as a chronic sequelae of rheumatic fever).

"Senile" Calcific Aortic Stenosis

Calcific aortic stenosis is the most common valve abnormality in patients presenting in their eighth to ninth decades of life (70–80 years of age). In 48% of patients presenting over 70 years of age, the underlying valve is a normally formed, tricuspid valve that suffers wear-and-tear changes over time leading to deposition of calcium on the arterial surfaces of the valve cusps. The calcium deposits lead to stiffness and immobility over time and create a narrowed (stenotic) opening to blood flow.

Pathology: Grossly, from above, the valve has three cusps with normal relationships with the aorta. The arterial surfaces of the cusps are covered by islands of firm, rigid, calcific deposits that prevent flexibility of the valve cusps. These rock-hard deposits prevent the cusps from completely retracting to the aortic wall and from completely closing. In addition to the valve changes, the left ventricle becomes thickened (hypertrophic) in response to the obstruction and the need to maintain adequate cardiac output (Figure 7-57).

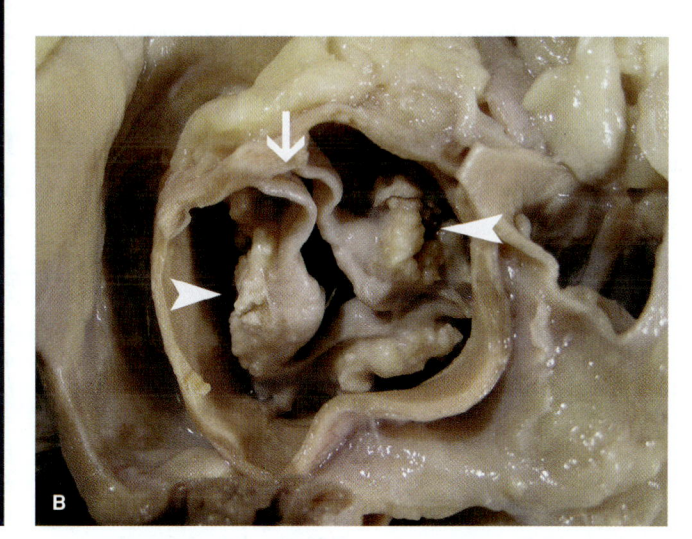

FIGURE 7-57 **Calcific aortic stenosis. (A)** Gross view of calcification of aortic valve is indicated (arrow). From Department of Pathology and Laboratory Medicine, University of North Carolina at Chapel Hill. **(B)** Congenitally bicuspid aortic valve with dystrophic calcification (arrowheads) over arterial surfaces causing stenosis. Congenital raphe is at the base of the conjoined cusp. From Kemp WL, Burns DK, Brown T. The Big Picture Pathology. New York, NY: McGraw-Hill Lange; 2008. Figure 10-24, page 125.

Histology shows destruction of the valve structure by calcification with islands of chronic inflammation and organized thrombus amidst the calcium.

Clinical features: The clinical features vary depending on the factors discussed earlier. The patients may present with angina, chest pain, fainting (syncope), dizziness, fatigue, shortness of breath, and/or symptoms of congestive heart failure. Like atherosclerotic coronary heart disease, the first symptom may be sudden death. The symptoms most commonly are exacerbated with exertion as cardiac output cannot be increased sufficiently to meet increased need. Typical angina chest pain is due to decreased cardiac output reducing flow to the coronary arteries leading to myocardial ischemia regardless of the patient's atherosclerotic state.

Physical examination demonstrates a systolic murmur at the level of the aortic valve due to the significant turbulence created by the obstruction to flow.

Patients with symptoms who are not treated have a very poor prognosis. Fifty percent (50%) of patients presenting with angina will die within 5 years without treatment. Fifty percent (50%) of patients with symptoms of congestive heart failure will die within 2 years without treatment.

Treatment: The crucial outcome of treatment is relief of the outflow obstruction accomplished by percutaneous or surgical procedures. Aortic valve replacement using either a surgical or transcatheter approach is preferred. Percutaneous valvuloplasty is an alternative palliative approach in patients with significant surgical risk.

Calcific Stenosis of a Congenitally Bicuspid Aortic Valve

Approximately 1% to 2% of the population is born with a congenitally abnormal aortic valve, making it one of the most common types of CHD. The congenitally bicuspid aortic valve may be an isolated finding or may be associated with other lesions of CHD. Bicuspid aortic valve may be transmitted in an autosomal dominant pattern, may occur sporadically, or can be seen in specific associations. Bicuspid aortic valves are commonly associated with coarctation of the aorta (50% of cases) and Turner syndrome (30% of patients).

Pathology: The normal, tricuspid aortic valve has three equal cusps and three commissures that connect the edges of the cusps to the aortic wall. The congenitally bicuspid aortic valve has two commissures with two, unequal sized cusps and a raphé (Figure 7-52). (The raphé is a seam-like ridge or seam that is found at the base of the conjoined cusp indicating the site of the abortive commissure that does not reach the aortic wall.) The right and left cusps are most frequently fused (75%–85%) with right and left commissures, creating an anterior, larger, conjoined, and posterior cusps with a central fibrous ridge (raphé) at the base of the anterior cusp. Less frequently, the right and noncoronary cusps (12%) and the left and noncoronary cusps (3%) are not separated. Of note, the coronary arteries arise from their usual, anterior locations.

The three cusps of a normal, tricuspid aortic valve completely retract to the aortic wall when open and meet in the middle of the opening when closed. The unequal size of the cusps and the fibrous ridge at the base of the conjoined cusp in the bicuspid aortic valve prevent the larger cusp from completely retracting to the aorta and from meeting the smaller cusp to close.

The valve is NOT stenotic initially; however, these hemodynamic changes cause turbulence at the level of the valve that leads to degenerative changes and calcium deposits similar to those seen with senile aortic valve stenosis. These degenerative changes and calcification occur earlier than those seen with a tricuspid valve. The gross pathology shows calcification of a valve with only two commissures and cusps (Figure 7-52B).

Clinical features: Initially, the valve causes no symptoms. On physical examination, an ejection sound or a click with a brief ejection murmur may be heard. As the stenosis worsens, the patient may exhibit the same symptoms as described earlier. Patients with a bicuspid aortic valve will **present much earlier (45–55 years of age)** compared to those with senile calcific aortic stenosis (70–80 years of age).

Treatment: Patients with a bicuspid aortic valve are routinely monitored for signs and symptoms of progressive valve dysfunction with echocardiography being performed at intervals. As patients with a bicuspid aortic valve present 10 to 20 years earlier than those with calcific aortic stenosis, the decision to proceed with surgical intervention is a significant decision. Surgical placement of a mechanical prosthetic valve leads to a life of anticoagulation therapy. Implantation of a bioprosthesis may lead to additional surgeries as the typical lifespan of the typical bioprosthesis is approximately 15 years and may be shorter in young adults.

BICUSPID AORTIC DISEASE (BAD): Patients with a congenitally bicuspid aortic valve are also known to have an increased risk for acute aortic dissection due to an inherent medial weakness. These patients require surveillance for aortic valve dysfunction and changes of the ascending thoracic aorta. In a study of the International Registry of Acute Aortic Dissection (IRAD), 9% of patients with an acute aortic dissection < 40 years old had a bicuspid aortic valve compared with 1% > 40 years old.

Mitral Valve Stenosis/Rheumatic Valvular Heart Disease

Mitral stenosis is caused by only one process: that of a postinflammatory type. Therefore, any disease process that causes inflammation of the mitral valve can lead to mitral stenosis. The disease that is most commonly associated with mitral stenosis is acute rheumatic fever (ARF) that leads to rheumatic valvular heart disease many (20–30) years later.

Acute rheumatic fever is an acute, delayed, immune-mediated multisystem inflammatory disease process that occurs 10 days to 6 weeks after a Group A β-hemolytic streptococcal (GAS) pharyngitis or "strep throat." The disease may present with multiple symptoms that can include arthritis, carditis, chorea, subcutaneous nodules, and erythema marginatum. Acute rheumatic fever can occur at any age, but most commonly affects those 5 to 15 years old.

Worldwide, there are approximately 470,000 new cases of rheumatic fever and 233,000 deaths attributable to rheumatic fever or rheumatic heart disease (RHD) each year. The incidence of ARF is approximately 19 per 100,000. Most of these cases are in developing countries where ARF and RHD are much more common and affect nearly 20 million people as the most common cause of cardiovascular death during the first five decades of life. In the United States and other developed countries, the incidence of ARF is much lower (approximately 2–4 cases per 100,000). This decreased incidence is most likely due to routine antibiotic treatment of acute pharyngitis caused by GAS.

Some studies have identified "rheumatogenic" strains of GAS implicated in outbreaks of ARF in the United States that included a few M serotypes (types 3, 5, 6, 14, 18, 19, 24, and 29). However, it appears that any streptococcal strain able to cause acute pharyngitis is capable of causing ARF.

Pathogenesis: The exact underlying mechanism of the development of ARF after GAS pharyngitis is unknown. The development of outbreaks of ARF after epidemics of streptococcal pharyngitis or scarlet fever associated with pharyngitis, the decrease of ARF with adequate treatment of GAS pharyngitis, and the fact that appropriate antimicrobial treatment prevents recurrence in patients with ARF emphasize the initiating role of bacterial infection. However, the rate of isolation of GAS from the oropharynx of patients with ARF is extremely low, even in populations without access to antibiotics. A genetic susceptibility linked to HLA-DR2 and DR4 may play a role in those who develop ARF after pharyngitis.

Streptococcal pharyngitis is the only streptococcal infection that has been associated with ARF. This may be related to the M protein of GAS strains associated with pharyngitis. Impetigo strains do colonize the pharynx; however, they do not appear to illicit as strong an immunologic reaction as pharyngitis strains.

Molecular mimicry is thought to be the underlying process by which the streptococcal pharyngitis leads to ARF. Antibodies to specific streptococcal antigens cross-react with host antigens as a result of molecular mimicry. Streptococcal M protein has been shown to share specific epitopes with cardiac myosin. A monoclonal antibody isolated from a patient with ARF was shown to cross-react with cardiac myosin, a prominent carbohydrate antigen of GAS, was cytotoxic to EC lines and reacted strongly with human valvular endothelium. In animal studies, monoclonal antibodies that cause Sydenham-like chorea (see below) also bind to the carbohydrate antigen of GAS and human lysoganglioside. Patients also have T cell clones that react with myosin, valve-derived proteins, and streptococcal M5 proteins, supporting a role for cellular immunity in the disease.

Diagnosis: The diagnosis of ARF is made clinically, most commonly in children 5 to 15 years of age. It is rare in children under 3 years and in adults. The American Heart Association has established specific criteria for the diagnosis of ARF (see Table 7-5).

Arthritis, most commonly the earliest symptom of ARF seen in 80% of patients, involves inflammation affecting several joints in a relatively short time; each is affected for days to weeks. The knees, ankles, elbows, and wrists are most common with the lower extremities usually involved first. The pain from the migratory arthritis rapidly subsides with nonsteroidal anti-inflammatory drug treatment.

Sydenham chorea (or "St. Vitus dance") can occur as late as 8 months postinfection. Patients with central nervous system manifestations may not exhibit any other symptoms, but cardiac involvement should be evaluated. The chorea presents as a series of abrupt, nonrhythmic, involuntary movements. Muscular weakness and emotional lability can also present.

Erythema marginatum is a pink or faintly red, nonpruritic rash involving the truck and extremities but not the face. The lesions extend outward from the center. Individual lesions may appear, disappear, and reappear in a matter of hours. The rash may persist or recur when all other symptoms have disappeared.

Subcutaneous nodules in ARF are firm, painless, usually symmetric lesions that vary in size and are located over boney surfaces or prominences or near tendons along extensor surfaces. In current outbreaks of ARF, only approximately 5% of patients exhibited subcutaneous nodule formation.

Acute rheumatic fever causes **a pancarditis**, affecting all layers of the heart (the epicardium, the myocardium, and the endocardium). Approximately 30% to 70% of patients with ARF have cardiac involvement with their first attack and in 73% to 90% of patients with all attacks including recurrences.

Pathology of Acute Rheumatic Fever

In the acute phase, small, uniform, fibrinous vegetations can be seen grossly along the valve surface. The myocardium most commonly appears normal. The epicardial surface may show a fibrinous pericarditis (Figure 7-58).

Histology of the acute phase of rheumatic fever shows small, 1 to 2 mm, fusiform or spherical, perivascular areas of fibrinoid necrosis with lymphoplasmacytic and macrophage inflammation known as **Aschoff nodules** (Figure 7-59). Macrophages create multinucleated giant cells and may become **Anitschkow** (or "caterpillar") cells. The Aschoff nodule (or body) is pathognomonic for ARF and can be seen in all layers of the heart.

TABLE 7-5 The American Heart Association Criteria for the Diagnosis of Acute Rheumatic Fever.

Acute rheumatic fever is characterized by group A streptococcal infection followed by clinical manifestations (major and minor) including:

- Major manifestations
  - Migratory arthritis (predominantly large joints)
  - Carditis and valvulitis (e.g., pancarditis)
  - Central nervous system involvement (e.g., Sydenham chorea)
  - Erythema marginatum
  - Subcutaneous nodules
- Minor manifestations
  - Arthralgias
  - Fever
  - Elevated acute phase reactants (erythrocyte sedimentation rate, C-reactive protein)
  - Prolonged PR interval

The diagnosis of ARF is likely in the presence of two major manifestations or one major and two minor manifestations.

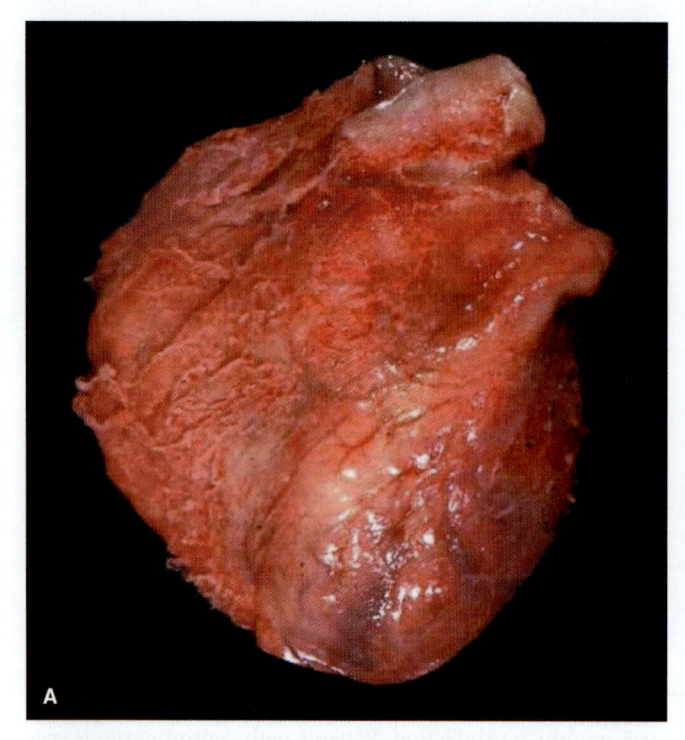

FIGURE 7-58 Acute rheumatic fever. **(A)** Rheumatic pericarditis (bread and butter pericarditis). From Department of Pathology and Laboratory Medicine, University of North Carolina at Chapel Hill.

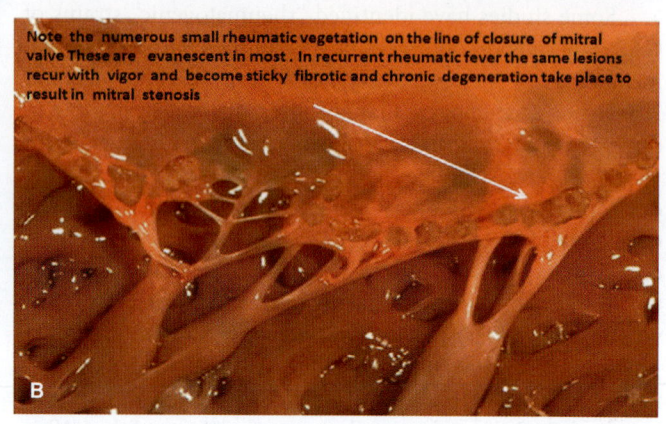

(B) Mitral valve vegetations along the line of valve closure. From Peter Anderson, D.V.M., Ph.D., PEIR Digital Library Image 1146.

Prognosis: Rheumatic heart disease is the most common and severe sequelae of ARF and can lead to severe valve scarring that develops over months to years; usually 20 to 40 years in developed countries. Symptomatic mitral stenosis can occur in those less than 20 years of age in underdeveloped countries due to ineffective use of antibiotics and/or an increased virulence of the organism. The number of patients who develop the long-term complications of RHD with a history of ARF is variable; of those who had evidence of cardiac involvement during the acute phase, approximately 50% will develop a murmur later in life as a manifestation of RHD. Rheumatic heart disease is the most frequent (99%) cause of mitral stenosis. With RHD, the mitral valve alone is most commonly affected in 65% to 70% of cases. The mitral and aortic valves are affected together in approximately 25% of cases. Rheumatic mitral stenosis is more common in women (2:1). Most patients are in their fifth to sixth decades at presentation.

Symptoms of Rheumatic Valvular Heart Disease

Patients are initially asymptomatic. The disease is slowly progressive and the mean interval between ARF and the onset of symptoms is 16 years with progression from mild to severe disability taking an average of 9 years. The resultant mitral stenosis causes a significant pressure gradient between the left atrium and ventricle in diastole. The elevated left atrial pressure and volume is reflected backwards into the lungs causing an increase in pulmonary venous, capillary, and arterial pressures and resistance (pulmonary hypertension). Over time, the right ventricle becomes hypertrophic secondary to the increased vascular resistance.

Once patients are symptomatic, there is no more than a 15% 10-year survival rate without treatment. Patients develop signs and symptoms of shortness of breath (dyspnea), fatigue, pulmonary edema, hemoptysis (coughing up of blood), thromboembolus, and right heart failure if the disease follows its natural course. Overall mortality increases as the patients' functional status decreases. Poor prognosis indicators include

FIGURE 7-59 Aschoff body with Anitschkow cells (arrow). From Department of Pathology and Laboratory Medicine, University of North Carolina at Chapel Hill.

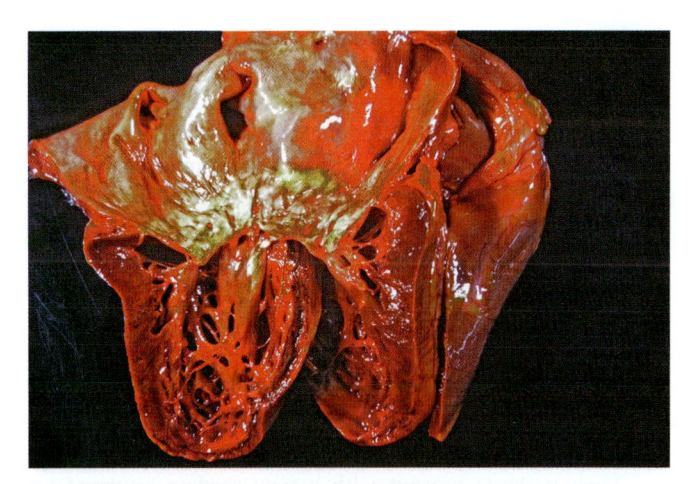

FIGURE 7-60 Gross pathology of rheumatic heart disease. Left ventricle has been cut open to display characteristic severe thickening of mitral valve leading to stenosis, thickened, fused leaflets and chordae tendineae showing scarring and calcification.
From Department of Pathology and Laboratory Medicine, University of North Carolina at Chapel Hill.

atrial fibrillation and progression to severe pulmonary hypertension. The mean survival of patients with pulmonary hypertension who did not undergo surgical repair was 2 years.

Pathology of rheumatic valve disease: Grossly, the valves are markedly scarred and thickened with fusion of the commissures with areas of calcification. The chordae tendineae are markedly shortened and fused. Due to the distorted shape of the valve orifice, it has been likened to a fish mouth, wedding ring, or sewing bobbin. If involved, the aortic valve will show marked fibrotic scarring, thickening, commissural fusion, and mild calcification (**Figure 7-60**). The valve histology shows marked fibrosis with loss of typical valve layers, scattered collections of chronic inflammation, and infiltration by thin- and thick-walled blood vessels.

Treatment: Pure mitral regurgitation is usually well tolerated, and the patients can remain asymptomatic for years. Signs and/or symptoms of left ventricular systolic dysfunction in patients with severe mitral regurgitation are indications for surgical replacement or repair. Mitral stenosis patients need to be evaluated for treatment as soon as symptoms develop. Percutaneous mitral balloon valvuloplasty (PMBV) is preferable to surgery in patients with favorable valve features. Patients undergoing PMBV have excellent results. Surgical repair or valve replacement is indicated in patients with moderate to severe mitral stenosis with moderate to severe regurgitation, persistent left atrial thrombus or valve morphology not favorable for PMBV.

Causes of Acquired Valvular Insufficiency

As discussed earlier, valvular insufficiency may be due to a primary valve abnormality or due to changes in valve support structures/geometry (secondary insufficiency). Causes of valve insufficiency that will be discussed include infective endocarditis, mitral valve prolapse, and carcinoid heart disease.

Infective Endocarditis

Several factors need to be considered when discussing infective endocarditis, including the types of organisms involved, the prior state of the valve, the condition of the patient, and the source of the infection. Infective endocarditis is separated into the following categories:

- Native valve endocarditis (NVE): By definition, the infective process forms on a native valve. NVE is subdivided into acute and subacute types.
- Prosthetic valve endocarditis (PVE): The infective process forms on a prosthetic valve. PVE is subdivided into early and late types.
- Intravenous drug abuse endocarditis: The infective process is associated with intravenous drug abuse.
- Health-care associated infective endocarditis (HCIE): The infective process is associated with recent health-care treatment or exposure. HCIE includes all non-hospital health-care environments.
- Nosocomial infective endocarditis (NIE): Defined as infective endocarditis that manifests within 48 hours of hospitalization, or that is associated with a hospital (such as a procedure done within 4 weeks of onset of symptoms).

Varieties of infective endocarditis (IE) that were uncommon in the early antibiotic era are becoming more common. Current changes in underlying valvular pathology and the significant increase in the number of intravascular procedures and devices have changed the types of and clinical presentation of IE. In the United States, 10,000 to 15,000 new cases of IE are diagnosed each year. The incidence rates for IE range from 0.6 to 6.0 cases per 100,000 person-years. Several factors have been identified that increase the risk of IE including:

- **Age >60 years.** More than 50% of IE cases occur in persons in this age group. It is felt that this is due to the change in the underlying cause of valve pathology from RHD to degenerative valve disease. As RHD has become less frequent in the United States, the number of cases of RHD-associated IE has decreased significantly from 39% to 6%. The number of patients with degenerative valve disease has replaced RHD as the primary underlying valve pathology leading to IE with approximately 50% of IE patients having calcific aortic stenosis (see earlier) as their underlying pathology.
- **Male gender.** Men are more frequently affected with IE with ratios varying from 3:2 to 9:1.
- **Intravenous drug abuse (IVDA).** IVDA increases the risk of IE due to the seeding of blood by bacteria from the skin and/or organisms that contaminate the drug or paraphernalia injected directly into the bloodstream. Some illicit drugs directly injure vascular endothelium predisposing to subsequent infection.
- **Poor dentition and dental infections.** Due to the significant bacterial numbers found in the mouth of these patients, this is a presumed risk. Routine dental cleaning does not have an increased risk for IE; however, dental surgeries that involve manipulation of the gingiva and perforation of the oral

mucosa can increase the IE risk. Patients with underlying structural heart disease or prosthetic valves should receive antibiotics pretreatment for invasive dental procedures.
- Comorbidities that significantly increase the risk for IE include:
  - **Structural heart disease:** Approximately 75% of patients have structural heart disease at the time they develop IE.
  - **Valvular disease:** Mitral valve prolapse (see later) with regurgitation or mitral annular calcification has an increased risk for IE. Mitral prolapse was the underlying cardiac lesion in about 25% of cases. The risk of IE in patients with mitral valve prolapse with regurgitation is five to eight times higher than patients with a normal mitral valve. However, patients with MVP without regurgitation have only a slightly increased risk of IE. Aortic valve disease is present in 12% to 30% of cases.
  - **CHD:** Aortic stenosis, bicuspid aortic valve, VSD, patent ductus arteriosus, and coarctation of the aorta are the CHDs most associated with an increased risk of IE. IE occurred most frequently in cases of VSDs and aortic stenosis.
  - **Prosthetic valves:** Prosthetic valve endocarditis accounts for 10% to 20% of cases of IE. Eventually, 5% of all prosthetic valves will develop IE.

Pathophysiology: All cases of IE arise from a common process. Cardiac abnormalities lead to hemodynamic dysfunction and endothelial injury. Endothelial injury, indwelling catheters, or prosthetic valves are sites predisposed to the formation of sterile fibrin thrombi. The introduction of bacteria into the blood through dental, medical, or surgical procedures, a preexisting infection elsewhere or injection of contaminated materials (bacteremia), allows the bacteria to settle on the valve with subsequent development of endocarditis. The organisms that most frequently cause IE possess a specific fibronectin receptor that is expressed on the surface of platelet-fibrin thrombi.

A large variety of microorganisms cause infective endocarditis with *Staphylococci* and *Streptococci* responsible for the majority of the cases. Viridans streptococci, a usually indolent group of normal oral flora, are seen in 50% to 60% of IE in patients with a preexisting cardiac abnormality. Viridans streptococci account for a total of 17% of total IE cases. *Staphylococcus aureus*, a usual skin inhabitant, is much more virulent and can attack deformed and previously normal valves. *Staphylococcus aureus*, responsible for approximately 30% of the total cases of IE, is the most common organism in IE occurring in intravenous drug use. The virulence of *S. aureus* is related to its production of destructive enzymes and adherence factors, and its ability to directly invade ECs (endotheliosis) where it can increase the cell's production of adhesion molecules and procoagulant factors. Other organisms known to cause IE include enterococci, HACEK group (*Haemophilus, Actinobacillus, Cardiobacterium, Eikenella,* and *Kingella*), all oral flora, gram-negative bacilli, rickettsiae, chlamydia, and fungi. In approximately 10% of cases, no organism can be isolated from the blood ("culture-negative" endocarditis) due to prior antibiotic treatment or difficulty in isolating the offender.

Clinical features: Infective endocarditis has been classified into an acute or subacute process based on the acuity and severity of the clinical course. The two types are distinguished by the virulence of the organism and the presence (or absence) of a preexisting cardiac abnormality. In **acute infective endocarditis**, the patient appears gravely ill with fevers, chills, and weakness due to a highly virulent organism affecting a previously normal cardiac valve. These patients suffer significant morbidity and mortality even with appropriate treatment including surgery. In **subacute IE**, the patients may present with nonspecific symptoms including weight loss, arthralgias, myalgias, and intermittent fevers.

Most patients present with a new cardiac murmur on physical examination (found in 90% of patients with left-sided lesions) and with stigmata of emboli including splinter hemorrhages of the fingernails, petechial hemorrhages, small (few millimeters), nodular, nontender lesions of the palms or soles (Janeway nodules), Osler nodes (painful, red lesions of the palms and soles due to immune complex deposition), and Roth spots (retinal hemorrhages). The diagnosis is confirmed with blood cultures positive for organisms that typically cause IE (those listed earlier) and echocardiographic findings.

Pathology: Friable, bulky growths (vegetations) are seen on the valve surface in all forms of the disease (Figure 7-61). The mitral and aortic valves are the most commonly affected sites of infection. The tricuspid valve may frequently be infected in IE due to intravenous drug abuse. The vegetative growths can be single or multiple and may involve more than one valve. The bacterial collections can erode through the valve leading to insufficiency or through the valve annulus leading to an abscess cavity (ring abscess); these complications are more likely with more virulent organisms. Due to the friable nature of the vegetations, fragments can embolize to distant organs. As there are large numbers of bacteria in the emboli, abscesses can form in these distant sites leading to the formation of septic infarcts or mycotic aneurysms.

Histology of the vegetations in active or acute endocarditis shows dense collections of bacteria, fibrin, platelets, and acute inflammation. In subacute endocarditis, histology may show evidence of healing or organization with chronic inflammation and fibrosis.

Prognosis: Complications due to IE are not uncommon with 57% of patients suffering at least one complication. Cardiac complications are the most frequent including heart failure, perivalvular abscess, pericarditis, and aortic mycotic aneurysm formation. Embolization of fragments of the vegetation is a common complication of IE. Several studies have shown that the risk of systemic embolization decreases after effective treatment has begun. Predictors of embolization include size of the vegetation (>10 mm), significant mobility of the vegetation, left-sided versus right-sided vegetation, microorganism type, and location on the valve.

Left untreated, infective endocarditis is generally fatal. With appropriate, long-term (6 weeks or more) antibiotic

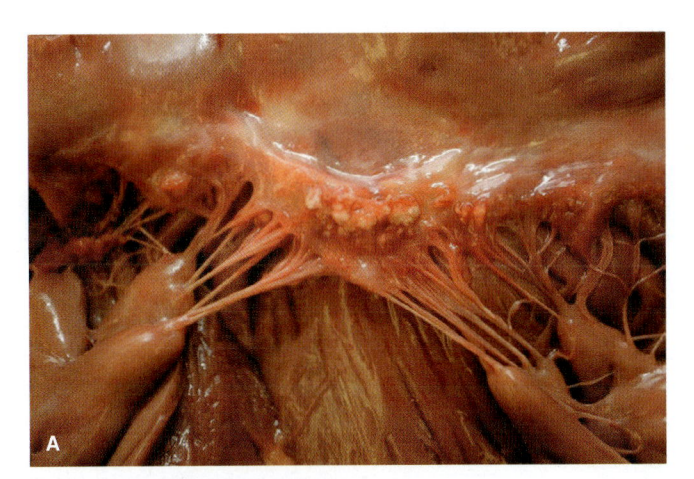

FIGURE 7-61 Bacterial endocarditis. **(A)** Gross view of vegetations on mitral valve composed of bacterial colonies and fibrin. From Karen Kelly MD Department of Pathology ECU Medical School

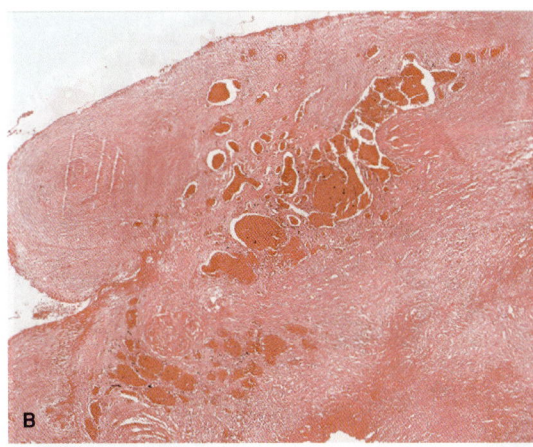

(B) Microscopic view of compacted fibrin and bacterial colonies on a damaged mitral valve. From Department of Pathology and Laboratory Medicine, University of North Carolina at Chapel Hill.

therapy and/or surgical management, morbidity and mortality are lessened. Multiple studies have shown an in-hospital mortality of between 18% and 23% with a 6-month mortality of between 22% and 27%. Increased mortality is associated with increased age, aortic valve involvement, congestive heart failure, central nervous system complications, and underlying disease (e.g., diabetes mellitus). The type of microorganism is also predictive of mortality: *S. aureus* infection, not due to intravenous drug abuse, is associated with a higher mortality rate (30%–40%). Streptococcal infective endocarditis is associated with a 10% mortality rate.

Streptococcal (*Streptococcus viridans* and *Streptococcus bovis*) infections have a 98% cure rate with appropriate medical and surgical therapies. Enterococci and *S. aureus* (in IVDA) infective endocarditis have a 90% cure rate. The cure rate for IE on prosthetic valve is approximately 10% to 20% lower.

Noninfective Endocarditis

No cardiovascular pathology section can be complete without the discussion of noninfective endocarditis.

***Nonbacterial Thrombotic Endocarditis* (NBTE)** is characterized by the presence of multiple, small (1–5 mm) masses of fibrin and platelets along the line of closure of valves (Figure 7-62). Histology of these lesions shows an admixture of platelets and fibrin without inflammation or organisms. These sterile, nondestructive lesions are most commonly found in patients with an underlying malignancy, burns, and disseminated intravascular coagulation. It is thought that the hypercoagulable state of these diseases leads to deposition of fibrin and platelets onto the valve. While the lesions are locally not significant, they have the potential for embolization leading to systemic complications. They are also a rich nidus for the development of infective endocarditis. If the lesions heal, there are no long-term sequelae to the valve.

***Endocarditis of SLE* (or Libman–Sacks Endocarditis)** primarily affects the tricuspid and mitral valves in patients with systemic lupus erythematosis (SLE). Like NBTE, these vegetations are composed of sterile, 1- to 4-mm, pink, granular masses. They are located adjacent to areas of inflammation and fibrinoid necrosis associated with immune complex deposition. These lesions can occur on any portion of the valve, on the chords, or over the atrial endocardial surfaces. As the immune complex deposition causes valve injury, healing and scarring can lead to valve deformity similar to rheumatic valve disease.

Mitral Valve Prolapse

Myxomatous degeneration of the mitral valve (mitral valve prolapse) is the most common valve abnormality, affecting approximately 2% to 3% of the population in the United States. Women are slightly more commonly affected than men and the disease is found in all ages. Mitral valve prolapse is most commonly sporadic,

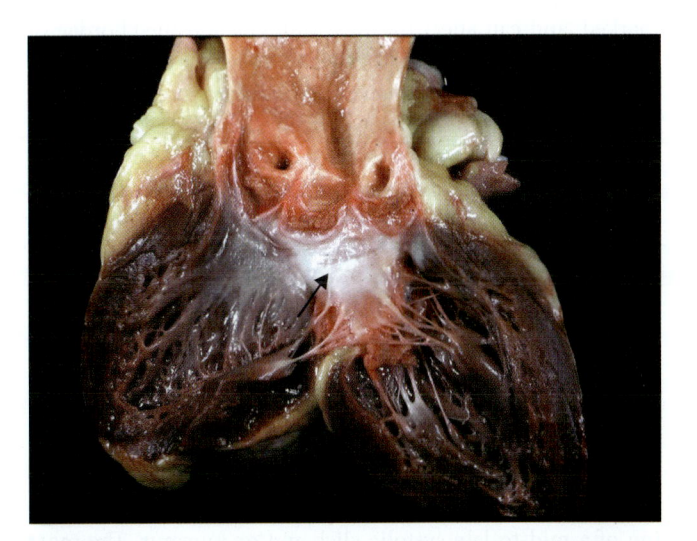

FIGURE 7-62 Nonbacterial thrombotic endocarditis (NBTE). Note the presence of multiple small masses of fibrin and platelets visible along the line of valve closure (arrow). From Department of Pathology and Laboratory Medicine, University of North Carolina at Chapel Hill.

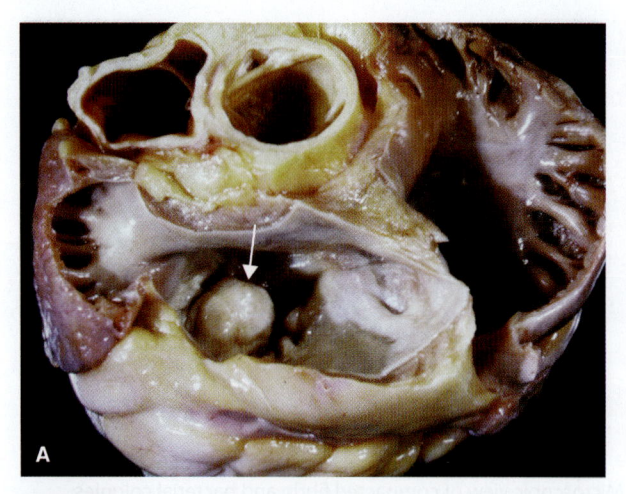

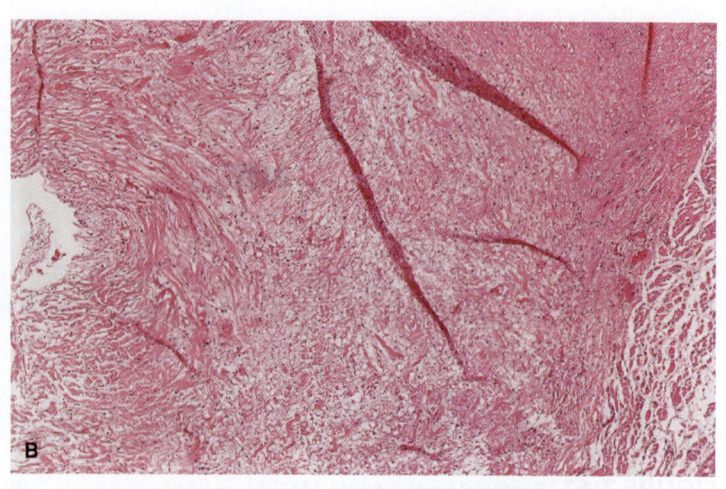

FIGURE 7-63 Mitral valve prolapse. **(A)** Billowing leaflet as seen from the left atrium (arrow). **(B)** Focal myxomatous change in the prolapsed mitral valve. From Department of Pathology and Laboratory Medicine, University of North Carolina at Chapel Hill.

although familial cases are inherited in an autosomal dominant pattern with incomplete penetrance. Three loci have been mapped to chromosomes 16, 11, and 13, although the genetic defects are currently unknown. X-linked transmission has also been described. The majority of patients (90%) with mitral valve prolapse are asymptomatic with a benign prognosis and normal life expectancy.

Pathogenesis: The specific mechanism of primary myxomatous degeneration is unknown, however, it is believed to be associated with an underlying intrinsic connective tissue abnormality. It is currently thought that isolated myxomatous degeneration of the mitral valve is one end along the spectrum of connective tissue diseases with Marfan syndrome, Ehlers–Danlos syndrome, osteogenesis imperfecta, and pseudoxanthoma elasticum at the "most affected" end. In the inherited form of the disease, the increased deposits of glycosaminoglycans are generalized throughout the valve structure, may be marked, and can affect the valve annulus and the chordae of the atrioventricular valves. In the most severe cases, the deposition of increased myxomatous material can affect all cardiac valves. Most commonly, however, the left-sided (specifically the mitral valve) valves are affected.

Secondary myxomatous degeneration is often focal, but can be more generalized in some cases. Due to abnormal hemodynamics, the added stress and stain can lead to a reactive deposition of myxomatous material within the valve leaflets. These changes can be seen in any situation that leads to abnormal valve function, including secondary chronic insufficiency due to ventricular dilatation or dysfunction due to ventricular outflow obstruction.

Clinical features: The majority of patients with MVP are asymptomatic with the valve abnormality found incidentally on physical examination with the classic auscultatory finding of a mid-to-late systolic click and/or murmur. The most common complications of mitral valve prolapse include severe mitral valve regurgitation, infective endocarditis, embolic events, and sudden death. Conventional wisdom has long known that "mitral regurgitation begets mitral regurgitation." Mitral regurgitation will continue to worsen eventually leading to congestive heart failure. The chordae tendineae of the valve structure can also be affected by the increased myxomatous deposition, leading to increased weakness and the possibility of rupture. The sudden onset of severe mitral regurgitation may be seen in patients who suffer from a ruptured chord.

Pathology: Generally, the mitral leaflets are thickened, redundant, hooded, or ballooned with a glistening, myxoid gross appearance **(Figure 7-63A)**. The cut surface shows a moist, gelatinous, gray thickening of the leaflets. The hooded or ballooned leaflets may bulge toward the atrium (Figure 7-57). Fibrin thrombi may be seen over the atrial surface of the valve leaflets. Chordae tendineae may be elongated and thinned. Ruptured chords may show thin, whisker-like ends that may reattach to the valve or other chords. The end of a ruptured chord may also appear bulbous and retracted. In the presence of a ruptured chord, there may be focal areas of endocardial thickening of the left atrium in the area of the "jet lesion." The presence of a ruptured chord allows focal regurgitation at its site that can "jet" into the left atrium. The repeated injury caused endocardial thickening of the left atrium opposite the ruptured chord.

Histology of mitral valve prolapse shows widening of the spongiosa or middle, flexible layer of the valve by increased amounts of glycosaminoglycan and loss of normal collagen and elastic fibers (Figure 7-57B). This myxomatous material also invades and disrupts the underlying fibrosa. The interruption and disruption of the fibrosa create a more flexible leaflet with wider excursion and less stability.

Calcification of the Mitral Valve Annulus

Calcification at the mitral valve annulus is a common condition frequently seen in women more than 60 years of age. The deposition of dystrophic calcium can be seen easily on chest radiograph. This calcification usually does not cause symptoms as it does not usually affect valve function. On cut section, a

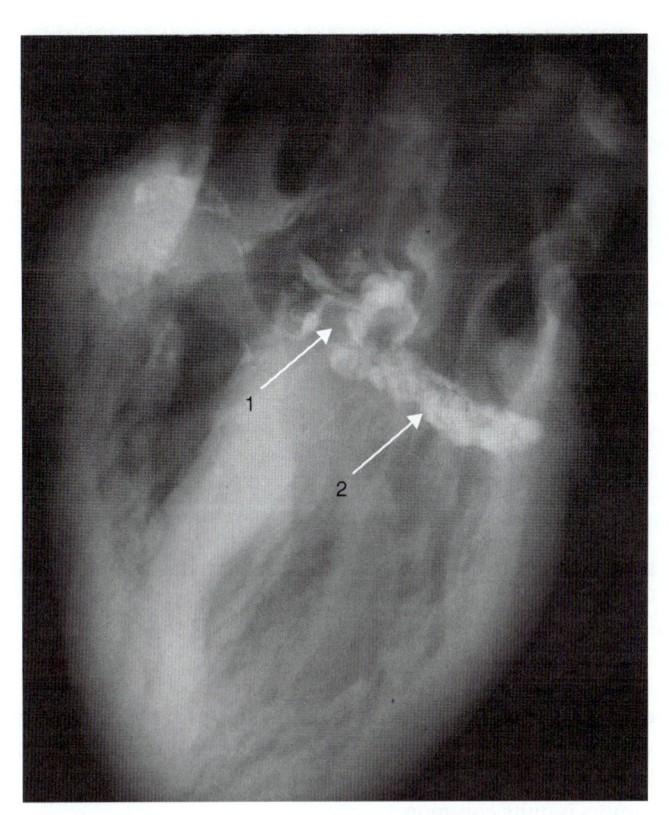

FIGURE 7-64 **Annular calcification of the mitral valve.** A radiograph of annular calcification of the mitral valve ring (arrow 2), an aging phenomenon that can cause mitral regurgitation. Age-related calcification of the aortic valve is also present (arrow 1). From Department of Pathology and Laboratory Medicine, University of North Carolina at Chapel Hill.

mass of yellow-white calcium is seen at the mitral annulus beneath the posterior mitral valve leaflet. This calcium deposition may occasionally cause retraction of the posterior leaflet and lead to valve insufficiency (Figure 7-64).

Carcinoid Valve/Heart Disease

Carcinoid heart disease occurs frequently in patients who have a carcinoid tumor of the gastrointestinal tract with metastases of organs that drain directly into the systemic venous circulation. The clinically significant endocardial and valve lesions are usually limited to the right heart affecting the tricuspid and pulmonary valves. Tricuspid regurgitation and pulmonary stenosis are most common, although the valve dysfunction is usually mixed. If the disease is inoperable, the carcinoid heart disease is often fatal. Grossly, the tricuspid valve shows thickening of the ventricular valve surface. The pulmonary valve shows thickening of the arterial face of the cusps. Histology shows normal valve layers with "stuck-on" plaques that are rich in proteoglycans. Older lesions are composed of dense collagen.

While the specific mechanism of the formation of the valve changes is unknown, it has been shown that patients with carcinoid heart disease have higher levels of plasma serotonin (5-hydroxytryptamine) and urinary 5-HIAA (5-hydroxyindole acetic acid, the main metabolite of serotonin) than those without cardiac effects. Other potential vasoactive substances that are elevated include neuropeptide K, substance P, and atrial natriuretic peptide. Of interest, the morphologic features of carcinoid heart disease are similar to those seen in patients taking methylsergide, ergot derivatives, and phentermine-fenfluramine. These drugs have also been shown to elevate plasma serotonin levels.

Prosthetic Heart Valves

Two types of prosthetic heart valves are currently in use: mechanical prosthesis and bioprosthetic valves. Each of the prosthetic valves has its advantages and disadvantages in replacing native valves.

The mechanical valve prosthesis is more durable than the bioprosthetic valve and has an expected durability of 20 to 30 years. Due to their construction, mechanical valves have areas of stasis. This stasis combined with the nonphysiologic surfaces potentiates thrombus formation, requiring patients with mechanical valves to receive lifetime anticoagulation therapy to lessen the risk of thromboembolic complications.

Bioprosthetic valves have cusps composed of human or animal valve or nonvalve tissue. The chemically preserved heterograft tissues have stable, several-year shelf lives with minimization of immunologic reactions. As the hemodynamics of a bioprosthetic valve are similar to a native valve, patients do not require lifetime anticoagulation, providing a viable option for patients in whom anticoagulation is contraindicated. Xenograft and allograft bioprostheses have been shown to have a higher rate of degeneration with a durability of approximately 15 years. In patients <65 years of age, the degeneration occurs more quickly and reoperation may be required.

Complications of valve prostheses include thrombosis, thromboembolus, bleeding events, prosthetic valve infective endocarditis, structural valve deterioration, and valve stenosis due to exuberant tissue reactivity.

CARDIAC TUMORS

While cardiac tumors are infrequent and are rarely identified at autopsy (prevalence of 0.02% to 0.25%), they are often surgically resected as primary lesions. Surgical pathologists are thus required to make a histologic diagnosis of these cardiac masses. Cardiac tumors may be symptomatic or may be identified incidentally on examination for seemingly unrelated findings. The majority of cardiac tumors are benign, but due to their ability to impair cardiac function, the likelihood of embolization and possible conduction system involvement, they require prompt evaluation and treatment.

Cardiac Myxoma

The cardiac myxoma, the most common tumor of the adult heart, is a distinctive tumor that arises exclusively in the endocardium, usually near the fossa ovalis. The cell of origin of the myxoma is unknown, but myxoma cells display

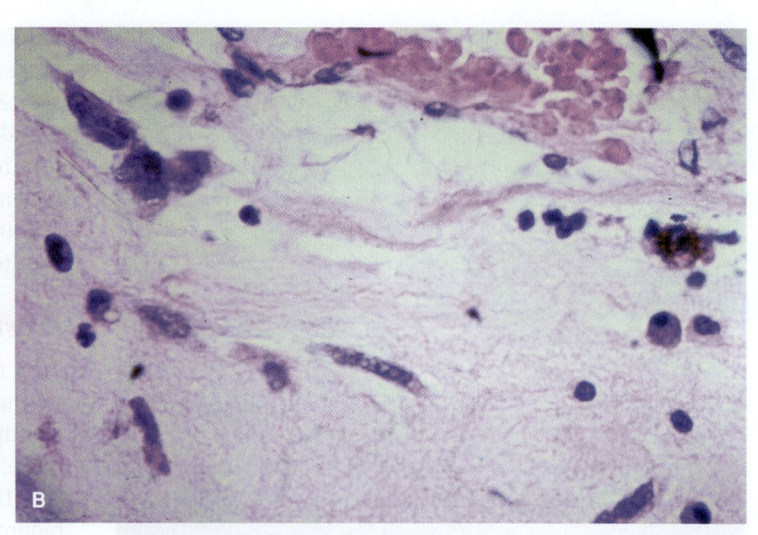

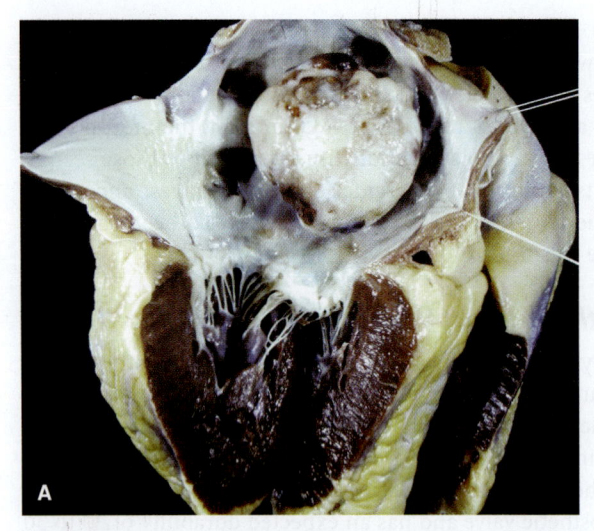

FIGURE 7-65 Cardiac myxoma. (A) Gross view shows a gelatinous tumor attached by a stalk to the left atrium. The tumor nearly fills the atrium. **(B)** A micrograph demonstrates the myxoid structure of the tumor and the stellate cells which characterize it. From Department of Pathology and Laboratory Medicine, University of North Carolina at Chapel Hill.

pluripotentiality and express a variety of antigens. It is believed that myxoma cells originate from mesenchymal elements capable of differentiating into neural and endothelial components. The tumors are composed of a variety of cellular elements including stromal and inflammatory cells.

Clinical features: Cardiac myxomas most commonly present in middle-aged patients (>50 years of age). Women are more frequently affected then men (6–7:1). The clinical features of a cardiac myxoma will depend on the tumor's location. Symptoms are usually related to flow obstruction, embolization, and/or elaboration of hormonal elements. Approximately 67% of patients present with cardiovascular symptoms suggestive of mitral valve dysfunction including palpitations, syncope, congestive heart failure, or sudden death. Auscultation abnormalities are found in up to 64% of patients. The classic "plop" is infrequent (<15%). Up to 33% of patients suffer from systemic embolization with 20% having neurologic defects. While women are more frequently affected by myxomas, men with the tumor are more likely to suffer from embolization. Various cell types in the tumor produce multiple humoral elements including growth factors and cytokines that can lead to significant nonspecific constitutional symptoms in up to 64% of patients such as weight loss, fever, myalgias, and arthralgias, symptoms which can be mistaken for a connective tissue disorder.

Echocardiography plays a fundamental role in diagnosis of cardiac myxomas. Once the diagnosis is established, surgical intervention should occur promptly due to the risk of embolization. Surgery is curative in the majority of cases. Recurrence can occur in 2% to 5% of patients. Those with recurrent tumors should be evaluated for the possibility of familial occurrence.

Pathology: Cardiac myxomas most frequently arise from the endocardium of the left atrium (75%). The remainder of the tumors arise in the right atrium and rarely in the ventricles. The tumors vary largely in size (from 1 to 15 cm and 15 to 180 g) and arise from a stalk near the fossa ovalis of the atrium. The external gross appearance may be smooth, shiny, friable, or villous. (Figure 7-59A) The 35% of villous and friable tumors have a higher likelihood of embolization. Calcification of the tumors is quite common.

Histology of the tumor shows extensive cellular heterogeneity with scarring, thrombosis, and hemorrhage. The diagnostic element is the polygonal, stellate myxoma cell that frequently forms cords, nests, or rings in a loose myxoid stroma containing abundant proteoglycans (Figure 7-65B). Toward the endothelial surface, the myxoma cells are often associated with capillaries. A rare number of tumors contain glandular elements that appear and stain identically to intestinal glands. Calcification, scarring, and metaplastic bone can be seen. Hemorrhage and organizing thrombus are frequent and can be a helpful diagnostic feature.

Carney complex: Ten percent of cardiac myxomas are seen in this autosomal dominant disorder characterized by multiple tumors including atrial and extracardiac myxomas, schwannomas, and endocrine tumors. The cardiac myxomas in these patients are typically found earlier and have a high tendency to recur. Patients with this disease also have pigmentation abnormalities including pigmented lentigines and blue nevi on the sclerae, face, lips, neck, and trunk. The most frequent endocrine disease is primary pigmented nodular adrenocortical disease. The diagnosis of this disease requires two or more major manifestations.

Cardiac Sarcomas

Primary malignant tumors are unusual in the heart and comprise approximately 15% of tumors. Malignant sarcomas are most common. Like benign cardiac tumors, the symptoms of malignant cardiac tumors depend on the size and location of the tumor, rather than the tissue type. Rhabdomyosarcomas make up approximately 20% of malignant sarcomas of the heart, occur most often in adults, and are usually multifocal.

Angiosarcomas are composed of malignant cells that form vascular spaces and arise primarily in the right atrium. Rare fibrosarcomas are white, fleshy masses that replace the ventricular myocardium made up of spindled cells. Areas of necrosis and hemorrhage can be seen with fibrosarcomas.

Sarcomatous tumors of the heart proliferate rapidly causing myocardial replacement and can lead to widespread metastatic disease. If the tumor is surgically resected, the patients may die of recurrence and most have a 6- to 12-month life expectancy. Other modalities including adjuvant chemotherapy and cardiac transplantation have been used to extend patients' lives.

Secondary Cardiac Tumors

Secondary tumor metastases involve the heart 100 times more often than primary cardiac tumors. Tumors metastasize to the heart by direct extension, lymphatic invasion, and vascular seeding. The solid tumors that most commonly involve the heart include lung and breast cancers, soft-tissue sarcomas, renal cell carcinoma, esophageal cancer, hepatocellular carcinoma, and thyroid cancer. Interestingly, there are several malignancies that preferentially metastasize to the heart including leukemias, lymphomas, and malignant melanoma. The cardiac involvement and its subsequent symptoms may lead to the initial diagnosis of disease. As with other cardiac tumors, patients' symptoms will depend on location and severity of tumor involvement. Tumor metastases affect the right side of the heart in 25% to 30% and the left side of the heart in 10% to 33% and are diffuse or bilateral in 30% to 35% of cases.

PERICARDIAL DISEASES

The pericardium is a fibroelastic tissue sac surrounding the heart. The **fibrous pericardium** is the outermost layer, which anchors the heart to the mediastinum. The **serous pericardium** is composed of a single layer of mesothelium lining the pericardial cavity. It is divided into the **parietal layer** applied to the inner face of the fibrous pericardium and the **visceral layer** (epicardium) immediately external to the heart surface. The pericardial cavity normally contains a small amount of serous fluid (20–30 mm). Because of the limited elasticity of the fibrous pericardium, accumulation of larger amounts of fluid can result in **cardiac tamponade** (Figure 7-9B), mechanical compression of the heart limiting normal cardiac movement (see later). *Diseases of the pericardium are associated with diseases of the heart or surrounding structures or secondary to systemic disease processes. Isolated pericardial disease is unusual* (Figure 7-66).

Acute Pericarditis

Primary pericarditis is uncommon and is usually caused by viral infection and may be associated with coexistent myocarditis. In most cases, acute pericarditis is secondary to cardiac disorders including acute transmural myocardial infarct, thoracic or systemic disorders (SLE, rheumatoid arthritis (RA)), radiation, metastatic tumors, or postoperative trauma. One common cause is uremia in patients with chronic kidney disease. Acute pericarditis most often resolves completely without sequelae. Rarely, it may lead to pericardial effusion in reaction to the inflammation or results in pericardial adhesions (scar).

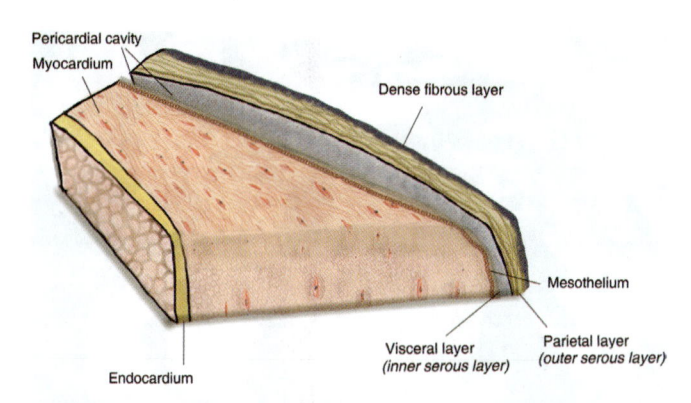

FIGURE 7-66 The anatomy of the pericardium. From Department of Pathology and Laboratory Medicine, University of North Carolina at Chapel Hill.

Clinical symptoms of acute pericarditis usually present as chest pain (not related to exertion) that worsens with lying flat and is relieved with sitting forward. A prominent friction rub is heard with auscultation.

Pathology: Gross examination of a heart with acute pericarditis due to viral infection or uremia shows a shaggy, irregular, ragged pericardial surface ("bread and butter" pericarditis). Bacterial infection will result in a purulent pericarditis with frank pus. Bacterial infections can involve the pericardial space by direct extension, seeding of the blood, lymphatic extension, and direct introduction. Pericarditis associated with tuberculosis infection may demonstrate areas of caseation. Histology of a viral-associated acute pericarditis shows altered fibrin material admixed with acute inflammatory cells (neutrophils). The other types will show changes consistent with their underlying etiology (Figure 7-58B).

Hemorrhagic pericarditis is seen occasionally in patients with malignant metastases or postoperative trauma. In these cases, the pericarditis is invested with numerous vascular elements that can bleed freely and can rarely lead to a hemopericardium.

Pericardial effusion is a collection of fluid in the pericardial space that can vary in composition depending on the underlying disease process. The fluid can be composed of clear, straw-colored fluid (effusion), blood (hemopericardium), or infectious/purulent fluid. The most important factors in the patient's ability to tolerate a pericardial effusion are the volume of the fluid and its rate of accumulation. Massive fluid accumulations can be long tolerated, if it occurs slowly over time. If the fluid accumulation is rapid, even a small volume of fluid cannot be tolerated and rapidly leads to cardiovascular symptoms.

In patients with congestive heart failure, pericardial effusions can accumulate over a long period of time. Radiographs may show a markedly enlarged cardiac silhouette due to large pericardial fluid accumulations. Patients with rupture of an acute myocardial

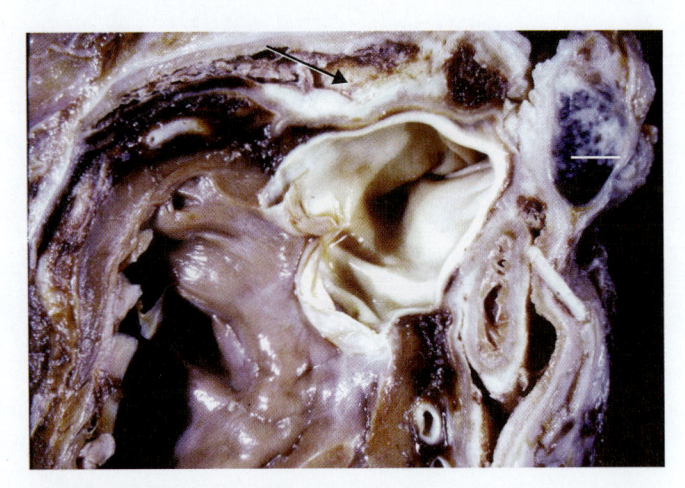

FIGURE 7-67 Constrictive pericarditis. Adult heart showing a late stage of tuberculous pericarditis. The pericardial space is widened and contains areas of caseation (arrow). A tuberculous node is also present (line). From Department of Pathology and Laboratory Medicine, University of North Carolina at Chapel Hill.

infarct or aortic dissection can suffer from a *hemopericardium*. The rapid accumulation of a small volume of blood (200–300 mL) into the inelastic pericardial sac causes *cardiac tamponade* and sudden death. The blood within the pericardial sac compresses the inferior and superior vena cavae preventing blood return into the right heart. The blood surrounding the heart also causes compression preventing relaxation during diastole and influx of blood into the heart. Cardiac output is affected, decreasing blood flow to the brain, leading to collapse.

Constrictive Pericarditis

Constrictive pericarditis involves encasement of the heart by dense fibrosis and/or fibrocalcific scar (concretio cordis) that prevents diastolic relaxation and decreases cardiac output (Figure 7-67). The condition is often a result of a chronic inflammatory process, potentially the sequelae of acute disease. Clinically, this process may appear similar to restrictive and hypertrophic obstructive cardiomyopathic processes. During the cardiac work-up, these diseases must be excluded as their treatment is significantly different. Treatment of constrictive pericarditis is surgical resection of the pericardium resulting in complete resolution of symptoms. Historically, tuberculosis was the most common cause of constrictive pericarditis. The most frequent cause of constrictive pericarditis is now idiopathic in 50% of cases. Radiation therapy to the chest and cardiothoracic surgery also may produce constrictive pericarditis.

CHAPTER 8

Pulmonary Pathology

William K. Funkhouser, M.D., Ph.D.

NORMAL LUNG ANATOMY AND PHYSIOLOGY

Normal Lung Development

Normal adult lung is a sophisticated system of conducting airways and gas exchange surfaces. The foregut develops a ventral outpouching that progressively bifurcates to create branch points ("carinas") for conducting airways (bronchi, then bronchioles, then alveolar ducts). Conducting airways form during the "pseudoglandular" phase by 15 weeks' gestational age, and proto-alveoli are evident in loose mesenchyme during the "canalicular" phase by 24 weeks' gestational age. The mesenchyme is progressively excluded or flattened between developing alveoli, such that an adult lung has back-to-back alveolar airspaces separated by elastin-rich, capillary-rich interstitial stroma.

In parallel with the development of the functional adult lung structure, the critical type II epithelial cell matures and begins to excrete surfactant, a natural detergent that breaks the water tension of the thin layer of water that covers the alveolar wall. Without type II cell surfactant, the newborn cannot generate enough mechanical force to inflate the alveoli, and will rapidly fatigue and arrest. *The probability of surfactant deficiency varies inversely with fetal age, such that surfactant deficiency will be seen in >50% of fetuses <28 weeks' gestational age. The fetal age at which 95% of fetuses can ventilate normally after delivery is 36 weeks.* Fetuses delivered before that age are monitored aggressively and treated promptly with synthetic surfactant if they have persistent atelectasis (collapse of lung tissue) and begin to tire.

Adult Lung Anatomy

The anatomy of the adult lung is best described starting at the larynx and proceeding toward the alveoli. The *trachea* and *bronchi* are encircled by near-circumferential cartilage rings that prevent collapse of these large-caliber airways during the expiratory phase of the ventilatory cycle. These airways show lush surface cilia and submucosal glands that excrete mucin. Moving distally in the conducting airways, the cartilage rings and submucosal glands are lost; these small-caliber airways are called *bronchioles*. Like the trachea and bronchi, bronchioles have lush surface cilia. The bronchi and bronchioles run adjacent to pulmonary artery branches of similar caliber. *Alveolar ducts* lose the cilia, as one enters the grapelike clusters of *alveoli*, the critically important sites for countercurrent exchange of inhaled O_2 and RBC-bound CO_2. Incomplete ridges subdivide this surface area into intersecting spheres that in tissue sections look like incomplete circles separated by thin, delicate, capillary-rich *alveolar septae*. The alveoli are lined by a watertight monolayer of type I cells. Efficient gas exchange requires minimal diffusion distance, and evolution has left us with a fused basement membrane in common between the alveolar surface type I epithelial cells and the underlying capillary endothelial cells. The capillaries within the alveolar septae are surrounded by abundant elastin, and together comprise the *interstitium* (Figure 8-1).

> **QUICK REVIEW**
> **Adult Lung Physiology**
>
> Ventilation volumes, flow rates, ventilation:perfusion (V:Q) matching, and gas exchange are important to the pulmonologist, whereas structure:function correlation and three chemical components (surfactant, elastin, and mucin) of the pulmonary system are important to the pathologist. The normal respiratory tree has unobstructed conducting airways, clean/dry alveoli, and thin delicate alveolar septae. Upon ventilation and perfusion of these alveoli, gas exchange occurs. Surfactant allows water tension in the alveoli to be broken. Elastin provides elastic recoil to keep lungs from overinflating. Mucin traps inspired dust before it reaches the alveoli.
>
> Lungs could not inflate unless type II epithelial cells make *surfactant* that serves as a detergent. Without surfactant, the surface tension of the water layer in the 3×10^8 alveoli comprising 80 m^2 of alveolar surface could not be overcome to allow inflation of the adult lung, and certainly that of the newborn lung.
>
> The lung, removed from the chest, would collapse because of the large amount of *elastin* in its interstitium. In vivo, vacuum pressure in the pleural space maintains the inflated state of the normal lung. If you lacerate the parietal pleura with a knife, the vacuum will be broken, and the lung will collapse. When present, elastin allows

effortless expiration during the ventilatory cycle. When elastin is absent, alveoli overinflate and rupture, leading to increased expiratory work, increased endexpiratory volumes, and histologic changes called *emphysema* (discussed later in the chapter). Therefore, normal ventilation requires surfactant to break the surface tension of water in the alveoli, a vacuum in the pleural space, and sufficient mechanical force by the chest wall and diaphragm to draw air into the alveoli.

Bronchial submucosal glands excrete *mucin* into ducts that lead to the ciliated surface of the airway. This mucin acts to catch inhaled dust and debris before it can reach the clean and dry alveoli. Surface cilia are powered by ATP to beat in a coordinated unidirectional fashion, sweeping the normally thin mucin layer with its dust and debris up/proximally/centrally, so that the mucin can be swallowed or coughed out. The net result is that the alveoli are protected from receiving or accumulating a burden of dust, debris, or mucin that would interfere with gas exchange.

Countercurrent diffusion between alveolar air O_2 and capillary RBC hemoglobin CO_2 is referred to as *gas exchange*, and occurs across two attenuated cell types (type I epithelium and endothelium) and a shared/fused basement membrane. O_2 and CO_2 diffuse according to their relative concentration gradients, unique diffusion characteristics for each molecule, and the diffusion distance, according to Fick's law. Anything that interferes with ventilation (e.g., blood, pus, pond water, or fibrin), small molecule diffusion (e.g., septal fibrosis), or capillary blood flow (e.g., thromboemboli and heart failure) interferes with this gas exchange, and can lead to *V:Q mismatch*. Mismatch in which the lung is perfused but not ventilated is called *shunting*. Mismatch in which the lung is ventilated but not perfused is called *dead space*. Ideally, there is physiologic autoregulation of V:Q. V:Q mismatch can be measured by the pulmonologist.

CASE 8-1

Clinical: A 65-year-old man with 30 pack-year smoking history, with new bloody sputum.

Radiology: Posteroanterior (PA) chest X-ray shows a solitary right upper lobe mass. CT scan shows the lung mass and hilar lymphadenopathy. Superimposed PET scan showed FDG signal in the lung mass and in the nodes.

Course: A transbronchial biopsy was performed.

Pathology: Hematoxylin and eosin (H&E)-stained section shows an invasive malignant neoplasm with cell–cell cohesion, focal desmosome formation, and focal cytoplasmic keratin accumulation (Figure 8-2). These features support squamous differentiation. The final diagnosis is **invasive squamous cell carcinoma**. Metastasis should be excluded. A computer search for previous biopsy material from this patient would be performed to formally exclude primary squamous carcinoma in another organ (e.g., head/neck mucosa or uterine cervix (if a female patient)) that could have metastasized to the lung.

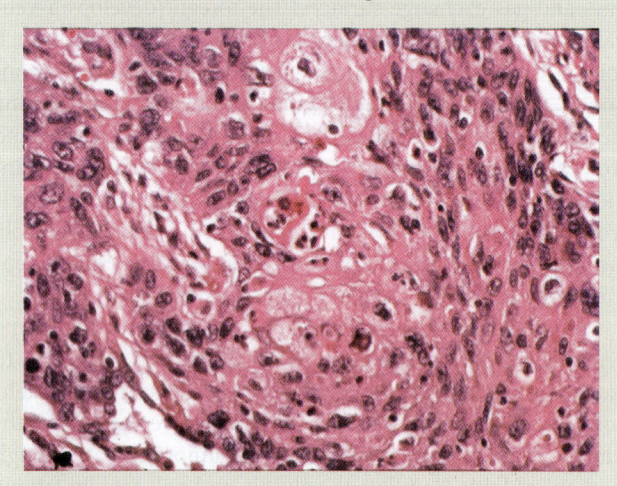

FIGURE 8-2 Invasive squamous cell carcinoma. Cytoplasmic keratin, crisp plasma membranes, and desmosomes (inter-cellular bridges) are diagnostic features.

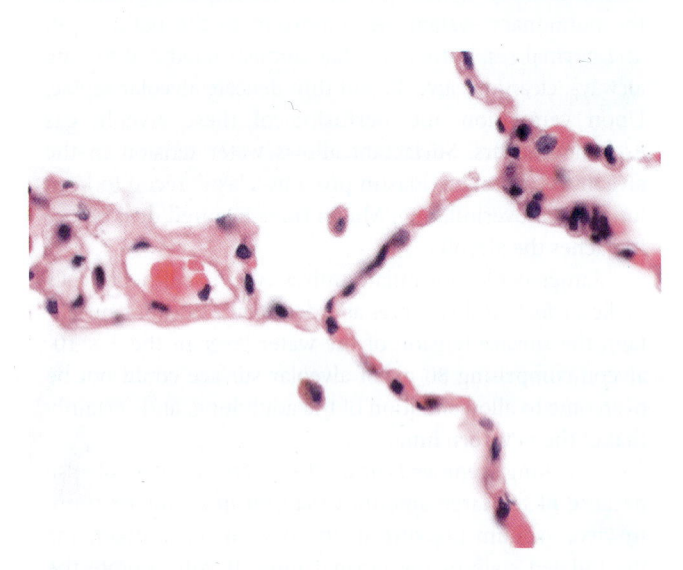

FIGURE 8-1 Normal alveolar parenchyma. Thin, delicate alveolar septae facilitate bidirectional gas exchange between alveolar gas and capillary red blood cell hemoglobin.

LUNG NEOPLASMS

Most neoplasms in the lung are malignant neoplasms of epithelial derivation, that is, *carcinomas*. Almost all (>85%) lung carcinomas are causally associated with cigarette smoking. We know this because of the above association between lung carcinoma incidence and smoking, but more importantly because the relative risk of lung carcinomas increases with cigarette smoking exposure, and decreases following smoking cessation.

What are the clinical implications of cigarette smoking as it relates to lung carcinomas? Roughly 200,000 new cases of lung carcinoma are expected in the United States next year. Hence, a legal, commercial product resulted in about 170,000 [(200,000)(0.85)] new patients with a potentially lethal malignancy. Given the 20% average 5-year survival rate for lung carcinoma, 136,000 of these newly diagnosed smokers with lung carcinoma will die within the next 5 years, possibly unnecessarily, in spite of best clinical efforts to manage their disease. With the adoption of smoking by women, lung carcinoma incidence and mortality rates for women have risen proportionately over the last 30 years, such that lung carcinomas are now the most common cause of death from neoplasm in women the United States. Few realize that lung carcinomas kill 50% more women each year than breast carcinoma. These are striking examples of unnecessary morbidity and mortality in America resulting from etiologic agents that are components of a commercial product. As an aside, if tobacco were made as expensive as designer drugs, consumption would decrease, and lung carcinomas, head/neck squamous carcinoma, chronic bronchitis, and emphysema would likely become orphan diseases in the United States.

Primary lung carcinoma is typically a unifocal clonal proliferation, recognizable microscopically as one of a limited number of types. Most primary lung carcinomas grow as dominant masses within the lung, and can be recognized with noninvasive radiographic techniques. Carcinoma can obstruct a large conducting airway, with development of either sterile or infectious pneumonias distal to the airway obstruction. Invasive carcinoma can erode into pulmonary arterial branches, and can result in exsanguination. Most commonly, carcinomas cause morbidity and mortality by metastasizing via blood vessels to other organs (e.g., brain, bone, liver, adrenal, and even skin). It is usually the disruption of normal function of other organs late in the course of the disease, as well as accompanying pain and cachexia, that lead to death.

Non-Small Cell Lung Carcinomas (NSCLC)

Squamous cell carcinoma of the lung is a disease of cigarette smokers, people breathing second-hand smoke, uranium miners, and rare patients with laryngeal human papillomavirus (HPV) infection. Roughly 20% of US adults (both men and women) smoke, whereas there are very few uranium miners, so most lung squamous cell carcinoma patients have a smoking history. Primary lung squamous cell carcinomas account for roughly 35% of all new lung carcinoma cases.

Most squamous cell carcinomas of lung develop in the bronchi, hence the old name, "bronchogenic" (born in the bronchus) carcinoma. Radiographically, these bronchial primaries are central in location. Squamous cell carcinoma develops from preexisting squamous cell carcinoma in situ, that is, full-thickness dysplasia developing in a background of squamous metaplasia (Figure 8-3). The presumed pathogenesis is that hot gases and entrained irritants in inhaled cigarette smoke cause the normal ciliated respiratory epithelium to change to squamous mucosa (squamous metaplasia). Continued exposure to entrained organic chemicals, particularly polyaromatic hydrocarbons, leads to the accumulation of mutations and DNA copy number changes, reflected in morphologic features of dysplasia (architectural disarray, nuclear pleomorphism, nuclear membrane irregularities, nuclear hyperchromasia, and increased mitotic rate). Squamous cell carcinoma confined to the surface epithelium and delimited by the basement membrane (squamous cell carcinoma in situ) has no metastatic potential, because it does not have access to either lymphatics or blood vessels deep to the basement membrane. However, once the malignant clone invades across the basement membrane (invasive squamous cell carcinoma) (Figure 8-2), it now has the potential to invade into lymph or blood vessels,

> **WHAT WE DO**
>
> Lung carcinomas are a heterogeneous group of neoplasms that the pathologist can distinguish morphologically by identifiable features of squamous carcinoma (desmosomes and/or keratin production), adenocarcinoma (glandular/papillary architecture +/− mucin production), or neuroendocrine neoplasms (coarse chromatin, neuroendocrine protein expression). Well- and moderately differentiated carcinomas are those that manifest recognizable features that allow subcategorization into squamous cell carcinoma, adenocarcinoma, or neuroendocrine neoplasms. Poorly differentiated or undifferentiated carcinomas may result in a differential diagnosis that includes not only carcinoma but also melanoma and lymphoma, requiring a panel of immunostains and mucin stains to clarify lineage and subtype. Because of major differences in clinical presentation and clinical therapies, the main clinical categories are "**non-small cell carcinomas**" (including squamous cell carcinoma, adenocarcinoma, adenosquamous carcinoma, large cell undifferentiated carcinoma (LCUC), sarcomatoid carcinoma, carcinoid tumors, salivary gland type carcinomas) and "**small cell carcinoma.**" Descriptions of these different neoplasms follow.

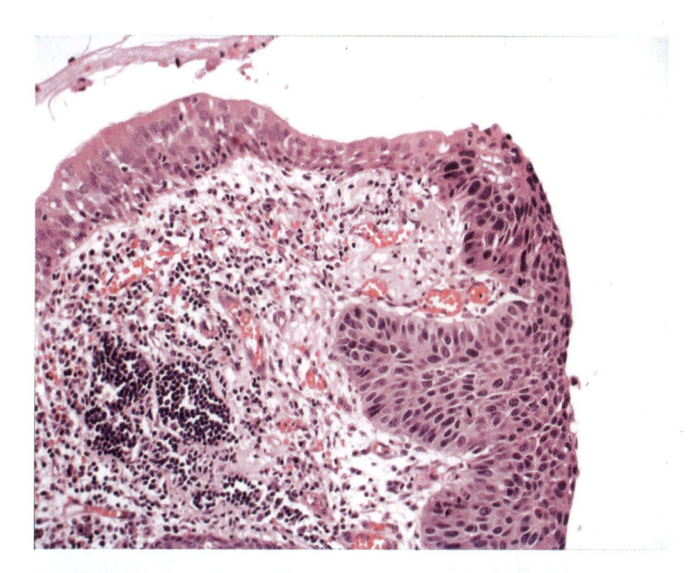

FIGURE 8-3 Squamous cell carcinoma in situ. Normal respiratory mucosa segues into progressively dysplastic squamous metaplasia; full-thickness dysplasia is known as squamous cell carcinoma in situ.

and to metastasize to regional nodes (via lymphatics) or to distant organs (via systemic blood flow). Well- to moderately differentiated invasive squamous cell carcinoma is identified by virtue of *desmosome* formation (intercellular bridges) and cytoplasmic accumulation of *keratin* [cytokeratin (CK)], an intermediate filament protein. At the protein level, over 95% of squamous cell carcinomas express CK 5/6 and P63, whereas few express thyroid transcription factor-1 (TTF-1) or aspartic protease napsin A, each of which can be detected by immunohistochemical (antibody-based) stains. At the molecular level, most squamous cell carcinomas show *P53* mutations and disruption of the *RB* pathway, but fewer *KRAS* mutations than are seen in adenocarcinomas.

The prognosis of squamous cell carcinoma, like other common NSCLC, is predicted based on *stage* (extent of disease, including size of the primary (T), extent of local invasion, presence of regional nodal metastases (N), and presence of distant metastasis (M)), *performance status*, and *weight loss history*.

Adenocarcinoma of the lung is a disease of both smokers and nonsmokers. If you are a lifelong nonsmoker with a new primary lung carcinoma, adenocarcinoma is the most likely diagnosis. Roughly 30% of new lung carcinomas will be diagnosed as adenocarcinomas.

Most adenocarcinomas present as distal/peripheral lung masses, in contrast to the central location of most squamous cell carcinomas. At the histologic level, there is an early group of adenocarcinomas that are limited to surface epithelial involvement. These have traditionally been called **bronchioloalveolar carcinomas (BAC)**. BAC can show either mucinous or nonmucinous differentiation. Neoplasms with this architecture that are <3 cm in size are now considered to be *adenocarcinoma in situ* (BAC/ACIS), with expected 5-year survival of 100% following negative-margin resection. Tumors <3 cm in size that are associated with invasion across the basement membrane, with resulting stromal response and remodeling of lung parenchyma, are considered *minimally invasive adenocarcinomas* if the invasive component is <0.5 cm. Tumors are considered *invasive* adenocarcinomas if the invasive component is >0.5 cm or the total tumor diameter is >3 cm.

Large cell undifferentiated carcinoma (LCUC) of the lung is the least common of the major types of NSCLC, comprising roughly 10% of patients with new lung carcinomas. These carcinomas can develop peripherally or centrally. The cell of origin for LCUC is unclear. At the histologic level, carcinoma cells are undifferentiated, with large nucleoli, more cytoplasm than expected for small cell carcinoma, and without any of the identifiable features of squamous cell carcinoma or adenocarcinoma (**Figure 8-6**). Molecular studies suggest that LCUC is a distinct disease entity, rather than just an undifferentiated form of more easily recognized NSCLC.

Other Non-Small Cell Lung Cancer: The remaining 5% of new lung tumor diagnoses are a potpourri of unusual

IN TRANSLATION

Invasive well- to moderately differentiated adenocarcinomas can be diagnosed by virtue of papillary, glandular/acinar (**Figure 8-4**), or solid architecture, as well as by mucin production (**Figure 8-5**). At the protein level, roughly 75% of adenocarcinomas express TTF-1 and napsin A, and few express CK5/6 or P63 by immunohistochemical stains. At the cytogenetic and molecular level, most lung adenocarcinomas have some combination of mutations (*EGFR, KRAS, BRAF, and P53*), and/or fusion gene formation (*EML4/ALK* inversion translocation). *The recent availability of small molecule inhibitors for mutant gene products of EGFR, BRAF, and ALK has made screening for these mutations an important aspect of case workup.*

FIGURE 8-4 Adenocarcinoma of lung. Discrete clusters with peripheral community borders and focal gland formation are noted.

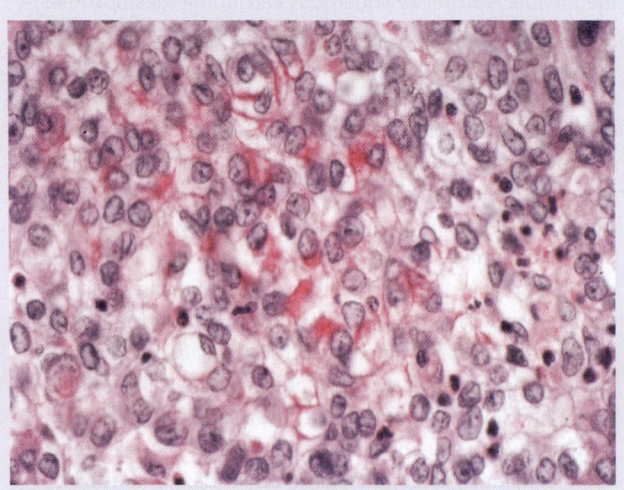

FIGURE 8-5 Adenocarcinoma of lung. Mucin stains [PAS after diastase digestion (PASd) or mucicarmine] can be used to detect intracytoplasmic mucin.

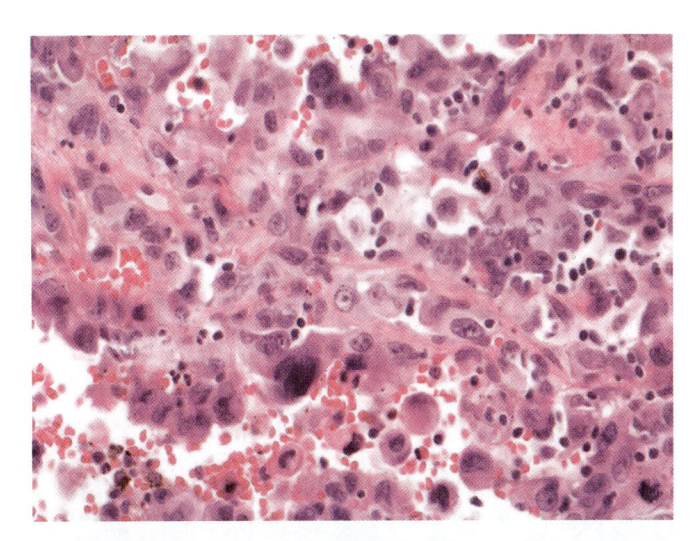

FIGURE 8-6 Large cell undifferentiated carcinoma of lung. This non-small cell carcinoma shows no squamous differentiation, neuroendocrine differentiation, or features of adenocarcinoma.

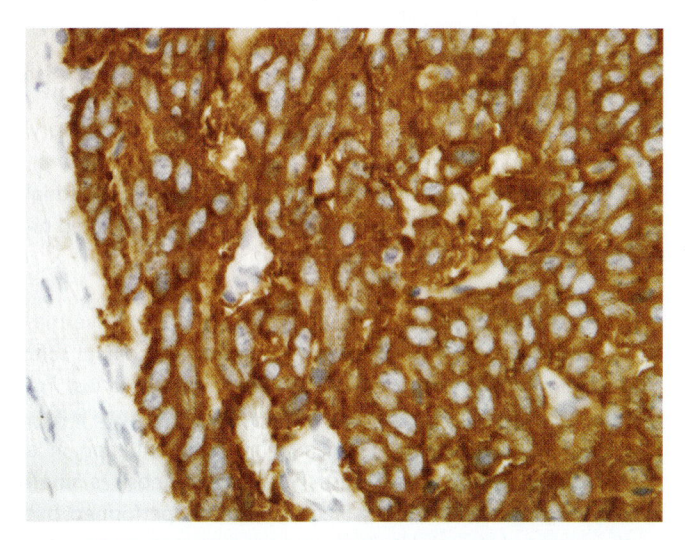

FIGURE 8-8 Mature carcinoid tumor, positive synaptophysin immunostain. Neuroendocrine neoplasms show variable reactivity for neuroendocrine proteins, including synaptophysin, chromogranin, and CD56.

neoplasms. Carcinomas that show prominent spindle cell or giant cell component are called "**sarcomatoid**" carcinomas. Carcinomas that mimic salivary gland carcinomas (**adenoid cystic carcinoma**, **mucoepidermoid carcinoma**) can arise from submucosal glands in the central tracheobronchial submucosa. Finally, there are three neuroendocrine neoplasms that are not small cell carcinomas (small cell carcinoma is discussed separately below). **Mature carcinoid tumor** typically presents in a young adult as a nested submucosal mass with airway obstruction, but is unlikely to metastasize, so can be treated with surgical resection alone. It is recognizably neuroendocrine, with nested growth, coarse chromatin (Figure 8-7), and with immunoreactivity for chromogranin and synaptophysin (Figure 8-8). However, it does not have prominent nucleoli or coagulative tumor cell necrosis, and it shows low mitotic activity and low growth fraction (as detected with Ki-67 antibody (Figure 8-9)). Carcinoid tumors with nucleolar prominence, focal mitotic activity, and focal coagulative tumor cell necrosis are called **atypical carcinoid tumors**. These have increased risk of metastasis, so may be considered for adjuvant chemotherapy following resection. At the high grade end of the neuroendocrine neoplasm spectrum is **large cell neuroendocrine carcinoma**, recognizable as a neuroendocrine carcinoma, with similar features (high mitotic rate, frequent apoptosis, frequent coagulative necrosis) to small cell carcinoma, but with significant cytoplasm and prominent nucleoli (unlike small cell carcinoma).

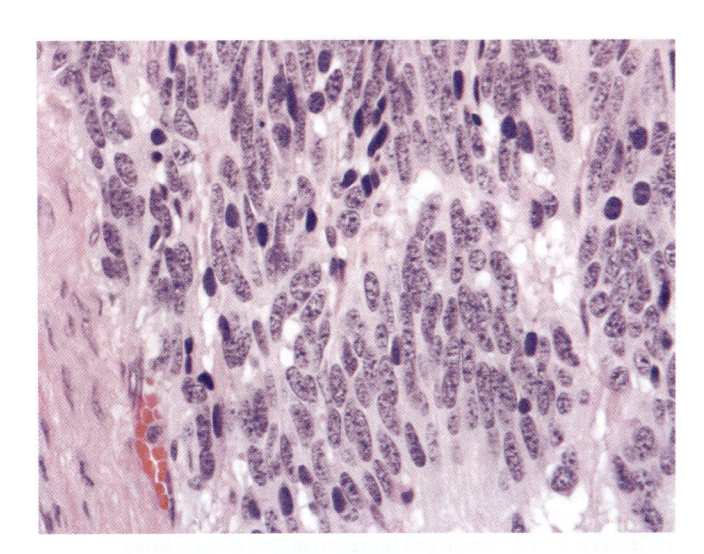

FIGURE 8-7 Mature carcinoid tumor. Clusters of neoplastic cells with coarse ("salt-and-pepper") chromatin show no nucleolar prominence, mitotic activity, or coagulative necrosis.

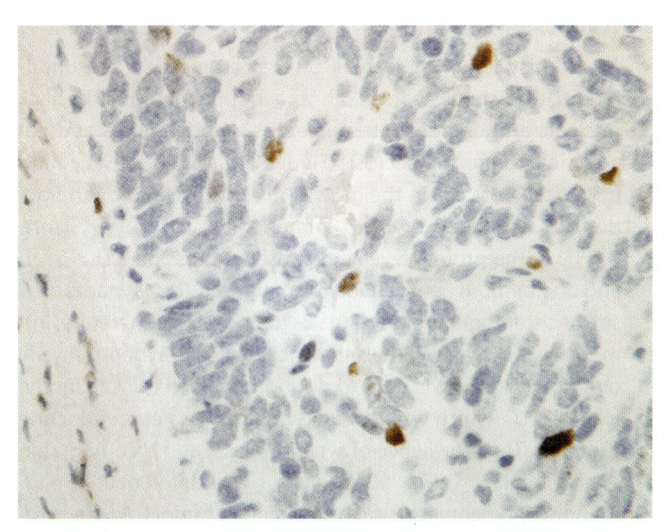

FIGURE 8-9 Mature carcinoid tumor, Ki-67 immunostain. The percentage of cells in the growth-division cycle ("growth fraction") can be estimated using the antibody, Ki-67. The growth fraction of mature carcinoid tumor is low.

CASE 8-2

Clinical: An 80-year-old man with 50 pack-year smoking history, with new bloody sputum.

Radiology: PA chest X-ray shows a hilar and mediastinal mass. CT scan shows the central lung mass with associated hilar/mediastinal lymphadenopathy.

Course: A transbronchial biopsy was performed.

Pathology: H&E-stained section shows an invasive malignant neoplasm with hyperchromatic nuclei, coarse "salt-and-pepper" chromatin, absent nucleoli, high N:C ratios, frequent mitotic figures, and coagulative necrosis (Figure 8-10). These features support neuroendocrine differentiation in a high-grade malignant neoplasm. The final diagnosis is **small cell lung carcinoma (SCLC)**. Staging should be performed, but the expected stage is late/high, and the expected prognosis is poor.

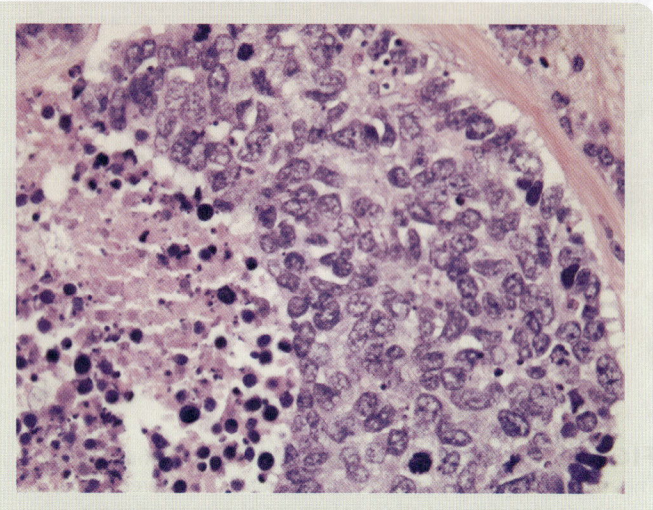

FIGURE 8-10 Small cell lung carcinoma (SCLC). This neuroendocrine neoplasm shows high N:C ratio cells, frequent mitotic figures, and coagulative tumor cell necrosis.

Small Cell Lung Carcinomas (SCLC)

Small cell carcinoma deserves a separate category within the lung carcinoma classification, based on its unique clinical presentation and differences in clinical management. Small cell carcinoma is unique because it typically metastasizes early, thereby presenting as late-stage disease in the majority of cases. Patients presenting with late-stage disease are treated with systemic chemotherapy to kill clinical/subclinical metastases and the primary, as well as radiotherapy for additional local control of the primary. Small cell carcinoma accounts for roughly 20% of newly diagnosed cases of lung carcinoma. It has some features in common with squamous cell carcinoma, that is, smoking history and central location of the primary. A subset of these carcinomas generates bioactive hormones, such that an SCLC patient might present with Cushing syndrome secondary to ectopic ACTH production. Like squamous cell carcinoma and adenocarcinoma, metastases can traffic via lymphatics to regional lymph nodes, and can traffic to distant sites via the systemic bloodstream.

IN TRANSLATION

At the histologic level, small cell carcinoma cells are undifferentiated, show coarse "salt and pepper" chromatin, lack nucleoli, and demonstrate numerous mitotic figures and coagulative tumor cell necrosis (Figure 8-10). SCLC shows a high percentage of cells in the growth-division cycle (growth fraction), as estimated by Ki-67 immunohistochemistry (Figure 8-11). At the protein level, most cases express pan-CK, TTF-1, and one or more neuroendocrine markers (CD56, synaptophysin, or chromogranin) (Figures 8-12 and 8-13). Therefore, immunohistochemical panels that include CD56, synaptophysin, or chromogranin will help to distinguish small cell carcinoma from NSCLC (which typically does not express neuroendocrine proteins). The prevalence of synaptophysin and chromogranin expression is lower for SCLC than for well-differentiated neuroendocrine neoplasms such as carcinoid tumors. At the cytogenetic level, there is aneuploidy with marked copy number variation across multiple chromosomes. At the molecular level, P53 mutation and myc amplification are common.

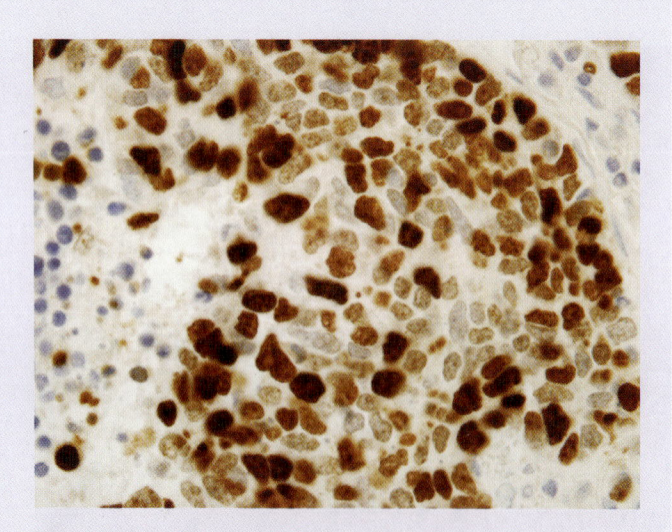

FIGURE 8-11 Small cell lung carcinoma (SCLC), Ki-67 immunostain. The growth fraction of SCLC is high, as estimated by Ki-67 immunostaining.

PULMONARY PATHOLOGY 223

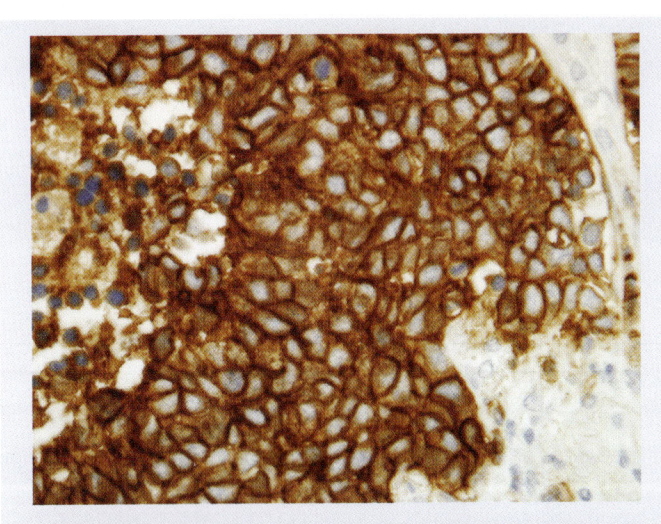

FIGURE 8-12 **Small cell lung carcinoma (SCC), positive CD56 immunostain.** Like other neuroendocrine neoplasms, SCLC shows reactivity for some or all of the neuroendocrine marker proteins, including CD56.

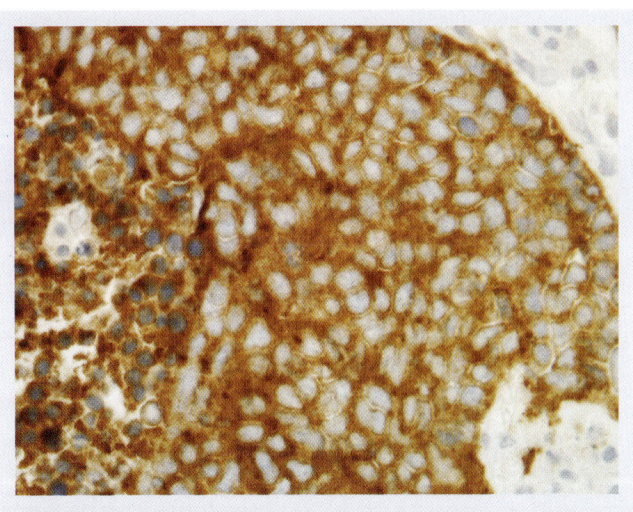

FIGURE 8-13 **Small cell lung carcinoma (SCC), positive synaptophysin immunostain.** Synaptophysin reactivity is noted in this example of SCLC, but SCLC reactivity for synaptophysin and chromogranin is variable.

The cell of origin for small cell carcinoma is unclear, but the occurrence of combined SCLC/NSCLC suggests that it may arise from a pluripotent cell type in the bronchi. By definition, small cell carcinoma is an undifferentiated neoplasm that demonstrates neuroendocrine features by H&E and immunohistochemistry.

Like the non-small cell carcinomas, prognosis for small cell carcinoma is related to *stage* at presentation, and to *performance status*. Genetic factors are not currently of use as prognostic variables. Because most small cell carcinomas present at a late stage (i.e., with distant metastases), overall prognosis for patients with small cell carcinoma is poor, with roughly 5% 5-year survival rates. In spite of this dismal prognosis, modern chemoradiotherapy has improved initial response rates and significantly prolonged survival, now averaging 18 months.

PLEURAL NEOPLASMS

Malignant Mesothelioma

Malignant mesothelioma was a relatively rare neoplasm prior to the use of mined asbestos starting in the early 20th century.

CASE 8-3

Clinical: A 72-year-old man nonsmoker with progressive dyspnea. PMHx (+) for previous employment as a pipefitter in a shipyard during World War II.

Radiology: PA chest X-ray shows a large pleural effusion. CT scan shows circumferential pleural thickening associated with pleural effusion.

Course: A video-assisted thoracoscopic surgery (VATS) biopsy was performed.

Pathology: H&E-stained section shows a stromal-invasive malignant neoplasm with epithelioid cytology, without specific features of NSCLC (Figure 8-14). These features support a diagnosis of carcinoma or mesothelioma. Immunostains show reactivity for calretinin (Figure 8-15) and CK5/6, with no reactivity for TTF1 (Figure 8-16) or P63. The final diagnosis is **epithelioid malignant mesothelioma**.

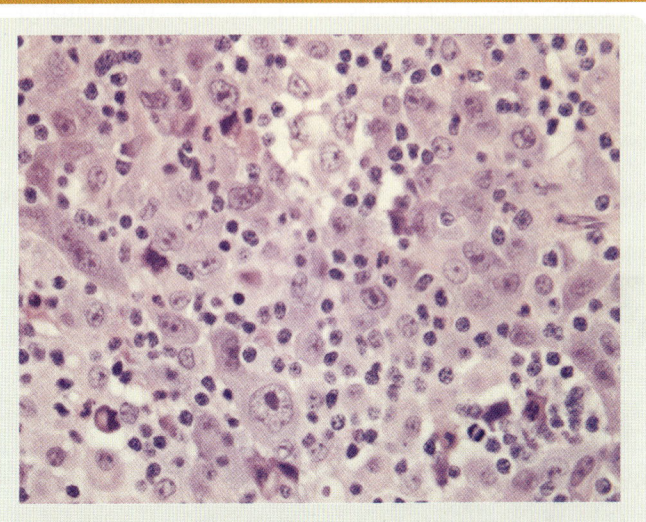

FIGURE 8-14 **Epithelioid mesothelioma.** This pleural-based mesothelial neoplasm could easily be confused with a peripherally located adenocarcinoma, so diagnosis requires radiographic correlation and tissue immunophenotyping for accurate diagnosis.

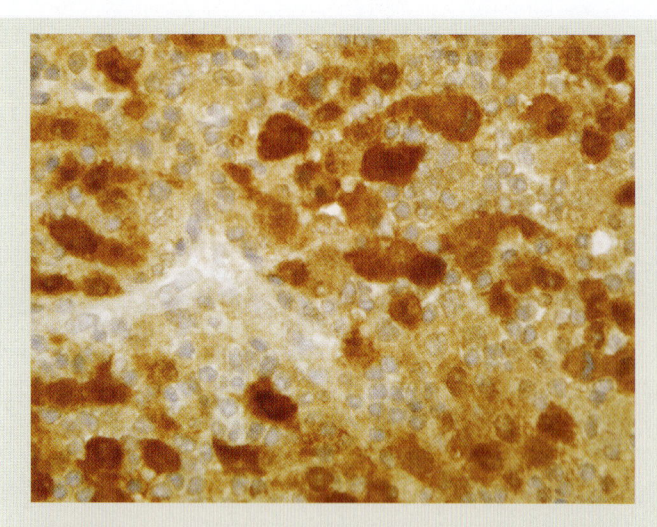

FIGURE 8-15 **Epithelioid mesothelioma, positive calretinin immunostain.** Calretinin reactivity is expected in mesothelioma, and would be unexpected in adenocarcinoma of lung.

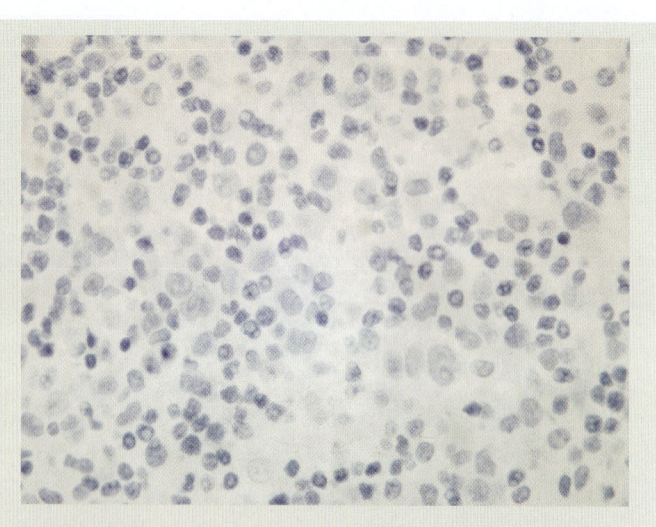

FIGURE 8-16 **Epithelioid mesothelioma, negative TTF-1 immunostain.** TTF-1 reactivity is expected in adenocarcinoma of lung, but would be unexpected in mesothelioma.

Purified asbestos was heavily used in the manufacturing trades as a flame retardant and thermal insulator, and found high demand during World War II in the shipbuilding industry. Unfortunately, increased numbers of asbestos workers presented with pleural fibrous plaques and malignant neoplasms 20–40 years following exposure to inhaled asbestos. This increased relative risk of pleural plaques and malignant mesothelioma was causally associated with asbestos, and led to the demise of the asbestos industry in the western world. Patients have a poor prognosis without treatment. Combination surgery, chemotherapy, and radiotherapy are currently used to manage these patients.

Both the fibrous plaques and the invasive malignant mesothelioma are frequently associated with asbestos fibers (**asbestos bodies** when seen in tissue) (Figure 8-17) from inhaled dust that migrated out to the subpleural stroma. The mechanism of malignant transformation is unknown, but these fibers presumably predispose the patient not only to a fibrous stromal response but also to the risk of transformation of mesothelial cells into a clonal neoplasm with invasive potential, that is, mesothelioma. At the histologic level, there is overlap in the cytologic features of reactive mesothelial atypia and malignant mesothelioma cells, so the pathologist requires evidence of definite stromal invasion and supportive radiographs to be confident in the diagnosis of invasive malignant mesothelioma.

Not all pleural effusions represent mesothelioma. The mesothelial surface is a simple monolayer that encases the lung in an airtight sac. Under normal physiologic conditions, the space between the visceral and parietal pleura is comprised of opposing monolayer mesothelial surfaces, with minimal fluid, no inflammatory cells, and a vacuum compared with atmospheric pressure. Under conditions of increased hydrostatic pressure, such as severe congestive heart failure, lymph can leak (as a low-protein transudate) into the pleural compartment. High-protein (exudative) pleural effusion can develop in the setting of lung/pleural infections

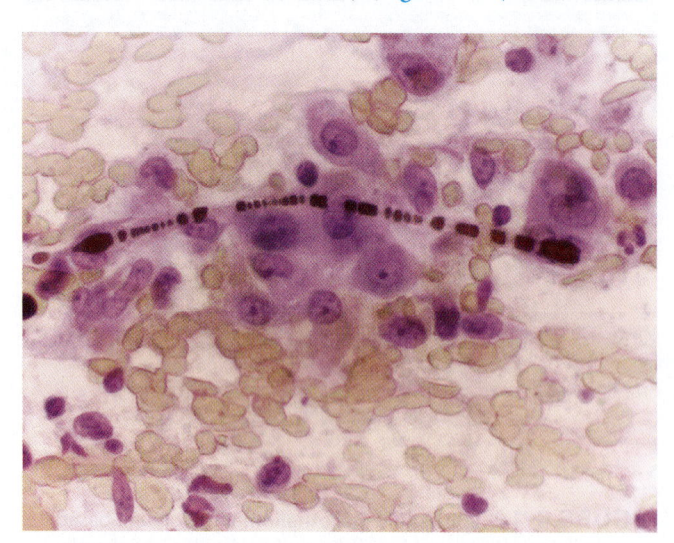

FIGURE 8-17 **Asbestos body.** Many but not all patients with mesothelioma have a history of dust exposure to the fibrogenic dust, asbestos.

> **IN TRANSLATION**
>
> At the protein level, most mesotheliomas express *calretinin* and *CK5/6*. At the cytogenetic level, there is copy number variation in mesothelioma cell lines, with frequent homozygous loss of 9p, which includes the locus *CDKN2A/ARF* that encodes P16/INK4A and P14/ARF. There is a global decrease in DNA methylation. Growth fraction (percentage of neoplastic cells in the growth division cycle) correlates inversely with patient survival. VEGF receptor and HIF-1-alpha signaling pathways are potential targets for customized therapy.

PULMONARY PATHOLOGY 225

(**empyema/pyothorax**), adjacent lung carcinoma, or neoplastic metastases to the pleural surface. Thoracentesis can be studied for cells and protein levels to determine whether the fluid represents a transudate or an exudate, and exudates can be studied by culture for microorganisms if infectious, and by cytopathology staining and diagnosis if neoplastic.

LUNG AND PLEURAL INFECTIONS

Bacterial Pneumonias

Bacterial pneumonias are a common cause of morbidity (5 million cases/year in the United States), and mortality (about 80,000 cases/year in the United States) and constitute about 10% of US hospital admissions. Risk factors include either reduced bone marrow production of neutrophils, neutrophils with intrinsic functional defects, defective ciliary function, cystic fibrosis (CF), indwelling endotracheal tube, lack of a cough reflex, and splenectomy. However, normal children and adults can also become infected. Most bacterial pneumonias can be treated with antibacterial drugs, but some species acquire resistance elements that predispose to multidrug resistance and chronic infection.

The primary defense mechanisms for the lung include the cough reflex, normal mucus, normal ciliary function, and normal macrophages. The failsafe defense is circulating neutrophils, which traffic to areas of infection to phagocytose and destroy bacteria. In settings where normal neutrophil

CASE 8-4

Clinical: A 90-year-old woman with shaking chills, fever, and productive cough.

Radiology: PA chest X-ray shows patchy infiltrates with air bronchograms.

Course: The patient died in the emergency room, and was received for autopsy exam.

Pathology: The lungs were multifocally consolidated (**Figure 8-18**). Tissue sections from the consolidated lung show alveolar filling by neutrophils (**Figure 8-19**). Bacterial Gram stain showed diplococcus (**Figure 8-20**), and cultures grew *Streptococcus pneumoniae*.

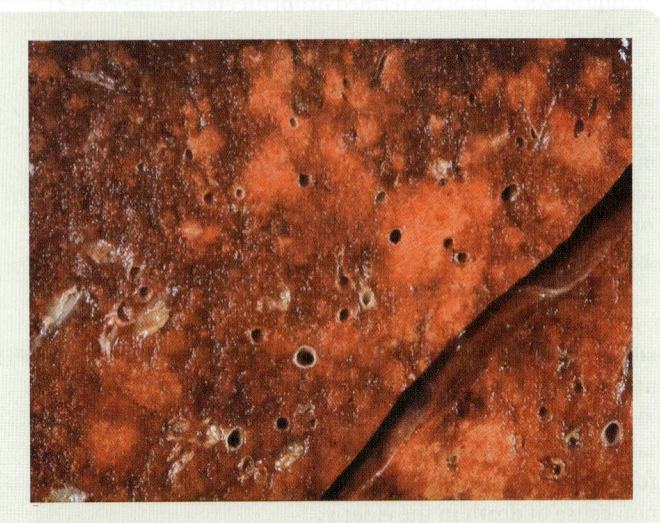

FIGURE 8-18 **Acute bronchopneumonia.** Patchy consolidation is noted grossly.

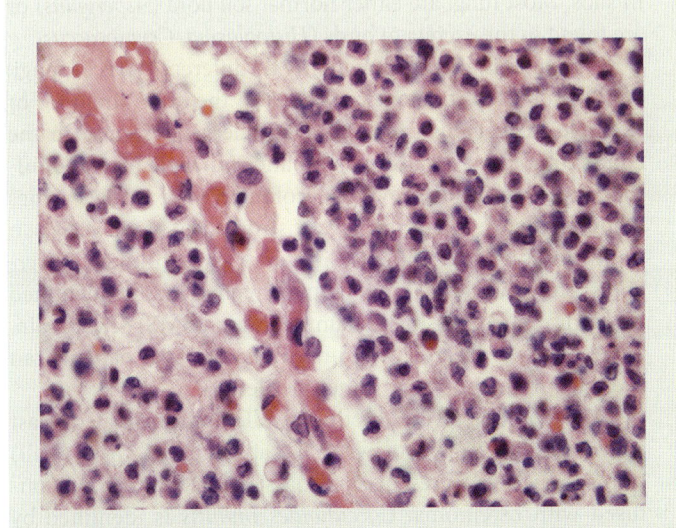

FIGURE 8-19 **Acute bronchopneumonia.** This case of bacterial bronchopneumonia generated a host response of sheets of neutrophils filling and expanding the alveolar air spaces.

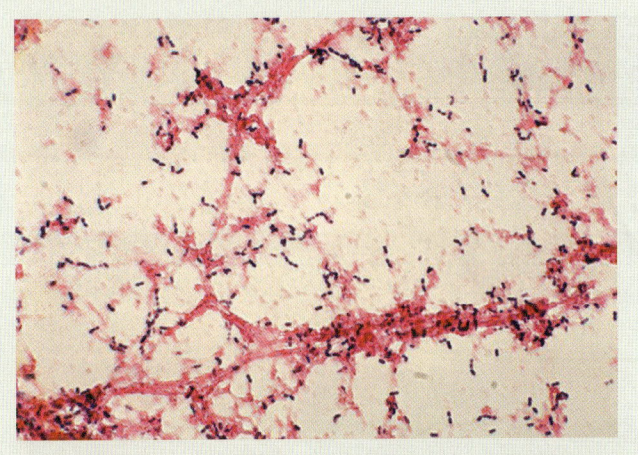

FIGURE 8-20 **Gram stain.** Gram stain can be used to identify bacteria in smears and sections, in this case diplococcus (*S. pneumoniae*) (courtesy of Dr. P. Gilligan). Source: http://phil.cdc.gov/phil/details.asp image number2896

production is impaired, for example, following marrow-ablative systemic chemotherapy, circulating neutrophil counts can drop to the point where bacterial infections proliferate unchecked. Certain congenital diseases such as **chronic granulomatous disease** feature defects in the neutrophils' ability to kill phagocytosed bacteria, resulting in an inadequate response to bacterial infection, with chronic abscess formation. At the level of the conducting airway, a bacterial inoculum will be responded to by neutrophils, leading to mucopurulent debris associated with the respiratory mucosal epithelium. If the ciliary function and mucin are normal, then this bacterial inoculum will be moved proximally and cleared. However, in patients with defective ciliary function (e.g., **primary ciliary dyskinesia**, PCD), or defective overly viscous mucin (e.g. **cystic fibrosis**, CF), the bacterial inoculum is not easily cleared and can form an obstructing plug of infected mucous producing inflammation, scarring, and irreversible dilation of the conducting airway, a process termed **bronchiectasis (Figure 8-21)**.

Radiographs are commonly used to determine the extent of infection. The common bacterial pneumonias present as radiodense **consolidation** of alveolar parenchyma that is grossly firm to palpation. Consolidation can be lobar (**lobar pneumonia**) or patchy/focal (**bronchopneumonia**). If the waterdense neutrophils and bacteria fill the alveoli, but not the conducting airways, "air bronchograms" will result, a useful radiographic sign for alveolar filling processes.

The most common bacterial species to infect the lung is *S. pneumoniae*. The organism is normal flora found in roughly half of us. Infection of the lung may be preceded by a viral infection that alters the ability of the lung to protect its mucosal epithelium from serving as a portal of entry for bacterial infection. Streptococcal pneumonia can be either patchy (focal) or lobar. Streptococcal bronchopneumonia is a common cause of death in the elderly.

Other community-acquired bacterial infections include *Pseudomonas sp.*, *Klebsiella sp.*, *Haemophilus sp.*, *Staphylococcus aureus*, and anaerobic *Streptococcus sp.* Within the hospital setting, drug-resistant strains are increasingly common, and can lead to chronic bacterial infections. For example, certain drug-resistant *P. aeruginosa* in CF patients may be impossible to eradicate. Some bacterial infections are more likely to cause parenchymal necrosis, abscess formation, and scarring in survivors, for example, *P. aeruginosa*, *Klebsiella pneumoniae*, *S. aureus*, and anaerobes.

Cultures and sensitivity testing are performed routinely using aerobic and anaerobic conditions in the clinical laboratory. Molecular methods are beginning to supplant culture-based methods for speciation and resistance element detection.

Mycoplasma Pneumonia

M. pneumoniae is a prokaryote without a cell wall, and is the smallest freely living organism (0.1×2 microns). It infects ciliated respiratory epithelium, leading to a denuding bronchitis/bronchiolitis. *M. pneumoniae* initially affects the conducting airways, leading to luminal exudates and possibly airway obstruction with distal atelectasis (collapse of lung tissue) observable on radiographs. The organism is highly transmissible through airborne spread, and is a common cause of community-acquired tracheobronchitis and bronchopneumonia. Normal children and adults are susceptible, typically presenting with tracheobronchitis and a nonproductive cough. Elevated titer of cold agglutinins may be measured in the serum. The infection is easily treated with antibiotics. Mortality from *M. pneumoniae* is rare.

Fungi

Fungal infections are predominantly seen in immunosuppressed individuals. Exceptions are indolent fungal infections in farmers exposed to high fungal loads in the inhaled air, for example, in silos. Most fungi are either normal soil flora (*Aspergillus*) or are found in the excreta of birds (*Histoplasma*, *Cryptococcus*).

The lung is affected differently by different types of fungi, and can develop different responses to the same fungus. For example, *Aspergillus* can trigger an allergic response in the conducting airway walls of asthmatics (**allergic bronchopulmonary aspergillosis**, ABPA), colonize preexisting cavities (**aspergilloma**), or can also invade stroma and blood vessels in immunosuppressed patients (**invasive aspergillosis**). *Aspergillus* grows as branching septate hyphae, easily identified by H&E or Gomori-methenamine silver (GMS) silver stain. Angioinvasive *Aspergillus* in immunosuppressed patients can present with hemoptysis, sometimes lethal.

Cryptococcus grows as thick-walled, encapsulated yeast forms, easily confirmed by PAS (capsule) and GMS (wall) stains, which can present as a mass lesion that can be confused with carcinoma. *Coccidioides immitis* is identified by virtue of its large spherules containing endospores. *Blastomyces* is identified by virtue of very large yeast forms ($25\ \mu$), with broad-based budding. *Histoplasma* grows as 3–$5\ \mu$ diameter yeast forms that trigger macrophage infiltrate and

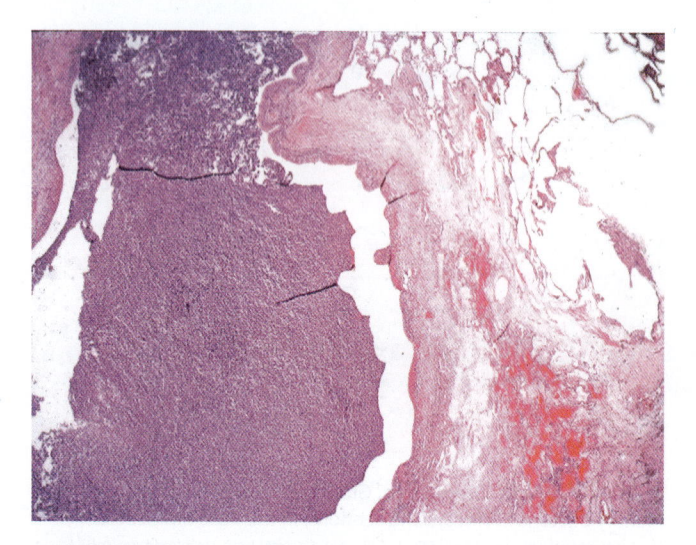

FIGURE 8-21 **Bronchiectasis.** The bronchial airway is dilated, with corrugated surface, with filling by mucopurulent debris, and with mural fibrosis and inflammation.

CASE 8-5

Clinical: A 43-year-old woman with HIV and new fever, cough, and dyspnea.
    Radiology: Patchy ground-glass infiltrates.
    Course: Wedge biopsy. Prompt response to sulfa antibiotic.

Pathology: Alveolar filling by a frothy exudate (Figure 8-22). Gomori-methenamine silver (GMS) (silver) stain positive for organisms (Figure 8-23). The diagnosis is *Pneumocystis carinii* pneumonia.

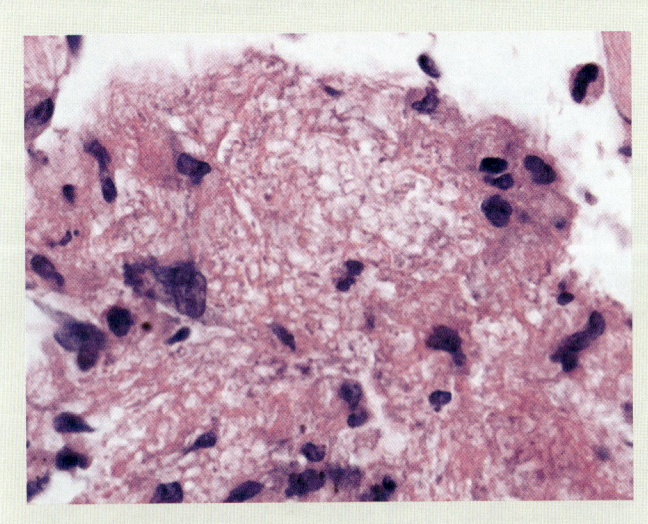

FIGURE 8-22 *Pneumocystis carinii* pneumonia (PCP). PCP infection generates a foamy exudate in the alveolar air spaces. Organisms are difficult to identify by H&E stain alone (Image used with permission from Dr. K. Volmar).

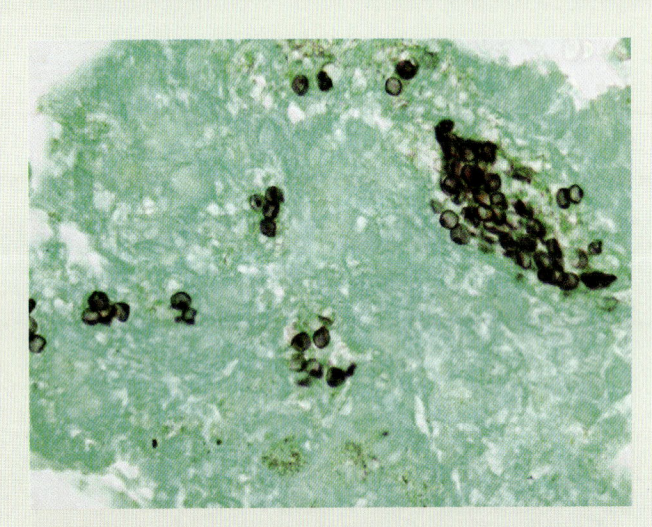

FIGURE 8-23 *Pneumocystis carinii* pneumonia. Organisms can be identified by silver (GMS) histochemical stain (Image used with permission from Dr. K. Volmar).

granuloma formation. *Pneumocystis* has a characteristic "teacup" appearance by silver stain such as GMS. The background of intraalveolar exudates can be mistaken for pulmonary edema or pulmonary alveolar proteinosis. GMS silver stains are used to identify the cell walls of all fungi because they do not stain background normal cells and thus have a high signal:noise stains for detection of fungi.

The host response to fungal infection is usually granulomatous, and it can exhibit the central coagulative-type necrosis also seen in the response to tuberculosis. Therefore, special stains for both fungi and TB are used when screening for infectious agents in patients whose tissue sections show necrotizing granulomatous inflammation.

Mycobacteria

Mycobacterium tuberculosis is responsible for an age-old disease that is alive and well in all parts of the world. Although it may be more common in developing countries, it appears frequently in the United States, and can lead to infections in both immunocompetent and immunocompromised hosts.

Most (>90% of) patients with primary aerosol exposure to tuberculosis (**primary TB**) are asymptomatic, with the only sign of this exposure being a solitary radiodense nodule in the upper lobe (**Ghon focus**), and conversion to a positive purified protein derivative (PPD) tuberculin skin test. Sections of this radiodense nodule will show granulomatous inflammation, which over time becomes fibrotic and calcified. The remaining (<10% of) patients with primary TB develop **progressive tuberculosis**, which can lead to hematogenous (**miliary**) spread to other organs.

Patients previously exposed to tuberculosis can develop **"secondary" TB** following re-exposure to infectious tuberculosis, or due to reactivation of the organisms within the Ghon focus. This can be seen in patients newly immunosuppressed by virtue of chemotherapy or HIV. Patients with secondary tuberculosis may develop cavities within the lung (**"cavitary TB"**), and can develop hematogenous dissemination to other organs (miliary TB).

The host response to mycobacteria involves a distinctive form of macrophages called an **epithelioid histiocyte**. Focal accumulation of epithelioid histiocytes is called a **granuloma**. Mycobacteria typically cause central coagulative necrosis within these granulomata (**caseating granulomas** named for their "cheese-like" gross appearance). Hence, the expected morphologic appearance of tuberculosis infection is necrotizing granulomatous inflammation (Figure 8-24).

Although epithelioid histiocytes can phagocytose mycobacteria, the organisms cannot be digested easily or completely, so remain viable but quarantined. Therefore, necrotizing granulomata should be considered infectious, a point that is relevant to

CASE 8-6

Clinical: A debilitated 80-year-old man with night sweats
Radiology: Calcified upper lobe nodule, multiple other nodules
Course: Wedge biopsy

Pathology: Necrotizing granulomatous inflammation (Figure 8-24)
Acid-fast bacilli (AFB) stain positive for short beaded rods (Figure 8-25)
Cultures (+) for *Mycobacterium tuberculosis*

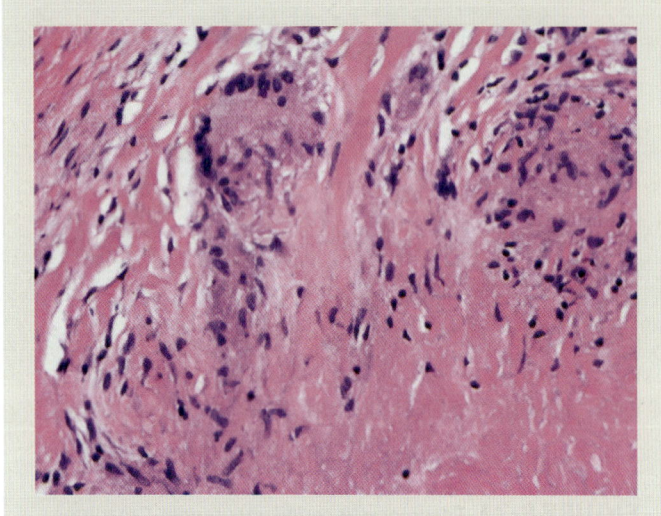

FIGURE 8-24 Tuberculosis. *M. tuberculosis* generates a host response of centrally necrotic granulomatous inflammation in immunocompetent individuals (Image used with permission fromf Dr. K. Volmar).

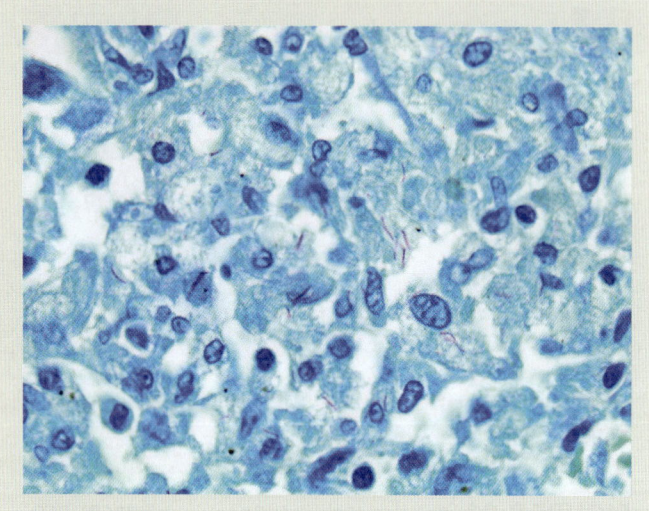

FIGURE 8-25 Tuberculosis. *M. tuberculosis* is a short-beaded rod that can be detected as red acid-fast bacilli (AFB) with histochemical stains (Image used with permission from Dr. K. Volmar).

the practice of surgery and pathology, as well as to the exposure of physicians and nurses in pulmonary medicine wards and clinics.

Although most tuberculosis can be treated with a standard three-drug regimen, multidrug-resistant organisms from other countries are being introduced into American society, such that chemosensitivity testing should be considered for new infections.

Immunocompromised patients (HIV, marrow-suppressive chemotherapy, post-transplantation) are at risk of other mycobacterial species as well. Before the advent of uniform pasteurization of milk, species from cattle (*M. bovis*) were associated with the development of necrotizing granulomata within cervical lymph nodes (*scrofula*). In the HIV era, infection with bird species (*M. avium*) is seen. Because patients with HIV do not have normal immune responses, these patients may have florid mycobacterial infection with few or no granulomas.

Viruses

Most of us are exposed to the common viruses in child- and young-adulthood, including Epstein–Barr virus (EBV), CMV, adenovirus, and herpes simplex virus. Individuals with competent specific immune responses can clear or control levels of proliferation of these viruses, such that they sustain limited clinical infections. In contrast, immunosuppressed individuals are at increased risk of either reactivation or new infection by these viruses, and their specific immune responses are now insufficient to control the infection.

The viruses mentioned above can infect conducting airway mucosal epithelium and/or alveolar epithelium, with accompanying mural and interstitial lymphocytic infiltrates in immunocompetent patients. Bacterial superinfection can complicate a viral infection of the lung, such that consolidating bacterial pneumonia can occur as a secondary event.

CMV is one of the most commonly identified viral pathogens in immunosuppressed individuals. Infection of the host leads to alveolar lining cells with enlarged nuclei, punched-

CASE 8-7

Clinical: A 25-year-old man now 4 months post lung allograft for CF. New positive serology for cytomegalovirus (CMV).
Radiology: Normal.
Pathology: Transbronchial biopsy positive for enlarged cells with discrete nuclear inclusions (Figure 8-31). The diagnosis is CMV.

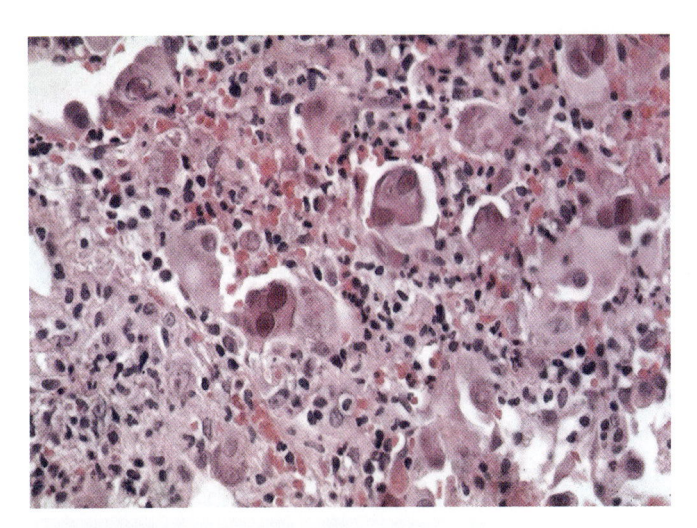

FIGURE 8-26 **Cytomegalovirus (CMV).** CMV is a DNA virus, so generates nuclear inclusions. CMV inclusions are discrete, and are identifiable by H&E stain (Image used with permission from Dr. K. Volmar).

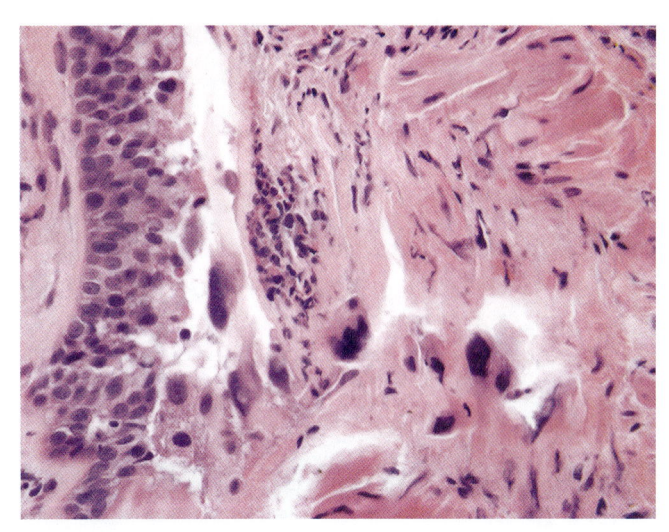

FIGURE 8-28 **Adenovirus.** Adenovirus is also a DNA virus, but shows a smudgy inclusion, usually identifiable by H&E stain.

out nuclear inclusions, cytomegaly, and sometimes cytoplasmic inclusions (Figure 8-26). This distinct morphology can be recognized on H&E stain. Parenchymal necrosis is unusual. *Adenovirus* also results in a distinctive nuclear inclusion, but it is "smudgy" without the discrete borders of CMV, and is typically associated with parenchymal necrosis. *Herpes simplex virus* infection is characterized by multinucleated giant cells, with marginated chromatin, hence the catchphrase "multinucleation, margination, and molding" to describe the viral cytopathic effect (Figure 8-27). Like adenovirus (Figure 8-28), herpes simplex virus infection typically leads to parenchymal necrosis. *HPV* as a primary infection in the lung is uncommon, but can develop in conducting airways as a result of aspiration of aerosolized live virus from the larynx in patients with **laryngeal squamous papillomatosis**. When involving the lung, these HPV-infected sites develop squamoproliferative lesions that are capable of being transformed into clonal squamous cell carcinoma. *EBV* has infected B lymphocytes of most individuals by young adulthood. It can be reactivated in the setting of immunosuppression. It is not associated with an identifiable viral cytopathic effect. However, it triggers a brisk immunoblastic proliferation of B and T lymphocytes in immunocompetent individuals. In the immunosuppressed, neither immunoblasts nor viral cytopathic effect will be clues for ongoing EBV infection. About 5–10% of patients chronically immunosuppressed after allograft transplantation will develop polyclonal or monoclonal B-cell proliferations, some morphologically identical to diffuse large B-cell lymphoma. These EBV-driven B cell proliferations are called **post-transplant lymphoproliferative disorders (PTLD)**. EBV can be identified in formalin-fixed tissue sections by in situ hybridization for EBV-associated nuclear RNA (EBER).

NON-NEOPLASTIC, NONINFECTIOUS LUNG AND PLEURAL DISEASES

Conducting Airway Diseases

Asthma

Roughly 3–5% of Americans are predisposed to *asthma*, a recurring, reversible bronchoconstriction due to hyperreactivity of airways. A variety of triggers for asthma have been described, including stress, allergies, infections, and exercise. Patients present with clinical wheezing (expiratory phase whistling sounds), which is usually controllable with medications. Rare cases of **status asthmaticus** are a recognized cause of death in uncontrolled asthma.

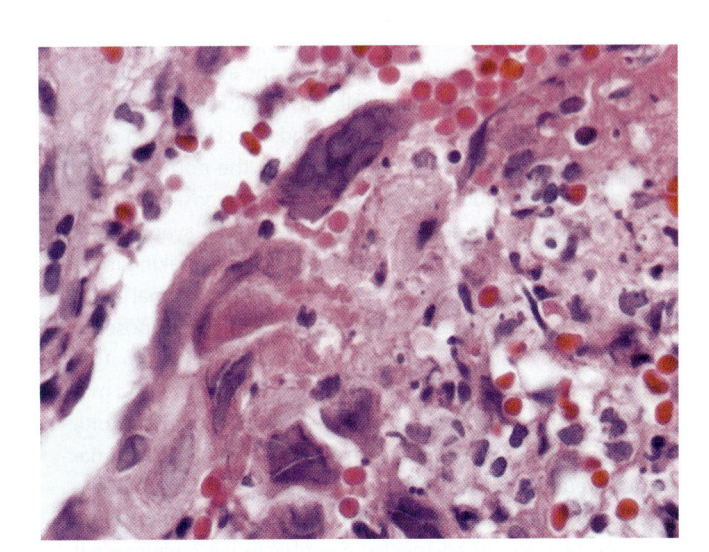

FIGURE 8-27 **Herpesvirus.** Herpesvirus is also a DNA virus, and is characterized by multinucleated nuclear inclusions, with margination of normal chromatin to the periphery of the nuclei, with molding of adjacent nuclei (the 3 Ms of herpes) (Image used with permission from Dr. K. Volmar).

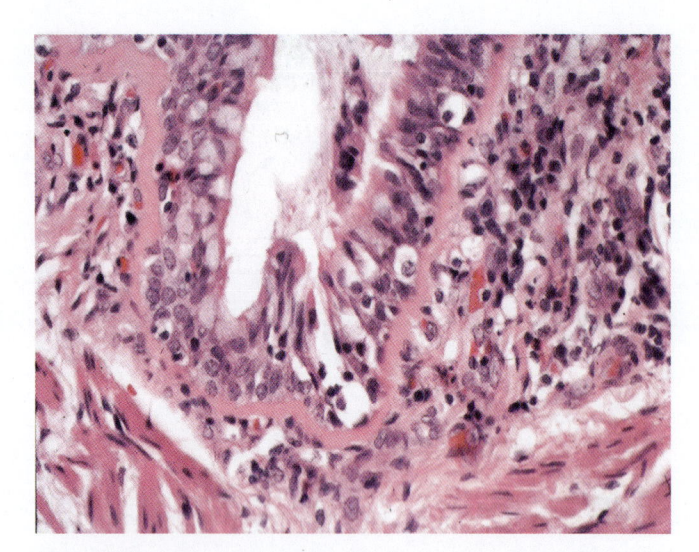

FIGURE 8-29 **Asthma.** Asthma is characterized by excess, including excess smooth muscle, thickened basement membrane, increased number of surface mucous cells, increased inflammatory cells within submucosa, and lumenal debris.

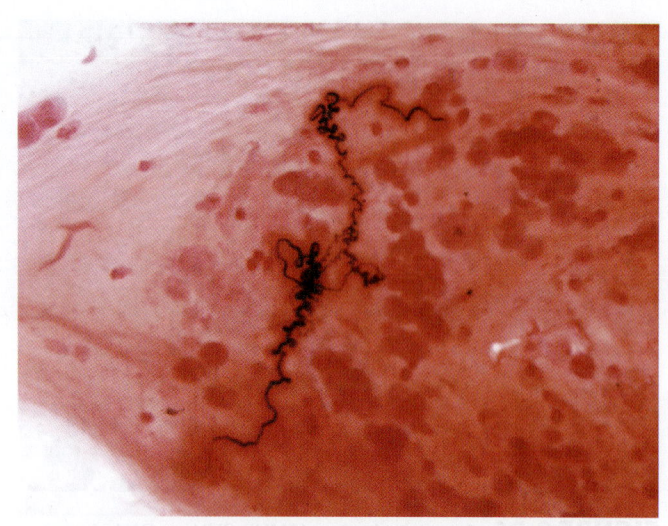

FIGURE 8-31 **Asthma, Curschmann spirals.** These are viscous mucin casts of small conducting airways from asthmatic patients.

Because it is a straightforward clinical diagnosis, it would be unusual to perform radiographs on patients with asthma. With severe bronchoconstriction, radiographs would show variable hyperinflation or hypoinflation (atelectasis) of different segments of the lung. Patients with status asthmaticus may have near-total obstruction of conducting airways, due to a combination of bronchoconstriction and mucous plugging. Patients with chronic asthma, or particularly those who died with status asthmaticus, may be studied at the histologic level. Airways from these individuals show thickening of basement membranes, hyperplasia of submucosal smooth muscle cells, hyperplasia of mucosal epithelial mucocytes, and accumulation of free mucin within the airway lumen **(Figure 8-29)**. In patients who have allergic triggers, eosinophils may be numerous, both within the wall of the airway and within the luminal mucinous debris. Eosinophil degranulation may be so prominent as to lead to crystallization of granule contents, recognized as spindle-shaped "Charcot–Leyden" crystals **(Figure 8-30)**. The mucous plugs within bronchioles can form mucin casts that can be coughed out and reviewed as cytology specimens, called "Curschmann spirals" **(Figure 8-31)**.

Cystic Fibrosis

Cystic fibrosis (CF) is a heritable single gene disorder due to loss of function of the CF transmembrane conductance regulator

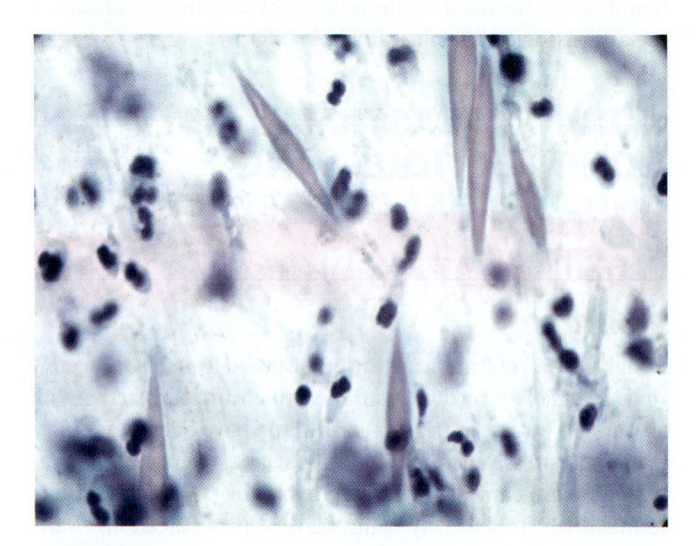

FIGURE 8-30 **Asthma, Charcot–Leyden crystals.** These crystals form in sites of excess eosinophil degranulation.

IN TRANSLATION

Loss-of-function mutations in the *CFTR* gene result in failure to transport bioactive CFTR protein to the apical membrane of the respiratory epithelial cell. This lack of bioactive CFTR protein in the apical membrane leads to changes in sodium, chloride, and free water content of the normally well-hydrated, thin mucus layer overlying the mucosal cilia, with resultant drying and thickening of the mucin layer in these patients. The mucin becomes thick and viscid, making it difficult or impossible to be moved proximally by normal ciliary unidirectional torque. This thick, viscid mucin predisposes to infection by bacteria, with a secondary acute inflammatory response. Inflammation of the wall promotes increased mucin production, which acts as a feed-forward process, ultimately leading to accumulation of large amounts of bacteria-rich, neutrophil-rich viscous mucin within the lumen of the conducting airway. Hence, the old name for CF, "mucoviscidosis." Modern broad-spectrum antibacterials have made it possible for these individuals to survive to reproductive age, and many now receive lung allografts at the time of end-stage lung disease.

CASE 8-8

Clinical: A 18-year-old woman with progressive bronchiectasis.
Radiology: Bronchiectasis, bronchopneumonia.
Pathology: Low power: Dilated, corrugated bronchi with luminal debris (Figure 8-21) (Figure 8-32). High power: Lumenal debris is rich in mucin and neutrophils (Figure 8-33).

Mol Gen Path: Homozygous for ΔF508 mutation in the CFTR locus (Figure 8-34).

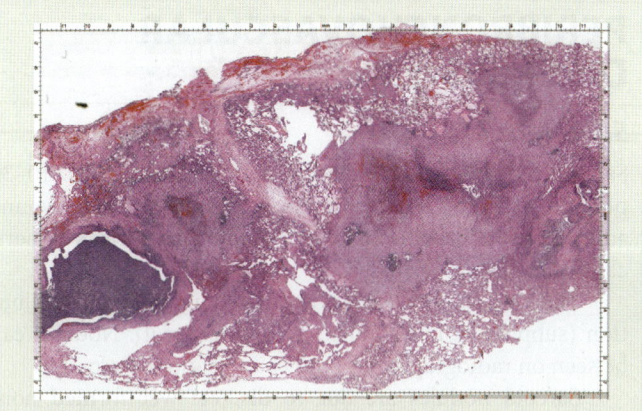

FIGURE 8-32 Cystic fibrosis (CF), lung (low power). It demonstrates bronchiectasis, bacterial superinfection, mural inflammation, and extensive damage to parenchyma.

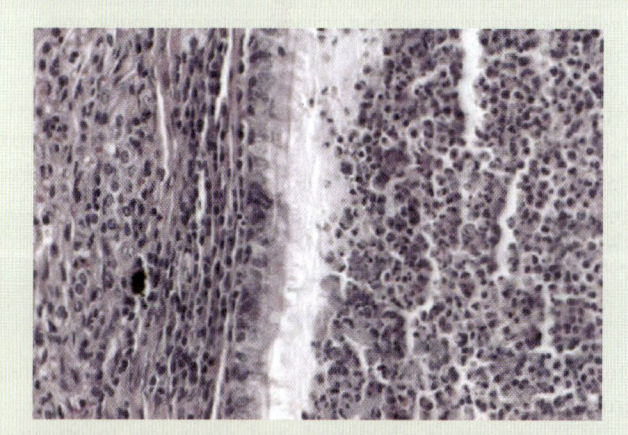

FIGURE 8-33 Cystic fibrosis, bronchiectasis. High-power shows markedly inflamed submucosa to the left, with mucopurulent luminal debris to the right.

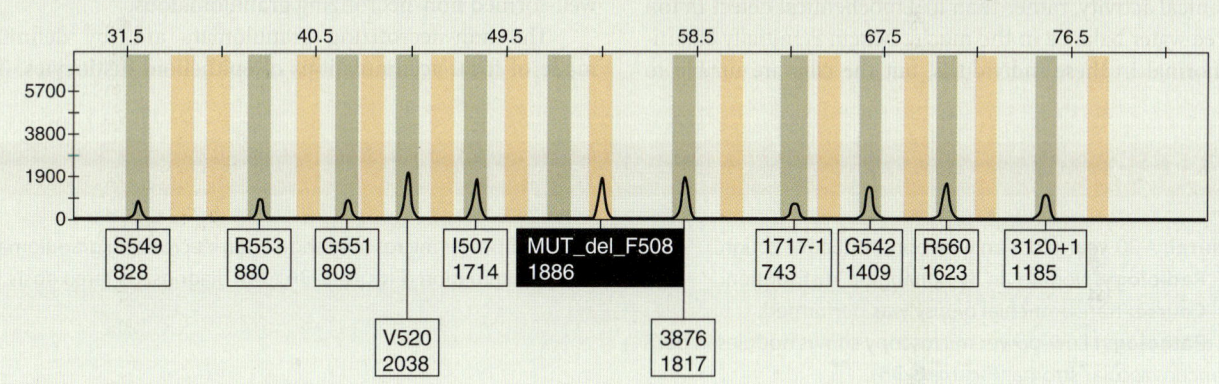

FIGURE 8-34 Molecular diagnosis. Oligo ligation assay can be used to detect the etiologic deleterious mutations of the CFTR gene, in this case the most common mutation, del F508.

protein, CFTR, encoded by the *CFTR* gene. It is more frequent in families of European ancestry. The incidence in US whites is roughly 1 per 3200. Inheritance is autosomal recessive, requiring loss-of-function mutations in both alleles.

Clinical progression of usual CF involves a stepwise process of mucus plugging of large airways, ultimately leading to irreversible dilation and corrugation of large airways, called **bronchiectasis**. This can be recognized easily, since the diameter of normal conducting airway is expected to be similar to the diameter of the adjacent pulmonary arterial branch. Postobstructive bacterial pneumonia is common. Thus, the affected lung in a patient undergoing lung transplantation for CF typically shows bronchiectasis, with foci of remodeling due to previous pneumonia, with foci of gross consolidation and active bacterial bronchopneumonia.

Because this is a single gene disorder, carrier screening and diagnostic testing are now routinely performed in molecular genetic pathology laboratories, with 30–40 mutations recognized as etiologic. ΔF508 (a 3-base deletion leading to loss of the codon translated into phenylalanine at amino acid position number 508) is the most common. Different mutations have different effects on the protein, and are correlated with different phenotypes.

Primary Ciliary Dyskinesia

Primary ciliary dyskinesia (PCD) is a heritable defective cilia phenotype due to a variety of mutations in a number of axonemal dynein arm and radial spoke genes. Like CF, PCD is more common in families of European ancestry, shows

IN TRANSLATION

About half of inherited ciliary defects have been mapped to *dynein* genes, a family of genes whose gene products serve as the ATP-driven motors that generate ciliary axonemal torque. Loss of function of these dynein arm proteins results in an uncoordinated, ineffective motion of the cilia, with measurable loss of mucociliary transport of mucin and debris up and out of the lung, and with male sterility due to ineffective sperm flagella. Like CF, mucus stasis results in bacterial superinfection, inflammation, and bronchiectasis. Bronchiectasis can be recognized radiographically and grossly, since the diameter of normal conducting airway is expected to be similar to the diameter of the adjacent pulmonary arterial branch.

autosomal recessive inheritance, and is associated with chronic inflammation of the lung leading to bronchiectasis.

PCD presents in childhood, and progresses to mucus plugging, bronchiectasis, and postobstructive bronchopneumonia. Unlike CF, the defect in PCD is due to defective ciliary mechanical activity, rather than to a biochemical defect in ion and free water balance in the mucin. Mucin is initially chemically normal in these individuals, but the cilia are unable to generate torque in a coordinated fashion to move the normal mucus layer up and out. However, the net result is similar to that of CF, in which stagnant mucous becomes infected by bacteria, accumulates, results in acute and chronic bronchitis, and ultimately leads to bronchiectasis, chronic bronchopneumonia, and end-stage lung failure.

PERIBRONCHOVASCULAR DISEASES

Sarcoidosis

Sarcoidosis is a common disease in the United States (10–30 per 100,000). The etiology is unknown. It presents in young adults, and is three times more common in African-Americans than in Caucasians.

The lung shows nodules that map the lymphatic distribution (subpleural, interlobular, and periarterial). Nodules can be seen on radiographs, and can be seen and felt grossly.

Sarcoid nodules are due to discrete well-formed non-necrotizing (non-caseating) granulomata. In addition to the lymphatic distribution in the lung parenchyma, the draining lymph nodes are also involved, and show identical discrete well-formed non-necrotizing granulomatous.

The non-necrotizing granulomata are (by definition) made of focal accumulations of epithelioid histiocytes. They

CASE 8-9

Clinical: A 30-year-old man with nonproductive cough.
Radiology: Nodules in "lymphangitic" distribution.
Course: Transbronchial biopsy was performed.
Pathology: Low-power microscopy shows nodules in peribronchovascular stroma (**Figure 8-35**).

High-power microscopy shows non-necrotizing granulomatous inflammation (**Figure 8-36**). The diagnosis is sarcoidosis.

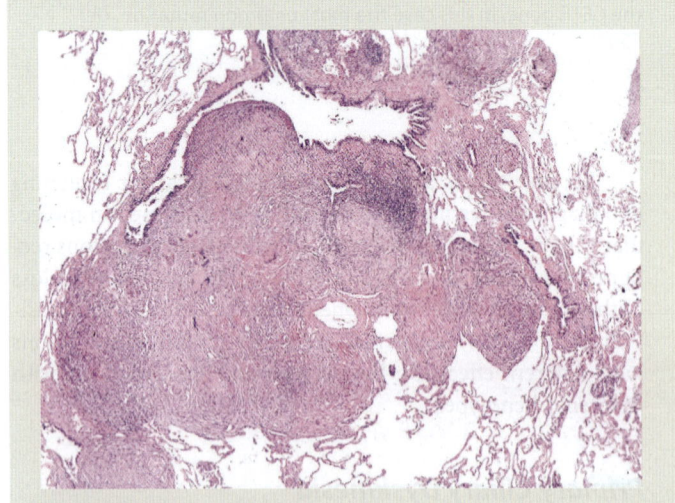

FIGURE 8-35 Sarcoidosis. Low-power view shows peribronchovascular expansion by discrete collections of epithelioid histiocytes.

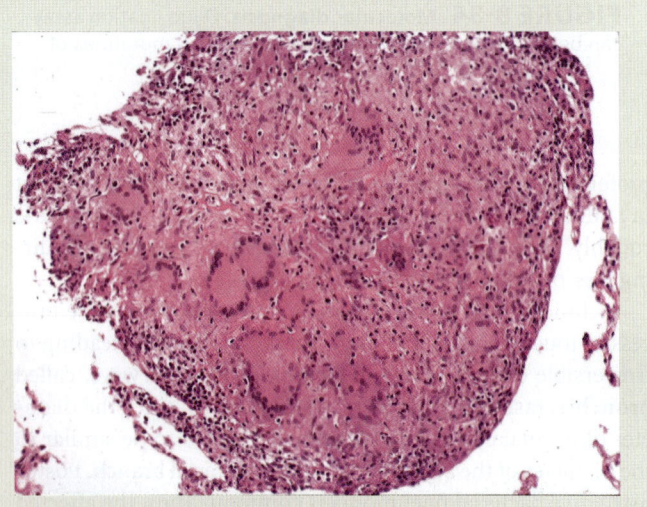

FIGURE 8-36 Sarcoidosis. High-power view shows discrete unencapsulated collections of epithelioid histiocytes with admixed Langerhans-type multinucleated giant cells.

may contain nonspecific material, including **Schaumann bodies, asteroid bodies**, and **Hamazaki–Wesenberg bodies**. Special stains for fungi and AFB (mycobacteria) are negative. Although sarcoidosis appears to be related to an extreme T-cell mediated response, possibly to an infectious agent, no particular etiologic agent has been reproducibly associated with sarcoidosis. Finding the etiology of sarcoidosis is an area of active research.

Hypersensitivity Pneumonia/Extrinsic Allergic Alveolitis

Hypersensitivity pneumonia/extrinsic allergic alveolitis reflects the host response to allergens. Because allergies are common in our society, extrinsic allergic alveolitis should be considered whenever an individual with an identifiable allergen exposure presents with pulmonary symptoms.

Lung radiographs may identify increased peribronchovascular radiodensities corresponding to the mixed inflammatory infiltrates described below. Histologic sections of the lung show bronchiolocentric mixed inflammatory infiltrates, typically rich in lymphocytes, histiocytes, and eosinophils (Figure 8-37). Eosinophils are associated with allergic response to organic antigens, including medications. Loose granulomata can be found in roughly half of the cases, but are less well-formed than those of sarcoidosis.

Langerhans Cell Histiocytosis (LCH)

Langerhans cell histiocytosis (LCH a.k.a pulmonary histiocytosis X, a.k.a eosinophilic granuloma) is a peribronchiolar inflammatory disease of adult smokers. Most patients present with dyspnea or nonproductive cough.

Lung radiographs are expected to show upper lobe-predominant nodular peribronchovascular densities, corresponding to Langerhans cell proliferation. Histologic sections of LCH show a bronchiolocentric accumulation of Langerhans cells. These may show a stellate appearance in tissue sections. Individual cells vary from ovoid to elongate, and may have prominent nuclear membrane irregularities, including longitudinal grooves (Figure 8-38). These cells have a characteristic immunoreactivity for S100 (Figure 8-39) and CD1a. Unlike LCH of childhood, this disease is polyclonal, and is considered a reactive hyperplasia, rather than a clonal neoplasm. Adjacent accumulation of alveolar macrophages in respiratory bronchioles, alveolar ducts, and alveoli represents concurrent **respiratory bronchiolitis and interstitial lung disease** (RBILD) with or without **desquamative interstitial pneumonitis** (DIP).

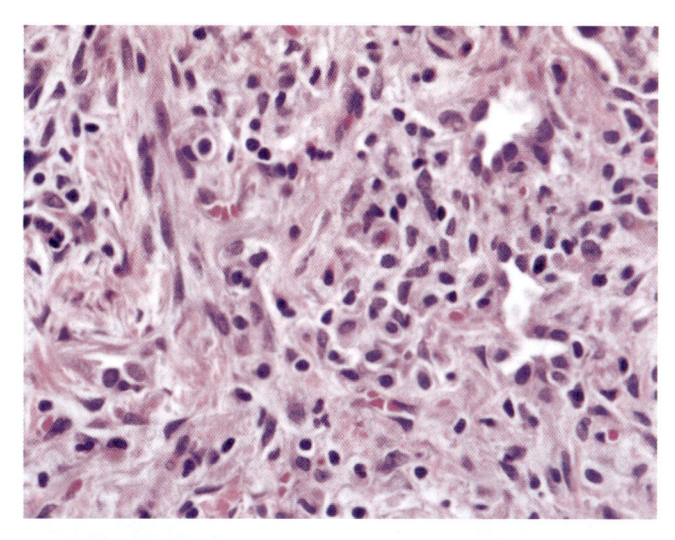

FIGURE 8-38 **Langerhans cell histiocytosis.** This cigarette smoke-associated disease results in airway-centric accumulation of nonclonal Langerhans cells, characterized by epithelioid and elongate spindled nuclei with nuclear membrane irregularities and grooves.

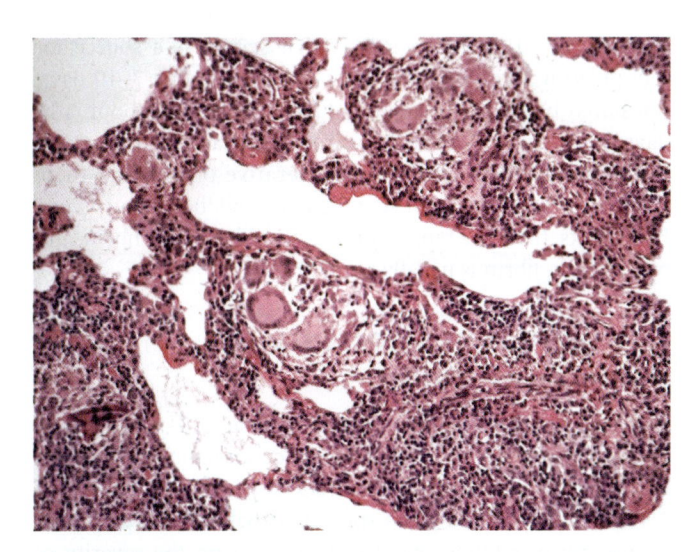

FIGURE 8-37 **Hypersensitivity pneumonia/extrinsic allergic alveolitis.** Airway-centric mixed inflammatory infiltrates, which can contain loose granulomata.

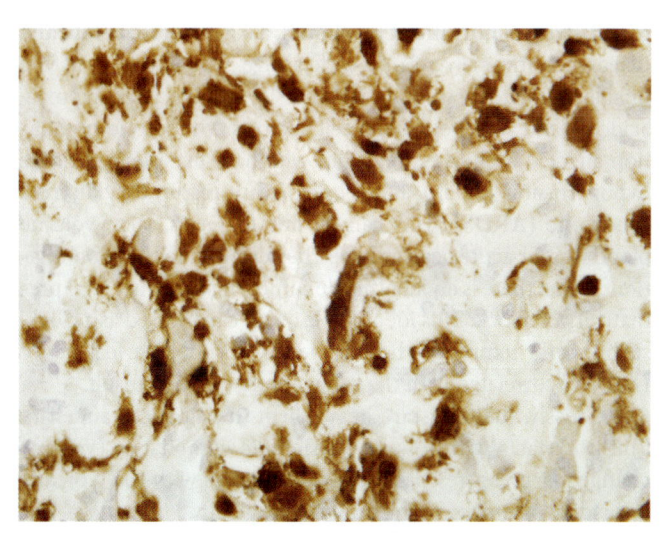

FIGURE 8-39 **Langerhans cell histiocytosis, positive S100 immunostain.** S100 and CD1a immunostains are used to identify Langerhans cells.

CASE 8-10

Clinical: A 60-year-old man in septic shock from acute pyelonephritis diagnosed 3 days before.
  Radiology: Diffuse alveolar filling process.
  Course: Multiorgan failure. Wedge biopsy of lung performed.

Pathology: Low power: Diffuse alveolar filling by hypocellular pink material (Figure 8-40). High power: Alveolar surface fibrin, type II cell prominence (Figure 8-41).
  Diagnosis: Diffuse alveolar damage, exudative phase.

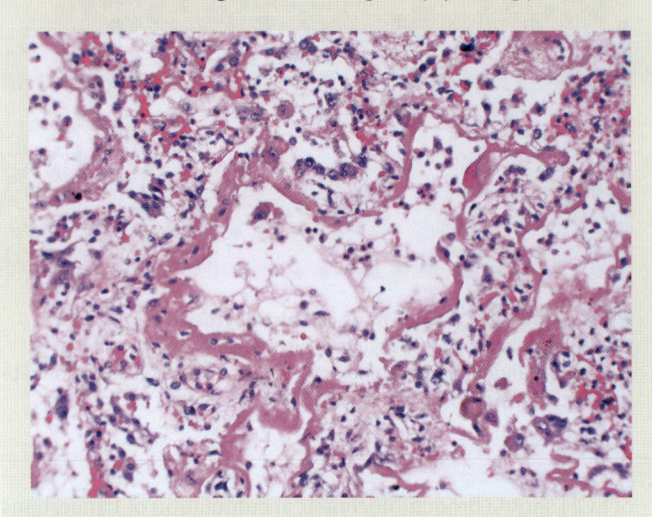

FIGURE 8-40 Diffuse alveolar damage (DAD), exudative phase. Serum coagulation cascade proteins are activated following alveolar injury, resulting in accumulation of fibrin in areas of denuded alveolar type I epithelium.

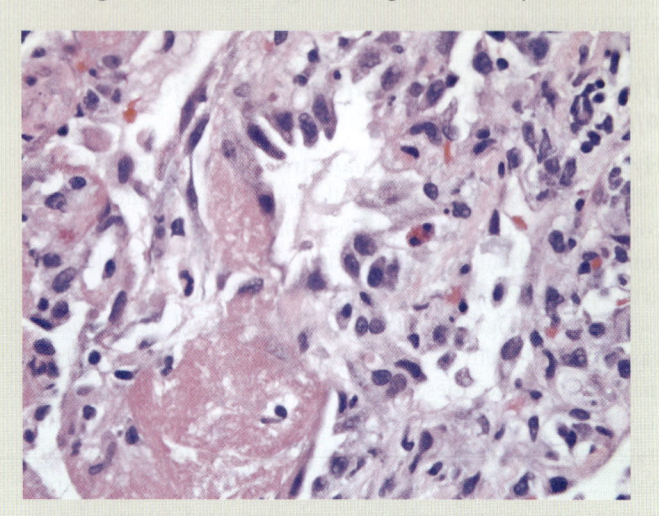

FIGURE 8-41 Diffuse alveolar damage, exudative phase. Type 2 cell hyperplasia is thought to be responsible for repopulation of the denuded type I epithelium.

ALVEOLAR AND ADJACENT INTERSTITIAL DISEASES

Diffuse Alveolar Damage (DAD)

Two distinct populations present with DAD. In newborns <36 weeks' fetal age, insufficiency of surfactant production prevents normal lung inflation. The probability of this disease (**respiratory distress syndrome of newborns**, a.k.a. **hyaline membrane disease**) is inversely related to fetal age. These newborns are unable to inflate their lungs, with persistent atelectasis, hypoxia, acidosis, and type I epithelial cell necrosis. The second population affected is children or adults who have experienced tissue hypoperfusion (shock), and is called **adult respiratory distress syndrome (ARDS)**. This can be due to sepsis, large volume blood loss, or acute heart failure. The key point for both populations is that there is an identifiable clinical insult, either fetal prematurity or shock. This identifiable insult can be used as a clock, such that the temporally homogeneous morphologic features of DAD are correlated with the timing of that clinical insult.

Grossly, the lungs are heavy, firm to palpation, and stiff. This correlates with loss of physiologic compliance (volume change per pressure change), and correlates with the typically diffuse involvement of the lung histologically.

Histologic sections of early DAD (<7 days after insult, known as **acute or exudative DAD**) show accumulation of fibrin, involving the alveolar airspace itself and/or the adjacent interstitium of the alveolar parenchyma. In premature infants without surfactant, this is associated with market atelectasis of the lung parenchyma. The morphologic features are identical in terms of the ratio of fibrin:fibroblasts from lobule to lobule.. This temporal homogeneity is expected for a disease triggered by an identifiable clinical insult at a single point in time.

When alveolar wall fibrin is present, it usually reflects denudation of the underlying type I epithelium (type I pneumocytes). Depending on the age of the lesion, there may be obvious type II cell hyperplasia that serves as a source for repopulating the type I cell layer. During the first 7–10 days, fibrin may be the only evidence of DAD. Starting at about 7–10 days, post-insult fibroblastic proliferation can usually be seen histologically (**organizing** or **proliferative** phase), and these fibroblasts either repair or scar the damaged lung in survivors. By 3 weeks, there are typically more fibroblasts than fibrin, and by 1 month, fibrin is usually scant or absent.

Desquamative Interstitial Pneumonia (DIP)

DIP is a disease of cigarette smokers, like LCH and RBILD. DIP is considered to be a reactive accumulation of alveolar macrophages in response to cigarette smoke dusts.

Radiographs and gross specimens will show a patchy or diffuse alveolar-filling process, depending on the severity of involvement. This corresponds to the accumulation of alveolar macrophages. Histologic sections show filling and expansion of alveolar air spaces by finely pigmented macrophages, so-called

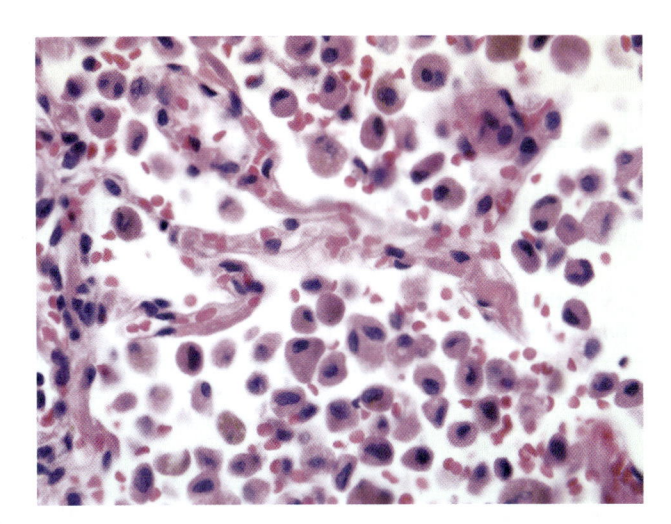

FIGURE 8-42 Desquamative interstitial pneumonia (DIP). This cigarette smoke-associated disease results in accumulation of finely pigmented "smokers-type" macrophages that fill and expand alveolar air spaces.

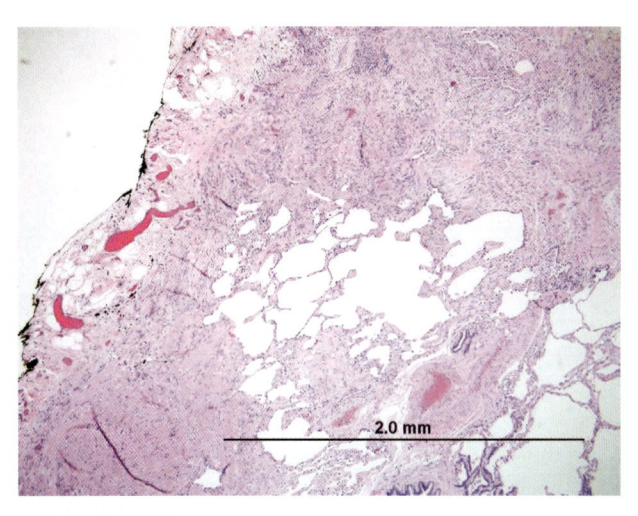

FIGURE 8-44 Usual interstitial pneumonia (UIP). This reaction pattern shows subpleural accentuation, with alternating zones of normal parenchyma, fibroblastic proliferation, and mature collagen-rich fibrosis.

"smoker's macrophages" (Figure 8-42). These macrophages are not Langerhans cells, and they are not the epithelioid histiocytes of sarcoidosis, TB, or fungal infection. They are probably a reactive accumulation in response to the dust load in smokers. These smoker's macrophages can fill adjacent conducting airways, called "respiratory bronchiolitis/interstitial lung disease (RBILD)" (Figure 8-43), such that DIP is likely part of a continuum with RBILD. The key point to remember is that all three diseases (LCH, DIP, and RBILD) are diseases of cigarette smokers, such that the diagnoses should not be entertained without a history of primary or secondary smoke exposure.

Usual Interstitial Pneumonia (UIP)

Usual interstitial pneumonia (UIP) is a disease of middle-aged and older patients, uncommon below 50 years of age. The etiology is unknown, that is, it is *idiopathic*. The prognosis is poor, with many patients dying of this disease. UIP patients may be candidates for lung transplantation if otherwise healthy.

Radiographs show patchy subpleural and interstitial radiodensities that are stable over time. Similar features can be seen in *autoimmune diseases* involving the lung, and in asbestosis. Grossly, there is subpleural fibrosis that is patchy in distribution. End-stage remodeling of parenchyma with visible cysts (**honeycomb change**) may be present.

Histologic sections show temporal heterogeneity, that is, variation from field to field with respect to the degree of fibroblastic proliferation and fibrosis. A typical case would show alternating fields of normal parenchyma, fibroblastic proliferation, and mature collagen-rich fibrosis (Figure 8-44). These findings can also be seen in other diseases, including rheumatoid lung diseases and asbestos pneumoconiosis, emphasizing the need for a careful clinical history, and getting tissue section iron stains for asbestos/ferruginous bodies, as a routine part of the pathologist's workup. When identifiable causes of this reaction pattern have been excluded, then this pathologic diagnosis, UIP, corresponds to the clinical diagnosis, "idiopathic pulmonary fibrosis" (IPF).

Pneumoconiosis

Pneumoconiosis is an exotic-sounding word that means accumulation of dust within the lung. This meaning has evolved, and currently refers to accumulation of non-biologic dusts (coal dust, asbestos, other silicates), some of which trigger parenchymal fibrosis (asbestos and other silicates). Therefore, this disease is usually seen in individuals with environmental exposure to high concentrations of inhaled non-biologic dust. The major fibrogenic dusts of interest are stone silicates (e.g., granite dusts) and asbestos fibers. Affected tradesmen would include stonemasons, sand blasters, miners, shipbuilders, and plumbers. Asbestos miners, shipbuilders, and plumbers were exposed to high asbestos dust loads in the era before asbestos was recognized as an etiologic agent for malignant mesothelioma, as previously discussed.

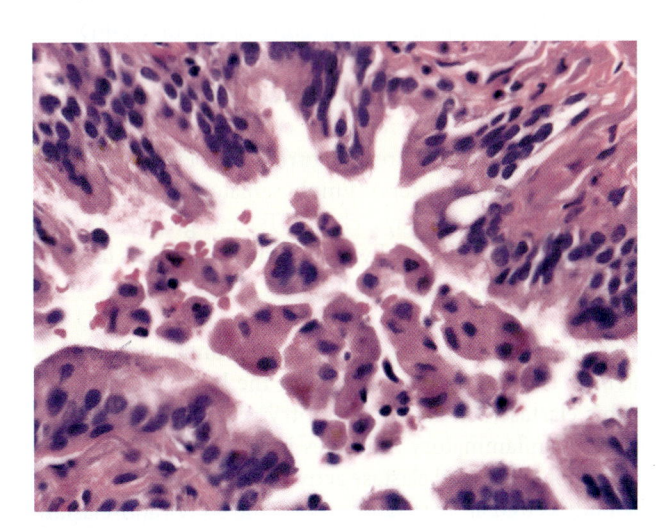

FIGURE 8-43 Respiratory bronchiolitis and interstitial lung disease (RBILD). Similar to DIP, above, this cigarette smoke-associated disease results in accumulation of smokers-type macrophages within the lumen of conducting airways.

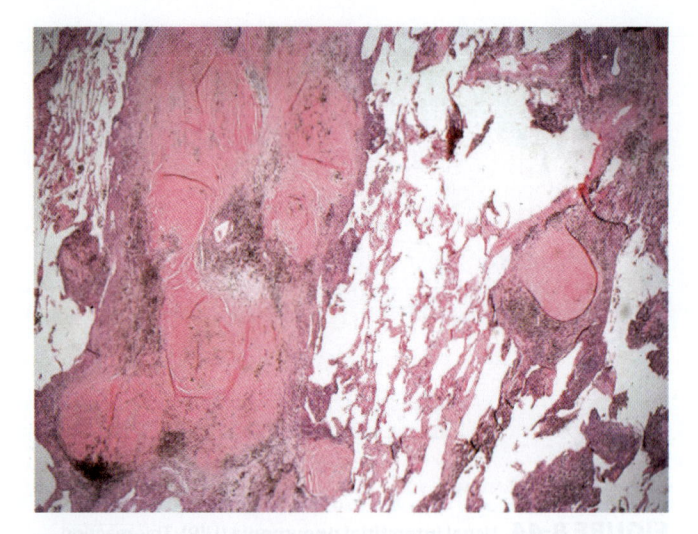

FIGURE 8-45 **Silicosis.** Silicate fibers are fibrogenic dusts; exposure can result in collagen-rich nodules within the lung parenchyma.

Grossly, silicosis presents as large nodules within the parenchyma of the lung, identifiable by radiographs and gross inspection. Asbestosis, on the other hand, presents as patchy subpleural fibrosis and pleural plaques.

Histologic sections from silicosis show an early brisk macrophage infiltrate that progresses to fibrotic nodules (**Figure 8-45**). Early asbestos may be unrecognized, presenting late with patchy subpleural fibrosis with admixed asbestos fibers (**Figures 8-46 and 8-17**).

The fibrous nodules of late silicosis are noninformative, as is the subpleural fibrosis of asbestosis. However, asbestos fibers can be identified by virtue of their propensity to have surface iron encrustation, forming so-called *ferruginous bodies* that can be identified with Prussian blue iron stains in tissue sections.

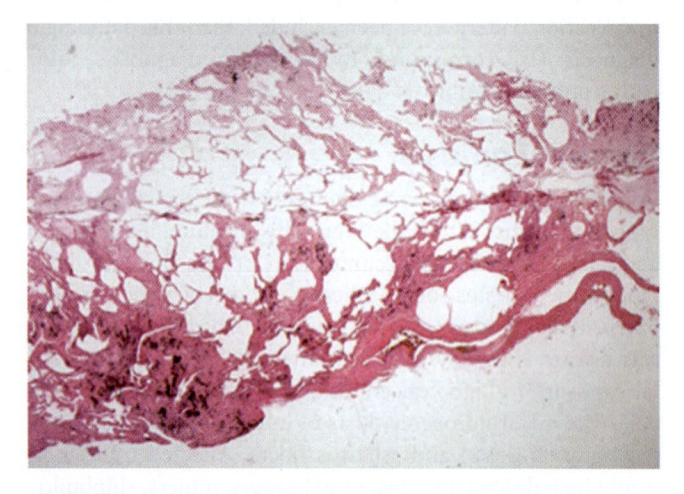

FIGURE 8-46 **Asbestosis.** Like silicates, asbestos dust is fibrogenic and nonmetabolizable; exposure can result in subpleural fibrosis that can mimic autoimmune disease and usual interstitial pneumonia (UIP). Image illustrates subpleural fibrosis.

CASE 8-11

Clinical: A 70-year-old man with 60 pack-year smoking history.
   Radiology: Upper lobe bullous changes, consistent with severe emphysema.
   Course: Upper lobe volume reduction surgery.
   Pathology: Septal destruction, centrilobular distribution (**Figure 8-47**).
   Diagnosis: Emphysema, chronic obstructive pulmonary disease (COPD)-associated.

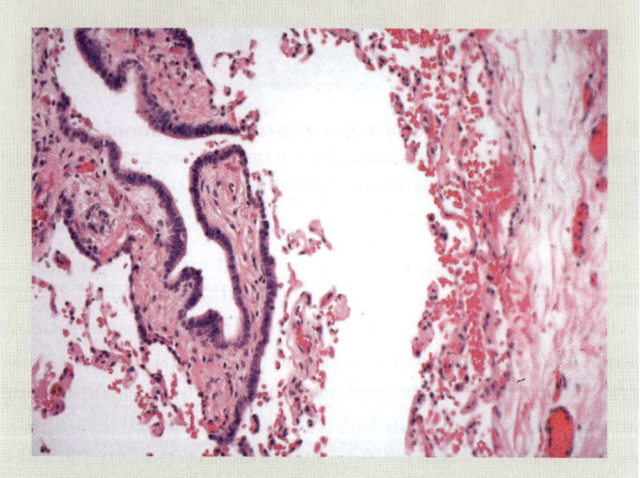

FIGURE 8-47 **Emphysema.** Damage to delicate alveolar septae can result in formation of progressively enlarged air spaces, with proportionate reduction in surface area for gas exchange. Centrilobular emphysema is a side effect of cigarette smoking, and is proportionate to exposure.

Emphysema

Two groups of individuals are affected by emphysema. The more common etiology is cigarette smoking (20% of Americans). Emphysema is a component of COPD, with severity proportional to pack-years of smoking.

Grossly, the lung is hyperinflated, due to destruction of interstitial elastin, with resulting coalescence of alveoli and loss of alveolar surface area (**Figure 8-47**). Fused alveoli can form large bullae (blisters). Emphysematous changes can be seen by plain chest X-rays, chest CTs, and grossly. In severe examples, the lung parenchyma minimally supports large volume bullae in the apex of the lung.

The final common pathway for both COPD and α_1-antitrypsin deficiency is a relative imbalance between intrinsic elastase production within the lung, and inhibition of this elastase activity by α_1-antitrypsin. Cigarette smoking increases inflammatory infiltrates in the lung, increasing the amount of neutrophil elastase activity in the lung. This exceeds the body's circulating α_1-antitrypsin (the body's anti-elastase). In α_1-antitrypsin deficiency, there is reduced circulating α_1-antitrypsin to block normal levels of lung elastase. The net result of both diseases is the destruction of elastin within the

IN TRANSLATION

The less common etiology (incidence 1:5,000 in the United States) is single gene loss-of-function mutations in the α_1-antitrypsin gene [SERPINA1, a.k.a. Pi (protease inhibitor)], leading to severe upper and lower lobe emphysema that begins in young adulthood. Patients with early onset emphysema warrant careful clinical history with respect to smoking and other affected family members. Laboratory workup includes serum levels of α_1-antitrypsin proteins, as well as mutational studies for the different germ line mutations in the SERPINA1 gene.

In α_1-antitrypsin deficiency, there are multiple described germ line loss-of-function mutations in the α_1-antitrypsin gene (SERPINA1). The most severe phenotype is associated with homozygosity for the Z allele. Mutations lead to folding abnormalities of the α_1-antitrypsin protein. The protein is produced in the liver. Misfolded α_1-antitrypsin protein is inefficiently excreted from the liver, so serum levels of α_1-antitrypsin protein are low, and the availability of the anti-elastase activity of this protein in the lung is insufficient to block normal and smoking-associated levels of elastase production in the lung. At the cellular level, a liver biopsy will show accumulation of α_1-antitrypsin protein. The lung will just show septal destruction.

interstitium of the lung, leading to progressive hyperinflation of the lung within the thorax.

The morphologic changes in emphysema are the sequelae of excess elastase activity in the lung. Emphysematous bullae show increased alveolar diameters and stubby residua of damaged alveolar septae. In smokers, background anthracotic pigment and smoker's macrophages may be present. COPD-associated emphysema typically begins around the small conducting airways ("**centrilobular emphysema**"), and in its most severe forms involves the entire lobule ("**panlobular emphysema**"). Alpha-1 antitrypsin deficiency typically presents with pan-lobular emphysema, and is accelerated by smoking.

CASE 8-12

Clinical: A 48-year-old man dies of myocardial infarct 15 days post-colectomy. Previous complaints of pleuritic chest pain

Radiology: Wedge-shaped, pleural-based water density.

Pathology: Autopsy lung gross appearance: wedge-shaped, pleural-based infarct (Figure 8-48) Tissue sections: thromboembolic occlusion of the pulmonary arterial branch at the apex of the wedge (Figure 8-49).

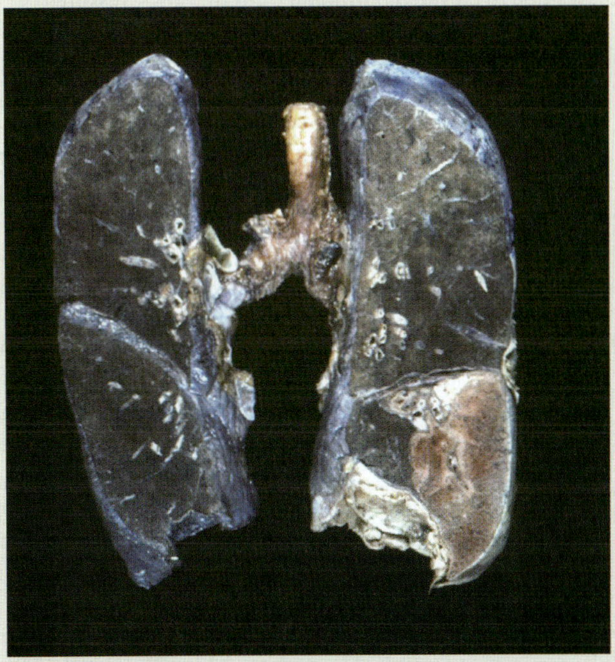

FIGURE 8-48 **Pulmonary embolism with infarction.** This autopsy specimen shows wedge-shaped, pleural-based infarct following pulmonary thromboembolism.

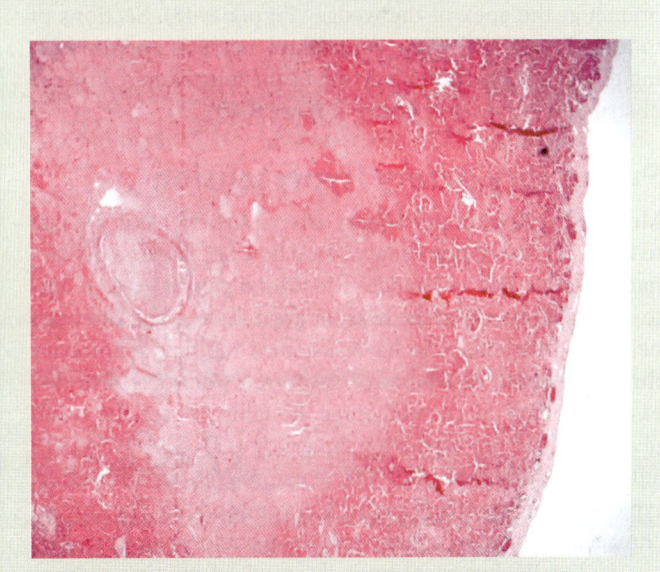

FIGURE 8-49 **Pulmonary embolism with infarction.** Many pulmonary emboli are thromboemboli, and these impact in pulmonary arterial branches in the periphery, leading to peripheral/distal ischemia, sometimes severe enough to infarct the parenchyma.

VASCULAR DISEASES

Pulmonary Emboli (PE)

Pulmonary thromboemboli (clinically **PE**) develop in patients with peripheral deep venous thrombi (DVT), typically originating within the lower extremities. These thrombi break loose and travel as emboli up the inferior vena cava, through the right heart, and finally plugging pulmonary arterial branches. These pulmonary thromboemboli can be asymptomatic, can be associated with acute onset shortness of breath, or can be a cause of sudden death, depending on the location and size of the pulmonary artery that is obstructed. Factors that predispose to DVT define the risk of development of PE, and include hypercoagulability due to factor II or factor V mutations, use of birth control pills, venous stasis, and local trauma.

Significant pulmonary thromboemboli can be seen grossly. However, they may not be seen on radiographs unless contrast is used. Contrast-enhanced CT scans are currently the screening study of choice. Severe thromboemboli associated with acute reduction in pulmonary blood flow create V:Q mismatch, and this can be detected using radionuclides in nuclear medicine studies. Equivocal cases may undergo right heart catheterization and angiograms to define the point of obstruction. In cases of sudden death due to PE, there will be no histologic abnormality of the parenchyma supplied by the obstructed pulmonary artery. If the patient survives the PE, the affected lung may show a downstream infarction that develops a wedge-shaped appearance grossly, based on the pleura, with the obstructed arterial branch at the apex of the wedge (**Figure 8-48**). Sections of infarcted lung will show coagulative necrosis corresponding to the wedge-shaped portion of the lung supplied by the obstructed pulmonary artery (**Figure 8-49**).

Pulmonary Artery Hypertension

Most cases (90%) of pulmonary arterial hypertension are due to either increased pulmonary blood flow or increased pulmonary vascular bed resistance. The former can be seen in left-to-right shunts within the heart or great vessels. The latter can be seen in patients who have sustained multiple pulmonary thromboemboli, or who have developed veno-occlusive disease secondary to chemotherapy. Roughly 5% are the result of an inherited predisposition, inherited as an GPA/Wegener's autosomal dominant trait. The remaining 5% are idiopathic, typically affecting otherwise healthy young adults. The current clinical classification scheme outlines 6 etiologic groups.

Unless PA hypertension is the result of multiple pulmonary thromboemboli, the lung may show no gross abnormality. If PA hypertension is the result of increased pulmonary blood flow, the lungs may be congested and heavier than normal.

Histologic sections of lung show a characteristic thickening of intima and media in the small arteries within the alveolar parenchyma itself (**Figure 8-50**). This is the resistance element that accounts for the elevated pulmonary artery blood pressure on wedge catheterization studies. Initial changes involve

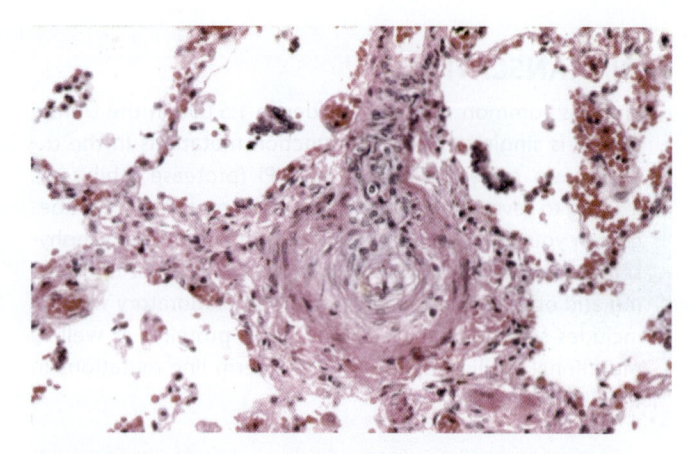

FIGURE 8-50 **Pulmonary arterial hypertension.** Pulmonary muscular arterial branches in the parenchyma show medial and intimal thickening, creating a resistance element at the level of pulmonary artery blood flow.

hyperplasia and hypertrophy of the media, followed by intimal hypertrophy, then intimal fibrosis, and ultimately complex **plexiform vascular lesions**. The last are indicative of an irreversible progression of disease. Other changes may reflect the etiology. For example, associated peripheral infarct would support a diagnosis of recurrent pulmonary thromboemboli. The presence of thickened or fibrotic pulmonary veins would support a diagnosis of pulmonary veno-occlusive disease. The key points are that the thickened muscular PA branches are the morphologic criterion for diagnosis of PA hypertension, and that there are multiple etiologies, with the majority of cases due to elevated pulmonary circuit flow/pressure.

Vasculitis

Pulmonary vasculitides are typically autoimmune diseases, some of which are systemic in nature such as **systemic lupus erythematosus (SLE)** and **granulomatosis with polyangiitis (GPA)** (formerly known as **Wegener granulomatosis**). **Goodpasture syndrome** is localized to the lung and kidney. The pulmonary vasculitides are more common in young adult women, but some of these diseases (e.g., SLE) can be seen in children. Serologic tests are available for the autoantibodies associated with these diseases, facilitating diagnosis in suspected cases. Diagnosis is relevant because of the need for immunosuppression, potentially life-saving in the case of GPA/Wegener's.

Gross abnormalities are noted within the lung following hemorrhage related to autoimmune vasculitis. This can range from patchy collections of fresh blood, to old blood with hemosiderin, to massive exsanguinating hemorrhage.

Histologic sections showing hemosiderin-laden macrophages indicate previously aspirated blood or local hemorrhage, supporting a diagnosis of vasculitis. When the disease is purely antibody-mediated (e.g., SLE and Goodpasture syndrome), there may be limited morphologic evidence of ongoing vasculitis, for example, fibrinoid necrosis of vessel wall or neutrophilic capillaritis. In contrast, GPA tends to generate geographic necrosis and granulomatous vasculitis (Figure 8-51), with elastica injury detectable by elastin stains. Although the inflammatory infiltrates of lupus and Goodpasture syndrome are nonspecific, GPA is characterized by accumulations of epithelioid histiocytes (granulomata), associated vasculitis, and frequent neutrophilic microabscesses. GPA is an ANCA-associated vasculitis with proteinase 3 (PR3) normally present in the neutrophil cytoplasm being the most common target resulting in the autoimmune c-ANCA reactivity. Strong evidence now correlates the anti-PR3 reactivity with the pathogenesis of the disease.

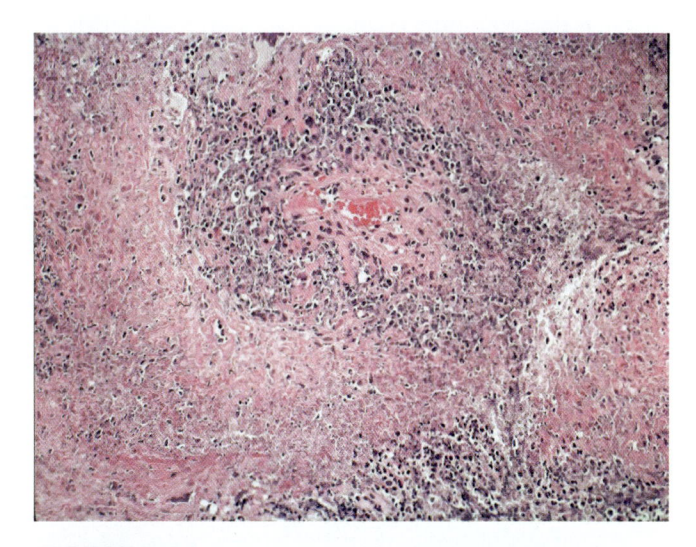

FIGURE 8-51 Wegener granulomatosis (granulomatosis with polyangiitis). The triad of coagulative necrosis, granulomatous inflammation, and vasculitis (of any vessel type) are diagnostic features of Wegener granulomatosis. Elevated c-ANCA antibody titers are found in the majority of patients with active disease.

CHAPTER 9

Pathology of the Gastrointestinal Tract

Kevin G. Greene, M.D. and Dimitri Trembath, M.D., Ph.D.

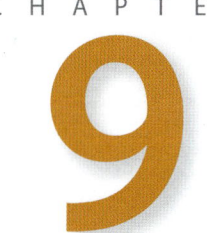

THE ESOPHAGUS

Normal Anatomy

The esophagus is a muscular tube that extends from approximately the level of the cricoid cartilage to its intersection with the stomach, known as the gastroesophageal (GE) junction. For clinical purposes, the distance to the GE junction is measured starting at the incisors and is generally about 25 cm in the adult.

Histologically, the esophagus consists of nonkeratinized squamous epithelium overlying lamina propria and submucosa. Beneath the submucosa is the muscularis propria, consisting of inner circular and outer longitudinal muscle layers. In the upper third of the esophagus, the muscularis propria consists of striated muscle that gives way to smooth muscle in the middle and lower thirds. There is no serosa to the esophagus that allows for spread of tumor into the posterior mediastinum; additionally, the submucosa contains a dense lymphatic system that allows tumors to metastasize to distant sites (**Figure 9-1**).

Pathology

Developmental Abnormalities

Developmental abnormalities involving the esophagus include atresia, fistulae, webs, and rings. Esophageal atresia occurs when there is incomplete separation between the trachea and esophagus, both of which develop from the primitive foregut, leading to incomplete formation of the esophagus. Frequently, esophageal atresia is accompanied by the development of fistula between the trachea and the esophagus. The most frequent anomaly is that of esophageal atresia with a distal tracheoesophageal fistula (**Figure 9-2**).

Other anatomic abnormalities of the esophagus are frequently secondary to a physical or environmental insult. Esophageal strictures/esophageal stenosis occurs when there is scarring of the esophageal wall following injury. Possible etiologies include gastroesophageal reflux disease (GERD), radiation/chemical injury (e.g., ingestion of alkaline substances such as lye), or autoimmune conditions such as scleroderma.

Esophagitis

Reflux Esophagitis

Reflux esophagitis is the most common variant of esophagitis, affecting approximately 10–20% of adults in the Western world. Men and women are affected equally and reflux esophagitis can be seen in all age groups. Typical symptoms include heartburn and dyspepsia.

Reflux is caused by dysfunction of the lower esophageal sphincter (LES) that allows gastric acid to reflux into the esophagus. Common reasons for dysfunction of the LES included anatomic abnormalities such as hiatus hernia, as well as dietary and environmental factors such as obesity, alcohol use, and tobacco abuse.

Grossly, the esophagus develops edema and hyperemia; continued reflux can lead to the development of mucosal erosions and ulcerations. Histologically, the squamous mucosa shows a combination of findings that point to a diagnosis of reflux including (1) basal cell hyperplasia, (2) elongation of the lamina propria papillae to greater than two-thirds of the overall height of the squamous epithelium, (3) spongiosis (intra- and extracellular edema, and (4) a variety of inflammatory cells including eosinophils, lymphocytes, and neutrophils (**Figure 9-3**).

Eosinophilic Esophagitis

Eosinophilic esophagitis (EoE) is less common than reflux esophagitis with an incidence of 0.1–1.2 per 10,000; nonetheless, it is the second most common form of chronic esophagitis. EoE is seen in both pediatric and adult populations. Children with EoE demonstrate failure to thrive and may complain of feelings of food "getting stuck" in their esophagus. Adults are more likely to present with symptoms similar to reflux esophagitis, including complaints of dyspepsia, nausea, and dysphagia.

At endoscopy, the esophagus may demonstrate mucosal rings, exudates, and/or linear furrows. Microscopically, as the name implies, the squamous epithelium shows infiltration by numerous eosinophils with accompanying eosinophilic microabscesses. Additionally, features similar to reflux esophagitis can also be present, including basal cell hyperplasia, lengthening of the lamina propria papillae, and an increase in intraepithelial lymphocytes. Given the overlap between the

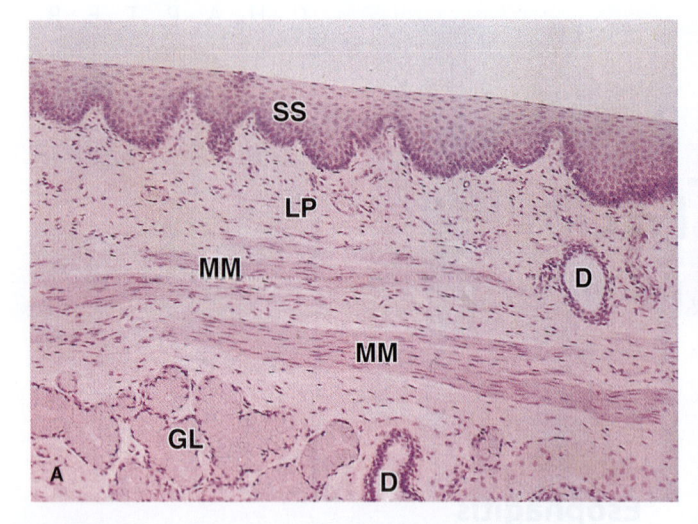

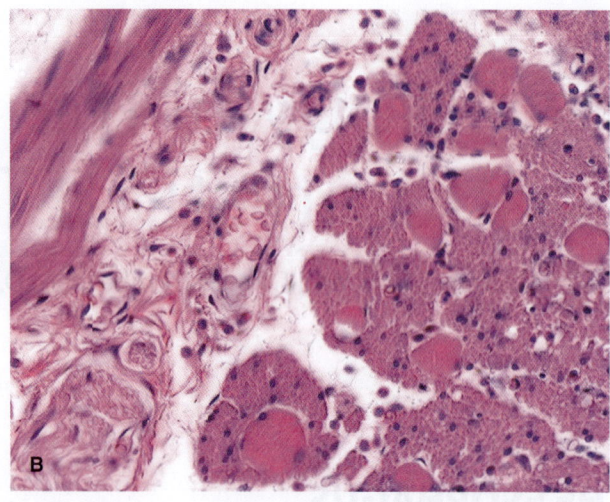

FIGURE 9-1 Histology of normal esophagus: **(A)** Longitudinal section of esophagus shows mucosa consisting of nonkeratinized stratified squamous epithelium (SS), lamina propria (LP), and smooth muscles of the muscularis mucosae (MM). Beneath the mucosa is the submucosa containing esophageal mucous glands (GL) that empty via ducts (D) onto the luminal surface. ×40. H&E. **(B)** Transverse section showing the muscularis halfway along the esophagus reveals a combination of skeletal muscle (right) and smooth muscle fibers (left) in the outer layer, which are cut both longitudinally and transversely here. This transition from muscles under voluntary control to the type controlled autonomically is important in the swallowing mechanism. ×200. H&E. Mescher AL. Junqueira's Basic Histology Text & Atlas, 12th ed. McGraw Hill Lange, New York: 2010. Page 260, Figure 15-14.

histologic features of reflux and EoE, it is recommended that patients first be tried on 2 months of high-dose proton pump inhibitor therapy to rule out reflux esophagitis before a diagnosis of EoE is considered (Figure 9-4).

Infectious Esophagitis

Infectious esophagitis is important predominantly in the immunocompromised populations. Appropriate communication between clinicians and pathologist is often the key to making the correct diagnoses in these patients.

Candida Esophagitis

Candida esophagitis is the most common form of infectious esophagitis. Patients are frequently immunocompromised or have preexisting conditions that predispose them to fungal infection. Concurrent oropharyngeal candidiasis is often found as well.

Patients with *Candida* esophagitis present with dysphagia and chest pain. Endoscopy demonstrates erythematous mucosa covered by white plaques that can be scraped away to reveal underlying ulcers. Histologic findings can be variable with some patients showing minimal changes

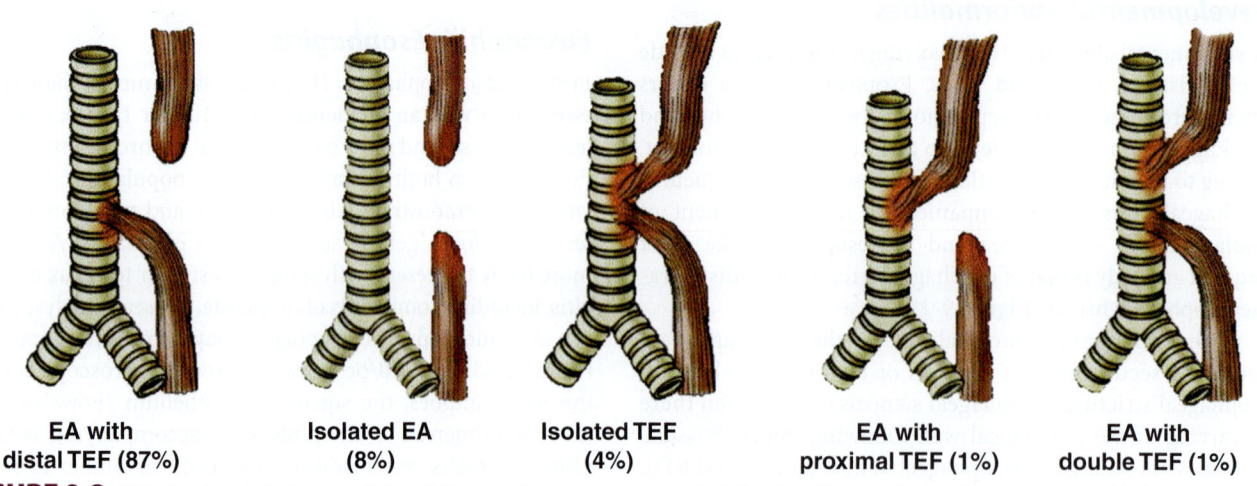

EA with distal TEF (87%) | Isolated EA (8%) | Isolated TEF (4%) | EA with proximal TEF (1%) | EA with double TEF (1%)

FIGURE 9-2 Developmental abnormalities of the esophagus: EA esophageal atresia, TEF tracheoesophageal fistula. Approximate frequency is indicated as a percentage of all observed cases. Source: Data from http://www.med-ed.virginia.edu/courses/rad/gi/esophagus/congen02.html © 2004 by the Rector & Visitors of the University of Virginia.

PATHOLOGY OF THE GASTROINTESTINAL TRACT

CASE 9-1

An overweight 40-year-old man presents to his local physician complaining of burning, gnawing chest pain. The pain is made worse by eating and is worse at night. At endoscopy, linear ulcers are seen in the distal esophagus with accompanying erythema. Biopsy results show squamous epithelium with reactive atypia, increased intraepithelial lymphocytes and rare eosinophils, edema, basal cell hyperplasia, and elongation of the papillae. The patient is counseled to lose weight and treated with proton pump inhibitors with resolution of his symptoms (Figure 9-3).

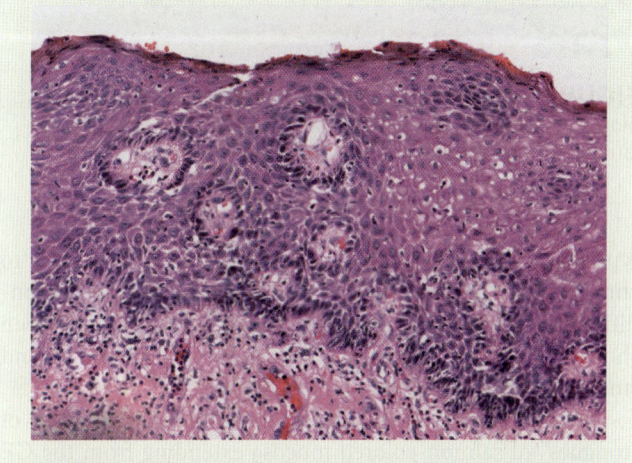

FIGURE 9-3 Microscopic findings of reflux esophagitis. Note the spongiosis secondary to edema, increased intraepithelial lymphocytes, basal cell hyperplasia, and increased papillae height.

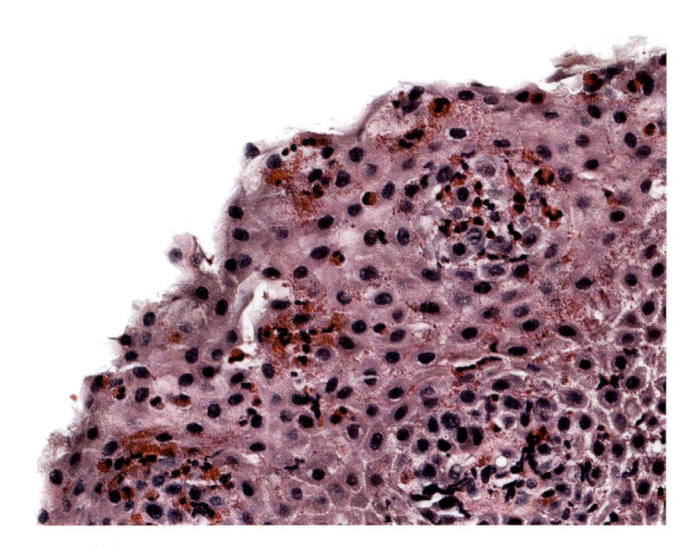

FIGURE 9-4 Eosinophilic esophagitis: Increased intraepithelial eosinophils are seen throughout the squamous epithelium accompanied by additional reactive changes including the presence of reactive lymphocytes and spongiosis.

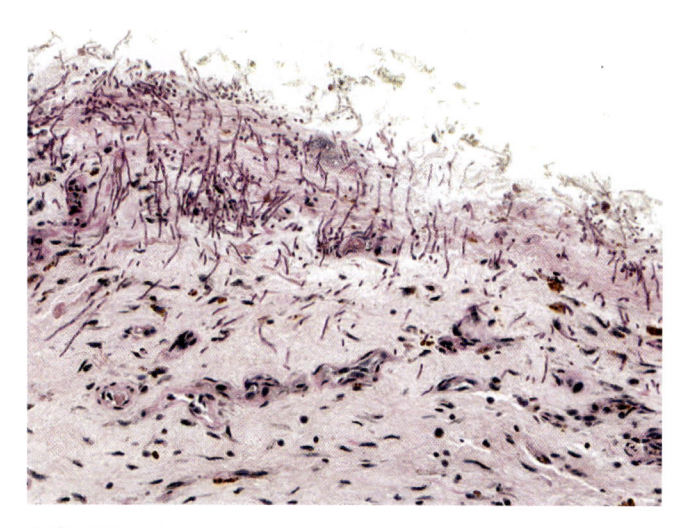

FIGURE 9-5 Candida esophagitis: Yeast forms and pseudohyphae are present along the surface and invading into the superficial mucosa.

to the squamous mucosa, while others have dense neutrophilic infiltrates, ulceration, and occasionally, granulomata (Figure 9-5).

CASE 9-2

A 35-year-old woman presents to her local emergency room for dysphagia. Pertinent past medical history includes positivity for HIV and prior noncompliance with retroviral therapy. Endoscopy reveals discrete, "punched out" ulcers along the length of the esophagus. Histologically, large, atypical cells are present both at the base of the ulcer and in surrounding endothelial cells with "owls-eye" inclusions in the nucleus. The patient is treated with antivirals and resumes her retroviral therapy with relief from her symptoms (Figure 9-6).

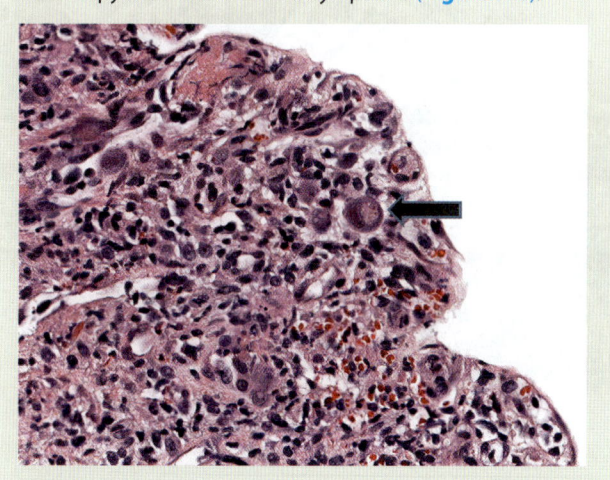

FIGURE 9-6 CMV esophagitis characterized by acute and chronic inflammation of the squamous epithelium. The arrow points to a CMV-infected cell; note the nuclear atypia with the typical "owls-eye" inclusion.

Cytomegalovirus Esophagitis

Patients with cytomegalovirus (CMV) esophagitis frequently present with dysphagia, nausea, and chest pain, similar to patients with reflux esophagitis. Unlike reflux esophagitis, however, patients with CMV and other forms of infectious esophagitis have concurrent fever as well. Endoscopy will frequently show ulcers of various types and possibly erosive esophagitis. Biopsies are best taken from the ulcer base, where microscopic examination demonstrates typical ulcer debris with cells containing the classic intranuclear "owl's eye" inclusions (Figure 9-6).

Herpesvirus Esophagitis

Herpesvirus (HSV) esophagitis is seen predominantly in patients who are immunocompromised. Similar to CMV, presenting symptoms include dysphagia accompanied by fever. Coexisting herpetic lesions in the genitalia or oral pharynx are seen in a minority of patients.

Grossly, HSV esophagitis shows erosive changes to the mucosa and frequently multiple superficial ulcers. Biopsies from the edge of the ulcer show, on histologic examination, ulcer debris with neutrophils and other inflammatory cells. HSV cytopathic effect is characterized by multinucleated cells demonstrating chromatin margination and ground glass nuclei (Figure 9-7).

Neoplasms and Precancerous Disease

Precancerous Lesions: Barrett Esophagus

Barrett esophagus (BE) is a term for a metaplastic, possibly precancerous condition that occurs when the squamous epithelium of the esophagus is replaced by columnar, intestinal-type epithelium with goblet cells. BE develops secondary to chronic injury and inflammation of the esophagus due to conditions such as reflux. The presence of hiatal hernia is also been shown to be a risk factor for BE, while the role of alcohol and smoking is less clear.

At endoscopy, BE is characterized by the presence of "tongues" of salmon-colored mucosa extending from the GE junction. Research has demonstrated that the length of BE seen at endoscopy correlates with risk of dysplasia and carcinoma. Microscopically, BE is characterized by the replacement of the normal squamous epithelium of the esophagus with intestinal-type epithelium demonstrating a mixture of goblet cells and gastric foveolar-type cells (Figure 9-8).

Case A case study of Barrett esophagus can be found in Chapter 2, Case 2-2.

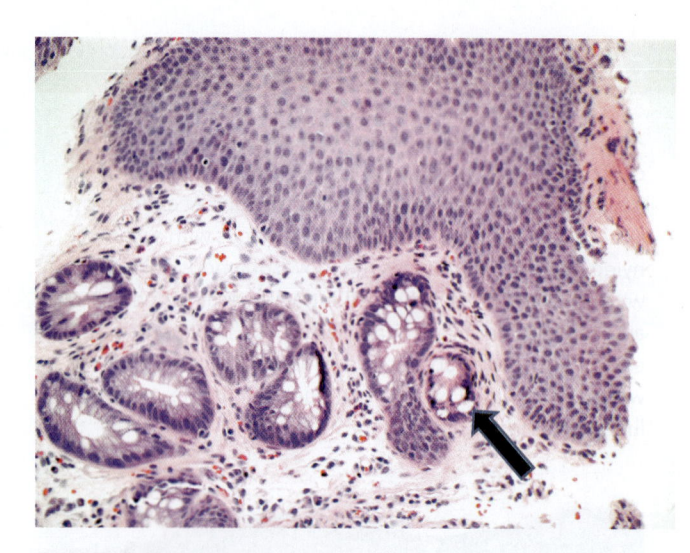

FIGURE 9-8 Barrett esophagus: Gastroesophageal junction biopsy demonstrating the intestinalized mucosa with goblet cells (arrow), consistent with Barrett esophagus.

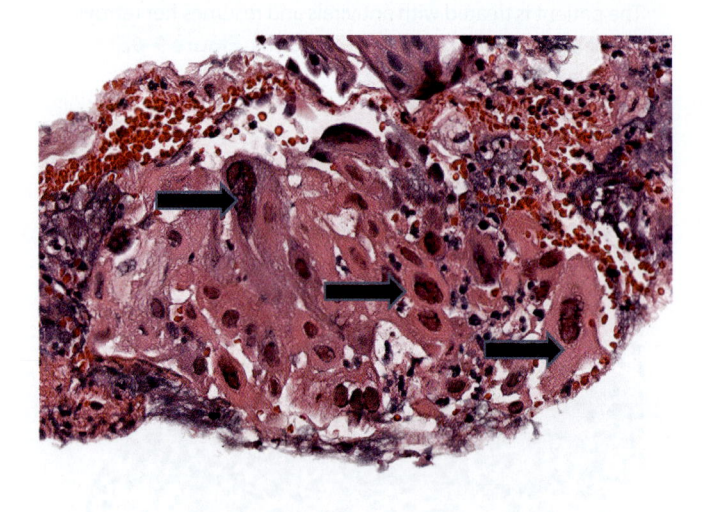

FIGURE 9-7 HSV esophagitis: Arrows point to typical multinucleated cells demonstrating viral nuclear inclusions characterized by a halo of residual chromatin. The cytoplasm has a ground glass appearance. The background is characterized by inflammation and ulceration.

Benign

Benign neoplasms of the esophagus are rare. Those benign tumors that do occur are usually submucosal in location and mesenchymal in origin. The most common is leiomyoma, a tumor arising from smooth muscle cells. Other infrequent tumors of the esophagus include squamous papilloma, inflammatory polyps, and granular cell tumors.

Malignant

Malignant tumors of the esophagus include squamous cell carcinoma and adenocarcinoma. Worldwide, squamous cell carcinoma is the most common form of esophageal carcinoma while adenocarcinoma is now the most common form of esophageal cancer in the United States.

Squamous Cell Carcinoma

There are worldwide geographic variations in the incidence of squamous cell carcinoma; the highest incidence rates are

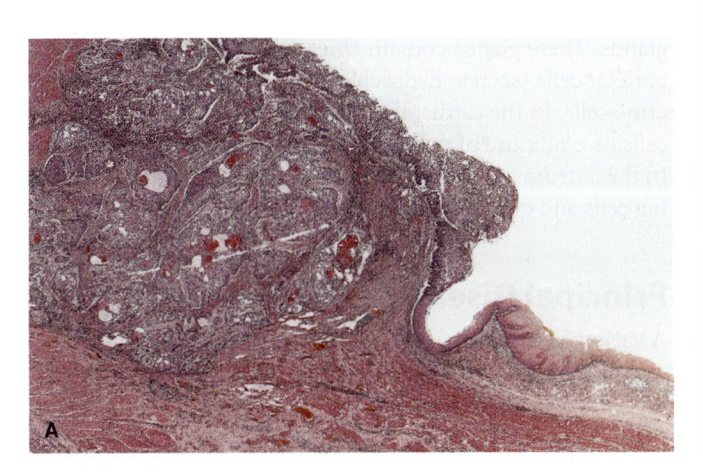

FIGURE 9-9 Squamous cell carcinoma: (A) (low power) Squamous cell cancer of the esophagus (left side of figure) characterized by islands of atypical squamous cells extending into the submucosa. **(B)** (high-power detail) Note keratin pearls (arrow). Cells demonstrate increased nuclear–cytoplasmic ratio, nuclear atypia, mitotic activity, and apoptotic debris.

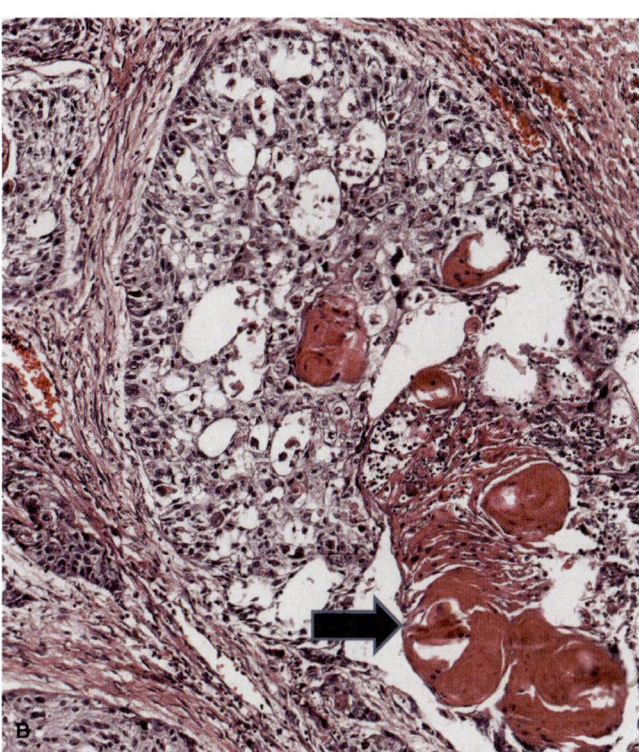

found in Asia and sub-Saharan Africa with the lowest rates in Europe and the United States. Major risk factors for the development of squamous cell carcinoma include smoking and alcohol abuse; lesser risk factors include poor nutrition and diets low in fruits and vegetables. Patients present with symptoms of dysphagia, weight loss, epigastric pain, and regurgitation.

Grossly, squamous cell carcinoma arises predominantly in the middle third of the esophagus, followed by the lower and upper third segments, respectively. The majority of tumors appear as fungating lesions with the remainder demonstrating an ulcerative or infiltrative appearance. Microscopically, squamous cell carcinomas appear similar to squamous cell carcinomas elsewhere in the body, consisting of well, moderately, or poorly differentiated tumors that show invasive nests and islands of squamous epithelium, frequently with generous keratinization. Invasion of the submucosa allows access to the region's rich lymphatic system, allowing metastases to regional lymph nodes, liver, and lung (Figure 9-9).

Case See Chapter 2, Case 2-2.

Adenocarcinoma

Adenocarcinoma of the esophagus is now the most common form of primary esophageal carcinoma in the United States with an incidence of 1 to 5/100,000 population per year in the early 2000s. BE is the single greatest risk factor for the development of adenocarcinoma. Meta-analysis has demonstrated that the incidence of adenocarcinoma in patients with BE is approximately 4/1000 person-years that translates to an approximately 10% risk in patients with BE. Given the relationship between GERD and the development of BE, it should come as no surprise that the clinical presentation of esophageal adenocarcinoma frequently overlaps with that of reflux.

As adenocarcinoma develops from BE, the tumor is therefore found predominantly at the GE junction. Adenocarcinoma typically appears as flat, ulcerated tumors with a minority having a fungating appearance. Residual tongues of BE can sometimes be seen near the tumor bed. Microscopically, esophageal adenocarcinoma is characterized by islands of invasive glands demonstrating various degrees of differentiation. A small number of adenocarcinomas are of the diffuse type and demonstrate signet ring morphology reminiscent of diffuse type gastric adenocarcinoma (Figure 9-10) (see also Chapter 2, Case 2-2).

STOMACH

Normal Anatomy and Histology of the Stomach

The stomach is a saccular organ located in the upper abdomen. The lumen is continuous with the esophagus at the GE

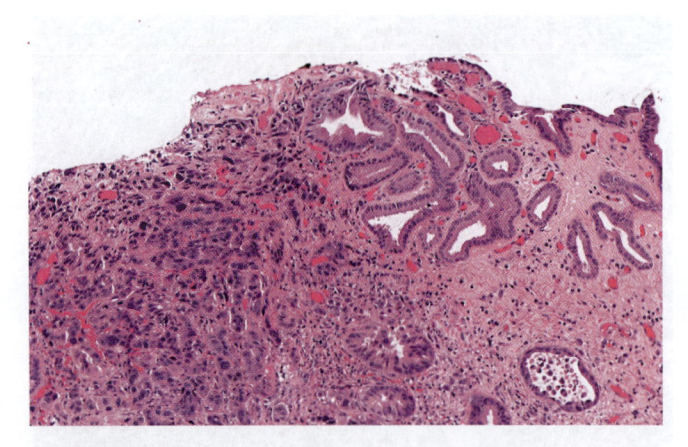

FIGURE 9-10 Adenocarcinoma of the esophagus. Islands of atypical glands with irregular architecture obliterate the mucosa and extend into the submucosa. Bizarre nuclei, mitotic activity, and apoptotic debris characterize the tumor cells.

junction and with the duodenum at the pyloric sphincter. The greater and lesser curvatures mark the left lateral and right lateral aspects of the stomach, respectively. The stomach is divided into five anatomic regions. The cardia is the most proximal region of the stomach and extends a very short distance from the GE junction (usually less than 5 mm). The fundus is the dome-shaped upper portion of the stomach, located to the left and above the GE junction. The body, or corpus, makes up the majority of the stomach and extends from the fundus to the antrum. The antrum makes up the distal third of the stomach and extends to the pylorus/pyloric sphincter, which is surrounded by a smooth muscle layer that controls the passage of food from the stomach to the duodenum. The gastric rugae are a series of mucosal folds that are prevalent in the fundus and body and allow the stomach to expand with a meal (Figure 9-11).

The gastric wall, from inside to outside, consists of the mucosa, submucosa, muscularis propria, and serosa. From the mucosal surface, gastric pits extend down to the secretory glands, providing a conduit for gastric secretions to enter the gastric lumen. The composition of gastric glands varies depending on the anatomic region of the stomach. The gastric body and fundus contain an abundance of oxyntic (fundic) glands. These glands contain chief cells (secrete pepsinogen), parietal cells (secrete hydrochloric acid), and scattered endocrine cells. In the cardia, the glands contain mucous secreting cells or a mixture of mucous secreting cells and oxyntic cells. In the antrum and pylorus, the glands contain mucous secreting cells and endocrine cells (Figure 9-12).

Principal Diseases of the Stomach

A variety of developmental disorders, inflammatory disorders, and neoplasms can be seen in the stomach.

Developmental Disorders

With the exception of pyloric stenosis, developmental disorders of the stomach are relatively rare and include congenital diaphragmatic hernias, duplications, diverticula, cysts, atresias, and congenital membranes.

Pyloric Stenosis

The pathologic hallmark of congenital pyloric stenosis is pronounced thickening of the inner circular layer of the muscularis propria of the pyloric sphincter. This thickening, likely in association with functional abnormalities of peristalsis, results in a narrowing of the pyloric canal that in turn obstructs the gastric outlet.

Clinically, this manifests as projectile vomiting during the first month of life. The ongoing loss of hydrochloric acid can lead to a hypochloremic metabolic alkalosis. The treatment of pyloric stenosis is surgical incision of the thickened pyloric smooth muscle (myotomy). Most patients have an excellent response to surgical intervention.

Inflammatory Disorders

Inflammatory disorders are an important category of stomach disease and are frequently encountered in the clinical setting.

Acute (Hemorrhagic) Gastritis

Acute hemorrhagic gastritis results from a breakdown in the mucosa's protective mucous-bicarbonate barrier, which leads to mucosal hemorrhage, erosion, and ulceration. The amount of hemorrhage can be quite substantial, and even fatal in some cases. Common causes include severe physiologic stress (e.g., burn injuries), aspirin and nonsteroidal anti-inflammatory use, and excessive ethanol consumption.

CASE 9-3

The patient is a 47-year-old healthy man who underwent an upper gastrointestinal (GI) endoscopy for mild dyspepsia. Endoscopic examination of the stomach revealed a few small superficial erosions within the gastric antrum. Representative lesions were biopsied for microscopic evaluation by a pathologist. Additional biopsies were obtained for *Campylobacter*-like organism (CLO) testing, which demonstrated the presence of urease activity. The following day, microscopic examination of the tissue showed mild active (neutrophilic) gastritis, severe chronic gastritis, and numerous *Helicobacter* organisms along the mucosal surface, consistent with *Helicobacter gastritis*. He was given prescriptions for antibiotics and a proton pump inhibitor, but failed to complete the treatment. Several years later, he underwent a follow-up upper GI endoscopy that showed multiple shallow gastric ulcers and prominent gastric folds. Biopsies were obtained and showed the presence of gastric marginal zone B-cell lymphoma, which has arisen from mucosa-associated lymphoid tissue (MALT) in the presence of chronic *Helicobacter* gastritis (see section "Marginal Zone B-cell Lymphoma" and Figure 9-20).

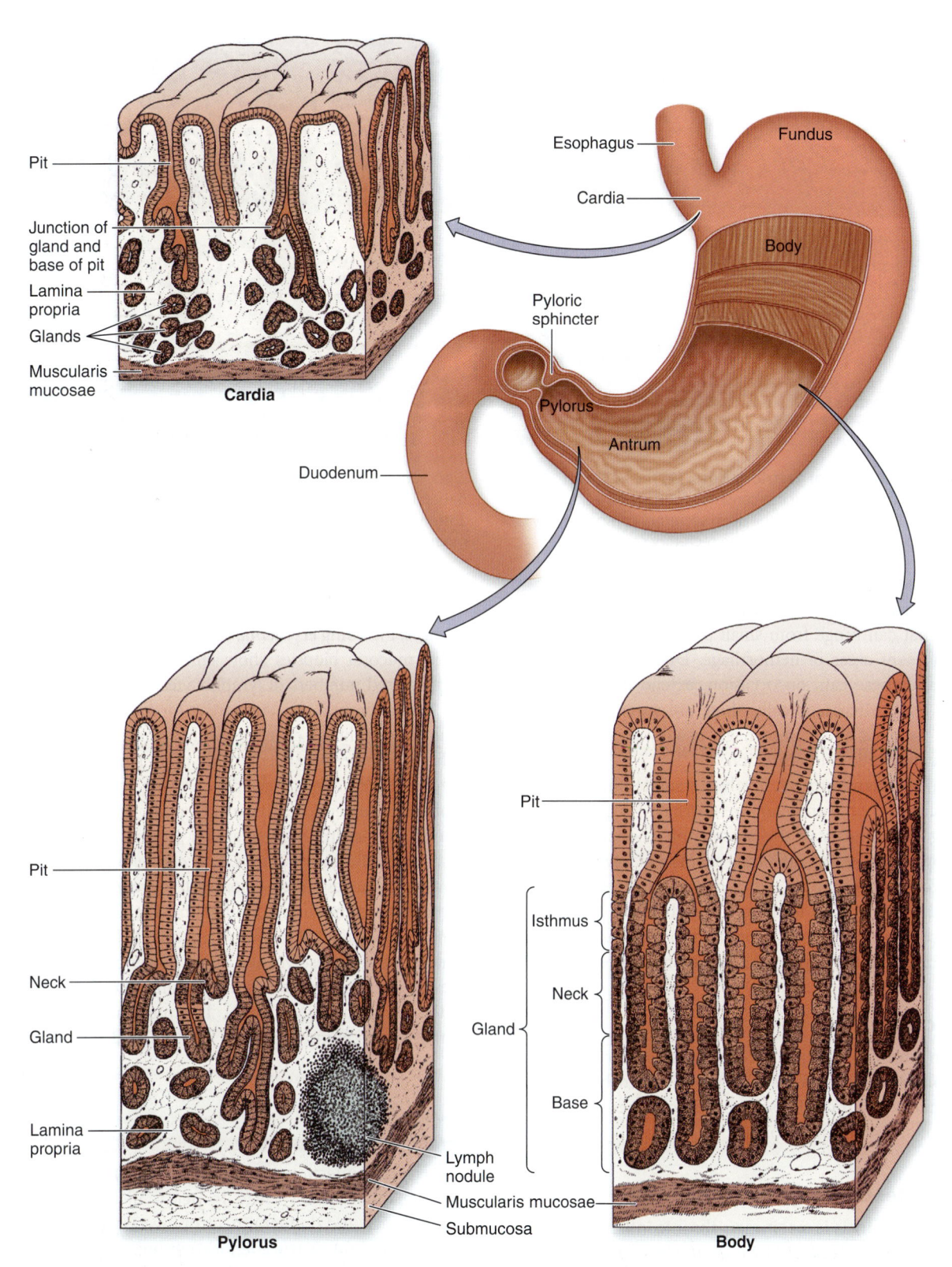

FIGURE 9-11 Regions of the stomach. The stomach is a muscular dilation of the digestive tract where mechanical and chemical digestion occurs. The muscularis consists of three layers for thorough mixing of the stomach contents as chyme: an outer longitudinal layer, a middle circular layer, and an inner oblique layer. The stomach mucosa shows distinct histological differences in the cardia, the fundus/body, and the pylorus. Cells that secrete HCl and pepsin are restricted mainly to the body and fundus regions. Glands of the cardia and pylorus produce primarily mucus. Source: Mescher AL. Junqueira's Basic Histology Text & Atlas, 12th ed. McGraw Hill Lange, New York: 2010. Page 261, Figure 15-15.

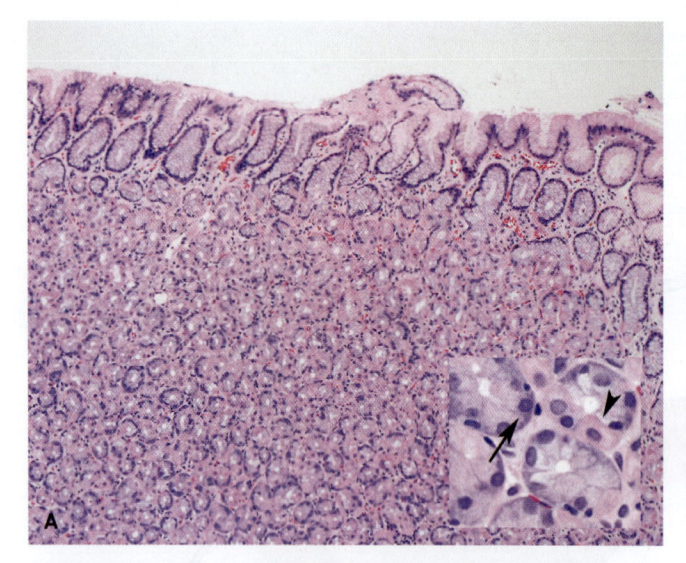

FIGURE 9-12 **Normal gastric mucosa. (A)** The epithelial component of the gastric mucosa consists of surface foveolar epithelium that is connected to the deep secretory component by gastric pits. In the body and fundus, the secretory component is predominantly made up of oxyntic glands. The inset highlights a parietal cell (arrowhead) and a chief cell (arrow). **(B)** In the cardia, antrum, and pylorus, the secretory component is predominantly made up of mucous secreting cells.

Examination of the stomach shows areas of mucosal hemorrhage that can range from small petechial hemorrhages to large confluent areas of hemorrhage. Discrete ulcers can be present and these can, on occasion, extend deeply into the stomach wall. Microscopically, there are variable degrees of mucosal necrosis and hemorrhage, usually accompanied by acute (neutrophilic) inflammation.

Clinical management involves maintaining hemodynamic stability, if significant hemorrhage is present, and restoring the integrity of the mucous-bicarbonate protective barrier by removing any offending agents and lowering gastric acid secretion through the use of histamine receptor antagonists and proton pump inhibitors. Prophylactic use of histamine receptor antagonists is common in the management of hospitalized patients to protect against "stress ulcers."

Chronic Gastritis

The term "chronic gastritis" encompasses a spectrum of stomach disorders, which are usually accompanied by a chronic inflammatory infiltrate. These disorders can present with dyspepsia but are often asymptomatic.

Helicobacter Gastritis

Helicobacter gastritis is a common chronic inflammatory disorder of the stomach caused by infection by *H. pylori*, and less commonly *H. heilmannii*. In addition to chronic gastritis, *H. pylori* infection can lead to peptic ulcer disease of the stomach and duodenum, atrophic gastritis, gastric MALT lymphoma, and gastric adenocarcinoma. Infection results from the ingestion of *Helicobacter* organisms, which are spiral-shaped gram-negative rods. Infection rates increase with age and are highest in developing parts of the world.

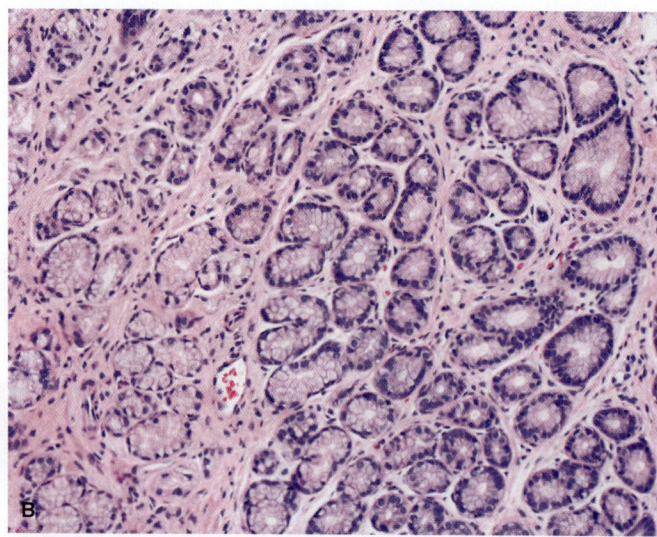

Examination of the stomach shows nonspecific mucosal changes, including erythema, erosions, and atrophy. Microscopically, mucosal biopsies show chronic gastritis, characterized by increased numbers of lymphocytes and plasma cells within the lamina propria (i.e., supportive loose connective tissue surrounding epithelial elements within the mucosa). Lymphoid follicles with germinal centers are often present and are highly specific for *Helicobacter* gastritis. During active infection, there is often an element of active (neutrophilic) gastritis. Neutrophils can be seen infiltrating the lamina propria, surface epithelium, gastric pits, and gastric glands. *Helicobacter* organisms are a non-invasive pathogen. They colonize the protective mucous layer and adhere to the surface epithelium. The neutrophilic component resolves quickly following treatment. The chronic inflammatory infiltrate resolves at a much slower pace and can still be present in endoscopic biopsies, even after successful eradication of the infection (**Figure 9-13**). Treatment involves a combination of proton pump inhibitors, bismuth, and antibiotics.

QUICK REVIEW
Helicobacter Gastritis

- *H. pylori* infection is a common cause of chronic gastritis.
- Infection can also lead to peptic ulcer disease of the stomach and duodenum, atrophic gastritis, MALT lymphoma, and gastric adenocarcinoma.
- Acute inflammation and lymphoid infiltrates with germinal centers are highly suggestive of infection.

Atrophic Gastritis

Atrophic gastritis is a gastric disorder characterized by progressive loss of normal gastric glands with replacement by

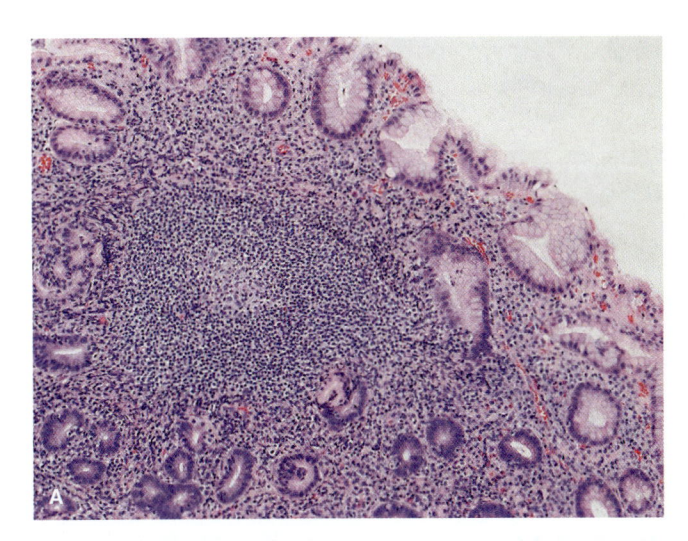

FIGURE 9-13 *Helicobacter* **gastritis. (A)** Note the dense lymphoplasmacytic infiltrate in the lamina propria with a characteristic germinal center. **(B)** A higher magnification view shows *H. pylori* organisms (arrows) within the superficial portion of the gastric pit. Note the associated intraepithelial neutrophils.

fibrous tissue and metaplastic intestinal epithelium. There are two major categories: autoimmune gastritis and multifocal atrophic gastritis. Both forms can result in dyspepsia, prompting endoscopic evaluation; however, they are most commonly asymptomatic and can be discovered during the work-up of other upper GI complaints. Atrophic gastritis, regardless of the etiology, increases a person's chances of developing gastric carcinoma. Intestinal metaplasia is thought to be a precursor lesion for dysplasia and carcinoma, similar to the sequence seen in Barrett esophagus (Figure 9-14).

Autoimmune Gastritis

Autoimmune gastritis is a form of atrophic gastritis that involves the body and fundus and is associated with serum autoantibodies to parietal cells and intrinsic factor. The precipitating factor that leads to the development of autoimmune gastritis is uncertain. Autoantibody-mediated destruction of parietal cells leads to progressive parietal cell loss and hypochlorhydria. Achlorhydria can occur in advanced cases. Chief cell loss also occurs, resulting in decreased pepsin activity. In response to decreased acid secretion, G cell hyperplasia occurs in the gastric antrum. G cells secrete gastrin in an effort to increase acid secretion. Gastrin also stimulates endocrine cells (i.e., enterochromaffin-like cells) in the gastric body to proliferate. Thus, neuroendocrine cell hyperplasia and neuroendocrine tumors and carcinomas can occur in autoimmune atrophic gastritis. Autoantibodies to intrinsic factor, a glycoprotein that plays a critical role in vitamin B_{12} absorption, can lead to pernicious anemia, a megaloblastic anemia resulting from decreased intrinsic factor-mediated absorption of vitamin B_{12}.

Multifocal Atrophic Gastritis

This form of atrophic gastritis was formerly known as environmental metaplastic atrophic gastritis. In contrast to autoimmune gastritis, multifocal atrophic gastritis predominantly involves the gastric antrum with possible spillover into the adjacent gastric body. As the name implies, involvement of the antrum tends to occur in a more patchy distribution. Mild hypochlorhydria is possible; however, achlorhydria and pernicious anemia are not encountered. Gastrin secretion is not typically elevated to a significant degree, thus neuroendocrine cell hyperplasia and neuroendocrine tumors are not a usual component. Chronic *H. pylori* infection is a common cause.

Gastric Ulcers

A mucosal erosion is a loss of the superficial portion of the mucosa due to injury and inflammation. Similarly, an ulcer is the loss of mucosa due to injury and inflammation; however,

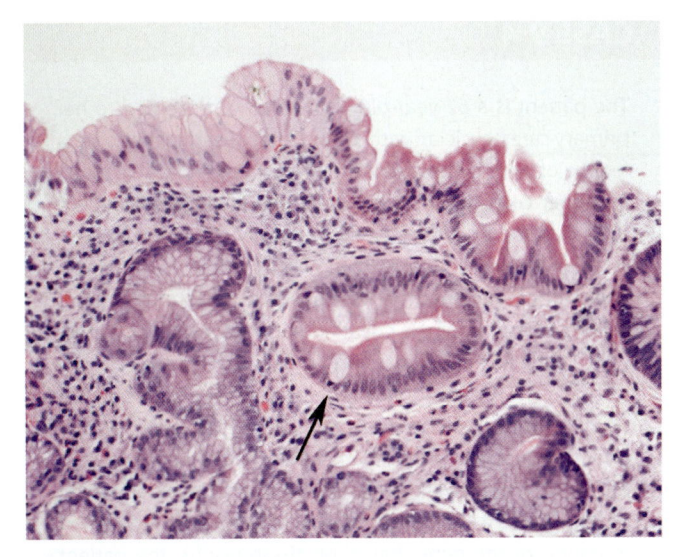

FIGURE 9-14 **Atrophic gastritis.** Normal gastric epithelial elements have been replaced by intestinal type epithelium in the center and upper right aspect of the image. Note the characteristic intestinal type goblet cells (arrow).

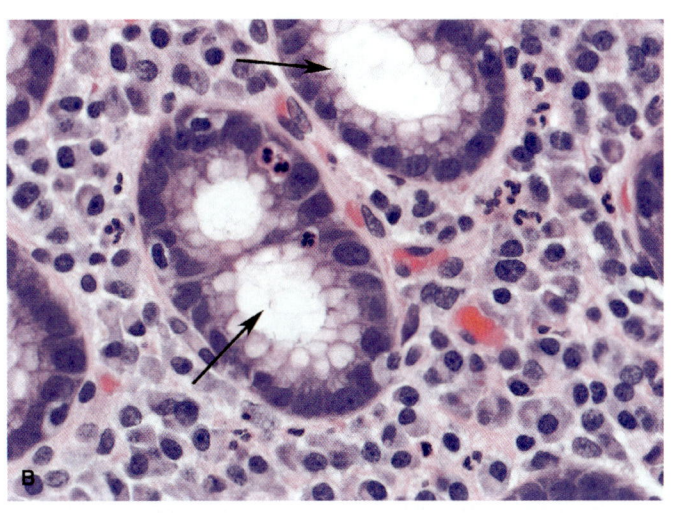

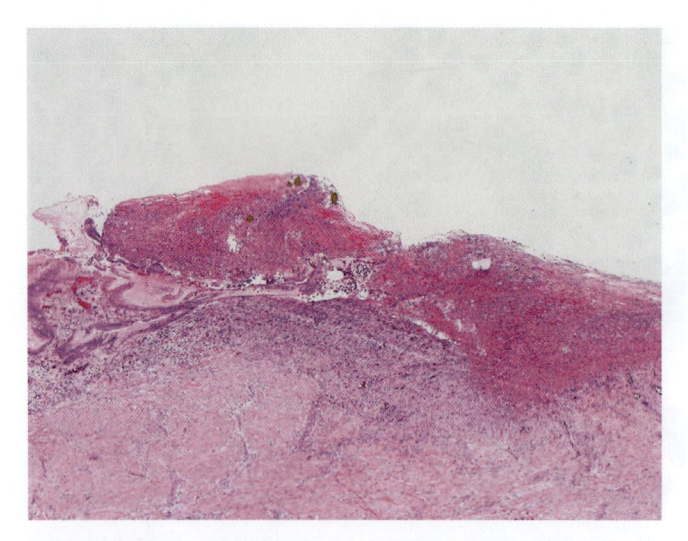

FIGURE 9-15 Gastric ulcer. This section of an ulcer margin shows a loss of the mucosa associated with acute and chronic inflammatory cells, fibrin, and necrotic debris.

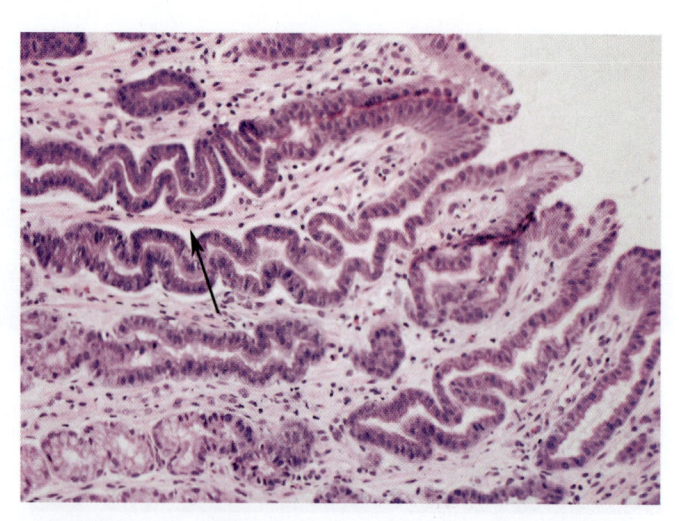

FIGURE 9-16 Reactive gastropathy. Several features of reactive gastropathy can be seen, including foveolar hyperplasia, lamina propria edema, minimal inflammatory cells, and lamina propria smooth muscle hyperplasia (arrow).

the loss involves the full thickness of the mucosa and may extend deeply within the wall of the stomach. Peptic ulcers are a form of acute and chronic ulceration resulting from breakdown of the mucous-bicarbonate barrier and subsequent gastric secretion-mediated injury. Environmental factors (e.g., smoking, aspirin and NSAIDs use), infection (e.g., *H. pylori*), systemic illness (e.g., cirrhosis, chronic renal failure), and genetic factors can play a role. Peptic ulcers can occur in the stomach or duodenum. Dyspepsia (i.e., indigestion) and epigastric pain are the most common symptoms. Severe hemorrhage, stomach perforation, and gastric outlet obstruction due to scarring can sometimes occur.

Grossly, gastric ulcers are well-delineated areas of gastric tissue loss, often with characteristic heaped-up tissue at the margin of the lesion. Microscopically, gastric ulcers are characterized by necrosis, an overlying exudate containing necrotic debris and acute inflammatory cells, and granulation tissue and fibrosis at the deep aspect of the lesion (Figure 9-15). It is important to note that gastric ulcers occasionally harbor occult malignancies, which are usually poorly differentiated gastric adenocarcinomas.

Reactive (Chemical) Gastropathy

Reactive gastropathy is a form of pauci-inflammatory mucosal injury that can occur in response to mucosal exposure to certain substances. Common offending agents include NSAIDs, bile (i.e., duodenogastric reflux), and alcohol.

Grossly, the gastric mucosa is often congested and edematous, and may have focal erosions. Microscopically, there is foveolar hyperplasia that imparts a characteristic corkscrew appearance to the gastric pits, lamina propria edema, vascular congestion, and smooth muscle proliferation within the interglandular stroma. There are occasionally superficial erosions with reparative epithelial changes (Figure 9-16).

Gastric Neoplasms

Adenocarcinoma

The overall rates of gastric adenocarcinoma in the United States are much lower than those seen in other parts of the world, such as Japan. However, gastric adenocarcinoma is still an important cause of cancer-related mortality in the United States.

The depth of invasion at the time of diagnosis can be used to stratify tumors into two categories: early gastric cancer and advanced gastric cancer. Early gastric cancer refers to invasive adenocarcinoma confined to the mucosa or submucosa. This earlier stage of invasion is being detected with greater

CASE 9-4

The patient is a 62-year-old woman who presented to her primary care physician with a complaint of early satiety (i.e., a feeling of early fullness when eating). As part of the workup, an upper GI endoscopy was performed, which showed an area of tissue bulging into the lumen of the stomach with intact overlying mucosa. Several biopsies were obtained. The pathologist made a diagnosis of GI stromal tumor (GIST). A CT scan of the chest and abdomen was obtained, which showed a 5 cm mass originating from the wall of the stomach, as well as multiple metastases to the liver. Because of the advanced stage of disease, a decision was made to treat the patient with chemotherapy. DNA sequencing of the *KIT* gene (encodes a tyrosine kinase) was performed on the patient's biopsy material, showing an activating mutation of the gene. Based on these results, the patient was started on imatinib, a tyrosine kinase inhibitor (see section "Gastrointestinal Stromal Tumor" and Figure 9-19).

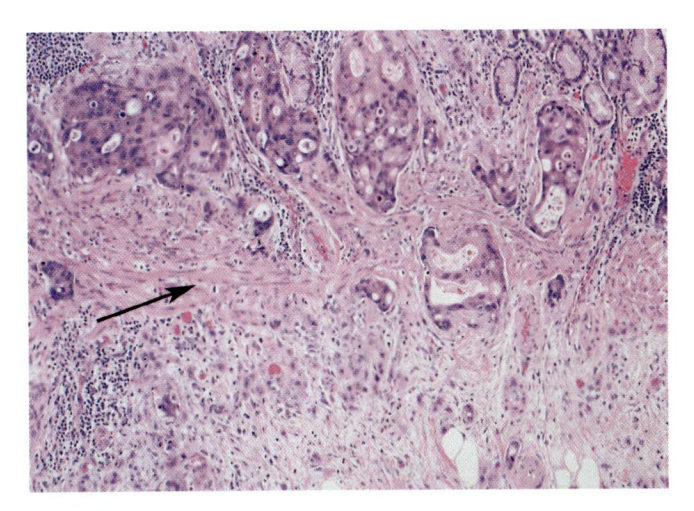

FIGURE 9-17 Intestinal-type adenocarcinoma. Several groups of gland forming carcinoma are present at the top of the image. To the right, invasion through the muscularis mucosa is evident (arrow marks muscularis mucosa).

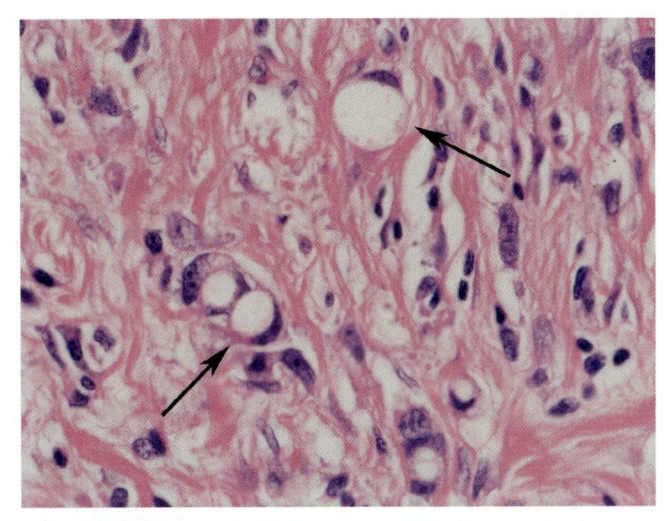

FIGURE 9-18 Signet ring cell carcinoma. Accumulation of mucin within the cytoplasm has pushed the nucleus to the edge of the tumor cell, imparting a signet ring appearance.

frequency due to the increased usage of upper endoscopy. Early gastric cancer has a much better 5-year survival rate than its counterpart advanced gastric cancer, which refers to invasive adenocarcinoma that has invaded into the muscularis propria or beyond.

Morphologically, gastric adenocarcinomas are broadly separated into two subtypes: intestinal type and diffuse type. Intestinal-type adenocarcinomas are gland-forming malignant neoplasms. In general, these tumors develop in older people, and chronic *H. pylori* infection is a common etiologic factor. The development of these tumors usually follows a sequence of atrophy to intestinal metaplasia to dysplasia to carcinoma (**Figure 9-17**). Diffuse-type adenocarcinomas, on the other hand, are composed of single cells or small groups of cells, without significant gland formation, and often develop in younger people. Signet ring cell carcinoma is an important subtype of diffuse-type adenocarcinoma and is composed of infiltrating cells with mucinous distension of the cytoplasm that compresses the nucleus to the edge of the cell, forming a characteristic signet ring appearance (**Figure 9-18**).

Intestinal-type adenocarcinomas are more likely to present as early gastric cancers, and diffuse-type adenocarcinomas are more likely to present as advanced gastric cancers, but there can be significant overlap.

QUICK REVIEW
Gastric Adenocarcinoma
- Early gastric cancer (i.e., tumor confined to the mucosa or submucosa) has a much better prognosis than advanced gastric cancer.
- Intestinal-type adenocarcinomas are gland forming malignancies that are more likely to present as early gastric cancer.
- Diffuse-type adenocarcinomas are composed of single cells or small groups of cells without significant gland formation and are more likely to present as advanced gastric cancer.
- Signet ring cell carcinoma is an important subtype of diffuse-type gastric adenocarcinoma.

Gastrointestinal Stromal Tumor

GIST is a mesenchymal tumor that can occur anyway in the GI tract; however, most tumors arise within the stomach. The cell of origin is the interstitial cell of Cajal, which plays a role in peristalsis. GIST development is usually sporadic and driven by mutations in either the *KIT* or the platelet-derived growth factor receptor alpha (*PDGFRA*) genes. These mutations lead to uncontrolled tyrosine kinase activity with resultant tumor cell proliferation. This tumor most commonly occurs in older people, but can occur at any age. The treatment of choice is surgical resection.

Grossly, the epicenter of these tumors is the submucosa or muscularis propria. Microscopically, spindle cell and epithelioid patterns are recognized. Staining for the immunohistochemical marker CD117 (c-kit) is seen in the vast majority of tumors. Tumor size is the greatest predictor of metastatic potential in GISTs of the stomach, with the majority of

IN TRANSLATION
For unresectable tumors (e.g., metastatic disease), treatment with tyrosine kinase inhibitors, such as imatinib, can result in at least a partial response in a significant number of patients, and a disease-free interval in some of these patients. Additional mutations in the *KIT* and *PDGFRA* genes can lead to resistance to tyrosine kinase inhibitors. Gene sequencing can be helpful in predicting the likelihood of a response to drug therapy.

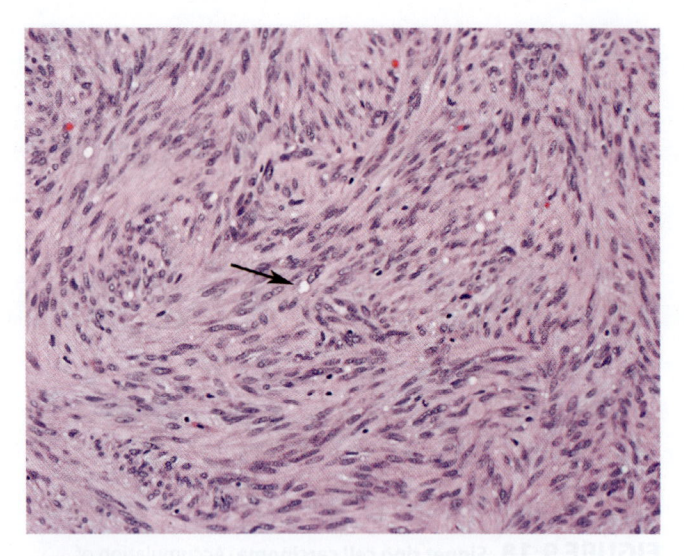

FIGURE 9-19 **Gastrointestinal stromal tumor.** This is an example of the spindle cell subtype. Perinuclear vacuoles (arrow) are frequently seen in this subtype of GIST.

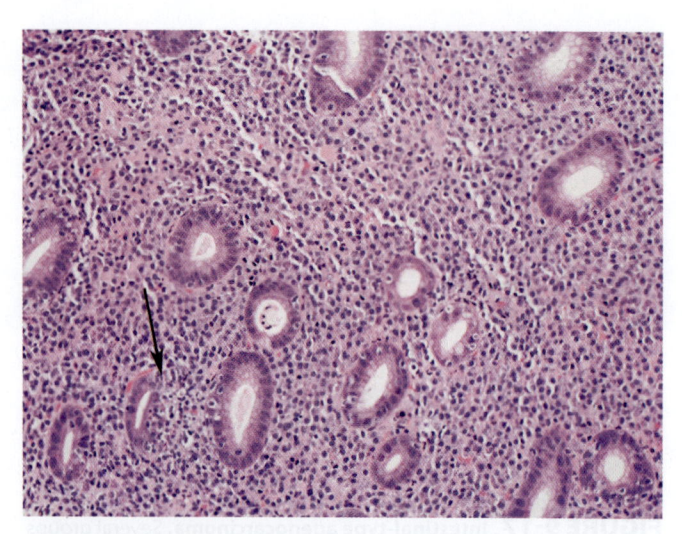

FIGURE 9-20 **Marginal-zone B-cell lymphoma.** The lamina propria is expanded by an atypical lymphoid infiltrate that results in effacement of the epithelial compartment. Note the lymphoepithelial lesion (arrow). *H. pylori* organisms are detectable at higher magnification.

tumors greater than 10 cm in diameter developing metastases (Figure 9-19).

Marginal-Zone B-cell Lymphoma

The stomach is the most common site for the development of extranodal marginal-zone B-cell lymphoma. This form of lymphoma develops from MALT. It is most common in older people, but can be seen in younger adults and rarely in adolescents. The majority of cases are driven by chronic *H. pylori* infection with chronic antigenic stimulation, resulting in the emergence of a clonal proliferation of neoplastic lymphoid cells.

Grossly, the gastric mucosa is often erythematous, eroded, or has thickened gastric folds. The appearance can mimic gastritis. Less commonly, discrete mucosal masses can be seen. Microscopically, there is a diffuse or vaguely nodular infiltrate of mildly atypical lymphoid cells that expand the lamina propria. Clusters of lymphoid cells can often be seen infiltrating and disrupting gastric glands, a finding referred to as lymphoepithelial lesions (Figure 9-20). Some cases show conspicuous plasma cell differentiation. Immunohistochemical stains are valuable in establishing the diagnosis. The neoplastic B-cells are CD20+, CD5–, CD10–, bcl6–, and cyclin D1–, and express monotypic surface immunoglobulin. CD43 is sometimes aberrantly coexpressed.

Eradication of the *H. pylori* infection can lead to regression of the lymphoma in some cases. More advanced cases are treated with chemotherapy and/or radiation therapy.

THE SMALL INTESTINE

Basic Anatomy/Histology

The small intestine develops during weeks 5 through 8 of embryonic development, connecting the distal stomach to the cloaca. Eventually, the small intestine will extend from the distal end of the stomach (the pylorus) to the ileocecal valve. Geographically, the small intestine is divided into three segments: the duodenum, which extends to the ligament of Treitz, the jejunum, generally considered to be the proximal 30% of the small intestine after the duodenum, and the ileum, the remaining 60–70% of the small intestine.

The small intestine demonstrates four layers: mucosa, covered by villi, fingerlike projections of epithelium whose primary purpose is to radically increase the absorptive area of the small intestine; submucosa, predominantly connective tissue with a rich blood supply; muscularis propria, consisting of an outer longitudinal and an inner circular layer of muscle; and finally a serosal surface, predominantly connective tissue and mesothelial cells.

Villi are covered by a mixture of columnar cells with microvilli on their surface (frequently referred to as a "brush border" when viewed microscopically), goblet cells, which contain acidic mucins and serve to distinguish intestinal epithelium from that of the stomach and esophagus, and brightly eosinophilic Paneth cells that are part of the gut's immune system. The center of villi consists of connective tissue, blood vessels, fibroblasts, and smooth muscle cells with a generous population of lymphocytes and eosinophils intermixed. At the base of the villi are the crypts of Lieberkühn that is the source of stem cells necessary for repairing the surface epithelium after injury. Also present within the duodenum are numerous submucosal Brunner glands, a type of mucous gland that releases bicarbonate ions, proteases, and glycoproteins (Figure 9-21).

Developmental Disorders

Meckel Diverticulum

Meckel diverticulum occurs when there is a persistent remnant of the vitelline duct next to the bowel wall. Meckel diverticulum exists in 2% of the population and most are found 40 cm proximal to the ileocecal valve. The "rule of

PATHOLOGY OF THE GASTROINTESTINAL TRACT   253

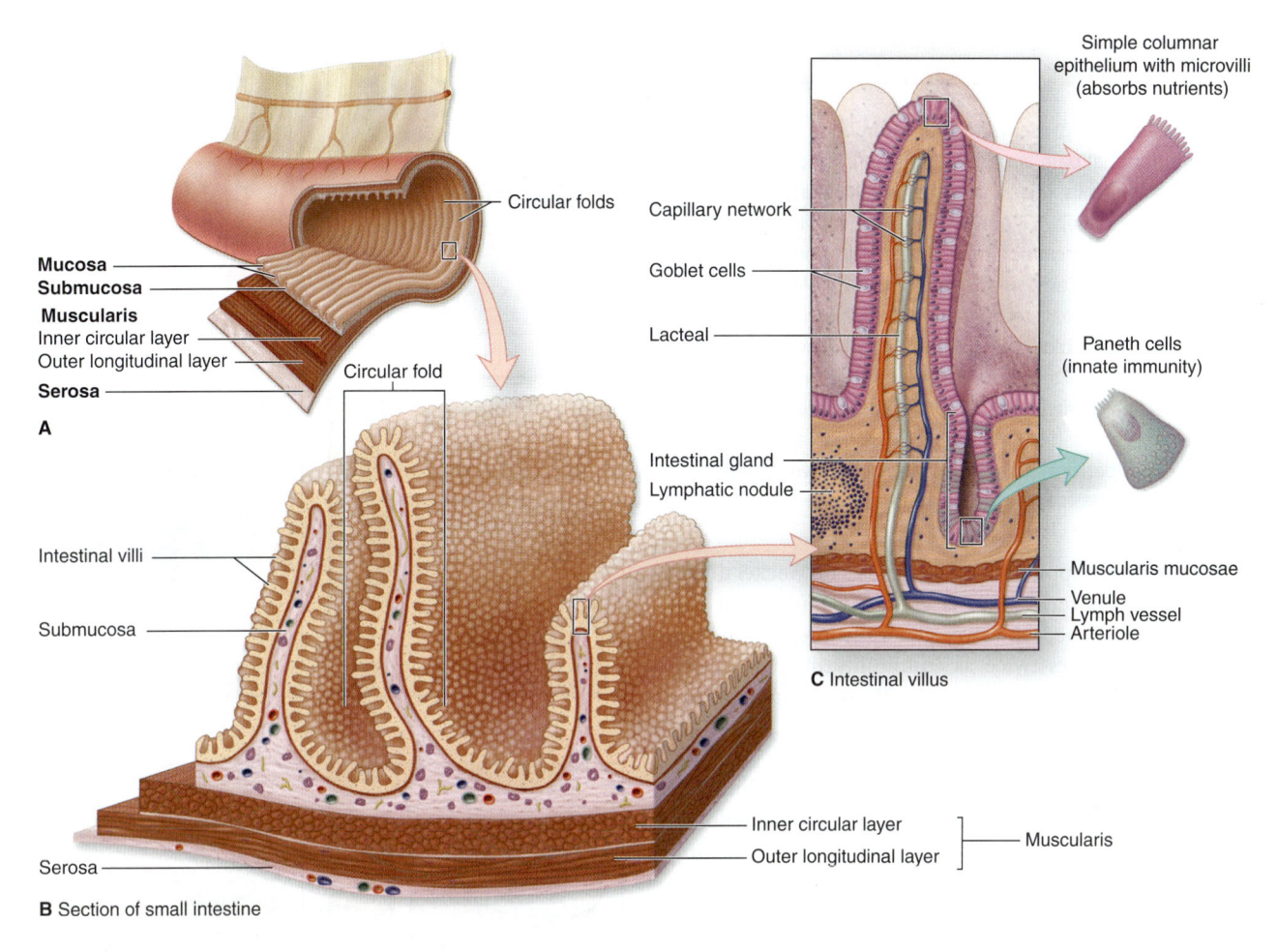

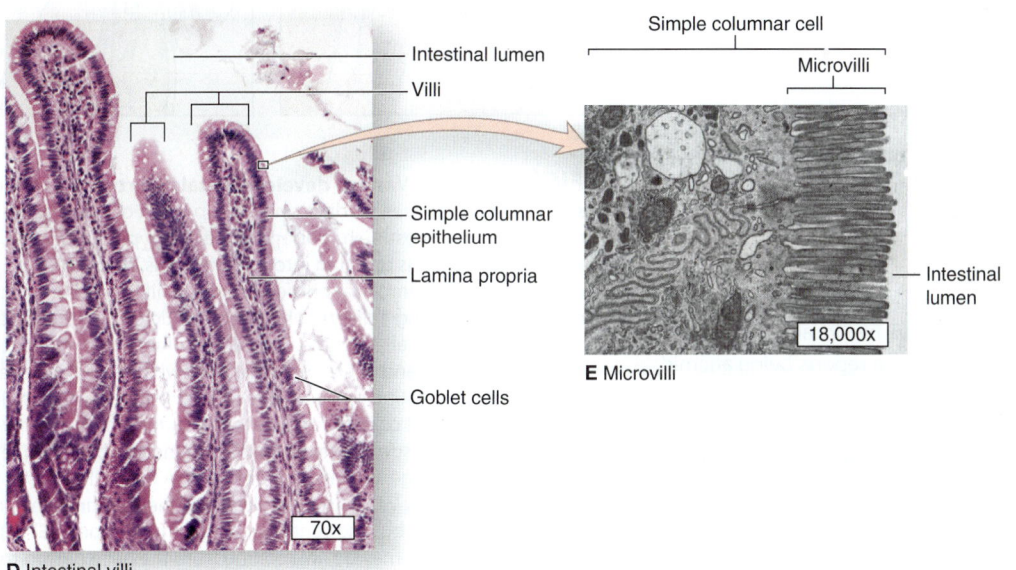

FIGURE 9-21 Absorptive surface of the small intestine.
(A) The mucosa and submucosa are the inner two of the gut's four concentric layers. (B) They form circular folds or plicae circulares, which increase the absorptive area. (C, D) They are lined by a dense covering of fingerlike projections called villi. Internally each villus contains lamina propria connective tissue with microvasculature and lymphatics called lacteals. Villi are covered with a simple columnar epithelium composed of absorptive enterocytes and goblet cells.

(E) At the apical cell membrane of each enterocyte are located dense microvilli, which serve to increase greatly the absorptive surface of the cell. Between the villi the covering epithelium invaginates to form short tubular intestinal glands or crypts, which include stem cells for the epithelium and Paneth cells that prevent intestinal flora from becoming concentrated in these glands where damage to the stem cells could occur. Source: Mescher AL. Junqueira's Basic Histology Text & Atlas, 12th ed. McGraw Hill Lange, New York: 2010. Page 270, Figure 15-25.

CASE 9-5

An 8-year-old boy presents to the emergency room with severe abdominal pain and vomiting. There is no history of diarrhea, fever, chills, recent travel, or family illness. There is no prior history of any GI abnormality in the child or in the family. The patient cannot tolerate clear liquids, suffering from coffee ground emesis and then vomiting blood. Physical examination reveals temperature of 38.5°C, heart rate of 130 beats/min, and blood pressure of 120/85. The child demonstrates abdominal tenderness with guarding and rebound tenderness, particularly in the periumbilical region. CBC demonstrates a left shift. Following a CT scan, an exploratory laparoscopy is performed, removing a Meckel diverticulum.

twos" is commonly applied to the diagnosis of Meckel diverticulum: Meckel diverticulum is generally found two feet proximal to the ileocecal valve, generally presents before 2 years of age, occurs twice as commonly in males compared with females, and is found in 2% of the population (Figure 9-22).

Patients with symptomatic Meckel diverticulum generally present with symptoms related to obstruction, bleeding and possibly perforation, with GI bleeding being the predominant finding. Ectopic gastric tissue found in the diverticulum is often the etiologic agent, secondary to the extremely acidic secretions. Treatment consists of resecting the diverticulum via laparotomy or laparoscopy.

Malabsorption

Celiac Disease

Celiac disease (CD) is an autoimmune disorder that occurs in adults and children at an incidence of approximately 1%.

CASE 9-6

A 40-year-old woman presented to her local physician for workup of chronic anemia. The patient reports being anemic since her early 20s. Her past medical history and family history were unremarkable for bleeding disorders. A CBC confirmed a low hematocrit. Red blood cell indices were normal, although ferritin was slightly low. Her family physician scheduled the patient for a colonoscopy and an upper GI endoscopy to rule out sources of bleeding. Colonoscopy was unremarkable while the upper GI endoscopy demonstrated flattened mucosa within the small bowel. Biopsy revealed villous blunting, an increased crypt to villous ratio, and increased intraepithelial lymphocytes. Additional lab testing demonstrated elevated tissue transglutaminase (tTG) IgA levels. The patient was diagnosed with celiac disease and instructed to follow a gluten-free diet with resolution of her anemia.

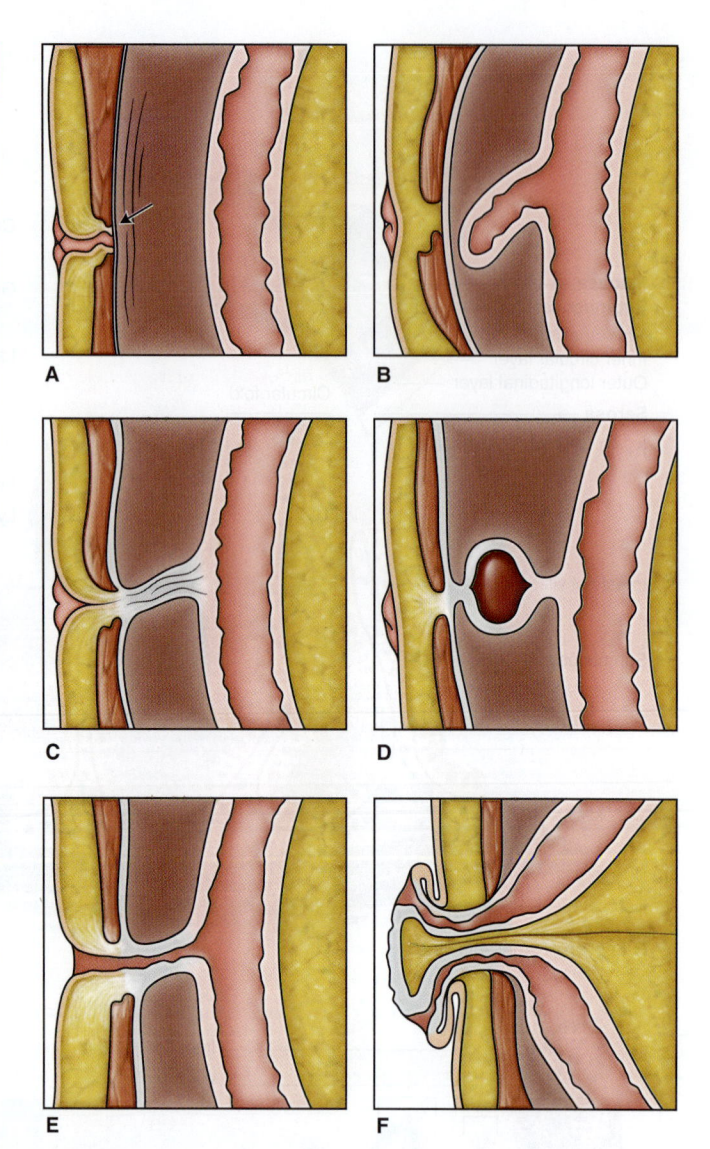

FIGURE 9-22 Various developmental diverticulitis of the small bowel. **(A)** Vitelline duct sinus. The portion of the vitelline duct attached to the intestine has disappeared as is typical. However, a sinus tract remains opening into the umbilicus. **(B)** Meckel diverticulum. The umbilical portion of the primitive vitelline duct has disappeared, leaving a diverticulum or outpouching communicating with the normal small intestine. The diverticulum can bleed, become inflamed, rupture, and act as the point from which an intussusception (the upstream intestine moves inside the downstream intestine) can occur. **(C)** Persistent cord of scar. The vitelline duct can be completely replaced by scar tissue; however, a twist around this band can result in intestinal blockage. **(D)** Vitelline duct cyst. A fluid-filled, cystic structure may occur when the umbilical and the intestinal ends of the duct disappear, but the central portion remains open. **(E)** Patent vitelline duct. There may be an opening from the belly button to the intestine that is characterized by passage of gas or drainage from the umbilicus. **(F)** Prolapse. Occasionally, the intestine may out-pouch through an open vitelline duct.

CD is seen in individuals predominantly of European origin; however, increased screening is now recognizing that CD has a similar prevalence rate in other parts of the world, including North Africa, the Middle East, and India. There appears to be a genetic predisposition to CD related to HLA class II genes as most individuals with CD are HLA-DQ2 positive with many other patients HLA-DQ8 positive.

In addition to genetics, however, environmental factors play a large role in the development of CD, specifically the exposure of susceptible individuals to gluten, a protein found in wheat. In individuals with CD, the tight junctions between epithelial cells covering the intestinal villi are compromised, allowing entry to gluten-derived peptides such as gliadin. These peptides induce an inflammatory response with accumulation of Th-1 cells that produce interferon gamma. This inflammatory response leads to damage of the villous surface of the small bowel, particularly within the duodenum.

Clinically, CD generally presents in infants and young children, but is increasingly recognized in older adults. Affected individuals, particularly children, present with diarrhea, abdominal distension, and failure to thrive. Older children and adults may present with extraintestinal manifestations including anemia and neurologic symptoms.

Diagnosis of CD has two requirements: (1) duodenal biopsy demonstrating the characteristic findings of CD and (2) remission of the disease when following a gluten-free diet. Histologically, CD is characterized by villous blunting, with an increased crypt to villous ratio. Generally, the villous to crypt ratio is 4:1 to 5:1; in CD, depending on the severity of the disorder, this ratio can be 2:1 or less, as the mucosa flattens and the villi disappear. Also present are increased numbers of intraepithelial lymphocytes (CD3-positive cells); the actual numbers vary, but most investigators agree that an increase of 30 or more intraepithelial lymphocytes per 100 epithelial cells warrants consideration of CD (Figure 9-23). Treatment consists of adhering to a gluten-free diet and rebiopsy after an appropriate period of time to demonstrate a return to normal or near-normal villous architecture. Complications of CD include intestinal adenocarcinoma, enteropathy-associated T-cell lymphoma, or refractory sprue.

Tropical Sprue

Tropical sprue (TS) is an acquired malabsorption syndrome seen in residents and tourists of tropical regions such as the Caribbean, Puerto Rico, Central America, South America, and West Africa. In affected regions, TS is thought to account for 40% of malabsorption in adults and children. The cause of TS is unclear. It may be secondary to persistent infection, although a specific etiologic agent has not been demonstrated.

Clinically, patients often present after visiting an area where TS is endemic. The patient experiences an acute illness consisting of non-bloody diarrhea, bloating, weight loss, and abdominal cramps. The initial illness subsides, but the patient continues to experience a chronic diarrhea that may be accompanied by weight loss and malaise. Infectious etiologies

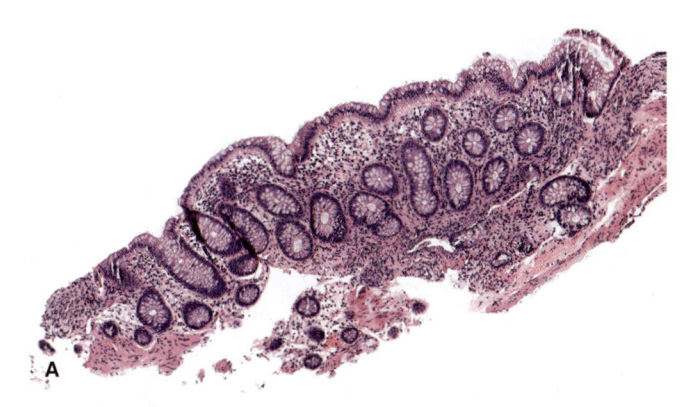

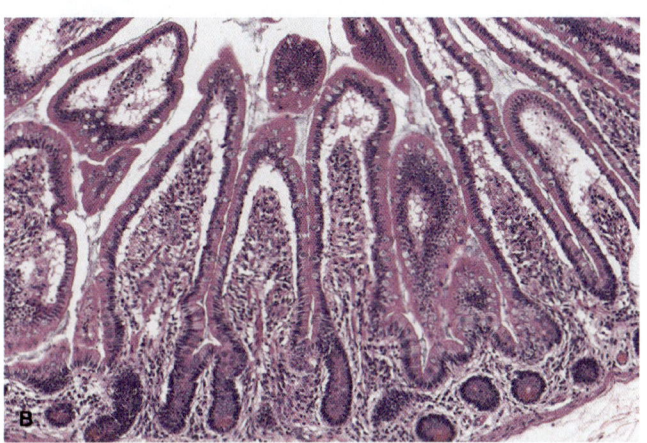

FIGURE 9-23 CD: **(A)** Intestinal biopsy specimen demonstrating CD. Note the marked blunting of villi producing a flattened mucosa. **(B)** shows a segment of normal small intestine with a normal villous to crypt ratio.

must be ruled out and small intestinal biopsy performed, the latter demonstrating findings similar to CD (villous blunting, increased intraepithelial lymphocytes, etc.); however, the entire length of the small bowel is generally affected while in CD the terminal ileum is generally spared. Treatment consists of supportive measures (restoring fluids and electrolytes), folate supplementation (to combat the macrocytic anemia that accompanies TS), and antibiotic therapy.

Inflammatory

Peptic Duodenitis

Peptic duodenitis (PD) exists on a continuum with peptic ulcer disease. PD describes a condition where there is acute and chronic inflammation of the duodenal mucosa, nearly always secondary to the effects of excessive gastric acid combined with loss of the mucus bicarbonate barrier. Patients with chronic *H. pylori* infections are at risk of PD as are patients who smoke and have chronic NSAID use.

Clinically, patients with PD are often indistinguishable from patients with peptic ulcer disease: both present with gnawing epigastric pain that is often relieved by eating or antacids. At endoscopy, patients with PD will frequently show erythema and friability to the duodenal mucosa, most

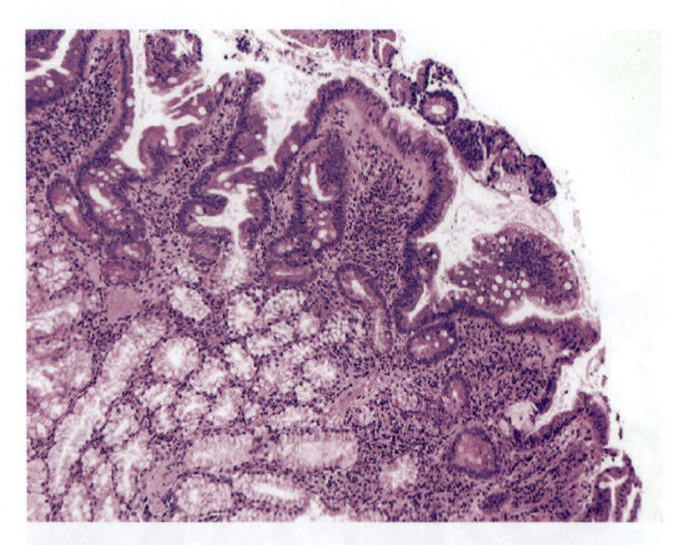

FIGURE 9-24 **Focal metaplasia in PD:** Enterocytes are replaced by foci of gastric-type mucus-secreting cells. Villi are shortened and blunted. The lamina propria shows an increase in the inflammatory cells (lymphocytes and plasma cells), associated with the hypertrophy and prolapse of Brunner glands. These features are typical of nonspecific chronic duodenitis. Source: Serra S, Jani PA. An Approach to Duodenal Biopsies. J Clin Pathol 2006;59:1133–1150. Figure 3, page 1137.

frequently at the duodenal bulb. Ulcers are similar to those seen elsewhere in the GI tract with penetration to the submucosa putting patients at risk of massive GI bleeding.

Histologically, there is overlap between PD and CD. Both will show villous blunting; significant differences are the lack of increased intraepithelial lymphocytes in PD, gastric foveolar metaplasia in response to mucosal injury in PD, and acute inflammation within the villi and crypts (Figure 9-24). The presence of foveolar metaplasia allows for colonization by *Helicobacter* that, in turn, leads to further foveolar metaplasia and inflammation via similar mechanisms (e.g., urease production) that *Helicobacter* employs in the stomach (see section "*Helicobacter* gastritis").

Treatment of PD consists both of lifestyle changes (patients with PD should stop smoking; if possible, patients using NSAIDs should cease their use) and medication. Patients with PD can be treated with H_2-blockers or proton pump inhibitors as well as antibiotic therapy if found to be colonized by *Helicobacter*.

Crohn Disease

The small intestine can be involved by inflammatory bowel disease as can the large intestine. The preferred site for Crohn disease is the terminal ileum, ulcerative colitis being limited to the colon. Inflammatory diseases of the bowel are discussed in greater detail in the section on the colon.

Infectious Diseases

Many infections of the small bowel also affect the colon and will be discussed in the chapter. Two that show preference for the small bowel are the parasitic infection by *Giardia lamblia*

and Whipple disease, caused by the bacterium *Tropheryma whipplei*.

Giardiasis

Giardia is found worldwide, infects both domestic and wild animals and is the most commonly diagnosed parasitic infection of the intestines. Infection is highest in children under 5 years of age and in patients in their fourth decade. *Giardia* infection occurs predominantly through exposure to contaminated drinking water.

The causative agent, *Giardia lamblia*, is a flagellated, binucleated protozoan parasite, which can exist in two forms: as an infectious cyst and as a mobile trophozoite. Infection occurs when the cyst is ingested, usually in contaminated water. Cysts pass through the stomach wall into the small intestine whereupon the trophozoites emerge and colonize the upper small intestine.

Following an incubation period of 1 to 2 weeks, patients with giardiasis typically present with abdominal cramps, nausea, and diarrhea. Malabsorption can occur, leading to failure to thrive. The majority of infections are self-limiting; however, chronic infections can occur and *Giardia* can be excreted in stool for months following initial infection, allowing for an extended period of infectivity.

Microscopically, biopsies from the small intestine demonstrate pear-shaped binucleated organisms near the epithelial surface of the villi (Figure 9-25). Host response can be varied, ranging from either normal villous architecture to villous atrophy and crypt hyperplasia reminiscent of CD. Diagnosis is usually based on immunologic assays to detect *Giardia* antigens in stool and treatment consists of antibiotic therapy.

Whipple Disease

Whipple disease (WD) is a rare infectious disease, caused by the bacterium *Tropheryma whipplei*, that can potentially affect all organ systems, but has a predilection for both the GI tract and CNS. Classically, WD occurs in middle-aged men in two stages: a prodromal stage characterized by arthralgias/arthritis followed

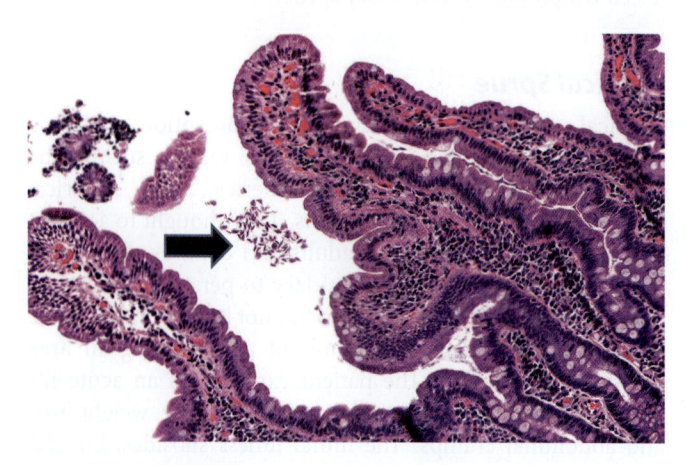

FIGURE 9-25 **Giardia trophozoites along the surface of the small intestine:** Note group of organisms (arrow).

PATHOLOGY OF THE GASTROINTESTINAL TRACT   257

> **CASE 9-7**
>
> A 45-year-old man presents to his local physician complaining of diarrhea and progressive weight loss, as well as arthralgias. There is no history of CD or inflammatory bowel disease. Workup reveals the patient is mildly febrile and has lymphadenopathy. Testing for HIV is negative. Upper GI endoscopy is performed and demonstrates yellowish plaques in the duodenum and jejunum. Microscopic findings show blunted villi expanded by numerous foamy macrophages in the lamina propria. Special stains demonstrate PAS-positive diastase resident bacterial rods within the macrophages. Polymerase chain reaction testing confirms the presence of the 16s ribosomal RNA genes of *T. whipplei*. Antibiotic therapy leads to resolution of the patient's symptoms.

by a second stage consisting of weight loss, diarrhea, and other manifestations depending on the organ systems affected.

At endoscopy, the duodenum frequently appears unaffected; a minority of cases demonstrates lymphangiectasia secondary to lymphatic obstruction by the organism and/or white-yellow plaques covering the mucosa. Microscopic examination demonstrates expansion of the lamina propria by numerous foamy macrophages containing the bacterium and surrounding dilated lymphatics (Figure 9-26). Numerous PAS-positive, diastase-resistant rod-like organisms can be demonstrated by special stains; however, additional diagnostic tools, such as immunohistochemistry using antibodies to *T. whipplei* or PCR to specific *T. whipplei* targets, such as the bacterium's RNA genes, are necessary to confirm the diagnosis.

Prior to antibiotic therapy, WD was fatal. Most patients now respond to antibiotics. CNS involvement is a serious consequence of infection with *T. whipplei* since patients can develop irreversible CNS damage including cognitive disturbances, epilepsy, and ataxia.

Neoplasms

Adenocarcinoma

Adenocarcinomas are the most common tumors of the small intestine, comprising up to 50% of all malignancies of the small bowel; however, compared with other organ systems, small intestine adenocarcinomas are still relatively rare, accounting for approximately 2% of GI tumors. The median age at time of presentation is 67 years with men affected slightly more often than women and African-Americans demonstrating a twofold increase in incidence compared with whites.

The duodenum is the most common site for small intestine adenocarcinomas, with tumors occurring most frequently around the ampulla of Vater. Like colorectal adenocarcinomas, the majority of small intestine adenocarcinomas are sporadic and appear to arise from preexisting adenomas; prognosis is dismal with a 5-year survival rate of 30%.

Small bowel adenocarcinomas are generally silent tumors until advanced enough to cause obstructive symptoms. Patients may present with occult GI bleeding causing anemia.

The gross appearance of small intestine adenocarcinomas depends extensively on the site; those tumors of the duodenum and ampulla are generally exophytic tumors, while more distal tumors display a more annular, stricturing appearance. Histologically, small intestine adenocarcinomas are very similar to their counterparts in the colorectum. Tumors show varying degrees of glandular architecture, ranging from well-differentiated tumors that appear similar to normal mucosa to extremely poorly differentiated tumors with minimal architectural detail. Even when well differentiated, nuclear pleomorphism is evident and the tumor cells demonstrate expanded nuclear–cytoplasmic ratios. Glands show cribriform architecture (Figure 9-27). Occasionally, tumors demonstrate more atypical histologic features such as squamous differentiation, although these features do not appear to have prognostic value.

Neuroendocrine Tumors

Neuroendocrine tumors of the small intestine have experienced a fluctuating classification system over the last decade; based on the current nomenclature of the World Health Organization, they consist of grade 1 neuroendocrine tumors (well-differentiated endocrine tumors or carcinoids), grade 2 neuroendocrine tumors (well-differentiated endocrine carcinomas), and neuroendocrine carcinomas (poorly differentiated endocrine carcinomas/small cell carcinoma). Overall, small intestine neuroendocrine tumors are rare tumors, comprising approximately 6–8% of neuroendocrine tumors of the GI tract. For tumors of the duodenum, there is a slight male predominance (1.5:1) with a mean age at presentation of 59 years. Approximately two-thirds of duodenal neuroendocrine neoplasms are gastrinomas, the remainder somatostatinomas. Tumors of the distal small intestine are predominantly found

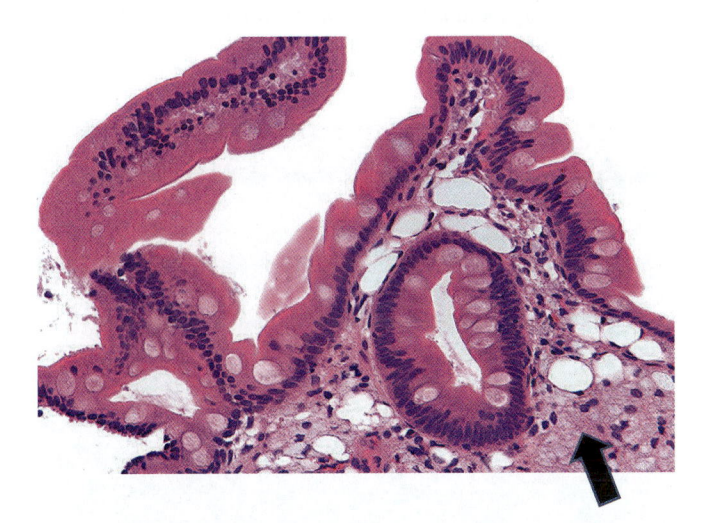

FIGURE 9-26 **Whipple disease:** Lamina propria demonstrates numerous foamy macrophages and dilated lymphatics (arrow).
Source: http://upload.wikimedia.org/wikipedia/commons/thumb/2/27/Whipple_disease_-a-_very_high_mag.jpg/1024px-Whipple_disease_-a-_very_high_mag.jpg

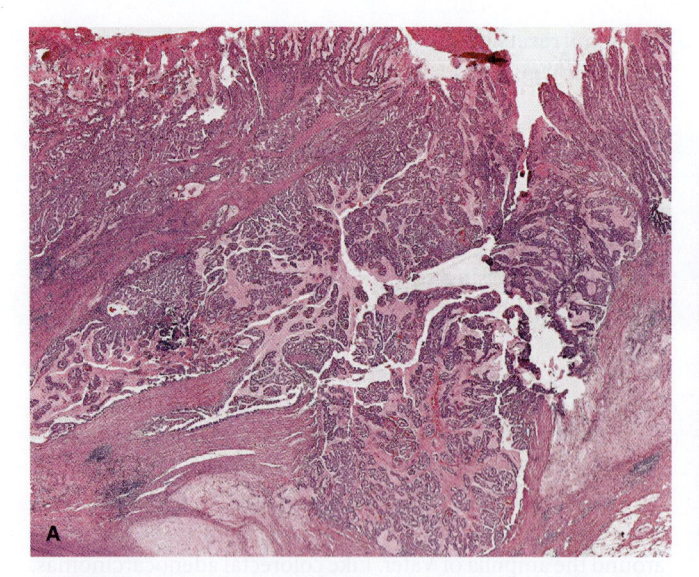

FIGURE 9-27 Adenocarcinoma of the duodenum: (A) Low-power view of invasive atypical glands. **(B)** High-power view of glands demonstrates nuclear atypia, increased nuclear cytoplasmic ratio, and cribriform (sieve-like) architecture.

in the ileum and most are enterochromaffin-cell serotonin producing carcinoids. Mean age at the time of diagnosis of distal tumors is 62 years and there is no sex predilection.

Most neuroendocrine tumors are discovered incidentally either by imaging or as the patient is undergoing endoscopy for other complaints. When patients do experience symptoms, it is generally due to local infiltration causing obstruction or hemorrhage; symptoms arising from secreted hormones are a less common occurrence.

Grossly, neuroendocrine tumors are small, well-demarcated lesions generally limited to the submucosa. Occasionally, the overlying mucosa may be ulcerated depending on how infiltrative the lesion is. Histologically, well-differentiated neoplasms (carcinoids) demonstrate round to oval nuclei with speckled, "salt and pepper" chromatin. Nucleoli are inconspicuous and mitoses infrequently identified **(Figure 9-28)**. In terms of immunohistochemistry, well-differentiated neoplasms demonstrate their neuroendocrine bona fides by the expression of markers such as synaptophysin, chromogranin and, depending on the tumor, specific peptides such as gastrin, somatostatin, or insulin. Tumors with increased mitotic activity qualify as grade 2 tumors. Neuroendocrine carcinomas are poorly differentiated tumors, morphologically similar to small cell carcinoma of the lung. Neuroendocrine carcinomas show small, dark nuclei surrounded by minimal cytoplasm; in the large cell variant they demonstrate large to intermediate cells with greater amounts of cytoplasm. Mitoses are frequent and necrosis is often seen. Similar to lower-grade tumors, carcinomas demonstrate expression of neuroendocrine markers (e.g., synaptophysin) via immunohistochemistry.

Prognosis is difficult to predict for neuroendocrine tumors. Best predictors appear to be invasion beyond the submucosa and metastases to lymph nodes or other distal sites. Neuroendocrine tumors of the distal small bowel have, in general, a worse prognosis than duodenal tumors.

COLON

Normal Anatomy and Histology of the Colon

The colon is the distal segment of the GI tract. It begins at the ileocecal valve, where it is continuous with the ileum of the small bowel, and ends at the anus. The colon is divided into several anatomic regions. The cecum is a pouch adjacent to the ileocecal valve. The appendix, a blind-ended tube, originates from the cecum at the appendiceal orifice. The lumen of the colon is continuous with that of the appendix. The cecum transitions to the ascending colon, which becomes the transverse colon at the hepatic flexure. The transverse colon becomes the descending colon at the splenic flexure. At the distal aspect of the descending colon is the sigmoid colon, which becomes the rectum **(Figure 9-29)**.

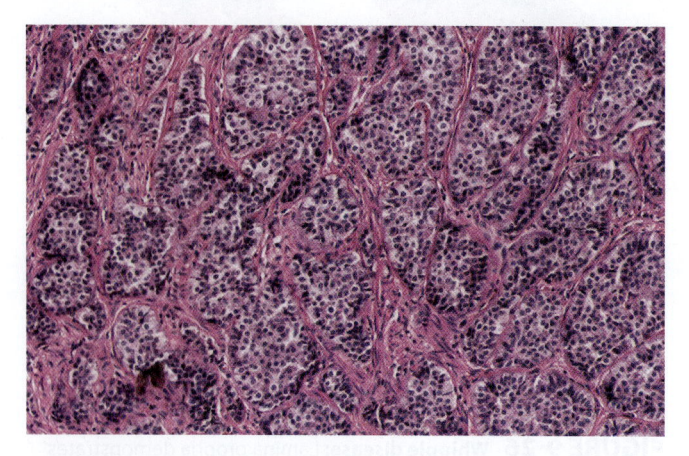

FIGURE 9-28 Carcinoid of the small intestine: High-power view shows round, regular tumor nuclei with "salt and pepper" chromatin. Note the lack of mitotic activity or nucleoli.

PATHOLOGY OF THE GASTROINTESTINAL TRACT

CASE 9-8

The patient is a 45-year-old woman who presented to her primary care physician with a complaint of rectal bleeding. Upon questioning, she reported that multiple family members had been diagnosed with colon cancer. A colonoscopy was performed and showed a large mass in the ascending colon. Biopsies of the mass were obtained and the pathologist rendered a diagnosis of "adenocarcinoma with mucinous features." Because of the patient's young age, presence of mucinous differentiation, and family history of colon cancer, the patient's oncologist requested additional pathologic studies, which revealed a loss of mismatch repair protein expression by immunohistochemistry and evidence of microsatellite instability. Based on these results, genetic testing was performed and the patient was diagnosed with Lynch syndrome. See section "Colorectal Carcinogenesis" and Figure 9-46.

The colonic wall, similar to other locations within the GI tract, consists of mucosa, submucosa, muscularis propria, and serosa. The muscularis propria has an inner circular layer and an outer longitudinal layer; however, unlike in other areas of the GI tract, the longitudinal layer is noncircumferential and consists of three longitudinal bundles called teniae coli. The rectum is invested by fibroadipose tissue and adjacent structures, without a serosal surface. This has important implications for surgical management of rectal cancer.

There are regular transverse folds of the mucosal surface. These dissipate toward the distal end of the colon. As opposed to the small bowel, which has surface villi, the mucosal surface of the colon is flat. From the mucosal surface, regularly spaced epithelial crypts extend down to the depths of the mucosa. The epithelium is composed of tall columnar cells with interspersed goblet cells. The tall columnar cells are responsible for water and electrolyte absorption, the primary function of the colon. The deep portions of the crypts contain reserve cells, which are responsible for epithelial growth and regeneration, and multiple types of neuroendocrine cells (**Figure 9-30**).

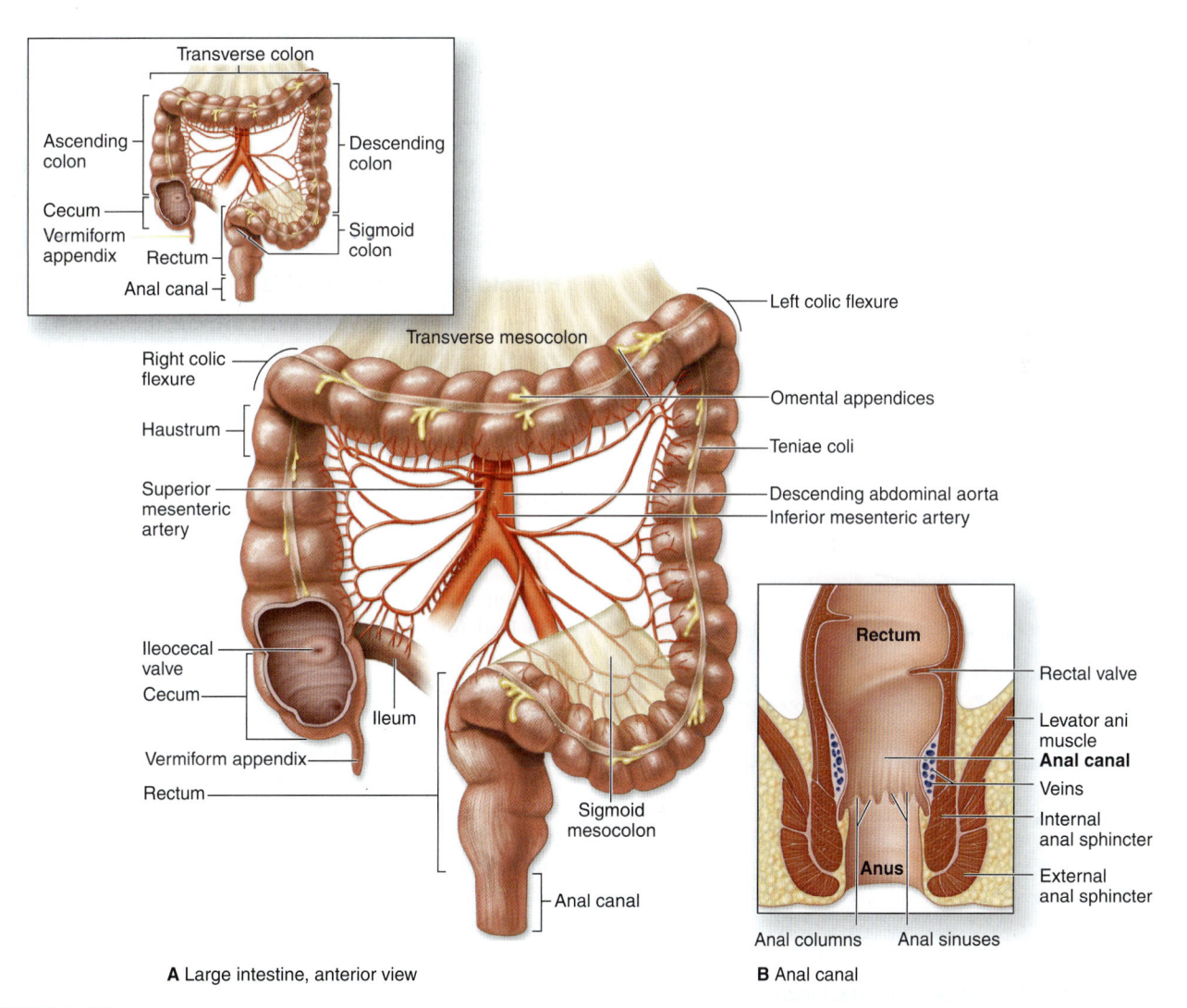

FIGURE 9-29 **Anatomy of the colon.** **(A)** Representation of the anterior portion of the colon. The right and left colic flexures are commonly referred to as the hepatic flexure and splenic flexure, respectively. **(B)** Anal canal. Source: Mescher AL. Junqueira's Basic Histology Text & Atlas, 12th ed. McGraw Hill Lange, New York: 2010. Page 278, Figure 15-36..

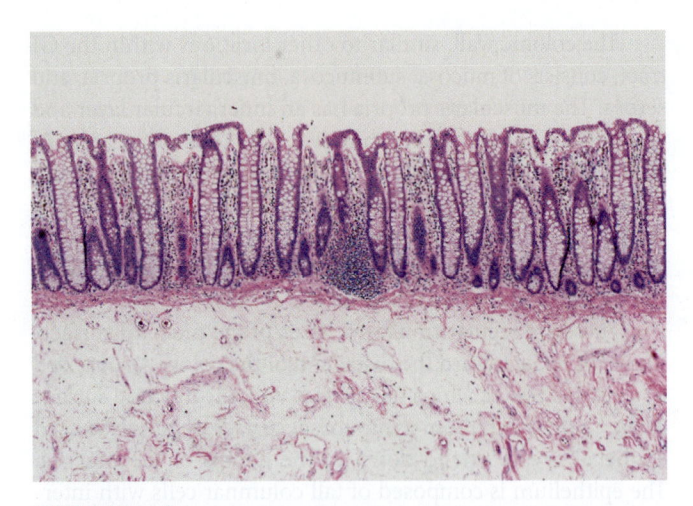

FIGURE 9-30 Normal colonic mucosa. The crypts in normal colonic mucosa are reminiscent of "test tubes in a rack" because of their shape and regular spacing. Lymphoid aggregates (center) are common in normal mucosa.

Principal Diseases of the Colon

The colon is the site of many important developmental, inflammatory, and neoplastic disorders.

Developmental Disorders of the Colon

The most common developmental disorders of the colon and rectum include Hirschsprung disease and a variety of anorectal malformations, ranging from mild stenosis to agenesis of the anorectal segment.

Hirschsprung Disease

Hirschsprung disease is a defect in the innervation of the distal colon, resulting from a failure of ganglion cell precursors to migrate from the neural crest to the anus during early development (Figure 9-31). Ganglion cells play a role is smooth muscle relaxation, thus allowing for relaxation of the colon and passage of intraluminal contents. Hirschsprung disease always involves the rectum and can extend for a variable degree proximally, depending on the point where ganglion cell migration terminates.

Classically, Hirschsprung disease presents shortly after birth with failure to pass meconium and signs of intestinal obstruction. In patients with very short aganglionic segments, constipation and intermittent fecal impaction may be the only manifestations of disease. Enterocolitis, bowel necrosis, and bowel wall perforation are serious complications that can occur as a result of severe colonic dilation.

Grossly, the aganglionic segment is strictured. Proximal to the strictured segment, the colon is dilated. Microscopic examination of biopsies obtained from the strictured segment reveals the hallmark of the disease, an absence of ganglion cells within the myenteric plexus between the circular and longitudinal layers of the muscularis propria and within the submucosa. Nerve fibers are often increased in sections from the aganglionic segment, a finding referred to as neural hyperplasia. Surgical resection of the aganglionic segment with primary anastomosis is the treatment of Hirschsprung disease.

Inflammatory Disorders of the Colon

In order to understand the pathology of inflammatory disorders of the colon, it is important to first develop an understanding of the concepts of active colitis and chronic colitis.

Histology of Active Colitis

When a neutrophilic infiltrate is present, the process is called active colitis. When neutrophils are present within the crypt epithelium, the pattern is called cryptitis. When neutrophils fill and distend a colonic crypt, the pattern is called a crypt abscess. On the more severe end of the spectrum of active colitis, there can be mucosal ulceration, which is usually accompanied by a neutrophilic infiltrate (Figure 9-32).

Histology of Chronic Colitis

Any inflammatory process that persists beyond a few weeks can lead to mucosal changes of chronic colitis. Classically, there is an increase in lamina propria chronic inflammation with distension of the lamina propria by lymphocytes and plasma cells. Plasma cells accumulate between the bases of the crypts and the muscularis mucosa, a finding known as basal plasmacytosis. The crypts lose the uniformity characteristic of normal mucosa. Many of the crypts no longer extend all the way to the muscularis mucosa. There is disarray in the distribution of crypts as the result of increased inflammation and foci of crypt injury and dropout. Branching toward the lower half of the crypts, occurring during crypt regeneration, is an important finding in chronic colitis. Finding Paneth cells, a specialized type of crypt cell thought to play a role in host defense, distal to the mid-transverse colon is also an indicator of chronic mucosal injury (Figure 9-33).

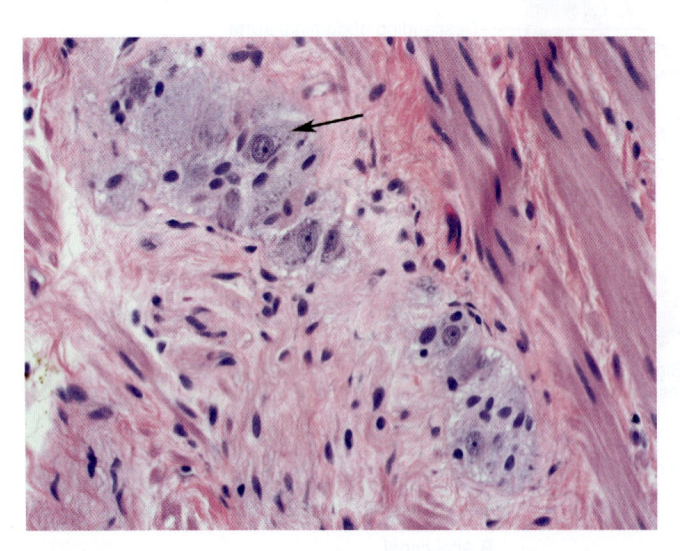

FIGURE 9-31 Mature ganglion cells. Hirschsprung disease occurs when ganglion cell precursors fail to migrate to the anus during early development. The arrow highlights a normal ganglion cell.

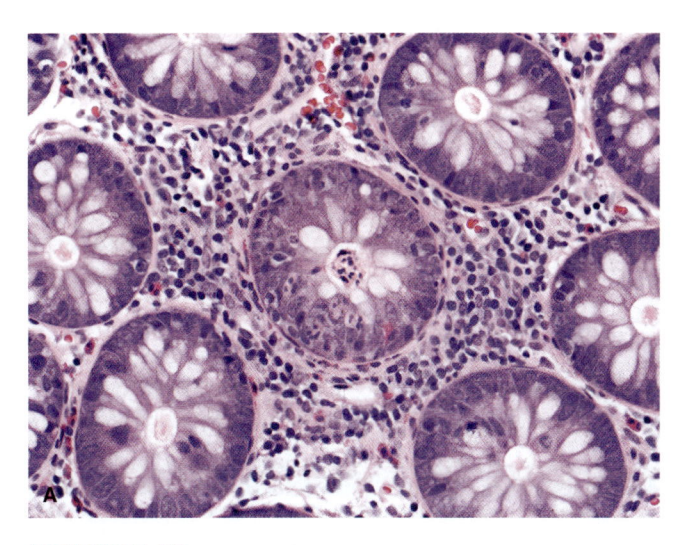

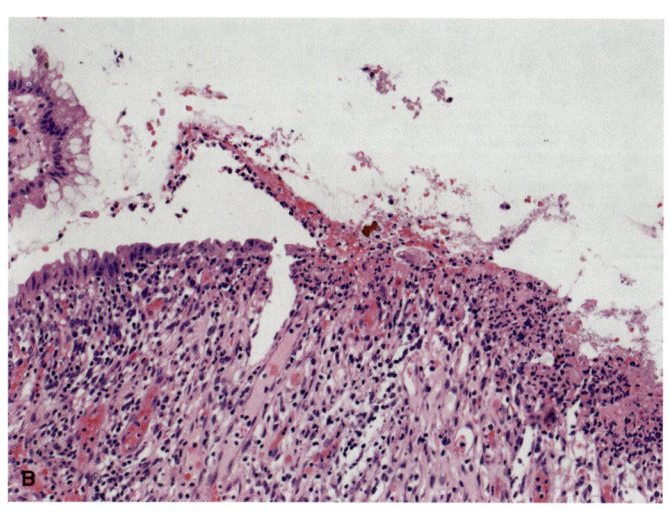

FIGURE 9-32 Active colitis. (A) The crypt epithelium in the center of this image is infiltrated by neutrophils (cryptitis). Note the early accumulation of neutrophils within the crypt lumen (crypt abscess). **(B)** Note the transition from intact surface epithelium (left) to denuded surface epithelium associated with acute inflammation and necrosis in this colonic ulcer.

Changes of active colitis and chronic colitis often coexist, a finding known as chronic active colitis. Infections, ischemia, drugs (commonly, NSAIDs), radiation, diverticular disease, and idiopathic inflammatory bowel disease can all lead to mucosal changes of active and chronic colitis, such that it is often not possible to establish a definitive cause by pathologic examination alone. In cases of colitis, correlation with all of the available information, including the clinical history, laboratory studies, microbiology studies, and endoscopic findings, is necessary to determine the etiology.

Infectious Colitis

A variety of bacterial, mycobacterial, fungal, parasitic, and viral pathogens can cause disease in the colon.

The most common bacterial organisms are *Escherichia coli*, *Salmonella*, *Shigella*, and *Campylobacter*. The source of infection is often contaminated food or water. Commonly, bacterial infections of the colon produce an "acute self-limited colitis" pattern of inflammation. This pattern is characterized by the histologic changes of active colitis without changes of chronic colitis. Sometimes the pathologic changes can suggest a particular pathogen. For instance, necrosis and hemorrhage can be seen with infection by enterohemorrhagic *E. coli* (O157:H7). Stool bacterial cultures play an important role in diagnosis.

Mycobacterium tuberculosis and *Mycobacterium avium* complex can both involve the colon. Fungal infections of the colon are usually seen in the setting of disseminated fungal disease. Several parasites can cause disease in the colon. *Entamoeba histolytica* infection leads to characteristic flask-shaped deep ulcerations.

CMV is a notable viral infection that can be seen in the colon. It is more frequently seen in immunocompromised people, but can be seen in the immunocompetent as well. People with HIV/AIDS or immunosuppression due to bone marrow transplant or immunosuppressive drug therapy are at increased risk. CMV often causes mucosal ulceration. Characteristic "owl's eye" cytopathic effect can be very focal and is typically seen in endothelial or stromal cells, and occasionally in epithelial cells (Figure 9-34).

Clostridium difficile Colitis

Clostridium difficile colitis is a unique form of infectious colitis that is characterized by the presence of mucosal surface exudates called pseudomembranes. While pseudomembranes are not entirely specific for *C. difficile* disease, the term "pseudomembranous colitis" is generally reserved for disease caused by this pathogen. Disease occurs when prior antibiotic exposure results in suppression of other normal gut flora, allowing

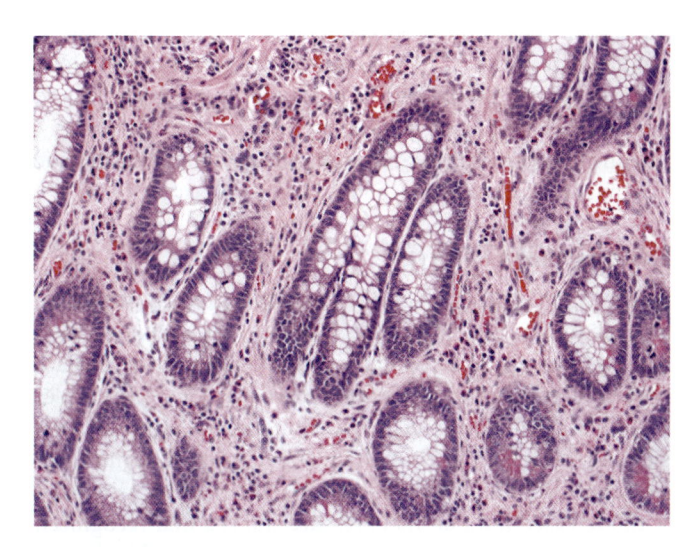

FIGURE 9-33 Chronic colitis. Branched crypts are a characteristic finding in chronic colitis. Note the irregular distribution of crypts (crypt disarray).

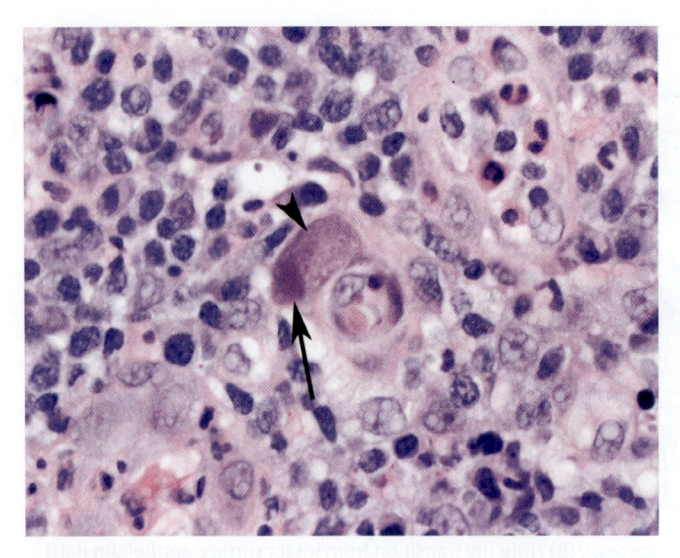

FIGURE 9-34 CMV colitis. Note the brightly eosinophilic nuclear inclusion (arrow) and smaller eosinophilic cytoplasmic inclusions (arrowhead) in this stromal cell infected with CMV.

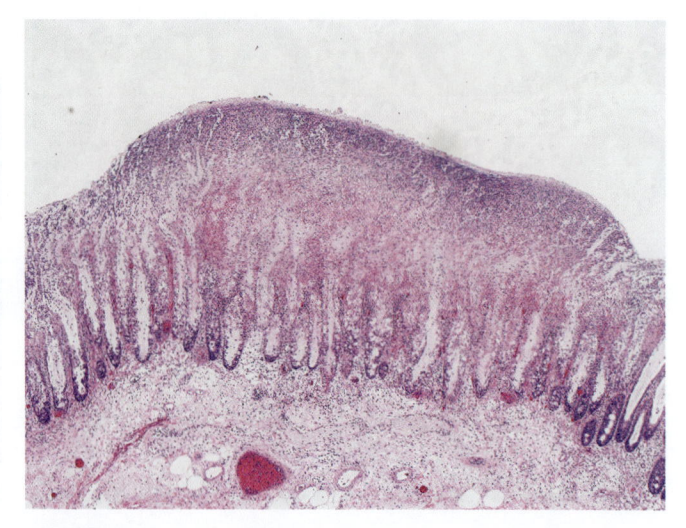

FIGURE 9-35 C. difficile colitis. This is an example of a pseudomembrane in a patient with a positive *C. difficile* stool assay. There is necrosis of the superficial halves of the crypts with an adherent laminated mixture of neutrophils, mucin, and fibrin.

C. difficile to thrive. The organism is not invasive, but rather causes disease by producing toxins that injure the colonic epithelium.

This infection is more common in older people, but can be seen in younger people as well. There is a spectrum of severity, ranging from mild diarrhea to severe diarrhea with abdominal pain, fever, leukocytosis, and even toxic megacolon with perforation. Diagnosis relies heavily on the detection of *C. difficile* toxin by stool assay. Supportive fluids and electrolytes and treatment with antibiotics with activity against *C. difficile* are usually effective. Surgical resection is necessary in cases complicated by ischemia or toxic megacolon.

Grossly, pseudomembranes appear as patchy yellow-white plaques adherent to the mucosal surface. The classic microscopic finding is the "volcano" lesion, which consists of vaguely laminated collections of neutrophils, fibrin, and mucin erupting from inflamed and distended crypts. This microscopic lesion is not always present. Sometimes only a minor exudate overlying distended crypts filled with neutrophils is present. There are varying degrees of mucosal necrosis (**Figure 9-35**).

Ischemic Colitis

Decreased blood flow to the colon, whether nonocclusive or occlusive, can result in mild mucosal ischemic injury or severe transmural infarction. The proximal portion of the colon is supplied by the superior mesenteric artery and the distal portion is supplied by the inferior mesenteric artery. The segment containing the distal transverse colon and splenic flexure is particularly susceptible to ischemic injury as this is a watershed area between the two major supplying arteries. Nonocclusive ischemic colitis is usually seen in the setting of acute blood loss or sepsis.

The clinical presentation depends on the severity of disease. Mild segmental injury may be asymptomatic or may cause rectal bleeding. Severe disease, as can be seen with acute thrombosis of one of the mesenteric arteries, can result in severe abdominal pain, abdominal distension, rectal bleeding, and even sepsis. Chronic ischemic colitis, as can be seen with atherosclerosis of the mesenteric arteries, can lead to intermittent crampy abdominal pain.

Grossly, the colon is edematous and may appear dusky and hemorrhagic if there is full-thickness necrosis. The mucosa is edematous and erythematous, and may show frank hemorrhage. Pseudomembranes, similar to those seen in *C. difficile* colitis, may be adherent to the mucosal surface. The microscopic appearance varies. Nonspecific features of active colitis may be present. More severe injury can lead to mucosal ulceration and transmural infarction. The superficial portions of the crypts are more susceptible to ischemic injury, thus there may be some preservation of the deepest portions of the crypts. The lamina propria often has a characteristic eosinophilic appearance in hematoxylin and eosin (H&E) stained sections due to the release of plasma proteins from injured capillaries, a finding referred to as lamina propria hyalinosis. Lamina propria fibrosis and crypt atrophy are characteristic findings seen in chronic ischemic colitis (**Figure 9-36**).

Diverticular Disease

A colonic diverticulum is a blind pouch composed of mucosa and submucosa that invaginates into the muscularis propria. It is lined by colonic mucosa that is in continuity with the surface mucosa. Diverticula are relatively uncommon in people under the age of 40 and become quite common in older people. The sigmoid colon is the most frequently involved segment. A low-fiber diet, common in Western societies, is associated with increased intraluminal pressure and is a well-recognized etiologic factor. Diverticula can become obstructed by inspissated mucous or fecal material, leading to distension, mucosal ischemia, and inflammation, a process now referred to as

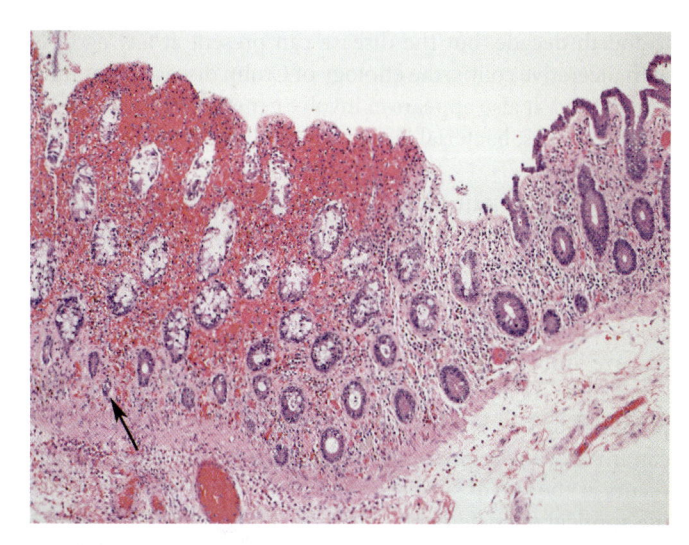

FIGURE 9-36 Ischemic colitis. This example of ischemic colitis shows mucosal hemorrhage, necrosis of the superficial portions of the crypts, and lamina propria hyalinosis. There is subtle atrophy of some of the crypts (arrow).

diverticulitis. Diverticulitis can lead to abscess formation, fistula formation, colonic perforation, and sepsis. Sometimes the associated fibrotic reaction can be so severe that it can result in a bowel obstruction (Figure 9-37).

Clinically, diverticulosis is usually asymptomatic. Diverticulitis, on the other hand, is associated with abdominal pain, fever, and leukocytosis. Some cases can be managed successfully with antibiotic treatment, but a significant number of patients require surgical intervention (e.g., abscess drainage, surgical resection).

Idiopathic Inflammatory Bowel Disease

Two diseases fall under the category of inflammatory bowel disease: ulcerative colitis and Crohn disease. Ulcerative colitis and Crohn disease share many similar features. There are also important differences. Principal differences include the distribution of disease within the GI tract and the presence or absence of inflammation involving the deeper layers of the bowel wall.

Ulcerative Colitis

Ulcerative colitis is a chronic inflammatory disorder of the colon and rectum, characterized by periods of exacerbation and remission. The disease usually first appears in adolescents and young adults, but there is a second smaller peak in older people. Until a few decades ago, the incidence had been on the rise, but it has since flattened out. The etiology is not fully understood, but is believed to involve a complex interplay between genetic factors, environmental factors, bacterial antigens, and disturbances of mucosal immunity.

While a series of intermittent flares is typically encountered, some people experience few flares separated by long periods of remission, while others suffer from continuous refractory disease requiring colectomy. The most common symptoms are bloody diarrhea, crampy abdominal pain, and tenesmus. More severe cases can be associated with systemic complications such as fever, dehydration, anemia, and electrolyte imbalances. There is an increased risk of colon cancer that is related to the extent and duration of disease. Surveillance colonoscopies are performed to monitor for the development of dysplasia. Toxic megacolon is an uncommon but important complication that occurs in some people with ulcerative colitis. In toxic megacolon, marked dilation of the colon leads to compromised perfusion, ischemic necrosis, and secondary bacterial infection, which can ultimately lead to sepsis. Systemic manifestations can be present in a minority of patients. These include arthritis, uveitis, skin lesions, and primary sclerosing cholangitis. If anti-inflammatory drugs, corticosteroids, and immunosuppressant therapy fail, total colectomy with ileoanal anastomosis has the potential to be curative.

Grossly, the involved mucosa is erythematous (red) and flattened. Small ulcers can coalesce to form larger areas of ulceration surrounding islands of regenerating mucosa. These regenerating islands have a polypoid appearance and are referred to as pseudopolyps. Importantly, these changes begin at the rectum and extend proximally (toward the cecum) in a continuous manner. The disease can be rectal only, or it can extend all the way to the cecum. This pattern of continuous involvement is different than that seen in Crohn disease (Figure 9-38). Of note, after the initiation of therapy, rectal sparing disease and skip lesions can be observed. The terminal ileum can occasionally show mild involvement, a condition referred to as "backwash ileitis".

Microscopically, there are nonspecific changes of active and chronic colitis. Importantly, the inflammatory infiltrates are restricted to the mucosa and superficial submucosa (Figure 9-39). Granulomas are absent, except for nonspecific mucin granulomas associated with crypt rupture.

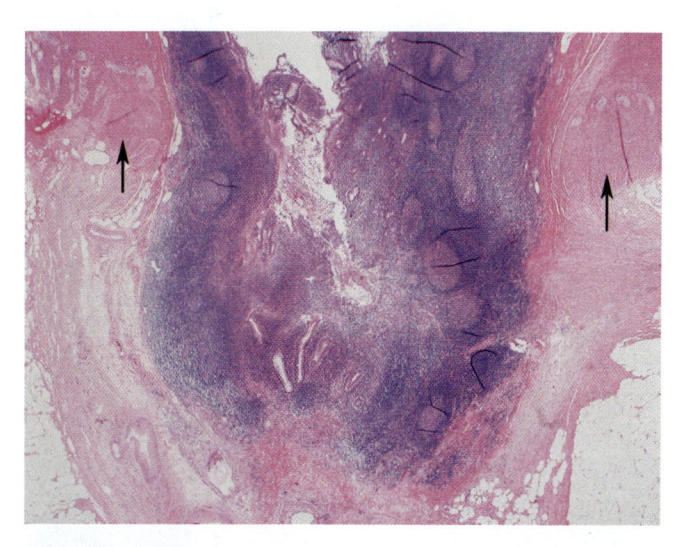

FIGURE 9-37 Diverticulosis. In diverticulosis, outpouchings of colonic mucosa and submucosa bulge through the muscularis propria at sites of colonic wall weakness. The muscularis propria is marked with arrows.

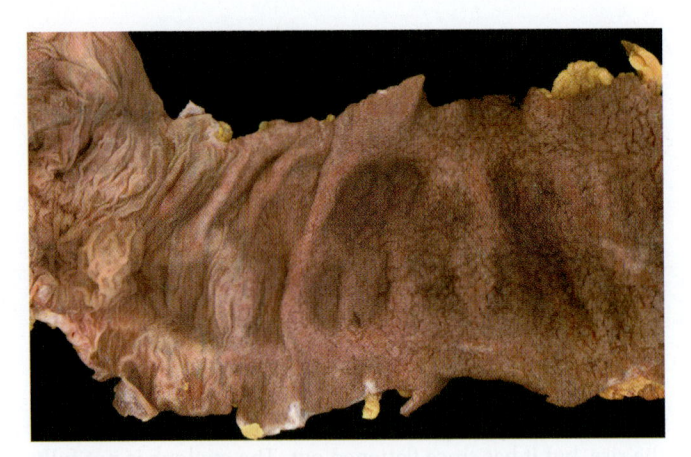

FIGURE 9-38 Ulcerative colitis. Note the continuous segment of mucosal erythema extending from the distal aspect of the specimen (right of image). This pattern of disease distribution is characteristic of ulcerative colitis.

> **QUICK REVIEW**
> **Ulcerative Colitis**
> - Idiopathic inflammatory disorder of the rectum and colon with periods of exacerbation and remission.
> - Classically involves the rectum and extends proximally in a continuous distribution.
> - Inflammation is mostly restricted to the mucosa.

Crohn Disease

Crohn disease is a chronic inflammatory disorder that most often involves the distal small bowel, but can involve any portion of the GI tract, including the colon. The incidence of Crohn disease is increasing. Peak incidence is in the second to fourth decade, but the disease can present at any age. As with ulcerative colitis, the etiology of Crohn disease is not fully understood. It also appears to involve genetic factors, environmental factors, bacterial antigens, and disturbances in mucosal immunity.

Abdominal pain, diarrhea, and fever are the main clinical manifestations. The severity of disease is highly variable, paralleling the variable location and extent of GI tract involvement. There is an increased risk of small bowel and colon cancer. Extraintestinal manifestations such as arthritis, eye inflammation, and primary sclerosing cholangitis can also be seen in Crohn disease. Surgical resection has less potential to be curative in Crohn disease since the disease can involve any segment of the GI tract. Crohn disease often recurs at the site of surgical anastomoses, further complicating surgical management.

Grossly, the involved mucosa is erythematous. Ulcers, including long linear ulcers, are common. Edematous mucosa is present in and around these ulcers, imparting a cobblestone appearance in many instances. Sectioning of the bowel wall shows fibrotic thickening, which is responsible for the strictures that can be seen with Crohn disease (**Figure 9-40**). In response to transmural inflammation, mesenteric fat extends around the outer circumference of the bowel and encases it, a process known as mesenteric fat wrapping. Strictures are common and fistulas can be seen in some cases. An important concept in Crohn disease is that these abnormalities are usually not continuous, that is, there are skip lesions with uninvolved segments located between diseased segments.

Microscopically, colonic involvement by Crohn disease is characterized by active colitis, chronic colitis, and mucosal ulceration. Small bowel disease is characterized by villous loss,

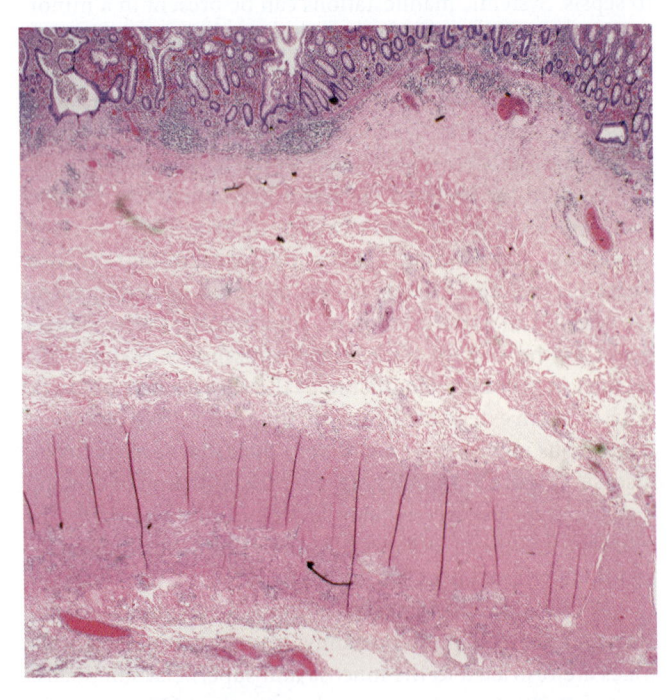

FIGURE 9-39 Ulcerative colitis. This low-power example of ulcerative colitis shows inflammation restricted to the mucosa and superficial submucosa and an absence of transmural inflammation.

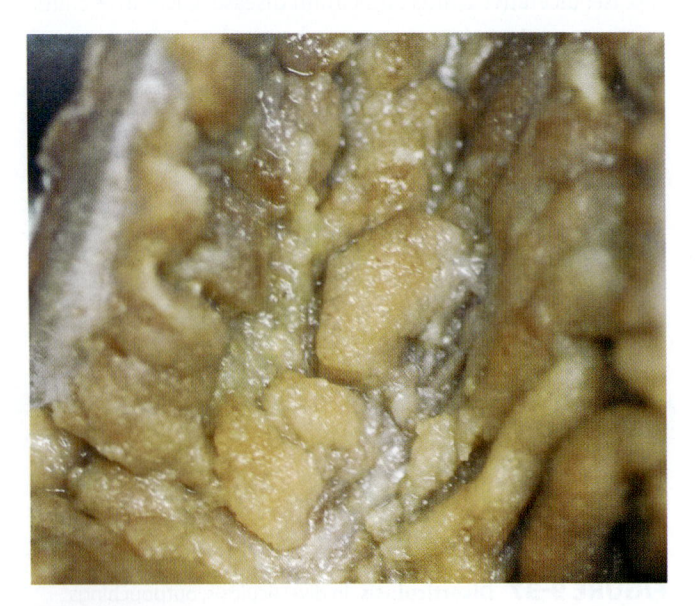

FIGURE 9-40 Crohn disease. Detailed view of a segment of resected colon from a patient with Crohn disease demonstrates a thickened colonic wall, linear ulcers, and a cobblestone appearance.

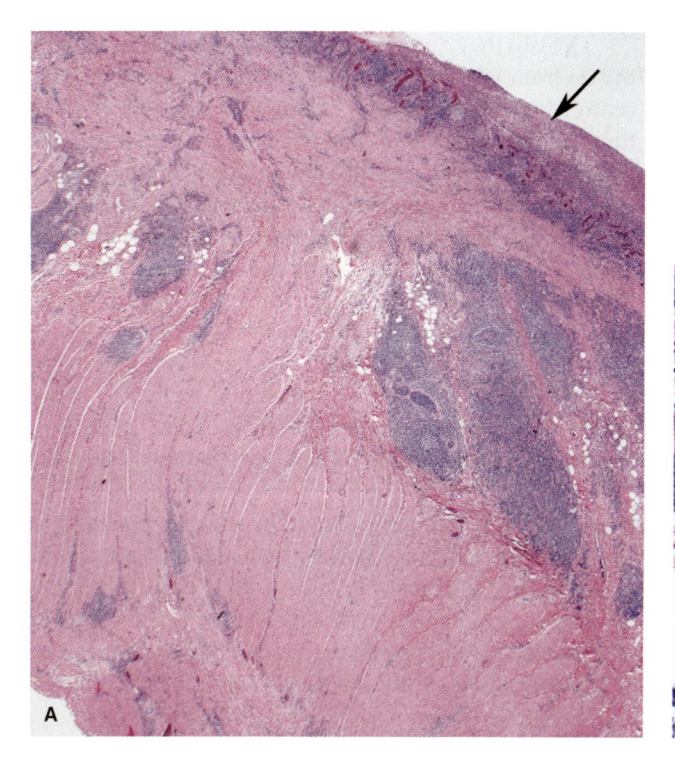

FIGURE 9-41 Crohn disease. **(A)** In contrast to ulcerative colitis, this low-power example of Crohn disease shows conspicuous transmural lymphoid aggregates. An ulcerated mucosal surface is noted by the arrow. **(B)** Epithelioid granulomas (arrow) are characteristic of Crohn disease.

mucosal ulceration, active (neutrophilic) cryptitis, and crypt hyperplasia and disarray. The presence of deep ulcers, fissures that extend into the submucosa, and transmural lymphoid aggregates is characteristic of Crohn disease and distinguishes it from ulcerative colitis. Epithelioid granulomas, not associated with crypt rupture, are also commonly seen in Crohn disease (Figure 9-41).

> **QUICK REVIEW**
> **Crohn Disease**
> - Idiopathic inflammatory disorder that can affect any segment of the GI tract (small bowel most common).
> - Skip lesions (i.e., intervening segments of uninvolved mucosa) are common.
> - Deep ulcers, granulomas, fissures, transmural lymphoid aggregates, fistulas, and mesenteric fat wrapping are classic findings.

Polyps and Neoplasms of the Colon

The term polyp simply refers to a mass that protrudes into the lumen of an organ. Polyps can be nondysplastic or dysplastic (i.e., preneoplastic). They can be classified based on the attachment to the mucosa as either pedunculated or sessile. Pedunculated polyps are attached to the mucosa by a discrete stalk, usually making for an easier resection. Sessile polyps are broad based and have no defined stalk. This can make resection more problematic and it often hinders the ability of the pathologist to evaluate the margins in dysplastic cases.

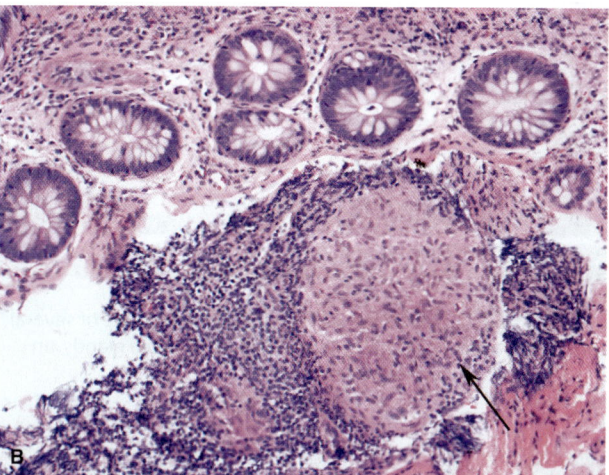

Inflammatory Polyps

Inflammatory polyps are areas of inflamed and regenerating mucosa that project above the mucosal surface. They can be seen in a variety of settings, but are especially common in inflammatory bowel disease. These lesions are nondysplastic (i.e., they are considered to have no malignant potential).

Hamartomatous Polyps

Hamartomatous polyps are nodules of benign but disorganized tissue. In the colon, they are usually made up of some degree of epithelial hyperplasia, crypt disarray and dilation, and proliferation and splaying of the muscularis mucosa. Hamartomatous polyps can be sporadic, in which case there is often only one polyp, or they can be part of a syndrome, where there can be over a hundred polyps throughout the GI tract. Dysplasia can develop in hamartomatous polyps and is more likely to occur with hamartomatous polyposis syndromes (Figure 9-42).

Precursor Lesions

Adenomatous polyps and certain types of serrated polyps have genetic abnormalities that put them on a pathway toward becoming carcinoma (i.e., a malignant epithelial neoplasm with invasive and metastatic potential).

Adenomatous Polyps

Adenomatous polyps are dysplastic lesions of the colonic epithelium. They are relatively common and are frequently encountered during screening colonoscopies.

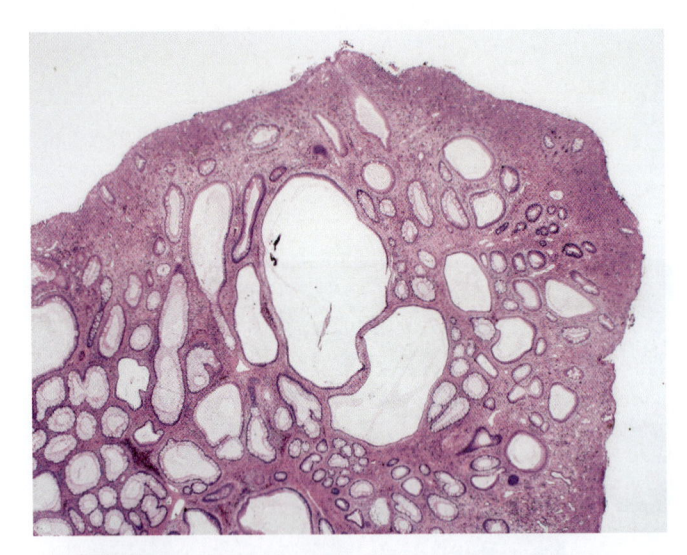

FIGURE 9-42 Juvenile polyp. This juvenile polyp, one of several types of hamartomatous polyps, shows cystically dilated glands, an inflamed stroma, and an ulcerated surface.

Grossly, they can be pedunculated or sessile and can range in size from just a few millimeters in diameter to well over a centimeter. Microscopically, there are two distinct architectural patterns: tubular and villous. Tubular adenomas consist of long tubules of dysplastic epithelium underlying a relatively smooth polyp surface. Villous adenomas are characterized by fingerlike projections of dysplastic epithelium that project above the mucosal surface. Many adenomatous polyps show a mixture of the two patterns and are referred to as tubulovillous adenomas. Villous architecture is associated with a higher risk of invasive carcinoma. There is a two-tiered system for grading dysplastic changes. Low-grade dysplasia is typified by enlarged, crowded, hyperchromatic (dark), and pseudostratified pencil-shaped nuclei. There is usually apoptotic debris present toward the base of dysplastic crypts. High-grade dysplasia is characterized by increased glandular architectural complexity associated with more severe nuclear atypia and a loss of nuclear polarity (i.e., some nuclei lose the normal perpendicular relationship to the epithelial basement membrane) (Figure 9-43). The presence of high-grade dysplasia indicates a much greater risk of concurrent or future invasive carcinoma.

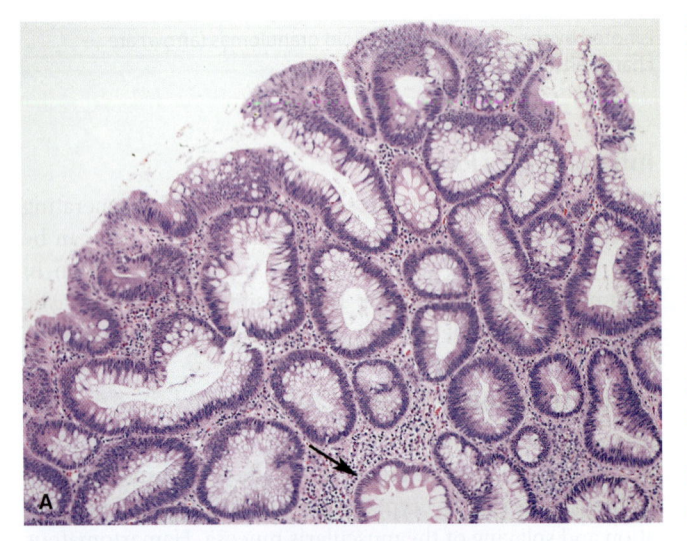

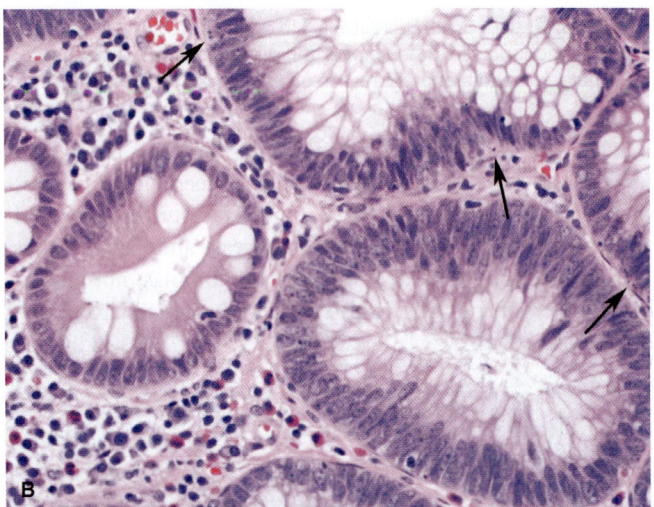

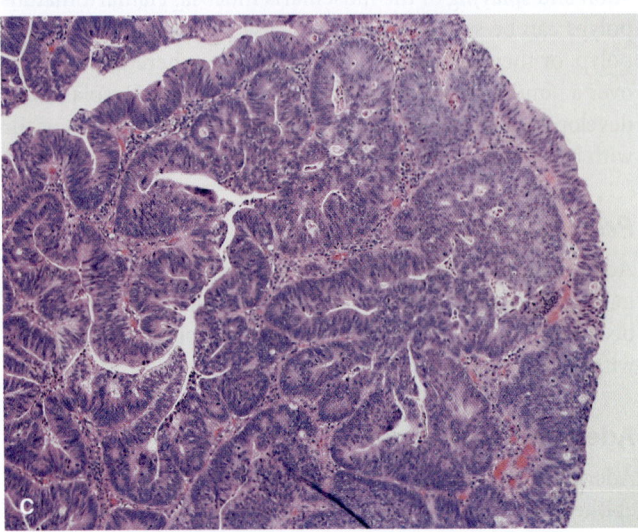

FIGURE 9-43 Adenomatous polyp. (A) In this adenomatous polyp with low-grade dysplasia, there is crowding of dysplastic crypts that are hyperchromatic due to an increase in nuclear size, nuclear pseudostratification, and a loss of cytoplasmic mucin. The arrow marks a nondysplastic crypt. **(B)** In this higher magnification view, note the contrast between the nondysplastic crypt on the left and the crypt with low-grade dysplasia on the right. Arrows mark foci of crypt cell apoptosis. **(C)** In high-grade dysplasia, there is increased glandular architectural complexity, increased nuclear atypia, loss of nuclear polarity, and increased mitotic activity.

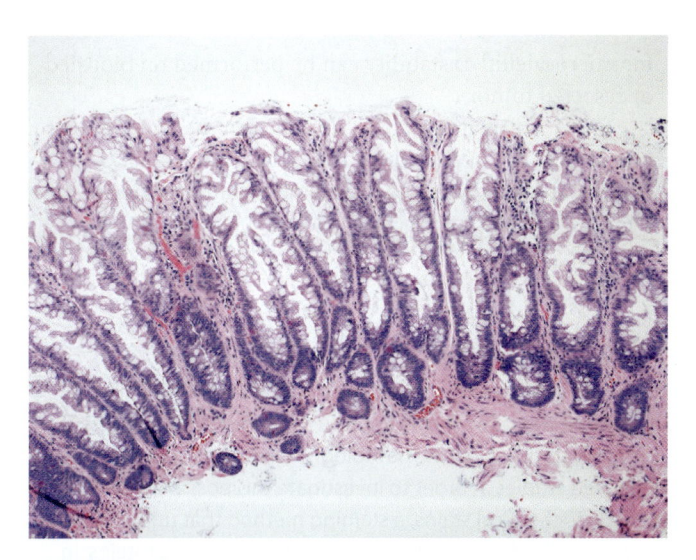

FIGURE 9-44 Hyperplastic polyp. Abnormal proliferation and cell turnover in hyperplastic polyps result in crowding of the superficial halves of the crypts, imparting a serrated appearance. Note that these changes do not extend to the crypt bases.

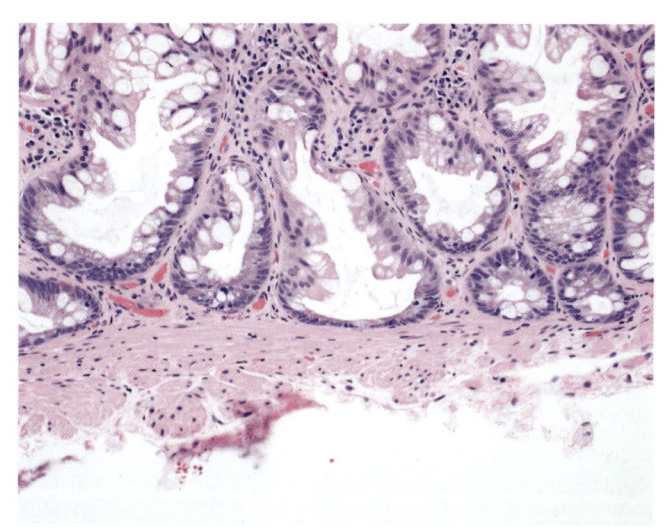

FIGURE 9-45 Sessile serrated polyp. In contrast to a hyperplastic polyp, notice how the crypt abnormalities extend to the crypt bases in a sessile serrated polyp. In the center of the image is a dilated crypt with early horizontal expansion of the crypt base creating the appearance of an inverted T.

Serrated Polyps

Recognized types of serrated polyps include hyperplastic polyps, sessile serrated polyps, mixed hyperplastic/adenomatous polyps, and traditional serrated adenomas.

Hyperplastic polyps are sessile polyps that form as the result of increased epithelial proliferation at the crypt bases coupled with slowed surface migration and sloughing. They are usually small and especially common in the rectum. Histologically, this manifests as dilation of the mid-to-upper aspects of the crypts, imparting a sawtooth or serrated appearance, with crowding of absorptive cells and goblet cells and surface tufting. Cytologic changes of dysplasia are not present (**Figure 9-44**).

Traditionally, hyperplastic polyps have been thought of as having no malignant potential. This may still be the case; however, emerging molecular data has shown at least a subset of hyperplastic polyps to exhibit genetic and cell cycle defects that theoretically could allow for malignant transformation.

Sessile serrated polyps (also known as sessile serrated adenomas) are a type of serrated polyp that morphologically resembles a hyperplastic polyp; however, the serrated changes involve all aspects of the crypts, including the bases, and the crypt bases can be branched or show horizontal expansion forming an inverted T (**Figure 9-45**). Sessile serrated polyps are usually larger (greater than 0.5 cm) and more commonly right sided. They are recognized as a precursor of invasive carcinoma.

Mixed hyperplastic/adenomatous polyps, perhaps more appropriately called sessile serrated polyps with dysplasia, are sessile serrated polyps in which conventional dysplasia has arisen due to the acquisition of additional genetic defects. Histologically, there are elements of sessile serrated polyp and adenomatous polyp.

Traditional serrated adenomas are polyps that have a vaguely serrated architectural pattern lined by conventional dysplastic epithelium.

Colorectal Carcinogenesis

Adenocarcinoma

Colorectal adenocarcinoma is one of the most common forms of cancer and is near the top of the list in terms of cancer-related mortality. The incidence increases with age, but colorectal cancer can be seen in younger people with long-standing inflammatory bowel disease or with a genetic predisposition, such as Lynch syndrome or familial adenomatous polyposis (FAP).

The clinical presentation is variable. Some cases are asymptomatic and discovered during routine screening colonoscopy. Occult blood loss or more significant rectal bleeding can occur. When the tumor is more advanced, abdominal pain and bowel obstruction can occur and diagnosis is sometimes made with discovery of metastatic disease. Surgical resection is the most realistic form of curative therapy with chemotherapy and radiation therapy being used in cases where there is unresectable disease or a high risk of recurrence after surgery.

Colorectal cancers are invasive carcinomas with a variable degree of gland formation (**Figure 9-46**). Some tumors have prominent mucin production with pools of extracellular mucin containing free-floating malignant epithelium (termed mucinous adenocarcinoma if this pattern occupies more than 50% of the tumor). The depth of invasion into the wall of the colon and the presence of metastatic disease are the two most important prognostic variables. Metastases commonly go to regional lymph nodes and to the liver.

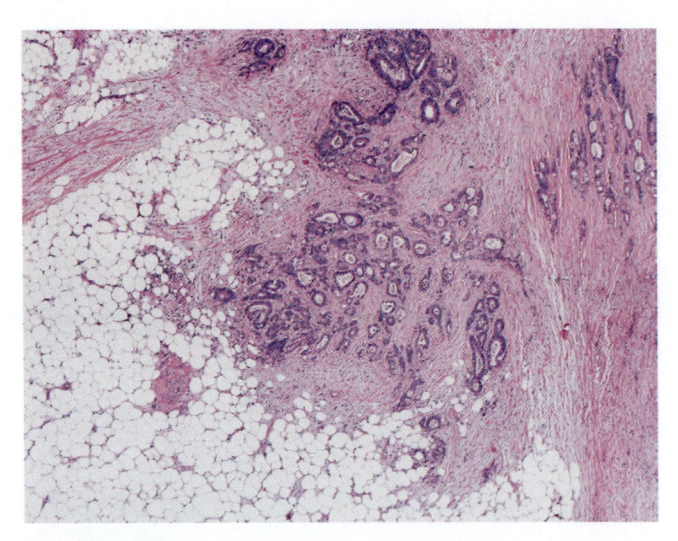

FIGURE 9-46 Invasive colonic adenocarcinoma. Malignant glands have invaded through the muscularis propria and into the subserosal adipose tissue. Note the surrounding fibroinflammatory stromal reaction (desmoplasia).

QUICK REVIEW
Molecular Models of Colorectal Carcinogenesis

The majority of colorectal cancers follow the chromosomal instability pathway of carcinogenesis. Mutations of the adenomatous polyposis coli (*APC*) gene occur early in the process, around the time of transition from normal to adenomatous epithelium. Late in the process, around the time of progression from adenoma to carcinoma, mutations of the tumor suppressor gene *TP53* occur. In between, mutations of other genes, such as the *RAS* oncogene, push the neoplastic epithelium further toward carcinoma.

People with FAP have a germ-line mutation of one of their *APC* genes and often have innumerable polyps within the colon, small bowel (duodenum, in particular), and stomach. Total colectomy with regular endoscopic surveillance is employed to detect advancement to invasive carcinoma.

A smaller percentage of colorectal cancers develop as the result of DNA mismatch repair defects (i.e., microsatellite instability pathway). The products of DNA mismatch repair genes are responsible for repairing errors in base pairing that occur during DNA replication. These errors commonly occur in repetitive sequences of DNA called microsatellites. When there is defective DNA mismatch repair, microsatellites tend to have varying numbers of repeats compared with the previously normal length, a phenomenon known as microsatellite instability. Certain clinical and histologic findings are suggestive of this defect. The tumors often occur in people under the age of 50. Microscopically, the tumors often display a high histologic grade, prominent mucinous differentiation, and sometimes are associated with a striking inflammatory reaction. Immunohistochemical stains to screen for a loss of DNA mismatch repair proteins and molecular testing to screen for microsatellite instability can be performed on biopsied or resected tumor.

DNA mismatch repair defects can be sporadic or hereditary. The hereditary form, Lynch syndrome, occurs when there is an inherited germ-line mutation of one of the DNA mismatch repair genes.

IN TRANSLATION

In cases of invasive colonic adenocarcinoma where there is a high index of suspicion for DNA mismatch repair defects, it is now common for the pathologist to perform more sophisticated studies in order to investigate this possibility. Immunohistochemical stains, a staining method that utilizes antigen–antibody interactions to identify specific proteins in tissue sections, can be used to evaluate for a loss of expression of mismatch repair proteins. Tissue sections can also be used to perform microsatellite analysis to identify tumors with microsatellite instability. Some institutions choose to perform this testing on all new colon cancer specimens.

APPENDIX

Normal Anatomy and Histology of the Appendix

The appendix is a tubular structure that attaches to the cecum. The average length is about 8 cm, but there can be quite a bit of variation. The appendiceal orifice is located at the site of attachment with the cecum and the lumen of the cecum is in continuity with that of the appendix. The appendiceal lumen closes at the appendiceal tip. The wall of the appendix is composed of the same layers that are seen in the colon (mucosa, submucosa, muscularis propria, and serosa). A portion of the appendix is invested by mesentery (i.e., the mesoappendix) (Figure 9-47).

Principal Diseases of the Appendix

Acute appendicitis is by far the most common disease of the appendix. Neoplasms can also be found in the appendix and these are sometimes found incidentally in appendectomies for acute appendicitis.

Acute Appendicitis

Acute inflammation of the wall of the appendix can result in abdominal pain, nausea, vomiting, fever, and leukocytosis. With transmural inflammation and mural necrosis, perforation can occur, which can be accompanied by sepsis. Children and adolescents are most commonly afflicted, but disease can occur at any age.

Many cases of acute appendicitis are caused by luminal obstruction, which leads to distension of the lumen distal

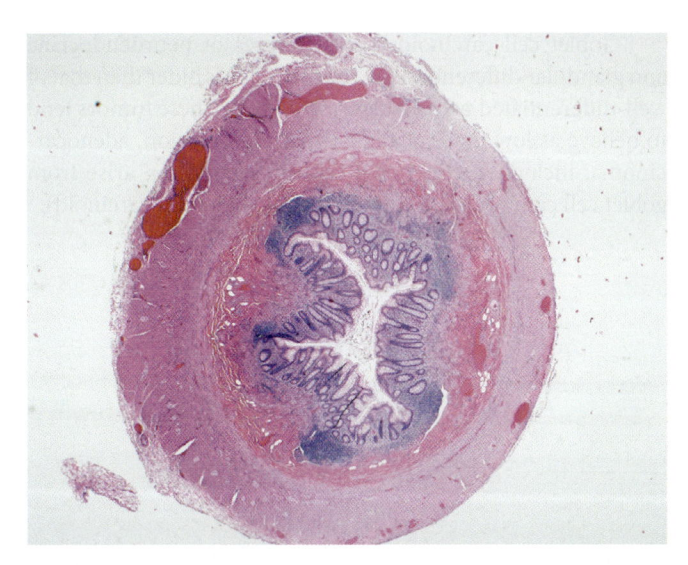

FIGURE 9-47 Normal appendix. This is a cross-section of a normal appendix. Note the mucosal and submucosal lymphoid aggregates.

CASE 9-9

The patient is a previously healthy 14-year-old boy who presented to the emergency department with abdominal pain and nausea. Physical examination showed a low-grade fever and an accentuation of the abdominal pain with deep palpation of the right lower quadrant. Laboratory studies showed a leukocytosis. A CT scan was performed, which showed a thickened appendiceal wall and periappendiceal changes suggestive of inflammation. A laparoscopic appendectomy was successfully performed. Pathologic examination showed acute inflammation of the appendiceal wall and a diagnosis of acute appendicitis was made (see section "Acute Appendicitis" and Figure 9-48).

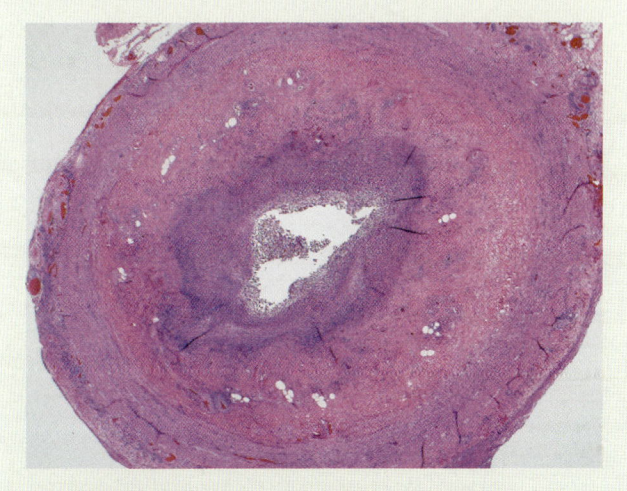

FIGURE 9-48 Acute appendicitis. In this low-power example of acute appendicitis, there is mucosal ulceration with a dense neutrophilic infiltrate present within the mucosa and superficial submucosa.

to the obstruction, increased intraluminal pressure, mucosal ischemia, and secondary bacterial infection. Fecaliths (i.e., hardened collections of feces), foreign bodies, tumors, pinworms (*Enterobius vermicularis*), and reactive lymphoid hyperplasia, sometimes due to viral infection, are the most common causes of luminal obstruction. In other cases, no obvious cause of luminal obstruction is identified.

Pathologically, acute appendicitis is characterized by varying degrees of neutrophilic infiltration and tissue necrosis. In cases with minimal acute inflammation, the appendix may appear grossly normal or may show congestion of serosal blood vessels. With increasing degrees of transmural inflammation, serosal exudates become apparent and perforation can be seen in severe cases (Figure 9-48).

Neoplasms of the Appendix

Generally speaking, the polyps and malignant neoplasms that occur in the colon can also be found in the appendix, though the incidences are much lower. A few neoplasms of the appendix deserve special attention.

Pseudomyxoma Peritonei

Pseudomyxoma peritonei refers to the presence of mucinous material in the abdominal cavity and on peritoneal surfaces. A large majority of cases are due to appendiceal neoplasms (e.g. low-grade mucinous neoplasm, high-grade mucinous adenocarcinoma). Malignant cells are typically found floating within pools of extracellular mucin.

Well-Differentiated Neuroendocrine Tumor (Carcinoid Tumor) and Goblet Cell Carcinoid

Well-differentiated neuroendocrine tumors arise within the deep mucosa or submucosa. They are often found

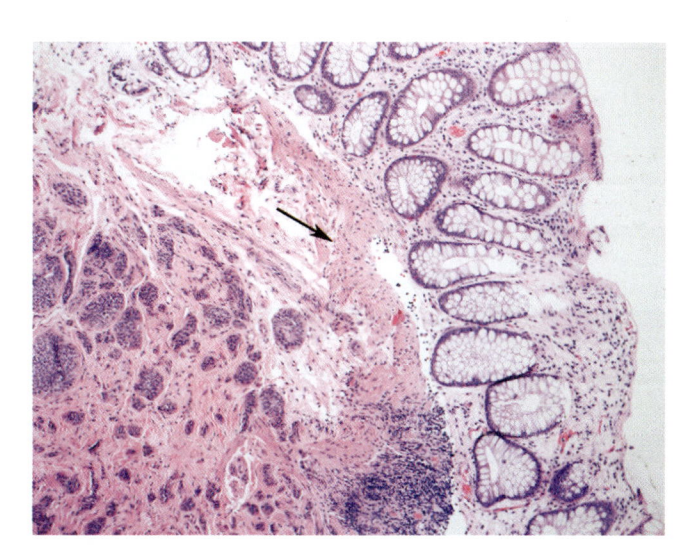

FIGURE 9-49 Well-differentiated neuroendocrine tumor of appendix. Deep to the muscularis mucosa (arrow), there is a proliferation of small nests of relatively bland appearing tumor cells that show a neuroendocrine phenotype by immunohistochemistry.

incidentally at the time of appendectomy for appendicitis. These tumors are most common in young adults, but can occur in children and older adults. Tumor staging is based on the size of the tumor and the presence or absence of invasion into adjacent structures (**Figure 9-49**).

Goblet cell carcinoids show features of neuroendocrine and glandular differentiation. The mean age is older than that of well-differentiated neuroendocrine tumors. These tumors tend to behave as low-grade malignancies. On occasion, adenocarcinoma, including signet ring cell carcinoma, can arise from goblet cell carcinoid (i.e., carcinoma ex-goblet cell carcinoid).

Pathology of the Liver, Gallbladder, and Extrahepatic Biliary Tract

CHAPTER 10

Kevin G. Greene, M.D.

LIVER

Introduction to the Functions of the Liver

The liver is a vital organ that performs a variety of important functions. It is unique among the internal organs for its ability to regenerate following tissue loss. Glucose homeostasis is maintained by the liver by way of glucose storage (as glycogen), glycogenolysis, and gluconeogenesis. In addition to glycogen, the liver is an important site for iron, copper, triglyceride, and lipid-soluble vitamin storage. A large number of serum proteins, such as albumin, clotting factors, and complement, are synthesized in the liver. Proper liver function is crucial for the catabolism of serum proteins and hormones and for the detoxification of exogenous substances, including many drugs. The liver is also the source of bile production, which is important for fat absorption within the small bowel.

CASE 10-1

The patient is a 46-year-old man who sought medical attention for vague complaints of fatigue, joint pain, and upper abdominal pain. Laboratory studies were performed as part of the patient's evaluation and showed elevations of serum iron, serum transferrin saturation, and serum ferritin. There were mild elevations of aspartate aminotransferase (AST) and alanine aminotransferase (ALT). Given these findings, a liver biopsy was performed and showed a prominent increase in iron accumulation within hepatocytes and early bridging fibrosis. A diagnosis of hemochromatosis was established. To evaluate for a genetic cause of hemochromatosis (i.e., primary hemochromatosis), analysis of the HFE gene was performed and showed a homozygous C282Y mutation, consistent with primary hemochromatosis (see section "Hemochromatosis" and Figure 10-16).

Normal Anatomy and Histology of the Liver

The liver is located in the right upper quadrant of the abdomen, immediately beneath the diaphragm. Two hepatic lobes are recognized: a larger right lobe and a smaller left lobe. The hepatic artery and portal vein provide the liver with a dual blood supply. The hepatic artery originates from the celiac axis and is the liver's source of more highly oxygenated blood. The portal vein is formed primarily by the convergence of the splenic vein and superior mesenteric vein. Because of its unique circulation, the portal vein provides the liver with metabolic substrates from the gut and provides a mechanism for ingested substances to be processed before entering the systemic circulation. The hepatic veins empty into the inferior vena cava and carry blood away from the liver and into the systemic circulation. The bile carrying ducts of the liver are called hepatic ducts. The right and left hepatic ducts empty into a common hepatic duct that merges with the cystic duct of the gallbladder to form the common bile duct (Figure 10-1).

From a microanatomical perspective, the liver is composed of structural units called hepatic lobules. It is easiest to think of the hepatic lobule as a two-dimensional hexagon arranged around a terminal hepatic venule (a.k.a. central vein). Portal tracts (a.k.a. portal triads) are located at the peripheral angles of the hexagon. Portal tracts contain branches of hepatic artery, portal vein, and hepatic duct and are supported by stroma. Surrounding the portal tract is a layer of hepatocytes called the limiting plate. The majority of the hepatic lobule is made up of plates of hepatocytes measuring 1–2 cells thick that radiate from the terminal hepatic venule to the periphery of the lobule. These hepatic plates are surrounded by hepatic sinusoids (Figures 10-2 and 10-3). A reticulin stain can be used to highlight the edges of the sinusoids.

Blood from branches of the hepatic artery and portal vein enters the sinusoids at the portal tracts. The blood flows through the sinusoid toward the terminal hepatic venule. Terminal hepatic venules drain into hepatic veins that, as previously noted, drain "processed" blood into the inferior vena cava. The sinusoid–hepatocyte junction is well suited to

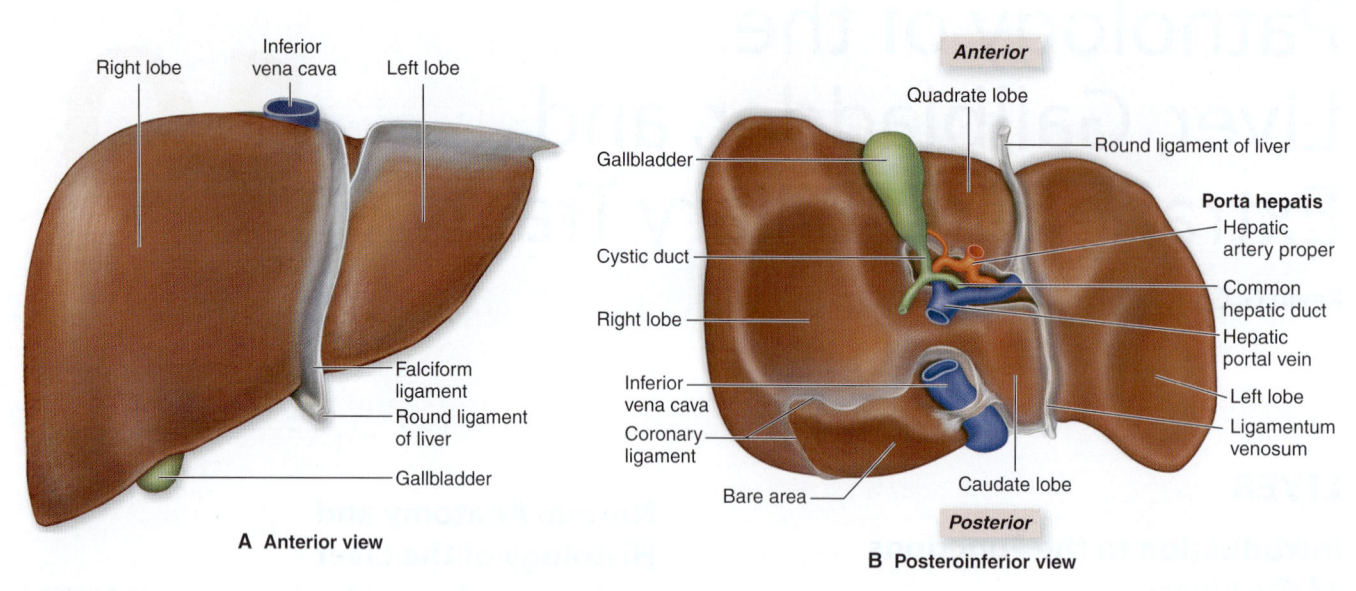

FIGURE 10-1 Anatomy of the liver. **(A)** Anterior and **(B)** posteroinferior. Source: Figure 26.18 in McKinley & O'Loughlin's Human Anatomy, 2nd ed.

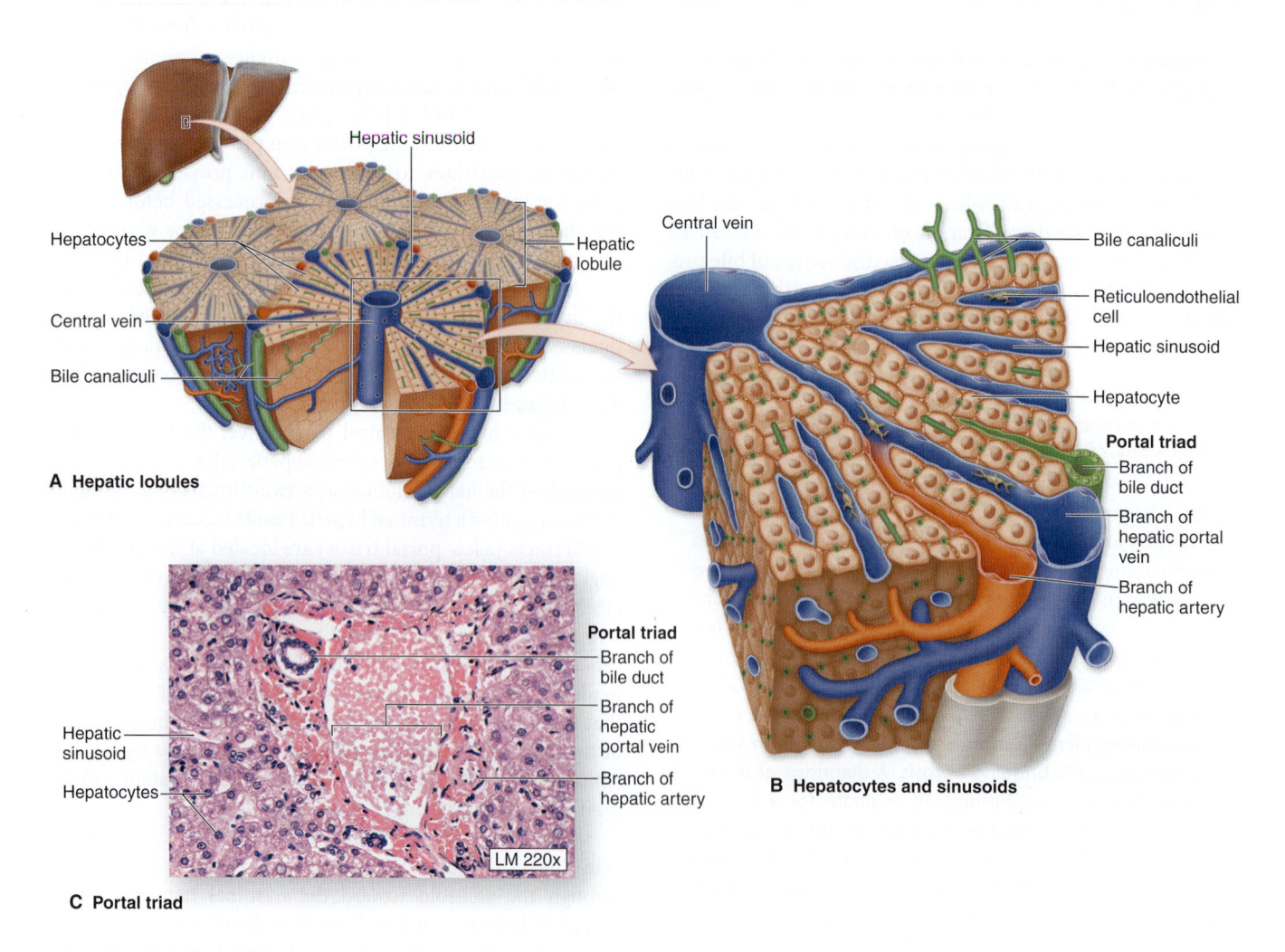

FIGURE 10-2 Anatomy of the hepatic lobule. **(A)** Depiction of multiple adjacent hepatic lobules. **(B)** Depiction of a portion of a hepatic lobule. **(C)** Photomicrograph of a portal tract. Source: Figure 26.19 in McKinley & O'Loughlin's Human Anatomy, 2nd ed.

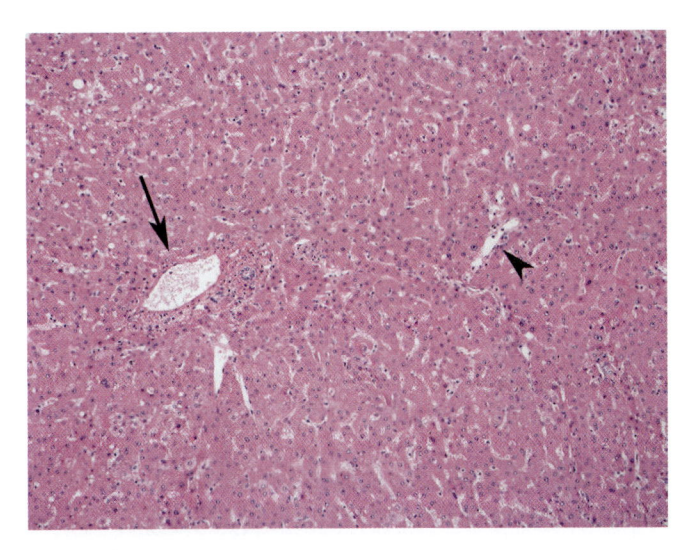

FIGURE 10-3 Hepatic lobule. In this section of liver, one portal tract (arrow) and one terminal hepatic venule (arrowhead) are present. The hepatocytes around the portal tract are referred to as zone 1 hepatocytes and the hepatocytes around the terminal hepatic venule are referred to as zone 3 hepatocytes. The hepatocytes in between are referred to as zone 2 hepatocytes.

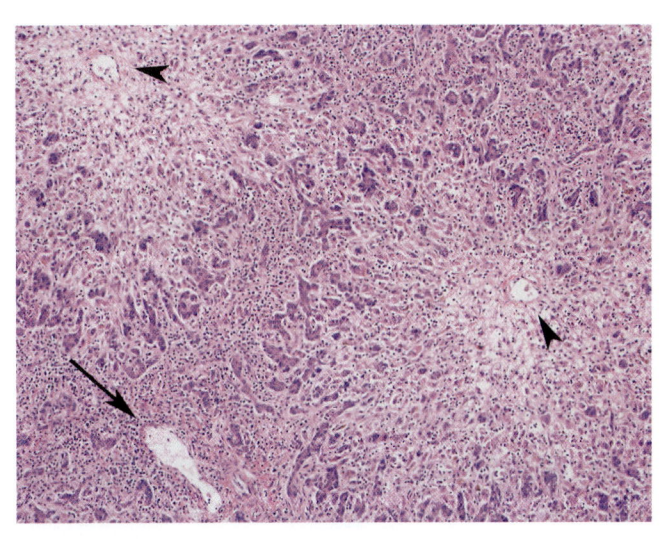

FIGURE 10-4 Fulminant liver failure. In this example of fulminant liver failure, there is panlobular hepatocyte necrosis. Bile duct-like structures are prominent and probably represent a proliferation of pluripotent cells in response to liver injury. The arrow marks a portal tract and the arrowheads mark terminal hepatic venules.

accommodate the free passage of plasma from the sinusoid to the hepatocyte, and vice versa.

Bile flows in the opposite direction. Bile is secreted by hepatocytes into spaces between adjacent hepatocytes called bile canaliculi. Bile flows from the bile canaliculi to the interlobular (portal tract) bile ducts though periportal bile ductules (a.k.a. cholangioles or canals of Hering).

Functionally, the liver is best thought of in terms of zones. Zone 1 is periportal, zone 3 is perivenular (i.e., around the terminal hepatic venule), and zone 2 is between zones 1 and 3. Zone 1 receives blood with the highest oxygen content, whereas zone 3 receives oxygen-poor blood and is most susceptible to ischemia. There are also metabolic differences between the zones.

Principal Diseases of the Liver

The liver is the site of a vast array of non-neoplastic and neoplastic disorders and pathologic evaluation of the liver can be intimidating. Histologically, some non-neoplastic and neoplastic disorders can closely resemble normal liver parenchyma, further complicating evaluation.

Liver Failure

Liver failure can be acute or chronic. Acute (fulminant) liver failure is most often caused by viral infection, drug/toxin injury, autoimmune hepatitis (AIH), or hepatic vein obstruction (Figure 10-4). The onset is rapid and, while some cases may be reversible, many cases require liver transplantation to avert death. Chronic liver failure is more insidious in onset and is usually seen in the setting of cirrhosis.

The clinical manifestations of liver failure are broad, which reflects the variety of liver functions outlined at the beginning of the chapter. Jaundice results from an inadequate clearance of bilirubin from the blood. Coagulopathy occurs in part due to reduced synthesis of coagulation factors. Decreased albumin synthesis results in edema due to albumin's effects on oncotic pressure. Hepatic encephalopathy, renal failure, pulmonary derangements, and endocrine derangements are also manifestations of liver failure.

Cirrhosis

Cirrhosis is the end-stage of several forms of chronic liver disease and is characterized by destruction of the normal liver tissue and the formation of scar tissue (i.e., bands of fibrosis) surrounding regenerative nodules of hepatocytes (Figure 10-5). The most common causes are hepatitis B, hepatitis C, and alcoholic and nonalcoholic steatohepatitis (NASH).

Vascular Disorders

Chronic Passive Congestion

Chronic passive congestion occurs when there is a physical or functional obstruction to the flow of blood through the hepatic vein. This occurs most commonly as the result of congestive heart failure, but can also occur with hepatic vein thrombosis (i.e., Budd–Chiari syndrome).

Grossly, the liver has a mottled cut surface that is said to resemble that of a nutmeg (nutmeg liver). Microscopically, there is dilation of the perivenular sinusoids, which are usually filled with red blood cells. This can cause atrophy of the adjacent zone 3 hepatocytes. Long-standing congestion can result in perivenular and zone 3 perisinusoidal fibrosis. Portal vein thrombosis can cause significant zone 3 hepatocyte necrosis (Figure 10-6).

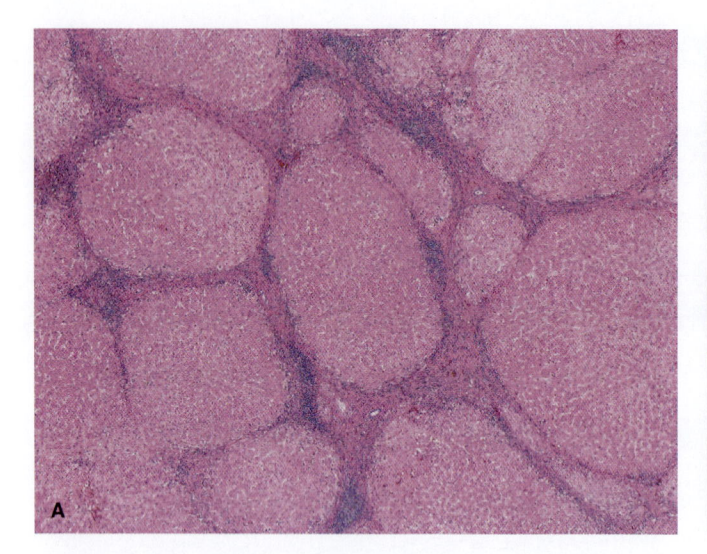

FIGURE 10-5 Cirrhosis. (A) Cirrhosis is a diffuse nodularity of the liver resulting from fibrous scarring and the formation of regenerative nodules of hepatocytes. **(B)** A trichrome stain is used to highlight collagen in the fibrous bands (blue staining).

Portal Hypertension

Increased pressure within the portal vein (i.e., portal hypertension) is caused by increased resistance to blood flow through the portal venous system and is most often the result of cirrhosis. Portal vein thrombosis, hepatic vein obstruction, and, in some parts of the world, hepatic schistosomiasis are other possible causes.

Esophageal varices are a potentially dangerous complication of portal hypertension, as they can rupture and result in massive GI bleeding. Esophageal varices form when increased pressure in the portal venous system causes a compensatory dilation of portal-systemic collaterals that are very small in diameter under normal circumstances. Splenomegaly, ascites, and spontaneous bacterial peritonitis are additional complications of portal hypertension.

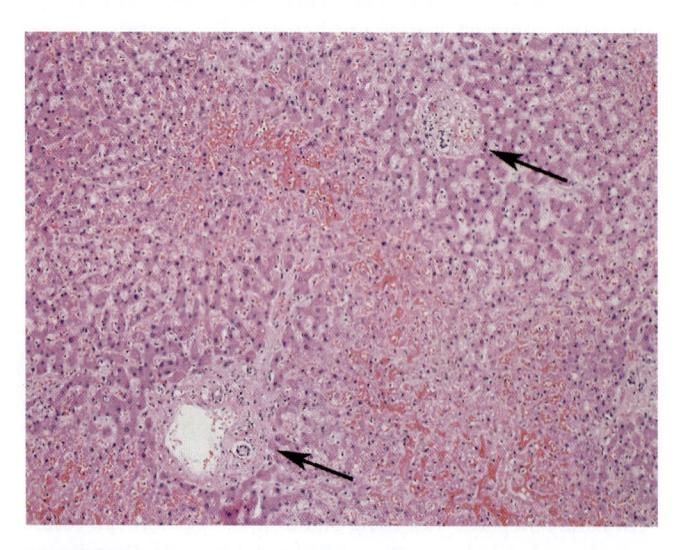

FIGURE 10-6 Centrilobular congestion. Note the accumulation of red blood cells within sinusoids in the centrilobular zone between two portal tracts (arrows mark portal tracts).

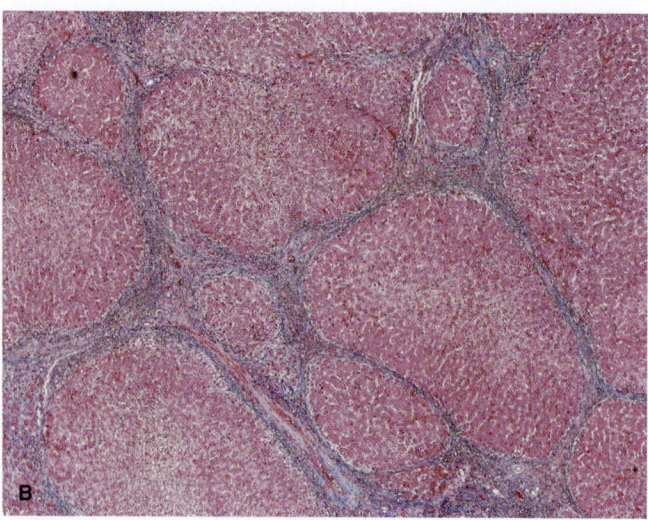

Infectious Disorders (Hepatitis)

Viral hepatitis is far and away the most common infectious cause of hepatitis and will be the focus of the following discussion. Bacterial and fungal infections of the liver are usually part of a broader systemic infection. A number of parasitic infections can occur in the liver and these are relatively rare in developed parts of the world.

Viral Hepatitis

Many viruses can show tropism for the liver. For example, yellow fever, a mosquito-borne infection, can cause severe hepatitis with a characteristic pattern of zone 2 hepatocyte necrosis. Herpes simplex virus can cause fulminant liver failure. Of course, any discussion of viral infections of the liver is going to center around the specific viral hepatitides.

Hepatitis A

Hepatitis A virus (HAV) is an RNA virus that usually results in an asymptomatic infection or an acute self-limited hepatitis. Fulminant liver failure occurs in a very small percentage of cases. HAV does not cause chronic hepatitis. Infection usually occurs through a fecal–oral route and is most common in environments with poor sanitation and contaminated food and water supplies. Infection results in the formation of antibodies. IgM antibodies develop during the acute phase of the illness and fall during recovery, while IgG antibodies develop during the recovery phase and remain present throughout life, conferring resistance to reinfection. The presence of serum anti-HAV IgM antibodies identifies HAV as the cause of acute hepatitis. A vaccine for HAV is available.

Pathology of Acute Viral Hepatitis: The most consistent findings seen in acute viral hepatitis are inflammatory infiltrates and hepatocellular injury. Cholestasis, bile duct injury, and endothelial injury are sometimes encountered.

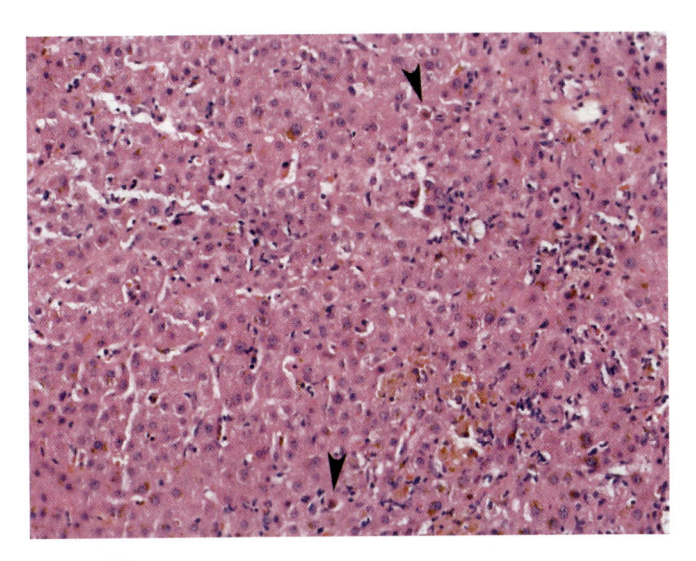

FIGURE 10-7 Acute viral hepatitis. Acute viral hepatitis is most commonly characterized by lymphocyte predominant inflammatory infiltrates and foci of hepatocyte injury and death. The arrowheads mark two apoptotic hepatocytes.

Early hepatocyte injury is in the form of cellular swelling and is thought to be reversible. Irreversible injury is recognized as hepatocyte apoptosis or hepatocyte dropout with replacement by inflammatory cells. The inflammatory infiltrates of acute viral hepatitis are predominantly lymphocytic. The inflammation and hepatocyte injury is found predominantly in zone 3; however, this is not always the case. There is usually less portal inflammation than is seen in chronic hepatitis (Figure 10-7).

Hepatitis B

Hepatitis B virus (HBV) is a DNA virus that can cause a spectrum of disease. Infection usually occurs via sexual transmission, sharing of contaminated needles, and vertical transmission from mother to child. Most infections in adults result in an asymptomatic infection or an acute self-limited hepatitis, similar to HAV. Approximately 5–10% of infections result in chronic hepatitis that can progress to cirrhosis and is a major risk factor for the development of hepatocellular carcinoma (HCC). A very small percentage of infections can result in fulminant liver failure. A higher percentage of children infected with HBV develop chronic hepatitis, including the majority of vertical transmission cases. The antigens and antibodies associated with HBV infection are summarized in Table 10-1. A vaccine for HBV is available.

Hepatitis C

Hepatitis C virus (HCV) is an RNA virus that causes chronic hepatitis in the large majority of infections. Many infections are asymptomatic. This can result in an extended period of indolent liver injury and unrecognized infectivity. Most infections are acquired through percutaneous exposure to infected blood. Vertical transmission and sexual transmission are much less common. Chronic HCV infection is the most common reason for liver transplantation and is a major risk factor for the development of HCC. Anti-HCV antibodies indicate exposure to HCV. A vaccine for HCV is not yet available.

Pathology of Chronic Viral Hepatitis: Classic findings in chronic viral hepatitis include portal inflammation, interface hepatitis (a.k.a. piecemeal necrosis), lobular necrosis, and varying degrees of hepatic fibrosis. The portal infiltrates are predominantly lymphocytic with lesser numbers of plasma cells, neutrophils, and eosinophils. The infiltrates can be restricted to the portal tracts or they can reach across the limiting plate and be associated with periportal hepatocyte necrosis (i.e., interface hepatitis). The earliest stage of fibrosis

TABLE 10-1 Antigens and antibodies associated with HBV infection

Antigen/Antibody	Definition	Application
Hepatitis B surface antigen (HBsAg)	Viral surface protein	• Present in blood during acute and chronic infections • Presence in blood is earliest indicator of HBV infection • Disappears with recovery
Hepatitis B surface antibody (anti-HBs)	Antibody produced in response to HBsAg	• Presence indicates recovery from infection or successful vaccination • Presence indicates immunity
Hepatitis B core antigen (HBcAg)	Viral core protein	• Present within hepatocytes only, not detectable in blood
Hepatitis B core antibody (anti-HBc)	Antibody produced in response to HBcAg	• Anti-HBc IgM is the first antibody produced after infection • Marker of prior infection (persists in resolved and chronic cases)
Hepatitis B e-antigen (HBeAg)	Protein produced and released by actively replicating HBV	• Marker of infectivity or treatment effectiveness

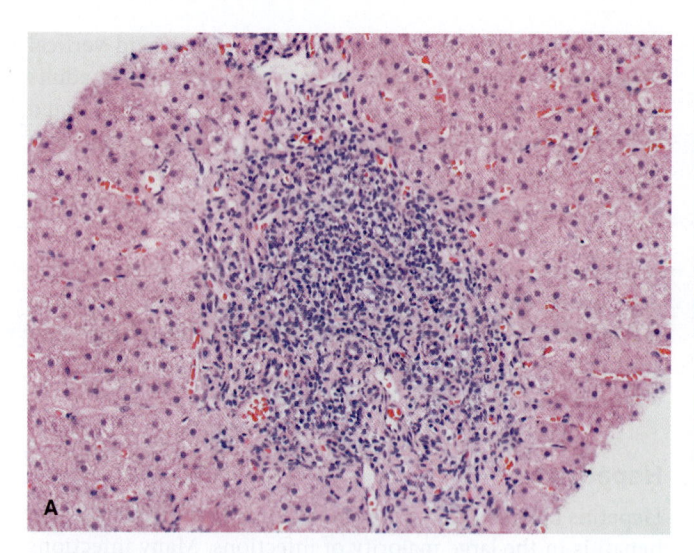

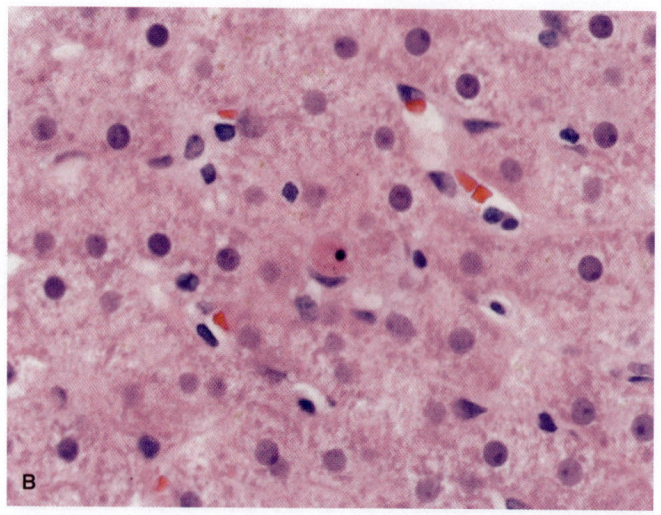

FIGURE 10-8 Chronic hepatitis C infection. **(A)** This expansive portal chronic inflammatory infiltrate, while not specific, is characteristic of hepatitis C infection. **(B)** Apoptotic hepatocytes (center) can be seen in several of the hepatitides, including viral hepatitis.

is portal fibrous expansion. With progression, fibrous bands extend from the portal tracts into the surrounding lobular parenchyma. When these bands connect with adjacent portal tracts, bridging fibrosis is present. Continued inflammation and injury can ultimately lead to cirrhosis **(Figure 10-8)**.

Chronic HCV infection is frequently associated with steatosis (i.e., fatty change of the liver). Expansive portal infiltrates with germinal center formation are more frequently seen in chronic HCV.

Hepatitis D and E

Hepatitis D is a defective RNA virus that requires the presence of HBsAg for propagation. Coinfection with HBV can result in a fulminant hepatitis or more severe chronic hepatitis.

Hepatitis E is an enteric RNA virus that is transmitted through a fecal–oral route and causes epidemics of acute self-limited hepatitis, usually in underdeveloped areas. Interestingly, mortality rates are higher in pregnant woman. Hepatitis E does not cause chronic hepatitis and there is no vaccine currently available.

Hepatitis (Noninfectious)

The most common causes of noninfectious hepatitis include fatty liver disease, AIH, and drug/toxin-induced liver injury.

> **IN TRANSLATION**
>
> HBV quantitative DNA testing can detect how much viral DNA is present in serum and is a useful gauge of infectivity, risk for progressive disease, and response to treatment. Similar testing can be performed to quantitate HCV.
>
> HBV and HCV genotype testing can help predict prognosis, including response to antiviral drugs.

Fatty Liver Disease

Fatty liver disease is an accumulation of excess lipids within hepatocytes that can lead to decreased liver function and, in some cases, cirrhosis. Fatty liver disease is broadly divided into two categories: alcoholic liver disease (ALD) and nonalcoholic fatty liver disease (NAFLD).

Alcoholic Liver Disease

The liver is the body's primary site of ethanol metabolism and increased ethanol consumption, whether in the form of binge drinking or chronic elevated intake, can lead to ALD. At the milder end of the spectrum, ethanol can cause a derangement in the liver's metabolism of dietary lipids, resulting in fat accumulation within the liver (i.e., steatosis). Ethanol-induced steatosis can disappear with ethanol cessation.

Alcoholic steatohepatitis is a more severe form of ALD, characterized by steatosis, hepatocyte swelling, lobular acute inflammation, and lobular fibrosis. These changes are found predominantly within zone 3. Hepatocyte swelling can be reversible or irreversible. Irreversible swelling is recognized histologically as ballooning degeneration. Hepatocytes that have undergone ballooning degeneration are enlarged and rounded, have wispy cytoplasm, and show nuclear pyknosis. Mallory's hyaline, an aggregate of cytokeratin filaments, can occasionally be found within the cytoplasm of injured hepatocytes **(Figure 10-9)**.

With chronic ethanol abuse, the ongoing liver injury, inflammation, fibrosis, and regeneration can ultimately lead to cirrhosis. Earlier stages of fibrosis show a characteristic perisinusoidal and pericellular pattern of fibrosis.

Nonalcoholic Fatty Liver Disease and Nonalcoholic Steatohepatitis

The patterns of injury in NAFLD are similar to those seen in ALD. The exact pathogenesis of NAFLD is uncertain; however,

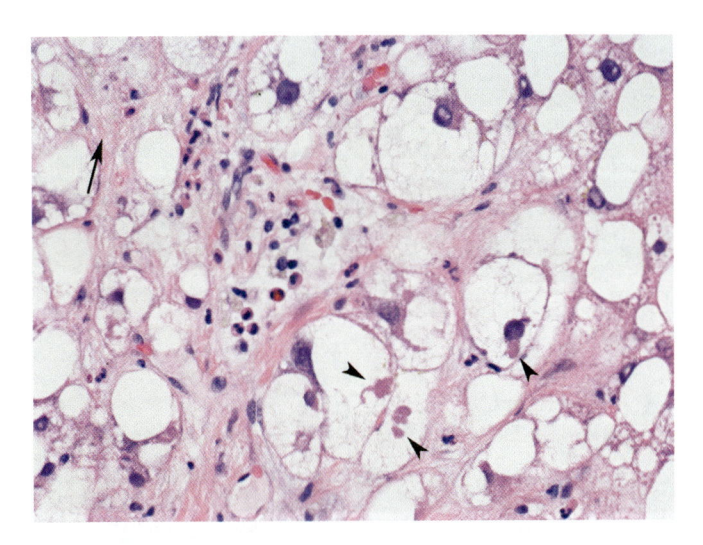

FIGURE 10-9 **Alcoholic steatohepatitis.** In this example of alcoholic steatohepatitis, note the conspicuous ballooning degeneration of hepatocytes, Mallory hyaline (arrowheads), and perisinusoidal fibrosis (arrow).

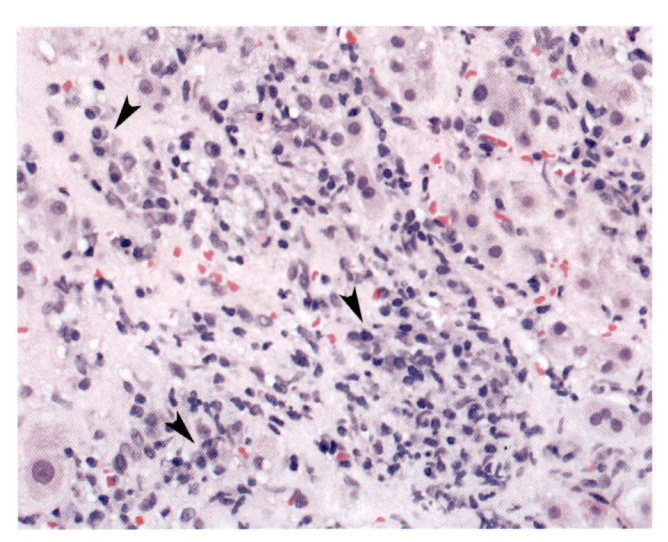

FIGURE 10-11 **Autoimmune hepatitis.** This high-magnification view of AIH shows a prominent inflammatory infiltrate with a conspicuous plasma cell component (arrowheads).

there are several well-recognized risk factors. Some risk factors include type 2 diabetes, hypertension, abnormal cholesterol levels, and obesity. Some drugs, such as methotrexate, can also cause NAFLD.

When NAFLD is associated with inflammation, hepatocyte injury, and fibrosis, it is referred to as NASH. Pathologically, NASH is very similar to alcoholic steatohepatitis except that NASH is often associated with more of a lymphocytic inflammatory infiltrate **(Figure 10-10)**.

The number of cases of NAFLD is increasing due to increased detection and a true increase in incidence, paralleling increases in obesity and type 2 diabetes. Many cases of "cryptogenic cirrhosis" are now believed to represent end-stage NAFLD.

Autoimmune Hepatitis

AIH is a form of chronic hepatitis where the immune system attacks the liver. It is associated with serum autoantibodies and an elevated total serum IgG. Most cases occur in young women; however, men and children can be affected. Most cases present as a chronic hepatitis, and progression to cirrhosis is common. Other cases present as an acute hepatitis or fulminant hepatitis. The histologic findings are variable and often show a severely active chronic hepatitis with prominent hepatocyte necrosis. Plasma cells are usually a conspicuous component of the inflammatory infiltrates **(Figure 10-11)**. AIH is treated with a combination of corticosteroids and immunosuppressants.

Drug- and Toxin-Induced Liver Injury

The number of drugs and toxins capable of causing liver injury and the spectrum of injury patterns caused by these chemicals are far too large to cover in great detail. It helps to think of these reactions as being either predictable (i.e., a specific chemical produces an expected injury pattern if given at a sufficient dose) or idiosyncratic (i.e., a chemical produces an unexpected reaction, often in a person with metabolic pathway polymorphisms). A classic example of a predictable liver injury is acetaminophen toxicity. At supratherapeutic doses, acetaminophen causes a distinctive pattern of centrilobular necrosis without significant inflammation **(Figure 10-12)**. With even greater doses, the entire lobule can be injured and death can occur due to fulminant liver failure.

Biliary Tract Disease

Bilirubin Metabolism and Jaundice

The liver is responsible for the transfer of bilirubin from blood to bile. Albumin-bound bilirubin is taken up from the hepatic

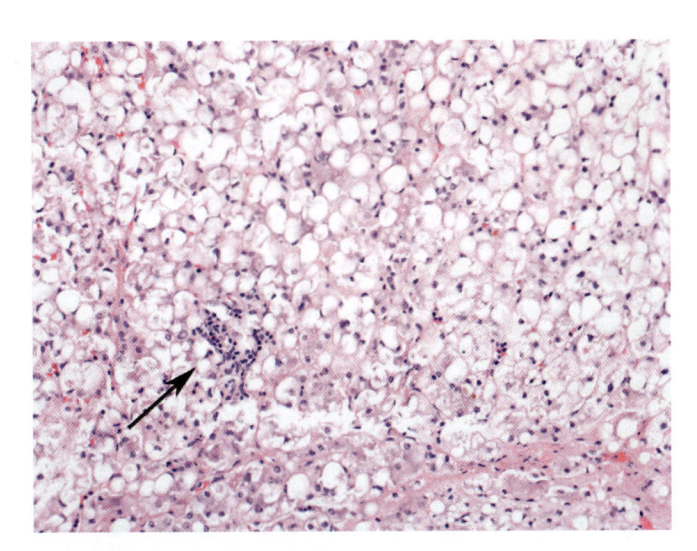

FIGURE 10-10 **Nonalcoholic steatohepatitis.** This is an example of NASH with a prominent steatosis component. The arrow marks a lobular lymphocytic infiltrate.

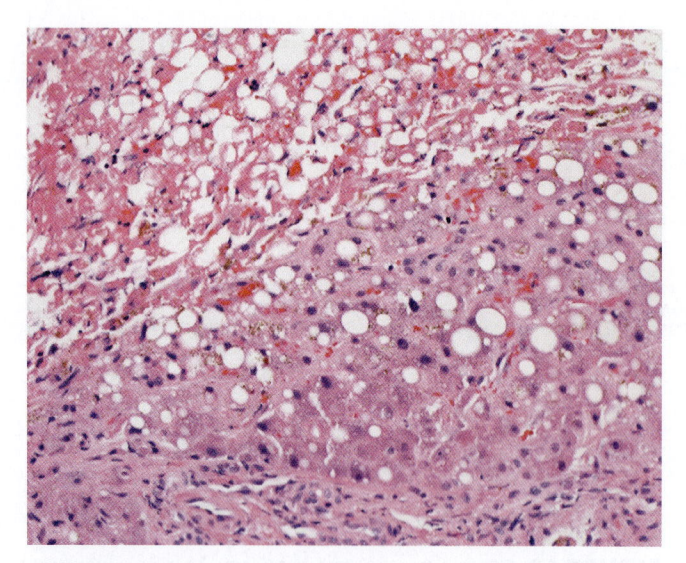

FIGURE 10-12 Acetaminophen toxicity. In this example of acetaminophen toxicity, the zone 1 and some of the zone 2 hepatocytes are viable (portal tract at bottom of image), whereas the centrilobular hepatocytes are necrotic (top of image). Note the paucity of inflammatory cells.

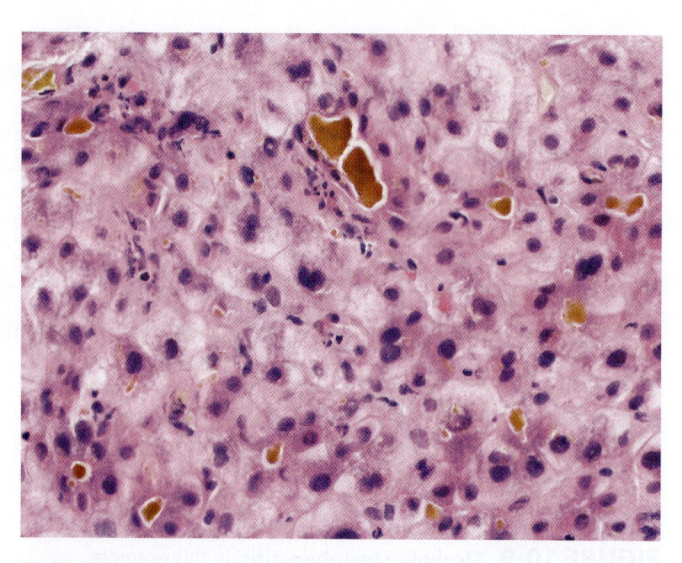

FIGURE 10-13 Cholestasis. Cholestasis is present in the form of plugs within bile canaliculi.

sinusoids by hepatocytes where it is conjugated into a water-soluble form and excreted into the bile canaliculi where it becomes part of bile.

Hyperbilirubinemia is the term for an elevated bilirubin level in the blood. With increasing bilirubin levels, the skin and sclerae become yellow. This finding is called jaundice or icterus. Defects at each step of bilirubin metabolism (e.g., bilirubin overproduction, decreased hepatic uptake of bilirubin, decreased bilirubin conjugation, and decreased excretion of conjugated bilirubin into bile) can result in hyperbilirubinemia and jaundice.

Cholestasis is a condition where the flow of bile from the liver is blocked, either functionally or mechanically. There are a variety of causes and these can occur within the liver (i.e., intrahepatic) or outside of the liver (i.e., extrahepatic). Cholestasis can be observed microscopically in the form of bile plugs within bile canaliculi and ducts (Figure 10-13). Bile pigment can sometimes be seen within hepatocytes. The accumulation of bile acids within hepatocytes is toxic to these cells.

Primary Sclerosing Cholangitis

Primary sclerosing cholangitis (PSC) is a chronic cholestatic disease of likely autoimmune etiology. PSC is more common in men and there is an apparent association with ulcerative colitis. The pathologic hallmark of PSC is periductal inflammation and fibrosis of intrahepatic and extrahepatic bile ducts with progressive obliteration of ducts (Figure 10-14). Over time, the disease can progress to cirrhosis. PSC has a relatively poor prognosis, often requiring transplantation, and is associated with an increased risk of cholangiocarcinoma.

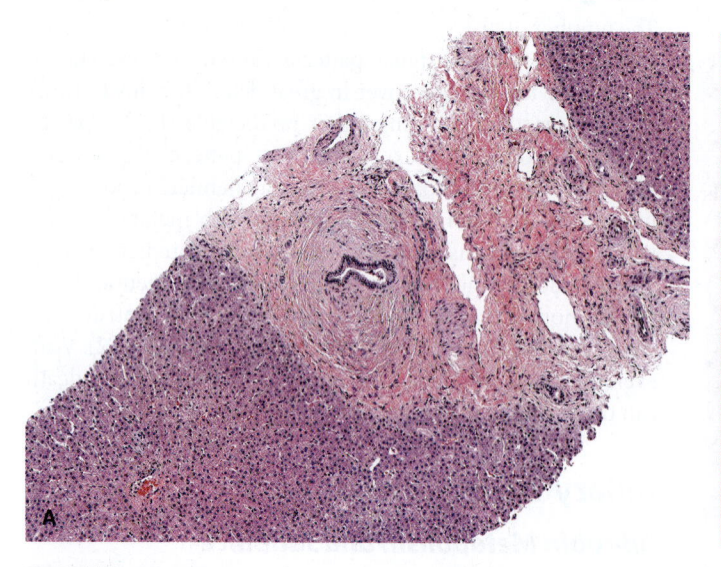

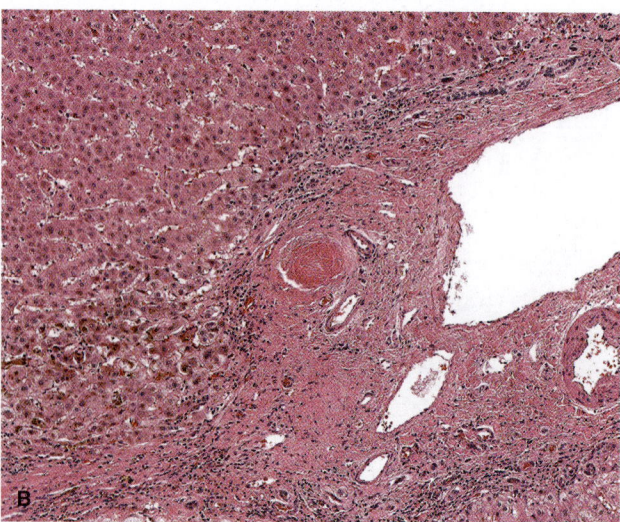

FIGURE 10-14 Primary sclerosing cholangitis. Periductal fibrosis **(A)** and fibro-obliterative bile duct scarring **(B)** are characteristic findings in PSC.

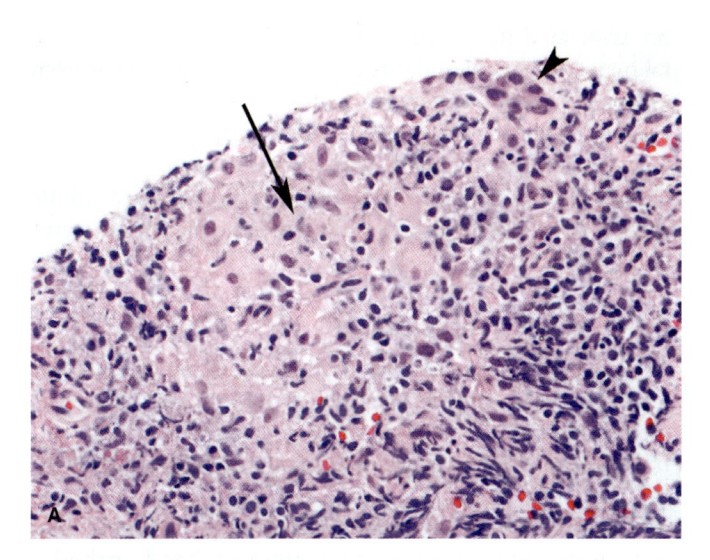

FIGURE 10-15 Primary biliary cirrhosis. **(A)** In this biopsy of a patient with PBC, note the poorly formed granuloma (arrow) adjacent to a bile duct (arrowhead). **(B)** Elsewhere, there are increased numbers of lymphocytes (arrowheads) within bile duct epithelium.

Primary Biliary Cirrhosis

Primary biliary cirrhosis (PBC) is another chronic cholestatic disease of likely autoimmune etiology. It is associated with an elevated serum IgM and the vast majority of patients have circulating antimitochondrial antibodies (AMA). AMA-negative PBC (a.k.a. autoimmune cholangitis) occurs in a small percentage of cases. There is a conspicuous female predominance. Fatigue and pruritus are common early symptoms. Pathologically, there is patchy lymphocyte-mediated destruction of small-to-medium-sized intrahepatic bile ducts that is often associated with granuloma formation (Figure 10-15). The decreased ability of the liver to secrete bile ultimately leads to hepatocyte injury and fibrosis. Progression to cirrhosis can occur, but does not do so uniformly. Transplantation is reasonably successful at treating late-stage PBC.

Metabolic Disorders

There are a variety of metabolic disorders that can affect the liver. A few classic examples are discussed below. Some metabolic disorders can lead to cirrhosis.

Hemochromatosis

Hereditary hemochromatosis (HH) is an autosomal recessive disorder of the HFE gene that results in increased intestinal absorption of iron with excessive accumulation of iron in the body. The classic signs of HH are cirrhosis, diabetes, cardiac disease, and skin pigmentation resulting from iron accumulation within the liver, pancreas, heart, and skin, respectively. Microscopic examination of the liver shows prominent iron accumulation within hepatocytes and sometimes bile ducts, which can be confirmed with a special stain for iron (Figure 10-16). If unrecognized, HH can lead to cirrhosis following an indolent clinical course. In cirrhosis resulting from HH, there is a high risk of developing HCC. The mainstay of treatment is the removal of iron from the body by repeat phlebotomy.

Secondary hemochromatosis is a form of iron overload that is not associated with a genetic mutation. It usually occurs in the setting of hematologic disorders and chronic blood transfusions.

> **IN TRANSLATION**
>
> As noted in the case of HH at the beginning of the chapter, molecular testing can be performed to look for mutations in the HFE gene. HH most commonly results from a homozygous mutation (C282Y) of the HFE gene.

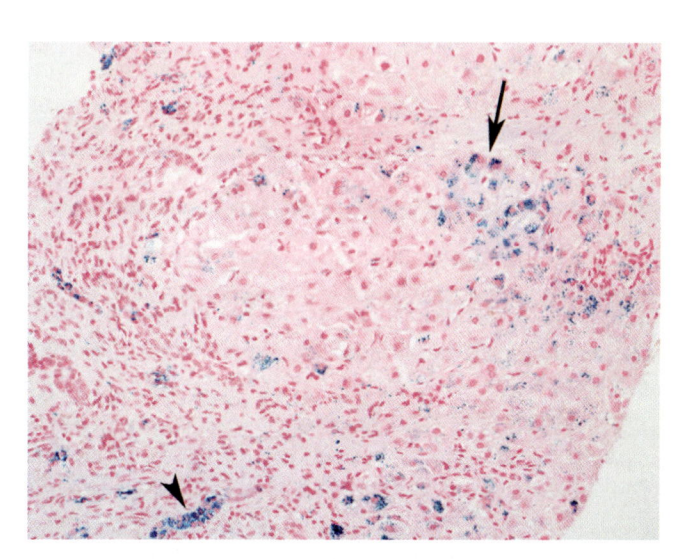

FIGURE 10-16 Hemochromatosis. This liver biopsy in a patient with hemochromatosis-induced cirrhosis shows increased iron accumulation within hepatocytes (arrow) and bile duct epithelium (arrowhead). Blue staining indicates the presence of iron in this iron stain.

Wilson Disease

Wilson disease is a rare autosomal recessive disorder of copper metabolism, resulting in copper accumulation within the liver and other organs. It typically results in a chronic hepatitis that can progress to cirrhosis, sometimes during childhood. Wilson disease is not believed to be associated with a substantial risk of HCC. Copper chelation therapy halts the progression of disease and can reverse copper deposits that are already present.

Alpha 1-Antitrypsin Deficiency

Alpha 1-antitrypsin (A1AT) deficiency, a disorder resulting from codominant inheritance of mutations of the *SERPINA1* gene, can involve the lungs and liver, causing emphysema and liver injury, respectively. A1AT is a protease inhibitor that has a protective effect in the lungs and liver. The existence of numerous gene isoforms allows for a broad spectrum of disease severity, ranging from no appreciable dysfunction to fatal neonatal hepatitis. The hallmark pathologic finding is that of eosinophilic periodic acid-Schiff (PAS)-positive cytoplasmic globules within hepatocytes (Figure 10-17). This disease often leads to cirrhosis and comes with a high risk of HCC.

Masses of the Liver

The liver is the site of several important mimickers of neoplasia, benign neoplasms, and malignant neoplasms.

Mimickers of Neoplasia

Nodular regenerative hyperplasia, focal nodular hyperplasia (FNH), bile duct hamartomas, and simple cysts are the most commonly encountered mimickers of neoplasia in the liver.

Nodular Regenerative Hyperplasia

Nodular regenerative hyperplasia is a non-neoplastic lesion characterized by hyperplastic liver nodules with little or no associated fibrosis. In some cases, it can result in portal hypertension. Nodular regenerative hyperplasia has been associated with a variety of medical conditions and medications, including oral contraceptive pills. Microscopically, vague nodules of hepatocytes compress adjacent parenchyma. The hepatic plates within the nodules are mildly thickened (2–3 cells thick) and there is no significant cytologic atypia.

Focal Nodular Hyperplasia

FNH is a non-neoplastic lesion that can occur in males or females of any age and is believed to form at sites of arterial malformation. There is no known association with oral contraceptive use. These lesions can become quite large (upwards of 15 cm in diameter). Grossly, FNH often has a characteristic central fibrous scar. Fibrous bands separate nodules of hepatocytes and impart an appearance of "focal cirrhosis." Microscopically, bands of chronically inflamed fibrous tissue containing thick-walled arteries and a proliferation of bile duct-like structures surround nodules of hepatocytes. Normal portal tracts are absent (Figure 10-18).

Benign Neoplasms of the Liver

A handful of benign neoplasms can occur in the liver. The two most commonly encountered are hemangiomas and hepatocellular adenomas.

Hemangioma

Hemangiomas are the most common benign tumors of the liver. These tumors are often found incidentally at the time of surgery, organ harvesting, or autopsy. On occasion, hemangiomas can grow to a large size, but spontaneous rupture is relatively uncommon. Grossly, hemangiomas are well-demarcated dark red tumors that clearly stand out against the background

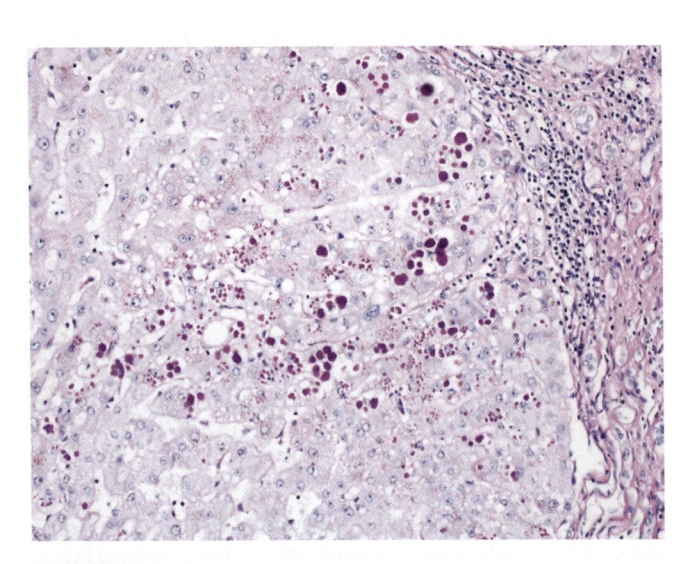

FIGURE 10-17 Alpha 1-antitrypsin deficiency. Intracytoplasmic globular inclusions are highlighted by a PAS stain.

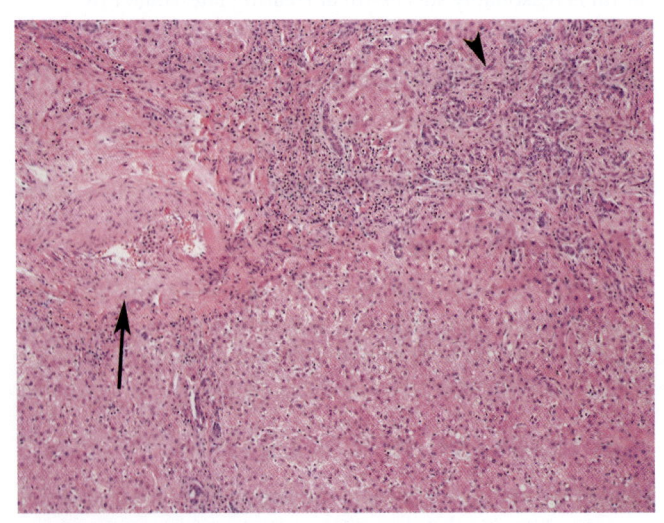

FIGURE 10-18 Focal nodular hyperplasia. In this example of FNH, a band of fibrous tissue containing a thick-walled artery (arrow) and a proliferation of bile duct structures (arrowhead) surrounds a nodule of hepatocytes (bottom right).

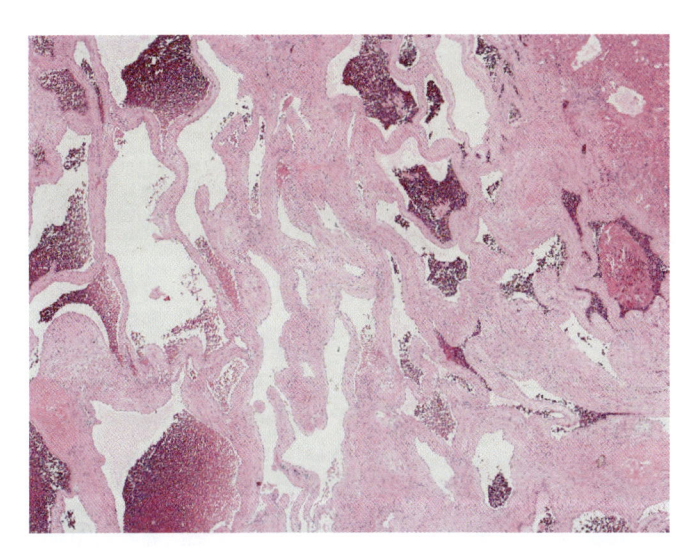

FIGURE 10-19 **Hemangioma.** In this example of a cavernous hemangioma, blood-filled spaces lined by flattened endothelial cells are supported by a fibrous stroma. Adjacent liver tissue is present in the upper right corner of the image.

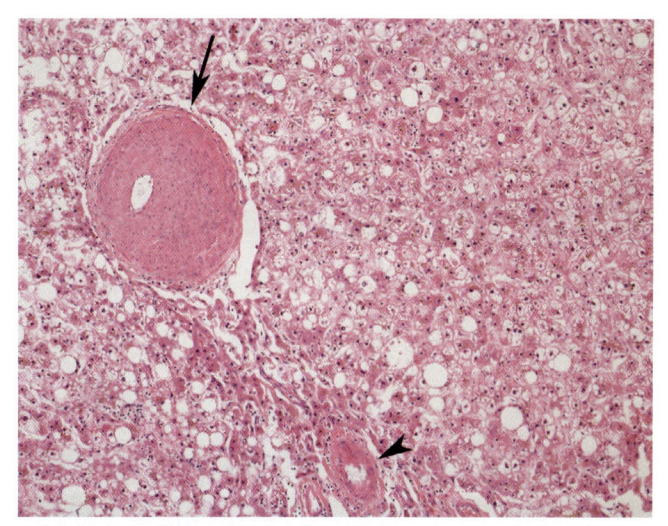

FIGURE 10-20 **Hepatocellular adenoma.** In this example of a hepatocellular adenoma, note the thick-walled blood vessel (arrow) and smaller arterial branch without associated portal tract structures (arrowhead). A subset of adenomas can show changes of steatohepatitis, like those seen in this example.

liver parenchyma. Microscopically, most hemangiomas are cavernous hemangiomas composed of endothelial-lined spaces supported by a fibrous stroma. Red blood cells are typically present within the spaces helping to separate these lesions from lymphangiomas (Figure 10-19). Severe sclerosis can sometimes occur making it difficult to recognize the prior existence of vascular spaces.

Hepatocellular Adenoma

Hepatocellular adenomas (hepatic adenomas or liver cell adenomas) are benign neoplasms of hepatocytes. They occur most commonly in women of childbearing age and are often associated with oral contraceptive use. When hepatocellular adenomas occur in men, they are often associated with anabolic steroid usage. These tumors can spontaneously rupture and hemorrhage into the abdominal cavity, resulting in a surgical emergency.

Hepatocellular adenomas are unencapsulated neoplasms that are well demarcated from the surrounding hepatic parenchyma. They are composed of a proliferation of bland hepatocytes with no more than rare mitotic activity. The neoplastic hepatocytes are arranged in trabeculae, which may be mildly thickened (e.g., 2–3 cells thick). Reticulin staining may be normal or mildly reduced; however, a pronounced loss of reticulin staining is uncommon and should raise concern for a well-differentiated HCC. Bile accumulation, steatosis, and features of steatohepatitis are not uncommon. Prominent arteries are present within the tumor and bile ducts and intact portal tracts are absent (Figure 10-20). The absence of bile ducts and portal tracts distinguishes these tumors from nodular regenerative hyperplasia and FNH. Hepatocellular adenomas associated with anabolic steroid use can show areas of blood-filled spaces called peliosis.

Malignant Neoplasms of the Liver

The two most common primary malignancies of the liver are HCC and cholangiocarcinoma. Hepatoblastoma is a rare but important malignancy in young children. Metastatic cancer involving the liver is common.

Hepatocellular Carcinoma

HCC ranks as one of the most common malignancies worldwide (high incidence in portions of Africa and Asia) and most commonly arises in cirrhotic livers of older people; however, cirrhosis is not always present. Alpha-fetoprotein levels are usually elevated in HCC and can be used to monitor for disease recurrence.

People with chronic HBV infection have a high risk of developing HCC. The increasing prevalence of HBV vaccination is expected to have a positive impact on the worldwide incidence of HCC. Coinfection with hepatitis B and C results in an even greater risk of HCC than infection with either virus alone. Alcoholic cirrhosis, hemochromatosis, A1AT deficiency, and aflatoxin exposure are also well-established risk factors for HCC. HCC may occur in a small percentage of people with NASH; however, this association is not entirely clear.

HCC is believed to undergo a multistep sequence of carcinogenesis; however, the exact sequence of histologic and molecular changes is not entirely understood. Precursor lesions (e.g., dysplastic nodules) are sometimes encountered.

Grossly, HCC can appear as a tan or green mass. The latter occurs if there is bile present. HCC has a tendency to invade portal or hepatic vein branches. Intravenous extension into the inferior vena cava is occasionally seen. The microscopic appearance can be quite variable. Some tumors are difficult to distinguish from benign hepatocyte proliferations. Others are so poorly differentiated that it is difficult to recognize a

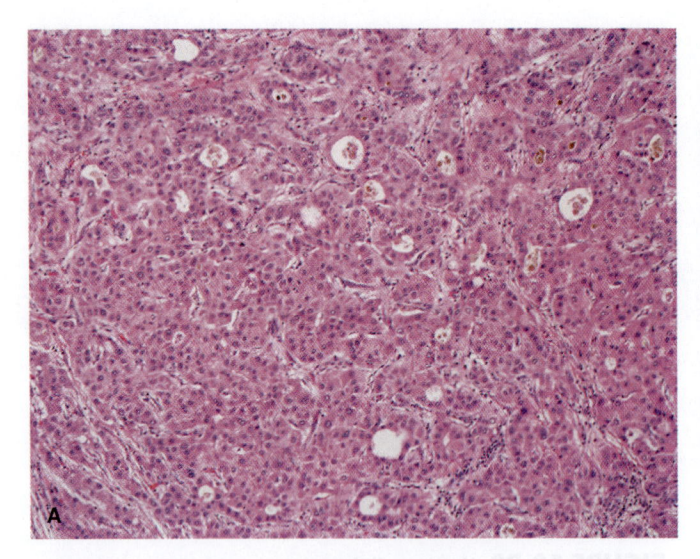

FIGURE 10-21 **Hepatocellular carcinoma. (A)** This example of HCC is notable for abnormal trabeculae of neoplastic hepatocytes, foci of pseudogland formation, and focal bile accumulation. **(B)** A higher magnification view shows moderate nuclear pleomorphism and increased mitotic activity (arrow).

hepatocyte origin. Trabecular and pseudoglandular growth patterns are most common. The trabecular pattern consists of thickened plates, or trabeculae, of hepatocytes that are often greater than 3 cells thick **(Figure 10-21)**. There is usually a decrease in reticulin staining and there are abnormal vascular channels between the trabeculae that are lined by endothelial cells that express CD34.

If complete tumor resection or ablation is not possible, HCC has a poor prognosis, often with survival times shorter than 1 year. This is due, in part, to the frequent presence of coexisting cirrhosis. These tumors tend to respond poorly to chemotherapy and radiation therapy. Metastases can occur and are most commonly seen in the portal lymph nodes and lungs.

Fibrolamellar Variant of HCC

The fibrolamellar variant of HCC is most commonly seen in the noncirrhotic livers of older children and young adults. These tumors have a characteristic microscopic appearance with trabeculae of tumor cells separated by parallel fibrous bands. The tumor cells have abundant eosinophilic cytoplasm and enlarged nuclei with prominent nucleoli **(Figure 10-22)**. These tumors have a better prognosis due to a greater likelihood of complete resection and an absence of cirrhosis.

> **QUICK REVIEW**
> **Hepatocellular Carcinoma**
> - Malignant neoplasm of hepatocytes that is most commonly seen in the setting of cirrhosis following years of liver inflammation and injury.
> - Variable histologic appearance; trabecular and pseudoglandular patterns are most common.
> - Very poor prognosis for usual type HCC if complete resection is not possible.

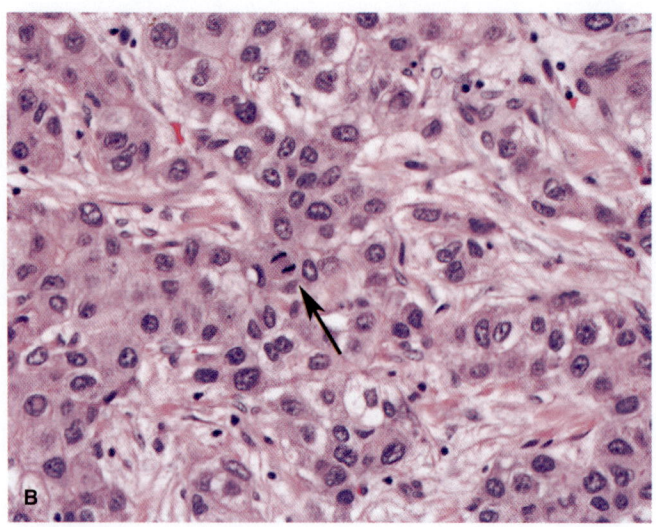

Cholangiocarcinoma

Carcinoma arising from intrahepatic bile ducts is called cholangiocarcinoma. When it occurs at the bifurcation of the common hepatic duct it is referred to as a Klatskin tumor. Cholangiocarcinoma usually occurs in older people and most cases arise in the setting of PSC, congenital bile duct cysts, or liver fluke (Clonorchis sinensis) infection. Cholangiocarcinoma is not typically associated with cirrhosis.

There are two main growth patterns recognized: mass forming type and periductal infiltrating type. The mass forming type shows radial growth with invasion into adjacent hepatic parenchyma. The periductal infiltrating type spreads longitudinally along intrahepatic bile ducts. Some tumors show a combination of both subtypes. The periductal infiltrating type

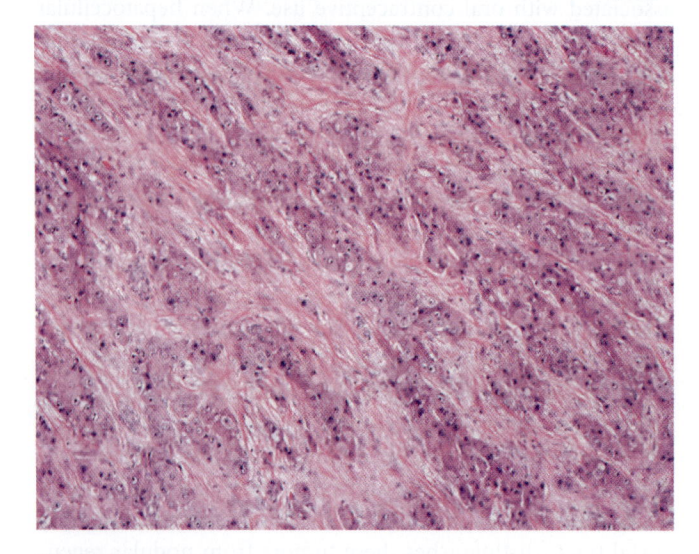

FIGURE 10-22 **Fibrolamellar variant of HCC.** This distinctive variant of HCC is characterized by trabeculae of tumor cells separated by parallel bands of fibrous tissue. The tumor cells have abundant granular cytoplasm and prominent nucleoli.

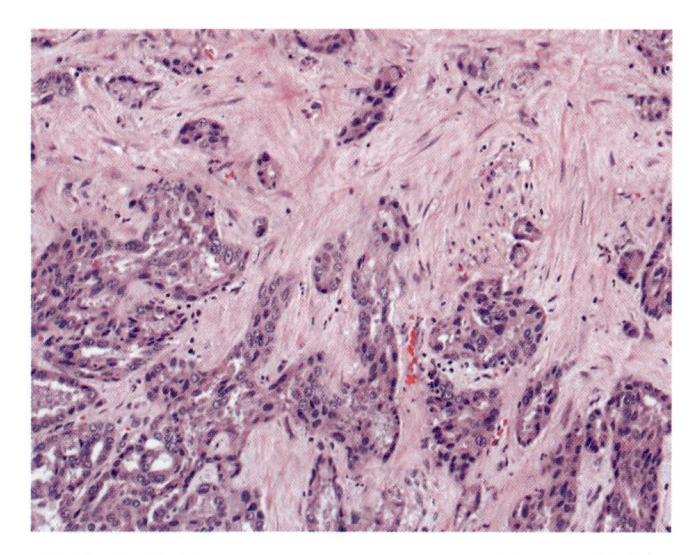

FIGURE 10-23 Cholangiocarcinoma. Cholangiocarcinoma is a gland forming malignancy of bile ducts. In this example, irregular infiltrating glands have elicited a prominent fibrotic stromal reaction.

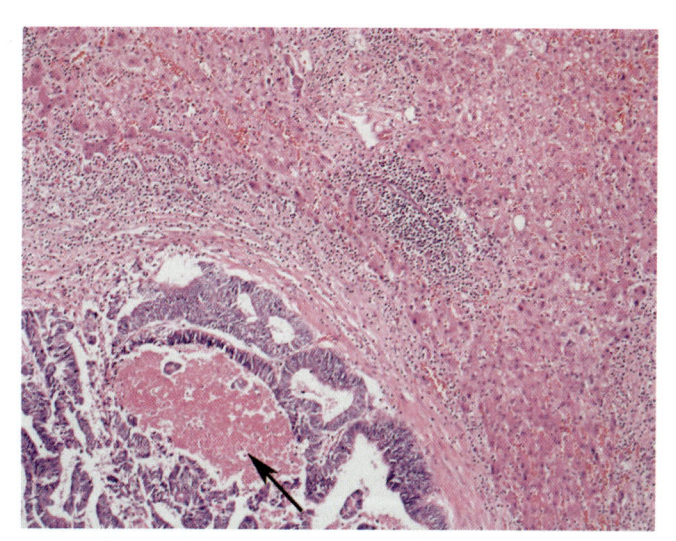

FIGURE 10-24 Metastatic colon cancer. "Dirty necrosis" (arrow) is typical of colorectal cancer. There are often nonspecific inflammatory changes adjacent to focal lesions in the liver.

is associated with a worse prognosis, as there is a lower likelihood of complete resection. Microscopically, these are gland-forming neoplasms, although gland formation may not be discernible in poorly differentiated tumors. Some tumors may be difficult to differentiate from the pseudoglandular pattern of HCC (Figure 10-23). The clinical history and special stains usually allow this distinction to be made. Similarly to HCC, these tumors often portend a poor prognosis.

Combined Hepatocellular–Cholangiocarcinoma

Some tumors can show distinctive areas of HCC and cholangiocarcinoma, so called combined hepatocellular–cholangiocarcinoma. These tumors are almost always the result of divergent differentiation within a single tumor.

Hepatoblastoma

Hepatoblastomas are pediatric tumors that can be seen at birth or within the first few years of life. Abdominal distension and failure to thrive are common presenting signs and alpha-fetoprotein is almost always elevated. The prognosis depends on the resectability and histologic subtype with the anaplastic variant having the worst prognosis.

Metastatic Cancer

Overall, metastases are the most common malignant tumors found in the liver. Colorectal adenocarcinoma is the most common metastasis to the liver and metastatic breast cancer, lung cancer, pancreatic cancer, and melanoma are also common (Figure 10-24). With sufficient tumor burden, portal hypertension and jaundice can occur.

Liver Transplantation

Allogeneic liver transplantation can be used in many people to treat advanced-stage liver disease. Liver allografts are suscepti-

ble to injury caused by the recipient's immune system. Typical findings of acute allograft rejection include mixed inflammatory infiltrates of the portal tracts, including increased numbers of eosinophils, lymphocytic infiltration and damage of interlobular (portal tract) bile ducts, and lymphocytic infiltration of portal vein branches and terminal hepatic venules with associated endothelial injury.

Chronic allograft rejection is characterized by a loss of bile ducts (vanishing bile duct syndrome) and a form of vascular occlusion known as obliterative endarteritis.

Acute allograft rejection is potentially reversible, while the changes of chronic allograft rejection are considered irreversible.

GALLBLADDER AND EXTRAHEPATIC BILIARY TRACT

Normal Anatomy and Histology of the Gallbladder and Extrahepatic Biliary Tract

The gallbladder is a thin-walled saccular organ attached to the inferior surface of the liver at the gallbladder fossa. Its function is to store and concentrate bile. Following stimulation by a meal, bile exits the gallbladder through the cystic duct. The cystic duct merges with the common hepatic duct to form the common bile duct, which opens into the duodenum along with the main pancreatic duct at the ampulla of Vater. While this is the most common duct configuration, some variation exists (Figure 10-25).

The wall of the gallbladder is composed of mucosa, muscularis propria, and adventitia. The portion of the gallbladder not adherent to the liver is covered by peritoneum (Figure 10-26).

CASE 10-2

The patient is a 44-year-old woman who presented to the emergency department with intermittent epigastric and right upper quadrant pain that was sometimes worsened following meals. Given the patient's demographics and her symptoms, an abdominal ultrasound was performed that showed objects in the gallbladder consistent with gallstones. A laparoscopic cholecystectomy was performed. Pathologic examination of the gallbladder showed several gallstones and microscopic changes consistent with chronic cholecystitis (see section "Cholecystitis" and Figure 10-28).

Principal Diseases of the Gallbladder and Extrahepatic Biliary Tract

Cholelithiasis and cholecystitis are the most commonly encountered diseases of the gallbladder. Congenital anomalies (e.g., choledochal cyst) can occur and gallbladder carcinoma, sometimes discovered incidentally, has an overall dismal prognosis.

Cholelithiasis

The presence of stones within the gallbladder is called cholelithiasis. Gallstones can be separated into two large categories: cholesterol stones and pigment stones. Cholelithiasis can be asymptomatic or it can result in biliary colic, which is an episodic right upper quadrant pain often exacerbated by meals and caused by obstruction of the cystic duct or common bile duct. Obstruction of the common bile duct can lead to obstructive jaundice, cholangitis (i.e., infection of the bile ducts), and pancreatitis. Cholecystectomy, often done laparoscopically, is the definitive treatment.

Cholesterol Stones

Cholesterol stones are the more common type and form as the result of increased cholesterol within bile and bile stasis. Bile with a higher concentration of cholesterol is more likely to precipitate. Some recognized risk factors include increasing age, obesity, female gender, high-cholesterol diet, premenopausal status in females, and oral contraceptive pills. Grossly, cholesterol stones are yellow and round or bosselated, ranging from less than a centimeter to a few centimeters in diameter (Figure 10-27).

Pigment Stones

Pigment stones can occur in the setting of malnutrition, hemolytic anemia, cirrhosis, and bacterial or parasitic biliary tract infections. Pigment stones tend to be smaller in diameter.

Cholecystitis

Cholecystitis is inflammation of the gallbladder.

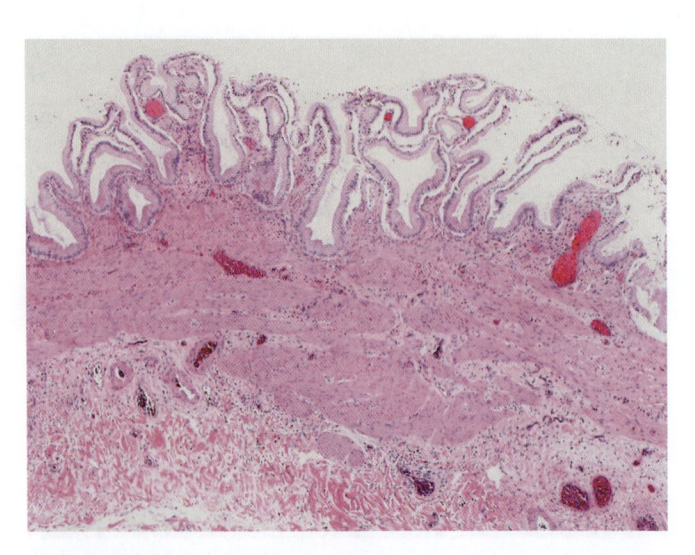

FIGURE 10-26 Normal gallbladder. This section of gallbladder shows the layers of the gallbladder wall (mucosa, muscularis propria, and adventitia).

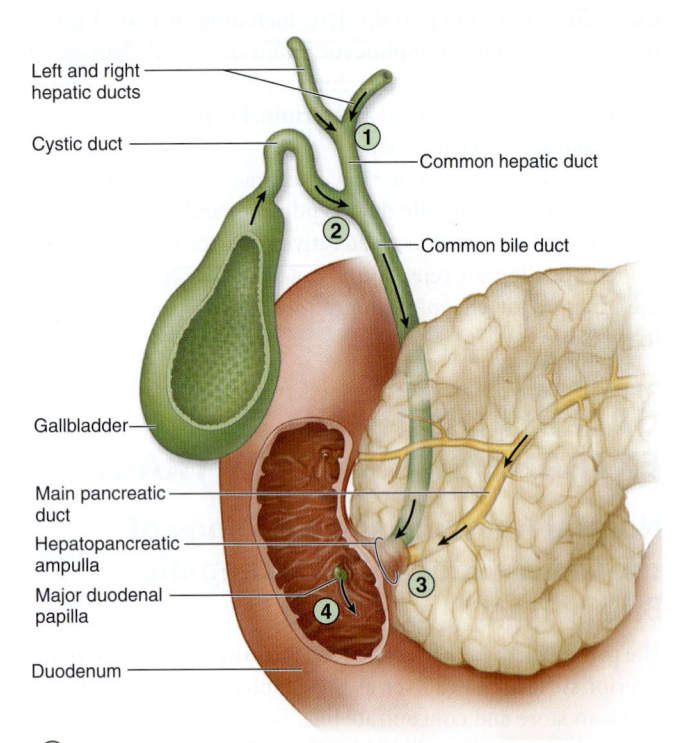

① Left and right hepatic ducts merge to form a common hepatic duct.
② Common hepatic and cystic ducts merge to form a common bile duct.
③ Pancreatic duct merges with common bile duct at the hepatopancreatic ampulla.
④ Bile and pancreatic juices enter duodenum at the major duodenal papilla.

FIGURE 10-25 Anatomy of the gallbladder and extrahepatic biliary tract. Source: Figure 26.21 in McKinley & O'Loughlin's Human Anatomy, 2nd ed.

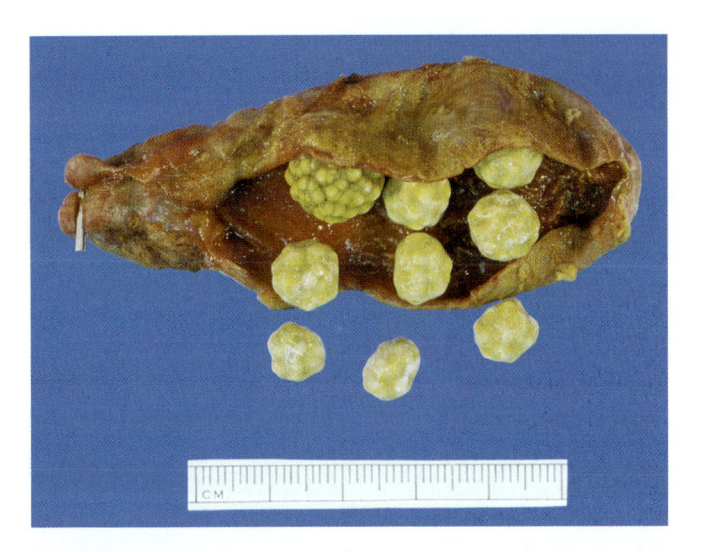

FIGURE 10-27 Cholesterol stones. Several cholesterol stones within a partially opened gallbladder. Source: McKinley & O'Loughlin's Human Anatomy, 2nd ed., page 804.

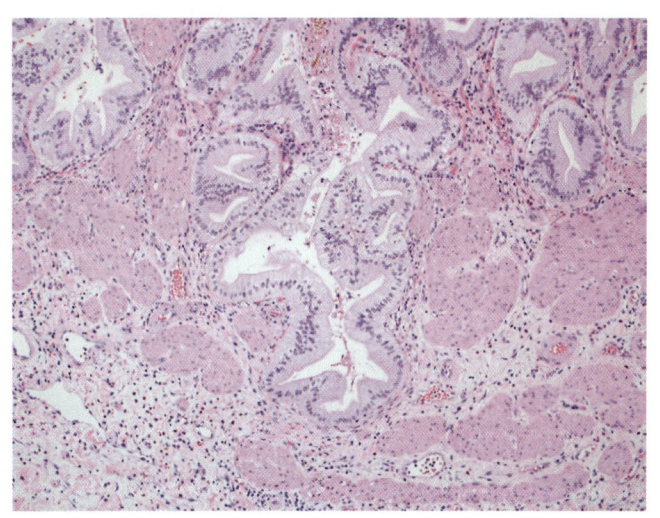

FIGURE 10-28 Chronic cholecystitis. This high-magnification view of chronic cholecystitis shows an outpouching of gallbladder mucosa extending into the muscularis propria. These Rokitansky–Aschoff sinuses are characteristic of chronic cholecystitis.

Acute Cholecystitis

Acute cholecystitis is usually caused by gallstones and often occurs in the setting of obstruction. It can present with abdominal pain, jaundice, fever, and leukocytosis. Grossly, the outer surface of the gallbladder is congested and erythematous and a surface exudate is common. The gallbladder wall is edematous and the mucosa is erythematous. Microscopically, there is acute and chronic inflammation with occasional ulceration or necrosis of the mucosa.

Chronic Cholecystitis

Chronic cholecystitis occurs in the setting of cholelithiasis or repeated episodes of acute cholecystitis. The clinical manifestations are typically those of cholelithiasis. Grossly, the gallbladder wall is firm and often thickened. Microscopically, there are lymphocytic infiltrates and outpouchings of mucosa extending into the muscularis propria (Rokitansky–Aschoff sinuses) (Figure 10-28). The latter finding develops as the result of increased intraluminal pressure.

Masses of the Gallbladder and Extrahepatic Biliary Tract

Benign neoplasms of the gallbladder and extrahepatic biliary tract are rare and can result in obstruction.

Gallbladder Carcinoma

Gallbladder carcinoma is a malignancy arising from the gallbladder mucosa. It is considered more common in women and often occurs in the setting of cholelithiasis and chronic cholecystitis. The prognosis is usually very poor as direct invasion of adjacent organs, lymph node metastases, and perineural invasion are common. Cancer-free survival is much more likely with early-stage tumors discovered incidentally at the time of cholecystectomy for gallstones.

Grossly, there is either a discrete mass or an area of firmness and thickening of the gallbladder wall. Adenocarcinoma, either with intestinal or gastric foveolar differentiation, is the most common subtype of carcinoma (Figure 10-29). The invasive carcinoma tends to elicit a prominent fibrotic stromal reaction, thus accounting for the gallbladder wall changes.

Bile Duct Adenocarcinoma

Extrahepatic bile duct adenocarcinoma is an invasive carcinoma of extrahepatic bile ducts (common hepatic duct, cystic duct, and common bile duct). The histologic findings and prognosis are comparable to intrahepatic cholangiocarcinoma.

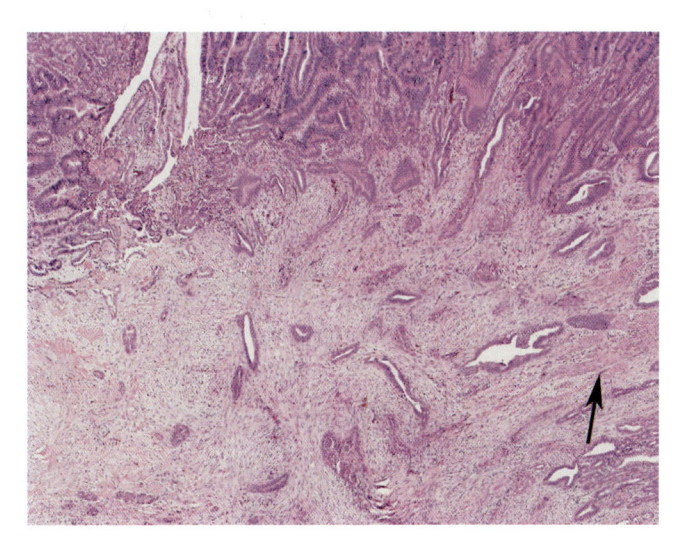

FIGURE 10-29 Gallbladder adenocarcinoma. In this deeply invading gallbladder adenocarcinoma, the tumor has invaded from the mucosal surface (top), through the muscularis propria (arrow), and into the adventitia.

CHAPTER 11

Pathology of the Pancreas

Kevin G. Greene, M.D.

INTRODUCTION

The pancreas contains two distinctive types of glandular tissue, an exocrine component and an endocrine component, which allow the organ to perform two different functions. Exocrine glands secrete their products into a duct system. The ducts, in turn, transport these secretions to a specific target. Acini are the functional units of the exocrine pancreas. Endocrine glands secrete their products directly into the blood, rather than into a duct system. Islets of Langerhans are the functional units of the endocrine pancreas.

NORMAL ANATOMY AND HISTOLOGY OF THE PANCREAS

Gross Anatomy

The pancreas is a retroperitoneal organ located in the upper abdomen and surrounded by a number of important organs and blood vessels. Although the pancreas is one continuous organ, it is thought of as having three anatomic regions based on its spatial relationship to surrounding structures. There are also minor functional differences between the anatomic regions, and certain diseases have a predilection for one region versus another.

The **head of the pancreas** is nestled within the curvature of the duodenum that abuts the right lateral and right inferior borders of the pancreas. The right borders of the superior mesenteric vessels, which lie directly posterior to the pancreas, mark the transition to the **body of the pancreas**. The body of the pancreas encompasses the majority of the pancreas and transitions distally into a tapered **tail of the pancreas**. In addition to the superior mesenteric vessels, the aorta and inferior vena cava lie posterior to the pancreas. Other organs that lie in close proximity to the pancreas include the stomach (anterior to the pancreas), spleen (at the distal tip of the pancreas), and left kidney (posterior to the tail of the pancreas) **(Figure 11-1)**.

Histology

Before discussing the anatomy of the pancreatic ductal system, it is helpful to first develop a working knowledge of the microscopic anatomy of the pancreas. Low-power examination of the pancreas reveals an organ composed of lobules of tissue **(Figure 11-2)**.

Exocrine tissue makes up the vast majority of the lobule. The functional unit of the exocrine pancreas is the acinus (pl. acini). Acini are organized collections of secretory cells that surround a central lumen. Acinar cells have peripherally located nuclei and abundant granular cytoplasm and secrete a variety of active enzymes and inactive proenzymes into the acinar lumen **(Figure 11-3)**. These secretion products are carried from the acini to the duodenum via the ductal system. Proenzymes are converted to active enzymes in the duodenum. A summary of some of the important pancreatic enzymes is included in **Table 11-1**.

Dotting a sea of exocrine tissue are the islets of Langerhans, the functional units of the endocrine pancreas. In hematoxylin and eosin-stained sections, islets appear paler than their more abundant exocrine counterparts **(Figure 11-4)**. A summary of some of the important islet produced hormones is included in **Table 11-2**.

Pancreatic Ductal System

Acinar cell secretions are collected in the acinar lumen and are transported to the duodenum through a series of progressively enlarging pancreatic ducts. Intralobular ducts are small ducts present within pancreatic lobules. Interlobular ducts are larger ducts present between lobules. Interlobular ducts drain into the main pancreatic duct, which usually merges with the common bile duct just proximal to the ampulla of Vater, the site where bile and pancreatic secretions enter the duodenum. In some people, a separate accessory pancreatic duct is present and empties directly into the duodenum, separate from the ampulla of Vater. Pancreatic duct epithelial cells secrete bicarbonate, which helps to neutralize the highly acidic material entering the duodenum from the stomach **(Figures 11-5 and 11-6)**.

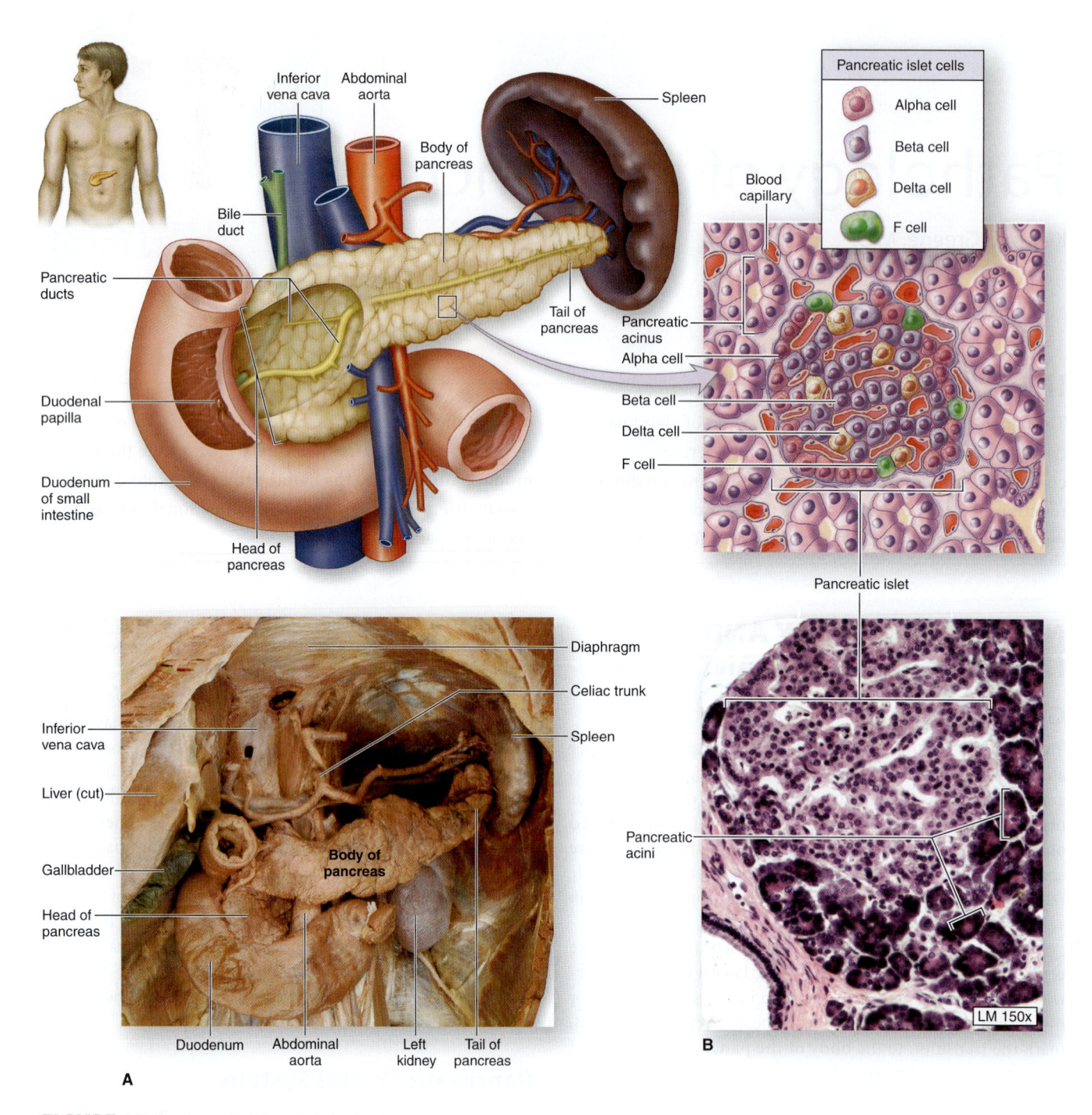

FIGURE 11-1 **Anatomy of the pancreas.** Source: McKinley M. and O'Loughlin. Human Anatomy, 2nd ed. New York: McGraw Hill 2007. Figure 20.14.

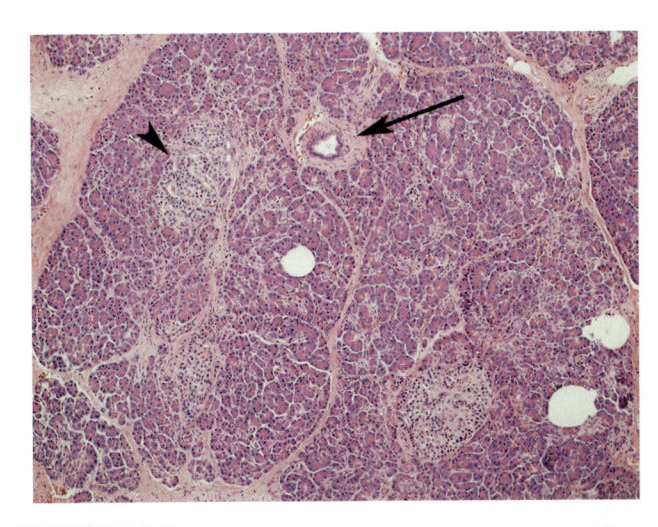

FIGURE 11-2 Pancreatic lobule. Grossly and microscopically normal pancreatic tissue has a lobular architecture. The majority of the lobule is composed of acinar tissue. Islets of Langerhans (arrowhead) and a pancreatic duct branch (arrow) are also present.

TABLE 11-1 Pancreatic enzymes.

Enzyme	Proenzyme	Function
Trypsin	Trypsinogen	Digestion of protein
Chymotrypsin	Chymotrypsinogen	Digestion of protein
Amylase	None	Digestion of starch
Lipase	None	Digestion of triglyceride

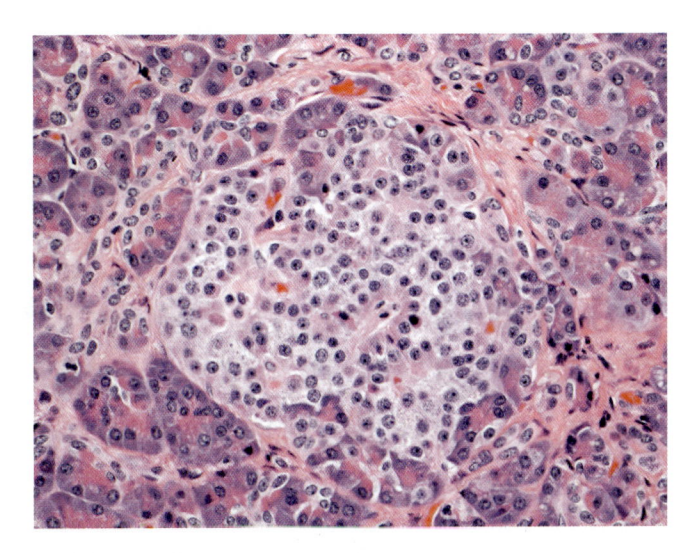

FIGURE 11-4 Islets of Langerhans. Islets of Langerhans, the functional units of the endocrine pancreas, consist of "islands" of neuroendocrine cells that secrete hormones into the blood for widespread distribution throughout the body.

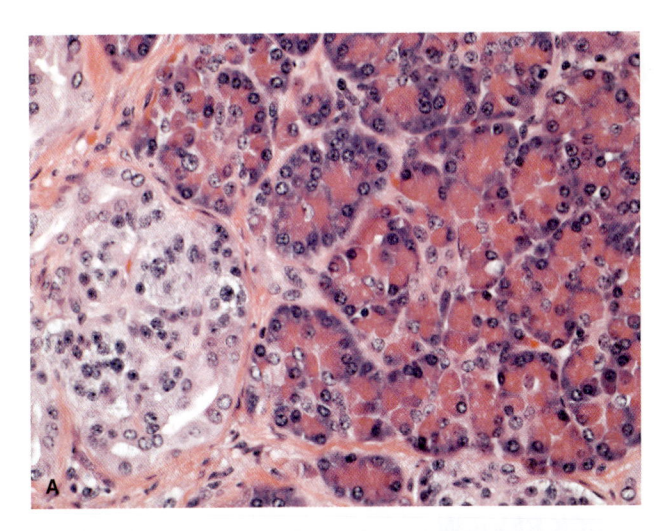

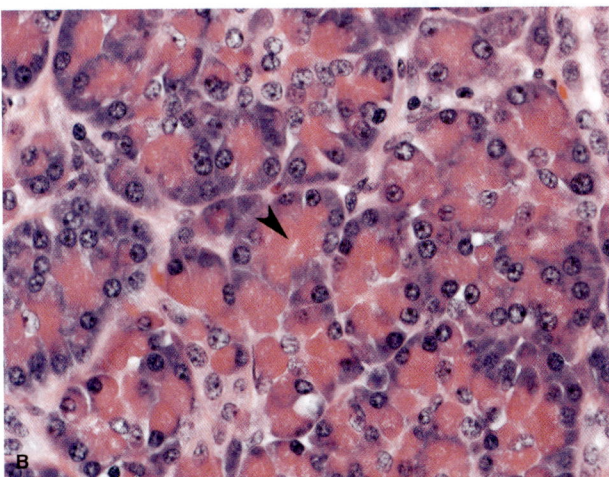

FIGURE 11-3 Pancreatic acini. (A) In contrast to islets of Langerhans (left), acini consist of exocrine glandular structures organized around a central lumen. **(B)** Acinar cells contain distinctive eosinophilic cytoplasmic zymogen granules. An acinar lumen is indicated by the arrowhead.

TABLE 11-2 Pancreatic hormones.

Hormone	Cell of Origin	Function
Insulin	Beta cells	• Regulation of carbohydrate and fat metabolism • Causes uptake of blood glucose into the liver, skeletal muscle, and fat (lowering blood glucose)
Glucagon	Alpha cells	• Regulation of carbohydrate metabolism • Causes conversion of liver glycogen to glucose (raising blood glucose)
Somatostatin	Delta cells (a.k.a. D cells)	• Inhibits the release of a variety of other peptide hormones
Pancreatic polypeptide	PP cells	• Regulation of pancreatic exocrine and endocrine secretions

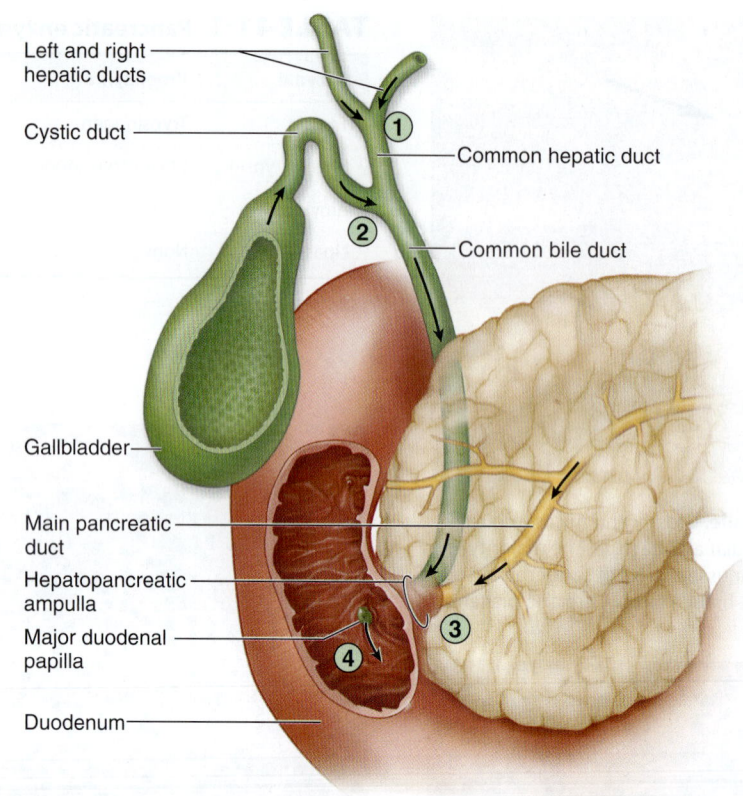

FIGURE 11-5 Diagram of the pancreatic ductal system. Source: McKinley M. and O'Loughlin. Human Anatomy, 2nd ed. New York: McGraw Hill 2007. Figure 26.21.

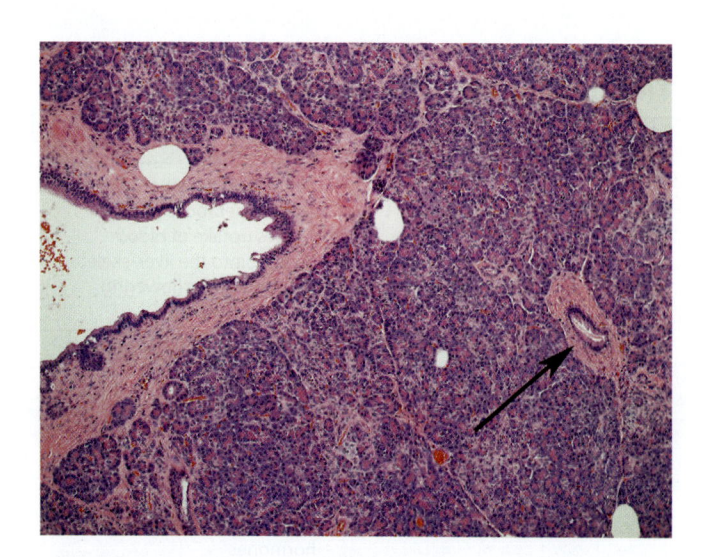

1. Left and right hepatic ducts merge to form a common hepatic duct.
2. Common hepatic and cystic ducts merge to form a common bile duct.
3. Pancreatic duct merges with common bile duct at the hepatopancreatic ampulla.
4. Bile and pancreatic juices enter duodenum at the major duodenal papilla.

FIGURE 11-6 **Intralobular and interlobular pancreatic ducts.** Acinar secretions pass from intralobular pancreatic ducts (arrow) into interlobular pancreatic ducts (left) on their way to the duodenum.

QUICK REVIEW

- Anatomically, the pancreas is subdivided into a head, body, and tail.
- The pancreas contains two distinctive types of glandular tissue: an exocrine component and an endocrine component.
- Exocrine pancreas: Acini secrete digestive enzymes into the pancreatic ducts for transport to their site of function in the duodenum.
- Endocrine pancreas: Islets of Langerhans secrete hormones (e.g., insulin and glucagon) directly into the blood.

PRINCIPAL DISEASES OF THE PANCREAS

A diverse collection of neoplastic and non-neoplastic diseases can affect the pancreas. This chapter will focus on the more common diseases, including pancreatitis, diabetes mellitus, and neoplasia.

CASE 11-1

The patient is a 48-year-old female who sought medical attention for a rapid onset of upper abdominal pain and vomiting. A physical examination performed in the emergency department showed an acutely ill female in obvious distress and with a blood pressure of 96/58. Laboratory studies were performed as part of the evaluation and showed elevated levels of serum amylase and lipase. Given this constellation of physical and laboratory findings, a diagnosis of acute pancreatitis was rendered. An abdominal ultrasound revealed a stone within the common bile duct and a dilated pancreatic duct.

Acute Pancreatitis

Acute pancreatitis is an inflammatory disease of the pancreas that is usually associated with a rapid onset of upper abdominal pain, classically radiating to the back. Patients often complain of anorexia, nausea, and vomiting. Eating tends to worsen the discomfort. Fever, hypotension, and tachycardia are common physical examination findings. Flank ecchymosis (**Grey Turner sign**) and periumbilical ecchymosis (**Cullen sign**), if present, are indicative of retroperitoneal hemorrhage.

Establishing a diagnosis of acute pancreatitis is usually straightforward. In addition to the characteristic signs and symptoms, the release of amylase and lipase from injured acinar cells results in elevated serum levels of these enzymes.

There are numerous potential causes of acute pancreatitis. Gallstones and ethanol abuse are the two most common causes in Western societies. Other recognized factors include medication toxicity, metabolic derangements (e.g., hypercalcemia), other obstructive processes (e.g., tumor), and trauma. Regardless of the etiology, a common sequence in the pathogenesis of acute pancreatitis involves the release of enzymes and proenzymes from injured acinar cells. The proenzymes undergo premature activation (i.e., prior to reaching their target in the duodenum) resulting in autodigestive necrosis of pancreatic and peripancreatic tissues.

Mortality rates are relatively low in uncomplicated interstitial acute pancreatitis, but approach one out of every three patients in acute hemorrhagic pancreatitis complicated by secondary bacterial infection.

PATHOLOGY

Grossly, the pancreas is pale and edematous in mild acute pancreatitis (a.k.a. interstitial acute pancreatitis) and hemorrhagic in severe acute pancreatitis (a.k.a. acute hemorrhagic pancreatitis). Chalky white deposits, characteristic of fat necrosis, form within peripancreatic adipose tissue due to an interaction between lipase, triglycerides, and calcium. Microscopically, acute pancreatitis is characterized by varying degrees of acute inflammation, hemorrhage, pancreatic necrosis, and peripancreatic fat necrosis (**Figure 11-7**).

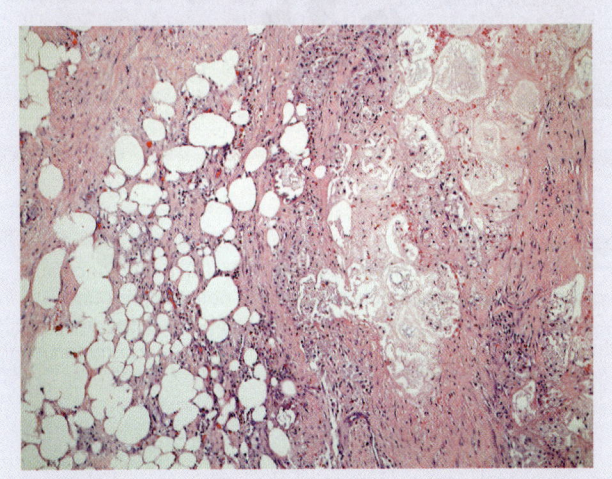

FIGURE 11-7 Acute pancreatitis. In this case of acute pancreatitis, spillage of activated digestive enzymes has resulted in peripancreatic fat necrosis (right).

Pseudocyst

Episodes of acute pancreatitis can be complicated by pseudocyst formation. A pseudocyst is a cystic collection of pancreatic enzymes, necrotic tissue, and blood that is surrounded by a fibrous wall. The prefix "pseudo" is applied to indicate the absence of a true epithelial lining. Although rare, pseudocysts can become infected or can rupture. They can also be mistaken clinically and radiologically for a cystic neoplasm (**Figure 11-8**).

Chronic Pancreatitis

Chronic pancreatitis is a chronic fibroinflammatory disease of the pancreas that results in a progressive loss of pancreatic parenchyma and replacement by fibrosis. Chronic pancreatitis can be associated with upper abdominal and back pain. As the disease worsens, the resulting insufficiency in pancreatic exocrine secretions can lead to malabsorption, steatorrhea, vitamin deficiency, and weight loss. Loss of a substantial percentage of the total acinar cell volume must occur before signs and symptoms of exocrine insufficiency are seen. Endocrine insufficiencies can occur in some patients; however, in chronic pancreatitis, islets of Langerhans are relatively preserved compared with acini and are lost in large numbers only very late in the disease progression.

Serum amylase and lipase may or may not be elevated. Establishing a diagnosis of chronic pancreatitis is usually facilitated by imaging studies, including abdominal X-ray, CT scan, endoscopic retrograde cholangiopancreatography (ERCP), magnetic resonance cholangiopancreatography (MRCP), and endoscopic ultrasound. Characteristic radiologic findings include glandular atrophy, pancreatic duct dilation, and calcifications.

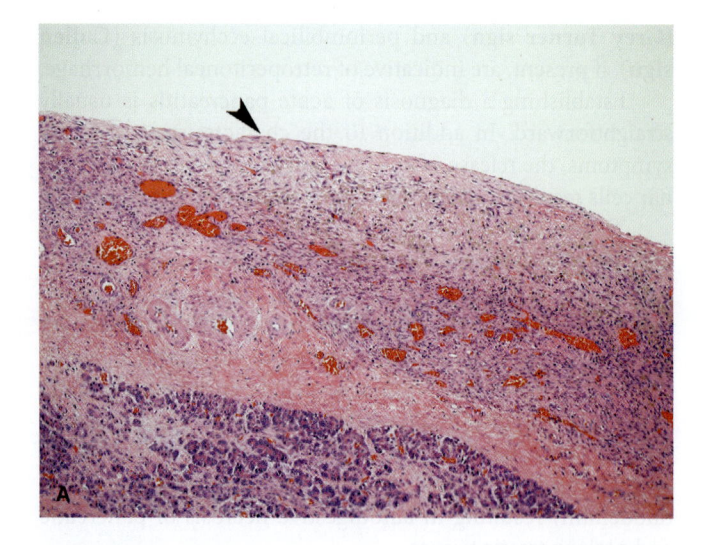

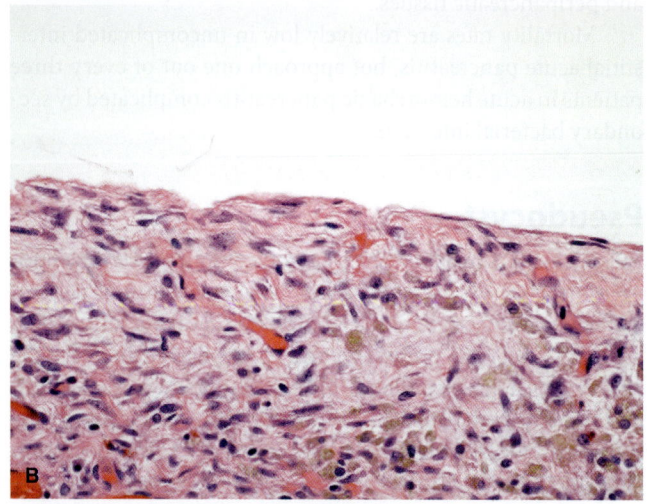

FIGURE 11-8 Pseudocyst. (A) The wall of a pseudocyst is composed of inflamed fibrous tissue. The arrowhead indicates the lining of the cyst. The central cavity of the cyst is present in the top of the image, and adjacent pancreatic parenchyma is present in the bottom of the image. **(B)** In this higher magnification view, note the absence of an epithelial lining.

Chronic ethanol abuse is the most common cause of chronic pancreatitis. There are a variety of additional factors that can lead to chronic pancreatitis including chronic mechanical obstruction of the pancreatic duct (e.g., stone or tumor) and autoimmune disease (i.e., autoimmune pancreatitis). Idiopathic chronic pancreatitis is a form of chronic pancreatitis in which risk factors for pancreatitis are not identified. In many patients, repeated episodes of clinically recognized acute pancreatitis lead to progressive parenchymal loss and fibrosis. In other patients, the disease is insidious and not recognized until pancreatic insufficiency develops.

Diabetes Mellitus

Diabetes mellitus is a group of disorders of glucose homeostasis that is caused by derangements in insulin production or utilization, leading to hyperglycemia. Over time, diabetes

PATHOLOGY

In well-developed chronic pancreatitis, the pancreas is shrunken and firm. The cut surface shows distorted architecture with a loss of the normal lobular appearance. The pancreatic ducts are commonly dilated as the result of chronic obstruction secondary to stones, inspissated secretions, or duct strictures. Calcifications are common. Microscopic examination shows chronic inflammation and a loss of pancreatic parenchyma with replacement by fibrosis. Acinar cells are most susceptible to injury and are lost earlier than islet cells. Pancreatic ducts are often dilated and occasionally contain inspissated secretions (**Figure 11-9**).

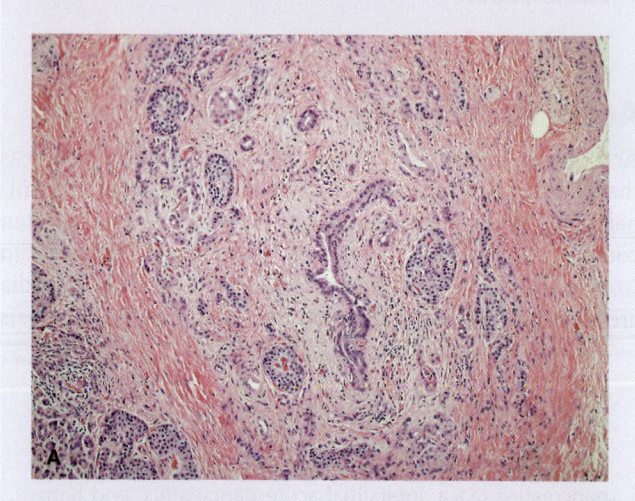

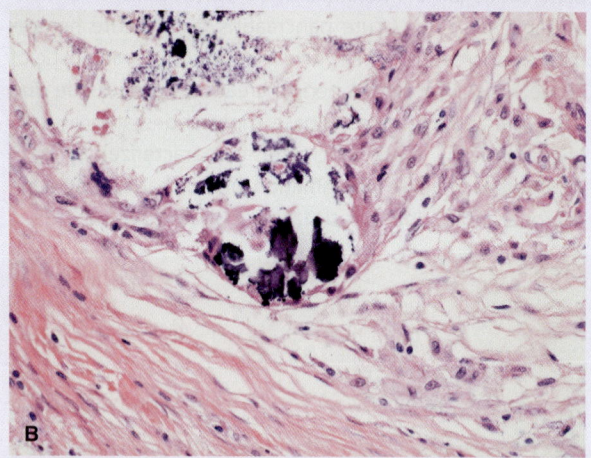

FIGURE 11-9 Chronic pancreatitis. (A) In this pancreatic lobule involved by chronic pancreatitis, note the profound loss of acinar tissue, the replacement by fibrous tissue, and the relative preservation of islets. **(B)** Calcifications are common in chronic pancreatitis.

can cause end-organ damage of the retina (i.e., diabetic retinopathy), kidney (i.e., diabetic nephropathy), and peripheral nerves (i.e., diabetic neuropathy). Diabetes is also a major risk factor for atherosclerotic cardiovascular disease, leading to myocardial infarctions and complications from peripheral vascular disease.

Type 1 Diabetes Mellitus

Type 1 diabetes is caused by autoimmune destruction of the beta cells of the islets of Langerhans, which leads to a profound drop in insulin production and secretion. This form of diabetes classically, though not always, presents as an acute metabolic decompensation characterized by severe hyperglycemia and ketoacidosis. Diabetic ketoacidosis occurs when fatty acids are utilized as an energy source rather than glucose. This fatty acid metabolism produces ketone bodies. A period of polyuria (increased urine output), polydipsia (increased thirst), and polyphagia (increased hunger) may occur prior to an acute episode of ketoacidosis. Type 1 diabetes typically presents at a younger age, classically around the time of puberty.

The treatment of type 1 diabetes involves the administration of exogenous insulin in order to maintain a healthy range of serum glucose. Without treatment, death would eventually occur due to ketoacidosis.

PATHOLOGY

As with most non-neoplastic diseases of the pancreas (autoimmune pancreatitis being a notable exception), biopsies are not typically part of the evaluation; however, having an understanding of the pathologic changes in diabetes is useful in terms of gaining a broader understanding of the overall disease process.

Early during the course of the disease, there is a lymphocytic infiltrate of pancreatic islets. This lesion is called "insulitis." As the disease progresses, there is continued destruction of beta cells until these cells are virtually absent. This absence can be demonstrated by an immunohistochemical stain specific for insulin. Some degree of acinar atrophy can be present, as well as intralobular and interlobular fibrosis.

QUICK REVIEW
Type 1 Diabetes
- Caused by autoimmune destruction of pancreatic islet beta cells.
- Often presents with ketoacidosis, a medical emergency.
- The hallmark histologic finding is insulitis.

Type 2 Diabetes Mellitus

The etiology of type 2 diabetes is more multifactorial and involves a combination of genetic susceptibility, impaired utilization of insulin by target tissues (i.e., insulin resistance), and an inadequate secretion of insulin by the pancreas. This form of diabetes classically develops in obese older adults; however, there is an increasing prevalence in younger persons coinciding with a rise in childhood obesity.

The management of type 2 diabetes is multifaceted. Lifestyle modifications to reduce body weight are important. A variety of oral medications are available that target different aspects of the pathophysiology. Some patients with refractory disease require insulin therapy.

PATHOLOGY

Microscopic examination of the pancreas is unremarkable in many patients with type 2 diabetes. In other patients, there are variable degrees of islet fibrosis, islet amyloid deposition, and beta cell loss. Insulitis is not a typical feature of type 2 diabetes.

QUICK REVIEW
Type 2 Diabetes
- Caused by a combination of insulin resistance and inadequate insulin secretion.
- Typically has an insidious onset in obese adults.
- Islet fibrosis and amyloid deposition are present in some patients.

Gestational Diabetes

Gestational diabetes is a transient form of diabetes that occurs in pregnant women due to increased insulin resistance during pregnancy. In uncomplicated cases, the hyperglycemia resolves during the postpartum period. Some cases mark the onset of type 2 diabetes or predict the future development of type 2 diabetes.

NEOPLASMS OF THE PANCREAS

By a wide margin, the two most common neoplasms of the pancreas are invasive ductal adenocarcinoma and well-differentiated pancreatic endocrine neoplasm. A sampling of other, less common epithelial neoplasms of the pancreas is listed in Table 11-3.

TABLE 11-3 Less common pancreatic neoplasms (WHO 2010 Classification).

Benign   • Serous cystadenoma, NOS
Premalignant lesions   • Pancreatic intraepithelial neoplasia (PanIN)   • Intraductal papillary mucinous neoplasm (IPMN)   • Mucinous cystic neoplasm (MCN)
Malignant lesions   • Adenosquamous carcinoma   • Acinar cell carcinoma   • Solid-pseudopapillary neoplasm   • Serous cystadenocarcinoma   • Pancreatoblastoma

CASE 11-2

The patient is a 62-year-old male with a long history of smoking cigarettes who sought medical attention for worsening upper abdominal pain. During the course of his evaluation, it was revealed that he had lost 25 pounds over the past 3 months. He had not been intentionally trying to lose weight. As part of his workup, an abdominal CT scan was obtained and showed an ill-defined mass in the head of the pancreas. An endoscopic ultrasound-guided fine-needle aspiration revealed malignant cells, consistent with adenocarcinoma. In addition, a peripancreatic lymph node was sampled and showed metastatic adenocarcinoma. Despite medical therapy, he died from his disease 8 months later.

Invasive Ductal Adenocarcinoma

Invasive ductal adenocarcinoma is a gland-forming malignant neoplasm of pancreatic ducts and is by far the most common neoplasm of the pancreas, benign or malignant. The incidence of disease is highest in adults over the age of 50, but occasional cases occur before the age of 50. Patients usually present with upper abdominal pain and precipitous weight loss. Tumors arising within the head of the pancreas can obstruct the common bile duct and cause jaundice, which is sometimes the presenting sign.

A variety of possible risk factors are recognized, including smoking, high dietary fat intake, diabetes, and chronic pancreatitis. Invasive ductal adenocarcinoma can arise within intraductal papillary mucinous neoplasms or mucinous cystic neoplasms, or can arise from dysplasia of pancreatic ducts.

The prognosis of invasive ductal adenocarcinoma is very poor. The majority of patients die less than 1 year after

PATHOLOGY

The diagnosis of invasive ductal adenocarcinoma is usually established by radiologic studies with or without the assistance of fine-needle aspiration cytology. Core biopsies to establish the diagnosis are rare. Pathologic tissue evaluation is usually reserved for staging of resections.

Grossly, invasive ductal adenocarcinoma appears as an irregular, firm, and tan-white effacement of the normal parenchyma. This appearance is due, in large part, to the significant degree of fibrosis that occurs in the tumor. In fact, it is often difficult to make the distinction between chronic pancreatitis and invasive ductal adenocarcinoma by gross examination, and chronic pancreatitis is often present surrounding these tumors.

Microscopic examination typically shows a haphazard infiltration of highly atypical glands, cell clusters, and individual cells within a fibrotic stroma. The malignant cells show a striking degree of nuclear pleomorphism (i.e., variation from one cell to the next) with a fourfold difference in nuclear size between cells within the same gland. Invasion of nerves (perineural invasion) and blood vessels (lymphovascular invasion) is common (**Figure 11-10**).

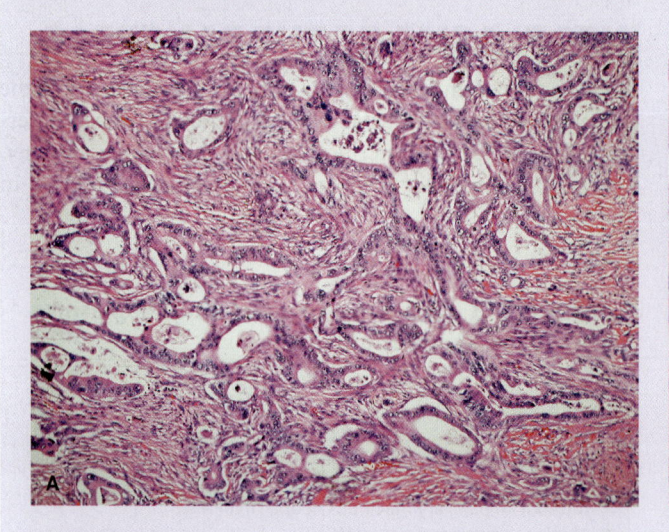

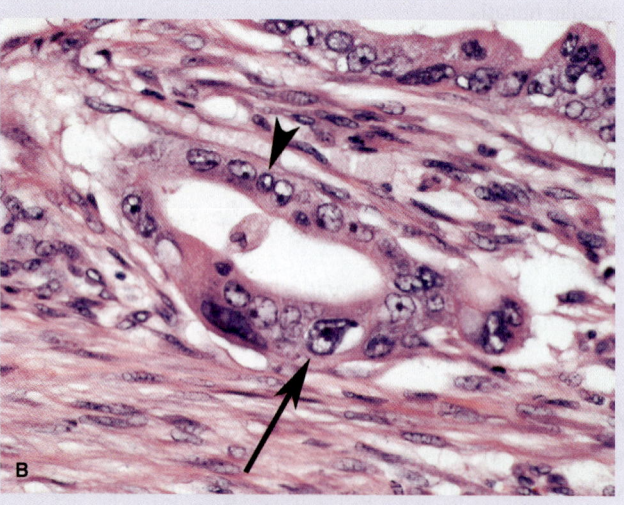

FIGURE 11-10 Invasive ductal adenocarcinoma. **(A)**, A haphazard infiltration of highly atypical glands within a fibrotic stroma is characteristic of invasive ductal adenocarcinoma. **(B)** Note the extreme pleomorphism between the two designated tumor cells of this malignant gland.

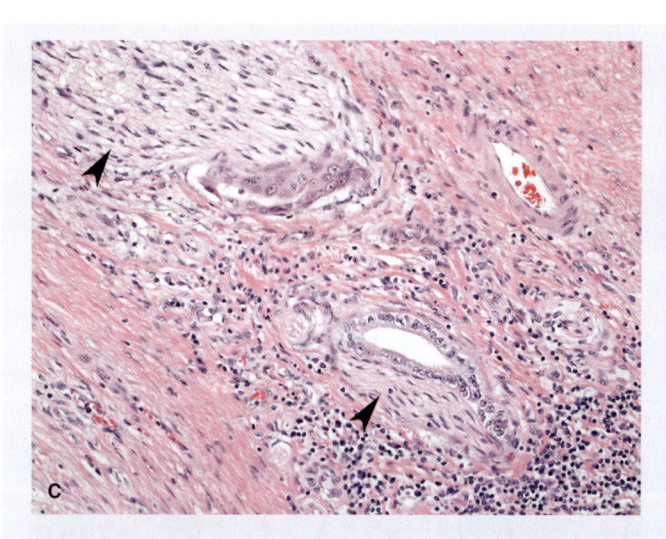

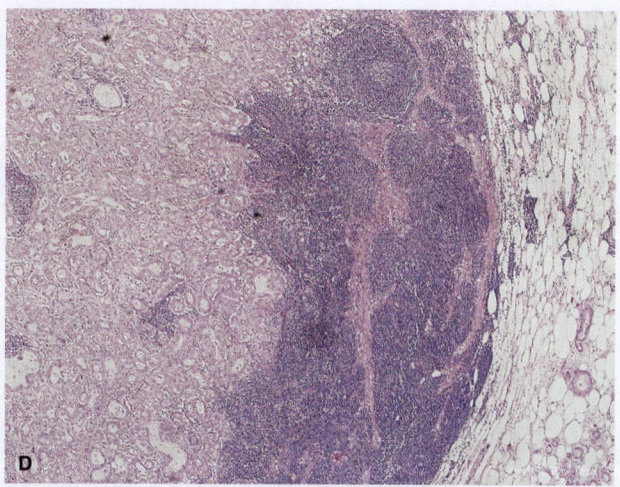

FIGURE 11-10 *(Continued)* Perineural invasion **(C)** is common (arrowheads mark peripheral nerves) as are lymph node metastases **(D)**.

receiving the diagnosis. This is due in large part to the growth characteristics of the tumor. Early invasion beyond the pancreas, early lymph node and liver metastases, and perineural invasion eliminate the possibility of surgical cure in the majority of cases.

Well-Differentiated Pancreatic Endocrine Neoplasm

Well-differentiated pancreatic endocrine neoplasms are a distinctive class of pancreatic tumors that, by definition, show neuroendocrine differentiation (i.e., neurosecretory granules can be demonstrated by electron microscopy). These tumors are the second most common tumors of the pancreas, behind only invasive ductal adenocarcinoma. It is believed that these tumors arise from pluripotent cells within the pancreatic ducts. Signs and symptoms present at evaluation depend in large part on whether the tumor is nonfunctioning or functioning.

Nonfunctioning Versus Functioning Tumors

Well-differentiated pancreatic endocrine neoplasms are broadly divided into two categories: nonfunctioning and functioning. Nonfunctioning tumors do not produce a hormone, produce only a small quantity of hormone, or lack a functional apparatus to secrete a hormone into the blood. Functioning tumors produce a hormone and secrete that hormone into the blood in a sufficient quantity to cause a paraneoplastic syndrome. A list of the functioning well-differentiated pancreatic endocrine neoplasms and their associated paraneoplastic syndromes is found in Table 11-4.

In general, benign or malignant behavior cannot be accurately predicted by microscopic features. A diagnosis of malignancy requires the documentation of invasion into peripancreatic tissues or the presence of metastatic disease. If a paraneoplastic syndrome is present, the hormone product produced can often predict the likelihood of malignancy. The vast majority of insulinomas do not invade beyond the pancreas or metastasize, while the remaining types of functioning tumors (e.g., somatostatinoma) tend to behave in a malignant fashion.

TABLE 11-4 Functioning well-differentiated pancreatic endocrine neoplasms.

Tumor	Hormone Product	Paraneoplastic Syndrome
Insulinoma	Insulin	Unregulated insulin secretion leads to hypoglycemia
Glucagonoma	Glucagon	Mild diabetes, migratory skin rash, anemia, venous thrombosis, and infection
Somatostatinoma	Somatostatin	Mild diabetes, gallstones, steatorrhea, and hypochlorhydria
Gastrinoma	Gastrin	Zollinger–Ellison syndrome: gastric hypersecretion with severe peptic ulcer disease and elevated serum gastrin
VIPoma	Vasoactive intestinal polypeptide	Severe, intractable watery diarrhea

PATHOLOGY

Well-differentiated pancreatic endocrine neoplasms tend to be well-circumscribed masses that may or may not be confined to the pancreas. A densely fibrotic stroma is not as commonly encountered as it is in invasive ductal adenocarcinoma.

Microscopic examination shows a neoplastic proliferation of relatively uniform tumor cells arranged in one or more characteristic growth patterns: nested, trabecular, acinar (not to be confused with exocrine acinar tissue), or solid. The tumor nuclei often have a characteristic speckled chromatin staining pattern referred to as a "salt and pepper" appearance (**Figure 11-11**). Neuroendocrine differentiation can be demonstrated by immunohistochemical stains for CD56, chromogranin, and synaptophysin.

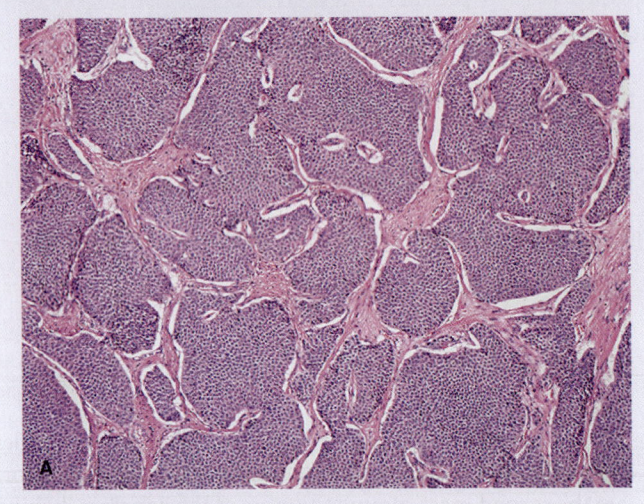

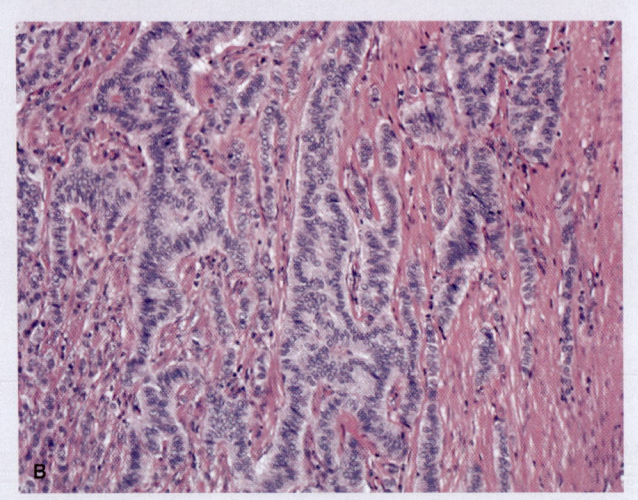

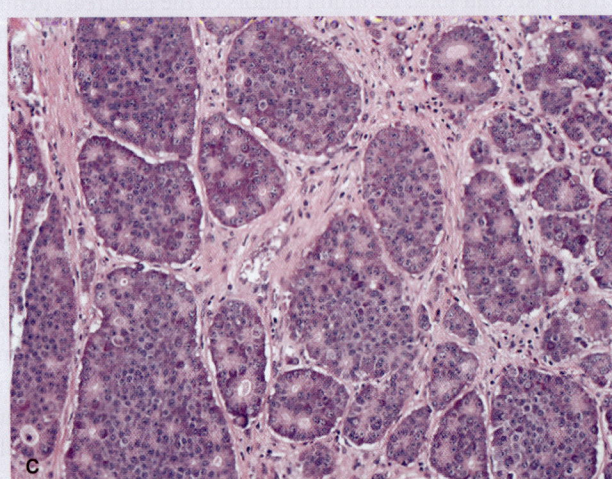

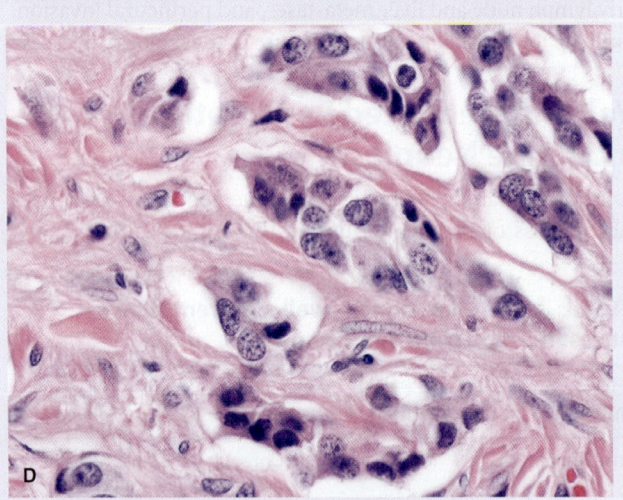

FIGURE 11-11 Well-differentiated pancreatic endocrine neoplasm. Three growth patterns are typical of well-differentiated pancreatic endocrine neoplasms. **(A)** The nested pattern consists of solid nests of tumor cells separated by stroma. **(B)** The trabecular pattern consists of thin ribbons or cords of tumor cells separated by stroma. **(C)** The acinar pattern is similar to the nested pattern, but contains rosettes of tumor cells mimicking acini. **(D)** Tumor nuclei appear speckled, an appearance referred to as "salt and pepper" chromatin.

IN TRANSLATION

A subset of well-differentiated pancreatic endocrine neoplasms arises in the setting of multiple endocrine neoplasia 1 (MEN1). MEN1 occurs in patients with germline mutations of one of their MEN1 genes, which predisposes them to neoplasms of the parathyroid gland, pancreas, and pituitary gland. The resulting pancreatic endocrine neoplasms are often multicentric.

CHAPTER 12

Pathology of Medical Renal Disease

J. Charles Jennette, M.D. and Adil M. Hussein Gasim, M.B.B.S.

INTRODUCTION

The clinical management of kidney diseases is divided primarily between specialized internists (nephrologists) and specialized surgeons (urologists). Similarly, the pathologic evaluation of kidney diseases is divided between specialized pathologists (nephropathologists) who specialize in kidney diseases that are managed by nephrologists, and pathologists (urologic pathologists) who specialize in kidney diseases that are managed by urologists. Nephrologists and nephropathologists focus on so-called medical renal disease, which includes non-neoplastic diseases that affect the renal parenchyma. Urologists and urologic pathologists focus on diseases that can affect any level of the urinary system from kidneys to urethra, including congenital, infectious, and neoplastic diseases. This chapter will deal with the many forms of medical renal disease, and Chapter 13 with urologic kidney disease.

WHAT WE DO
Medical Renal Disease Versus Urologic Disease and the Role of Nephropathologists

Nephrologists work closely with nephropathologists (renal pathologists) in the management of medical renal disease that requires renal biopsy. *Many medical renal diseases, especially glomerular diseases, can only be definitively diagnosed by evaluating renal biopsy specimens.* Further, repeat renal biopsies are important in the follow-up management of some patients to assess response to therapy, and to determine the degree of disease activity versus chronicity.

Kidney biopsies are most often obtained by percutaneous needle biopsy. The biopsy needle, usually with ultrasound guidance, is inserted into the patient's flank. Because most medical renal diseases have diagnostic features only in the cortex, the goal is to obtain enough renal cortex for a definitive pathologic diagnosis. Renal biopsy specimens are routinely evaluated by light microscopy, immunofluorescence microscopy (or immunohistochemistry), and electron microscopy. Renal biopsies are the only major type of surgical pathology specimen that is routinely processed for electron microscopy. Immunofluorescence microscopy uses fluorochrome-labeled reagent antibodies to detect deposition of IgG, IgA, IgM, C3, C1q, kappa light chains, lambda light chains and fibrin in renal tissue, especially glomeruli. Special immunohistochemistry is required for some specimens, for example, to detect genetically determined protein abnormalities [e.g., abnormal glomerular basement membrane (GBM) collagen caused by mutations of collagen 4 genes], protein deposits other than immunoglobulin (e.g., amyloid A and myoglobin), and infectious pathogens (e.g., polyoma virus). Electron microscopy is able to detect ultrastructural changes that are not discernible by light microscopy but are essential for precise diagnosis. The importance of immunofluorescence microscopy and electron microscopy will become apparent as the diagnostic features of renal diseases are presented in this chapter.

GLOMERULAR AND VASCULAR DISEASES

QUICK REVIEW
Normal Glomerular and Vascular Anatomy and Histology

The kidneys are highly vascularized organs with numerous vessels of many types that are the targets for multiple diseases.

At the hilum of the kidney, the main renal artery branches into anterior and posterior branches that feed into interlobar arteries that enter the renal parenchyma on either side of each papillary tip. The interlobar arteries feed into the arcuate arteries that run between the outer medulla and the cortex and give rise to interlobular arteries that run perpendicularly toward the renal capsule and give off multiple arterioles that become the afferent arterioles that enter glomerular tufts. Blood exits glomeruli via the efferent arterioles and subsequently provides sustenance to cortical and medullary tubules via peritubular capillaries. *Thus, whenever there is glomerular injury, secondary tubular injury may occur and can be a conspicuous histopathologic feature in addition to the primary glomerular lesions.*

Glomerular disease accounts for a high proportion of medical renal diseases, and thus a clear understanding of glomerular structure and function is essential to understand many of the diseases discussed in this chapter. The glomerulus is a ball (*Glomus*) formed by interconnected capillaries (Figure 12-1). The glomerular capillaries (Figure 12-2) are supported by a stalk of mesangial cells that are highly specialized smooth muscle cells that have multiple functions in addition to providing support for the glomerular capillaries including regulation of capillary blood flow, and clearance of debris from the circulation and subendothelial zone. Glomerular capillaries are lined by specialized endothelial cells that are fenestrated, and thus allow relatively unimpeded access to the underlying GBM (Figure 12-2). Adjacent to the mesangium, the endothelial cell sits directly against the mesangial matrix. In the remainder of the capillary wall, the endothelial cell lies adjacent to the GBM.

GBM is produced primarily by the overlying epithelial cells (podocytes). The GBM surrounds the peripheral capillary wall and, at the juncture with the mesangium, splays out over the mesangium as the paramesangial GBM (Figure 12-2). Thus, the GBM does not completely

FIGURE 12-1 Normal glomerulus. Light microscopy of a glomerulus with the hilum at the bottom. The periodic acid–Schiff (PAS) stain accentuates collagen in GBMs, mesangial matrix, Bowman capsule basement membrane, and tubule basement membranes (PAS stain).

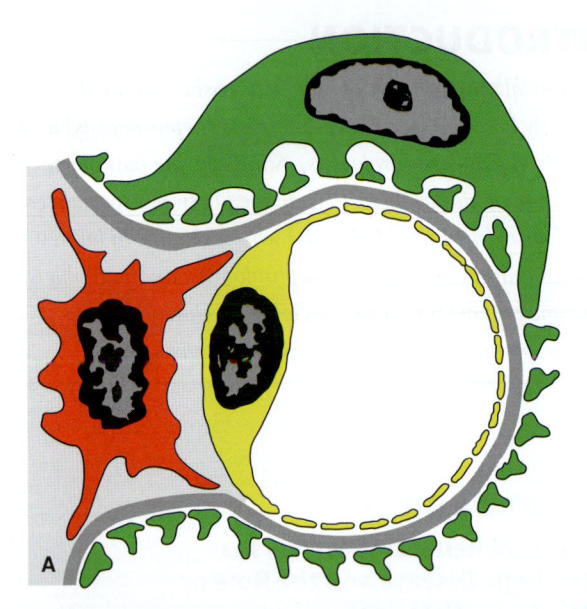

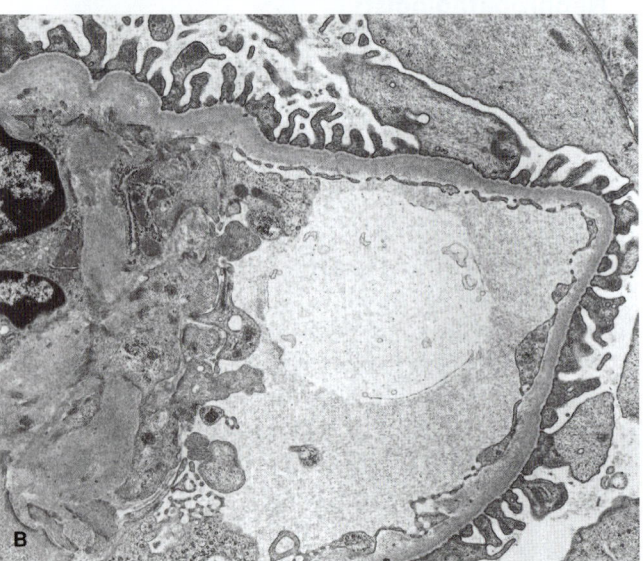

FIGURE 12-2 Diagram (A) and electron micrograph (B) of a normal glomerular capillary. The diagram depicts a podocyte (green) with foot processes extending to the GBM (dark gray), an endothelial cell with fenestrations (yellow), and a mesangial cell (red) surrounded by mesangial matrix (light gray).

surround the glomerular capillary lumen, which allows direct entry of materials from the plasma and the subendothelial zone into the mesangium.

The outer surface of the GBM is covered by podocytes that have foot processes that sit on the urinary space surface of the GBM (Figure 12-2). Extending between each foot process is a very thin slit diaphragm that resembles an adherens-like intercellular junction and provides the most selective barrier to the passage of proteins from the plasma into the urinary space. Integrity of the slit diaphragm appears to be the major determinant of capillary wall permeability to proteins.

GLOMERULAR DISEASE SYNDROMES

Injury to glomeruli causes a variety of clinical signs and symptoms because of disturbance of the many homeostatic functions of glomeruli. Disturbances in capillary wall integrity, especially injury to podocytes, result in increased permeability to proteins with resultant increased levels of protein in the urine (**proteinuria**). Injury to capillary walls that allows the cellular elements of blood to spill into the urine results in hematuria. Substantial impairment of blood flow through glomeruli, for example, caused by inflammation or scarring, results in reduced glomerular filtration that causes an elevation in blood urea nitrogen, increase in serum creatinine, and a reduction in glomerular filtration rate. Disturbance of blood pressure regulation and volume regulation results in hypertension.

Different forms of glomerular disease and different severities of glomerular injury tend to produce different combinations of signs and symptoms (Table 12-1). Patients with relatively mild glomerular disease may have asymptomatic proteinuria or asymptomatic hematuria or both, which is detected only by urinalysis. Diseases that cause severe proteinuria (greater than 3 g/24 hours) result in the **nephrotic syndrome**. Diseases that cause overt glomerular inflammation (**glomerulonephritis**) present with prominent hematuria often accompanied by hypertension, renal insufficiency, and proteinuria that usually are less severe than in patients with nephrotic syndrome. If glomerulonephritis results in a rapid loss of renal function, for example, requiring dialysis within 1 month, the disease is referred to as **rapidly progressive glomerulonephritis** (RPGN). Glomerular diseases may progress to chronic kidney disease, and, in some instances, to end-stage kidney disease. *In the United States, diabetic nephropathy is the leading cause of end-stage kidney disease, hypertensive arterionephrosclerosis is the second leading cause, and all other forms of glomerular disease are the third leading cause.* As will be discussed later in this chapter, glomerular injury is a major component of diabetic nephropathy and of hypertensive nephropathy.

Nephrotic Syndrome

The nephrotic syndrome results from severe proteinuria (>3g/24 hours) with resultant edema, hypoproteinemia including hypoalbuminemia and hyperlipidemia including hypertriglyceridemia (Table 12-1). The edema of nephrotic syndrome is most often found in a periorbital and ankle distribution, but the edema can be widespread and even associated with **anasarca** (severe and generalized edema). In addition to proteinuria, patients with nephrotic syndrome often have **lipiduria** with lipids and lipoproteins in the urine, sometimes configured as **oval fat bodies** or **fatty casts** that can be seen by microscopic examination of urine. Mild proteinuria does not produce overt manifestations of nephrotic syndrome and is only detected by urinalysis. Although hematuria, hypertension, and renal insufficiency are more conspicuous features of the glomerulonephritic syndrome, all of these features may be present to some degree in patients with the nephrotic syndrome. Likewise, patients with a clear-cut glomerulonephritic syndrome with extensive hematuria, hypertension, and renal insufficiency virtually always have some degree of proteinuria and may have edema. The edema formation in glomerulonephritis is caused more by sodium retention, whereas the edema in nephrotic syndrome is caused primarily by reduced oncotic pressure in the plasma because of hypoproteinemia.

Some glomerular diseases most often present with nephrotic syndrome, whereas others most often present with glomerulonephritic (nephritic) syndrome and some tend to have overlapping features of both syndromes (Table 12-2). *Glomerular diseases are categorized as primary when they are not associated with a systemic disease process or secondary when they are caused by (secondary to) a systemic disease.* The primary glomerular diseases that most often present with the nephrotic syndrome include **minimal-change glomerulopathy** (minimal-change disease), **membranous glomerulopathy**, and **focal segmental glomerulosclerosis** (FSGS). **Diabetic glomerulosclerosis** and **renal amyloidosis** are example of secondary forms of glomerular disease that present with the nephrotic syndrome. *Of the primary glomerular diseases that cause the nephrotic syndrome, minimal-change glomerulopathy is the most common cause of nephrotic syndrome in young children, membranous glomerulopathy is the most common cause of primary nephrotic syndrome in Caucasian adults, and FSGS is the most common cause of nephrotic syndrome in African-Americans.*

TABLE 12-1 Glomerular diseases often present clinically with either nephrotic or nephritic (glomerulonephritic) syndrome, which have overlapping signs and symptoms.

	Nephrotic Syndrome	Nephritic Syndrome
Edema	+ to +++	o to ++
Proteinuria	++ to +++	+ to ++
Hypoproteinemia	+ to +++	o to +
Hematuria	o to ++	++ to +++
Hyperlipidemia	++ to +++	o to +
Azotemia	o to ++	o to +++
Hypertension	o to +	o to +++

CASE 12-1

A 35-year-old Caucasian male developed periorbital edema and swollen ankles. His primary care physician confirmed the edema. Blood pressure was normal. Point-of-care laboratory testing in the office revealed 4+ (out of 0-4+) protein and 1+ hematuria in the urine. He was referred to a nephrologists and further evaluation confirmed the edema and normal blood pressure. Laboratory findings included 4+ proteinuria with urine protein to creatinine ratio 4.7, 1+ hematuria with 5–10 dysmorphic red blood cells (RBCs)/hpf, 0–5 white blood cell (WBC)/hpf, serum creatinine 1.2 mg/dL, serum albumin 3.1 g/dL, serum cholesterol 355 mg/dL, and normal C3 and C4. Serologic testing for lupus, hepatitis B, and hepatitis C was negative.

A renal biopsy was performed and was diagnostic for membranous glomerulopathy (Figures 12-3 and 12-4).

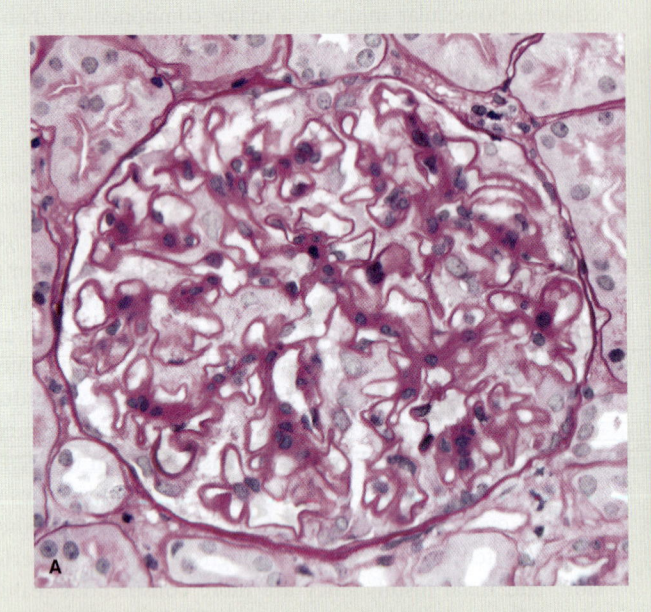

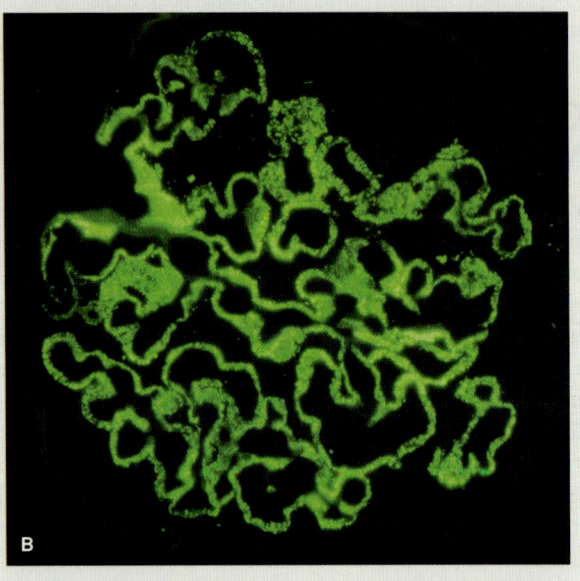

FIGURE 12-3 Membranous glomerulopathy with thick capillary walls but no hypercellularity by light microscopy (**A.** PAS stain, compare with Figure 12-1), and granular capillary wall staining for IgG by immunofluorescence microscopy (**B**).

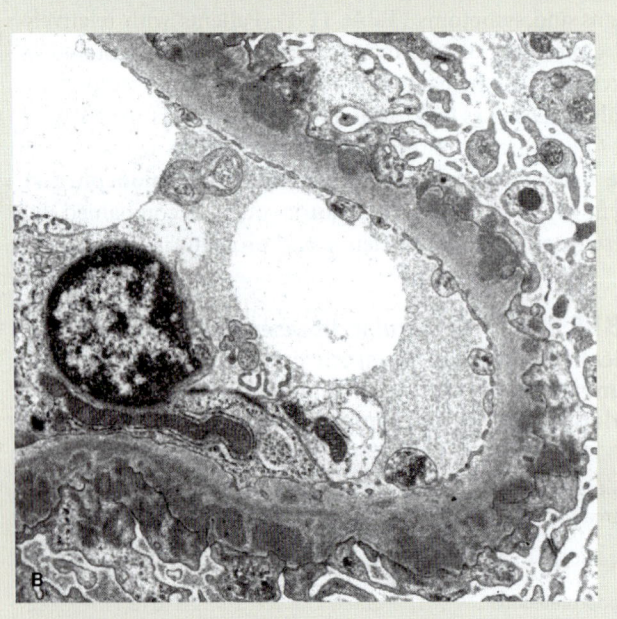

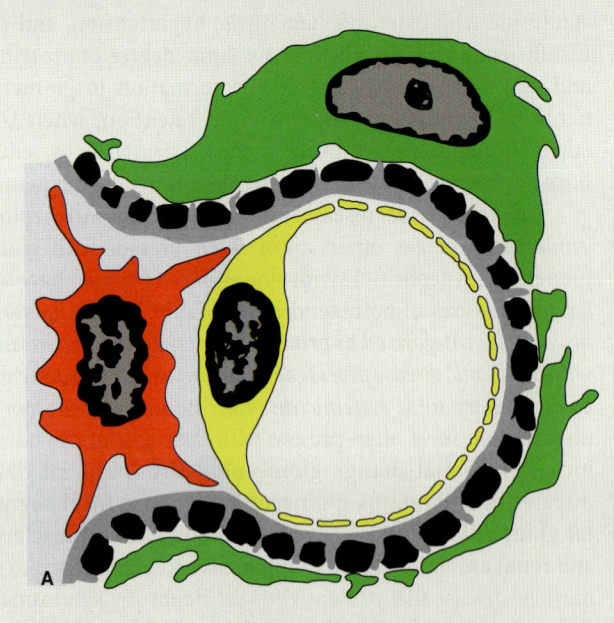

FIGURE 12-4 Diagram (A) and electron micrograph (B) of membranous glomerulopathy. Electron microscopic features of membranous glomerulopathy include numerous subepithelial electron-dense deposits that correspond to the immune complexes seen by immunofluorescence microscopy, and effacement of podocyte foot processes. Compare with Figure 12-2 (key as in Figure 12-2).

TABLE 12-2 Likelihood of different clinical presentations of glomerular diseases.

	Nephrotic Syndrome	Asymptomatic Hematuria or Proteinuria	Acute or Recurring GN	Rapidly Progressive GN
Minimal-change glomerulopathy	++++	o	o	o
FSGS	+++	++	o	o
Membranous GN	+++	+		
MPGN/DDD	+++	+	+++	+
Alport syndrome	o	+++	+++	o
Thin GBM lesion	o	++++	o	o
IgA nephropathy	+	+++	+++	+
Acute postinfectious GN		++++	o	o
Lupus GN		+	+++	++
ANCA GN		+	++	++++
Anti-GBM GN		o	+	++++

Membranous Glomerulopathy

By light microscopy, membranous glomerulopathy is characterized by thickening of capillary walls in the absence of increased glomerular cellularity (hypercellularity) (Figure 12-3A). By electron microscopy, the capillary wall thickening is seen to be caused by the deposition of electron dense immune complex aggregates in the subepithelial zone between podocytes and GBM (Figure 12-4A and B). There may be deposition of varying amounts of GBM material between and around the deposits. There is effacement of podocyte foot processes overlying the deposits. Immunofluorescence microscopy demonstrates granular staining of glomerular capillaries with antibodies specific for immunoglobulin, especially IgG (Figure 12-3B), and complement, including C3. The subepithelial immune complexes form in situ in the subepithelial zone and are composed of antibodies from the circulation and antigens derived either from podocytes or from the circulation.

Approximately 75% of patients with membranous glomerulopathy have immune complexes composed of autoantibodies directed against antiphospholipase A2 receptor proteins that are produced by podocytes. The autoantibodies reach the subepithelial zone from the plasma and bind to antigens released by podocytes to form the subepithelial immune complex deposits. Membranous glomerulopathy also can be caused by (secondary to) antigens derived from systemic sources including infections (e.g., hepatitis B), cancer (e.g., carcinoma), and drugs (e.g., penicillamine). Membranous glomerulopathy also can be one of many phenotypes of glomerular injury caused by systemic lupus erythematosus. The nature of circulating autoantibodies and antigens in lupus determines whether a patient will develop a membranous glomerulopathy or a more inflammatory form of lupus glomerulonephritis that will be discussed later.

Minimal-Change Glomerulopathy

Minimal-change glomerulopathy (minimal-change disease) has no discernible histologic abnormalities by light microscopy, or only minimal increase in mesangial matrix or cellularity. By immunofluorescence microscopy, there is no staining for immunoglobulins or complement. The only consistent pathologic abnormality is seen by electron microscopy and is extensive effacement of podocyte foot processes (Figure 12-5). Instead of multiple individual foot processes normally lined up along the urinary surface of capillary walls, there is a more continuous layer of cytoplasm on the urinary surface of capillary walls. Even though the podocyte cytoplasm appears more continuous after foot process effacement than when the foot processes are intact, the podocytes are much more permeable to the passage of protein. Normally, there is a slit membrane between each podocyte that has low permeability to proteins, especially more positively charged larger proteins. In nephrotic syndrome, these adherens-like junctions between adjacent podocytes have increased permeability. Any form of glomerular disease with substantial proteinuria will have foot process effacement. However, in minimal-change glomerulopathy, the foot process effacement is the only pathologic lesion with none of the features of other glomerular diseases that are described in this chapter. Thus, the pathologic diagnosis of minimal-change glomerulopathy is a diagnosis of exclusion.

Focal Segmental Glomerulosclerosis

In the context of glomerular disease, focal indicates that less than 50% of glomeruli have a histologic abnormality, whereas diffuse indicates that 50% or more of glomeruli have a histologic abnormality. Segmental indicates that only a portion of a glomerular

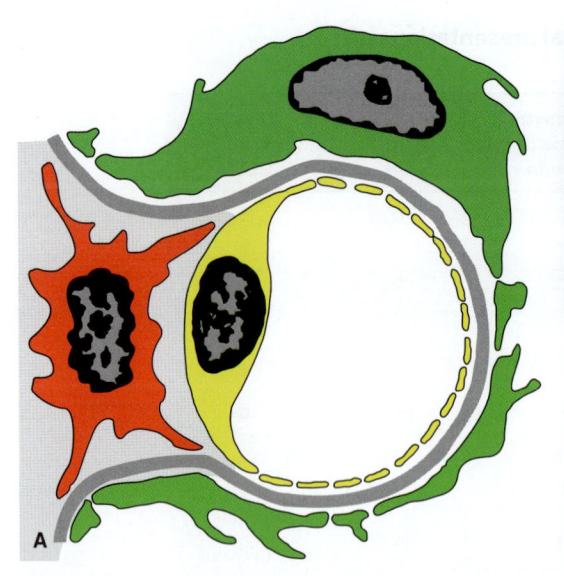

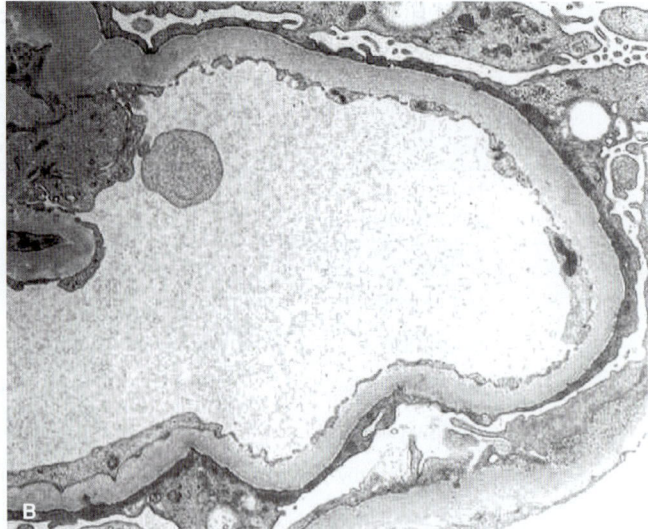

FIGURE 12-5 Diagram (A) and electron micrograph (B) of minimal-change glomerulopathy. Electron microscopic features of minimal-change glomerulopathy include effacement of podocyte foot processes in the absence of ultrastructural features of other diseases. Compare with Figure 12-2 (key as in Figure 12-2).

tuft has histologic injury, whereas global indicates that an entire glomerular tuft is injured. Thus, FSGS indicates that, at least at the beginning of the disease, only a portion of glomeruli have lesions by light microscopy and only a portion (segment) of the involved glomerular tufts have lesions. The term **sclerosis** indicates that there has been an accumulation of collagenous matrix at a site of injury. This is in essence a scar. In the setting of glomerular disease, the term sclerosis is used rather than fibrosis because the collagen is released by mesangial cells, endothelial cells, and podocytes rather than by fibroblasts.

FSGS is characterized by focal segmental glomerular consolidation and sclerosis (scarring) (Figure 12-6). Many different forms of injury result in localized glomerular scarring. Therefore, to diagnose FSGS, other glomerular diseases that cause glomerular scarring must be ruled out, for example, focal segmental glomerulonephritis that has caused segmental scarring (sclerosis). By immunofluorescence microscopy, there is no evidence of immune complex deposition, and by electron microscopy, there is foot process effacement but no immune complex dense deposits. *FSGS has many different etiologies and pathogenic mechanisms.* As with other glomerular diseases, FSGS may occur as a primary (idiopathic) disease confined to the kidney, or can be secondary to a systemic process or a recognized etiology (Table 12-3).

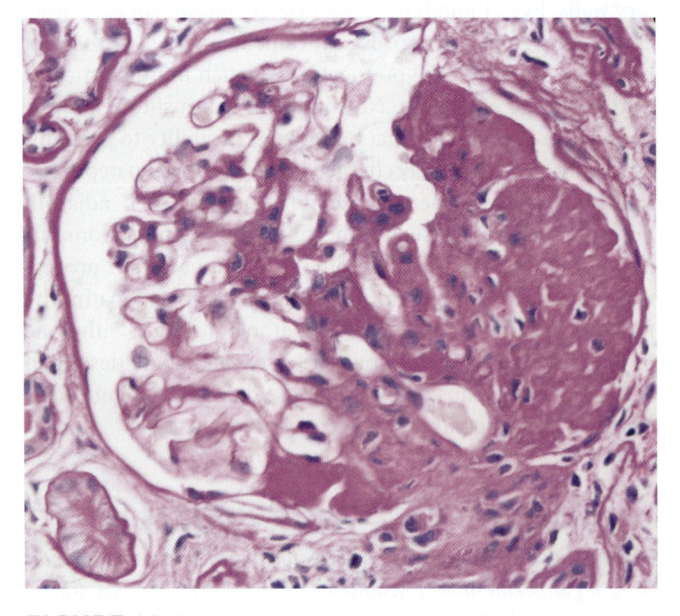

FIGURE 12-6 Focal segmental glomerulosclerosis. Glomerulus with segmental sclerosis (PAS stain). Compare with Figure 12-1.

TABLE 12-3 FSGS categories based on etiology and pathogenesis.

PRIMARY (IDIOPATHIC) FSGS
SECONDARY FSGS
VIRUS-ASSOCIATED
HIV-1 ("HIV-associated nephropathy")
Parvovirus B-19
FAMILIAL FSGS
Mutations in α-actinin 4 gene
Mutations in NPHS2 gene for podocin
Mutations in TRPC6 gene for a cation channel
DRUG TOXICITY
Heroin ("Heroin nephropathy")
Pamidronate
Interferon
MEDIATED BY ADAPTIVE STRUCTURAL RESPONSES
Reduced renal mass
Obesity
Cyanotic congenital heart disease
Sickle cell anemia

IN TRANSLATION
Pathogenesis and Etiology of Focal Segmental Glomerulosclerosis

FSGS is pathologically, etiologically, pathogenetically, and clinically very heterogeneous (Table 12-3). Most FSGS is idiopathic with no known cause. However, in recent years a number of etiologies have been identified. The podocyte is the primary target of injury in some patients. This has been clearly demonstrated in patients with hereditary forms of FSGS who have mutations in genes that produce podocyte proteins, for example, nephrin, which is a major component of podocyte slit membranes. Overwork of glomeruli also can cause FSGS. One mechanism for overwork is compensatory hypertrophy in response to reduced renal tissue, for example, if one kidney and a portion of the other kidney are removed for cancer. The residual renal tissue undergoes hypertrophy and is at risk of development of focal FSGS. Fortunately, removal of one kidney is not sufficient to increase the risk of FSGS in the contralateral kidney, which allows living donors to provide kidneys for transplantation. Another mechanism for glomerular overwork is marked obesity, which results in compensatory glomerular hypertrophy and risk of development for FSGS. *Not surprisingly, there is a marked increase in obesity-associated proteinuria and FSGS in parallel with the increasing incidence of obesity.*

Diabetic Glomerulosclerosis

Diabetic glomerulosclerosis underlies the clinical syndrome of **diabetic nephropathy**, which is characterized by proteinuria, progressive decline in glomerular filtration rate and hypertension. Early mild diabetic glomerulosclerosis produces only very low levels of asymptomatic albuminuria (**microalbuminuria**). As diabetic glomerulosclerosis progresses, proteinuria becomes more severe and can reach nephrotic range. With further progression, there is loss of renal function.

The early pathologic lesion of diabetic glomerulosclerosis is thickening of GBMs and increase in mesangial matrix that can be so mild that it is only identifiable by electron microscopy (**Figure 12-7**). With progression, there is more and more mesangial matrix increase and thickening of GBMs. Eventually, the increase in mesangial matrix results in the formation of well-defined nodules called **Kimmelstiel–Wilson nodules** that can be seen by light microscopy (**Figure 12-8**). Similar glomerular changes occur in patients with type I and type II diabetes mellitus, although the glomerular disease in type II diabetes mellitus is more often complicated by changes of hypertensive injury in addition to the diabetic changes.

Amyloidosis and Monoclonal Immunoglobulin Deposition Disease

The clinical differential diagnosis in any patient with the nephrotic syndrome who has reached 60 years of age should include amyloidosis. *Amyloidosis results from the accumulation of monotypic proteins in tissue in a unique configuration that results in the formation of randomly arranged fibrils.* Different types of amyloid are caused by more than 20 different

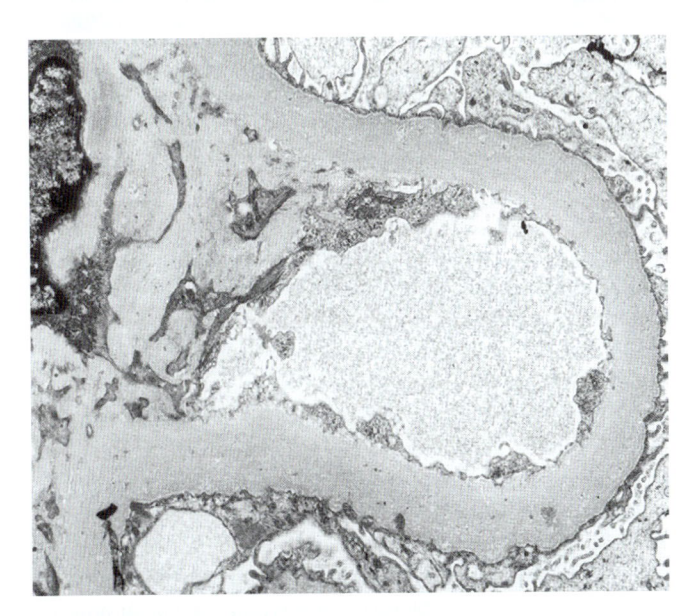

FIGURE 12-7 **Diabetic glomerulosclerosis.** Electron micrograph showing markedly thickened GBM and increased mesangial matrix. Compare with Figure 12-2B.

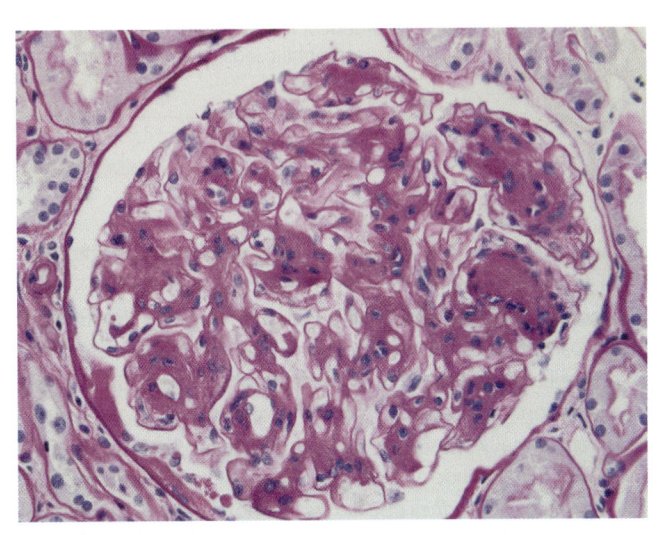

FIGURE 12-8 **Diabetic glomerulosclerosis.** Light microscopy showing segmental increase in mesangial matrix, including Kimmelstiel–Wilson nodules. Compare with Figure 12-1.

CASE 12-2

A 65-year-old Caucasian male developed periorbital edema and swollen ankles. His primary care physician confirmed the edema. Blood pressure was 155/97 mmHg. Point-of-care laboratory testing in the office revealed 4+ protein and 1+ hematuria in the urine. He was referred to a nephrologists and further evaluation confirmed the edema and hypertension. Laboratory findings included 4+ proteinuria with urine protein to creatinine ratio 4.9, trace hematuria with <5 dysmorphic RBCs/hpf, 5–10 WBC/hpf, serum creatinine 3.2 mg/dL, serum albumin 3.4 g/dL, serum cholesterol 320 mg/dL, and normal C3 and C4. Serum and urine protein electrophoresis and immunofixation revealed monoclonal IgG lambda. Serum-free lambda/kappa/ light chain ratio was markedly elevated. A bone marrow biopsy revealed slightly increased plasma cells but was not definitive for multiple myeloma.

A renal biopsy demonstrated amyloid light chain (AL) amyloidosis composed of lambda light chains, but no light chain cast nephropathy (Figures 12-9 and 12-10).

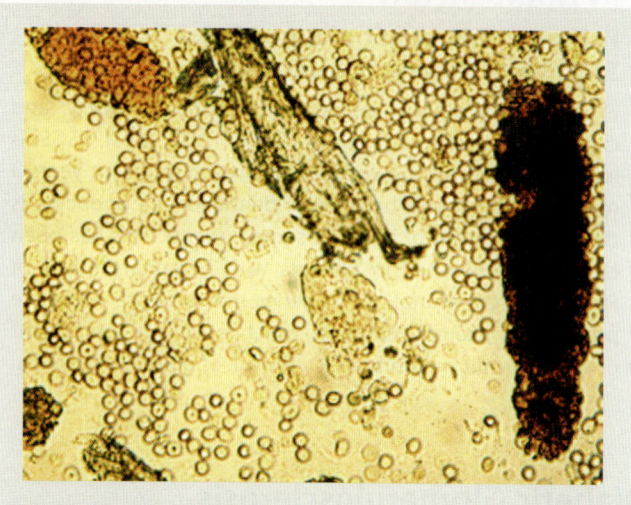

FIGURE 12-10 RBC casts. Microscopic examination of urine demonstrating RBC casts (upper left and right).

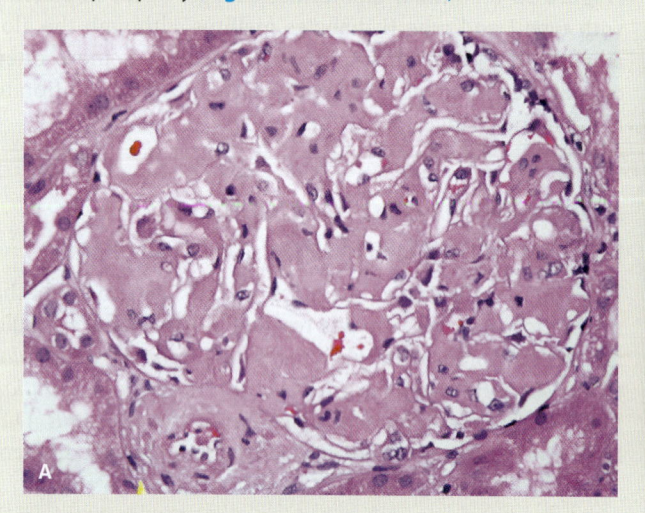

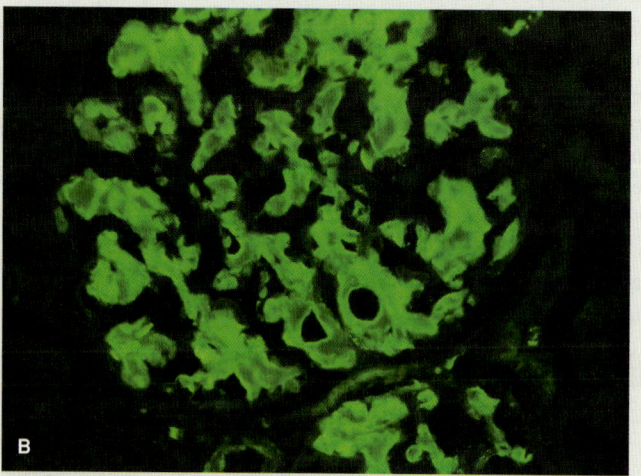

FIGURE 12-9 AL amyloidosis. By light microscopy, amyloidosis causes replacement of normal glomerular architecture by amorphous acidophilic (eosinophilic) material (A, hematoxylin and eosin stain, H&E stain). Immunofluorescence microscopy of AL amyloid demonstrates deposits of monoclonal immunoglobulin light chains (B, anti-lambda).

IN TRANSLATION
Monoclonal Immunoglobulin Pathogenesis

AL amyloid is caused by a B-cell dyscrasia that produces large amounts of monoclonal light chains resulting in amyloid deposits if the proteins have amyloidogenic biophysical properties. Lambda light chains cause AL amyloidosis more often than kappa light chains. Rare cases of amyloidosis are caused by abnormally truncated monoclonal heavy chains (AH amyloid). *Not all monoclonal immunoglobulins have the same capability of causing kidney disease.* As just noted, some monoclonal immunoglobulins cause AL amyloidosis with fibrillary deposits, whereas others cause a form of glomerular monoclonal immunoglobulin deposition with granular deposits (usually caused by kappa light chains), cast formation in tubular lumens resulting in acute tubular epithelial injury, accumulate in the cytoplasm of proximal tubular epithelial cells resulting in a **tubulopathy**, and are not associated with any kidney disease. There is evidence from experimental animal studies and tissue culture studies that different monoclonal immunoglobulins have different pathogenic capabilities based on as yet poorly understood differences in their biophysical characteristics. Because of this pathogenic variability, the differential diagnosis in a patient with kidney disease associated with monoclonal immunoglobulins in the blood or urine is broader than AL amyloidosis alone.

proteins. The two types of amyloid that most often cause glomerular disease are AL amyloid composed of immunoglobulin light chains and AA amyloid composed of amyloid A protein. In developed countries, most amyloid that causes kidney disease is AL amyloid, whereas, in developing or undeveloped countries, most amyloid that causes kidney disease is AA amyloid. The higher frequency of AA amyloidosis is the result of chronic inflammatory and infectious diseases that are more prevalent in these settings.

Asymptomatic Hematuria and Nephritic Syndrome

The glomerular diseases discussed thus far do not have overt inflammatory changes with an obvious influx of inflammatory cells. This is in contrast to glomerular diseases that usually present with more glomerulonephritic clinical features including prominent hematuria, and varying degrees of hypertension and renal insufficiency, and usually proteinuric of <3 g/day. The most characteristic feature of the glomerulonephritic (nephritic) syndrome is the presence of glomerular hematuria (Table 12-1). Asymptomatic hematuria without other clinical manifestations of glomerular disease tends to occur in mild or early glomerular disease.

More than 90% of all patients who have hematuria do not have glomerular hematuria. Most hematuria is the result of urinary tract disease and not glomerulonephritis. Common causes of urinary tract hematuria are urinary bladder infection, urethritis, prostatitis, urolithiasis, nephrolithiasis, and urinary tract neoplasms. Urinary tract hemorrhage other than glomerular hemorrhage is usually red or pink grossly, and microscopic examination during urinalysis demonstrates predominantly round RBCs often with a normal concave appearance. When it can be seen grossly, glomerular hematuria is tea-colored or coke-colored and by urinalysis there are many dysmorphic RBCs that have multiple blebs on the surface sometimes looking like Mickey Mouse ears. Another very distinct feature of glomerular hematuria is the presence of RBC casts in the urine that results from the accumulation of RBCs in the lumens of distal tubules where they become embedded **Tamm–Horsfall protein** to form a cylindrical cast that spills into the urine (Figure 12-10). The presence of these casts indicates that the hemorrhage has come from high up in the nephrons and not from the urothelial surface. If hematuria is caused by glomerulonephritis, there is almost always some degree of proteinuria, although this is usually less than nephrotic range (less than 3g/24 hours). Urologic hematuria is not accompanied by significant proteinuria. Depending on the nature of the underlying glomerular disease, glomerular hematuria may occur in the setting of

1. Asymptomatic hematuria
2. One episode of acute glomerulonephritis with or without acute renal failure (ARF)
3. Recurring episodes of acute glomerulonephritis
4. RPGN with rapid renal failure
5. Progressive chronic renal failure

TABLE 12-4 Likelihood of different clinical presentations in patients with different histopathologic patterns of antibody-mediated glomerulonephritis (GN).

	Asymptomatic Hematuria	Acute or Recurring GN	Rapidly Progressive GN
No lesion by light microscopy	++++	0	0
Mesangioproliferative GN	+++	+++	+
Proliferative GN	+	+++	+
Crescentic GN	+	++	++++

Pathologically, inflammatory glomerular diseases (glomerulonephritides) typically have glomerular hypercellularity resulting from both influx of inflammatory cells, such as neutrophils, monocytes, and macrophages, and proliferation of glomerular cells, including mesangial cells, endothelial cells, and epithelial cells.

Pathologic diagnosis of glomerular disease required two components. One component is based on the pattern and severity of glomerular injury and is designated by descriptive terms such as mesangioproliferative glomerulonephritis, proliferative glomerulonephritis, necrotizing glomerulonephritis, and crescentic glomerulonephritis. The clinical presentation is influenced by the pattern of glomerular injury (Table 12-4). A second component of the diagnosis indicates the etiology or pathogenesis of the glomerular disease and includes terms such as IgA nephropathy, lupus glomerulonephritis, anti-GBM glomerulonephritis and antineutrophil cytoplasmic autoantibody (ANCA) glomerulonephritis. The etiologic and pathogenic category of glomerular disease correlates with the propensity to cause a certain pattern of glomerular injury, which in turn influences the likelihood of a particular clinical presentation (Table 12-2).

Lupus Glomerulonephritis

Systemic lupus erythematosus is an autoimmune disease that most often affects young African-American women but may occur in patients of any age or race. Virtually any organ of the body can be affected. The kidneys are one of the most frequent sites of injury and renal disease is a major cause of morbidity and mortality.

Lupus glomerulonephritis is caused by glomerular localization of immune complex deposits composed of autoantibodies of multiple specificities bound to the respective autoantigens and associated with activated complement components.

Lupus glomerulonephritis has many different clinical presentations and severities determined by the nature,

IN TRANSLATION

Pathogenesis of Antibody-Mediated Glomerulonephritis

The inflammation that causes most forms of glomerulonephritis is mediated by antibodies. Antibody-mediated glomerulonephritis can be divided into

1. Immune complex-mediated glomerulonephritis
2. Antiglomerular basement membrane antibody (anti-GBM)-mediated glomerulonephritis
3. ANCA-mediated glomerulonephritis

These categories can be distinguished by immunofluorescence microscopy (Figure 12-11), because

1. Immune complex-mediated glomerulonephritis has prominent granular deposits of immunoglobulin and complement in glomerular capillaries or mesangium or both (Figure 12-11A, left panel)
2. Anti-GBM disease has linear staining of GBMs for immunoglobulin (Figure 12-11B, middle panel)
3. ANCA-mediated glomerulonephritis has circulating ANCA with little or no immunoglobulin staining in glomeruli (Figure 12-11C, right panel)

Immune complexes that deposit or form in situ in glomeruli mediate inflammation by activating complement, and by activating leukocytes via Fc gamma receptor engagement. There are multiple categories of immune complex-mediated glomerulonephritis characterized by different locations and different compositions of the immune complexes, including membranoproliferative glomerulonephritis (MPGN), IgA nephropathy, postinfectious glomerulonephritis, lupus glomerulonephritis, and many others.

Anti-GBM antibodies bind directly to GBMs, in essence forming immune complexes in situ, and mediate inflammation by activating complement, and by activating leukocytes via Fc gamma receptor engagement.

ANCAs mediate inflammation by binding to target antigens (proteinase-3 or myeloperoxidase) that are displayed at the surface of circulating neutrophils causing them to adhere to small vessels (such as glomerular capillaries), undergo activation, and release destructive enzymes and oxygen radicals that injure vessel walls.

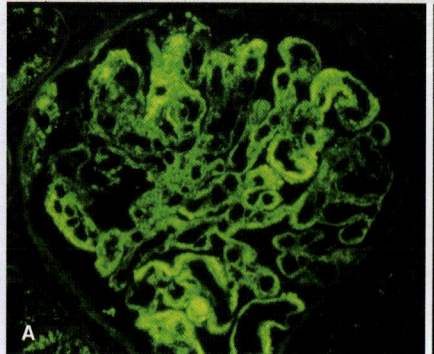

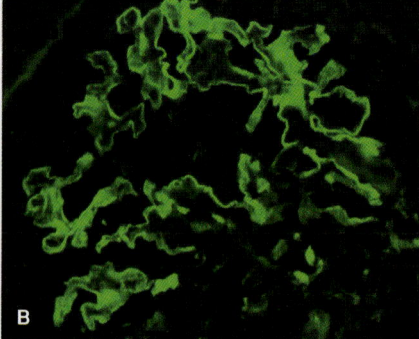

FIGURE 12-11 By immunofluorescence microscopy, immune complex-mediated glomerulonephritis has prominent granular deposits of immunoglobulin and complement in glomerular capillaries or mesangium or both (**A**, left panel), anti-GBM disease has linear staining of GBMs for immunoglobulin (**B**, middle panel), and ANCA-mediated glomerulonephritis has circulating ANCA with little or no immunoglobulin staining in glomeruli (**C**, right panel) (immunofluorescence with anti-IgG).

WHAT WE DO

Pathologic Patterns of Glomerulonephritis: Proliferative, Necrotizing, Crescentic, and Sclerosing Glomerulonephritis

The pathologic diagnosis of glomerulonephritis includes both a descriptive term that characterizes the nature and severity of the histopathologic injury and a designation that indicates either the immunopathogenesis or etiology of the glomerulonephritis. The possible histopathologic patterns of glomerulonephritis are similar in all pathogenic categories; however, different pathogenic categories have different likelihoods of causing one type of histologic lesion versus another. The histopathologic patterns of injury in glomerulonephritis are determined by the severity of injury, the type of injury, and also the temporal stage of the disease with respect to acuity, chronicity, progression, and resolution.

As shown in Table 12-4, the clinical manifestations of glomerular disease correlate to a degree with the pattern of injury, and some categories of glomerulonephritis are more likely to produce particular patterns of glomerular injury rather than others. The crescentic glomerulonephritis category of injury that often is accompanied by RPGN clinically is important to recognize quickly and to diagnose accurately because timely and aggressive institution of immunosuppressive therapy is critically important for long-term preservation of renal function and optimum patient outcome.

No Lesion by Light Microscopy: With mild glomerular injury, immunofluorescence and electron microscopy may reveal a pathogenic process that is not detectable by light microscopy (i.e., glomeruli look normal by light microscopy). In this circumstance, patients usually have very mild clinical manifestations of glomerular disease such as asymptomatic hematuria, asymptomatic proteinuria or both.

Mesangioproliferative Glomerulonephritis (Figure 12-12A): Another relatively mild expression of glomerular injury is the presence of mesangial hypercellularity in the absence of other glomerular lesions. Mild mesangioproliferative glomerulonephritis may manifest with asymptomatic hematuria or proteinuria, or may have more overt clinical features of glomerulonephritis.

Proliferative Glomerulonephritis (Figure 12-12B, 12C): Overt inflammation of glomeruli results not only in mesangial hypercellularity but also proliferation of endothelial cells and influx of leukocytes including monocytes, macrophages, and neutrophils. This pattern of injury is referred to as endocapillary proliferative glomerulonephritis or simply proliferative glomerulonephritis. However, the term "proliferative" in this context should be understood to refer to hypercellularity

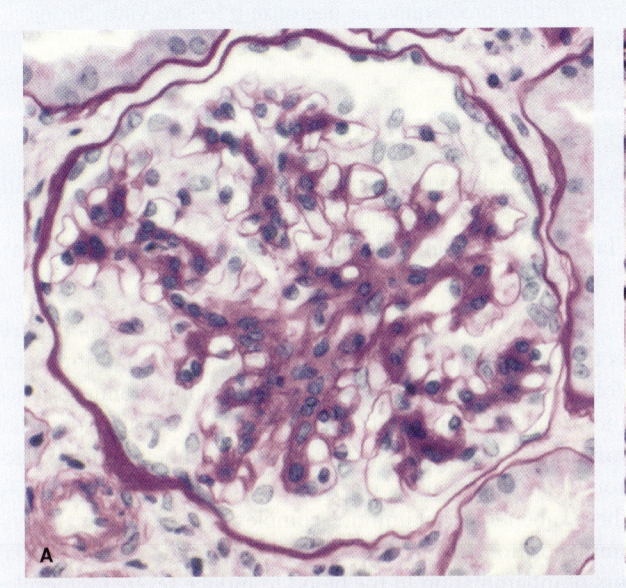

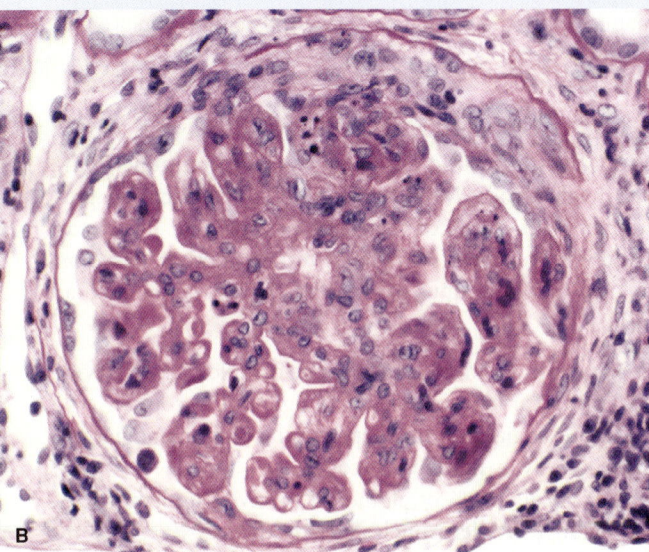

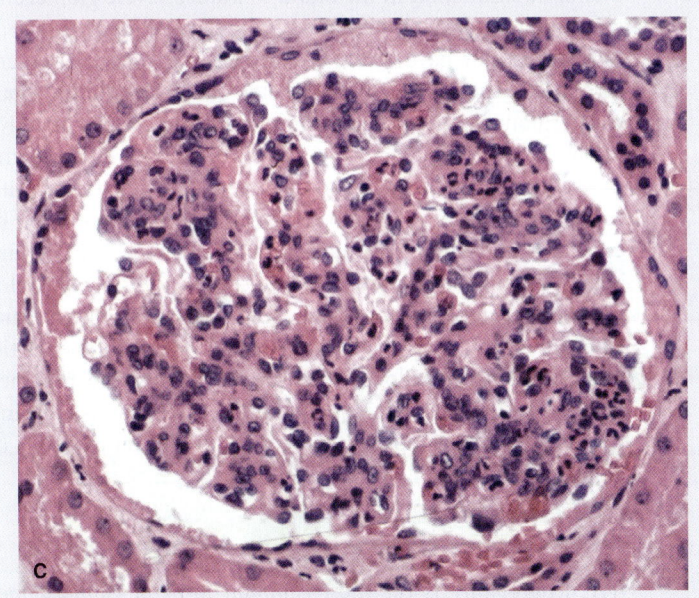

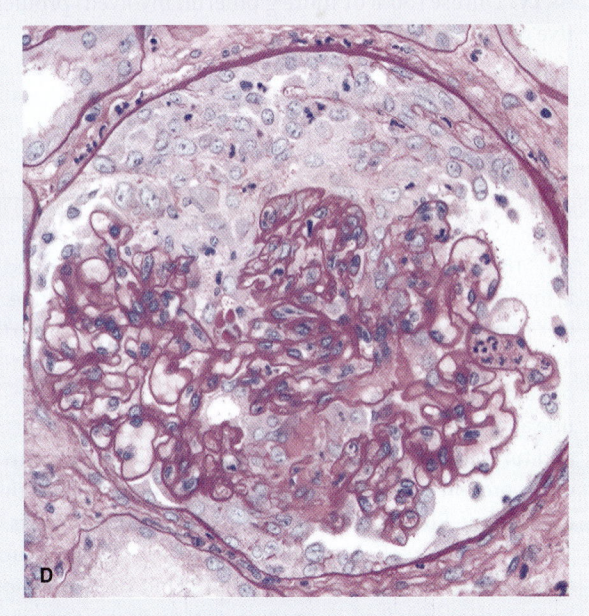

FIGURE 12-12 Common histopathologic patterns of glomerular inflammatory. (A) IgA nephropathy with mesangioproliferative glomerulonephritis with mesangial hypercellularity (PAS stain). (B) Proliferative (class IV) lupus glomerulonephritis with complex endocapillary hypercellularity caused by proliferation of mesangial and endothelial cells and influx of leukocytes, thick capillary walls caused by immune complex deposition, and a small cellular crescent (extracapillary hypercellularity) 11:00 to 3:00 (PAS stain). (C) Acute postinfectious (post-streptococcal) glomerulonephritis with numerous polymorphonuclear leukocytes in capillary lumens (H&E stain). (D) ANCA crescentic glomerulonephritis with a large cellular crescent from 10:00 to 2:00 composed predominantly of proliferating epithelial cells (PAS stain).

caused not only by proliferative of glomerular cells but also to influx of leukocytes.

Crescentic Glomerulonephritis (Figure 12-12D): Extensive inflammation can result in the rupture of capillary walls with spillage of inflammatory mediators into Bowman space where they incite a cellular reaction with both the proliferation of epithelial cells and the influx of leukocytes including macrophages. This cellular reaction within Bowman cell is called a crescent, because times the section through this cellular lesion has the shape of a crescent when looked at in two dimensions. Crescent formation is not specific for a specific etiology or pathogenic mechanism, but rather is a marker for severe glomerular inflammatory injury. Severe inflammatory injury also can produce segmental necrosis in glomeruli especially in the most aggressive forms of glomerulonephritis, anti-GBM glomerulonephritis, and ANCA glomerulonephritis.

Chronic Glomerulonephritis: Any form of glomerular disease can progress to varying degrees of glomerular scarring (sclerosis). Advanced diffuse global glomerular sclerosis is characteristic of end-stage kidney disease secondary to glomerulonephritis. All of the patterns of glomerular injury can occur as focal or diffuse, and segmental or global lesions. In patients who have had recurring bouts of active glomerular injury with intervening intervals of relative quiescence will have an admixture of acute proliferative or necrotizing lesions with chronic sclerotic lesions.

amount, and distribution of nephritogenic immune complexes in glomeruli. Most histopathologic patterns of glomerulonephritis can occur in lupus patients and there may be evolution over time from one pattern to another. Based on pathologic findings, lupus glomerulonephritis is classified as follows:

Class I: Exclusively mesangial immune complex deposits with no glomerular lesion observed by light microscopy.
Class II: Mesangial immune deposits and only mesangial hypercellularity by light microscopy.
Class III: Focal (<50% of glomeruli involved) inflammatory proliferative or sclerosing lesions.
Class IV: Diffuse (50% or more glomeruli involved) proliferative or sclerosing lesions.
Class V: Predominantly membranous glomerulopathy with numerous subepithelial immune complex deposits.
Class VI: More than 90% global glomerular sclerotic indicating end-stage kidney disease.

Patients with class III and class IV lupus glomerulonephritis typically have extensive glomerular deposition of immunoglobulin and complement detected by immunofluorescence microscopy (Figure 12-11A), and numerous subendothelial immune complex deposits that appear as subendothelial electron dense material by electron microscopy (**Figure 12-13**). These subendothelial immune complex deposits are in an optimum position to interact with humoral and cellular mediators of inflammation in the blood to induce severe glomerular inflammation. Patients with class III or class IV lupus glomerulonephritis may have severe enough disease to cause crescent formation. The severity (Class) helps guide therapy for lupus glomerulonephritis. Patients who have the most severe active inflammatory disease (active Class III or Class IV) receive the most aggressive immunosuppressive therapy. Patients with active lupus glomerulonephritis usually have consumption of complement resulting in hypocomplementemia. MPGN and acute postinfectious glomerulonephritis as well as lupus glomerulonephritis are associated with hypocomplementemia, whereas IgA nephropathy, anti-GBM glomerulonephritis, and ANCA glomerulonephritis are not. Thus, the presence or absence of hypocomplementemia is useful in establishing the differential diagnosis in patients with clinical evidence of glomerulonephritis.

IgA Nephropathy and IgA Vasculitis

IgA nephropathy is the most common form of glomerulonephritis in industrialized countries. In less developed countries, proliferative and MPGN caused by acute or chronic infections are more common. *The defining feature of IgA nephropathy is the presence of IgA-dominant or IgA co-dominant mesangial immune deposits in a renal biopsy specimen*, that is, immunofluorescence microscopy demonstrating that staining for IgA is more intense, or at least as intense as staining for IgG and

CASE 12-3

An 18-year-old African-American female developed arthralgias, a rash on her cheeks, and tea-colored urine. Her primary care physician confirmed the malar rash and joint tenderness. Blood pressure was 145/91 mmHg. Point-of-care laboratory testing in the office revealed 3+ proteinuria and 4+ hematuria. She was referred to a nephrologists and further evaluation demonstrated 4+ proteinuria with urine protein to creatinine ratio 2.6, 4+ hematuria with dysmorphic RBCs too numerous to count and RBC casts, 10–20 WBC/hpf, serum creatinine 3.2 mg/dL, serum albumin 3.5 g/dL, and serum cholesterol 198 mg/dL. Serologic testing demonstrated a positive anti-nuclear antibody assay (ANA) at a titer of 1:320, positive anti-DNA, positive anti-Sm, serum C3 65, and serum C4 8.

A renal biopsy was performed and was diagnostic for diffuse proliferative lupus glomerulonephritis (class IV lupus glomerulonephritis) (Figure 12-12B).

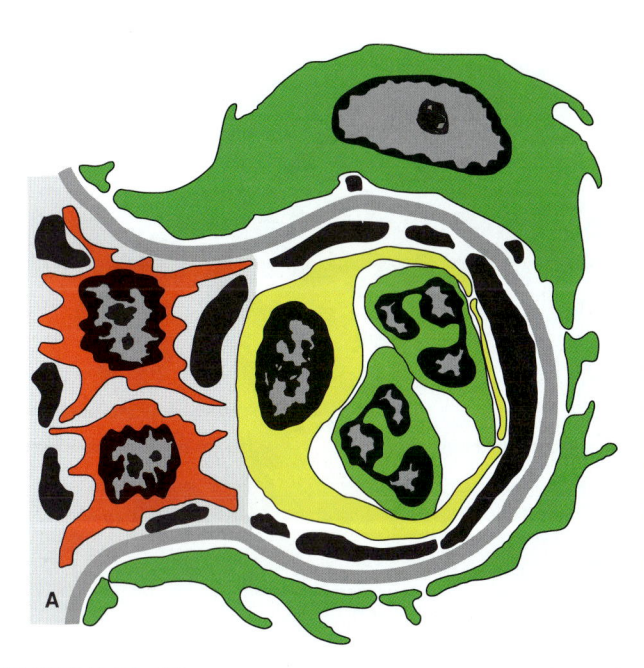

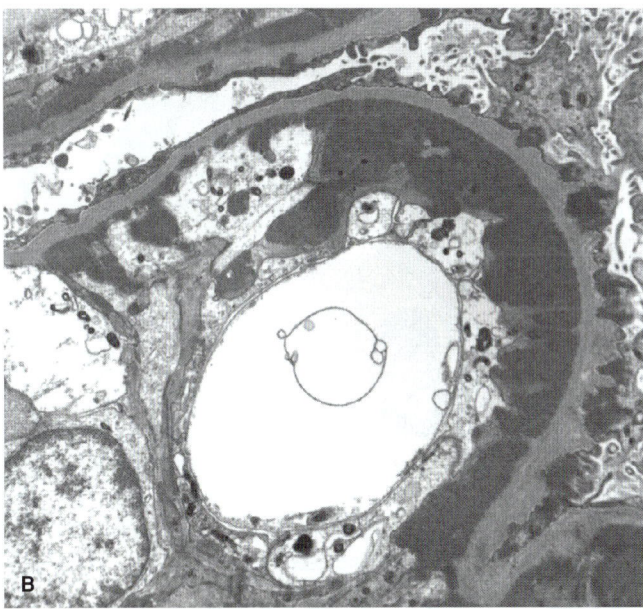

FIGURE 12-13 Diagram (A) and electron micrograph (B) of proliferative lupus glomerulonephritis. By electron microscopy, diffuse proliferative (class IV) lupus glomerulonephritis has extensive subendothelial as well as mesangial and scattered subepithelial immune complex electron dense deposits. Compare with Figure 12-2 (key as in Figure 12-2).

IgM (Figure 12-14). There also is substantial staining for C3 indicating that complement activation is playing a role in the pathogenesis of the glomerular injury.

The clinical presentation of patients with IgA nephropathy can be extremely varied depending on the nature of the underlying glomerular lesions. Similar to lupus glomerulonephritis, by light microscopy, IgA nephropathy may have no discernible glomerular changes, mesangioproliferative changes, focal or diffuse proliferative changes, and varying degrees of glomerular sclerosis. Severe cases may have crescent formation. By electron microscopy, the most frequent finding is mesangial dense deposits corresponding to the IgA-dominant immune deposits (Figure 12-15). Severe cases often have at least some capillary wall dense deposits.

A characteristic presentation is onset of features of glomerulonephritis at the same time as the onset of an upper

CASE 12-4

An 18-year-old Caucasian male developed pharyngitis and fever, and the following day noticed that his urine was very dark (tea-colored). His primary care physician confirmed the fever and pharyngitis, and noted that there was no rash. The patient gave a history of noticing transient dark urine in the past. There was no family history of renal disease. Blood pressure was 140/88 mmHg. Point-of-care laboratory testing in the office revealed 2+ proteinuria and 3+ hematuria. He was referred to a nephrologists and further evaluation demonstrated 2+ proteinuria with urine protein to creatinine ratio 1.8, 3+ hematuria with >50 dysmorphic RBC/hpf, serum creatinine 1.7 mg/dL, serum albumin 4.1 g/dL, and serum cholesterol 187 mg/dL. Serologic testing demonstrated a negative ANA, negative anti-DNA, serum C3 130, serum C4 29, negative ANCA, and normal ASO titer.

A renal biopsy was performed and was diagnostic for IgA nephropathy (Figures 12-14 and 12-15).

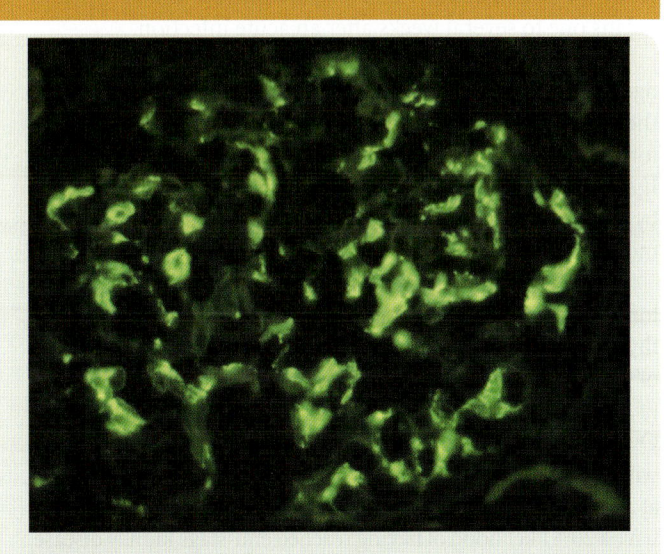

FIGURE 12-14 IgA nephropathy. Immunofluorescence microscopy demonstrating intense mesangial staining for IgA, but no staining of capillary walls. Compare with Figure 12-3B, which has capillary wall staining.

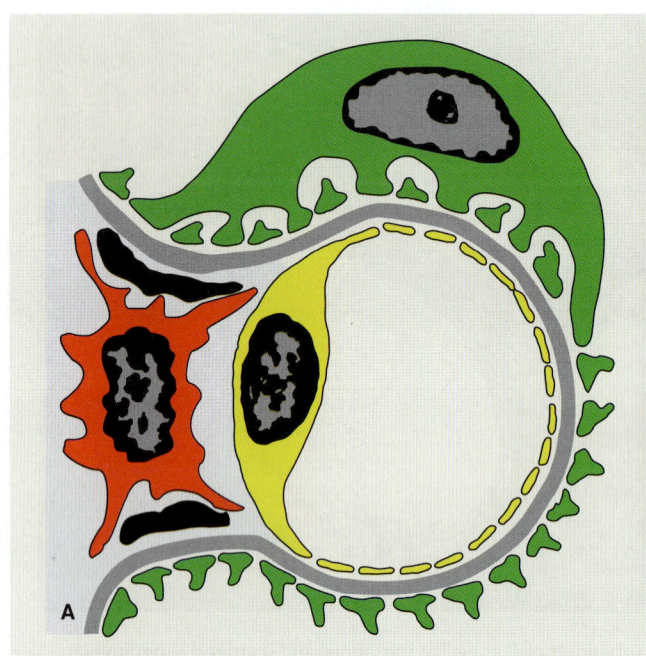

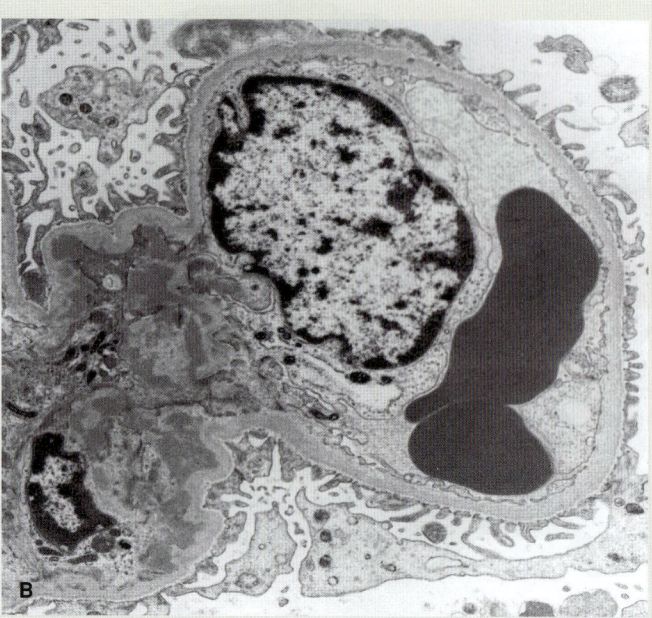

FIGURE 12-15 **Diagram (A) and electron micrograph (B) of mesangial dense deposits.** A specimen with mesangial staining for immune deposits by immunofluorescence microscopy showing mesangial electron dense deposits but no capillary wall dense deposits by electron microscopy. This can be seen with IgA nephropathy, lupus glomerulonephritis (class I and II), and other immune complex-mediated glomerulonephritis (key as in Figure 12-2).

respiratory tract infection. For example, a patient may develop a pharyngitis and at the same time will notice discoloration of the urine that is found to be glomerular hematuria, usually accompanied by other features of glomerulonephritis such as subnephrotic proteinuria, hypertension, and renal insufficiency. This presentation is called synpharyngitic (syn, with or together) and is distinct from the postpharyngitic presentation of postinfectious glomerulonephritis, which typically begins one to several weeks after an acute infection.

IgA nephropathy may be diagnosed as a result of the recognition of glomerular hematuria in asymptomatic patients at the time of a routine physical examination or an examination for insurance or induction into the military. In this setting, IgA nephropathy and thin basement membrane lesion caused by a genetic abnormality in GBM collagen are the most commonly identified glomerular diseases at the time of biopsy.

Although synpharyngitic glomerulonephritis and asymptomatic hematuria are common presentations for IgA nephropathy, patients may present with any of the clinical manifestations of glomerular disease including isolated acute glomerulonephritis, RPGN, or indolent progressive chronic glomerulonephritis. Overall, the outcome of IgA nephropathy is extremely variable with the risk of developing advanced renal insufficiency accruing at approximately 1% per year, thus after 20 years a patient would have a 20% likelihood of having reached end-stage kidney disease.

IgA nephropathy usually occurs as a renal limited process but can occur as a component of a systemic small vessel vasculitis, IgA vasculitis (**Henoch–Schönlein purpura**). Patients with IgA vasculitis often present with lower extremity purpura that results from IgA-dominant immune complexes localizing within small dermal vessels and causing vascular inflammation and hemorrhage. Abdominal pain caused by small vessel vasculitis in the gut and arthralgias also is a frequent manifestation of IgA vasculitis. IgA vasculitis is more common in children than adults and the initial clinical episode usually is self-limited, although some patients have persistent and eventually progressive glomerular disease.

Acute Postinfectious Glomerulonephritis

Acute postinfectious glomerulonephritis is characterized by the acute onset of clinical features of glomerulonephritis approximately 1–2 weeks following the onset of an acute infectious process, most often either bacterial pharyngitis or bacterial pyoderma. Streptococcal or staphylococcal infections are the most frequent etiologies. The pathogenic mechanism involves either the generation of nephritogenic immune complexes containing antigens derived from the infectious pathogen or the release of complement activating factors by the infectious pathogen that result in the accumulation of activated complement components within glomeruli, which mediated recruitment of inflammatory cells, especially polymorphonuclear leukocytes.

In the acute phase of the disease, the characteristic histopathologic finding is marked glomerular hypercellularity caused predominantly by the influx of numerous polymorphonuclear neutrophils (Figure 12-12C). Immunofluorescence microscopy demonstrates coarsely granular immune

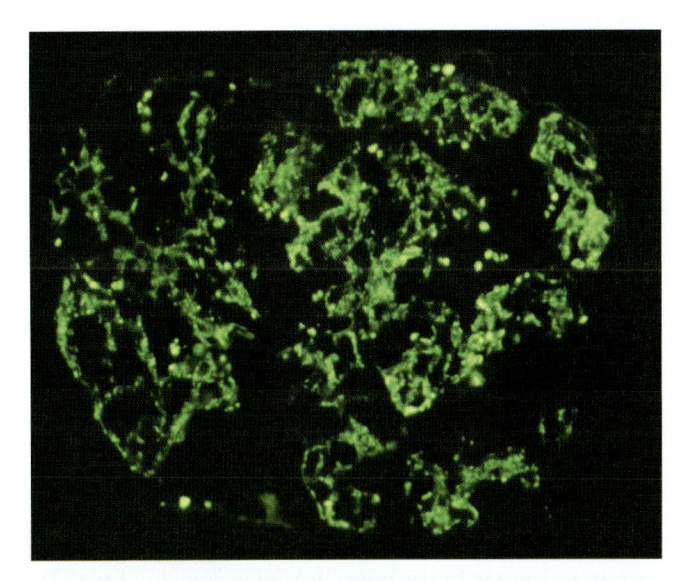

FIGURE 12-16 Acute postinfectious glomerulonephritis. Coarsely granular capillary wall and mesangial staining for C3.

deposits that staining predominantly for C3 (Figure 12-16). By electron microscopy, the coarsely granular immune deposits correspond to variably sized subepithelial dense deposits, some of which have a hump-like appearance (Figure 12-17). Subendothelial and mesangial electron dense deposits also occur and are probably more important in mediating the inflammation. Acute postinfectious glomerulonephritis usually is self-limited. Greater than 90% of patients have complete resolution within weeks to months with no subsequent adverse effects.

Membranoproliferative Glomerulonephritis

MPGN is a category of inflammatory glomerular disease that can present clinically either as nephrotic syndrome or glomerulonephritic syndrome or a mixed nephrotic and glomerulonephritic features. A laboratory finding that increases the likelihood of MPGN in a patient with glomerular disease is the presence of hypocomplementemia, especially a reduction in C3 without a comparable reduction in C4. Other glomerular diseases that have hypocomplementemia include acute postinfectious glomerulonephritis and lupus nephritis, whereas glomerular diseases that do not have a reduction in C3 or C4 are IgA nephropathy, anti-GBM glomerulonephritis, and ANCA glomerulonephritis.

By light microscopy, MPGN is characterized by thick capillary walls and by glomerular hypercellularity (Figure 12-18). The thick capillary walls result from the deposition of either immune complexes or activated complement proteins and the resultant matrix and cellular remodeling induced by these deposits. The hypercellularity results from proliferative of glomerular cells, especially mesangial cells, as well as the influx of leukocytes, especially monocytes and macrophages.

There are two major variants of MPGN:

1. Immune complex MPGN
2. C3 glomerulopathy MPGN.

In both variants, the pathogenic mechanism involves the activation of complement within glomeruli resulting in the mediation of inflammation, including the influx of

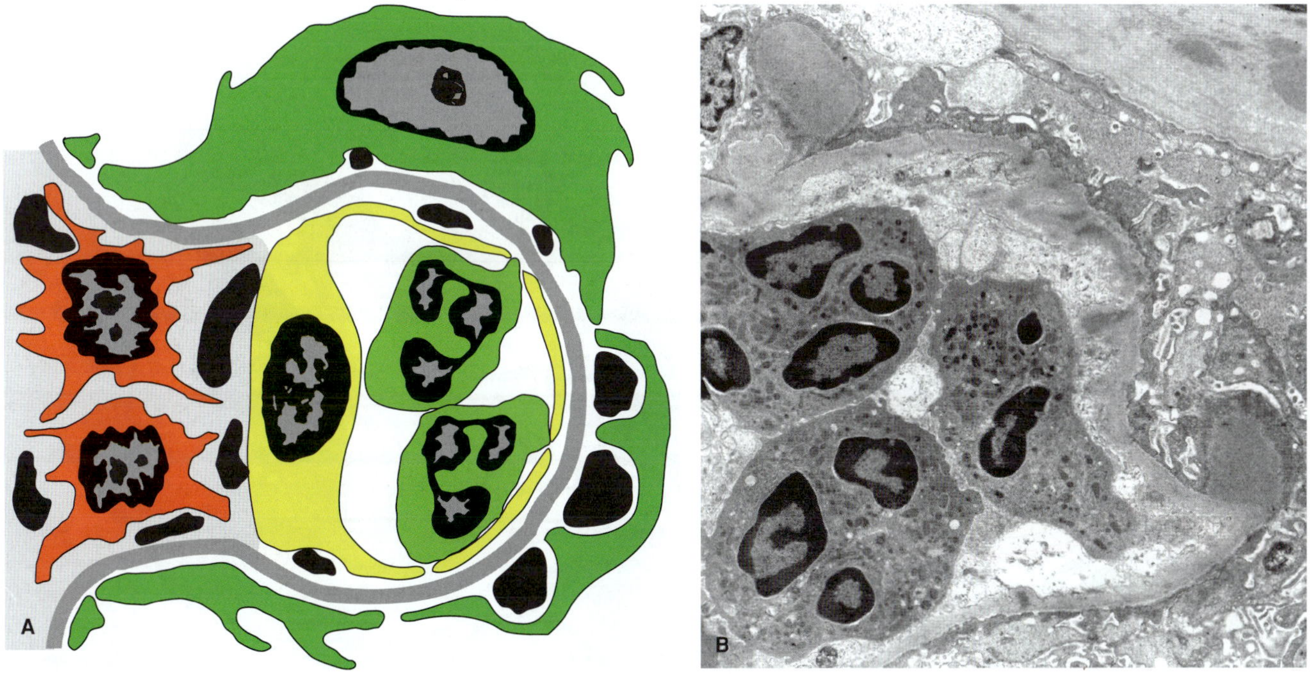

FIGURE 12-17 Diagram (A) and electron micrograph (B) of acute postinfectious glomerulonephritis. Electron microscopy shows scattered, variably sized subepithelial electron dense hump-like deposits, as well as scattered, small subendothelial and mesangial dense deposits, often accompanied by neutrophils in the capillary lumens (key as in Figure 12-2).

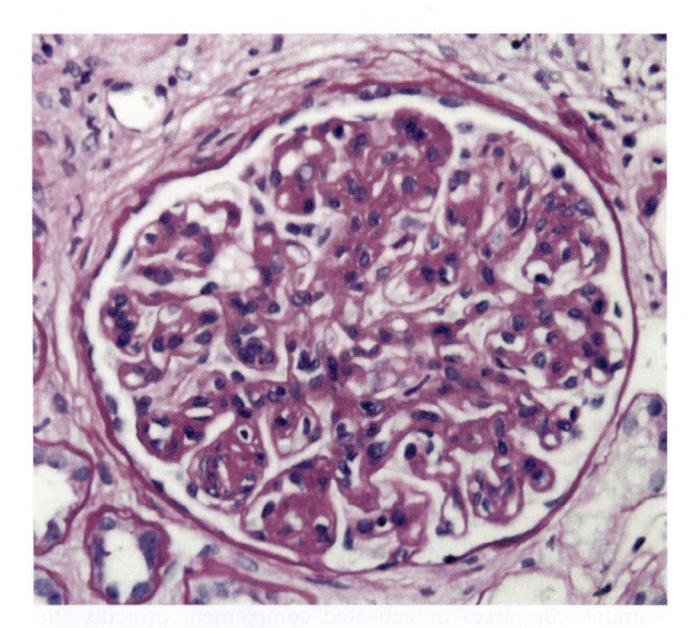

FIGURE 12-18 MPGN. Light microscopy (PAS stain) showing thick capillary walls with GBM remodeling and replication, as well as mesangial hypercellularity and increased mesangial matrix.

inflammatory cells. Glomerular lesions are characterized by both a thickening of capillary walls and hypercellularity. The thickening of capillary walls and the hypercellularity are induced by the inflammatory mediators generated either by accumulation of immune complexes or of activated complement in the absence of immunoglobulin.

The pathogenic complement-rich deposits mediate the infiltration of leukocytes, promote proliferation of glomerular cells including mesangial cells and endothelial cells, and induce increased deposition of subendothelial basement membrane material and mesangial matrix material (Figure 12-18). Electron microscopy reveals scattered subendothelial and mesangial electron dense deposits with varying numbers of subepithelial dense deposits representing either the accumulation of immune complexes or activated complement components (Figure 12-19). A less common ultrastructural appearance that is restricted to patients with glomerulonephritis secondary to complement dysregulation (C3 glomerulopathy) is characterized by bands of electron dense material within GBMs and is referred to as **dense deposit disease** (DDD) (Figure 12-20).

Anti-GBM Glomerulonephritis

The most aggressive form of glomerulonephritis is caused by anti-GBM antibodies. Anti-GBM antibodies are directed against an epitope in the noncollagenous domain of type IV collagen. This same epitope also is present in the basement membranes of pulmonary alveolar capillaries. The epitope appears to be hidden in normal basement membranes but can be exposed by conformational alterations in the type IV collagen that exposes the cryptic epitope. Immunofluorescence microscopy reveals linear GBM staining in biopsy specimens with anti-GBM disease (Figure 12-11B).

Approximately half of patients with anti-GBM disease have renal limited disease and the remainder have pulmonary-renal syndrome with both glomerulonephritis and injury to pulmonary alveolar capillaries causing pulmonary hemorrhage and hemoptysis. Combined pulmonary hemorrhage and glomerulonephritis caused by anti-GBM antibodies is called **Goodpasture syndrome**. However, most pulmonary

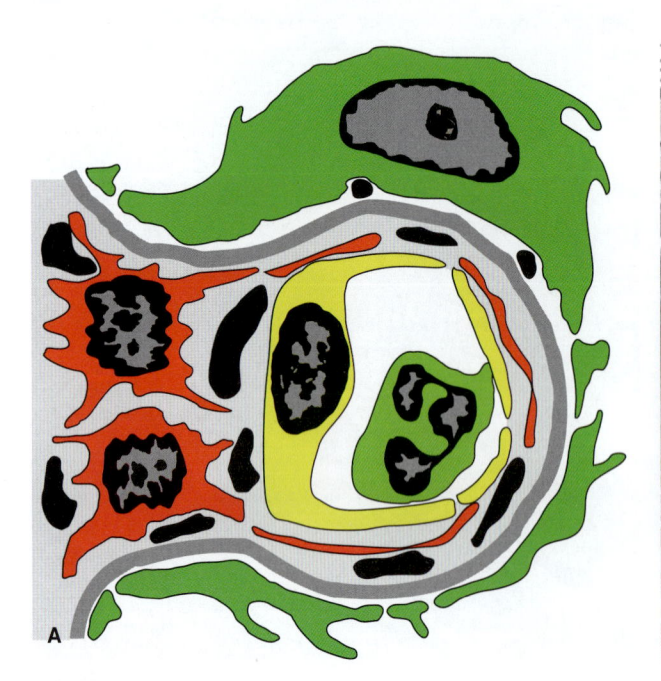

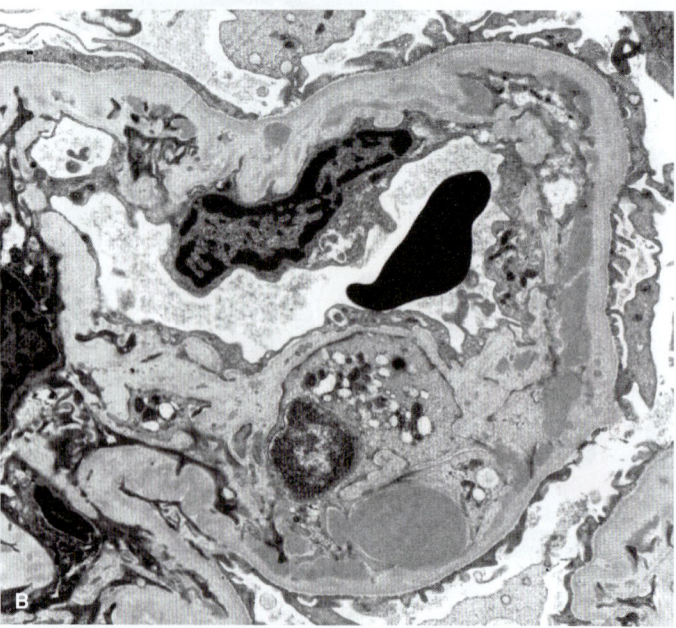

FIGURE 12-19 Diagram (A) and electron micrograph (B) of **MPGN.** Electron microscopy demonstrating subendothelial electron dense deposits with thickened capillary walls caused not only by the deposits but also by interposition of mesangial cytoplasm and deposition of additional matrix material (key as in Figure 12-2).

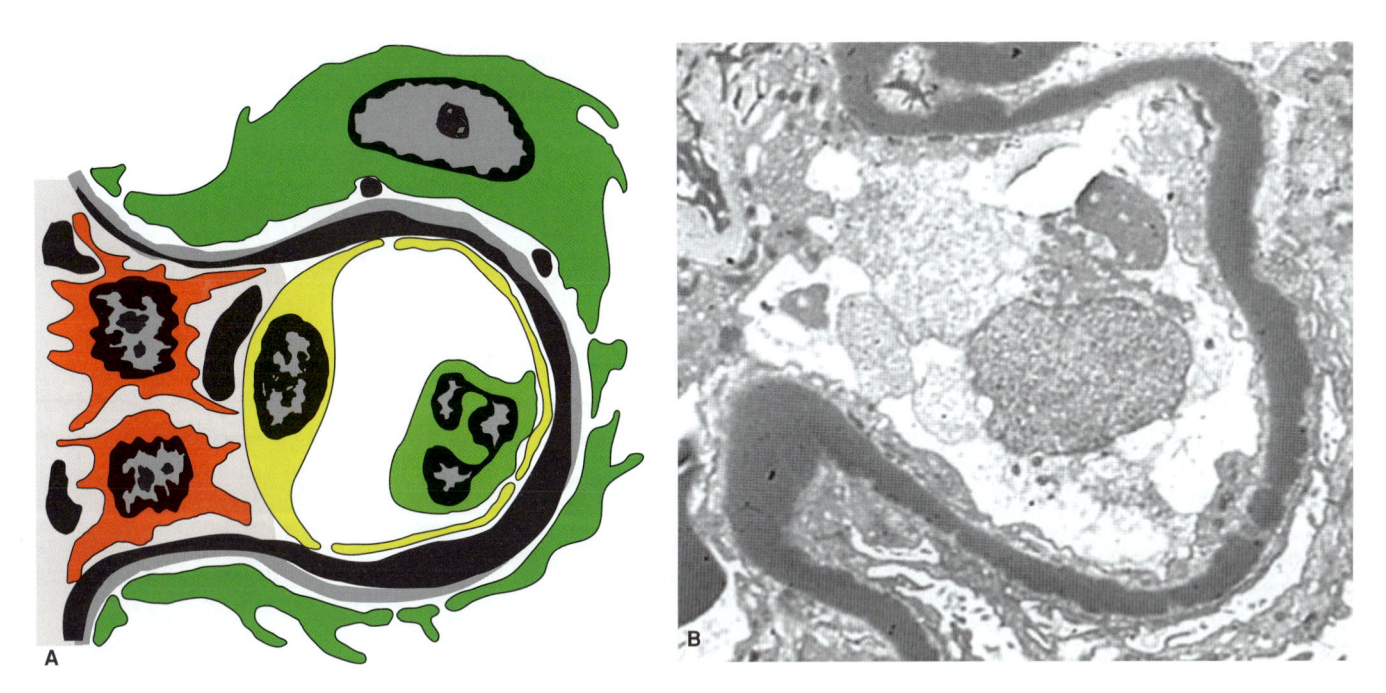

FIGURE 12-20 Diagram (A) and electron micrograph (B) of DDD. Electron microscopy demonstrating bands of electron dense material within GBMs (key as in Figure 12-2).

renal syndrome is caused by ANCA disease rather than anti-GBM disease.

Renal biopsy specimens in patients with anti-GBM glomerulonephritis demonstrate glomerular crescent formation (Figure 12-12D) in over 90% of patients, and many patients have extensive crescentic glomerulonephritis pathologically and RPGN clinically. In the acute phase of injury, there typically is extensive glomerular necrosis as well as crescent formation. Extensive glomerular necrosis results in extensive glomerular scarring and chronic renal failure or end-stage kidney disease. Patients with anti-GBM disease are treated with aggressive immunosuppression including apheresis to remove circulating nephritogenic anti-GBM antibodies.

ANCA Glomerulonephritis

ANCA glomerulonephritis is the most common form of aggressive glomerulonephritis in adults, especially older adults. Although the clinical presentation is varied, many patients with ANCA glomerulonephritis present with severe, often

IN TRANSLATION
Pathogenesis of MPGN

MPGN that results from complement dysregulation (C3 glomerulopathy) is mediated predominantly by uncontrolled activation of the alternative pathway of complement activation. All three complement activation pathways (classical, alternative, lectin) produce a complex of proteins with C3 convertase activity that activates C3 and the subsequent steps in the generation of inflammatory mediators. The C3 convertase of the alternative pathway is composed of activation fragments of C3 (C3b) and complement factor B (Bb) stabilized by properdin. Alternative pathway activation is occurring at a very low level at all times and is held in check by regulatory proteins including complement factor H and complement factor I.

Immune complex glomerulonephritis can be caused by chronic infections (e.g., chronic bacterial osteomyelitis, mastoiditis, or subacute bacterial endocarditis), autoimmune disease (e.g., cryoglobulinemia, which in turn is often caused by hepatitis C virus infection), or malignancy (e.g., carcinoma, sarcoma or lymphoma).

The C3 glomerulopathy variant of MPGN can be caused by either genetic mutations that result in reduced alternative pathway control and resulting increased activation or by autoantibodies that similarly result in reduced control and increased activation. For example, genetic mutations that reduce the amount or function of complement factor H or complement factor I can cause MPGN, and autoantibodies that stabilize the alternative pathway C3 convertase or autoantibodies that reduce the amount and effectiveness of complement factor H or complement factor I can cause the C3 glomerulopathy variant of MPGN. In addition to an MPGN pattern of injury, patients with C3 glomerulopathy caused by complement dysregulation may have other patterns of focal or diffuse proliferative glomerulonephritis.

The treatment of MPGN is very different if the cause is a chronic infectious disease (e.g., antimicrobial therapy) versus an autoimmune process (e.g., immunosuppression) versus a genetic abnormality (e.g., plasma replacement therapy).

CASE 12-5

A 67-year-old Caucasian female presented to an emergency room with hemoptysis and severe dyspnea. Examination confirmed the hemoptysis and revealed, fever, purpuric rash on the lower extremities and buttocks, joint tenderness in multiple fingers, and unilateral weakness and reduced sensation in the left lower extremity and right hand. The eyes, ears, nose, and mouth were unremarkable except for blood in the nares with underlying unremarkable mucosa. She gave no prior history of similar signs or symptoms. Blood pressure was 150/94 mmHg. Laboratory results included 2+ proteinuria with urine protein to creatinine ratio 2.3, 4+ hematuria with >50 dysmorphic RBC/hpf and RBC casts, serum creatinine 5.7 mg/dL, serum albumin 3.8 g/dL, and serum cholesterol 228 mg/dL. Serologic testing demonstrated a negative ANA, negative anti-DNA, serum C3 120, serum C4 21, negative anti-GBM, negative PR3-ANCA, and positive myeloperoxidase ANCA (MPO-ANCA).

A renal biopsy was performed and was diagnostic for pauci-immune necrotizing and crescentic glomerulonephritis, and also demonstrated necrotizing arteritis affecting small interlobular arteries (Figure 12-21). The pathology report also included a comment that the clinicopathologic correlation was indicative of MPO-ANCA microscopic polyangiitis.

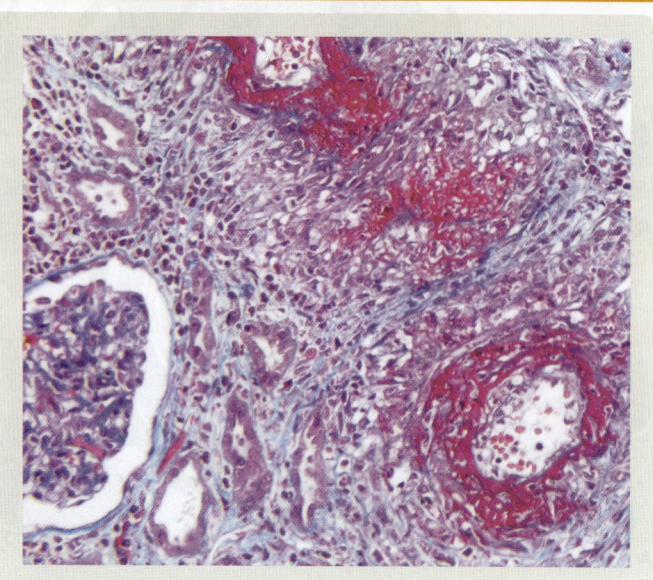

FIGURE 12-21 **ANCA vasculitis.** Light microscopy of a renal biopsy specimen from a patient with microscopic polyangiitis showing inflammation and fibrinoid necrosis of interlobular arteries (Masson trichrome stain).

rapidly progressive, glomerulonephritis. Approximately three-quarters of patients with ANCA glomerulonephritis also have systemic small vessel vasculitis accompanying the glomerulonephritis. Virtually any organ in the body can be affected by ANCA small vessel vasculitis. Common manifestations include purpura caused by inflammation of small dermal vessels, asymmetrical peripheral neuropathy caused by inflammation of epineural arteries, pulmonary hemorrhage caused by either hemorrhagic capillaritis or necrotizing granulomatous inflammation, upper respiratory tract inflammation including necrotizing ulcerative mucosal lesions in the nose and sinuses, and ocular manifestations of vasculitis.

There are four major clinicopathologic variants of ANCA disease.

1. **Renal limited ANCA Glomerulonephritis:** No accompanying features of systemic vasculitis.
2. **Microscopic Polyangiitis (MPA):** Small vessel vasculitis in multiple organs but no evidence of granulomatous inflammation, no history of asthma and no eosinophilia.
3. **Granulomatosis with Polyangiitis (GPA) (formerly called Wegener granulomatosis):** Glomerulonephritis and/or vasculitis as well as necrotizing granulomatous inflammation, which occurs most often in the upper or lower respiratory tract.
4. **Eosinophilic Granulomatosis with Polyangiitis (EGPA) (formerly called Churg–Strauss syndrome):** Glomerulonephritis and/or vasculitis and necrotizing granulomatous inflammation, as well as tissue and blood eosinophilia, and a history of asthma.

In addition to categorization based on clinical and pathologic manifestations, patients with ANCA disease also are categorized based on the specificity of the autoantibodies for either proteinase 3 (PR3-ANCA) or MPO-ANCA or the uncommon absence of ANCA (ANCA-negative). Any of the ANCA specificities can be observed in any of the four clinicopathologic variants; however, MPO-ANCA is most often associated with renal limited disease and MPA, PR3-ANCA is most often associated with GPA, and patients with EGPA are usually ANCA-negative if there is no glomerulonephritis and are usually MPO-ANCA-positive if there is glomerulonephritis.

ANCA disease is treated with aggressive immunosuppression. *For optimum patient outcome, ANCA-disease must be diagnosed early and accurately so that appropriate therapy can be initiated quickly.*

Hereditary Nephritis and Thin Basement Membrane Lesion

In addition to the inflammatory glomerulonephritis, the differential diagnosis of glomerular hematuria includes genetic abnormalities in the GBMs that result in leakage of RBCs into the urine. The two major pathologic expressions of hereditary basement membrane nephropathies are hereditary nephritis (Alport syndrome) and thin basement membrane nephropathy.

A major constituent of the GBM is type IV collagen. Type IV collagen is composed of interwoven alpha 3, alpha 4, and alpha 5 heterotrimers. This type of collagen is present in aural and ocular basement membranes as well as GBMs.

CASE 12-6

A 31-year-old Caucasian male visited an audiologist complaining of difficulty hearing. The audiologist detected sensorineural hearing loss most severe for high tones. The patient gave a history of an uncle with severe hearing impairment who also developed kidney failure requiring dialysis. The audiologist referred him to a nephrologists because he suspected Alport syndrome. The nephrologist elicited additional history that the patient had multiple diagnoses of urinary tract infection since childhood. He did not recall noticing discolored urine. He was not aware of any kidney, hearing, or eye disease in his family other than his uncle. Physical examination was unremarkable except for blood pressure of 148/92 mmHg. Laboratory results included 2+ proteinuria with urine protein to creatinine ratio 2.6, 3+ hematuria with 20–30 dysmorphic RBC/hpf but no RBC casts, serum creatinine 1.9 mg/dL, serum albumin 4.1 g/dL, serum cholesterol 232 mg/dL, negative ANA, negative anti-DNA, serum C3 130, serum C4 31, and negative PR3-ANCA and MPO-ANCA.

A renal biopsy was performed and was diagnostic for Alport syndrome with focal glomerular sclerosis, absence of GBM immunostaining for alpha 3 and alpha 5 type IV collagen (Figure 12-22), and GBM lamination by electron microscopy (Figure 12-23).

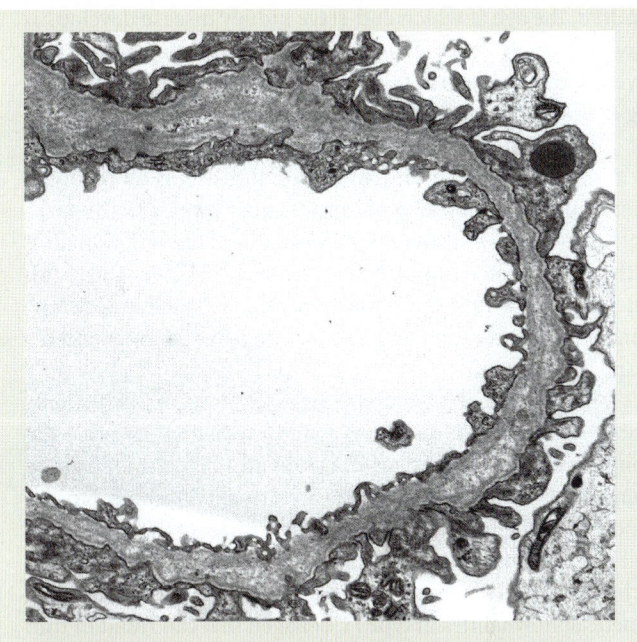

FIGURE 12-23 Alport syndrome. Electron microscopy demonstrating abnormal GBM lamination. Compare with Figure 12-2B.

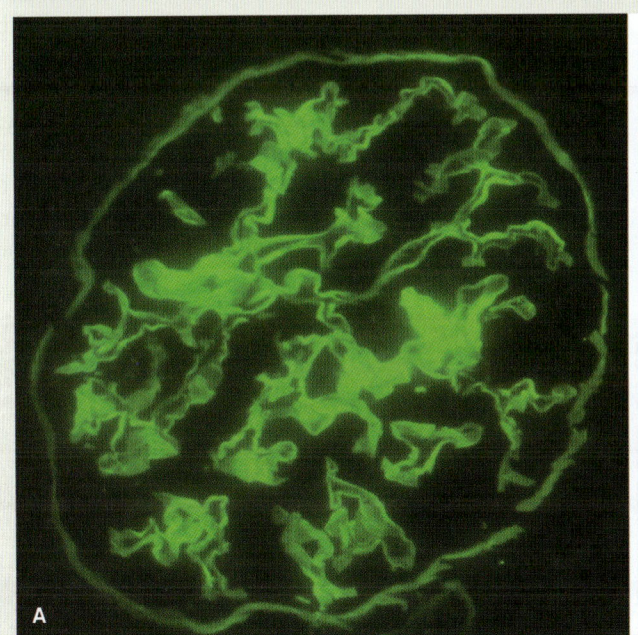

FIGURE 12-22 Alport syndrome. Immunofluorescence microscopy demonstrating appropriate GBM staining of a normal control specimen (A) and absence of GBM staining for alpha 5 type IV collagen in the patient glomerulus (B).

Patients with the Alport syndrome have abnormalities in glomeruli, ears, and eyes. Symptoms include bilateral high frequency hearing loss, a variety of ocular abnormalities, and glomerular hematuria with progressive development of renal failure.

Approximately 85% of Alport syndrome is X linked, 15% autosomal recessive, and only very rarely autosomal-dominant. X-linked disease most often targets the alpha 5 chain of type IV collagen. In the most common X-linked form of hereditary nephritis, males have hematuria from birth and develop progressive renal failure reaching end-stage disease at different ages in different kindreds; however, within a specific kindred, the age at which end-stage kidney disease develops is similar. Females with heterozygous X-linked disease are less severely affected with only about a quarter of patients developing end-stage kidney disease, usually after 50 years old.

By light microscopy, Alport syndrome causes progressive focal segmental and eventually more diffuse and more global glomerular sclerosis as renal insufficiency worsens. By electron microscopy, GBMs are abnormal and show lamination with a moth-eaten appearance (Figure 12-23). Females with heterozygous X-linked disease more often have a marked thinning of the GBM rather than lamination (thin basement membrane lesion).

Thin basement membrane lesion also occurs in patients who do not have typical Alport syndrome but rather have only nonprogressive glomerular disease with hematuria. Family members may share this genetic abnormality, resulting in the syndrome of benign familial hematuria. Many of these kindreds will have heterozygous mutations within the alpha 3 or the alpha 4 chain of type IV collagen, although there are a great variety of genetic abnormalities in type IV collagen that can result in thin basement membrane lesion and benign familial hematuria.

Hypertensive Arterionephrosclerosis

Hypertensive arterionephrosclerosis is second only to diabetic glomerulosclerosis as a cause of end-stage kidney disease in North America. The most common form of hypertensive nephropathy occurs gradually in patients who are in the upper portion of the distribution curve for blood pressure in a given population.

Hypertension has been characterized as either lower level benign or higher level malignant hypertension. Initially, nonmalignant hypertension is not associated with end organ damage; however, chronic hypertension eventually causes damage in many organs including the kidneys.

Malignant hypertension is characterized by diastolic blood pressure greater than 140 mmHg usually with systolic blood pressure greater than 210 mmHg with associated retinal vascular changes, papilledema, encephalopathy, and acute renal impairment. The clinical and pathologic manifestations of nephropathy caused by malignant hypertension are very similar to those occurring in other forms of thrombotic microangiopathy and will be discussed later along with those diseases.

Chronic hypertensive nephropathy (**arterionephrosclerosis**) is characterized clinically by slow progression of renal insufficiency with only minimal or minor proteinuria and no glomerular hematuria. The kidneys become progressively smaller as a result of parenchymal atrophy and scarring, and the surface of the kidney has a fine granular appearance because of alternating depressions caused by scarring and bulges caused by compensatory hypertrophy. Histologically, the most severe parenchymal injury is in a subcapsular distribution with zones of interstitial fibrosis, tubular atrophy, and glomerular sclerosis alternating with adjacent zones of hypertrophy of residual intact nephrons. Conceptually, the subcapsular areas of atrophy and scarring are the result of reduced profusion at the terminal end at the vascular tree as a result of narrowing of the lumens of arteries and arterioles caused by arteriolosclerosis and arteriosclerosis.

Hypertensive arteriosclerosis affects arteries of all sizes, including lobar, arcuate, and interlobular arteries. The ubiquitous feature is fibrotic thickening of the intima with resultant narrowing of the lumen (Figure 12-24A). There may also be focal atrophy and sclerosis of the arterial muscularis. Arterioles have hyalinosis with the accumulation of proteinaceous,

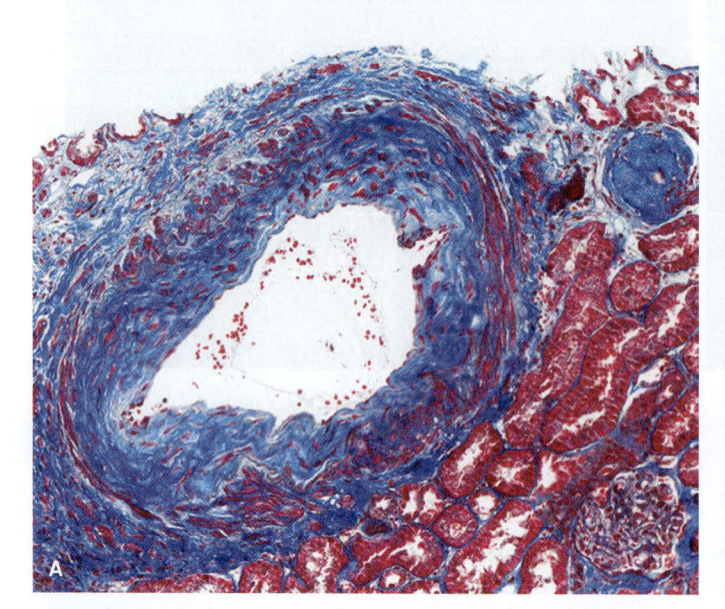

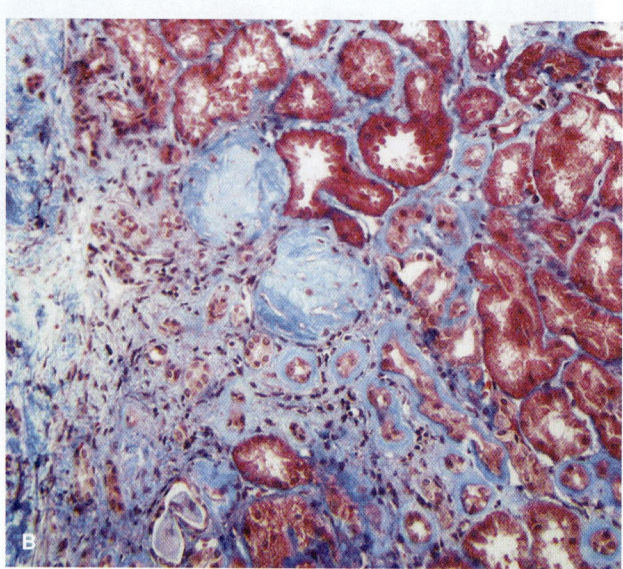

FIGURE 12-24 Hypertensive arterionephrosclerosis. Light microscopy showing severe arteriosclerosis of an arcuate artery **(A)** with marked intimal fibrosis and atrophy and sclerosis of the muscularis, and subcapsular global sclerosis of glomeruli with adjacent tubular atrophy and interstitial fibrosis **(B)**. This Masson trichrome stain stains collagen blue.

glassy appearing (hyaline) material beneath the endothelial cells. Arteriolar hyalinosis results in narrowing of the lumen. Especially in the zones of subcapsular atrophy, glomeruli have progressive wrinkling and contraction of the glomerular tufts with eventual scarring and loss of cellularity. There also is progressive interstitial fibrosis and tubular atrophy adjacent to the globally sclerotic glomeruli (Figure 12-24B). Initially, there is compensatory hypertrophy both structurally and functionally in unaffected nephrons, but over time the progressive process leads to more and more parenchymal atrophy and fibrosis.

Adequate control of blood pressure is the primary management strategy for preventing the onset and progression of hypertensive arterionephrosclerosis.

Eclampsia and Preeclampsia

Eclampsia and preeclampsia comprise a hypertensive disorder of pregnancy (**toxemia of pregnancy**). Preeclampsia is characterized by pregnancy-induced hypertension and proteinuria. Eclampsia is defined by the development of tonic–clonic seizures in a patient with features of preeclampsia. Placental abnormalities are the underlying cause of the condition, and removal of the placenta ameliorates the condition.

The major pathologic feature of preeclampsia/eclampsia is marked swelling of glomerular capillary endothelial cells, resulting in narrowing of capillary lumens (**endotheliosis**) (Figure 12-25). There may also be localized expansion of the subendothelial zone sometimes containing proteinaceous material. By light microscopy, the swollen endothelial cells obliterate the capillary lumens (Figure 12-26).

Treatment of preeclampsia involves prevention of seizures (usually using magnesium sulfate) and control of hypertension. If other measures are not successful in controlling the disease, termination of pregnancy may be required to avert multiorgan damage.

> **IN TRANSLATION**
>
> **Pathogenesis of Eclampsia/Preeclampsia**
>
> The renal target of the disease is the glomerulus, and mediation of the glomerular injury involves the vascular endothelial growth factor (VEGF) family of vasoactive proteins. The VEGF family also is involved in placental events. There is evidence that increased levels of circulating antagonists of VEGF receptors in glomeruli induce preeclampsia/eclampsia. Support for this comes from the use of antiangiogenic drugs in cancer therapy that block VEGF function and result in proteinuria caused by glomerular lesions that closely resemble the lesions of preeclampsia/eclampsia.

Thrombotic Microangiopathies

The thrombotic microangiopathies are characterized clinically by hypertension, renal insufficiency, microangiopathic hemolytic anemia (MAHA), and thrombocytopenia. MAHA has circulating fragmented RBCs (schistocytes) resulting from fragmentation as the erythrocyte as they flow through injured small vessels. Thrombotic microangiopathies can be divided into two pathogenetically distinct categories:

1. Thrombotic thrombocytopenic purpura (TTP) mediated by abnormalities in von Willebrand factor (vWF)
2. Hemolytic uremic syndrome (HUS) mediated by a variety of mechanisms of renal vascular endothelial injury.

Thrombotic Thrombocytopenic Purpura

Patients with TTP typically have fever, severe hypertension, MAHA, thrombocytopenia, neurologic dysfunction,

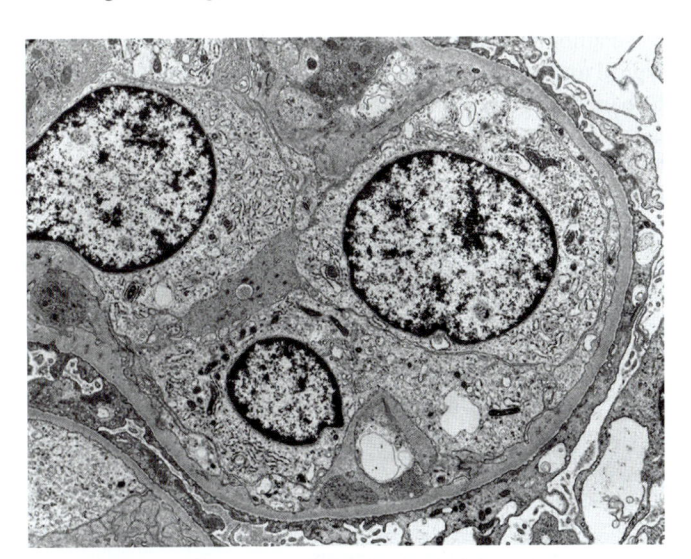

FIGURE 12-25 Preeclampsia. Electron microscopy showing obliteration of a glomerular capillary lumen by endothelial swelling. Compare with Figure 12-2B.

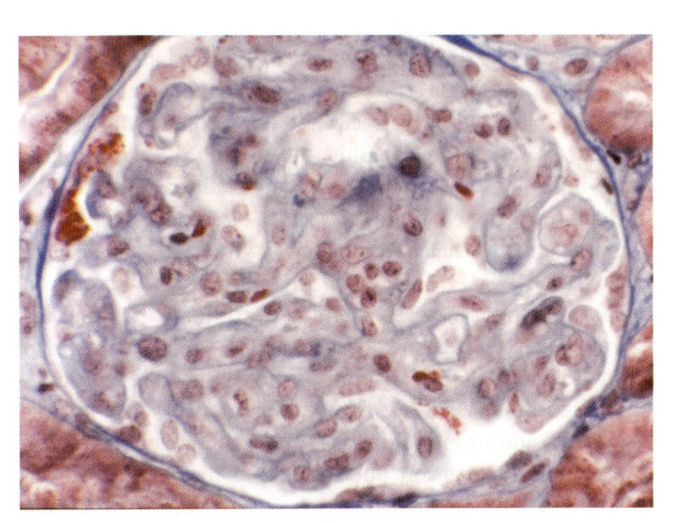

FIGURE 12-26 Preeclampsia. Light microscopy (Masson trichrome stain) obliteration of glomerular capillary lumens by swollen endothelial cells.

and bleeding that is manifested in the skin as petechiae or purpura. However, patients with TTP usually have less frequent and less severe renal failure than patients with HUS.

TTP is caused by abnormalities in endothelial vWF. Normal vWF is displayed on the surface of endothelial cells as large multimers. The length of these multimers is regulated by proteolysis by a vWF cleaving metalloproteinase (ADAMTS13). Abnormalities in the amount or function of ADAMTS13 result in abnormally long vWF multimers that predispose to microvascular platelet-rich thrombosis. Abnormalities in ADAMTS13 activity can result from genetic mutations or can be acquired by the development of autoantibodies to ADAMTS13.

Patients with TTP develop platelet-rich thrombi in small vessels in virtually every organ of the body (Figure 12-27). Thrombi in the brain produce the neurologic manifestations of TTP and thrombi in the kidneys produce the renal manifestations. The histopathologic manifestation of TTP in the kidney is the presence of scattered capillary thrombi in glomeruli as well as occasional thrombi in arterioles. These thrombi often are accompanied by remodeling in adjacent vessel walls. In glomerular capillary walls, there is replication of GBMs and expansion of the subendothelial zone and endothelial swelling.

Treatment of TTP often involves plasma exchange, which replaces ADAMTS 13 in patients with genetic abnormalities and removes autoantibodies in patients with antibodies to ADAMTS13.

Hemolytic Uremic Syndrome

Patients with HUS often have features that overlap with the clinical presentation of TTP, including severe hypertension, thrombocytopenia, MAHA, and renal insufficiency. However, cutaneous purpura and petechiae and prominent neurologic manifestations are rare.

HUS is caused by endothelial injury, primarily of endothelia in glomerular capillaries, arterioles, and small arteries. HUS may be divided into typical HUS and atypical HUS (Table 12-5). Typical HUS is caused by infection, usually *E. coli* O157:H7, which usually is acquired from contaminated food or water. *E. coli* produces a Shiga-like toxin (SLT) (verotoxin) that is injurious to endothelial cells, especially endothelial cells in small renal vessels. Patients with *E. coli* infection develop a hemorrhagic diarrhea and thus this form of HUS also is designated D+HUS. Typical (D+positive) HUS is most common in children and is a life-threatening condition with a mortality rate of 5–10%. Atypical HUS (D-HUS) has been defined as any form of HUS that is not secondary to an SLT-producing infection. D-HUS has many different etiologies, including drugs, autoimmune diseases and genetic abnormalities. Malignant hypertension often is caused by HUS. However, in some patients, malignant hypertension appears to be the cause of the HUS.

A subset of atypical HUS is caused by dysregulation of the alternative complement pathway as a result of genetic

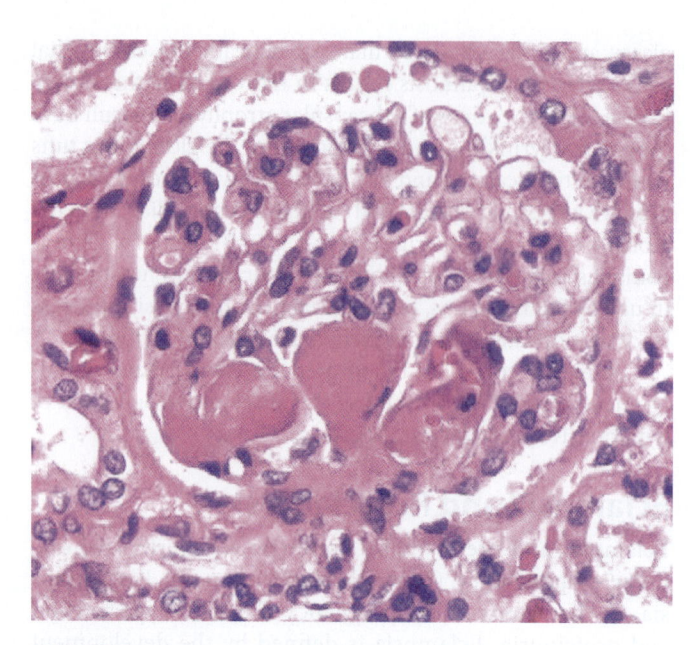

FIGURE 12-27 TTP. Thrombi in glomerular capillaries at the hilum (H&E stain).

deficiencies in or autoimmune interference with regulatory mechanisms. The term atypical HUS is restricted by some to HUS resulting from complement dysregulation. Atypical HUS can be induced by mutations in complement factor H, complement factor I, membrane cofactor protein (MCP), and complement factor B, thrombomodulin or C3. Atypical HUS also can be induced by autoantibodies directed against complement controlled proteins, for example, antibodies against complement factor H. Patients with these abnormalities often have a reduction in circulating C3; however, serum C4 is normal because the abnormal activation targets primarily the alternative complement pathway. Plasma exchange and plasma therapy have been used to treat atypical HUS secondary to disturbance in complement regulation.

Pathologic abnormalities are indistinguishable between typical and atypical HUS. The most constant finding is a disturbance of glomerular capillary endothelial cells with loss

TABLE 12-5 Causes of HUS-type TMA.

D+ Typical HUS
Shiga-like toxin-induced HUS (e.g., *E. coli*, Shigella)
D- Atypical HUS
Familial/genetic HUS (e.g., complement factor H mutations)
Autoantibodies to complement control proteins (e.g., antifactor H)
Neuraminadase-induced HUS (e.g., *Streptococcus pneumoniae*)
Drug-induced HUS (e.g., calcineurin inhibitor and anti-VEGF)
Bone marrow transplantation-induced HUS
Radiation-induced HUS
Pregnancy associated HUS
Systemic sclerosis renal crisis HUS
Malignant hypertensive nephropathy
Antiphospholipid antibody syndrome (APS) with HUS
Idiopathic HUS

PATHOLOGY OF MEDICAL RENAL DISEASE   319

CASE 12-7

A 6-year-old girl developed fever and abdominal pain, followed a day later by severe diarrhea contain bloody streaks. The fever, pain, and diarrhea persisted, and she was taken to an emergency room where she received IV fluids for dehydration. Laboratory findings included normal urinalysis, serum creatinine 0.9 mg/dL, and elevated WBC with increased neutrophils. She returned home and over the next several days the amount of diarrhea decreased, although there was persistent blood in the stool. She continued to feel ill and developed nausea and vomiting, and noticed dark urine. She was taken to the emergency room again. Laboratory findings included 2+ hematuria, 2+ proteinuria with urine protein to creatinine ratio 2.8, serum creatinine 2.6 mg/dL, anemia with schistocytes on the blood smear, and thrombocytopenia. A stool sample was sent to the laboratory for analysis. The following day, the clinical laboratory reported that an assay for Shiga toxin was positive, and cultures were positive for Shiga toxin-producing *Escherichia coli* (STEC).

A renal biopsy was not performed in this patient because the clinical and laboratory findings were diagnostic for typical (diarrhea-positive) HUS caused by STEC. If a biopsy had been performed, it would have shown the findings in **Figures 12-28** and **12-29**.

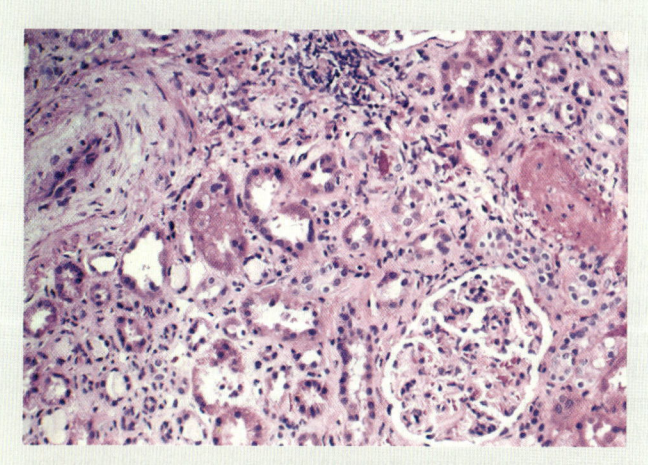

FIGURE 12-29 HUS. On the right side of the image is an arteriole with fibrinoid necrosis of the wall and a thrombus in the lumen. On the left of the image is an interlobular artery with an edematous intima that has obliterated the lumen. There also is diffuse ischemic injury to the tubules and intestinal edema (H&E stain).

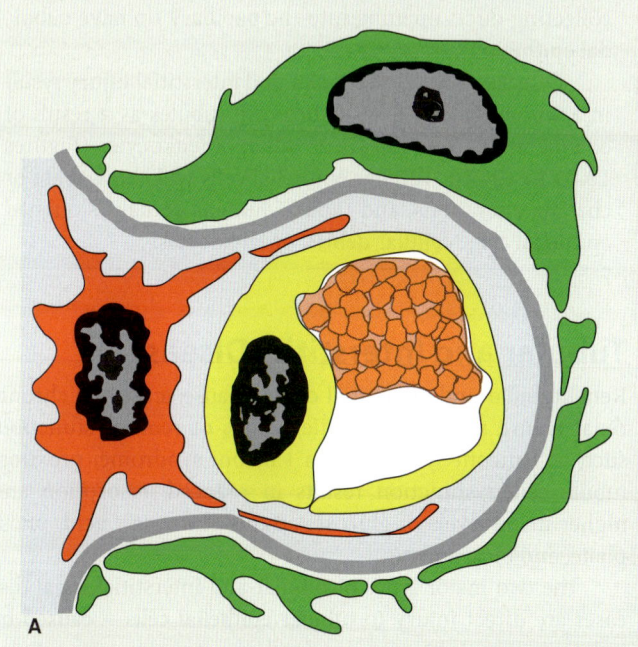

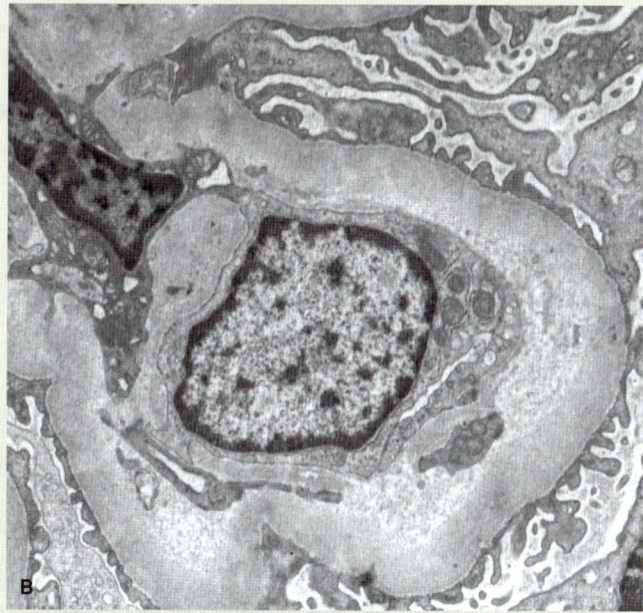

FIGURE 12-28 HUS. Diagram (A) and electron micrograph (B) of HUS. Electron microscopy showing glomerular capillary endothelial cell swelling and separation from the GBM, resulting in an expanded electron lucent subendothelial zone. The diagram depicts a platelet-rich thrombus that is not seen in the electron micrograph. Compare with Figure 12-2A (key as in Figure 12-2).

of fenestrations, swelling, and separation from the GBM resulting in an expanded electron lucent subendothelial zone (Figure 12-28). Superimposed glomerular capillary platelet-rich thrombosis may occur but is not a constant finding in biopsy samples. Extensive glomerular capillary injury results in segmental glomerular necrosis or lysis of mesangial areas (**mesangiolysis**). These acute changes can evolve to more chronic capillary wall alterations with basement membrane remodeling and replication.

Pathologic changes also often occur in arterioles and small arteries. Afferent arterioles may develop fibrinoid necrosis in the wall with insudation of plasma into injured arteriolar walls and formation of fibrin (Figure 12-29). Lumens of arterioles may be occluded by platelet-rich thrombi. Interlobular and arcuate arteries may have a marked edematous thickening of the intima with varying degrees of fibrinoid necrosis (Figure 12-29). Platelet-rich thrombi also may occur in the lumens of these vessels. Chronic lesions in arterioles and arteries are characterized by deposition of layers of collagen producing an onion skin appearance in the thickened intima. The acute glomerular, arteriolar, and arterial lesions may include scattered fragments of RBCs (schistocytes) in the walls of the injured vessels and embedded in thrombi.

Atheroembolization

Atherosclerosis is an inflammatory vascular disease associated with lipid accumulation in the walls of the aorta and major arterial branches. Atherosclerosis in the wall of the aorta can impair the orifice of the main renal artery and can affect the wall of the main renal artery, resulting in renal artery stenosis with **renovascular hypertension** and reduced renal function due to ischemia.

Atherosclerosis also can cause renal disease by the embolization of fragments of plaques into the renal artery with showering of the distal small vessels, resulting in acute and chronic renal failure. This may happen at the time of catheterization of the aorta during angiography or may occur as a spontaneous process in patients with severe aortic atherosclerosis.

Histologically, scattered emboli with cholesterol crystals are present in small arteries, arterioles, and glomerular capillaries (**Figure 12-30**). The cholesterol is dissolved in the preparation of histologic slides, but cholesterol clefts are left behind that can be identified histologically. Atheroembolization can be associated with hypocomplementemia and blood eosinophilia. Thus, atheroembolic renal disease can be confused with acute hypersensitivity tubulointerstitial nephritis or acute glomerulonephritis. Atheroembolization also can cause lower extremity purpura that mimics small vessel vasculitis.

> ### QUICK REVIEW
> #### Normal Renal Tubular and Interstitial Histology
> In the renal cortex, there is normally only a very small amount of interstitium except in advential areas adjacent to larger vessels. The cortical tubules appear to be almost back-to-back separated only by peritubular capillaries and a small amount of fibrous interstitial tissue (**Figure 12-31**). In the cortex, most cross sections of tubules are of proximal convoluted tubules with fewer admixed distal tubules. Proximal tubular epithelial cells have abundant cytoplasm and well-defined brush borders lining the tubular lumen.
>
> The medulla has a greater proportion of interstitial tissue and tubules with cuboidal epithelial cells without conspicuous brush borders or flat epithelium. The distal collecting ducts opening into the papillary tip have cuboidal epithelium.
>
> Diseases that cause tubular and interstitial injury result in a widening of the space between tubules as a result of edema, interstitial fibrosis or influx of leukocytes (Figures 12-31 to 12-36). Tubular epithelial cells will show acute or chronic alterations, and tubular lumens contain sloughed epithelial cells, cellular debris, or leukocytes.

Tubular and Interstitial Diseases

Renal tubular and interstitial disease cause acute and chronic renal failure and other manifestations of renal dysfunction, such as Fanconi syndrome. In Fanconi syndrome, proximal tubule cell dysfunction results in reduced absorption and higher urine levels of glucose, amino acids, uric acid, phosphate, and bicarbonate.

The two major types of tubular and interstitial renal diseases are direct injury to tubular epithelial cells— caused by ischemia or nephrotoxins—and inflammatory injury to tubules and interstitium—caused by infection or hypersensitivity.

Renal disease caused by glomerular injury is accompanied by hematuria with dysmorphic RBCs or RBC casts in the urine and proteinuria (usually >1 g/day). Renal disease caused by tubular or interstitial disease only rarely has dysmorphic hematuria and very rarely causes >2 g/day proteinuria. On urinalysis, patients with acute tubular epithelial injury have dirty (muddy) brown casts in the urine that result from sloughing of cytochrome pigment laden tubular epithelial cell cytoplasm into the urine, epithelial cells, and epithelial cell casts. Tubular injury releases intracellular tubular epithelial cell proteins into

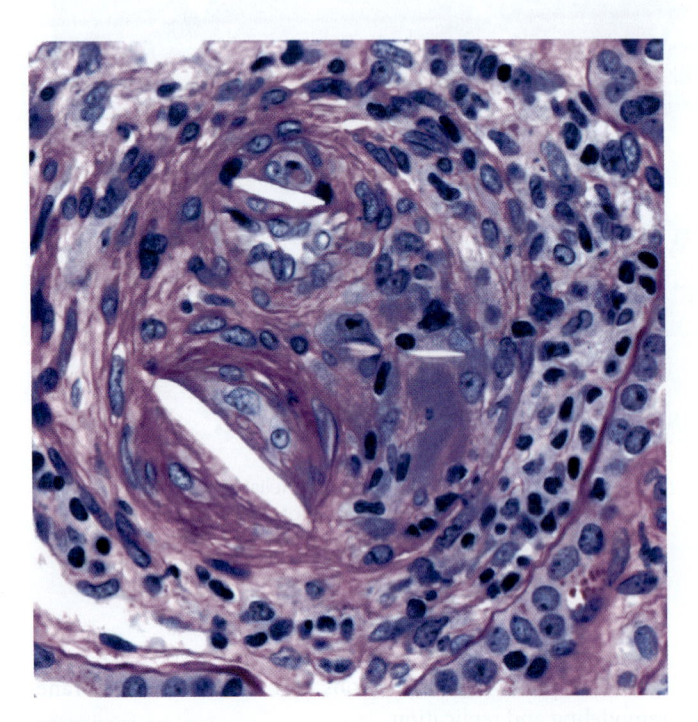

FIGURE 12-30 Atheroembolization. Cholesterol clefts in a small interlobular artery that was occluded by an atheroembolus. There has been a chronic inflammatory response to the embolus with macrophages and fibrosis surrounding the clefts (PAS stain).

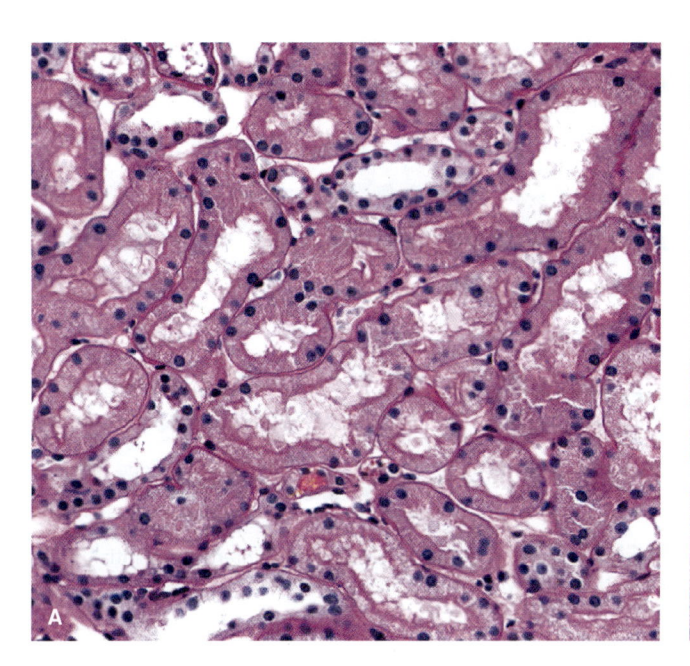

FIGURE 12-31 **Cortical tubules. (A)** Normal cortical tubules that are almost back-to-back separated only by peritubular capillaries and a small amount of fibrous interstitial tissue. This PAS stain demonstrates the well-defined brush border on the proximal tubules, which comprise most of the field of view. **(B)**. Cortex with a zone of chronic tubulointerstitial injury with atrophic tubules with thickened basement membranes, interstitial fibrosis, and interstitial influx of chronic inflammatory cells.

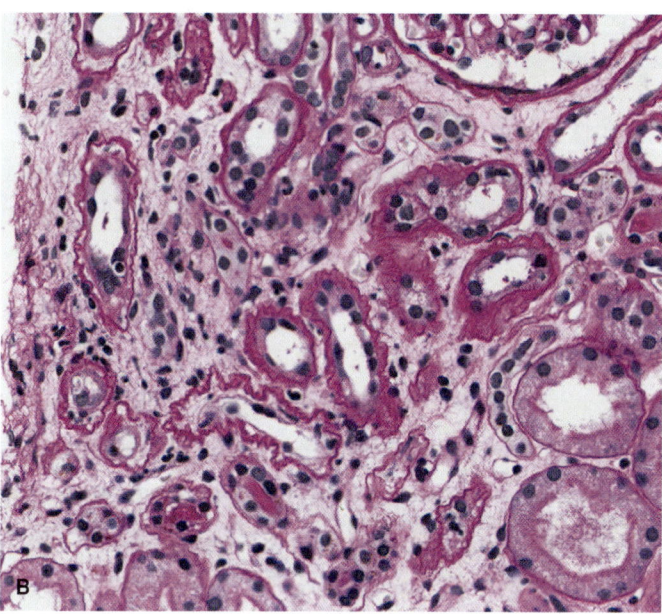

the urine that can be measured as markers of injury, such as kidney injury molecule 1 (KIM-1) and human neutrophil gelatinase-associated lipocalin (NGAL). Patients with tubulointerstitial nephritis have leukocytes and WBC casts in the urine.

> **QUICK REVIEW**
> **Acute Kidney Injury**
>
> Acute kidney injury (AKI), formerly called ARF, is rapid loss of renal function with a rapid rise in serum creatinine of >0.3 mg/dL or a 50% or greater increase in absolute creatinine value. AKI may be accompanied by anuria or severe oliguria (less than 0.5 ml/kg/h for greater than 6 hours). AKI is classified as follows:
>
> 1. **Prerenal:** AKI caused by systemic processes, such as dehydration or severe hemorrhage, which produce functional renal failure but not observable pathologic lesions.
> 2. **Postrenal:** AKI caused by urinary tract obstruction, for example, by urinary tract stones, urinary tract neoplasms or urethral obstruction from prostatic hyperplasia.
> 3. **Renal:** AKI caused by injury to the intrinsic renal parenchyma, including glomeruli, tubules, or vessels.

ACUTE TUBULAR EPITHELIAL INJURY

Acute tubular epithelial injury is the most common cause of intrinsic renal AKI. However, acute tubulointerstitial nephritis as well as glomerular and vascular diseases cause AKI. For example, severe acute proliferative glomerulonephritis such as severe acute postinfectious glomerulonephritis, crescentic glomerulonephritis such as crescentic anti-GBM or ANCA glomerulonephritis, and thrombotic microangiopathy including HUS and TTP cause AKI.

The two major categories of tubular AKI are ischemic AKI and nephrotoxic AKI. *Prerenal* ischemic AKI differs from *renal* ischemic AKI based on the extent of tubular epithelial injury and the reversibility of the failure. Prerenal AKI is quickly reversed with correction of the prerenal abnormality and is accompanied by no identifiable histopathologic changes in tubules. In contrast, ischemic renal AKI requires a latent period of tissue repair before recovery of function and is characterized pathologically by tubular epithelial changes and interstitial edema.

Causes of Tubular AKI:

1. Ischemic AKI: Hemorrhage, shock, burn, dehydration, diarrhea, and heart failure.
2. Nephrotoxic AKI: drugs (e.g., aminoglycosides), organic solvents (e.g., ethylene glycol, carbon tetrachloride), and poisons (e.g., paraquat).

In the past, ischemic AKI was designated acute tubular necrosis (ATN); however, this is not an appropriate designation for the pattern of injury that is seen most often with ischemic AKI. The most characteristic lesion is a flattening (simplification) of proximal tubular epithelial cells (Figure 12-32). This is accompanied by interstitial edema and early in the process by the presence of cytoplasmic debris within tubular lumens. Much of this cytoplasmic debris derives from the sloughing of apical cytoplasm into the urine, although there is a minor contribution from sloughing of dead cells or even viable cells into the

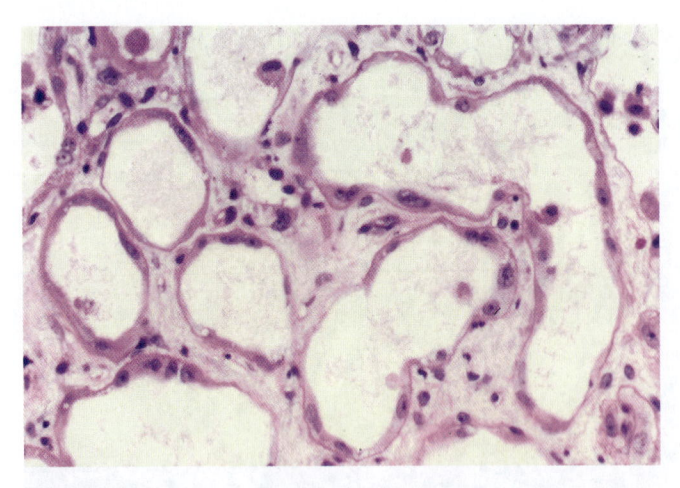

FIGURE 12-32 **Ischemic AKI.** Light microscopy demonstrating flattening (simplification) of proximal tubular epithelial cells and interstitial edema but no interstitial influx of inflammatory cells. Compare with Figure 12-31.

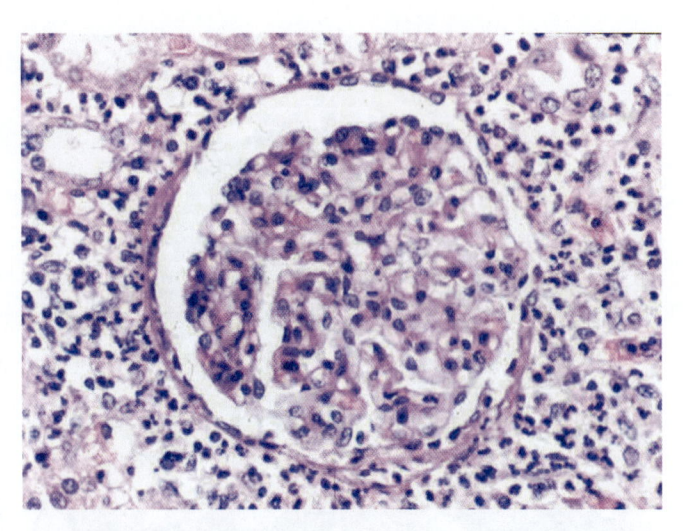

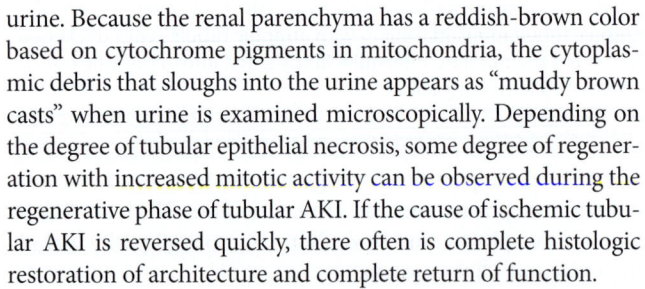

FIGURE 12-33 **Acute pyelonephritis.** Intense interstitial infiltration of polymorphonuclear leukocytes.

urine. Because the renal parenchyma has a reddish-brown color based on cytochrome pigments in mitochondria, the cytoplasmic debris that sloughs into the urine appears as "muddy brown casts" when urine is examined microscopically. Depending on the degree of tubular epithelial necrosis, some degree of regeneration with increased mitotic activity can be observed during the regenerative phase of tubular AKI. If the cause of ischemic tubular AKI is reversed quickly, there often is complete histologic restoration of architecture and complete return of function.

Nephrotoxic tubular AKI can be caused by a variety of agents including nephrotoxic drugs, for example, aminoglycosides. Nephrotoxic tubular AKI may have an appearance very similar to ischemic tubular AKI, although usually there is more overt tubular epithelial necrosis with more sloughing of cells into the urine and denudation of portions of tubular basement membranes. Severe tubular AKI may require an interval of renal replacement therapy with hemodialysis, although patient scan recover full renal function if the cause can be eliminated and the injury is reversible.

TUBULOINTERSTITIAL NEPHRITIS

Acute Tubulointerstitial Nephritis

Acute inflammation of tubules and interstitium can cause ARF, and if the inflammatory process persists this can evolve into chronic tubulointerstitial nephritis and chronic interstitial fibrosis and tubular atrophy with risk of progression to end-stage kidney disease. *Two major categories of acute tubulointerstitial nephritis are acute pyelonephritis and acute hypersensitivity tubulointerstitial nephritis.*

1. Acute pyelonephritis: Caused by bacterial infection most commonly *E. coli* infection.
2. Hypersensitivity tubulointerstitial nephritis: Caused by an allergic response, for example, to a drug or other substances that are ingested, such as herbal remedies.

By far the most common route of infection in acute pyelonephritis is an ascending infection in the urinary tract, for example, derived from a bacterial bladder infection. Much less common is hematogenous spread of bacterial infection to the renal parenchyma. Acute pyelonephritis is characterized by extensive influx of polymorphonuclear leukocytes within the interstitium, tubules (**tubulitis**), and lumens of tubules (WBC casts) (**Figure 12-33**). Because of the ascending origin of the infection, the medulla is characteristically involved as well the cortex. Acute and chronic pyelonephritis usually has a predisposing urinary tract condition such as persistent urinary tract infections, reflux, or **urolithiasis**.

With persistence or recurrence of acute pyelonephritis, the disease process evolves into chronic pyelonephritis, which usually is accompanied by marked erosion of the papillary tip resulting in dilation of the adjacent calyx (**caliectasis**), which can be observed in imaging studies. The most characteristic pathologic features of chronic pyelonephritis are the gross changes in the kidney with broad-based scars in the parenchyma overlying areas of cortical and medullary atrophy with adjacent caliectasis. The histopathologic features are relatively nonspecific with varying degrees of tubular atrophy, interstitial fibrosis, and interstitial infiltration by chronic inflammatory cells (Figure 12-31B). A distinctive but not specific alteration is a fragmentation of tubules with the fragmented segments forming spherical structures with cast material in their lumens that resemble thyroid follicles with colloid (**thyroidization**). In addition to antimicrobial treatment, the management of acute and chronic pyelonephritis requires correction of any urinary tract abnormality that predispose for bacterial infection.

A special uncommon form of chronic pyelonephritis is **xanthogranulomatous pyelonephritis**. This uncommon form of pyelonephritis is characterized by irregular accumulations of yellowish material in the renal parenchyma by gross examination that is found to be sheets of lipid-laden foamy macrophages (**xanthoma** cells) by histologic examination.

CASE 12-8

A 76-year-old Caucasian female who lived alone developed worsening malaise, nausea, and vomiting. Her daughter visited and was alarmed by her condition, which also included moderate disorientation, and took her to an emergency room. Physical examination revealed normal blood pressure, low-grade fever, normal neurologic exam except for mild cognitive impairment, no skin lesions, and no evidence of respiratory track disease. Laboratory results included mild anemia, mild leukocytosis with no increase in blood eosinophils, 2+ proteinuria with urine protein to creatinine ratio 1.6, 2+ hematuria with 10–20 dysmorphic RBC/hpf with no RBC casts, 10–20 WBC/hpf with no WBC casts, serum creatinine 4.9 mg/dL, serum albumin 3.5 g/dL, and serum cholesterol 288 mg/dL. Serologic testing demonstrated a negative ANA, negative PR3-ANCA, negative MPO-ANCA, serum C3 132, and serum C4 33.

A renal biopsy was performed and revealed hypersensitivity acute tubulointerstitial nephritis (Figure 12-34). Once the renal biopsy diagnosis was made, additional history was obtained that the patient had seen her primary care doctor 1 month earlier complaining for severe heartburn (dyspepsia), especially at night when she went to bed, and was given a prescription for the proton pump inhibitor Omeprazole (Prilosec). The drug was discontinued.

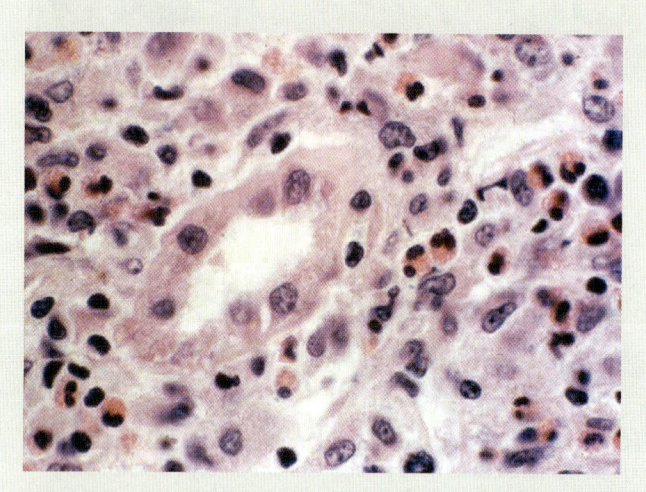

FIGURE 12-34 Acute hypersensitivity tubulointerstitial nephritis. Light microscopy showing interstitial infiltration by mononuclear leukocytes and numerous eosinophils with bilobed nuclei and granular reddish-orange cytoplasm (H&E stain).

This disease results from persistent infection with a number of different pathogens including proteus, pseudomonas, klebsiella, and *E. coli*.

Hypersensitivity Tubulointerstitial Nephritis

Hypersensitivity tubulointerstitial nephritis results from an allergic response, for example, to a drug. Drugs that can induce hypersensitivity tubulointerstitial nephritis include diuretics, antibiotics, especially beta-lactam antibiotics, nonsteroidal anti-inflammatory drugs, proton pump inhibitors, and many others. AKI caused by acute hypersensitivity tubulointerstitial nephritis usually occurs 2 or more weeks following the initiation of drug treatment. The classic triad of symptoms and signs are fever, rash, and blood eosinophilia; however, many patients do not have all of these clinical features.

Urinalysis demonstrates increased WBCs, often including eosinophils, as well as WBC casts. Systemic features of allergy such as fever and rash may be present as well as blood eosinophilia.

The histopathologic features of hypersensitivity tubulointerstitial nephritis are focal interstitial edema with interstitial infiltration by predominantly mononuclear leukocytes (lymphocytes, monocytes, macrophages) with varying numbers of admixed eosinophils that may be very conspicuous in some patients (Figure 12-34) and rare in others. Focal acute tubulitis is present with the interstitial infiltrates and is defined by the presence of lymphocytes on the epithelial side of tubular basement membranes. With persistence of a hypersensitivity tubulointerstitial nephritis, interstitial fibrosis begins and infiltrates may take on a granulomatous appearance with clustering of macrophages and occasional giant cell formation.

Acute hypersensitivity tubulointerstitial nephritis is generally reversible if the initiating exposure is identified and removed. The disease will recur with subsequent re-exposure to the inciting agent.

Light Chain Cast Nephropathy and Tubulopathy

Circulating monoclonal immunoglobulin from a B-cell dyscrasia can cause kidney injury through multiple mechanisms. Renal disease caused by AL amyloidosis and by monoclonal immunoglobulin deposition disease resulting in glomerular injury, nephrotic syndrome, and progressive renal failure was described earlier. *Monoclonal immunoglobulin, especially monoclonal light chains, also can cause tubular injury with two patterns of injury: light chain cast nephropathy and light chain tubulopathy.*

Light chain cast nephropathy is the most common form of kidney disease associated with circulating monoclonal immunoglobulin. It is characterized by the formation of casts within tubular lumens composed of the monoclonal immunoglobulin mixed with Tamm–Horsfall proteins. These casts often have an adjacent inflammatory response including multinucleated giant cells (Figure 12-35). The casts have a more angular, fractured, or crystalline appearance than nonspecific

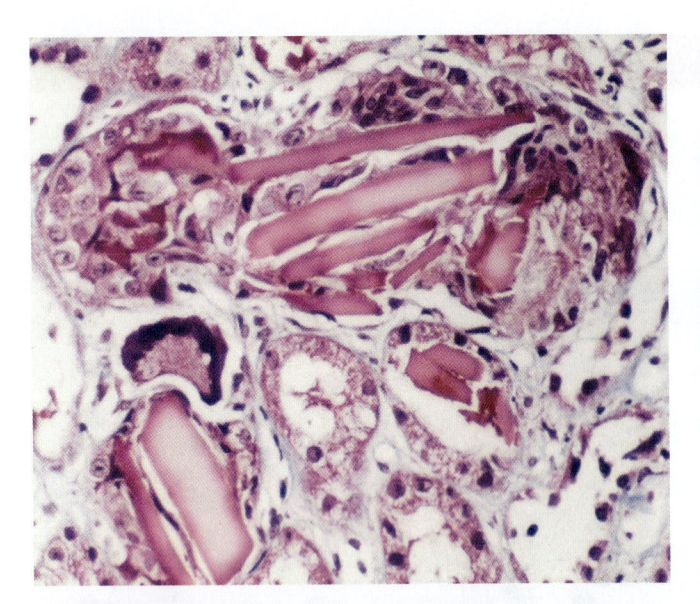

FIGURE 12-35 **Light chain cast nephropathy.** These angular, fractured casts have adjacent inflammatory cells including multinucleated giant cells (Masson trichrome stain).

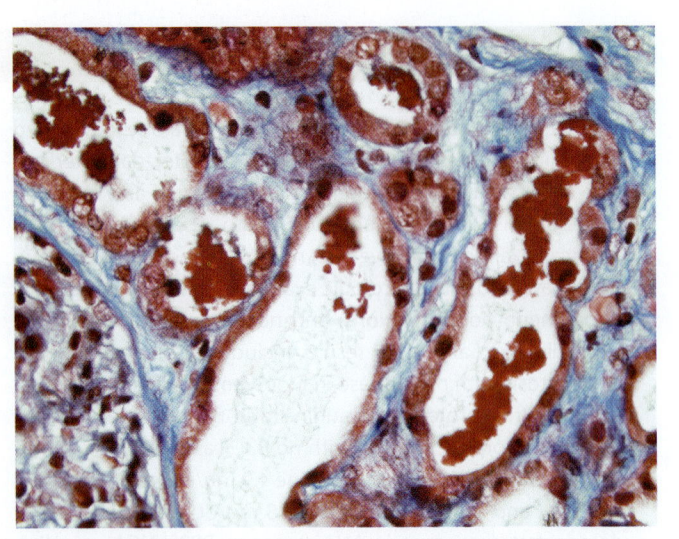

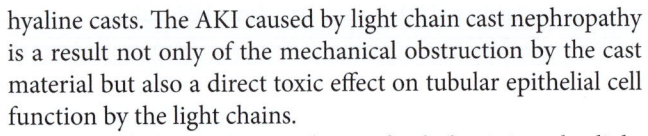

FIGURE 12-36 **Myoglobinuric cast nephropathy.** These myoglobin casts are coarsely granular and red with Masson trichrome staining. Immunohistochemical staining for myoglobin versus hemoglobin would be required to confirm that the casts are composed of myoglobin.

hyaline casts. The AKI caused by light chain cast nephropathy is a result not only of the mechanical obstruction by the cast material but also a direct toxic effect on tubular epithelial cell function by the light chains.

A much less common form of tubular injury by light chains is light chain tubulopathy in which proximal tubules have internalized large amounts of light chains resulting in engorgement of the cytoplasm by vacuoles filled with light chains, sometimes in a crystalline configuration. This leads to extensive dysfunction of tubules that can manifest clinically as **Fanconi syndrome**.

Myoglobinuric and Hemoglobinuric Cast Nephropathy

Excess excretion of myoglobin or hemoglobin in the urine can cause AKI and is characterized pathologically by conspicuous coarsely granular cast material composed of the myoglobin or hemoglobin in tubular lumens. As with light chain cast nephropathy, the AKI is a result of not only mechanical obstruction but also toxicity to tubular epithelial function. Myoglobinuria results from rhabdomyolysis produced by severe trauma, especially crush injury, and associated with alcohol and drug abuse, most likely because of prolonged pressure on muscles during episodes of immobilization. Hemoglobinuria and hemoglobinuric AKI result from extensive hemolysis.

Histologically, hemoglobin and myoglobin casts are not distinguishable from each other by routine staining (Figure 12-36); however, immunohistochemical staining for myoglobin versus hemoglobin is diagnostic. Management of hemoglobinuric and myoglobinuric AKI includes vigorous hydration and alkaline diuresis. The initiating cause must be corrected. Recovery of renal function is usual, although an interval of renal replacement therapy (dialysis) may be required.

RENAL TRANSPLANT PATHOLOGY

Renal transplantation is the preferred form of renal replacement therapy over chronic dialysis because of improved quality of life, and longer kidney and patient survival. Disease in renal transplants can be divided into disease caused by rejection and disease not caused by rejection. Disease caused by rejection can be categorized on the basis of mechanism as antibody-mediated versus T-cell-mediated, and on the basis of duration as acute versus chronic. However, patients may have concurrent combinations or antibody-mediated and cell-mediated rejection, and acute and chronic rejection.

Acute Cell-Mediated Rejection

Acute cell-mediated rejection is the most common form of acute rejection and occurs in up to 10% of renal transplants during the first year after transplantation. Acute cell-mediated rejection typically manifests as an acute rise in serum creatinine along with a reduction in urine output if the injury is severe enough. Acute cell-mediated rejection is mediated by alloreactive T cells specific for either MHC (HLA) or non-MHC antigens. Alloreactive T cells can target tubular epithelial cells, or endothelial cells in glomerular capillaries, peritubular capillaries, or arteries. The most common histologic manifestation is tubulointerstitial inflammation including tubulitis of nonatrophic tubules with T lymphocytes on the epithelial side of tubular basement membranes. Severe tubulitis results

CASE 12-9

A 35-year-old Asian male developed end-stage kidney disease secondary to biopsy-proven IgA nephropathy and received a living related donor kidney transplant. The transplant functioned well with a fall in serum creatinine to a baseline of approximately 1.4 mg/dL. However, 3 months after transplantation, the patient noticed a decrease in urine output and sensed very slight tenderness in his groin near the transplant. He visited his nephrologist who obtained the following laboratory results: serum creatinine 2.3 mg/dL, 1+ proteinuria with urine protein to creatinine ratio 0.7, and 5-10 RBC/hpf and 10-20 WBC/hpf in the urine.

A renal transplant biopsy revealed acute cellular tubulointerstitial rejection with endarteritis (C4d-negative) (Figures 12-37 and 12-38).

FIGURE 12-37 Acute cellular tubulointerstitial rejection. Light microscopy demonstrating tubulointerstitial inflammation with tubulitis with lymphocytes on the epithelial side of tubular basement membranes and focal disruption of tubular basement membranes (PAS stain).

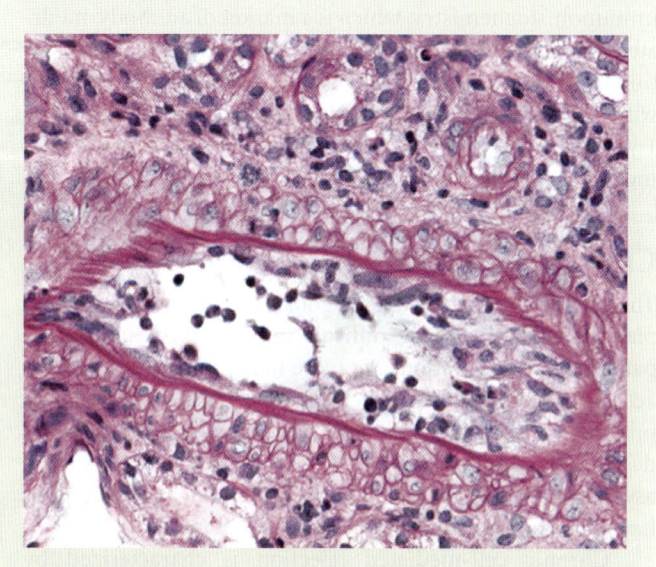

FIGURE 12-38 Acute cellular rejection with endarteritis. Light microscopy demonstrating endarteritis affecting an interlobular artery with mononuclear leukocytes beneath swollen endothelial cells, resulting in the accumulation of leukocytes within the intima. There also are leukocytes adhering to the activated endothelial cells (PAS stain).

in focal disruption tubules with rupture of tubular basement membranes (Figure 12-37).

Mild acute cell-mediated rejection affects only tubules with no apparent involvement of vessels. More severe cell-mediated rejection has injury to arteries with localized endarteritis (intimal arteritis) with infiltration of predominantly mononuclear leukocytes beneath endothelial cells, resulting in the accumulation of leukocytes within the intima (Figure 12-38). The most severe manifestation of cell-mediated rejection is extension of the arterial inflammation into the muscularis sometimes accompanied with fibrinoid necrosis. Glomeruli also may show evidence of increased margination of T lymphocytes and monocytes (**glomerulitis**). *Tubulitis alone is the most common manifestation of acute cell-mediated rejection and has a good 1-year graft survival of > 90%.* Approximately a third of specimens with acute cell-mediated rejection have endarteritis, which predicts a 1-year graft survival to approximately 75%. Less than 5% of acute cell-mediated rejection has a component of arteritis with fibrinoid necrosis, and these patients have less than 20% graft survival at 1 year.

Hyperacute and Acute Antibody-Mediated Rejection

A rare form of severe antibody-mediated rejection is hyperacute rejection. Hyperacute rejection results from the presence of preexisting circulating antibodies to donor endothelial cells at the time of transplantation. These antidonor antibodies may be directed against ABO blood group antigens or MHC antigens. In the current era of transplant management, this process is extremely rare. Once this process has occurred, there is in essence no treatment and the transplant is nonfunctioning. The transplant is cyanotic and hemorrhagic and will become overtly necrotic over time. Histologically, within hours there will be the development of numerous vascular thrombi and extensive margination and diapedesis of neutrophils. There is interstitial edema and hemorrhage and development of fibrinoid necrosis in arteries.

The most common form of acute antibody-mediated rejection manifests as rising serum creatinine, possibly accompanied by oliguria. Antibody-mediated rejection accounts for approximately a third to a quarter of episodes of acute renal transplant rejection. Approximately 90% of patients will have detectable circulating donor-specific antibodies to HLA class I or II. Histologic manifestations of acute antibody-mediated rejection include dilation of peritubular capillaries, accumulation of neutrophils in peritubular capillaries, glomerulitis with increased neutrophils and mononuclear leukocytes in capillary lumens, glomerular capillary thrombi, and the presence of diffuse staining of peritubular capillaries for C4d by immunofluorescence microscopy or immunohistochemistry, which is a marker of antibody-mediated complement activation. Acute antibody-mediated rejection has a worse prognosis than acute cell-mediated rejection with approximately 25% of patients having graft loss after 1 year compared with less than 5% graft loss after acute cell-mediated rejection.

Chronic Rejection

The clinical and pathologic diagnosis of chronic renal transplant rejection is more difficult because the clinical and pathologic manifestations are more nonspecific than those of acute rejection. Chronic rejection typically presents as slowly progressive chronic renal transplant failure, often with some degree of proteinuria and hypertension. Some patients will be asymptomatic clinically but found on surveillance biopsy to have substantial evidence of chronic rejection.

Chronic cell-mediated rejection is characterized by interstitial fibrosis, interstitial infiltration by chronic inflammatory cells, focal segmental and global glomerular sclerosis, and marked arterial intimal fibrosis. One of the better distinguishing features of chronic rejection is the presence of intimal fibrosis that is not accompanied by conspicuous lamination of elastica, which would be present if the fibrotic intimal thickening was caused by other mechanisms of intimal fibrosis, such as hypertension. There also may be more conspicuous mononuclear leukocytes within the thickened intima than is usually seen with other forms of arteriosclerosis. In contrast to chronic antibody-mediated rejection, there should be little or no staining for C4d in peritubular capillaries.

Conceptually, chronic antibody-mediated rejection results from persistent or recurrent episodes or antibody-mediated endothelial injury with resultant remodeling of vessel walls.

Chronic antibody-mediated rejection causes alterations in

1. Glomeruli: chronic transplant glomerulopathy
2. Peritubular capillaries: replication of basement membranes
3. Arteries: fibrotic intimal thickening

The arterial changes are similar to those caused by chronic cellular rejection. The glomerular changes include thickening of capillary walls resulting from expansion of the subendothelial zone with replication of basement membrane material in the absence of immune complex type electron dense deposits. Peritubular capillaries are seen by electron microscopy to have replication (lamination) of basement membranes indicative of recurring injury and stimulation of endothelial cells to lay down basement membrane collagen. There also may be increased numbers of mononuclear leukocytes within the lumens of peritubular capillaries. C4d staining is positive in some patients. Once features of chronic antibody-mediated rejection are present, especially chronic transplant glomerulopathy, there is a 50% or greater chance of graft loss within 5 years.

Renal Transplant Disease Not Caused by Rejection

Renal transplant disease not caused by rejection can be categorized as follows:

1. Donor disease
2. Recurrent native kidney disease
3. Disease related to treatment

Pretransplantation screening of donors and kidneys is intended to minimize the transfer of a systemic or renal disease from the donor to the recipient. This reduces but does not eliminate the risk of transferring an infectious, metabolic/genetic or neoplastic disease to the recipient. Some donor kidney disease, especially mild donor disease, can resolve once the transplant is placed in the recipient. For example, IgA nephropathy and diabetic glomerulosclerosis in a donor kidney can resolve after transplantation, especially if it is not advanced or severe. The donor disease that is most often seen in transplant kidney is hypertensive or age-related arterionephrosclerosis or arteriosclerosis alone. Implantation (zero hour) renal transplant biopsies are performed to assess any donor disease in the transplant. Arteriosclerosis, interstitial fibrosis, tubular atrophy, and chronic inflammation are important to identify so that it will not be misinterpreted later as the development of chronic transplant rejection.

Genetic and metabolic diseases that cause end-stage kidney disease can recur in renal transplants, for example, primary **hyperoxaluria, cystinosis,** and **Fabry** disease. Virtually any form of glomerular disease that is not caused by an intrinsic genetic abnormality in the native kidneys can recur in a kidney transplant, including FSGS, membranous glomerulopathy, MPGN, IgA nephropathy, lupus glomerulonephritis, amyloidosis, and ANCA glomerulonephritis. Anti-GBM disease rarely recurs unless the patient undergoes transplantation before circulating levels of anti-GBM antibodies disappear. In addition, any of these diseases can occur as de novo disease. Overall, when native glomerular disease recurs in a transplant, it causes graft loss in less than 20% of patients after 5–10 years.

Antirejection therapy produces risks to the transplant and to the patient. The extensive immunosuppression puts patients at risk of infections, including CMV, EBV, herpes simplex, hepatitis B, hepatitis C, and BK polyomavirus. Of particular significance to the renal transplant is the risk of BK polyomavirus nephropathy. The BK virus may be derived from either the recipient or the donor urinary tract where it is reactivated from a latent infection to cause overt renal BK virus nephropathy with tubulointerstitial nephritis. BK polyomavirus only causes disease in immunocompromised patients. BK virus nephropathy causes acute renal transplant failure, although it is responsible for less than 5% of acute failure in renal transplants. Histologically, overt, BK virus nephropathy causes tubulointerstitial inflammation with tubulitis and nuclear viral inclusions. Immunohistochemistry can confirm the presence of the virus in the renal parenchyma (Figure 12-39).

Drugs used in the management of renal transplants may cause renal transplant injury. A leading example is calcineurin inhibitors (immunosuppressive drugs, such as cyclosporine and tacrolimus), which cause both functional and structural injury to renal vessels especially arterioles. Calcineurin inhibitor toxicity is dose related. The mildest form of calcineurin inhibitor toxicity causes renal dysfunction by afferent arteriolar vasoconstriction, is reversible, and has no histologic features. The most common histologic abnormality is destruction of smooth muscle cells in afferent arterioles with replacement by glassy (hyaline) proteinaceous material. More severe injury results in a thrombotic microangiopathy with fibrinoid necrosis and thrombosis. This may be accompanied by changes in glomerular tufts ranging from segmental sclerosis to features of thrombotic microangiopathy. Tubular epithelial cell injury most often manifests as isometric vacuolation of proximal tubular epithelial cells. Identification of calcineurin inhibitory toxicity should lead to reduction or cessation of calcineurin inhibitory therapy.

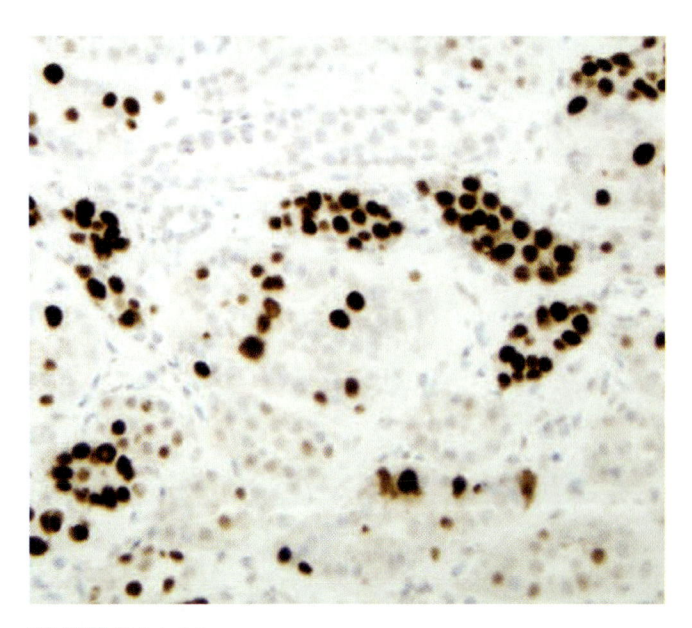

FIGURE 12-39 **BK polyomavirus nephropathy.**
Immunohistochemical staining of virions in the nuclei of tubules in a renal transplant with BK nephropathy.

Urologic Pathology of the, Lower Urinary Tract, Male GU System and Kidney

CHAPTER 13

Susan Maygarden, M.D.

REVIEW OF NORMAL HISTOLOGY OF THE LOWER URINARY TRACT "QUICK REVIEW"

The outflow of the kidneys (renal pelvis, ureters, bladder, and urethra) comprises the lower urinary tract (Figure 13-1). The basic histology is that all are lined by **urothelium** (transitional epithelium), which covers a connective tissue layer of lamina propria, a variably thick layer of smooth muscle (muscularis propria) and adventitia (Figure 13-2). Urothelium is specialized epithelium that is multilayered with large surface superficial cells (umbrella cells), which can change shape as the bladder dilates and contracts. These contain specialized cell junctions that are resistant to permeation by urine. Beneath this are five to six layers of smaller urothelial cells. The muscularis propria is well developed in the bladder, and coordinated contraction of this muscle (detrusor muscle) helps in emptying the bladder. Muscle is less prominent in the ureters and the urethra. The distal urethra is lined by squamous epithelium, which is continuity with the squamous epithelium of the external genitalia. Both the male and female urethra contain mucinous glands in their walls.

REVIEW OF LOWER URINARY TRACT AND NORMAL MALE GU DEVELOPMENT

The lower urinary tract develops from the anterior part of the cloaca. In early fetal development, this area of the cloaca becomes the urogenital sinus, and develops into the fetal urinary bladder, proximal urethra, and the urachus. The distal urethra develops from the urogenital membrane, and the proximal and distal structures fuse. The urachus is a temporary structure that connects to the umbilicus, and this involutes in later fetal life. The ureters develop as lateral buds from the bladder, grow cranially, and induce the formation of the kidney from the metanephric blastema.

Development of the male genital system is complex. The testes begin as intra-abdominal organs, from the genital ridges in the coelomic cavity. These contain primordial germ cells that are originally from the yolk sac and migrate into the genital ridges. Testes develop from this mixture of tissues, and they migrate from their intra-abdominal location into the inguinal canal and eventually the scrotum. During development in the abdomen, testes connect with

FIGURE 13-1 Gross image of kidneys, ureters, and bladder. Kidneys are shown in coronal section. The bladder has been opened to show oblique ureteral openings in the posterolateral wall. The neck of the bladder and the urethral opening are visible at the bottom of the figure.

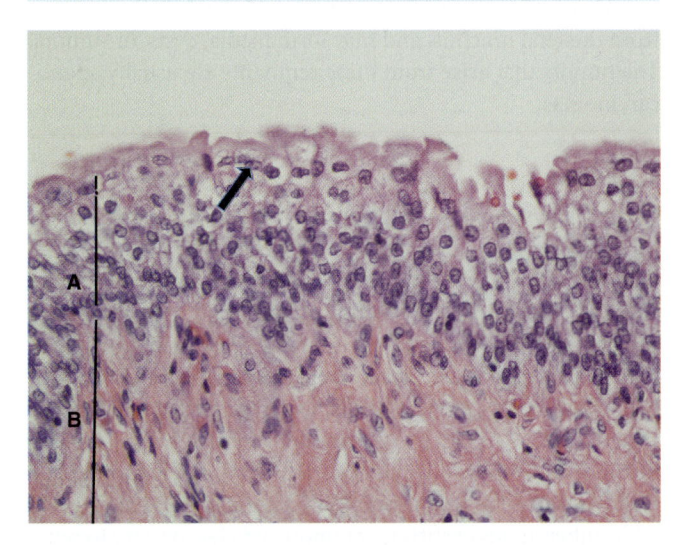

FIGURE 13-2 Photomicrograph of normal urothelium. Arrow indicates umbrella cell layer of urothelium epithelium. Line "A" indicates urothelium, and line "B" indicates lamina propria. The muscularis propria is not shown.

their outflow tracts derived from Wolffian ducts. These develop into the epididymis and vas deferens. The external male genitalia develop from the genital tubercle and the anterior urogenital sinus. The presence of testosterone allows development of these primordial tissues into the scrotum and penis.

URINARY BLADDER

Principal diseases of the bladder include congenital anomalies, inflammatory conditions, benign proliferative lesions, and tumors. Obstructive disease of the bladder is most commonly related to prostatic hypertrophy and will be discussed with the prostate.

Congenital Anomalies

The bladder is complex embryologically, and thus congenital anomalies are not uncommon.

Exstrophy of the bladder refers to absence of the anterior wall of the bladder (due to incomplete resorption of the anterior cloacal membrane), and in this condition the bladder is open on the abdominal skin. Urine drains freely out of the defect, and the open posterior bladder wall quickly becomes inflamed and undergoes squamous and glandular metaplasia. This condition is now currently corrected surgically early in life, but in past times patients with uncorrected exstrophy had a high risk of malignant transformation related to constant inflammation and irritation of epithelium. *However, even patients with corrected exstrophy are of increased risk because of the metaplasias present in the residual urothelium.*

Diverticula of the bladder are due to outpouchings of the urothelium and lamina propria through areas of weakness in the muscle layers, and the urothelium within these diverticula may become inflamed and stones may form.

Urachal remnants are persistent glandular structures from the fetal urachus, and may form fistula, cysts, or tumors. The tumors that arise from these remnants are usually adenocarcinomas.

Cystitis

Cystitis is inflammation of the bladder. It may be acute, chronic, or granulomatous, infectious or noninfectious. Risk factors include (1) being of female sex (because females have shorter urethras than males), (2) having urinary outflow obstruction causing stagnation of the urine (most commonly a result of benign prostatic hyperplasia (BPH) in males), (3) history of instrumentation of the bladder (such as catheterization or cystoscopy), (4) presence of bladder stones, and (5) history of diabetes, immunodeficiency, radiation, or chemotherapy. Coliforms are the most common bacterial pathogen. Worldwide, tuberculous cystitis is common and is secondary to renal tuberculosis.

Acute cystitis (Figure 13-3) shows acute inflammatory cells (neutrophils), edema, and hemorrhage of the epi-

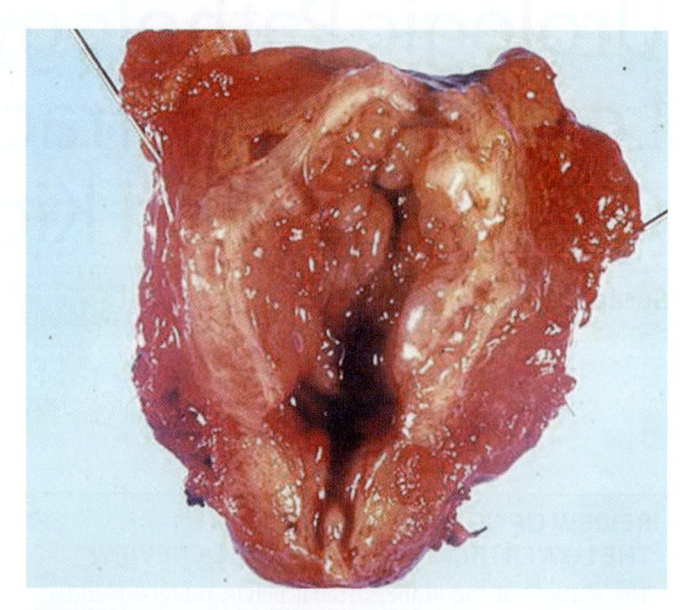

FIGURE 13-3 Gross photo of acute cystitis. The exposed mucosa is hyperemic and edematous.

thelium and lamina propria (Figure 13-4). Chronic cystitis shows an infiltrate with lymphocytes and plasma cells, and if long-standing fibrosis of the lamina propria. The chronic inflammatory cells may organize into lymphoid follicles with germinal centers (follicular cystitis). Granulomatous cystitis shows epithelioid macrophages and giant cells. This may be seen with tuberculosis and other mycobacteria, such as Bacillus Calmette–Guerin, which is instilled into the bladder as a treatment of some bladder cancers.

Malakoplakia is a rare inflammatory disorder identified by the accumulation of foamy macrophages. The aggregation of macrophages is often seen grossly as a yellow plaque or

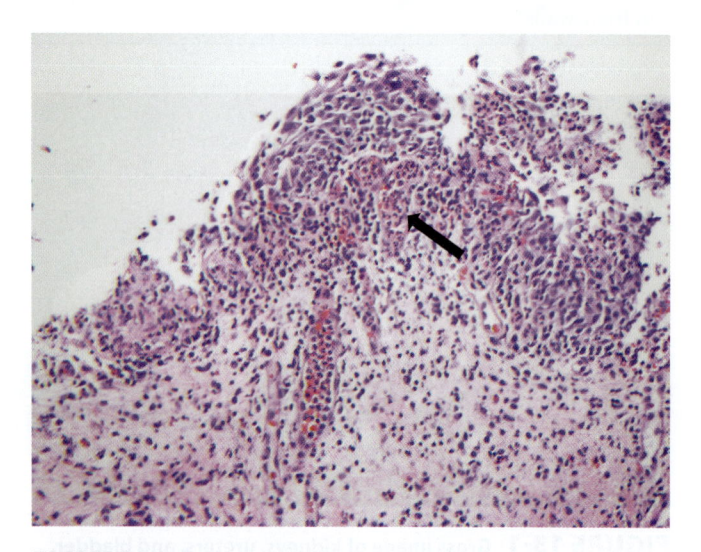

FIGURE 13-4 Photomicrograph of acute cystitis. The urothelial mucosa is infiltrated by neutrophils and the tissue is edematous. Small vascular channels are filled with acute inflammatory cells (arrow).

HUNTING FOR ZEBRAS

Schistosomiasis is a parasite endemic in North Africa and the Middle East. The organism enters through the skin, often in the lower leg, through contact with infected water. It causes marked chronic inflammation of the bladder wall secondary to organisms that settle in the veins of the bladder and provoke an intense inflammatory response. As a result the urothelium undergoes squamous metaplasia. *Patients with long-standing schistosomiasis are at increased risk of malignancy, which are usually squamous cell carcinomas.*

mass. The macrophages contain variable numbers of calcified, laminated inclusions that are known as **Michaelis–Gutmann bodies** (Figure 13-5 see case below). These structures are lysosomes that contain partially degraded bacteria. *Malakoplakia is thought to be a disorder associated with defective bacterial destruction by macrophages.* It is most often seen in immunosuppressed patients infected with *Escherichia coli*, although other bacteria may be implicated. The incompletely degraded bacteria and engorged lysosomes serve as a nidus of calcification. The most common site of malakoplakia is the bladder, although other sites both within and outside of the urinary tract may be involved.

Benign Proliferative Lesions

Benign proliferative and metaplastic lesions are common in the urinary tract. These are often associated with inflammation, but can also be seen with chronic irritation such as stones or an indwelling catheter. Bladder exstrophy is often associated with widespread proliferative lesions.

Brunn nests and Brunn buds are invaginations of the surface epithelium that may be either detached (nests) or attached (buds) to the surface. These are so common as to be variants of normal.

Cystitis cystica is cystic change within Brunn nests and buds. These may be seen grossly as clustered tiny cysts on the bladder surface. Glandular metaplasia to mucinous epithelium may occur within the epithelium of cystitis cystica, and this is termed **cystitis glandularis**.

Squamous metaplasia is transformation of the normal urothelium to squamous epithelium. It is common in the trigone of adult women and in this location is probably a variant of normal. It is less common in men, and is more likely to be associated chronic irritation and inflammation.

Nephrogenic metaplasia (nephrogenic adenoma) is a metaplastic change of urothelium to renal tubular type epithelium. It may produce clusters of tubules in the lamina propria or an exophytic papillary mass.

Patients with extensive metaplasia and long-standing inflammation are at increased risk of the development of malignancies,

CASE 13-1

Malakoplakia

A 52-year-old lung transplant patient complains of urinary tract symptoms of urgency and frequency. Cystoscopic examination of the bladder shows a 2 cm yellow plaque-like mass in the dome of the bladder. Biopsy of this mass **(Figure 13-5)** shows numerous macrophages with abundant granular cytoplasm with a sprinkling of neutrophils and lymphocytes. The macrophages are positive with periodic acid–Schiff stain. Some of the macrophages contain laminated basophilic structures that are positive with von Kossa stain for calcium.

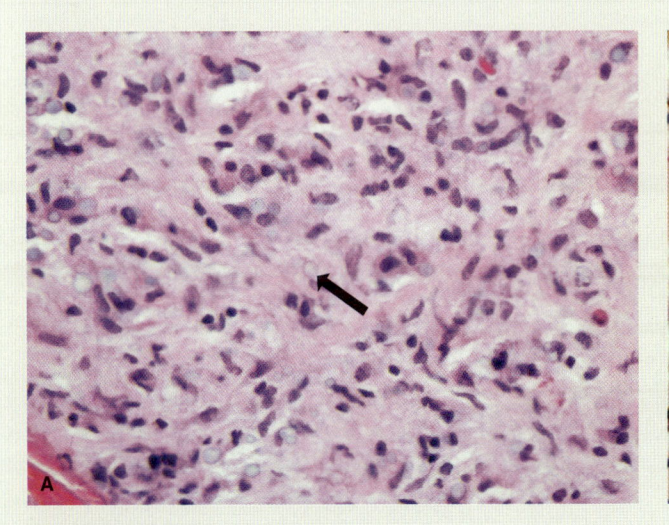

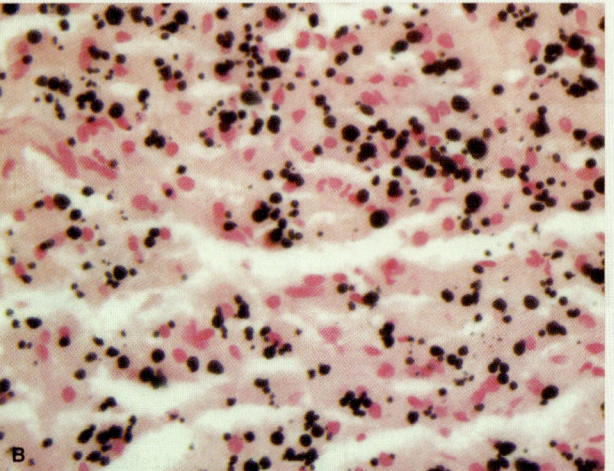

FIGURE 13-5 Photomicrograph of malakoplakia **(A)** The section stained with H&E shows poorly defined lucent inclusions within cells (arrow). **(B)** The section has been prepared using the von Kossa stain that highlights calcium deposits in black. The dark cellular inclusions represent Michaelis–Gutmann bodies, lysosomes engorged with partially degraded, and calcified bacteria.

and the malignancies that arise in these settings may be of the metaplastic tissue type. Thus, patients with extensive squamous metaplasia are at risk of development of squamous cell carcinoma (such as patients with schistosomiasis) and those with extensive cystitis glandularis are at risk of adenocarcinoma (such as is found in association with exstrophy).

Bladder Obstruction

Chronic obstruction of the bladder (such as by BPH) causes changes in the bladder including dilatation, muscle hypertrophy, trabeculation, and diverticula. Patients are often symptomatic with lower urinary tract symptoms (LUTS). This is discussed further in the section on benign prostate hyperplasia.

Bladder Tumors

The most common site of tumors of the urinary tract is the bladder. Bladder cancer is at least partially related to carcinogens present in the urine, and for that reason all of the urothelium (i.e., all cells bathed by urine) is at risk of development of malignancy in a patient with a urothelial tumor (resulting in the so-called **field effect** of urothelial malignancy). The bladder is the most frequently involved site, because (1) the majority of the urothelium is found in the bladder, (2) the bladder is the storage organ for urine, and hence (3) the bladder urothelium has the most intense exposure to any urinary carcinogens. Known carcinogens associated with urothelial tumors include benzene dyes (arylamines), some chemotherapeutic

CASE 13-2

Bladder Cancer Linked to Cytoxan (Cyclophosphamide) Exposure

A 40-year-old female visits her family practice physician with a complaint of gross hematuria. Her past medical history is significant for Hodgkin disease treated with chemotherapy (including Cytoxan) when she was a teenager. Urine culture is taken but is negative, but nevertheless the patient is given a course of antibiotics. The antibiotics do not clear the hematuria and the patient is referred to a urologist. Bladder cytology shows malignant cells (**Figure 13-6**), and cystoscopy shows a ragged tumor involving the left bladder sidewall (**Figure 13-7**). Biopsy of this tumor shows invasive high-grade urothelial carcinoma invasive into the muscularis propria (**Figure 13-8**).

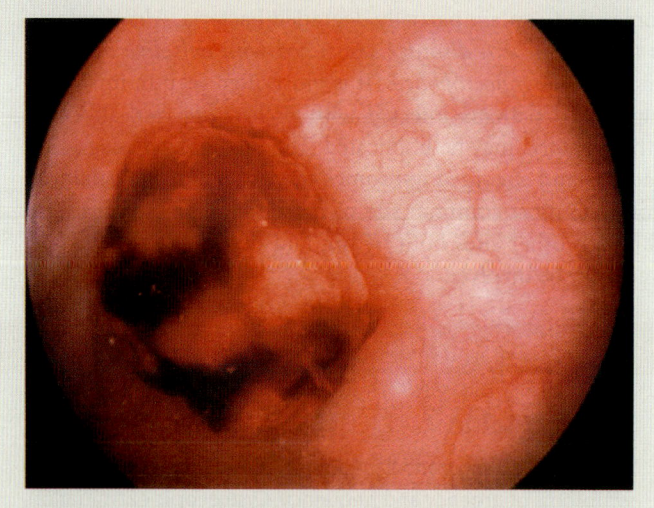

FIGURE 13-7 Cystoscopic image of invasive bladder cancer. Source: http://www.comiterpa.com/Comiterpa_v2.0/home2.html

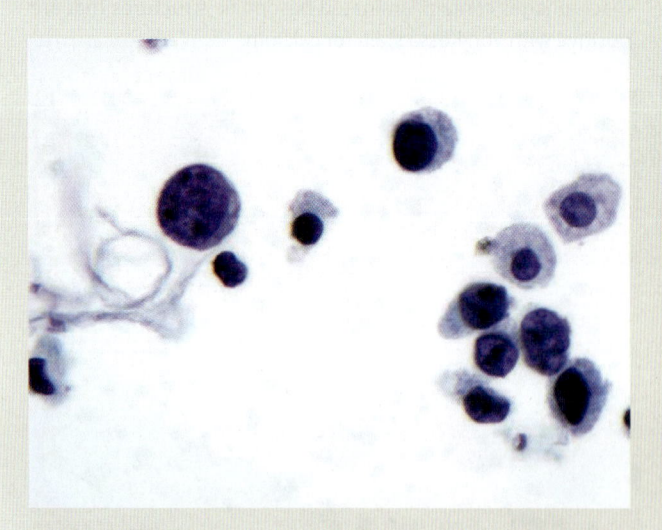

FIGURE 13-6 Urine cytology with malignant cells. Factors suggesting malignant urothelium include the following. Cells have markedly increased nuclear to cytoplasmic ratios with hyperchromatic nuclei. Intracytoplasmic vacuoles are common. Several cells are spindle shaped. Cells are discohesive. Abnormal cells are numerous

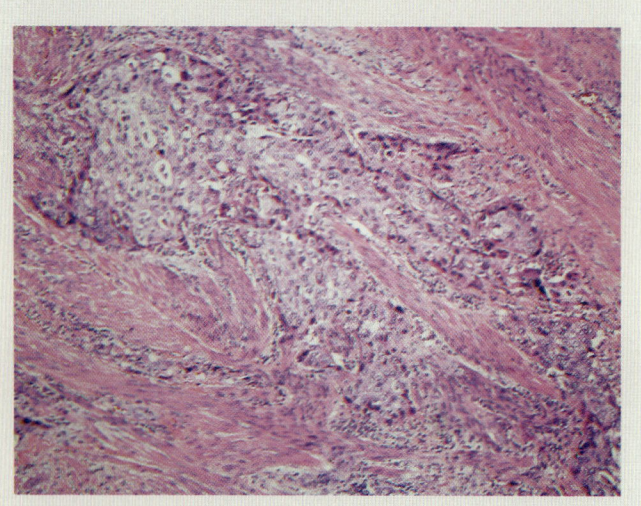

FIGURE 13-8 Photomicrograph of high-grade urothelial carcinoma. The pleomorphic tumor cells are shown invading the muscularis propria.

IN TRANSLATION
Molecular Based Screening Tests for Urothelial Carcinoma

The chromosomal abnormalities that are most commonly identified in bladder cancer have been exploited to develop molecular-based screening tests for urothelial cancer. The most common of these is a fluorescent in situ hybridization based test that can be done on urine (UroVysion™). Aneuploidy of chromosomes 3,7,17 and loss of the p16 locus on 9p12 are evaluated. The test is a helpful adjuvant to urine cytology and clinical follow-up of patients with signs and symptoms or a history of bladder cancer.

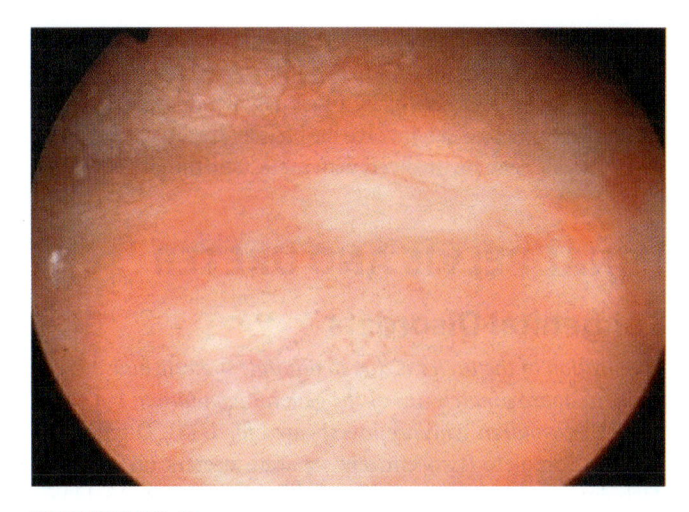

FIGURE 13-9 Cystoscopic image of urothelial carcinoma in situ. Reprinted from Sylvester RJ, van der Meijden A, Witjes JA, et al. High-grade Taurothelial carcinoma and carcinoma in situ of the bladder. Urology; 66:90–107, Copyright 2005, with permission from Elsevier.

agents (such as Cytoxan mentioned above), analgesics that are excreted in the urine, and cigarette smoking (since smoking related carcinogens are excreted in the urine). Historically, arylamines were the most common agent associated with bladder cancer. The concept of carcinogens in the urine being associated with urothelial cancer was first defined in textile workers in New England. Workers involved with the dyeing of cloth had an extraordinarily high incidence of bladder cancer in the late 19th and early 20th century, before environmental controls were in place. Currently, cigarette smoking is the most common risk factor for bladder cancer. Schistosomiasis is associated with bladder cancers, because of the chronic inflammation and squamous metaplasia associated with long-standing infection with this organism. A large number of chromosomal abnormalities have been identified in bladder cancer.

The most common types of bladder tumors are **urothelial (transitional cell) neoplasms.** These show a variety of growth patterns and degrees of cytologic atypia. There are basically three different presentations of bladder neoplasms.

Low-grade noninvasive papillary lesions (papilloma, low-grade carcinoma) *usually present with blood in the urine (hematuria).* Cystoscopy discloses single or multiple lesions having an exophytic, delicate papillary pattern of growth, which do not invade into the bladder wall. Microscopically, these tumors show increased number of layers of urothelial cells in a papillary architecture, and have only mild cytologic atypia. These are usually treated by simple excision. These lesions may recur but only rarely progress to high-grade invasive tumors. Patients undergo surveillance cystoscopy to look for recurrent tumors.

Urothelial carcinoma in situ is a flat lesion that contains malignant cells confined by the basement membrane of the epithelium without invasion, and does not have a papillary architecture. These are grossly seen as red patches or diffuse erythema of the bladder and mimic the gross appearance of cystitis. This lesion usually presents with hematuria and painful urination. Malignant cells may be seen in the urine when examined cytologically (Figure 13-6). *These lesions often progress to invasive tumors if left untreated.* Treatment is usually with topical immunotherapy using attenuated mycobacterium BCG instilled in the bladder or topical chemotherapy. In some cases the lesion regresses, but if it does not the patient usually undergoes cystectomy (see **Figures 13-9** and **13-10**).

Invasive carcinomas are almost always high-grade tumors, which often have invaded into the muscularis of the bladder at presentation. Patients usually present with hematuria, sometimes also with pelvic pain or obstruction of one or both ureters. Muscle invasive bladder cancer is aggressive and long-term survival is poor. Prognosis of bladder cancer depends on stage and grade. Stage is the most important factor, but within any given stage grade has a significant contribution.

Unusual variants of bladder cancer include **squamous cell carcinoma**, which is associated with schistosomiasis, and rarely in the setting of chronic urinary tract infections (UTIs) accompanied by squamous metaplasia, such as occurs in paraplegics with indwelling catheters. **Adenocarcinomas** are associated with glandular metaplasia, such as with exstrophy, or associated with urachal remnants. **Sarcomas**, which arise from the stroma of the

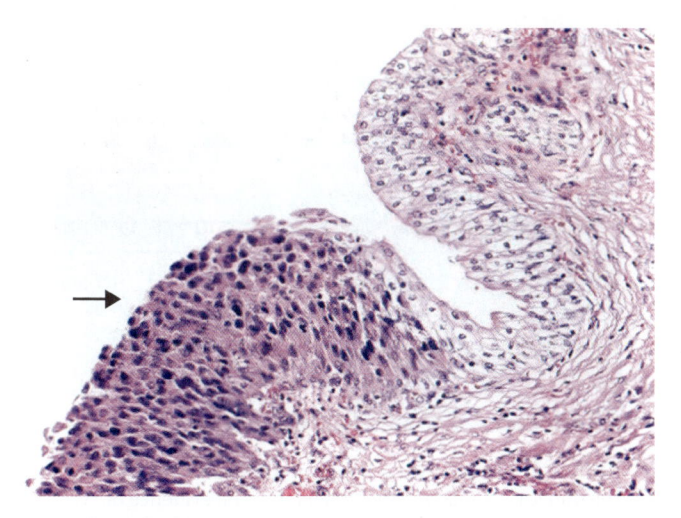

FIGURE 13-10 Photomicrograph of urothelial carcinoma in situ. Area of malignancy is shown by arrow. The upper portion of the field demonstrates normal urothelium for comparison.

bladder, are very rare in adults, but are relatively more common in children where **embryonal rhabdomyosarcoma** is the most frequent example. Occasionally, other pelvic tumors such as cervical or rectal cancer can involve the bladder by direct extension, or the bladder can be involved with metastatic tumors.

RENAL PELVIS AND URETER

Congenital Disorders

Duplication of the ureter is due to multiple ureteric buds, which occur in approximately 1% of the general population, but in up to 10% of children who are investigated for UTIs. Duplication may be complete (two entirely separate ureters on one side each entering the bladder independently see Figure 13-11) or incomplete (one ureter entering the bladder, branching before the collecting system). Complete duplication is more likely to be symptomatic, with obstruction of the upper pole ureter and incompetence (urine reflux) of the lower pole ureter the common presentation.

CASE 13-3

Duplication of the Ureter

A 2-year-old boy is referred to a pediatric urologist for multiple episodes of UTI. Abdominal ultrasound shows dilatation of the collecting system of the upper pole of the kidney with no dilation of the lower pole. Voiding cystoureterography shows reflex into the lower pole of the kidney. This suggests the possibility of duplication of the ureter with obstruction of the upper pole ureter and reflex of the lower pole ureters (Figure 13-11).

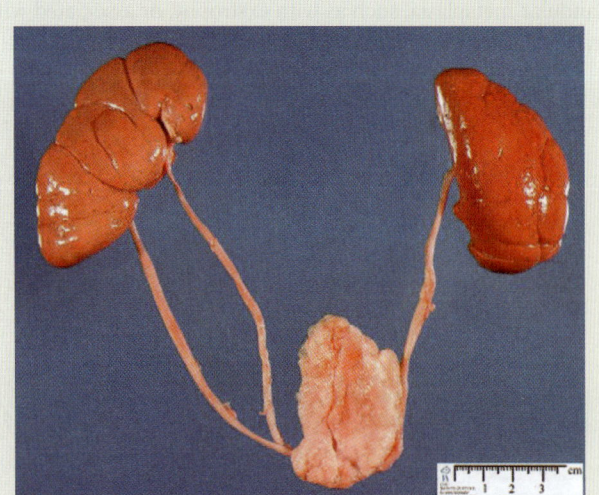

FIGURE 13-11 **Gross image of duplication of ureters.** The duplication is complete. Ureters show no evidence of obstruction. Source: http://www.humpath.com/spip.php?article3423&id_document=24321#documents_portfolio

Congenital Obstruction, particularly of the ureteropelvic junction, is a common cause of hydronephrosis in children. Abnormal amounts of smooth muscle or fibrous tissue replace the muscle of the ureteropelvic junction in such cases. Other causes of congenital obstruction are **ureteric valves** (transverse folds across the lumen of the ureters) or **congenital atresia (stenosis of the ureter)**. Agenesis of the ureter results in agenesis of the corresponding kidney, since the kidney is formed by induction of the mesonephric blastema by the ureteric bud. Congenital dilatation of the ureter, known as **congenital megaureter**, is due to an adynamic segment of ureter that fails to contract in a coordinated fashion to aid the flow of urine.

Obstruction

Obstruction of the ureter may intrinsic (within the lumen of the ureter) or extrinsic (outside the ureter). **Intrinsic** causes include tumors, stones, blood clots and inflammation, and fibrosis. **Extrinsic** causes include anything that partially or completely compresses the ureter, such as extraureteral tumors, fibrosis (especially idiopathic retroperitoneal fibrosis), endometriosis, and occasionally pregnancy.

Tumors

The most common tumor of the renal pelvis and ureter is urothelial carcinoma (transitional cell carcinoma). These are biologically similar to bladder urothelial carcinoma, and discussed in more detail in the bladder section above. Involvement of the ureter or renal pelvis is much less common than the bladder.

PRINCIPAL DISEASES OF THE TESTIS

QUICK REVEIW

Normal Anatomy and Histology

The testes begin intra-abdominally, but descend to the scrotum usually in the late intrauterine period. The scrotal location allows the testes to function at a lower temperature, which is necessary for normal sperm development. The testes are composed of coiled seminiferous tubules present in a loose stroma that contains Leydig cells. Within the seminiferous tubules sperm are produced from germ cells by meiosis. Germ cells progress from spermatogonia to primary spermatocytes to secondary spermatocytes to spermatids to spermatozoa, depending on the stage of meiosis. Also within the seminiferous tubules are Sertoli cells, which nourish sperm and secrete inhibin that helps regulate pituitary gonadotropins (FSH and LH). The stromal Leydig cells secrete testosterone, the male androgenic hormone. The testis is covered by a tough white fibrous capsule, the tunica albuginea. Adjacent to the testis is the epididymis, which is a storage sac for sperm. The outflow of sperm is through the vas deferens in the spermatic cord to the urethra (Figure 13-12).

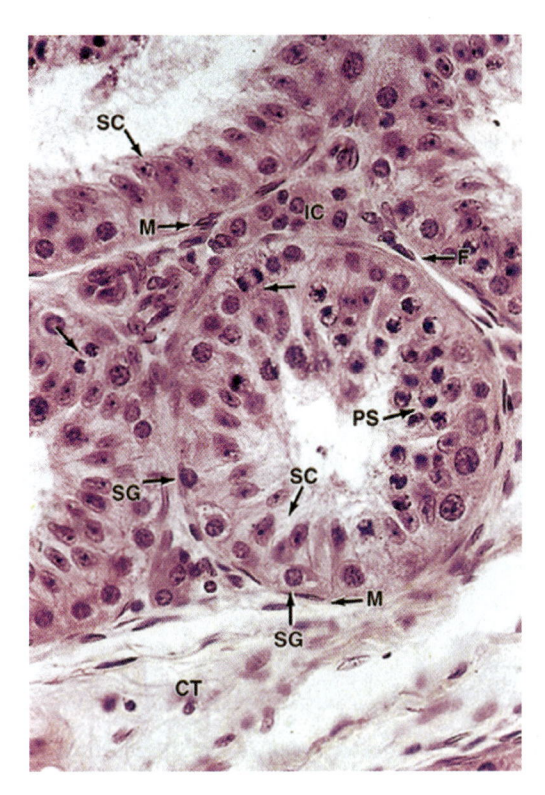

FIGURE 13-12 Photomicrograph of normal testis histology (detail of seminiferous tubule and interstitial cells). The micrograph shows seminiferous tubules surrounded by connective tissue (CT), containing many large rounded or polygonal interstitial cells (Leydig cells) (IC) secreting androgens. Immediately surrounding each tubule are flattened myoid cells (M), which contract to help move sperm out of the tubule, and layers of fibroblasts (F). Inside the tubule itself is a unique seminiferous epithelium composed of columnar supporting cells called Sertoli cells (SC), which usually have oval nuclei and distinct nucleoli, and germ cells of the spermatogenic lineage. Prominent among the latter are spermatogonia (SG), diploid cells always located near the basement membrane, and primary spermatocytes (PS) that are undergoing meiosis closer to the lumen of the tubule. At the upper left corner is a portion of a straight tubule, which lacks germ cells and consists solely of Sertoli cells. (Mescher et al. Junqueira's Basic Histology Text & Atlas, 12th edition. New York, NY: McGraw Hill Lange. 2008;374)

CASE 13-4

Germ Cell Aplasia

A 32-year-old married male visits a urologist because he and his wife have not been able to conceive after 3 years of trying. The patient's wife had been previously pregnant with a different partner. Physical examination shows no abnormalities, and past medical history and social history are unrevealing. Semen analysis shows no sperm present. Serum LH, FSH, testosterone, and prolactin are all normal. Transrectal and scrotal ultrasound show no abnormalities, specifically normal sized testis were seen with no evidence of varicocele or ejaculatory duct obstruction. Vasography shows patent excretory ducts bilaterally. Testicular biopsy is performed to further evaluate the testis and potentially retrieve sperm for in vitro fertilization. Biopsy shows normal sized seminiferous tubules with no germ cells and only Sertoli cells (Figure 13-13).

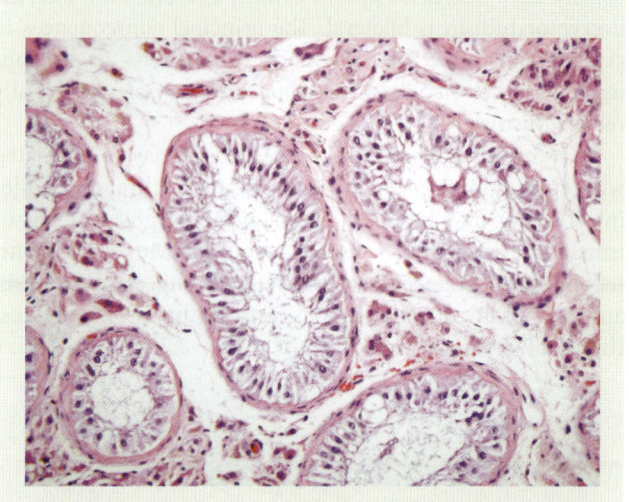

FIGURE 13-13 Photomicrograph of testis with germ cell aplasia. (A) Note complete absence of spermatogonia around periphery of the seminiferous tubules. Refer to Figure 13-12 (normal) for comparison of Histologic details.

Male Infertility

Male infertility is a complex topic, and only the high points will be touched on here. Male infertility can be divided into pretesticular causes (such as endocrine and metabolic causes), testicular causes (intrinsic to the testis), and post-testicular causes (blockages of the excretory ducts).

Pretesticular causes include disorders of the hypothalamus, pituitary, and peripheral organs that interfere with the hormone cascade necessary for normal testicular functioning. Common examples are (1) tumors involving the pituitary or impinging on the hypothalamus, (2) a systemic disease or medication that suppresses the release of hormones or has antiandrogenic effects, and (3) idiopathic failure of production of gonadotrophic releasing hormone by the hypothalamus (idiopathic hypogonadotropic hypogonadism).

Testicular causes of infertility are multifactorial and are both congenital and noncongenital. Cryptorchidism, the most common pediatric genital-associated defect, is associated with sterility when left untreated. Causes of cryptorchidism (see below) are generally multifactorial lacking well-defined genetic etiology. Infertility associated with chromosomal abnormalities includes Klinefelter syndrome [XXY], Y chromosome microdeletions, which may result in germ cell aplasia (Sertoli cell only syndrome see Figure 13-13), Down syndrome, and a number of single gene mutations. Examples of the latter include myotonic dystrophy, which may be associated with testicular atrophy and Noonan Syndrome, most often caused by an autosomal dominant condition resulting in cryptorchidism. Noncongenital causes of infertility include varicocele, trauma, chemotherapy, radiation, and inflammation of the testis (orchitis).

Post-testicular causes include problems with sperm transport through the excretory ducts of the testis, and include congenital and acquired blockages of the ducts, cystic fibrosis, and immotile cilia such as is seen with Kartagener syndrome.

Non-Neoplastic Testicular Lesions

Cryptorchidism is failure of one or both testes to descend into the scrotum. It is more common in premature than full-term infants. In many of these children, the testis will descend spontaneously in the first year of life. If it does not, the testis is usually placed in the correct position surgically (orchiopexy). Uncorrected cryptorchid testes are smaller than normal, contain smaller seminiferous tubules and fewer germ cells, and show a thickened basement membrane and increased stromal fibrosis (Figure 13-14). Patients with one cryptorchid testis usually have decreased sperm counts, and often are infertile if cryptorchidism is bilateral. The principal consequences of cryptorchidism are infertility and increased risk of developing a germ cell neoplasm. Orchiopexy may not significantly reduce this risk.

Orchitis is inflammation of the testis. It may be associated with **epididymitis**, occur secondary to a urethral or bladder infection, or may be due to hematogenous spread of organisms. Bacterial orchitis is usually associated with epididymitis secondary to gram-negative bacteria. Syphilis, tuberculosis, and mumps are other infectious diseases that involve the testis, usually hematogenously.

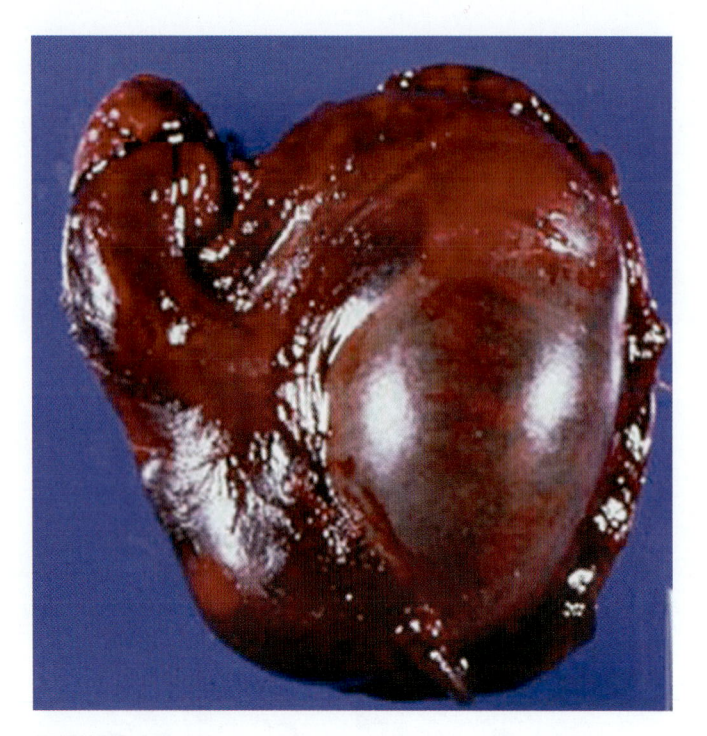

FIGURE 13-15 Gross image of infarcted, torsed testis.

Torsion of the testis is twisting of the spermatic cord within the scrotum, causing vascular compression of the vessels contained in the spermatic cord, which eventuates in hemorrhagic infarction of the testis (Figures 13-15 and 13-16). This is an exquisitely painful condition and a medical emergency. Torsion is most often seen in young men engaging in vigorous exercise. Surgery to untwist the spermatic cord and "tack down" the testis in the scrotum is undertaken if the condition is caught before the testis infarcts, otherwise the necrotic testis is removed.

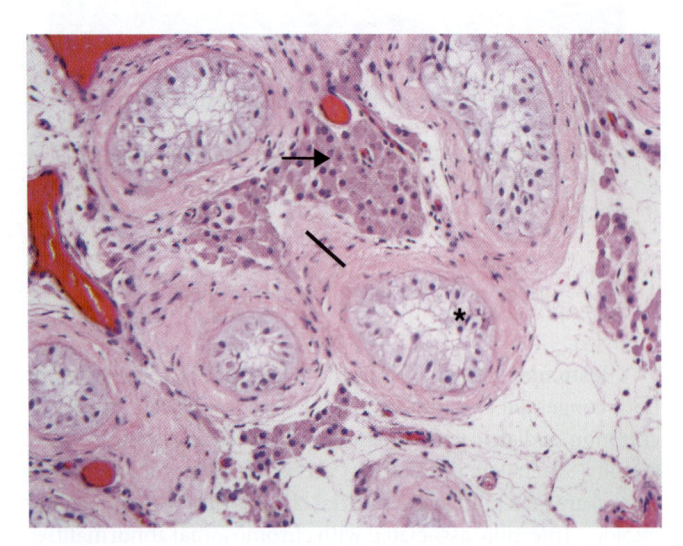

FIGURE 13-14 **Photomicrograph of cryptorchidism.** Seminiferous tubules are smaller than normal and contain few (if any) germ cells. Leydig cells are increased in number and hypertrophic having a vacuolated cytoplasm (arrow). There is increased stromal fibrosis and a thickened basement membranes of the tubules (line). Seminiferous tubules contain mostly immature Leydig cells having extensive cytoplasmic processes that fill the tubule (*).

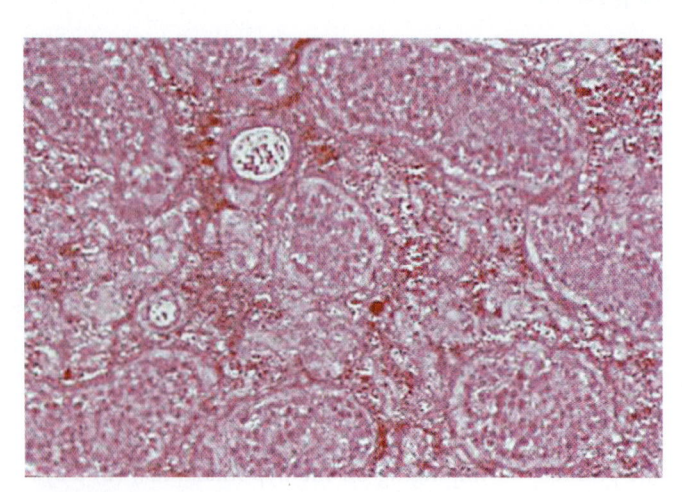

FIGURE 13-16 **Photomicrograph of infarcted testis.** The testis demonstrates coagulative focus with only stromal elements and hemorrhage visible.

Testicular Tumors

The most common tumors of the testis are germ cell tumors. Unlike most solid organ tumors, testicular germ cell tumors usually present in young adult life (especially age 25–45). Pathogenesis of testicular carcinoma is unknown in most cases. However, men who have or have had cryptorchidism or genetic syndromes that cause gonadal dysgenesis are at increased risk. The precursor lesion of testicular germ cell tumors is **intratubular germ cell neoplasia**, which consists of malignant germ cells within the seminiferous tubules without invasion of the stroma. Occasionally, this in situ lesion is found when the testis is biopsied for infertility.

Most primary testicular germ cell tumors are present as a painless solid mass within the testis. *A solid intratesticular*

CASE 13-5

Mixed Nonseminomatous Germ Cell Tumor of the Testis

A 23-year-old paratrooper presents to his medical officer with a unilateral 4 cm painless testicular mass. Ultrasound shows that the mass is solid and intratesticular. Serum tumor markers are drawn, and show that both the serum beta-human choriogonadotropin (β-HCG) and alpha-fetoprotein (AFP) are elevated (541 units and 370 units, respectively, with normal being less than 10 units and less than 5 units, respectively). The patient is taken to surgery and a radical orchiectomy is performed, which consists of an incision made into the inguinal area; the testis drawn up into the incision by the spermatic cord, the testis inspected, the spermatic cord clamped, and cut; and the testis with attached epididymis and spermatic cord removed and sent to pathology. Grossly, an intratesticular nodule is present, and microscopically a mixed germ cell tumor is seen, with components of embryonal carcinoma, yolk sac tumor, choriocarcinoma, and teratoma (**Figures 13-17** and **13-18**). After surgery the tumor markers remained elevated, and CT scan of the abdomen shows retroperitoneal lymphadenopathy. Three cycles of chemotherapy are given and the lymphadenopathy regresses and the tumor markers return to normal baseline.

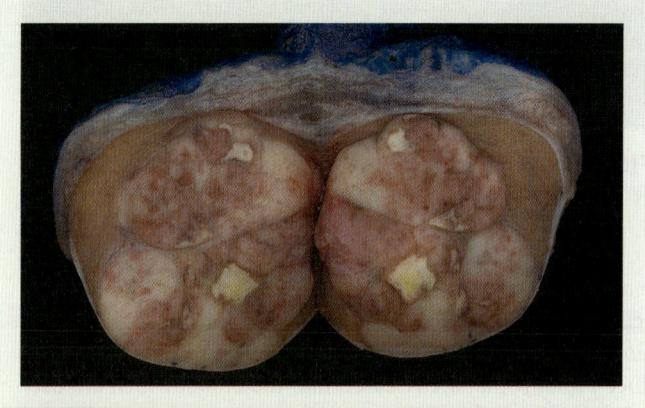

FIGURE 13-17 Gross photo of nonseminomatous germ cell tumor: Heterogeneous tumor components occupy almost all of this "bivalved" (transected and spread open) testis. The blue color (upper margin of specimen) represents "inking" (ink placed on the external margin) by the surgical pathologist.

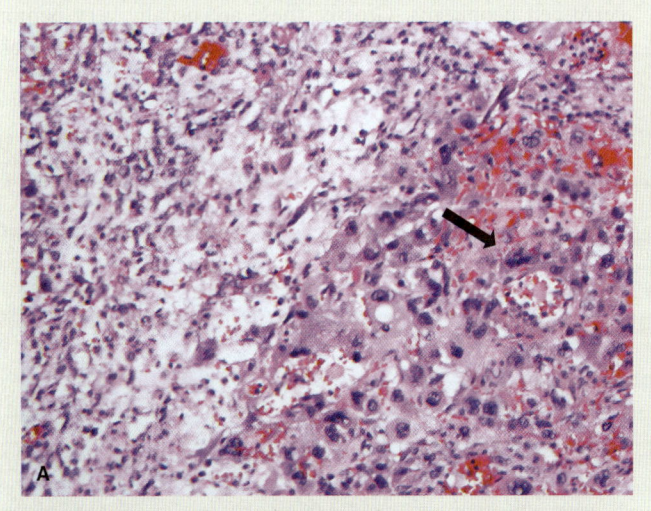

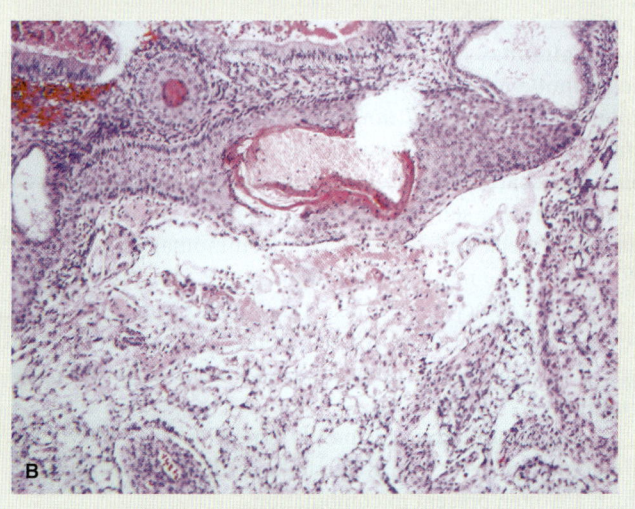

FIGURE 13-18 Photomicrograph of nonseminomatous germ cell tumor (containing teratoma, yolk sac tumor, and choriocarcinoma). **(A)** Multinucleate syncytiotrophoblastic cells of the choriocarcinoma component are easy to discern (arrow) in this area of the tumor (see also Figure 13-23). **(B)** The upper third of the field shows a disorganized mixture of benign-appearing tissue characteristic of teratomas. The lower two thirds show glandular and microcystic structures associated with yolk sac tumors (better described in Figure 13-22).

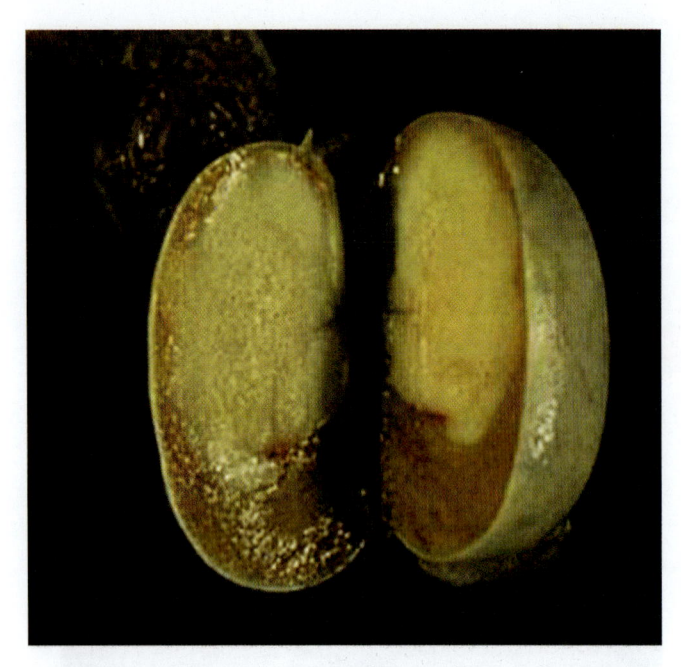

FIGURE 13-19 **Gross photo of seminoma:** Note the clearly demarcated white/tan tumor in the body of the testis.

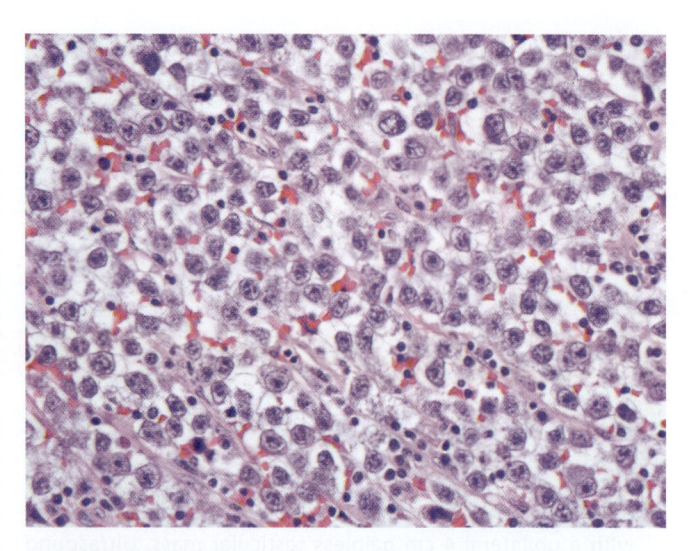

FIGURE 13-20 **Photomicrograph of seminoma.** The tumor cells are uniform and have a polygonal shape. Many of the nuclei appear vesiculated. The cytoplasm is often clear and difficult to see and may also contain vesicles. The cells are similar in appearance to spermatogonia.

mass is a malignant neoplasm until proven otherwise. Germ cells are pluripotential, and have the ability to differentiate along different embryonic lines. Some germ cell tumors produce proteins that are released into the blood, which are useful as tumor markers. The two principal markers are **AFP** and **β-HCG**. These can be helpful in classifying the tumors preoperatively, and following patients postoperatively. **Lactic dehydrogenase (LDH)** may also be elevated in testicular cancer. It is not specific to any particular type of testicular cancer or even to testicular cancer, but may serve as a marker of tissue injury and tumor burden.

Seminomas contain malignant germ cells that retain the phenotypic features of spermatogonia. *This is the most common pure germ cell tumor (40%).* The peak age of presentation is 30–40. Grossly, the tumors are white/tan, solid, and sharply demarcated from the surrounding testis. Microscopically, seminomas contain large, uniform malignant germ cells and lymphocytes. Seminomas are usually AFP and HCG negative. Seminomas are initially treated by radical orchiectomy. If these tumors become metastatic, they are very radiation sensitive. Chemotherapy may also be used. On the whole, seminoma has an excellent prognosis **(Figures 13-19 and 13-20).**

Nonseminomatous germ cell tumors include embryonal carcinoma, yolk sac tumor, teratoma and choriocarcinoma, which are often present in combination.

Embryonal carcinoma presents about a decade earlier than seminoma, usually in young men in their 20s. Grossly, these tumors are more heterogeneous than seminoma, and are often partially necrotic and may contain cysts or hemorrhage. Microscopically these tumors show highly pleomorphic cells in glands, cords, sheets, and papillae. Embryonal carcinomas are usually AFP and HCG negative **(Figure 13-21).**

Yolk sac tumor is usually a childhood tumor (under age 10) when pure, but is most commonly a component of adult mixed germ cell tumor. The gross appearance is often partially cystic and hemorrhagic. A variety of glandular patters (cysts, acini, papillae) are seen microscopically. These tumors are usually AFP positive, and massive elevations of serum AFP may sometimes occur. HCG is negative **(Figure 13-22).**

Choriocarcinoma is a very unusual as a pure testicular tumor, and is most commonly found as a component of mixed germ cell neoplasms. Grossly, these are usually very hemorrhagic or necrotic. Microscopically, these tumors contain

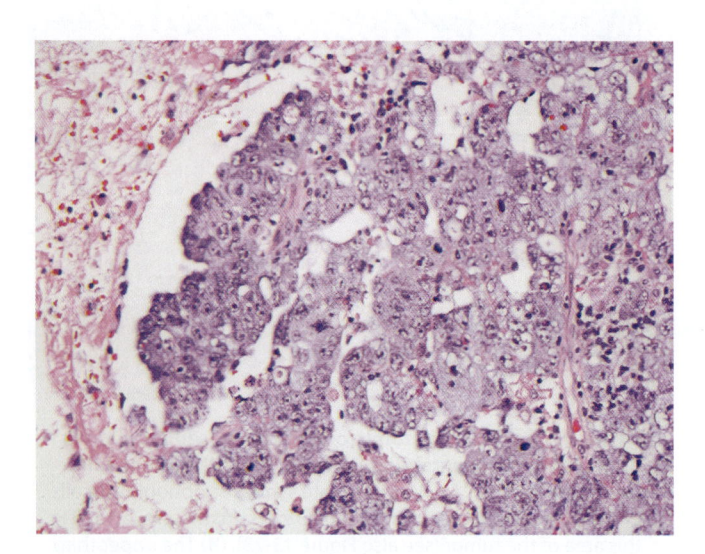

FIGURE 13-21 **Photomicrograph of embryonal carcinoma.** Tumor consists of sheets of pleomorphic undifferentiated cells.

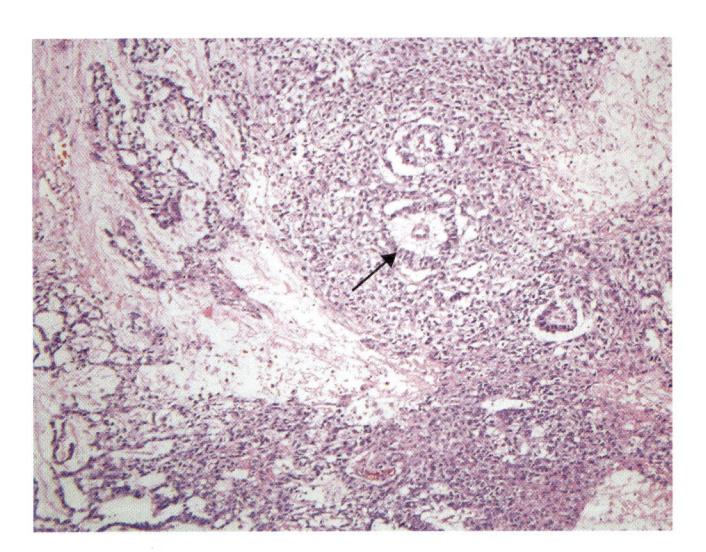

FIGURE 13-22 Photomicrograph of yolk sac tumor. Tumors have a glandular pattern and contain characteristic **Schiller–Duval bodies** (arrow), which are rounded masses of yolk sac tumor surrounded by a clear space. They mimic glomeruli in appearance.

malignant syncytiotrophoblast and cytotrophoblast, and mimic the development of the placenta. HCG levels are elevated, often greater than 10,000 mIU/mL, and AFP is negative (Figures 13-18A and 13-23).

Teratomas develop along somatic cell lines, and can show surprisingly normal-appearing tissues presenting in a disorganized fashion. Skin, GI epithelium, cartilage, and neural tissues are all common in teratomas, often jumbled together. Sometimes immature fetal-appearing tissues are present. Teratomas have a variable gross and microscopic appearance, depending on the tissues present. In children, pure teratomas are possible, but in adults they are usually part of a mixed germ cell tumor. Teratomas may have a benign course in children, but are malignant in adults as they represent terminal somatic differentiation in a malignant germ cell tumor. Teratomas are AFP and HCG negative (Figure 13-18B).

Mixed germ cell tumors are more common than any individual pure tumor. Any mixture is possible, but the most common is teratocarcinoma, which is mixed teratoma and embryonal carcinoma (Figure 13-18). The nonseminomatous germ cell tumors are initially treated with radical orchiectomy, and may also be treated up front with adjuvant chemotherapy because these tumors are aggressive. Spread to the lymph nodes of the retroperitoneum is the most usual site of metastasis but widespread hematogenous spread to other organs, especially the lungs and brain can occur. However, patients have a good prognosis even with widespread metastasis, because of advances in modern chemotherapy, one of the great success stories of modern medicine. Tumor markers are helpful in following patients with nonseminomatous germ cell tumors.

Gonadal Stromal/Sex Cord Tumors

Gonadal stromal and sex cord tumors are much less common than germ cell tumors, compromising less than 5% of testicular tumors. *They predominately arise from the Sertoli cells within seminiferous tubules and stromal Leydig cells. Most are benign.*

Leydig cell tumors have two age peaks: about 20% occur in childhood (usually between ages 5 and 10) and the remainder in adulthood. Many Leydig cell tumors are hormonally active. Either testosterone or estrogen may be produced by the tumor. Testosterone-producing Leydig cell tumors may give rise to precocious puberty in children. In adults, testosterone-producing tumors are less clinically apparent, and patients more often present with a clinical testicular mass. Estrogen-producing tumors may produce gynecomastia and other findings of feminization. Pathologically, Leydig cell tumors are

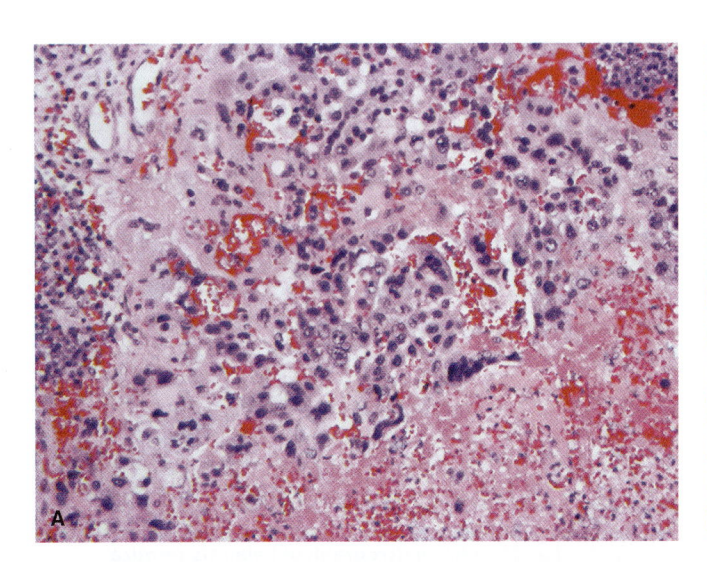

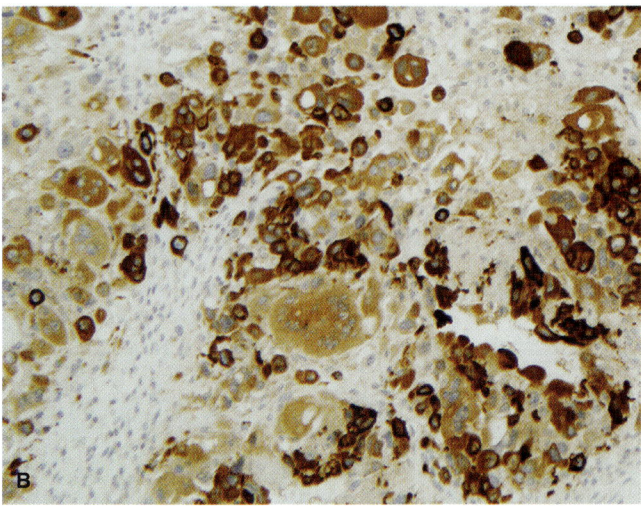

FIGURE 13-23 Photomicrograph of choriocarcinoma. **(A)** Choriocarcinoma contains distinctive multinucleated giant syncytiotrophoblasts and mononuclear cytotrophoblasts (see also Figure 18A). **(B)** The malignant cell population is highlighted using immunostaining for HCG (brown color).

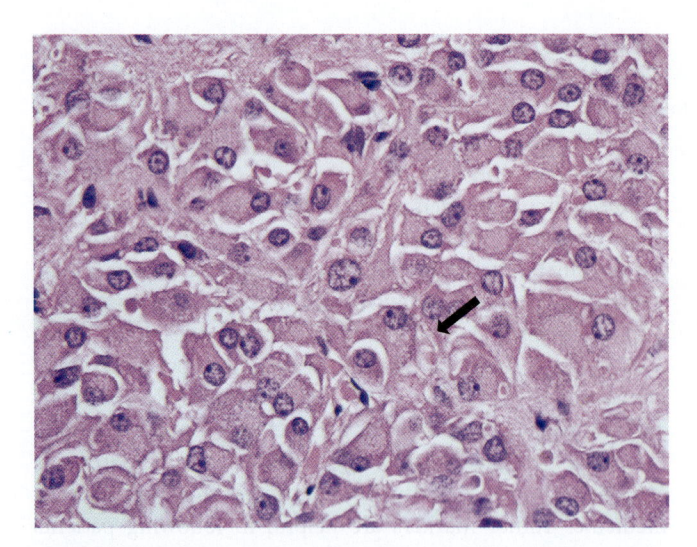

FIGURE 13-24 **Photomicrograph of Leydig cell tumor.** Tumor cells are uniform and have eosinophilic cytoplasm that may contain rod-shaped crystals of Reinke (arrow).

grossly seen as yellow-brown masses. They are composed of uniform cells with eosinophilic cytoplasm. Rod-shaped intracytoplasmic **crystals of Reinke** may be seen in up to 40% of cases **(Figure 13-24)**.

Sertoli cell tumors are less common than Leydig cell tumors. They are usually found in middle age and present with a mass, although estrogen production may occur. Sertoli cell tumors are composed of cells with scant cytoplasm arranged in cords or tubules **(Figure 13-25)**.

EXTERNAL GENITALIA

External male genitalia include the penis and the scrotum. The principal diseases of the external male genitalia are congenital, inflammatory, infectious, cysts of the scrotum, and neoplasms.

The most common congenital abnormalities in this area involve the urethra. **Epispadias** is congenital absence of the upper wall of the urethra, causing the urethral opening to appear on the dorsum of the penis. **Hypospadias** is much more common, and in this condition the urethra opens on the underside of the penis or on the perineum.

The most common noninfectious inflammatory condition in this area is **phimosis***, a condition in which the foreskin cannot be retracted behind the glans penis.* It may be seen in uncircumcised men at any age. Phimosis may be congenital or noncongenital. Acquired phimosis is usually due to chronic inflammation and fibrosis, often due to poor hygiene. The treatment of phimosis is circumcision.

Peyronie disease is a fibrosis of the shaft of the penis and can cause pain and penile curvature during erection. It is usually treated by surgical excision of the fibrosis. **Balanitis** refers to inflammation of the skin of the penis, resulting from virtually any dermatologic lesion or infection. **Balanitis xerotica obliterans** is penile lichen sclerosis (see Chapter 20 Pathology of the Skin). It is a chronic and atrophic condition of the skin and mucous membranes that commonly involves genital and perianal skin. The cause is unknown, but it may be related to autoimmune mechanisms. The disease can be grossly seen as an atrophic-appearing white patch on the glans penis or prepuce. Microscopically, the epidermis is atrophic with vacuolation of the basal cells and possibly surface hyperkeratosis. The dermis is edematous and the collagen in the dermis is present as a homogeneous band with a layer of chronic inflammatory cells beneath **(Figure 13-26)**. Balanitis xerotica obliterans may precede or coexist with penile cancer.

Sexually transmitted diseases are common and are only briefly reviewed here.

Syphilis is caused by the spirochete *Treponema pallidum*. The classic manifestation of primary syphilis is the chancre, which is an ulcer at the site of entry of the organism, and is

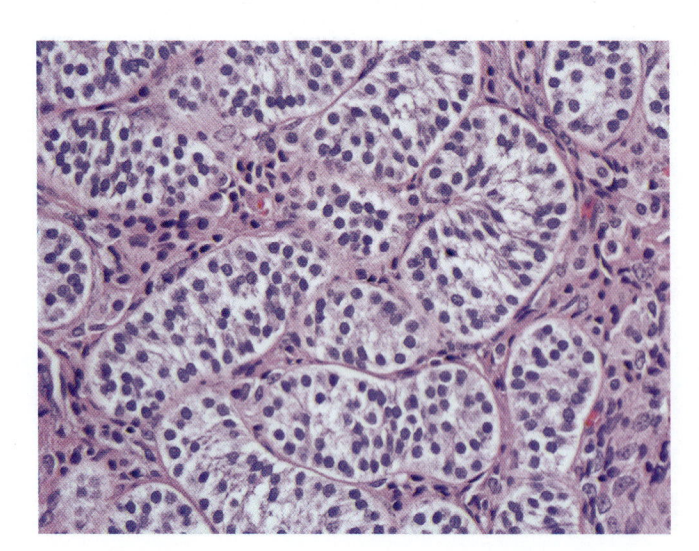

FIGURE 13-25 **Photomicrograph of Sertoli cell tumor.** Sertoli cell tumors form tubular structures strikingly similar to seminiferous tubules in cases of germ cell aplasia (as in Figure 13-13).

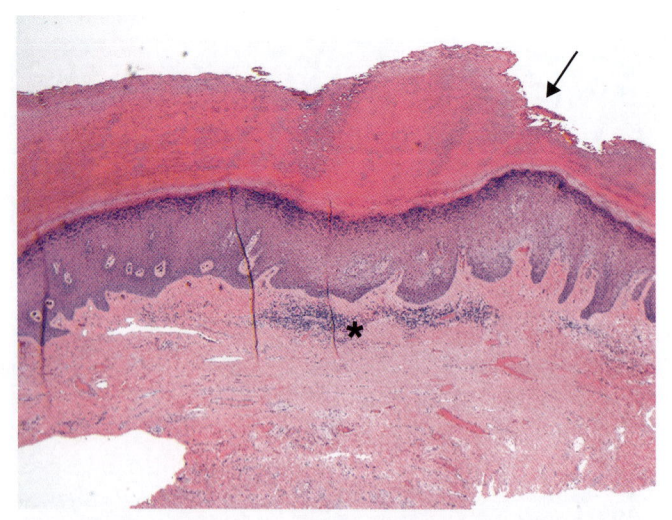

FIGURE 13-26 **Photomicrograph of balanitis xerotica obliterans.** The atrophic epidermis exhibits marked hyperkeratosis (arrow). There is lichenoid (band-like) inflammation in the dermis below the rete ridges (*).

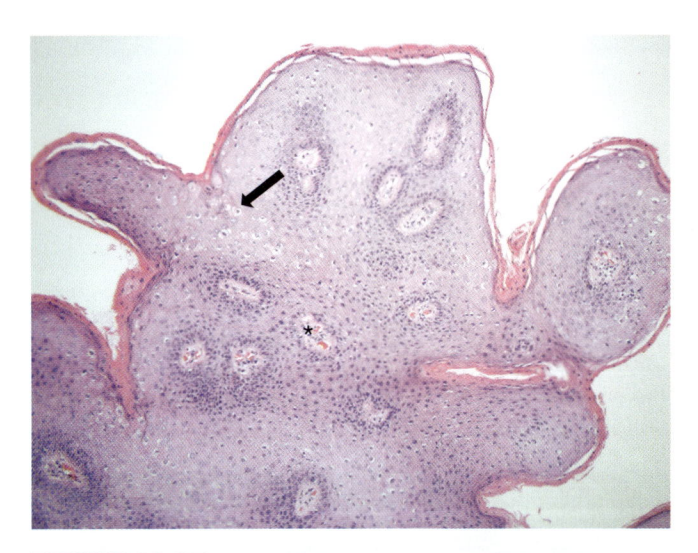

FIGURE 13-27 Photomicrograph of condyloma acuminatum of the penis. The lesion demonstrates marked epidermal hyperplasia and contains numerous small fibrovascular bundles (cut in cross section) (*). There is hyperkeratosis with parakeratosis. The characteristic koilocytosis (nuclear haloing) of HPV is visible in many areas (arrow).

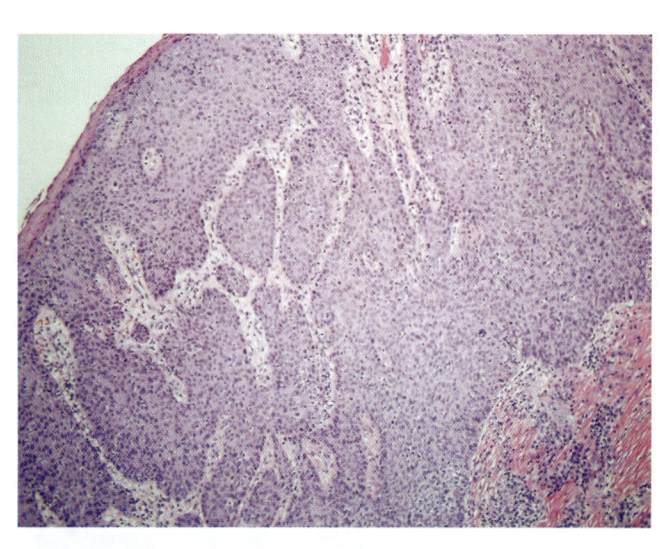

FIGURE 13-28 Photomicrograph of invasive squamous cell carcinoma of the penis. Cords of invasive squamous cells invade into the underlying fibrovascular tissue.

seen on the penis as well as the vulva, vagina, anus, or mouth. The organisms are present within the epidermis of the ulcer and in vessel walls. There is often endothelial proliferation. The external male GU organs may also be involved in **secondary syphilis** with the lesions **of condyloma lata**, which are white plaques on the perineum or scrotum (or vulva), microscopically corresponding to papillomatous hyperplasia of the epidermis with chronic inflammation in the underlying dermis and numerous spirochetes. These lesions are highly infectious.

Condyloma acuminatum (venereal wart) is due to Human papilloma virus (HPV) infection. Types 6 and 11 are the most common in this site. Grossly, warty lesions are present that microscopically show thickened squamous epithelium with a papillary architecture, and may show koilocytic nuclear atypia (Figure 13-27).

The cystic lesions that arise from the scrotal sac around the testis are the various "celes."

Hydrocele is accumulation of serous fluid in the space between the parietal and visceral tunica vaginalis. These may be idiopathic or associated with inguinal hernia or inflammatory conditions. **Hematocele** is accumulation of blood in this space, and often is associated with prior hydrocele. **Spermatocele** refers to what is actually an epididymal cyst. It is a dilatation of an efferent ductile of the head of the epididymis or the rete testis. It contains sperm originating from the epididymis. These three conditions are usually treated by simple surgical excision of cystic mass. **Varicocele** is a mass of dilated veins of the pampiniform plexus of the spermatic cord. The increased volume of blood in close proximity to the testis can cause testicular atrophy and infertility in the adjacent testis. Treatment is ligation of these vessels. *It is important to clinically distinguish these cystic lesions from true intratesticular masses, so as not to confuse these with testicular cancer.*

The most common neoplasm of the external genitalia is squamous cell carcinoma.

An interesting historical note is that scrotal squamous cell carcinoma was the first human cancer associated with a carcinogen. Chimney sweeps in the 18th and 19th century in England, constantly exposed to soot, developed squamous cell carcinoma of the scrotum because the rugae of the scrotal skin trapped soot with its many carcinogens. *Today, the most common tumor site of squamous cell carcinoma in the external genitalia is the penis, and the disease is almost always confined to uncircumcised men.*

A variety of names are used to refer to the different forms of this disease. Squamous cell carcinoma in situ is either **Bowen disease** if the shaft of the penis is involved, or **erythroplasia of Queyrat** if on the glans or foreskin.

Invasive squamous cell carcinoma is usually an exophytic mass, which may be minimally or extensively invasive. Spread is to inguinal lymph nodes (Figure 13-28). A variant of squamous cell carcinoma is **verrucous carcinoma** (formerly known as **giant condyloma of Buschke and Lowenstein**) that is very well-differentiated squamous carcinoma that may be locally destructive but does not metastasize.

PATHOLOGY OF THE PROSTATE

Review of Normal Anatomy, Histology, and Physiology

The prostate is a fibromuscular and glandular organ that sits in the pelvis distal to the urinary bladder (Figure 13-29). The primary function of the prostate gland is to secrete fluid that contributes to seminal fluid to nourish sperm, and prostatic fluid contains enzymes that play an important part in liquefying seminal fluid to promote spermatic motility. The

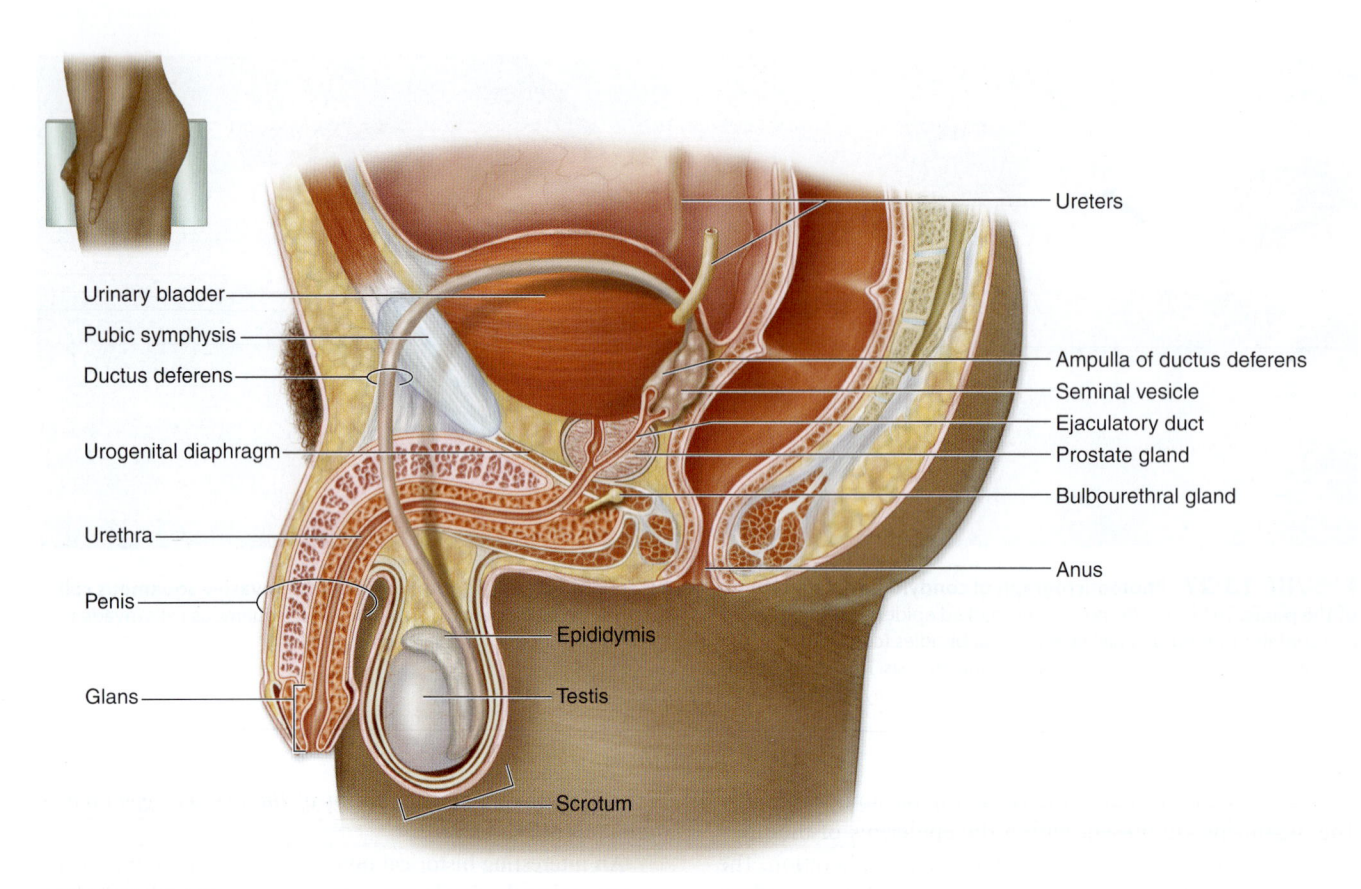

FIGURE 13-29 Diagram of location of the prostate in the pelvis. (Mescher et al. Junqueira's Basic Histology Text & Atlas, 12th edition. New York, NY: McGraw Hill Lange. 2010;372, Figure21-1.).

prostatic ducts drain into the urethra at the verumontanum. The prostate is shaped like an upside-down triangle, with the base of the prostate adjacent to the bladder, and the apex of the prostate pointing down into the pelvis. The urethra is completely enclosed within the prostate gland, and some diseases of the prostate (especially BPH) may compress the urethra, causing bladder outlet obstruction. Histologically, the prostate is composed of complex, branching glands set in a fibromuscular stroma. Approximately 65% of the volume of normal prostate is stroma (smooth muscle or fibrous tissue), and 35% are glands. The glandular epithelium is bilayered **(Figure 13-30A)**. The luminal cells are the secretory cells, and the basal cells play a role in support of the secretory cells and are the proliferative compartment of the prostate

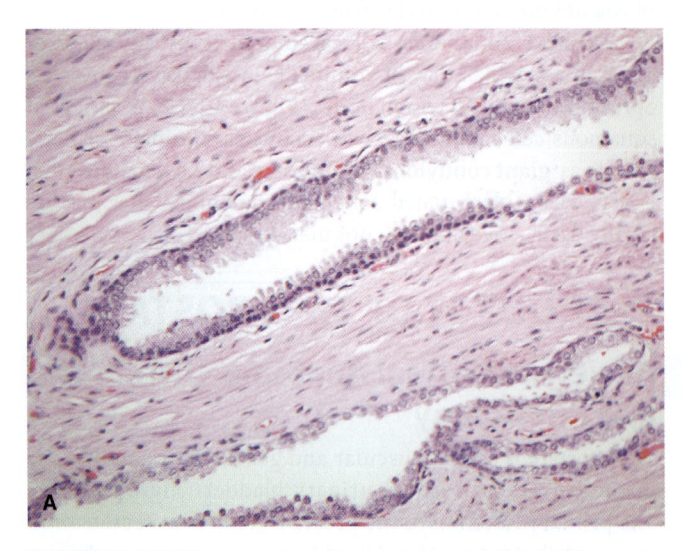

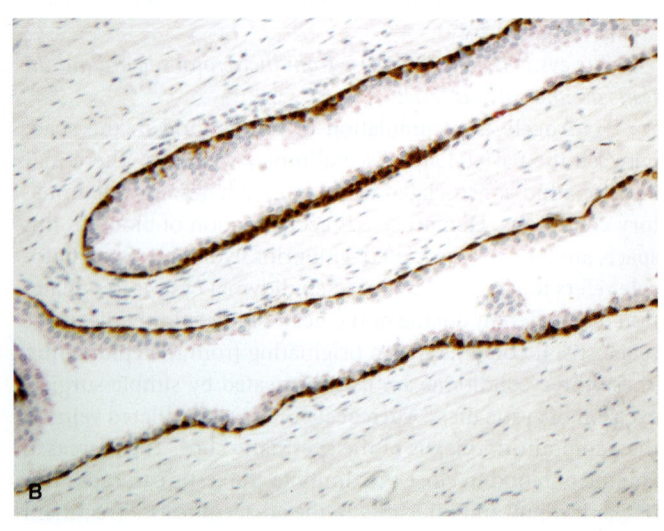

FIGURE 13-30 Photomicrograph of benign prostatic tissue. (A) Prostate glands are lined by bi-layered epithelium, consisting of a basal and secretory cell layer. The fibromuscular stroma surrounds the glandular elements. **(B)** Immunostain for high molecular weight keratin highlights basal cells in normal prostate (brown color).

glands. The secretory cells contain and secrete various proteins, and among them are prostatic-specific antigen (PSA) and prostatic acid phosphatase (PSAP). These two proteins are markers of both benign and malignant prostate epithelial cells, and these proteins may be detected by immunohistochemistry and measured in the serum as markers of prostate disease. PSA is a more sensitive marker than PSAP, and is the marker most used clinically. The basal cells lack PSA and PSAP, but contain high molecular weight cytokeratin (HWCK), which serves as an immunohistochemical marker for benign basal cells (Figure 13-30B). Both the glandular and stromal cells contain hormone receptors and are under hormonal control.

QUICK REVIEW
Zones of the Prostate and the Diseases Which are Most Likely to Occur in These Zones (Figure 13-31)

Different diseases have propensities to involve different parts of the prostate. Because of this, the prostate is functionally divided into three zones: the peripheral zone, the transition zone, and the central zone. The peripheral zone is the posterior-lateral portion of the prostate (against the rectum), and also extends to the apex and wraps around the distal urethra. This is the zone in which most carcinomas arise. Somewhat fortuitously, this is also the zone that is more easily examined by digital rectal examination. The transition zone is in the middle of the prostate in the periurethral location, and wraps around the proximal urethra. Unfortunately, this is the zone in which BPH arises, and this localization of hyperplasia exacerbates the tendency for hyperplasia to obstruct the urethra. The central zone is anterior and proximal, and is primarily fibromuscular tissue resistant to hyperplasia and carcinoma.

QUICK REVIEW
Major Points in the Hormonal Axis of the Prostate

The prostate is a hormonally controlled organ, and normal growth and development of the prostate is dependent having an intact hypothalamus/pituitary/testicular axis. The hypothalamus secretes lutenizing hormone releasing hormone (LHRH) that stimulates the pituitary gland to secrete lutenizing hormone (LH), which stimulates the Leydig cells of the testis to secrete testosterone. Testosterone is converted to dihydrotestosterone (DHT) by the enzyme 5-alpha reductase in the prostatic epithelial cells. DHT is the active form of the hormone. DHT binds to the androgen receptors of prostatic glandular cells and activates cell functions, especially cellular proliferation. DHT is required for development of prostatic hyperplasia and prostate carcinoma. Any interruption of this hormonal cascade will interfere with prostatic growth and development, and manipulations of these hormones are used for treatment of both benign hyperplasia and carcinoma of the prostate.

Hypothalamus $\xrightarrow{LHRH}$ Pituitary $\xrightarrow{LH}$ Leydig cells of testis $\rightarrow$ Testosterone $\xrightarrow{\text{5-alpha reductase}}$ Dihydrotestosterone

CASE 13-6

Chronic Prostatitis

A 45-year-old male complains of low back pain and pelvic pain, following a UTI 4 months ago. He describes a "dragging" sensation in his groin, slight burning with urination, and frequent urination. He visits a urologist, who diagnoses chronic prostatitis and prescribes a 6-week course of antibiotics (Figure 13-32).

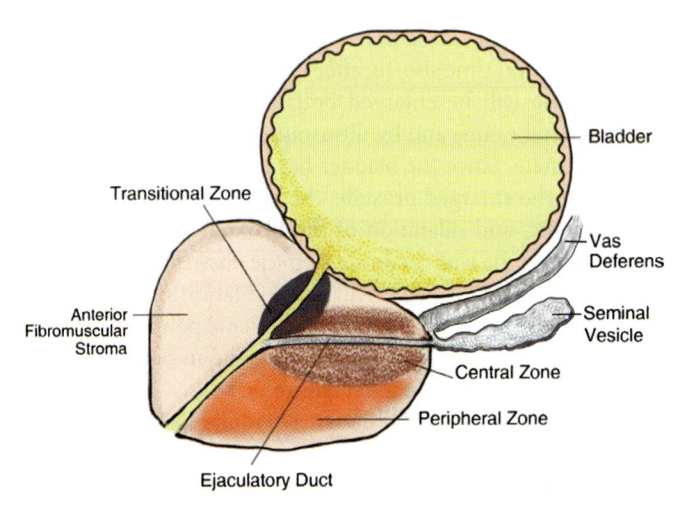

FIGURE 13-31 Diagram of the zones of the prostate.
Department of Pathology and Laboratory Medicine, University of North Carolina at Chapel Hill.

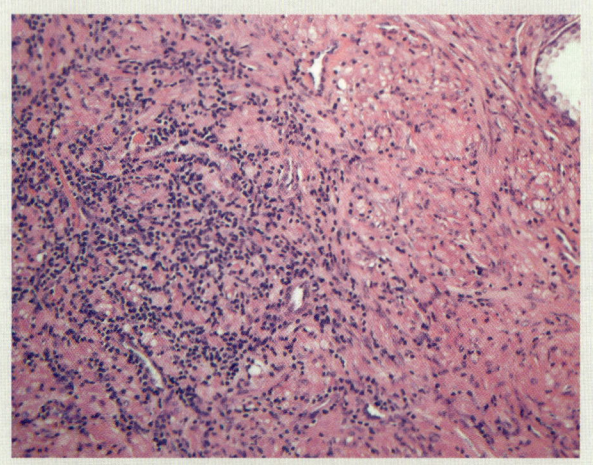

FIGURE 13-32 Photomicrograph of chronic prostatitis. There is infiltration of the stroma by mononuclear cells, predominantly lymphocytes.

PRINCIPAL DISEASES OF THE PROSTATE

The principal diseases of the prostate are prostatitis, benign hyperplasia, and carcinoma. All three of these entities may cause elevation of serum PSA.

Prostatitis

Prostatitis is inflammation of the prostate. As is true in all organs, inflammation may be acute, chronic, or granulomatous. **Acute prostatitis** shows neutrophils microscopically and is often a complication of a urinary tract infection (UTI). The most common organisms involved are coliform bacteria. **Chronic prostatitis** (Figure 13-32) shows mononuclear cells (lymphocytes and plasma cells, sometimes macrophages) and may or may not follow a UTI. Some cases are bacterial, but many also be due to other organisms, especially *Chlamydia*, *Mycoplasma*, and *Trichomonas*. Chronic prostatitis may also be due to obstructed ducts secondary to hyperplasia. **Granulomatous prostatitis** is often not infectious and shows histiocytes (macrophages) and giant cells (Figure 13-33).

All forms of prostatitis may cause elevation in serum PSA (see below)

> **QUICK REVIEW**
> **Major Causes of Prostatitis**
>
> Acute prostatitis: Usually bacterial, follows a UTI. Common infectious agents are coliform bacteria.
>
> Chronic prostatitis: May be the sequel of a UTI or an episode of acute prostatitis, and in these cases are bacterial (especially coliform bacteria). Other causes are *Chlamydia*, *Mycoplasma*, and *Trichomonas*.

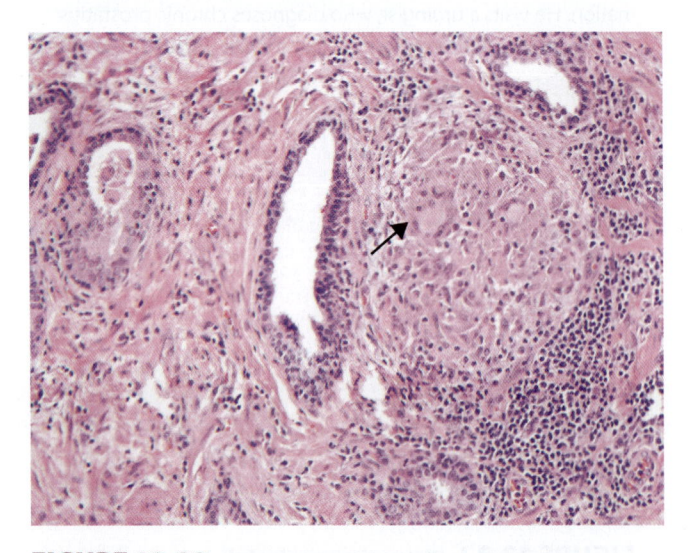

FIGURE 13-33 Photomicrograph of granulomatous prostatitis. A granuloma containing giant cells (arrow) is adjacent to a gland and surrounded by lymphocytes infiltrating the stroma.

> **HUNTING FOR ZEBRAS**
> **Granulomatous Prostatitis**
>
> While unusual, granulomatous prostatitis is clinically important due to its ability to mimic carcinoma. Granulomatous prostatitis may be due to rupture of prostatic ducts (often secondary to obstruction), with spillage of secretions into the stroma inciting a granulomatous response. Other causes are mycobacterial or fungal infections. Patients who are treated with BCG for bladder cancer usually have mycobacterial-associated granulomatous prostatitis. Granulomatous prostatitis may cause a markedly elevated PSA and may cause a very abnormal digital examination, raising concern for prostate cancer. The prostate will become hard and nodular, often in a asymmetric fashion. Biopsy is needed in such cases to exclude malignancy (Figure 13-33).

> Granulomatous prostatitis: Noninfectious causes: obstruction of ducts causing spillage of prostate secretions. Infectious causes: acid-fast bacilli (including BCG) and fungus.

Benign Prostatic Hyperplasia (BPH)

BPH is a very common disorder caused by enlargement of the transition zone of the prostate. The proliferation may be of glands and/or stroma. BPH usually begins around age 40, but often is not symptomatic until later in life. BPH is more common in the United States and Western Europe than elsewhere in the world, raising the possibility that the typical Western diet plays a part in the development of this condition. Development of BPH depends on an intact prostate hormonal axis (see above).

Patients with BPH usually present with lower urinary tract symptoms (LUTS), which include difficulty in initiating urination, dribbling at the end of urination, reduction in the force of the urinary stream, nocturia, and sensation of having to void a second time shortly after urination (double voiding). The prostate will be enlarged both by clinical examination (digital rectal exam) and by ultrasound estimation of the size of the prostate. Since the bladder has to work harder to force urine past the enlarged prostate, the bladder muscle becomes hypertrophic, and dilatation of the bladder lumen with trabeculations of the wall is common. If the obstruction is severe, the back pressure of urine will cause dilation of the ureters (**hydroureter**) and even dilation of the renal pelvis (**hydronephrosis**). The damage may be insidious, and in rare cases may cause partial or complete renal failure.

Microscopically, BPH shows a nodular proliferation of glands and stroma. Early in the disease, the transition zone is expanded by these nodules. As the disease progresses, the nodules compress the urethra and the normal peripheral zone. The hyperplastic glands often show infoldings of the epithelium,

CASE 13-7

A 75-year-old farmer visits his family practice physician with complaints of being tired because he has to get up four to five times a night to urinate. However, each time he only produces a small amount. He reports difficulty in initiating urination and dribbling at the end. Sometimes he urinates a small amount and within a few minutes feels like he has to go again and urinates about the same amount the second time. His physician refers him to a urologist, who tests his urine with normal results. He does an ultrasound examination of his bladder after the patient tries to completely empty his bladder, and 250 mL of urine remain (post-void residual). This is 5 to 10 times the normal amount. His prostate is enlarged with an estimated size 80 g (normal about 20 g). He is prescribed a 5-alpha reductase blocker with slight improvement in symptoms. The patient wishes for more relief of his symptoms, and in consultation with his urologist chooses to have a transurethral resection of the prostate. Examination of the resected prostate chips (Figure 13-34) shows BPH (Figure 13-35).

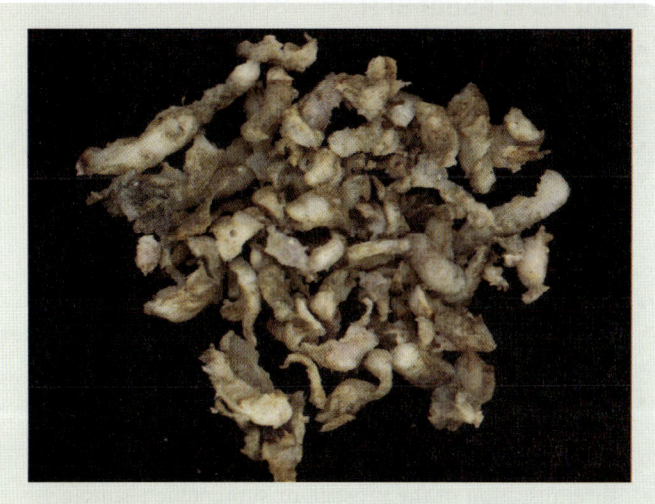

FIGURE 13-34 Gross photo of prostate chips. Prostate tissue from a transurethral resection submitted to surgical pathology for analysis.

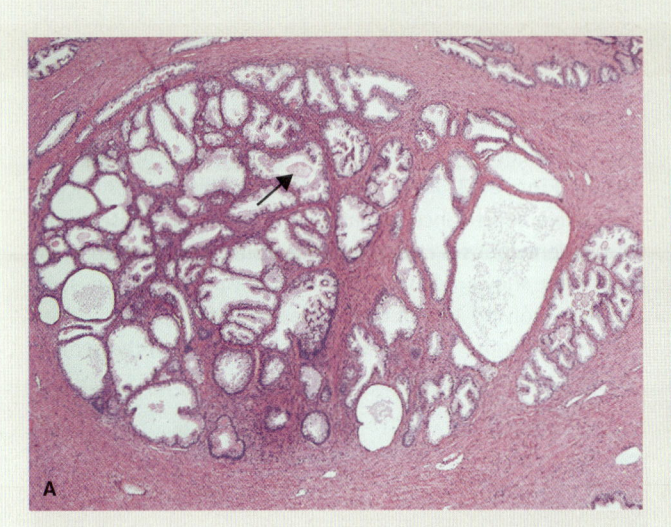

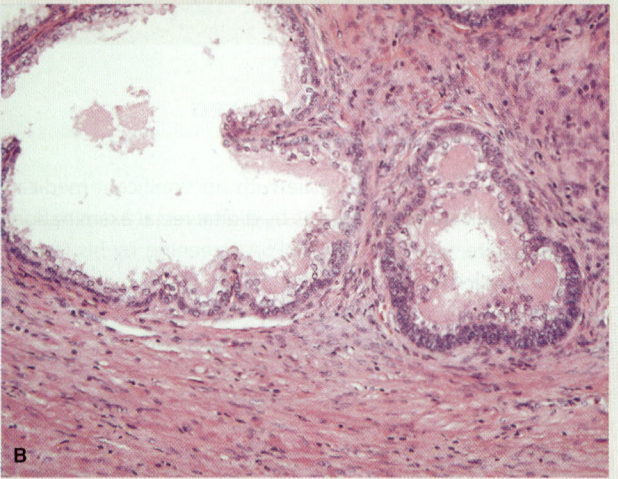

FIGURE 13-35 Photomicrograph of BPH. (A) Low power and (B) high power. At low power, a nodule containing multiple glands in a cribriform pattern is seen. The glands show multiple epithelial infoldings. One gland (arrow) contains a corpora amylacea (layered concretion). The increased stromal cellularity is easy to appreciate in the high-power view.

and the stroma is more cellular than usual. Chronic inflammation is often present in the stroma (Figure 13-35).

Since benign prostatic epithelium produces PSA, BPH can cause an elevation of serum PSA because a larger number of benign glands are present.

In the past, transurethral resection of the prostate was a common surgical procedure, and prostate "chips" were common specimens in surgical pathology. More advanced cases of BPH were treated by suprapubic prostatectomy, which is enucleation of the transition zone of the prostate in an open surgical procedure. Both of these surgeries target only the transition zone, and patients who have had these procedures do not have a decreased risk of subsequent prostate cancer because the peripheral zone of the prostate remains. In the modern era, most patients with BPH are treated medically with drugs that either inhibit the 5-alpha reductase enzyme to reduce prostate size or with alpha adrenergic blockers to decrease the smooth muscle tone of the prostate to "relax" the stroma and functionally reduce the obstruction. Occasional patients do not adequately respond to medical management, and surgical treatments are still used in this group of patients.

QUICK REVIEW
Major Facts About BPH

- Arises in the transition zone
- Due to a proliferation of glands and stroma in a nodular configuration
- Causes obstruction of the urethra
- Symptoms include difficulty starting and stopping urination, decrease in force of urinary stream, increased post-void residual (termed "Lower urinary symptoms" or "LUTS" by urologists)
- Bladder may have dilated lumen and/or trabeculations of the wall
- When severe, can cause hydroureter or hydronephrosis
- Usually treated medically with either/both 5-alpha reductase inhibitors or alphaadrenergic blockers
- Medically refractory cases may be treated with transurethral resection of the prostate or suprapubic ("simple") prostatectomy

Prostate Carcinoma

Prostate carcinoma is the most common cancer of American men, and the second most common cause of cancer death. The true frequency of prostate carcinoma is far more common than the clinical incidence, due to an extremely high rate of "latent" or "incidental" cancers that are biologically indolent and are only detected at autopsy or when prostate tissue is examined microscopically for clinically benign reasons (such as for BPH). This combination of facts makes prostate cancer unique among human cancers: it is a cancer that in most cases is not fatal, but it is still a very common cause of cancer death. Since it very difficult to predict the clinical course in any individual patient, it is a cancer that can be either under- and over-treated. Screening for prostate cancer is common, but is not very specific for malignancy and the diagnostic tests that are currently available are poor in predicting which cancers will be biologically aggressive.

The incidence of prostate cancer increases with age, and rises sharply after age 50. There is a marked worldwide

CASE 13-8

Prostate Carcinoma Diagnosed by Needle Biopsy

The patient is a 55-year-old male with no significant medical complaints and no abnormalities by digital rectal examination of the prostate, who has routine PSA screening by his family practice physician. The results of 5.5 ng/dL prompt a referral to a urologist, who takes 12 biopsies of the prostate (two each from the right and left apex, mid and base of the prostate) Both cores from the right mid prostate and one from the right base contain adenocarcinoma, Gleason combined score 7(3+4) (Figure 13-36A). After a discussion of options (including active surveillance, radiation and radical prostatectomy), the patient chooses radical prostatectomy. Examination of the specimen shows adenocarcinoma, Gleason combined score 7(3+4), involving 15% of the prostate with focal extraprostatic extension (Figure 13-36B), and no involvement of the seminal vesicles and negative surgical margin.

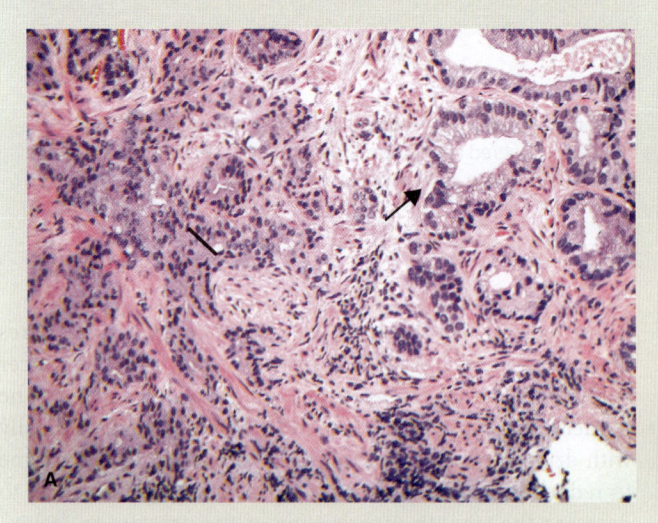

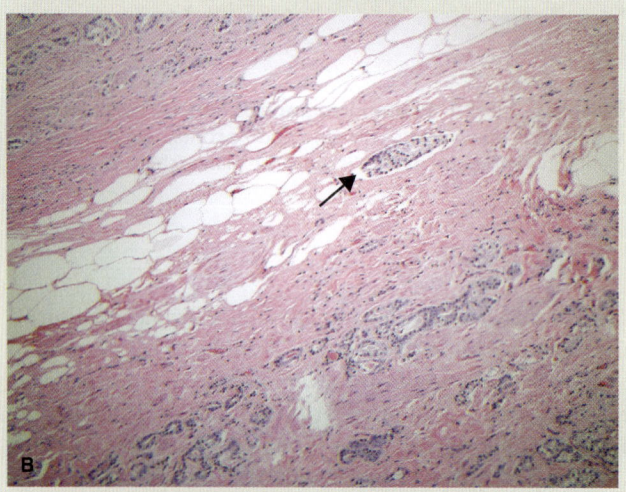

FIGURE 13-36 Adenocarcinoma, Gleason 7(3+4) in needle biopsy. **(A)** Two components (grade 3, arrow and grade 4 line) present in needle biopsy are indicated. **(B)** Extraprostatic extension of adenocarcinoma into adipose tissue (center of photo) and blood vessel (arrow).

variation in the incidence of the disease, with the United States and Western Europe being sites with the highest incidence. There are racial differences in the incidence of prostate cancer, and within the United States African-American men have a higher cancer rate than Caucasian men. There is also a familial component of the risk of prostate cancer, which is currently estimated to be fairly small. Diet and exposure to environmental carcinogens may play a part in the development of prostate cancer, but the evidence is conflicting and intense research is ongoing on these topics. Development of prostate cancer requires an intact hormonal axis.

*The most likely precursor of invasive prostate cancer is **prostatic intraepithelial neoplasia (PIN)**, which consists of prostate glands with cytologic atypia but without invasion into the stroma.* The basal cells in ducts that contain PIN are present but are frequently attenuated.

Screening for prostate cancer: The two principal screening methods for prostate cancer are digital rectal examination and serum PSA. PSA is secreted by both benign and malignant prostate epithelial cells. As mentioned above, elevated PSA may be seen in prostatitis, benign hyperplasia, and carcinoma. The reason for elevated PSA in prostatitis is probably that inflammation causes increased permeability of the cell membrane allowing more PSA to leak into the bloodstream. In BPH elevated PSA is related to the increased number of benign glands as compared with normal. In cancer, both greater numbers of malignant glands and their increased permeability are likely to be causes of elevation of PSA levels.

WHAT WE DO

The standard laboratory definition of an elevated PSA is greater than 4.0 ng/mL. However, a single cut-off value for normal PSA is not possible, and the normal PSA value changes with age. Younger men should normally have a very low PSA, and thus a PSA less than 4.0 might well represent an elevated level in that age group. The size of the organ and coexistent benign hyperplasia must also be taken into consideration, because a higher PSA would normally be expected in a large prostate due to the increase in glandular epithelial mass. Large numbers of false positive results occur with PSA screening, and the positive predictive value of a PSA of 4.0 ng/mL is approximately 25%. Thus, most patients with an elevated PSA in fact do not have cancer. Conversely, false negative PSA results also occur. This happens when prostate cancers are very small, or are very poorly differentiated and lack the ability to produce PSA.

It is apparent that the PSA level is a fairly insensitive screening test, but it is still the best that we currently have. Unfortunately, it may not be good enough. After decades of the US medical establishment recommending annual PSA screening to men over the age of 45 or 50 (depending on family history and/or race), the US Preventive Services Task Force in 2011 released a statement that PSA screening does not save lives and instead causes enormous harm. This recommendation was based on analysis of two large screening trials published in 2009, one from the United States and one from Europe. The taskforce's recommendations were based on numerous findings, including (1) many PSA levels are found to fall near the common action threshold of 2.5–4.0 ng/dL, causing multiple rounds of retesting in some patients; (2) if cancer is found, it is often impossible to predict which cancers with be lethal and should be treated and which are indolent and will never cause harm to the patient; (3) treatment of biologically indolent cancers can cause serious side effects, and (4) some of the aggressive cancers will be lethal in spite of treatment and even detecting them early will not change the natural history of the disease.

Another issue is the substantial costs of screening. The large European screening trial estimated that $5.2 million (US) would have to be spent on screening and the interventions that follow to prevent one death from prostate cancer. This figure does not include the costs of serial PSA testing in patients with borderline results. Many in the public health arena believe that the current PSA-based screening paradigm does not compare favorably with other health-care priorities. However, PSA screening will not disappear overnight. The PSA density (a mathematical calculation of the PSA level divided by the estimated size of the gland to account for BPH) is posited to compensate for the effect of differences in prostate mass and the PSA velocity (measuring and plotting the PSA level over time to determine how rapidly the PSA is increasing, with rapid elevations being more worrisome for cancer) are simple modifications that may help clarify PSA testing. However, PSA density measurement requires transrectal ultrasound and PSA velocity determination requires repeated PSA assay.

When prostate cancer is suspected, either by physical examination or because of an elevated PSA, biopsies are usually taken of the prostate for pathologic examination. Biopsies are concentrated in the peripheral zone of the prostate (the most likely site of prostate cancer), and usually 8–14 needle cores are taken of different areas to ensure a good sampling of the gland. Occasionally, other prostate tissues are submitted to pathology for presumed benign disease (such as "prostate chips from a transurethral resection for BPH). These are also examined microscopically, and prostate cancer is found in some of these specimens as well due to the fairly high incidence of prostate cancer in the United States.

> **QUICK REVIEW**
> **Facts About PSA Screening**
> - Along with digital rectal examination, PSA screening is currently the most used screening test for prostate cancer, but is not very specific for the disease.
> - PSA is made in prostate epithelial cells and leaks into the blood, and hence all conditions that cause increase in numbers of epithelial cells and permeability of the cells will elevate PSA. Prostatitis, BPH, and cancer will all cause elevations of PSA. Only about 25% of patients with elevated PSA will be shown to have cancer when biopsied.
> - PSA is expected to be lower in younger men.
> - PSA density and PSA velocity are modifications of the PSA level that may be more predictive of cancer
> - Some cancers are very poorly differentiated and may not produce much PSA, and hence false negative results may occur.

> **IN TRANSLATION**
> **Molecular Biomarkers for Prostate Cancer**
> New biomarkers are on the horizon for prostate cancer. Gene rearrangements have been reported in the gene for androgen-regulated transmembrane protease serine 2 (TMPRSS2), and this is currently being explored in clinical trials to determine if this rearrangement could be used as a cancer marker. Several other genes have been reported to be upregulated in prostate tumors and are considered candidates as tumor markers, but much work needs to be done before they can be used clinically.

The great majority of prostate cancers are adenocarcinomas, and arise from the ducts of the prostate. Other rare tumors of the prostate do occur, including transitional cell carcinoma from the overlying urothelium, sarcomas from the stroma, other rare carcinomas associated with metaplasia, or divergent differentiation of the glandular epithelium. Tumors that involve the prostate by direct extension (such as colon cancer) or metastasis (such as lymphoma or melanoma) also occur. However, when we talk about "prostate cancer" without specifying the type, we are usually referring to adenocarcinoma.

As previously noted, prostate cancer preferentially arises within the peripheral zone. Many cancers are small and are not detectable by physical examination or by gross examination of a specimen, but larger tumors will be felt as firm nodules and may be seen as yellow-white dense nodules when the organ is examined grossly. Microscopically, adenocarcinoma is composed of glands that are (1) smaller and more densely packed than normal, (2) lack a basal layer, (3) show nuclear enlargement, and (4) contain prominent nucleoli. The glands of carcinoma are PSA and PAP (prostatic alkaline phosphatase) positive, which is *not* helpful in distinguishing between benign and malignant lesions of the prostate (because the epithelium of both stain for these proteins). However, the absence of basal cells as shown by a negative HWCK stain is a useful finding.

Prostate cancer is graded primarily by architectural criteria. Low-grade tumors are composed of well-formed glands of uniform size with smooth edges to the groups of malignant glands. Intermediate-grade tumors show variability to the sizes of the glands, and show infiltration of the malignant glands in between benign glands. High-grade tumors show poor gland formation with only rudimentary or no glands and may contain necrosis. The current grading scheme for prostate carcinomas uses the **Gleason grading system**, which assigns numbers to the patterns of carcinoma from 1 (well differentiated) to 5 (poorly differentiated) **(Figure 13-37)**, and accounts for tumor heterogeneity by assigning a primary pattern and a secondary pattern (Figure 13-36). If only one pattern is present, this number is assigned twice. Thus, tumors are given an overall Gleason score ranging from 2 to 10. Most cancers have scores from 5 to 7. Higher score tumors, particularly those with a primary pattern of 4 or 5, have a less favorable prognosis.

> **QUICK REVIEW**
> **Major Facts About Prostate Cancer Gleason Grading**
> - Grade is assigned by architectural features, primarily the degree of gland formation and the crowdedness of the glands
> - Grades range from 1 (lowest) to 5 (highest)
> - To account for heterogeneity of the tumor, Gleason score is assigned. Score is the most predominant grade added to the second most predominant grade. Thus, the scores range from 2 to 10. The higher the score, the less favorable the prognosis (Figures 13-36, 13-37)

When carcinoma is detected on a needle biopsy, the tumor may be treated by surgery, radiation, or sometimes just by following the patient closely by physical examination and PSA level (known as "active surveillance," formerly known as "watchful waiting"), which is most often appropriate for older patients with a small amount of cancer having a low Gleason score, or with significant comorbidities. If surgery is chosen, a radical prostatectomy is performed. In this operation, the entire prostate is removed along with the seminal vesicles. In order to preserve sexual function, the nerves that run laterally to the prostate are spared if possible. The prostatectomy specimen is carefully "inked" so the surgical margins can be determined, and examined microscopically to evaluate the type and grade of the cancer, determine the extent of tumor within the gland, invasion of tumor to other organs, and determine the status of the margins. Obturator or pelvic lymph node

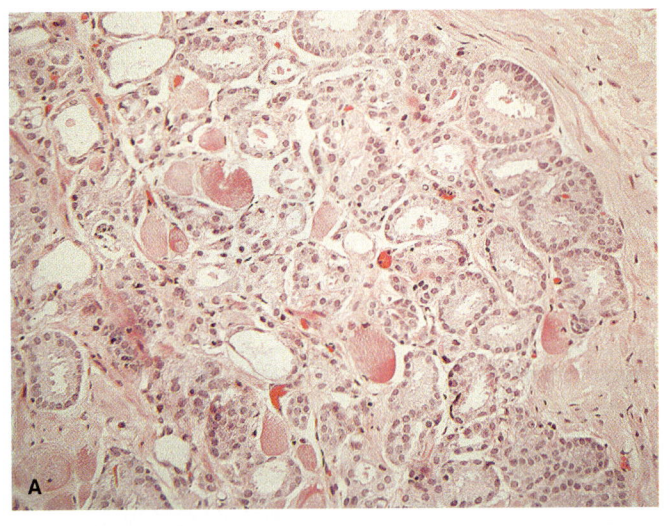

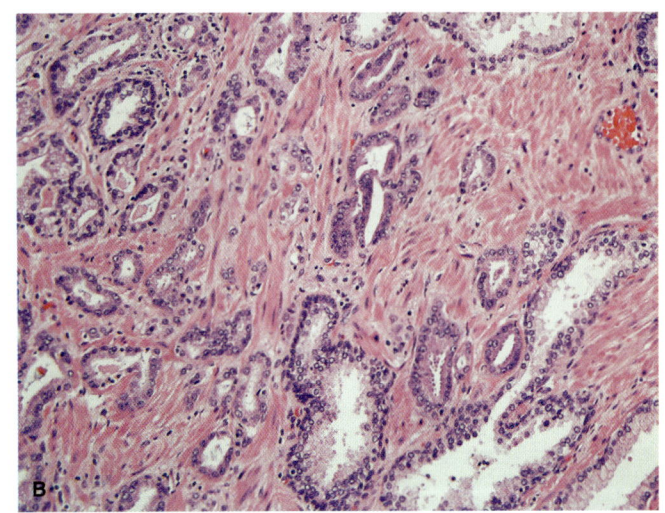

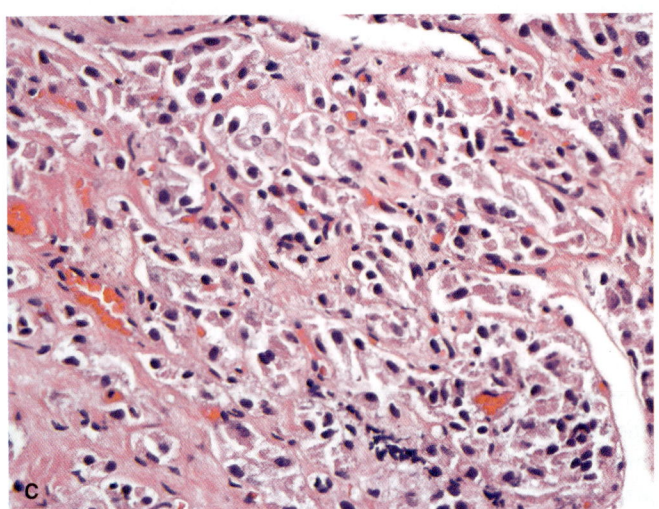

FIGURE 13-37 Photomicrographs of prostate adenocarcinoma differing in Gleason grade. **(A)** Gleason grade 1, **(B)** Gleason grade 3, and **(C)** Gleason grade 5.

dissection may also be done if the tumor contains a component of high-grade carcinoma. From this examination, pathologic staging of the specimen can be done.

Prostate cancer has a propensity to extend through the capsule of the prostate gland, often growing around nerves (perineural space invasion). Some cases involve the seminal vesicles by direct extension. Metastatic disease preferentially involves lymph nodes and bone. Early metastatic disease involves obturator and pelvic nodes, and later other abdominal nodes. Systemic metastatic disease is concentrated on bony metastases, especially involving the spine, ribs, and pelvis. The bone metastases are usually **blastic** (they appear dense and sclerotic on X-ray). This is different from most other metastases to bone, which are usually **lytic** (appear as lucent on X-ray). Bone scan is the usual method of surveillance for bone metastases (**Figure 13-38**). If metastatic disease is biopsied and there is uncertainty that the tumor is from the prostate, immunostains for PSA and PAP can be performed. Serum PSA is the most common way of monitoring patients for metastatic disease. After surgery or radiation therapy to the prostate gland, serum PSA should be essentially undetectable. If the PSA rises after surgery or radiation, this suggests recurrence or metastatic disease. The level of serum PSA often roughly correlates with tumor burden.

Hormone therapy is initially helpful in controlling tumor cell growth in patients with metastatic disease. Prostate cancer is hormonally responsive early in its course. Androgen deprivation (inhibition of release of testosterone), either by removing the testes or by LHRH agonists (such as Lupron, which shuts off release of LH by feedback inhibition) or more recently LHRH antagonists (which directly work on the pituitary to block LH secretion) will slow the progression of metastatic prostate cancer by removing hormonal stimulation. After several years, however, malignant populations of tumor cells that are hormone independent emerge and the tumor resumes growth once again. This is known by oncologists as **androgen-independent prostate cancer.**

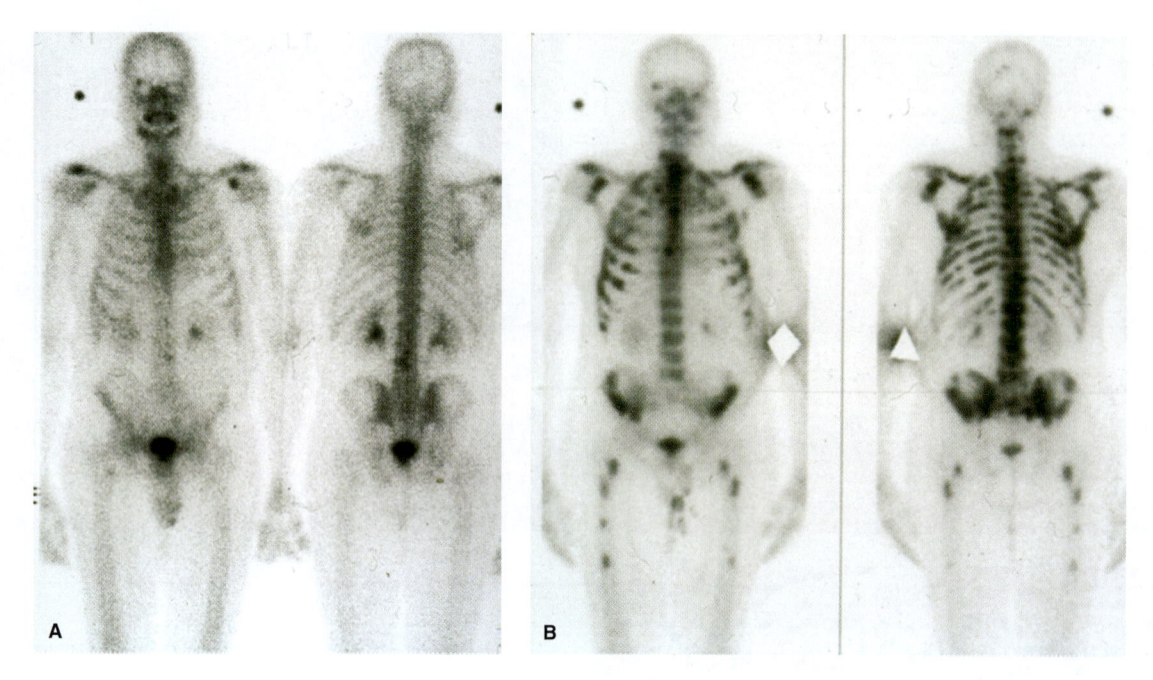

FIGURE 13-38 Images of gamma camera bone scans using a radiotracer (technetium Tc 99m methylene diphosphonate) that concentrates in metastases. **(A)** negative scan (tracer present largely in the kidneys and bladder as it is excreted) **(B)** Positive scan seen as dark spots in bone. Notice the metastases in the spinal column, ribs, pelvic bones and femurs.

CASE 13-9

Metastatic Prostate Cancer

A 65-year-old male presents to a chiropractor with back pain. The patient does not like going to the doctor and has not had a checkup in 15 years since his wife passed away. After several manipulations, the patient is not improving, and he is referred to an orthopedic surgeon. That physician obtains an MRI of the spine, which shows numerous blastic lesions throughout the vertebral bodies. A serum PSA is drawn, and the level is 1050 ng/dL (normal is < 4 ng/dL). The patient is referred to an oncologist for a presumptive diagnosis of metastatic prostate cancer. Because the patient's insurance company will not approve the reimbursement of hormone therapy for metastatic prostate cancer without a tissue diagnosis, a CT guided biopsy of one of the lesions is performed by a radiologist and shows metastatic adenocarcinoma that is positive by immunostaining for PSA **(Figure 13-39)**.

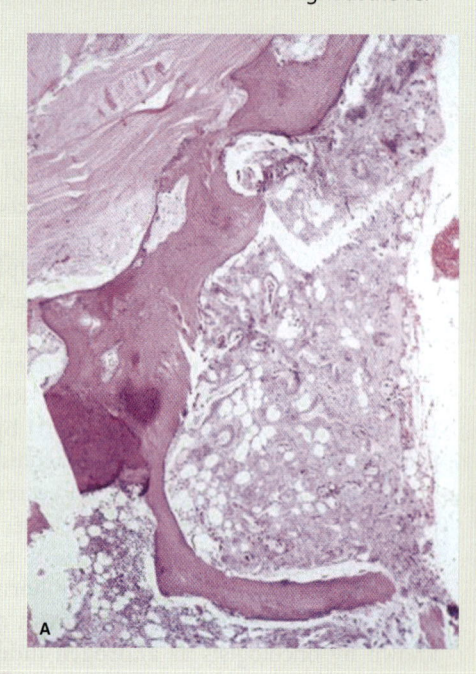

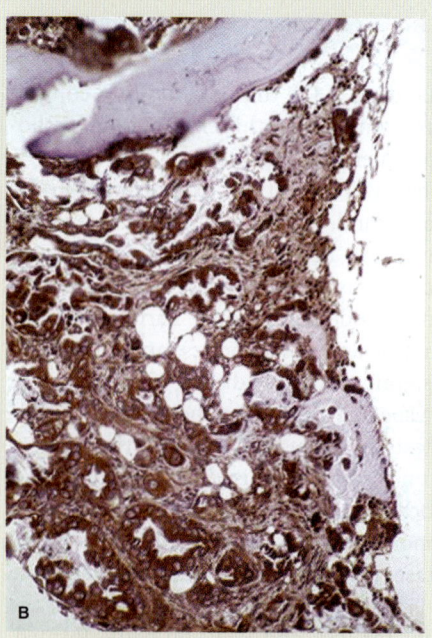

FIGURE 13-39 Photomicrograph of bone biopsy with metastatic prostate adenocarcinoma. **(A)** H&E staining and **(B)** positive immunostaining for PSA (brown color).

UROLOGIC PATHOLOGY OF THE KIDNEY

This section will cover the lesions of the kidney that are usually managed by urologists. Medical renal disease is covered in Chapter 12.

Congenital Anomalies of the Kidney and Ureter

A variety of congenital anomalies can involve the kidneys and ureters, and many of these are asymptomatic. These may come to clinical attention when CT scans are done at surgery. **Renal agenesis** is absence of one or both kidneys. Absence of one kidney is usually asymptomatic; bilateral agenesis is usually incompatible with life (**Potter syndrome or Potter sequence**). Infants with bilateral renal agenesis suffer the complications of oligohydramnios, since much of the volume of amniotic fluid is urine produced by the fetus in utero. With insufficient amniotic fluid, the fetus is compressed within the uterus and has facial and limb abnormalities. However, the most severe complication of Potter sequence is pulmonary hypoplasia, because amniotic fluid is necessary for proper development of the fetal lung. Infants are usually stillborn or suffer severe respiratory insufficiency after birth. **Renal hypoplasia** is a small but histologically normal kidney, and is usually inconsequential. **Ectopic kidney** is a normal kidney in an abnormal place (usually in the pelvis). This is usually asymptomatic, and only important when planning surgery or radiation so the kidney can be avoided. **Horseshoe kidney** is rotation and joining of both kidneys in the midline, also important to know when planning surgery. As in the section on renal pelvis and ureter above, obstruction of the ureter, usually at the ureteropelvic junction (**ureteropelvic junction obstruction**), is an important cause of childhood hydronephrosis and is usually corrected surgically (Figure 13-40).

Renal Cystic Diseases

This section will only discuss the major renal cystic diseases.

Renal dysplasia is only sometimes cystic. Renal dysplasia is a developmental disorder due to an abnormality in metanephric differentiation interfering with the interaction between the ureteric bud and the metanephric blastema. Most often the inciting event is a urinary tract abnormality that causes obstruction. Renal dysplasia can cause a variety of histologic appearances in the affected kidney or kidneys. One or both may be involved, and involvement may be all or part of the kidney. The affected kidney tissue may be small (aplastic) or large, cystic or solid. The pathologic hallmark is undifferentiated tubules and ducts, surrounded by collars of cellular undifferentiated mesenchyme (Figure 13-41), and may contain smooth muscle and cartilage. Sometimes entrapped or rudimentary glomeruli are present admixed with the cysts. One of the most common presentations of renal dysplasia is unilateral and cystic and is termed multicystic dysplasia. This usually is found as a mass in a newborn, and is often clinically concerning for malignancy. **The most common cause of an abdominal mass in a newborn is multicystic renal dysplasia.** Renal dysplasia may or may not be hereditary, and may be associated with anomalies in other organs. For that reason genetic counseling is often done with parents who have a child with renal dysplasia, especially for aplastic dysplasia and diffuse cystic dysplasia. Multicystic dysplasia is less likely to hereditary.

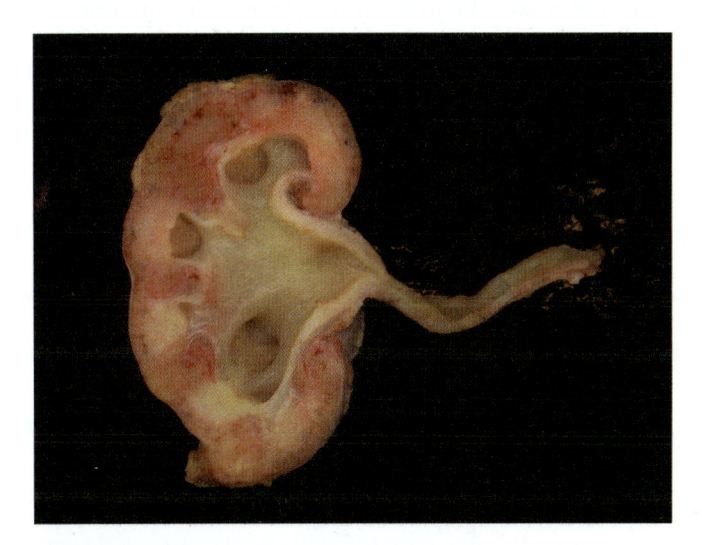

FIGURE 13-40 Gross image of hydronephrosis secondary to ureteropelvic junction obstruction. This gross image is of the kidney of a child that was found to be nonfunctional due to ureteropelvic junction obstruction. This fairly common congenital condition is due to a variety of causes such as intrinsic fibrosis of ureter wall, ureteral valves blocking the flow of urine, kinking of the ureter from high insertion of the ureter in the renal pelvis, or compression by crossing blood vessels. If unilateral, this may be asymptomatic and only found if an abdominal ultrasound is done showing hydronephrosis.

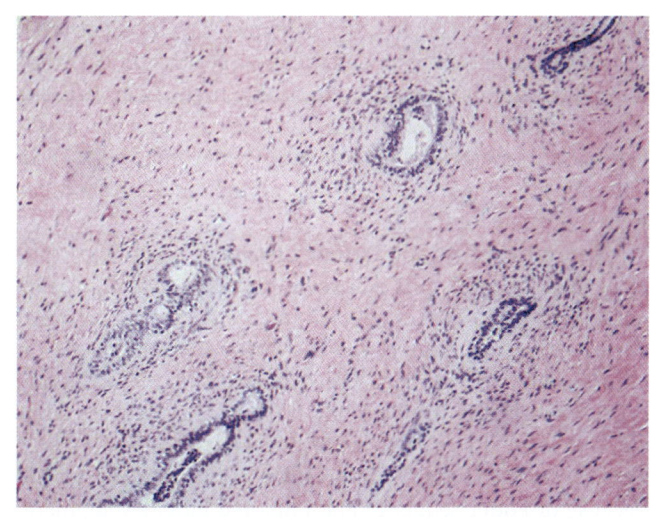

FIGURE 13-41 Photomicrograph of renal dysplasia. This example of renal dysplasia is solid, and consists of small primitive tubules surrounded by collars of undifferentiated mesenchyme.

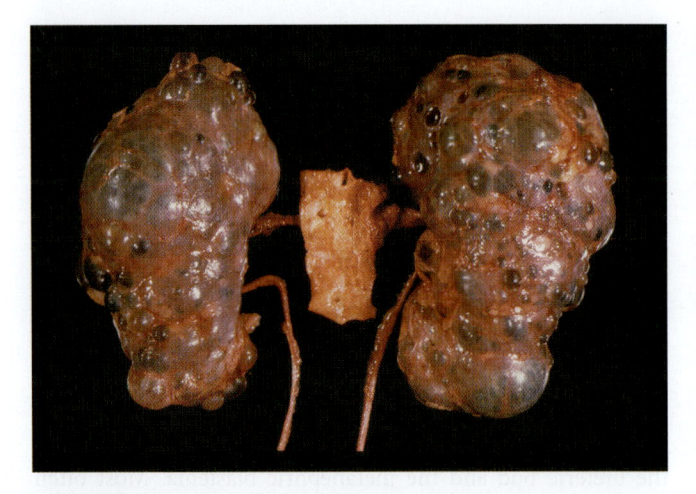

FIGURE 13-42 **Adult polycystic kidney disease.** This gross image at autopsy shows greatly enlarged kidneys that have the appearance of masses of cysts.

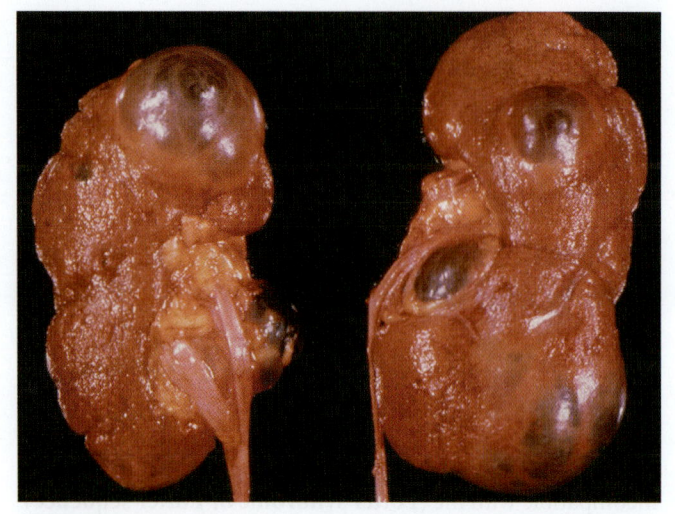

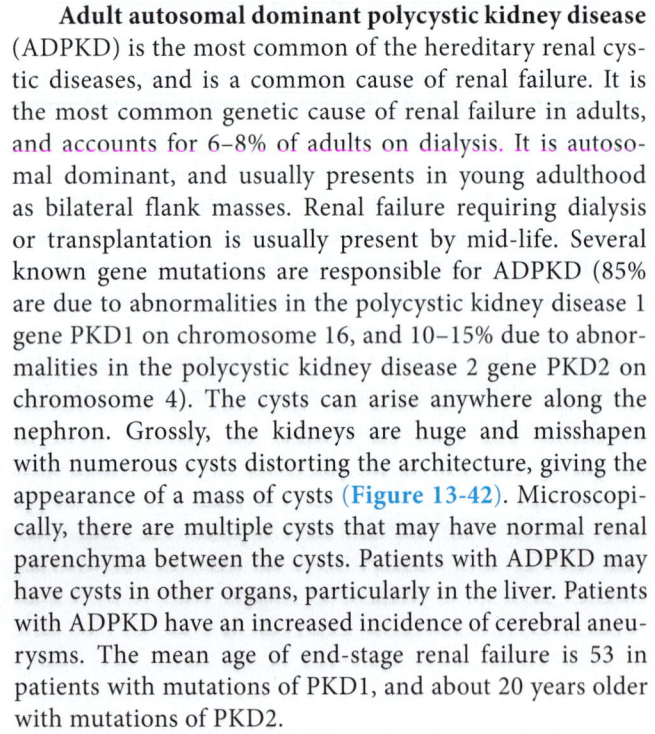

FIGURE 13-43 **Simple renal cysts.** This gross image shows bilateral kidneys at autopsy that each contains a few cortical cysts. This would have been asymptomatic and of no clinical consequence.

Adult autosomal dominant polycystic kidney disease (ADPKD) is the most common of the hereditary renal cystic diseases, and is a common cause of renal failure. It is the most common genetic cause of renal failure in adults, and accounts for 6–8% of adults on dialysis. It is autosomal dominant, and usually presents in young adulthood as bilateral flank masses. Renal failure requiring dialysis or transplantation is usually present by mid-life. Several known gene mutations are responsible for ADPKD (85% are due to abnormalities in the polycystic kidney disease 1 gene PKD1 on chromosome 16, and 10–15% due to abnormalities in the polycystic kidney disease 2 gene PKD2 on chromosome 4). The cysts can arise anywhere along the nephron. Grossly, the kidneys are huge and misshapen with numerous cysts distorting the architecture, giving the appearance of a mass of cysts (Figure 13-42). Microscopically, there are multiple cysts that may have normal renal parenchyma between the cysts. Patients with ADPKD may have cysts in other organs, particularly in the liver. Patients with ADPKD have an increased incidence of cerebral aneurysms. The mean age of end-stage renal failure is 53 in patients with mutations of PKD1, and about 20 years older with mutations of PKD2.

Infantile polycystic kidney disease is much less common than ADPKD. It is autosomal recessive, usually apparent at birth, and 75% of affected infants die in the perinatal period. It is due to abnormalities of the PKDHD1 gene on chromosome 6. The cysts are dilatations of the collecting ducts. Grossly, the disease is bilateral and causes enlarged but smooth kidneys that have the overall appearance of big kidneys. About a quarter of infants die in the neonatal period because of Potter sequence and impaired lung development. Patients with infantile autosomal recessive polycystic kidney disease also have congenital hepatic fibrosis associated with hyperplastic and cystically dilated bile ducts, and the ensuing hepatic dysfunction may be of more clinical significance than the kidney disease.

Simple renal cysts are extremely common, seen in at least half of adults over the age of 50. They are usually found incidentally when radiographic studies of the kidney are performed for another reason, or at autopsy. Simple cysts usually involve the renal cortex, are single or are present in small numbers (Figure 13-43), and lined by a single layer of flattened epithelium. They are either just followed, unroofed surgically, or may be excised (often by a partial nephrectomy) if there is concern for malignancy radiographically. Simple cysts are benign.

Acquired renal cystic disease is related to long-term dialysis for medical renal disease. At least 75% of dialysis patients will develop cysts in their kidneys. While the exact reason for cyst development is not known, one postulate is that cysts develop because a few nephrons are able to continue to produce urine, but the fluid often is entrapped within the scarred and distorted kidney and cystic dilatation ensues. Initially the cysts are lined by flattened epithelium, but epithelial proliferation and neoplastic transformation to renal cell carcinoma may develop, possibly related to concentrated toxins in the urine within the cysts. Because of the risk of carcinoma, patients on long-term dialysis are followed by radiographic studies, and solid areas in cysts are considered suspicious for malignancy and are usually excised.

QUICK REVIEW

The table reviews some of the salient points of the different types of common renal cystic disorders.

Name of Lesion	Heredity	Presentation	Gross Appearance	Microscopic Appearance
Renal dysplasia	May or may not be inherited	Usually at birth, often flank mass	Variable, unilateral or bilateral, partial or complete involvement, solid or cystic, large or small kidney	Primitive tubules and ducts, collars of mesenchyme, may have muscle or cartilage
Adult polycystic kidney disease	Inherited, autosomal dominant	Young adult to middle age, pain or bilateral flank masses	Bilateral, massively enlarged distorted kidneys	Cysts at any point along the nephron
Infantile polycystic kidney disease	Inherited, autosomal recessive	At birth or as an infant, bilateral flank masses	Bilateral, smoothly enlarged kidneys	Radial cysts representing dilatation of the collecting system
Simple cysts	Not inherited	Asymptomatic, detected incidentally, usually midlife or later	One or several cortical cysts	Cysts lined by simple epithelium
Acquired renal cystic disease	Not inherited	In patients on chronic dialysis, detected radiographically	Multiple cysts usually within scarred atrophic kidneys	Initially cysts lined by simple epithelium, epithelium may become atypical or multilayered, propensity to develop renal cell carcinoma in cysts

Obstructive Uropathy and Urinary Stones (Calculi)

Any obstruction of the urine outflow will cause **obstructive uropathy**. Causes of obstruction may be intrinsic (anything within the urinary system that obstructs urine flow, such as stones, blood clots, tumors, posterior urethral valves, strictures) or extrinsic (lesions outside the urinary tract that compress it, such as prostate hyperplasia, tumors that compress the ureters, retroperitoneal fibrosis, even pregnancy can cause mild obstruction). Dysfunction of kidney function by obstruction is termed **obstructive nephropathy**, dilatation of the collecting system of the kidney is **hydronephrosis**, and dilatation of the ureter is **hydroureter**. Chronic obstruction is an insidious cause of renal failure. Obstruction on one side can cause atrophy of the affected kidney, and can be entirely asymptomatic until renal function is lost on that side. Bilateral partial chronic obstruction can cause a slow, often clinically inapparent reduction of renal function until too late, and the patient develops chronic renal failure. Bilateral acute obstruction causes acute renal failure.

Urinary tract stones (calculi) are of several types. **Calcium stones** comprise approximately 75% of stones. These are seen radiographically. **Infection stones** are associated with urinary tract infections (Figure 13-44). The most common organisms are Proteus and Providencia, and these urea-splitting bacteria cause precipitation of magnesium ammonium phosphate (struvite) and calcium phosphate (apatite). The resulting stones are branched and complex and commonly fill the collecting system to form a cast. These are difficult to remove without nephrectomy, and cause infection, bleeding, and abscesses. **Uric acid stones** are seen in patients with hyperuricemia and gout. These stones are radiolucent. **Cystine stones** are rare, but relatively more common in childhood, and are associated with hereditary cystinuria.

Renal Tumors

Solid renal masses are considered malignant neoplasms until proven otherwise. At least 90% of solid masses are malignant, and radiology is usually not helpful in distinguishing benign from malignant masses. The exception is angiomyolipoma, discussed below.

Malignant Tumors

Most solid renal tumors are **renal cell carcinomas**, which are adenocarcinomas that may show a variety of patterns. Most

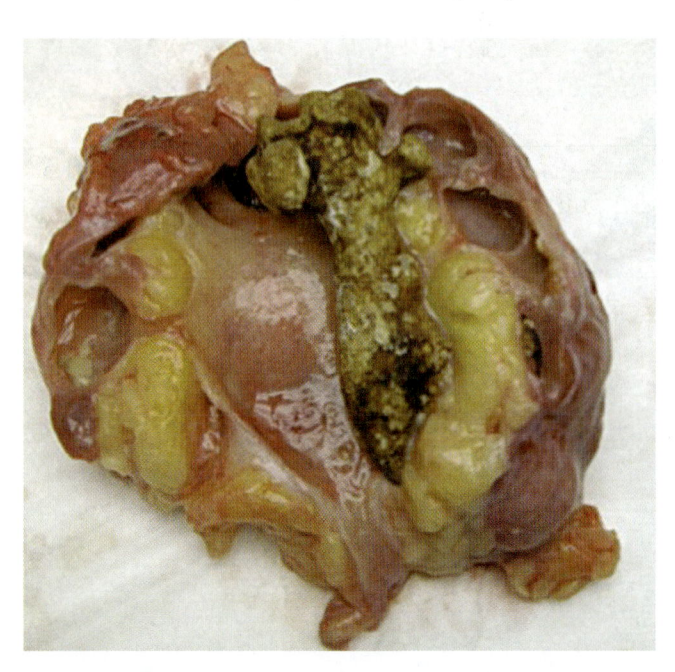

FIGURE 13-44 Nephrolithiasis (infection stones). This staghorn calculus fills the renal pelvis and calyceal system with a branching stone that has caused hydronephrosis.

arise from renal tubular epithelium from the renal cortex. The most common show clear cell morphology, and for that reason clear cell carcinoma is sometimes considered a synonym of renal cell carcinoma. This is not strictly true, as there are nonclear cell types of renal cell carcinoma, and not all clear cell carcinomas are from the kidney, and for these reasons the term renal cell carcinoma (RCC) is preferred.

Most RCCs are sporadic, but about 5% are hereditary. The etiology of sporadic RCC is complex and likely is associated with environmental toxins in many cases. The link between tobacco use and RCC is well established. Somewhat less certain is the relationship between industrial chemicals (especially arsenic, cadmium and trichloroethylene) and renal cell carcinoma. The risk of developing RCC related to tobacco use is directly associated with the amount and duration of exposure to tobacco in a dose-dependent fashion. Obese patients have an increased risk of renal cell carcinoma, possibly related to adipokines such as leptin, chronic tissue hypoxia, insulin resistance, or altered endocrine responses. Hypertension is also associated with RCC, and is independent of obesity.

Among the hereditary renal cancer syndromes, the best known of these is **von Hippel–Lindau** disease, an autosomal dominant cancer syndrome. It is characterized by hemangioblastomas in the brain, clear cell RCC, and pheochromocytomas, among other lesions. It is due to mutations in the VHL gene on chromosome 3p. Other hereditary cancer syndromes **are hereditary papillary renal cell carcinoma syndrome**, due to mutations in the MET oncogene on chromosome 7q, **Birt–Hogg–Dube** syndrome due to mutations in the BHD gene on chromosome 17, and **constitutional chromosome 3 translocation** causing translocation-associated RCC.

The most common subtype of RCC is **clear cell RCC** (approximately 70%). Less common subtypes are **papillary RCC** (15%), **chromophobe RCC** (5%), and rare subtypes such as **collecting duct RCC** and **medullary RCC** (each about 1%). **Sarcomatoid RCC** is a dedifferentiation that can be seen in any subtype, and conveys a less favorable prognosis. Some of the different subtypes are illustrated in Figure 13-45. Abnormalities in chromosome 3 are associated with clear cell RCCs (both sporadic clear cell RCCs and hereditary clear cell subtypes such as

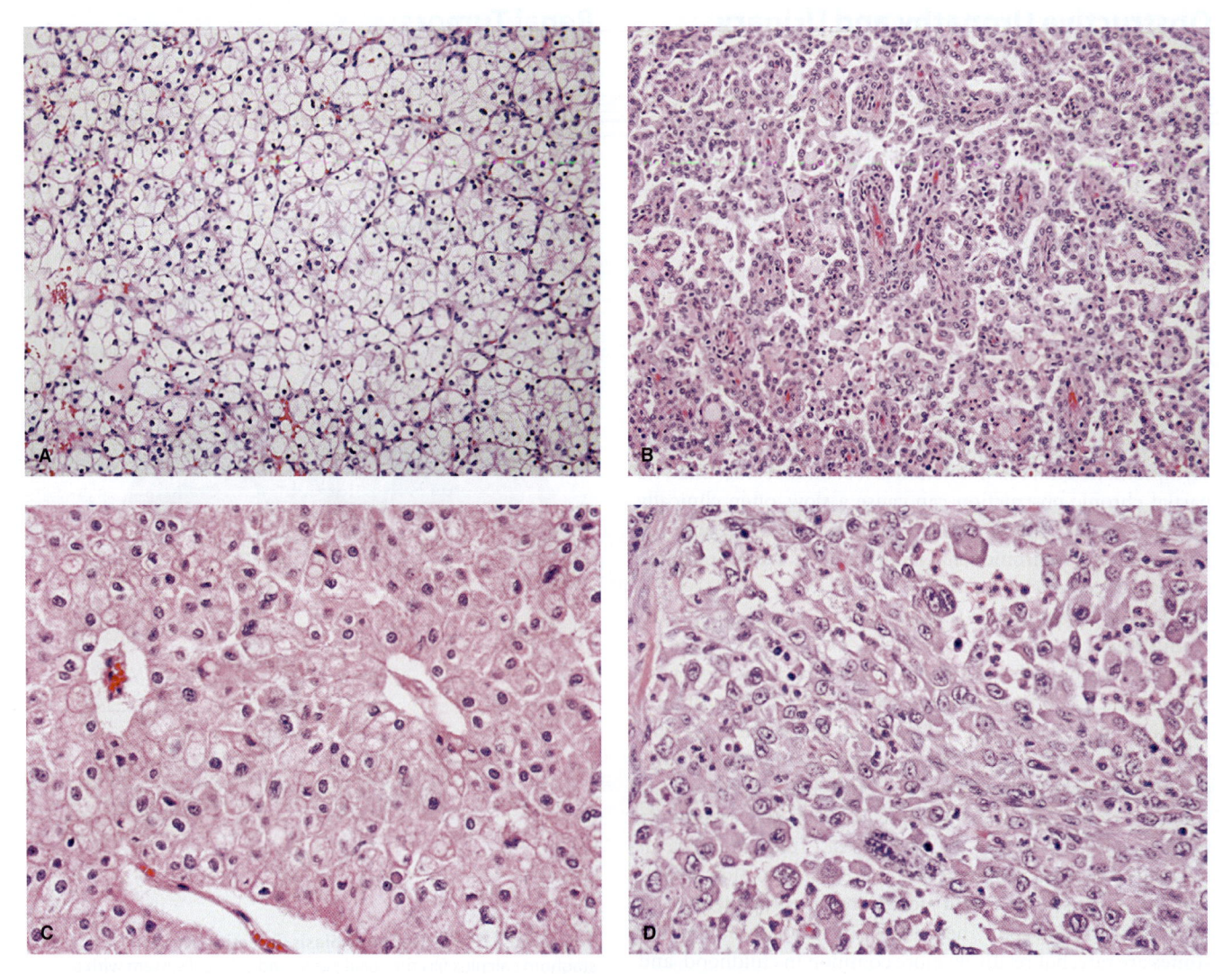

FIGURE 13-45 **Photomicrograph of histologic patterns of renal cell carcinoma. (A)** Clear cell renal cell carcinoma. **(B)** Papillary renal cell carcinoma. **(C)** Chromophobe renal cell carcinoma. **(D)** Sarcomatoid renal cell carcinoma.

those associated with von Hippel–Lindau disease and translocation-associated RCC). Chromosomal abnormalities in chromosome 7, 16, and 17 are associated with some papillary RCC.

The classic clinical presentation of RCC is the triad of an abdominal mass, flank pain, and hematuria, but less than 10% of patients present with these findings today. Currently, most RCCs are found incidentally when abdominal imaging is done for another reason. But RCC can present with ectopic hormone production, a paraneoplastic syndrome or as metastatic disease. A not uncommon presentation is the finding of multiple lung metastases found on chest CT scan, and when abdominal CT is done a renal mass is detected, and when biopsied is shown to be RCC.

The gross appearance of RCC is variable. Masses may be solid or partially cystic, may have a bright yellow cut surface, and hemorrhage and necrosis are common (Figure 13-46). Microscopically, tumor cells may be clear or granular, and may grow in a variety of patterns (glands, sheets, papillary structures, etc.). RCC is graded by nuclear size and pleomorphism, and staged by tumor size, whether or not the tumor is confined to the kidney, presence of vascular invasion, and involvement of lymph nodes and metastases. RCCs have a peculiar propensity for growing into the renal vein and forming tumor thrombi, which may extend into the vena cava or even into the right atrium of the heart.

The mainstay of therapy for RCC is surgery. Partial nephrectomies are performed most commonly to preserve renal function. Ablation of tumors by radiofrequency ablation or cryotherapy is a less invasive treatment modality. For patients with metastatic RCC, targeted therapy to growth receptors expressed by the tumor (such as VEGF) has promise in increasing life expectancy in these patients.

The most common childhood renal neoplasm is **Wilms tumor (nephroblastoma)**. This is one of the "small-, round-, blue-cell tumors" of childhood and is a tumor of the immature embryonal renal elements of the developing kidney. Wilms tumor is the most common abdominal solid tumor of infants and children. Median age of diagnosis is 3.5 years, and the usual presentation is that of an abdominal mass. Wilms tumors are solid, fleshy appearing tumors composed of the elements of fetal renal tissue (Figure 13-47). The elements are illustrated in Figure 13-48: (1) blastema (cellular zones of small round to oval cells with scant cytoplasm), (2) epithelium

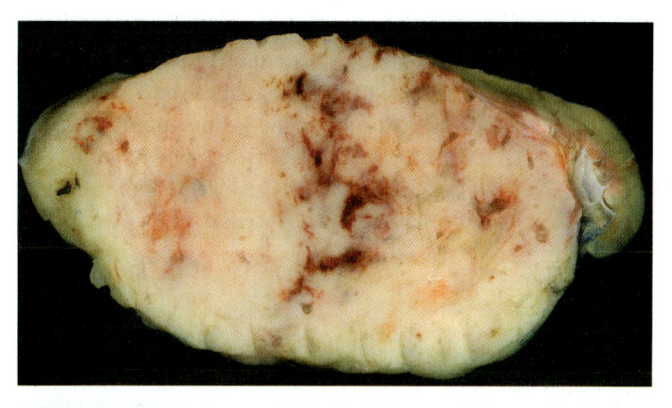

FIGURE 13-47 Gross image of Wilms tumor (nephroblastoma). The tumor is very large in relation to the size of the kidney (the small rim of normal tissue on the right side of the photo). It is a fleshy, solid, white mass with small areas of necrosis and hemorrhage.

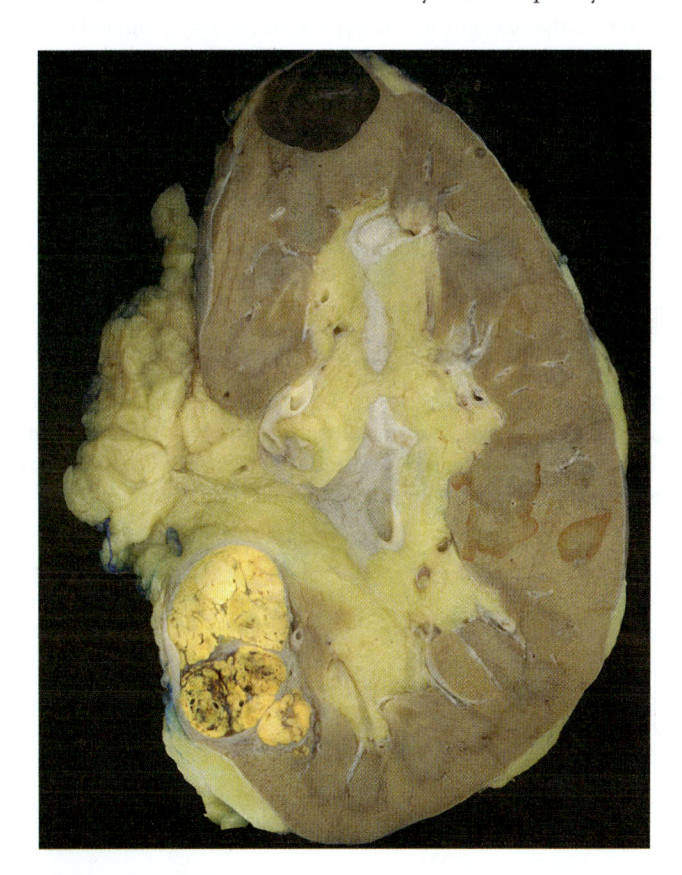

FIGURE 13-46 Gross image of renal cell carcinoma. The tumor is the bright yellow intraparenchymal mass in the lower pole of the kidney (arrow). A simple cyst is in the upper pole.

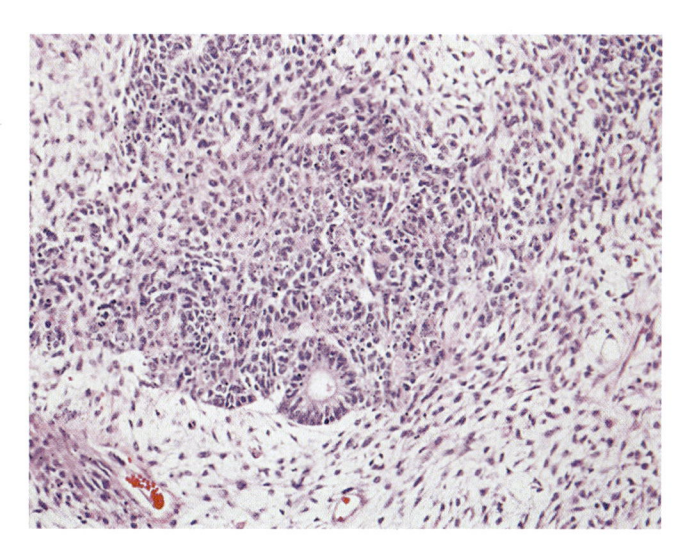

FIGURE 13-48 Photomicrograph of Wilms tumor (nephroblastoma). All three elements of nephroblastoma are seen in this image: epithelial (the tubule in the center of the photo), blastema (the crowded blue cells above the tubule), and stroma (the looser pale area containing long spindled cells below the tubule).

(tubular epithelial structures reminiscent of developing kidney tubules) and (3) stroma mesenchymal tissue composed of loose spindled cells that may show differentiation into smooth or skeletal muscle, cartilage, or fat. Some Wilms tumors have all three elements; some have only one or two. A portion of Wilms tumors have anaplasia, defined as large bizarre tumor cells at least three times the size of adjacent cells, or atypical mitotic figures. Anaplasia in a Wilms tumor is an unfavorable prognostic finding. Tumors are staged by their extent and whether the tumor is able to be removed intact without spillage in the abdomen and with negative surgical margins. The treatment of Wilms tumor is one of the success stories of modern medicine. Chemotherapy and radiation therapy added to surgical resection have dramatically improved the outcome of these patients.

IN TRANSLATION

While most Wilms tumors are sporadic, in about 10–15% of cases they are inherited and often but not always are associated with defined congenital syndromes. These include the following:

WAGR syndrome: **W**ilms tumor, **a**niridia, **g**enitourinary abnormalities, and mental **r**etardation. This syndrome has been shown to be associated with abnormalities in the short arm of chromosome 11 (11p13). One of the genes in this location is WT1, which encodes a gene essential to normal renal and gonadal development. In WAGR syndrome, the WT1 abnormalities are deletions.

Beckwith–Wiedemann syndrome: An overgrowth syndrome in which visceromegaly, macroglossia, gigantism, hemihypertrophy, and hyperinsulinemic hypoglycemia may be present. Patients with this syndrome are predisposed to have embryonal neoplasms, including Wilms tumor. This syndrome is associated with abnormalities on chromosome 11 near the WT1 locus at 11p15, the WT2 locus.

Denys–Drash syndrome: Congenital nephropathy associated with glomerular mesangial sclerosis, intersexual disorders, and Wilms tumor. This syndrome is due to dominant negative mutations in the WT1 gene, a different and more severe mutation seen in WAGR syndrome. The mutation is associated both with the development of Wilms tumors and the nephropathy seen in the non-neoplastic kidney tissue. Consequently, patients with Denys–Drash syndrome have severe kidney compromise as well as a high risk of development of Wilms tumor.

Patients with sporadic Wilms tumor rarely may have germline mutations of WT1 without either WAGR or Denys–Drash syndrome, and 10–20% of cases may have somatic mutations of WT1. Other somatic mutations that have been identified in sporadic Wilms tumor include the WTX mutation and mutations in the beta-catenin gene.

BENIGN TUMORS

Benign tumors of the kidney include oncocytoma and angiomyolipoma. **Oncocytoma** is a benign neoplasm composed of sheets and tubules composed of granular, eosinophilic cells with bland nuclei. These form solid masses in the kidney and by radiologic imaging are impossible to distinguish from renal cell carcinoma. Thus, these are usually biopsied or removed to exclude renal cell carcinoma, since solid renal masses are carcinoma until proven otherwise. **Angiomyolipoma** is a benign lesion of the renal capsule considered to be a hamartoma (an overgrowth of benign tissue in a place that the tissue is not normally found). These are strongly associated with tuberous sclerosis. The name comes from the three components of the lesion: blood vessels ("angio"), smooth muscle ("myo"), and adipose tissue ("lipoma"). Angiomyolipoma may be able to be recognized radiographically because of the characteristic capsular location and the fat density in the lesion by CT scan. If the radiologist is confident that a renal lesion is a small angiomyolipoma than the mass is usually only followed.

CHAPTER 14

Hematopathology

Cherie H. Dunphy, M.D., George Fedoriw, M.D., and Stephanie Mathews, M.D.

INTRODUCTION

WHAT WE DO

Hematopathology is one of the most diverse areas of pathology, since it represents a hybrid discipline involving clinical pathology (i.e., laboratory medicine) and anatomic pathology (surgical pathology of lymph nodes and extranodal tissues involved with hematolymphoid disorders). This field of pathology also uses cytomorphology and histology in combination with numerous ancillary tools (i.e., enzyme cytochemical and immunohistochemical staining, flow cytometric immunophenotyping, and cytogenetic and molecular techniques) in diagnosing and prognosticating hematolymphoid disorders. In some instances, the appropriate diagnosis of the hematolymphoid disorder also relies heavily on clinical and radiologic data.

For example, acute promyelocytic leukemia (APL) (as described later in this chapter) has characteristic, unique cytomorphological, enzyme cytochemical, and flow cytometric immunophenotypic features that are defined by the ever-present t(15;17)(q24;21) or similar variant. This translocation may be detected most rapidly by fluorescence in situ hybridization (FISH) performed in the cytogenetics laboratory. It is important to recognize this subtype of acute myeloid leukemia (AML) as soon as possible, since it is often associated with disseminated intravascular coagulation (DIC) and has a specific therapy (different from all other forms of AML).

In addition, for example, evaluation of plasma cell proliferations relies heavily on cytomorphological and histological features in combination with immunohistochemical and in situ hybridization studies for clonality. However, even with these techniques, the appropriate classification (and prognostication) of the plasma cell dyscrasia (PCD) must be based on close integration of the clinical and radiologic data (as well as cytogenetic and molecular data, respectively) in each case, as described again later in this chapter.

DISORDERS OF ERYTHROID CELLS

Anemias

Group of erythroid disorders, due to nonneoplastic and neoplastic etiologies, resulting in anemia.

Anemias represent a decrease in red cell mass or hemoglobin (Hgb) concentration, and often manifest with clinical features related to overall inadequate oxygen transport and/or volume depletion. The diverse underlying pathophysiologic mechanisms can be conceptually divided into three broad categories: decreased red cell production, increased destruction or turnover, and blood loss. In principle, the latter is most straightforward, but the source of bleeding is not always easily identified. Causes of decreased production, also referred to as hypoproliferative anemias, and increased destruction, can be related to a variety of neoplastic and nonneoplastic etiologies.

Common causes of anemia are listed in Table 14-1. A thorough history and physical examination along with an appropriately directed laboratory investigation are paramount to properly identifying the cause and guiding therapy.

Automated peripheral blood (PB) analyzers in clinical laboratories provide measurements of Hgb and hematocrit (HCT) concentration, or the percent of blood volume composed of red blood cells. However, these instruments output other important red cell characteristics, such as the mean corpuscular (or cellular) volume (MCV) and red cell distribution width (RDW). The MCV can be used to further define anemias as microcytic, normocytic, or macrocytic if the mean red blood cell volume is less than, equal to, or greater than normal, respectively. Ultimately, a manual review of the PB smear may provide additional information and insightful clues as to the underlying cause of anemia.

TABLE 14-1 Causes of anemia.

Microcytic	Normocytic	Macrocytic
Iron deficiency anemia	Blood loss	B12/folate deficiency
Thalassemia	Erythropoietin deficiency	Myelodysplastic syndrome
Sideroblastic anemias	Anemia of chronic disease	Liver disease
Lead poisoning		Hypothyroidism
Anemia of chronic disease		Chronic alcohol ingestion

CASE STUDY: Iron-Deficiency Anemia

Iron-deficiency anemia is a microcytic anemia due to a deficiency of iron, which is essential for the synthesis of Hgb

A 35-year-old woman presents to her primary physician with a several month history of slowly progressive fatigue.

CBC Data
WBC count: 10,900/μL
Hgb: 9.3 g/dL
MCV: 62
RDW: 19%
Platelet count: 399,000/μL

The PB smear (**Figure 14-1A**) demonstrates a hypochromic and microcytic anemia with numerous platelets in the background. The patient has a long-standing history of irregular and heavy menstrual cycles and previously identified uterine leiomyomata. Further laboratory studies reveal the following results:

Serum iron: 5 μg/dL (26-170 μg/dL)
Total iron binding capacity: 750 μg/mL (262-474 μg/dL)
Ferritin: 4 ng/mL (12–160 ng/mL)

The clinical and laboratory findings are classic for iron-deficiency anemia, likely resultant from chronic blood loss. Iron deficiency is a common cause of anemia worldwide, resulting from insufficient iron for appropriate Hgb synthesis.

In addition to the microcytic anemia, patients with iron deficiency can present with thrombocytosis and leukocytosis (as seen in this case). The serum iron levels are typically low, although may reflect recent iron intake rather than adequate iron stores. Total iron binding capacity is increased and the iron binding protein, transferrin, is similarly elevated. Levels of the intracellular iron regulatory protein, ferritin, effectively relate to the total systemic iron stores. Although rarely biopsied if clinically straightforward, cases refractory to iron replacement may necessitate a bone marrow (BM) evaluation. The findings in the BM are not specific and vary in severity (**Figure 14-1B**).

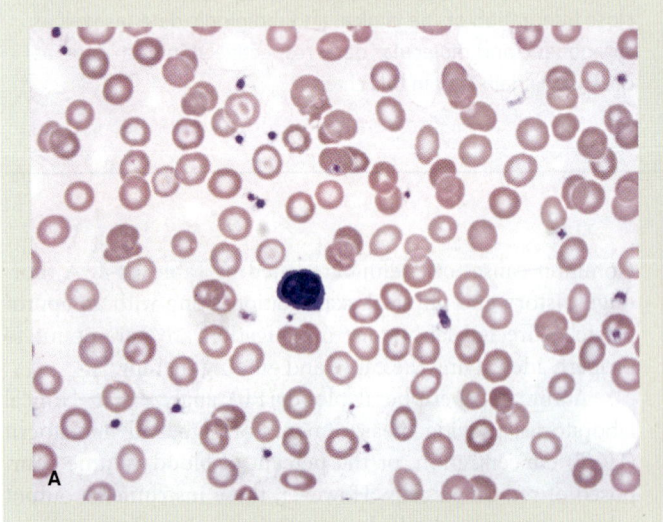

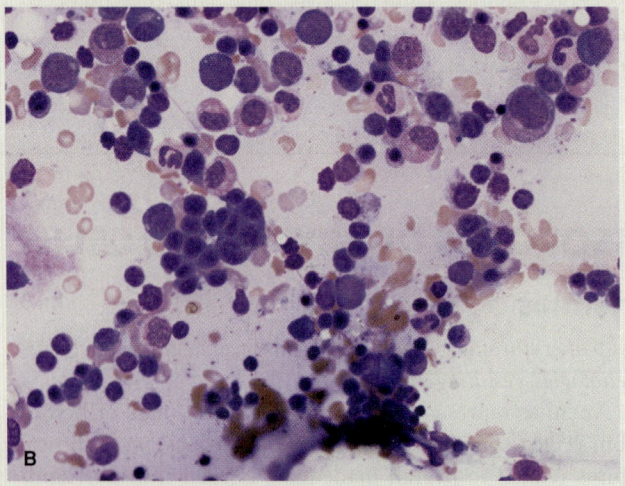

FIGURE 14-1 Iron deficiency anemia. The PB smear (**A**, Wright stain, ×1000) demonstrates a hypochromic microcytic anemia. A circulating lymphocyte, present in the center of the image, is available for size comparison. The Wright-Giemsa-stained BM aspirate (**B**, ×600) shows a normocellular BM with relative erythroid hyperplasia. Erythropoiesis is typically morphologically normal, although some dysplastic features may be identified. The iron stains would reveal absence of adequate iron stores.

CASE STUDY: Refractory Anemia [Refractory Anemia with Ring Sideroblasts (RARS)]

Refractory anemia falls within the group of myelodysplastic syndromes (MDS) due to ineffective erythropoiesis.

A 79-year-old man presents with a 4-year history of a macrocytic anemia, who is now transfusion dependent.

CBC Data
WBC count: 7200/μL
Hgb: 9.3 g/dL (after transfusion)
MCV: 100
RDW: 22.3
Platelet count: 275,000/μL

The BM aspirate and biopsy are hypercellular and demonstrate an erythroid hyperplasia with significant erythroid hyperplasia and dyspoiesis of the erythroid lineage (Figure 14-2A). Stains for iron demonstrate increased iron stores and numerous ring sideroblasts (Figure 14-2B). These clinical and morphologic features are consistent with myelodysplasia, specifically RARS.

MDS represent a heterogenous group of hematopoietic neoplasms with a variably increased risk of progression to AML. These malignancies typically present with otherwise unexplained PB cytopenia(s) that are a consequence of ineffective hematopoiesis. RARS represents a common form of MDS specifically affecting erythropoiesis. In contrast to other forms of MDS, refractory anemia has a relatively indolent clinical course and a low risk of progression to acute leukemia.

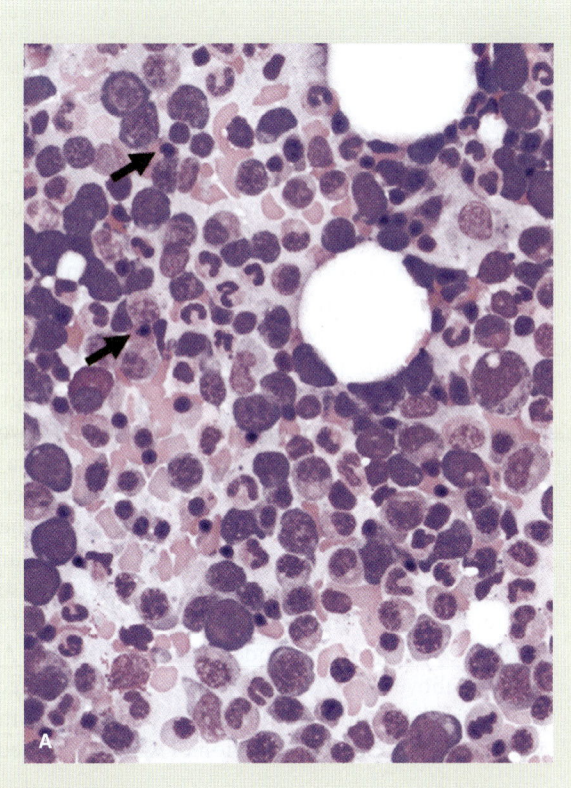

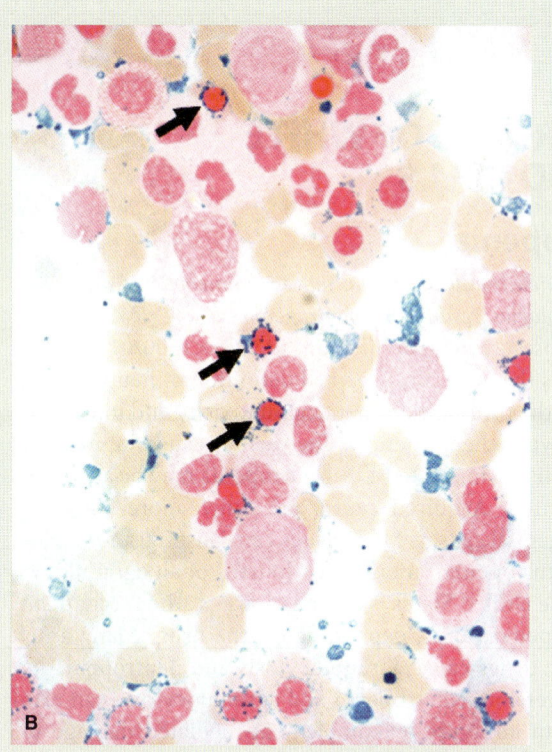

FIGURE 14-2 RARS. As is typical for most cases of MDS, the BM aspirate (**A**, Wright stain, ×600) is hypercellular. The erythroid series shows dyspoietic features including irregular nuclear contours with nuclear blebbing (arrows) and megaloblastoid changes. The granulocytic and megakaryocytic lineages are, by definition, morphologically normal. Iron stain of the aspirate (**B**, ×1000) shows abundant iron (blue) and many ring sideroblasts (arrows), representing mitochondrial iron deposition along the nuclear border.

Polycythemias

Group of erythroid disorders due to nonneoplastic and neoplastic etiologies resulting in polycythemia (Table 14-2).

Polycythemias, or elevated red cell mass, represent a group of erythroid disorders due to nonneoplastic and neoplastic etiologies. Clinical manifestations are typically related to underlying cause rather than the erythrocytosis itself.

TABLE 14-2 Causes of polycythemia.

Malignant (Primary)	Physiologic (Secondary)
Polycythemia vera	Chronic hypoxia
	Altitude related
	Iatrogenic
Genetic	
Inherited mutations of HIFs	
Rare hemoglobinopathies	

HIFs, hypoxia-inducible factors.

CASE STUDY: Copper-Deficiency Anemia

HUNTING FOR ZEBRAS

Copper deficiency is rare and may cause sideroblastic anemia (case of copper-deficiency anemia).

The patient is a 12-year-old boy with a history of microcytic hypochromic anemia.

CBC Data
WBC count: 3000/μL
Hgb: 8.0 g/dL (after transfusion)
MCV: 57
Platelet count: 250,000/μL

Laboratory testing and supplementation have excluded iron deficiency.

Although B12 and folate deficiency are most commonly considered, a variety of nutritional deficiencies can clinically manifest with signs and symptoms of anemia. Copper deficiency is a rare cause of anemia, and can present with neurologic manifestations. Although hereditary and several acquired causes have been identified, the etiology remains uncertain for many patients. PB manifestations are diverse and include micro-, normo-, and macrocytic anemia, leukopenia with neutropenia, and less commonly, thrombocytopenia. The BM in these patients demonstrates erythroid dyspoiesis, in many cases morphologically indistinguishable from primary MDS. Iron stains highlight ring sideroblasts, thus making copper deficiency a rare cause of sideroblastic anemia.

DISORDERS OF WHITE BLOOD CELLS

Neutropenia

Group of neutrophil disorders, due to nonneoplastic and neoplastic etiologies, resulting in neutropenia.

An absolute neutrophil count (ANC) <1500/μL (<1.5 × 10(9)/L) is the generally accepted definition of neutropenia, as well as the threshold for neutrophil toxicity and infectious risk following chemotherapy. The various causes of neutropenia are listed in Table 14-3. Neutropenia may be acquired or congenital. Acquired causes are much more common than congenital causes. Many drugs can cause agranulocytosis and neutropenia. About three-fourths of all agranulocytosis in the United States is related to drugs. The mechanism of neutropenia varies, depending on the drug. Many antineoplastic drugs cause agranulocytosis and neutropenia by BM suppression. Neutropenia and agranulocytosis can also result from antibody or complement-mediated damage to the stem cells. Some drugs may cause increased peripheral destruction of white cells. Procainamide, antithyroid drugs, and sulfasalazine are at the top of the list of drugs causing this problem. Most agranulocytosis is related to the direct effect related to its dose. Phenothiazines, semisynthetic penicillins, nonsteroidal anti-inflammatory drugs (NSAIDs), aminopyrine derivatives, benzodiazepines, barbiturate, gold compounds, sulfonamides, and antithyroid medications are the most common causes of neutropenia and agranulocytosis. The neutropenia manifests in about 1–2 weeks after exposure to these drugs. Degree of neutropenia depends upon the dose and duration of exposure. Recovery usually occurs within few days of stopping the drug. The marrow recovery may take 10–14 days. Sometimes, a rebound leukocytosis may occur. If the neutropenia is not very severe and the medication is an essential drug for the patient, the drug may be continued with under close monitoring. As long as ANC is above 500–700 and there is no active infection, the drug may be continued if needed. Some drugs may cause increased peripheral destruction of white cells. Neutropenia

CASE STUDY: Secondary Polycythemia Due to Hypoxia

Secondary polycythemia is a non-neoplastic condition of increased red blood cell mass.

Secondary polycythemia refers to the increased red blood cell mass not related to a primary erythroid neoplasm.

A 55-year-old female with a long-standing history of chronic obstructive pulmonary disease and sleep apnea presents to her primary physician for routine follow-up. She has been a heavy smoker for approximately 15 years.

CBC Data
WBC count: 10,000/μL
Hgb: 15.8 g/dL
MCV: 93
Platelet count: 400,000/μL

The morphologic features of the PB smear confirm increased numbers of red cells, but are otherwise unremarkable.

In this clinical context, the cause of the increased Hgb concentration is likely the result of increased erythropoietin production as a consequence of hypoxia. A similar mechanism is also responsible for altitude-associated polycythemia. Other secondary causes of increased red cell mass include paraneoplastic syndromes, hereditary disorders of Hgb and erythropoietin homeostasis, and rare hemoglobinopathies.

CASE STUDY: Polycythemia Vera

Polycythemia vera (PV) is a chronic myeloproliferative neoplasm characterized by red blood cell production independent of the mechanisms that normally regulate erythropoiesis.

A 54-year-old woman is referred to a hematologist for a several month long history of progressive headaches and erythromelalgia of the lower extremities. Physical examination reveals mild splenomegaly and facial plethora.

CBC Data
WBC count: 15,000/μL
Hgb: 18.5 g/dL
Platelet count: 500,000/μL

Other Laboratory Findings
Erythropoietin: 3 (ref range: 4–27 mU/mL)
PCR for V617F JAK2 mutation: POSITIVE

PV is a chronic myeloproliferative neoplasm characterized by red blood cell production independent of the mechanisms that normally regulate erythropoiesis. The identification of the acquired activating mutation of the JAK2 kinase (V617F) is identified in nearly all cases of PV, and along with decreased erythropoietin levels, supports this diagnosis. The BM (Figure 14-3) is typically hypercellular with expansion of all myeloid lineages. The erythroid morphology is normal. Hyperlobated and increased megakaryocytes are commonly identified, sharing morphologic features with other myeloproliferative neoplasms. The clinical course is generally indolent, but the risk of transformation to MDS or acute leukemia is not insignificant.

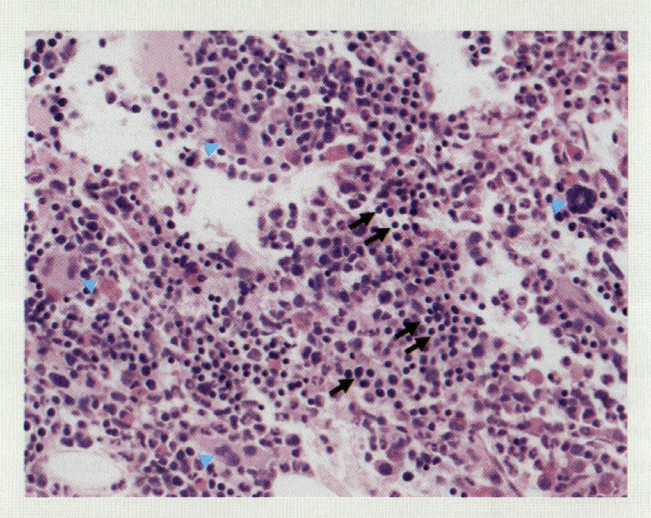

FIGURE 14-3 PV. The hematoxylin and eosin (H&E)-stained BM biopsy sections demonstrate a markedly hypercellular BM with expansion of the erythroid series (arrows) and appropriate granulopoiesis (×400). Numerous megakaryocytes are also present (arrow heads), although this feature does not effectively distinguish PV from some other myeloproliferative neoplasms.

TABLE 14-3 Causes of neutropenia.

Acquired
- Drug-induced neutropenia and agranulocytosis due to direct effect of drug dosage
- Autoimmune destruction of neutrophils (either as a primary immune disorder—typically presents in early childhood or associated with another disease—RA, SLE, Felty syndrome) or from drugs stimulating the immune system to attack the cells
- Infections (more commonly viral infections, but also bacterial or parasitic infections—HIV, tuberculosis, *Ehrlichia*, malaria, parvo B19, EBV, HepB, HCV, etc.)
- Hypersplenism
- Complement activation (2/2 ECMO, HD, cardiopulmonary bypass, etc.)
- PNH
- Bone marrow failure or disorders (i.e., leukemias, myelodysplastic syndrome, aplastic anemia, myelofibrosis, lymphomas, and multiple myeloma)
- Immunologic due to BMT or blood transfusion
- Medications that may damage the bone marrow or neutrophils, including cancer chemotherapy
- Radiation therapy
  - Nutritional deficiency (vitamin B12, copper, folate)

Congenital
- Neutropenias associated with immune defects
- Congenital neutropenia due to mutations
  - Cyclic neutropenia
  - Kostmann syndrome (severe congenital neutropenia) – typically die in early childhood
- Chronic benign neutropenia
- Neutropenia w/ phenotypic abnormalities
  - Shwachman–Diamond–Oski syndrome
  - Cartilage-hair hypoplasia syndrome
  - Dyskeratosis congenita
  - Barth syndrome
  - Chediak–Higashi syndrome
- Benign familial neutropenia
  - Do not mount leukocytosis to infection, but are able to mount fever and inflammatory response. Not associated with higher infection incidence
- Myeloperoxidase deficiency
  - Not a real neutropenia, and most often identified incidentally. Can occasionally be associated with recurrent infections

CASE STUDY: Neutropenia Due to Drug Therapy

Neutropenia may occur secondary to drug therapy and the most common drug-induced blood dyscrasia is a neutropenia.

A 52-year-old male with a kidney transplant a year previously presents with leukopenia. Medications include alemtuzumab, valganciclovir, trimethoprim, sulfamethoxazole, and mycophenolate mofetil. The patient has been undergoing plasmapheresis for recurrent membranous nephropathy.

CBC Data
WBC count: 700/μL
Hgb: 10.3 g/dL
Platelet count: 299,000/μL
ANC: 400/μL

The mycophenolate mofetil is decreased in dosage, and within 2 months the WBC count increases to 6100/μL with an ANC of 5200/μL. In addition, the Hgb level increases to 13.1 g/dL. This approach supports the most likely drug-induced neutropenia.

Other causes of acquired neutropenia should also be considered, including a possible primary BM disorder, particularly a MDS, especially in light of the associated anemia.

---

and agranulocytosis can also result from antibody or compliment-mediated damage to the stem cells. Neutropenia may also be immune mediated in association with an autoimmune disorder or secondary to a drug-induced neutropenia.

Infections may also cause neutropenia. Although most bacterial infections stimulate an increase in neutrophils, some bacterial infections such as typhoid fever and brucellosis and many viral diseases, including hepatitis, influenza, rubella, rubeola, and mumps, decrease the neutrophil count. An overwhelming infection can also deplete the BM of neutrophils and produce neutropenia.

Neutropenia Secondary to Myelodysplastic Syndrome

Neutropenia may occur alone or in association with anemia and/or thrombocytopenia in a MDS (i.e., refractory neutropenia or refractory cytopenia with multilineage dysplasia). As mentioned previously, acquired causes of neutropenia are much more common than congenital causes.

HUNTING FOR ZEBRAS
Cyclic Neutropenia

Cyclic neutropenia is a rare (1–2 per million,) typically autosomal-dominant inherited disorder with variable expression, usually presenting in the first year of life.

It is characterized by neutropenia that recurs every 14–35 days, although over 90% of patients exhibit a cycle period of 21 days. While the disease tends to be benign, several affected patients have died of infection. The disorder has been found to be due to germ line mutations in ELA2. ELA2 encodes neutrophil elastase. Interestingly, molecular studies have demonstrated that this protein represents an oncoprotein. Kostmann syndrome is also associated with ELA2 mutations as well as granulocyte colony-stimulating factor receptor (GCSF-r) mutations, and approximately 20% will go on to develop MDS and/or AML.

Refer again to Table 14-3 for the list of congenital causes of neutropenia.

Neutrophilia

Group of neutrophil disorders, due to nonneoplastic and neoplastic etiologies, resulting in neutrophilia.

Neutrophilia is defined as an increase in the ANC, which may vary depending on the normal range within the testing laboratory. Various causes of neutrophilia are listed in Table 14-4. Secondary causes of neutrophilia are much more common than primary causes. A true increase in neutrophil production most often reflects an infection, particularly an acute bacterial infection. Neutrophilia can occur from acute infections caused by cocci (e.g., staphylococci, pneumococci, streptococci, meningococci, and gonococci), bacilli (i.e., *Escherichia coli, Pseudomonas aeruginosa, and Actinomyces* species), certain fungi (i.e., *Coccidioides immitis*), spirochetes, viruses (i.e., rabies, poliomyelitis, herpes zoster, smallpox, and varicella), rickettsia, and parasites (i.e., liver fluke). Neutrophilia may also be seen with furuncles, abscesses, tonsillitis, appendicitis, otitis media, osteomyelitis, arthritis, cholecystitis, salpingitis, meningitis, diphtheria, plague, and peritonitis. Refer to Table 14-4 for the list of other secondary causes of neutrophilia.

Although secondary causes of neutrophilia are much more common than primary causes, a primary neutrophilia should be excluded. Neutrophilia may represent the initial finding in myeloproliferative neoplasms, particularly chronic myelogenous leukemia (CML).

Chronic Myelogenous Leukemia

Chronic myelogenous leukemia (CML) is a myeloproliferative neoplasm characterized by an initial major finding of neutrophilia. CML originates in an abnormal pluripotent BM stem cell and is consistently associated with the *BCR–ABL1* fusion gene located in the Philadelphia chromosome, which is found in all myeloid lineages.

Rarely, an absolute neutrophilia may also be associated with nonhematopoietic tumors (i.e., squamous cell

TABLE 14-4 Causes of neutrophilia and monocytosis.

Primary Neutrophilia
- Hereditary neutrophilia
- Familial myeloproliferative disease
- Familial cold autoinflammatory syndrome
- Down syndrome
- Leukocyte adhesion deficiency
- Pelger–Huet anomaly
- Amegakaryocytic thrombocytopenia
- Chronic idiopathic neutrophilia
- Myeloproliferative neoplasms, including chronic myeloid leukemia
- Chronic neutrophilic leukemia

Secondary Neutrophilia
- Acute infection
- Chronic inflammation
- Effect of proinflammatory cytokines
- Cigarette smoking
- Stress neutrophilia
- Exercise
- Physiologic neutrophilia is also seen in pregnancy, labor, and in newborns
- Epinephrine injection
- Acute myocardial infarction
- Burns
- Postoperative state
- Acute attacks of gout
- Acute glomerulonephritis
- Rheumatic fever
- Collagen vascular diseases
- Hypersensitivity reactions
- Diabetic ketoacidosis
- Preeclampsia
- Uremia
- Heatstroke
- Acute hemorrhage
- Glucocorticoids and other drugs
- Poisoning (lead, mercury, digitalis, camphor, antipyrine, phenacetin, quinidine, pyrogallol, turpentine, arsphenamine, and insect venoms)
- Differentiation syndrome (potentially fatal complication of induction chemotherapy in patients with acute promyelocytic leukemia)
- Marrow stimulation
- Marrow invasion and leukoerythroblastic reaction
- Nonhematologic malignancy
- Paraneoplastic leukemoid reaction
- Sweet syndrome
- Asplenia

Monocytosis
Reactive
- Acute and chronic infections (bacterial and viral infections, tuberculosis, malaria, Rocky Mountain spotted fever)
- Chronic ulcerative colitis, Crohn disease
- Sarcoidosis
- Connective tissue diseases
- Autoimmune disease (rheumatoid arthritis, SLE)
- Benign hematological disorders (hemolytic anemia, immune thrombocytopenic purpura)
- After administration of granulocyte-monocyte colony-stimulating factor (GM-CSF) or intravenous immunoglobulin therapy
- Recovery from chemotherapy, bone marrow injury, or chronic neutropenia
- Postmyocardial infarction
- Postoperative state
- Postsplenectomy

Malignant
- Leukemias (chronic myelomonocytic leukemia, juvenile myelomonocytic leukemia, acute myeloid leukemias with a monocytic component—AMML, and AMoL)
- Paraneoplastic phenomenon (Hodgkin and non-Hodgkin lymphomas, plasma cell dyscrasia, and rarely carcinoma-particularly lung, colorectal and renal carcinomas)

CASE STUDY: Neutrophilia Due to Arthritis

A 4-year-old male presents with 7–10-day history of high spiking fever, rash, and aching in the wrists and knees.

CBC Data
WBC count: 36,400/μL
Hgb: 10.6 g/dL
Platelet count: 662,000/μL
ANC: 32,100/μL (Figure 14-4)

He was diagnosed with juvenile idiopathic arthritis and begun on methotrexate, anakinra (IL-1 receptor antagonist), and prednisone (20 mg b.i.d. for total 40 mg daily). A follow-up visit 5 weeks after initial presentation revealed resolution of symptoms and a WBC count of 8800/μL with and ANC of 7000/μL.

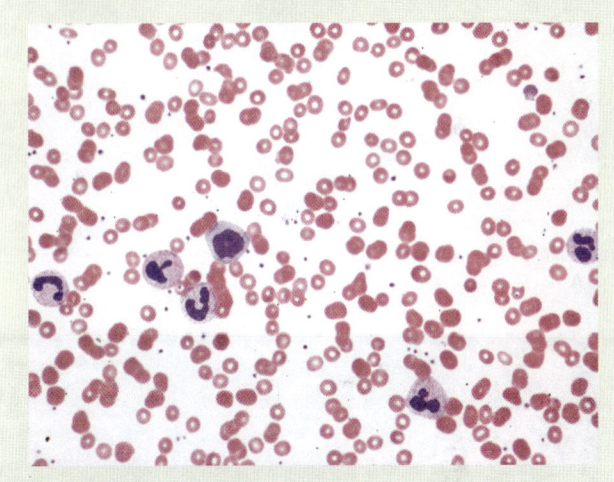

FIGURE 14-4 Neutrophilia. PB smear demonstrating leukemoid reaction with an increase in neutrophils and increased granulation within the cytoplasm (Wright stain, ×600).

carcinoma) as a paraneoplastic phenomenon secondary to cytokine production by the tumor.

Lymphocytoses

In adults, an absolute lymphocytosis is defined as an increase in the peripheral blood lymphocyte count (ALC) of greater than 4000/μL; in older children (up to 6 years of age), greater

HUNTING FOR ZEBRAS
Paraneoplastic Neutrophilia

Paraneoplastic leukemoid reaction is caused by nonhematopoietic tumor-producing hematopoietic growth factors, including GCSF (or other hematopoietic cytokines, such as IL-6), without BM involvement.

CASE STUDY: Chronic Myelogenous Leukemia

A 40-year-old male presents with a new onset of a diarrheal illness. He presented to a local physician and was noted on physical examination to have an enlarged spleen.

CBC Data
WBC count: 143,900/μL
Hgb: 11.9 g/dL
Platelet count: 589,000/μL
ANC: 122,300/μL

The PB smear reveals a marked leukocytosis with neutrophilia, a few myelocytes and promyelocytes, rare blasts, and a basophilia (4,300/μL) (Figure 14-5A). The BM aspiration and biopsy reveal a markedly hypercellular BM (99% cellular) with small megakaryocytic forms and a markedly increased M:E ratio of 29:1 (Figure 14-5B and C).

Cytogenetic analysis reveals a t(9;22)(q34;q11.2) and DNA studies reveal *BCR–ABL* p210 transcripts.

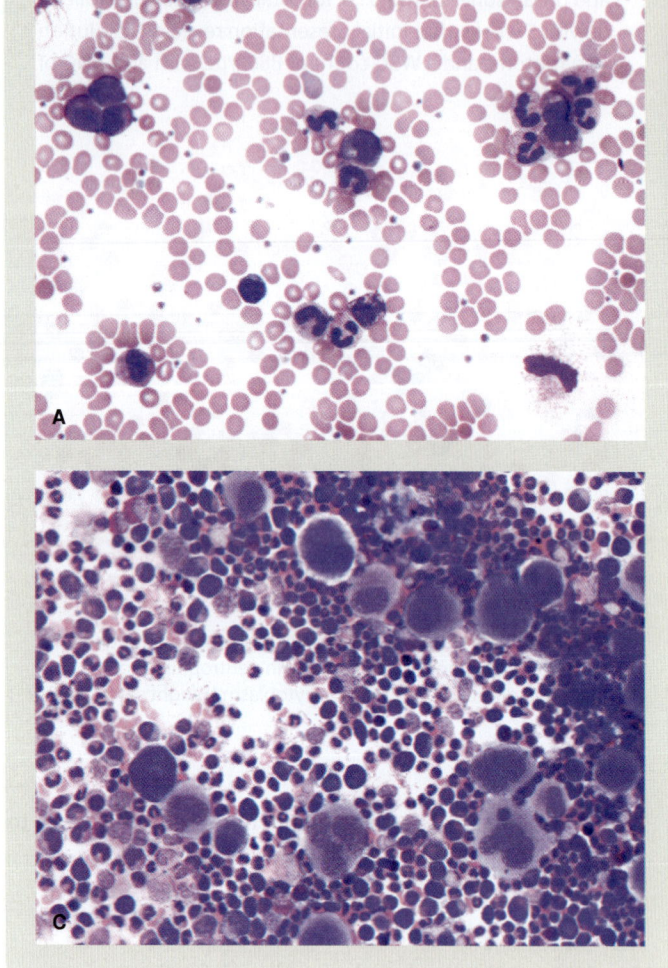

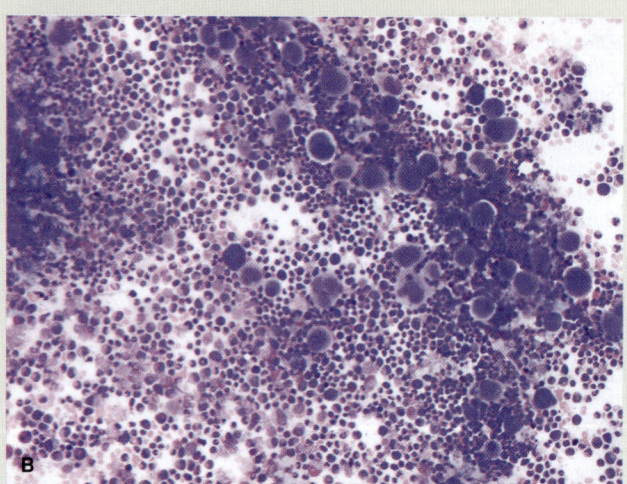

FIGURE 14-5 Chronic myelogenous leukemia. The PB smear (**A**, Wright stain, ×600) demonstrates an increase in neutrophils and granulocytic precursors. An occasional cell has basophilic granules within the cytoplasm. The BM aspirate (**B** and **C**, Wright stain; B- ×400; C- ×600) reveals a markedly hypercellular marrow with increased megakaryocytes (with clustering and numerous small forms), a predominance of granulocytic cells, markedly decreased erythroid elements, and scattered eosinophils and mast cells.

than 7000/μL; and in infants, greater than 9000/μL. A relative lymphocytosis occurs when there is a higher proportion (greater than 40%) of lymphocytes among the white blood cells (WBCs); however, the ALC is normal (less than 4,000/μL). A relative lymphocytosis is normal in children under the age of 2 years.

An absolute lymphocytosis in children and young adults most often reflects an infection, particularly a viral infection (i.e., infectious mononucleosis) or an infection with pertussis. In older adults with an absolute lymphocytosis, a chronic lymphoproliferative disorder should be considered and excluded. Various causes of an absolute lymphocytosis are listed in Table 14-5.

Lymphocytoses may be due to various reactive causes, including viral agents, as well as due to clonal proliferations, and are composed of mature lymphocytes.

TABLE 14-5 Causes of lymphocytosis.

Absolute Lymphocytosis
- Acute viral infections (i.e., infectious mononucleosis—EBV, cytomegalovirus infection, infectious hepatitis, HIV, and measles)
- Other acute infections (i.e., whooping cough—pertussis; typhoid fever—*Salmonella* typhi)
- Protozoal infections (i.e., toxoplasmosis and American trypanosomiasis—Chagas disease)
- Chronic bacterial infections (i.e., tuberculosis, brucellosis, or syphilis)
- Serum sickness
- Chronic lymphoproliferative disorders (i.e., CLL, Waldenström macroglobulinemia—WM, and large granular lymphocytosis/leukemia)
- Sezary syndrome
- Adult T-cell leukemia/lymphoma
- Prolymphocytic leukemia
- Peripheralizing lymphomas
- Acute lymphoblastic leukemia

Relative Lymphocytosis
- Age less than 2 years
- Autoimmune disorders (i.e., connective tissue diseases, collagen vascular diseases, Graves disease, and Addison disease) associated with chronic inflammation
- Inflammatory bowel disease (i.e., Crohn disease and ulcerative colitis)
- Allergic and hypersensitivity reactions
- Splenomegaly with splenic sequestration of granulocytes or splenectomy

Chronic Lymphocytic Leukemia

The most common chronic lymphoproliferative disorder presenting with an absolute lymphocytosis is chronic lymphocytic leukemia (CLL). CLL is also the most common leukemia of adults in Western countries.

T-Cell Prolymphocytic Leukemia

The morphologic features of CLL may also be confused with the malignant cells composing the small cell variant of T-cell prolymphocytic leukemia (T-PLL), which has a much more aggressive clinical course.

T-PLL is an aggressive T-cell leukemia characterized by the proliferation of small-to-medium-sized prolymphocytes with a mature post-thymic T-cell phenotype involving the PB, BM, lymph nodes, spleen, and skin. The morphology of the leukemic cells may range from those of typical prolymphocytes with a single prominent nucleolus to small forms with no apparent nucleolus (i.e., the small cell variant), which may mimic the cells of CLL.

T-PLL is rare, representing approximately 2% of cases of mature lymphocytic leukemias. It is important to distinguish it from CLL, as described above, since T-PLL has a much more aggressive clinical course and is treated differently.

Monocytopenia

Monocytopenia is relatively rare and defined as an abnormally low level of monocytes in the PB (i.e., less than 200/μL) and can be seen in non-neoplastic (i.e., HIV infection) and neoplastic (i.e., hairy cell leukemia) disorders.

Lymphocytosis Due to Infection with EBV

CASE STUDY: Infectious Mononucleosis

Infectious mononucleosis is due to a viral infection with Epstein–Barr virus (EBV), resulting in a reactive peripheral lymphocytosis, composed predominantly of T cells.

A 22-year-old college student presents with a recent history of sore throat, fever, and palpable cervical lymphadenopathy and splenomegaly.

CBC Data
WBC count: 63,600/μL
Hgb: 9.9 g/dL
Platelet count: 256,000/μL
ALC: 45,300/μL

Review of the PB smear reveals a marked increase in atypical lymphocytes (Figure 14-6). Flow cytometric analysis of the PB reveals 78% of cells within the lymphocyte region. Cells within the lymphocyte region are composed of 87% T cells (CD4:CD8 ratio is 0.7) without an aberrant immunophenotype, 8% polyclonal B cells, and 5% natural killer (NK) cells. The patient subsequently had a positive Mono spot test. The patient was diagnosed with infectious mononucleosis.

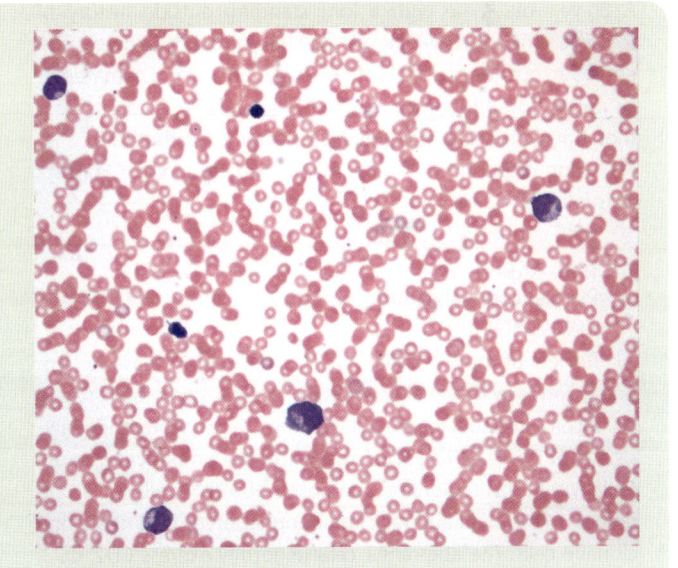

FIGURE 14-6 Reactive lymphocytosis. PB smear demonstrating a reactive lymphocytosis, composed of enlarged lymphoid cells with associated basophilic cytoplasm (Wright stain, ×600).

CASE STUDY: Chronic Lymphocytic Leukemia

CLL is a neoplasm composed of monomorphic and clonal small, round B lymphocytes. The cells usually coexpress CD5 and CD23. In the absence of extramedullary tissue involvement, there must be greater than 5000/µL peripheral monoclonal lymphocytes with a CLL phenotype.

A 49-year-old male is referred for the evaluation of possible CLL. He presented to his primary care provider with mild fatigue, but few other symptoms. A routine CBC showed a white count of 120,000 that were predominantly lymphocytes.

Upon presentation at referral, his CBC data is as follows:
WBC count: 149,500/µL
Hgb: 15.1g/dL
Platelet count: 119,000/µL
ALC: 123,200/µL

Review of the PB smear reveals a marked increase in the number of small, round, mature lymphocytes (Figure 14-7). Flow cytometric analysis of the PB reveals 92% cells within the lymphocyte region. Cells within this region are composed of 2% T cells (CD4:CD8 ratio is 1:1) without an aberrant immunophenotype, 96% monoclonal B cells, and 2% presumed NK cells. The monoclonal B-cells variably express CD19, CD20, CD23, CD79b, CD38, selective kappa surface light chains, aberrant CD5, and ZAP-70. They do not express CD10. This immunophenotype is characteristic of CLL, representing 88% of the peripheral WBCs. ZAP-70 expression is associated with a worse prognosis in CLL. Cytogenetic analysis reveals an abnormal karyotype: 46,XY,del(11)(q?14q?23),del(13)(q?12q?14)[1]/46,XY[4]. Del (13) is the most common abnormality identified in CLL by FISH analysis.

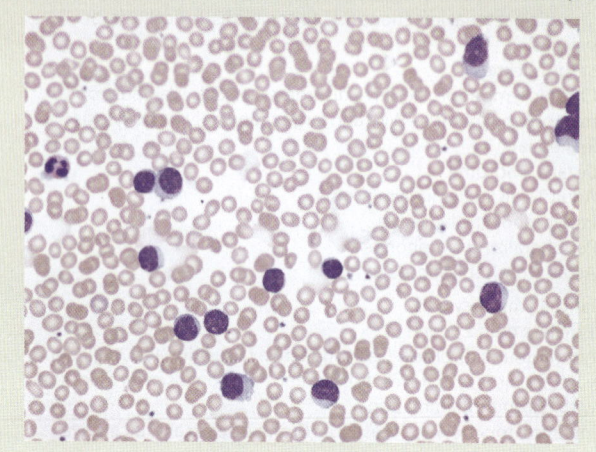

FIGURE 14-7 Chronic lymphocytic leukemia. PB smear demonstrating chronic lymphocytic leukemia, composed of a monotonous population of predominantly small, round, mature lymphocytes (Wright stain, ×600).

CASE STUDY: T-PLL

HUNTING FOR ZEBRAS

A 66-year-old male with a long-standing outside history of "chronic lymphocytic leukemia" (no chemotherapy to date) presents to an outside hospital with bloody diarrhea and hematemesis and is noted to have a markedly elevated WBC count. He is then transferred to a major medical center for further care.

Upon presentation at the major medical center, CBC data is as follows:
WBC count: 117,100/µL
Hgb: 9.2 g/dL
Platelet count: 45,000/µL
ALC: 90,400/µL

Review of the PB smear reveals a marked increase in lymphoid forms with variably irregular nuclear contours (Figure 14-8); prolymphocytes are not identified. Flow cytometric analysis of the PB reveals 90% of cells are within the lymphocyte region. Cells within this region are composed of 99% T cells (CD4:CD8 ratio is 1:1) with an aberrant immunophenotype and <1% polyclonal B cells. The aberrant T cells uniformly express CD2, CD3, CD4 and CD8, CD5, CD7, and CD25, and lack expression of CD10, CD1a, CD34, CD56, CD117, and myeloid or B-cell antigens. This immunophenotype is characteristic of a mature aberrant T-cell immunophenotype, representing 90% of the peripheral WBCs and consistent with the small cell variant of T-PLL.

Such a presentation of a reported history of CLL is not uncommon in this variant of T-PLL, due to the overlapping morphologic features with CLL. Such a case supports the importance of performing flow cytometric immunophenotyping in all cases suspected of "CLL."

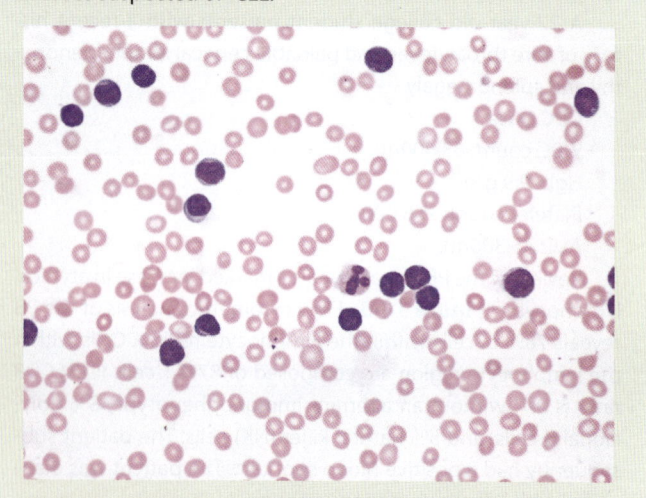

FIGURE 14-8 T-cell prolymphocytic leukemia. PB smear in case of T-PLL, demonstrating an increase in predominantly small lymphoid forms with variably irregular nuclear contours (Wright stain, ×600).

> **CASE STUDY: Monocytopenia in AIDS**
>
> A 48-year-old male with a history of HIV/AIDS presents with a 2-month history of progressive cough and fever. He also has a warm autoimmune hemolytic anemia (receiving weekly rituximab), resolving candidemia, splenomegaly, and worsening thrombocytopenia.
>
> **CBC Data**
> WBC count: 4600/μL
> Hgb: 6.6 g/dL
> Platelet count: 18,000/μL
> ANC: 4100/μL
> ALC: 400/μL (normal: 2000–4000/μL)
> Monocyte count: 0.

Monocytopenia Secondary to Hairy Cell Leukemia

Monocytopenia typically also occurs in hairy cell leukemia, and should be considered in patients presenting with unexplained pancytopenia in the appropriate clinical context.

Monocytoses

An absolute monocytosis is defined as a peripheral monocyte count greater than 1000/μL. The various causes of an absolute monocytosis are listed in Table 14-4.

Monocytoses may be due to various reactive causes as well as to clonal disorders. Reactive causes of an absolute monocytosis should be sought, particularly in adult patients. In an adult patient, an unexplained, persistent (greater than 3 months) absolute monocytosis should be considered a clonal process until proven otherwise.

> **CASE STUDY: Monocytosis Due to Bacterial Infection**
>
> *Postoperative states may be associated with a peripheral monocytosis.*
>
> A 83-year-old female with a history of fracture status-post hip replacement presents with leukocytosis and anemia post surgery.
>
> **CBC Data**
> WBC count: 52,900/μL
> Hgb: 10.8 g/dL
> Platelet count: 377,000/μL
> NEUT: 34,700/μL
> Monocyte count: 9200/μL
>
> Two months after presentation, the monocytosis had resolved. Thus, this original finding was attributed to postoperative infection. Unless proven otherwise, a persistent absolute monocytosis in an adult should be considered a clonal/neoplastic process.

Chronic Myelomonocytic Leukemia

Chronic myelomonocytic leukemia (CMML) is a neoplasm composed of monocytic cells at various stages of differentiation.

CMML is a clonal BM stem cell disorder in which monocytosis is a major defining feature. Diagnostic criteria for CMML are as follows:

1. Persistent PB monocytosis (>1000/μL)
2. No Philadelphia chromosome or *BCR–ABL* fusion gene
3. Fewer than 20% blasts (including myeloblasts or monoblasts) and/or blast equivalents (promonocytes: monocytic cells with a single prominent nucleolus) in the PB or BM
4. Dysplasia in one or more myeloid cell lines.

If myelodysplasia is absent or minimal, the diagnosis of CMML may still be made if the other requirements are met (i.e., an acquired, clonal cytogenetic abnormality is detectable in the BM cells or the monocytosis has persisted for 3 months or longer, and all other causes of monocytosis have been excluded).

If greater than 20% blasts and/or promonocytes are present in the PB or BM, the World Health Organization (WHO) classification diagnosis is AML.

CMML is further divided into CMML-1 and CMML-2, based on the percentage of blasts and/or promonocytes:

- In CMML-1, blasts and/or promonocytes represent fewer than 5% of peripheral WBCs (WBCs) and fewer than 10% of BM nucleated cells.
- In CMML-2, blasts and/or promonocytes represent between 5% and 19% of peripheral WBCs or between 10% and 19% of BM cells. CMML-2 may also be diagnosed when there are fewer than 20% blasts in the PB or BM if Auer rods are identified.

It should always be kept in mind that a diagnosis of CMML should never be based on PB findings only and without BM examination, since there may be a higher percentage of immature cells (blasts and/or promonocytes) in the BM, meeting the criteria for AML.

A persistent, absolute monocytosis may also be associated with lymphomas and more rarely carcinomas as a paraneoplastic phenomenon. *Paraneoplastic monocytosis is caused by non-hematopoietic tumor-producing hematopoietic growth factors, including GM-CSF, without BM involvement.*

DISORDERS OF PLATELETS

Thrombocytopenias

Group of platelet disorders, due to non-neoplastic and neoplastic etiologies, leading to thrombocytopenia.

Platelets are an integral part of the coagulation system and hemostasis. Their function is complex, and they serve to form a mechanical plug at sites of vascular injury, and as important reservoirs of other procoagulant factors. A variety of disorders are responsible for decreased numbers of platelets, or

CASE STUDY: CMML

This case demonstrates that although the "clonal" monocytic cells in CMML may appear mature morphologically, a combination of ancillary studies (FCI, and/or cytogenetic and molecular analyses) aids in distinguishing reactive from clonal processes.

A 76-year-old male presents with a 2-year history of "myeloproliferative disorder of unknown origin" associated with splenomegaly. He has been followed by a hematologist/oncologist since his diagnosis and multiple BM biopsies have failed to demonstrate any evidence of leukemia. Shortly after initial presentation he reports a 60-pound weight loss in less than 3 months. He has struggled with anemia as a result of his condition and its sequelae (fatigue, pallor, etc.). He currently reports the requirement of intermittent transfusions of PRBC to stabilize his Hgb and HCT levels, the most recent of which was a 2-unit transfusion.

CBC Data upon referral
WBC count: 27,200/μL
Hgb: 10.6 g/dL
Platelet count: 79,000/μL
MCV: 104
Monocyte count: 1700/μL

Review of the PB smear reveals a macrocytosis of the red blood cells, confirming the macrocytic anemia and a monocytosis composed of mature monocytes (**Figure 14-9A**). Flow cytometric analysis of the PB reveals 22% of cells in the monocyte region. Cells within the monocyte region are composed of aberrant monocytic cells expressing CD11b, CD13, CD14, CD33, CD64, and HLA-DR with significant loss of expression of CD15 by 42% of the monocytic cells (Figures 14-9B and C). They are negative for CD117, CD10, CD34, and CD56.

A persistent, unexplained absolute monocytosis with the aberrant flow cytometric findings supports a diagnosis of CMML in this elderly male. In this particular case, a BM examination was recommended to exclude a more acute process.

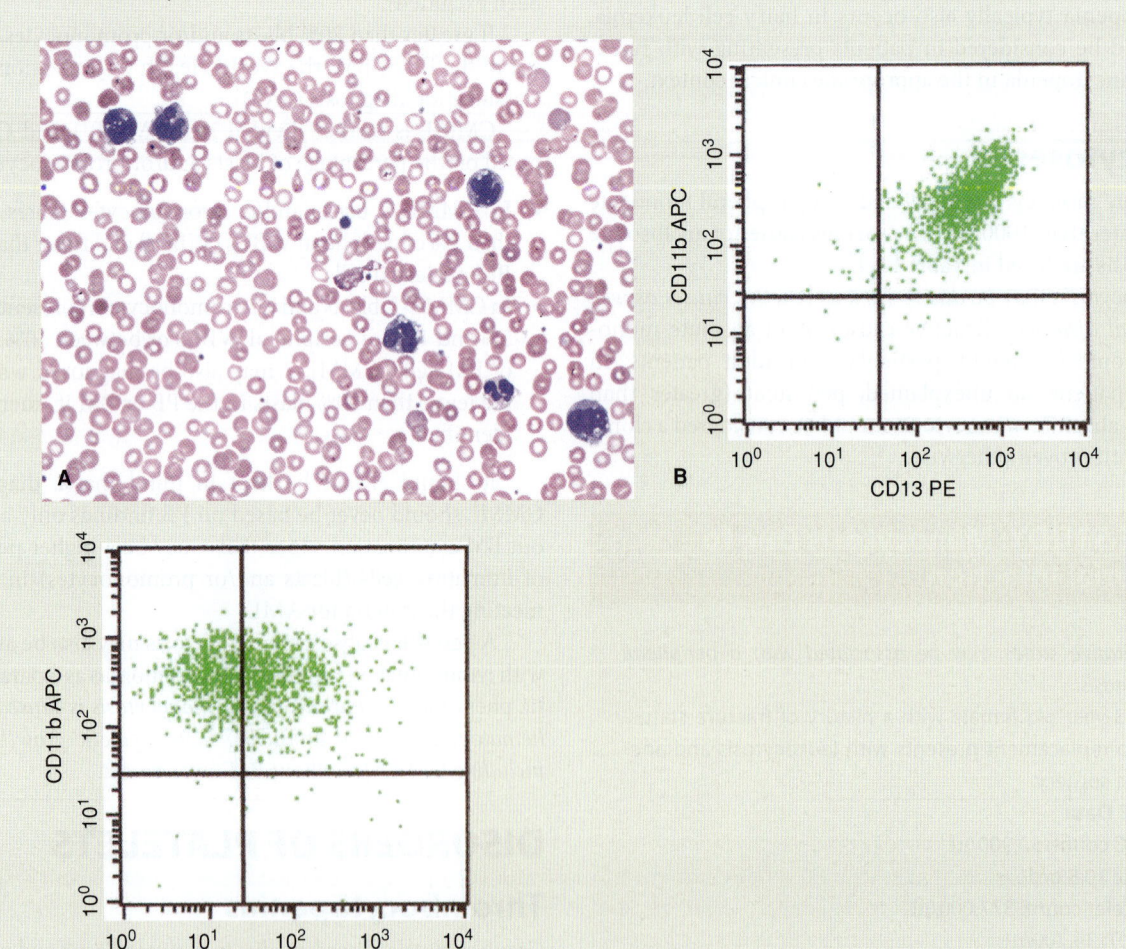

FIGURE 14-9 CMML. PB smear (**A**, Wright stain, ×600). This case of CMML demonstrates an increase in mature monocytes. The corresponding flow cytograms of the pB mature monocytes demonstrate strong expressions of CD13 and CD11b (**B**, upper right box), but loss of expression of CD15 on a significant population of the mature monocytes. (**C**) demonstrates cells expressing CD11b, but not expressing CD15 (upper left box).

TABLE 14-6 Causes of thrombocytopenia.

Quantitative		Qualitative
Decreased production	Destruction or sequestration	Congenital
Congenital	Splenomegaly	Bernard–Soulier syndrome
B12/folate deficiency	ITP	Glanzmann thrombasthenia
Aplastic anemia	DIC	Acquired
Myelodysplastic syndrome	Other autoimmune disease	Aspirin
Mass effect		Uremia
Bone marrow metastasis		Liver failure
Acute leukemia		
Myelofibrosis		

ITP, immune thrombocytopenic purpura; DIC, disseminated intravascular coagulopathy.

thrombocytopenia, but qualitative defects of platelet function have similar sequelae. Table 14-6 highlights both quantitative and qualitative platelet disorders resulting in thrombocytopenia. Clinical manifestations of thrombocytopenia typically include bleeding from mucosal sites and petechial hemorrhages on the skin.

Although the clinical and laboratory findings are classic for ITP, a BM biopsy may be necessary to exclude other etiologies. Cases of acute lymphoblastic leukemia present commonly in this age group and can be associated with marked thrombocytopenia. The BM findings in ITP are often subtle, with preservation of the myeloid and erythroid lineages, and variably increased numbers of megakaryocytes.

CASE STUDY: Idiopathic Thrombocytopenic Purpura (ITP)

ITP is a condition in which platelets are opsonised with antiplatelet autoantibodies and removed prematurely by the reticuloendothelial system, leading to a reduced PB platelet count. The etiology is obscure and the clinical course is variable and unpredictable.

A 9-year-old boy presented to the emergency department with a rapidly progressive history of easy bruising and epistaxis. He has no significant medical history and has otherwise felt well.

CBC Data
WBC count: 13,500/μL
Hgb: 14.1 g/dL
Platelet count: 3000/μL

CASE STUDY: Thrombocytopenia Due to a Lymphoproliferative Disorder (CLL)

A 85-year-old man with a long-standing history of CLL presents for regular follow-up. He was diagnosed over a decade prior, and did not require treatment until he was found to have splenomegaly and lymphadenopathy approximately 4 years ago. He has recently felt more tired, and petechial hemorrhages are noted over his lower extremities bilaterally.

CBC Data
WBC count: 45,500/μL
Lymphocytes: 76%
Hgb: 9.0 g/dL
Platelet count: 35,000/μL

A BM biopsy demonstrated significant involvement of his BM space by CLL. Minimal residual hematopoiesis was evident in the background. In this case, marrow replacement likely accounts for the decreased platelet count.

Thrombocytopenia associated with CLL is common and is seen in 50% of patients at presentation and becomes higher as the disease progresses. It is usually due to BM replacement by the malignant process and is an indication of therapy of the disease. In 2% of patients, the thrombocytopenia is immune mediated due to an autoantibody directed at platelet specific surface membrane antigens.

Thrombocytoses

Group of platelet disorders, due to non-neoplastic and neoplastic etiologies, leading to thrombocytosis (Table 14-7).

Most commonly, thrombocytosis is a reactive phenomenon and can be readily explained by the patient's history and straightforward laboratory assessment.

Thrombocytosis is the primary feature of essential thrombocythemia. However, a secondary cause of thrombocytosis must

TABLE 14-7 Causes of thrombocytosis.

Malignant (Primary)	Reactive (Secondary)
Essential thrombocytosis	Inflammation/infection
Chronic myelogenous leukemia	Hyposplenism/asplenia
Primary myelofibrosis	Iron deficiency anemia
Myelodysplastic syndrome with isolated del (5q)	Drug effect
RARS-t	

RARS-t, refractory anemia with ring sideroblasts associated with marked thrombocytosis.

CASE STUDY: Thrombocytosis Due to Iron Deficiency Anemia

Iron deficiency is often associated with a thrombocytosis, through an unclear mechanism.

A 55-year-old man with a history of hypertension presents with complaints of fatigue. He reports a 10-pound weight loss over the last 3 months.

CBC Data
WBC count: 9500/μL
Hgb: 10.0 g/dL
Platelet count: 45,6000/μL

The physical examination is generally unremarkable, but a rectal examination reveals occult blood-positive stool. Iron studies reveal a decreased serum iron and increased total iron binding capacity.

The clinical presentation is consistent with a primary adenocarcinoma of the colon. Likely long-standing blood loss is responsible for the associated iron deficiency anemia.

Refractory anemia with ringed sideroblasts associated with marked thrombocytosis (RARS-T) is a primary myeloid neoplasm that must be considered in all cases suspected of essential thrombocythemia. It is characterized by anemia and numerous ringed sideroblasts. Thus, an iron stain should be ordered in such cases.

RARS-T shares both myeloproliferative and myelodysplastic features. The clinical presentation relates largely to the associated anemia rather than the thrombocytosis, but the morphologic features in the BM are overlapping (Figure 14-11A). Iron stains are particularly useful and highlight numerous ring sideroblasts (Figure 14-11B).

OTHER PRIMARY BONE MARROW DISORDERS

Acute Leukemias

Acute leukemias are a group of neoplastic disorders composed of blasts or immature leukemic cells of myeloid, precursor B cell, or precursor T-cell lineage.

The lineage of the various acute leukemias is determined by immunophenotyping of the blasts/leukemic cells by either flow cytometry (preferred when there are leukemic cells in the PB or when a BM aspirate is able to be obtained) or by immunohistochemistry (in the absence of leukemic cells in the PB and only a BM biopsy). Acute leukemias of myeloid

be excluded, and the other myeloproliferative neoplasms, such as CML and primary myelofibrosis, and prefibrotic phase, must also be considered.

Refractory anemia with ringed sideroblasts associated with marked thrombocytosis.

CASE STUDY: Thrombocytotosis Due to a Myeloproliferative Neoplasm (Essential Thrombocythemia)

A 63-year-old woman presents with easy bruising, epistaxis, and fatigue for the past few months. Physical examination demonstrates scattered petechial hemorrhages on the upper and lower extremities, chest, and back.

CBC Data
WBC count: 5200/μL
Hgb: 11 g/dL
Platelet count: 855,000/μL

A BM biopsy is performed (Figure 14-10). Routine cytogenetic analysis reveals a normal female karyotype and FISH studies are negative for the t(9;22) (i.e., the Philadelphia chromosome). No JAK2 mutation is identified by molecular analysis. These findings are consistent with a diagnosis of essential thrombocythemia. Thrombocytosis is the primary feature of essential thrombocythemia. However, a secondary cause of thrombocytosis must be excluded, and the other myeloproliferative neoplasms, such as CML and primary myelofibrosis, prefibrotic phase, must also be considered. The clinical manifestations of essential thrombocythemia are highly variable. Although the platelet count is increased, both thrombus formation and bleeding are common, owing to abnormal or defective platelet function. Although negative in this case, mutations of JAK2 are identified in approximately 50% of patients.

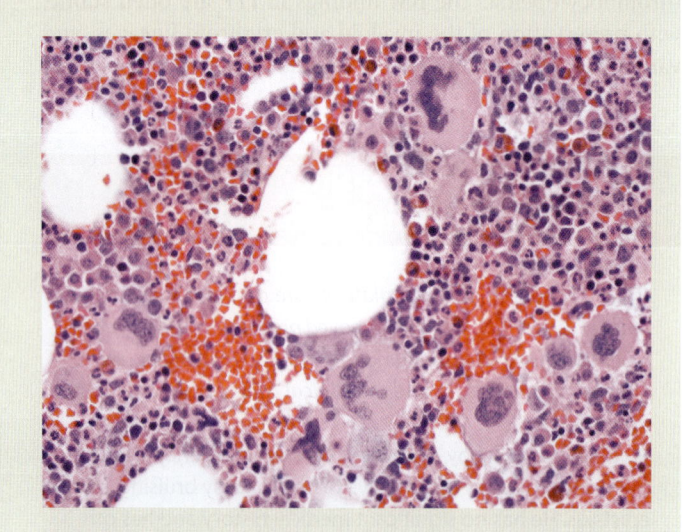

FIGURE 14-10 Essential thrombocythemia. The H&E-stained BM biopsy section reveals a slightly hypercellular marrow with marked expansion of the megakaryocytic lineage (×600). The megakaryocytes are typically larger than normal, with irregular nuclear lobulation. The erythroid and granulocytic lineages are relatively spared and significant fibrosis is not identified.

HEMATOPATHOLOGY 371

TABLE 14-8 Acute myeloid leukemia.

Classification
Acute myeloblastic leukemia, minimally differentiated (AML, M0)
Acute myeloblastic leukemia without maturation (AML, M1)
Acute myeloblastic leukemia with maturation (AML, M2) [AML with t(8;21)(q22;q22);(AML/ETO)]
Acute promyelocytic leukemia (AML, M3; APL) [AML with t(15;17)(q22;q12); (PML/RARα) and variants]
Acute myelomonocytic leukemia (AML, M4; AMML)
AMML, Eto [AML with inv(16)(p13q22) or t(16;16)(p13;q22);(CBFβ/MYH11)]
Acute monoblastic leukemia (AML, M5a)
Acute monocytic leukemia (AMLM5b) (Acute monoblastic leukemia and acute monocytic leukemia: AMoL) [AML with t(9;11)(p22;q23)(MLLT3-MLL)]
Acute erythroid leukemias Erythroleukemia (erythroid/myeloid) (AML, M6a) Pure erythroid leukemia (AML, M6b)
Acute megakaryoblastic leukemia (AML, M7) Variant: Acute myeloid leukemia/transient myeloproliferative disorder in Down syndrome
B Lymphoblastic Leukemia Classification
B lymphoblastic leukemia/lymphoma, NOS
B lymphoblastic leukemia/lymphoma with t(9;22)(q34;q11.2)(BCR/ABL-1)
B lymphoblastic leukemia/lymphoma with rearrangement of 11q23 (MLL)
B lymphoblastic leukemia/lymphoma with t(1;19)(q23;p13.3) [E2A/PBX1-(TCF3-PBX1)]
B lymphoblastic leukemia/lymphoma with t(5;14)(q31;q32)(IL3/IGH)
B lymphoblastic leukemia/lymphoma with t(12;21)(p13;q22); TEL-AML1 (ETV6-RUNX1)
B lymphoblastic leukemia/lymphoma with hyperdiploidy
B lymphoblastic leukemia/lymphoma with hypodiploidy
T Lymphoblastic Leukemia Classification
T lymphoblastic leukemia/lymphoma

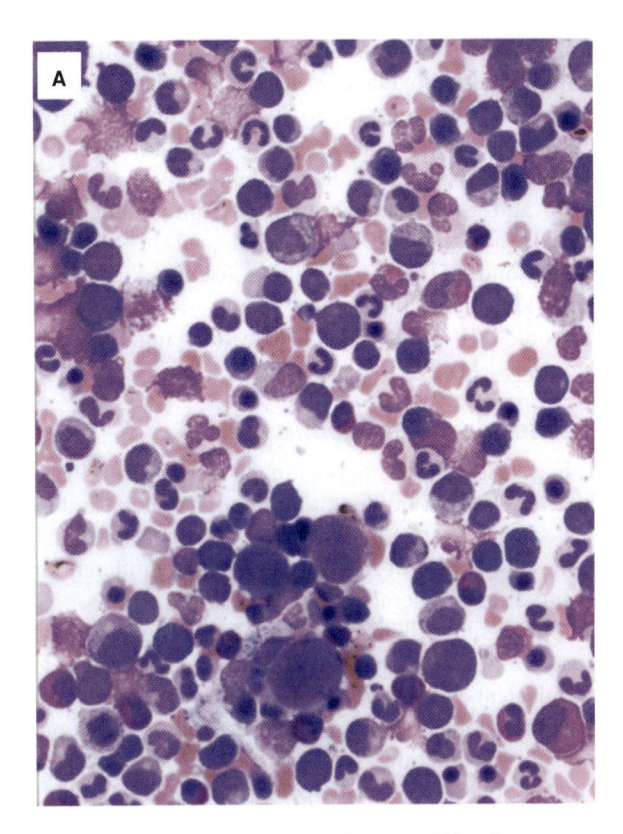

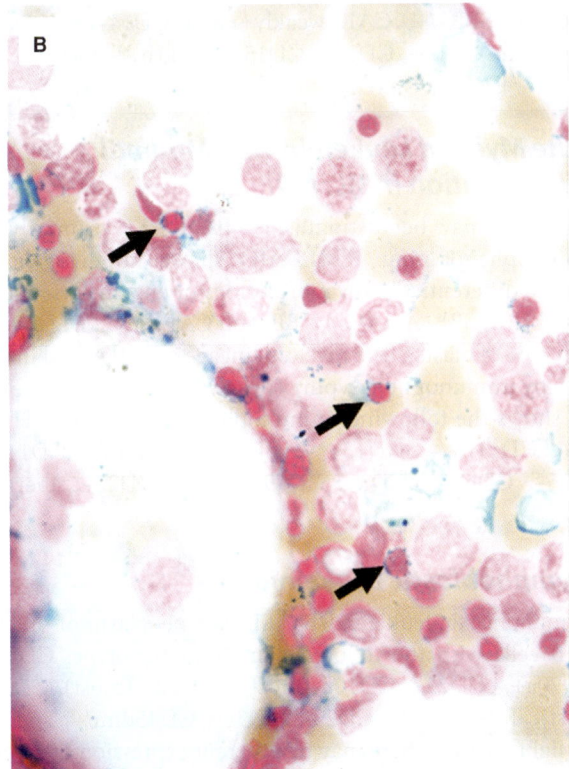

FIGURE 14-11 RARS with marked thrombocytosis. In these cases, the BM aspirate (**A**, Wright stain, ×600) demonstrates primarily dyspoietic features of the erythroid lineage as seen in RARS. Iron stained aspirate smears (**B**, ×1000) show numerous ring sideroblasts in keeping with that diagnosis. However, there is thrombocytosis noted in the PB, and occasionally expansion of the megakaryocytic lineage is identified in the BM.

lineage (i.e., AMLs) are defined as greater than 20% leukemic cells in the PB or BM. The various subtypes of AML are listed in Table 14-8. The abnormal promyelocytes in AML, M3 (APL) and the promonocytes in AML, M5b (acute monocytic leukemia, AMoL) are considered "blast equivalents" for diagnostic purposes. Those AMLs that may morphologically resemble acute leukemias of lymphoid lineage (i.e., AML, minimally differentiated: AML, M0) are distinguished primarily by immunophenotyping. Acute leukemias of precursor B-cell lineage (B-ALL) and precursor T-cell lineage (T-ALL) are defined in therapeutic protocols as greater than 25% blasts in the PB or BM. The various subtypes of B-ALL and T-ALL are also listed in Table 14-8. The B-ALL is primarily subclassified, based on cytogenetic and/or molecular findings. Those acute leukemias, that show no clear evidence of single lineage differentiation, are classified as acute leukemias of ambiguous lineage.

Acute Myeloid Leukemias

Certain recurring cytogenetic abnormalities have been identified in some myeloid leukemias such as t(8;21)(q22;q22)(AML/ETO); t(15;17)(q22;q12)(PML/RARα); inv(16)(p13q22) or (16;16)(p13;q22)(CBFβ/MYH11); or t(9;11)(p22;q23)(MLLT3-MLL). If one of the recurring cytogenetic abnormalities is identified, then the AML is classified as such. APL (AML, M3) is only diagnosed when the associated recurring cytogenetic abnormality is identified. In addition, the finding of t(8;21)(q22;q22); (AML/ETO); t(15;17)(q22;q12); (PML/RARα); inv(16)(p13q22) or (16;16)(p13;q22); (CBFβ/MYH11) defines AML in these cases *regardless of the blast cell count*. So, even if the percentage of blasts or leukemic cells (in the case of APL) is less than 20%, a diagnosis of the appropriate AML may be reached. Cases with t(9;11)(p22;q23) and fewer than 20% blasts must be monitored closely for development of more definitive evidence of AML. However, recurring cytogenetic abnormalities have not been identified in other myeloid leukemias such as AML, M0, M1, M2, M4, M5, M6, and M7 (Table 14-8).

Subclassifying AML using recurring cytogenetic abnormalities is of diagnostic, prognostic and therapeutic importance. The recurring cytogenetic abnormalities, including (8;21)(q22;q22); (AML/ETO); t(15;17)(q22;q12); (PML/RARα); and inv(16)(p13q22) or (16;16)(p13;q22); (CBFβ/MYH11), are all generally associated with a good prognosis. AML with t(9;11)(p22;q23) has an intermediate prognosis. In addition, APL is clinically associated with DIC and has a particular sensitivity to treatment with all-trans retinoic acid (ATRA). It is thus important to recognize this subtype prior to therapy.

Acute Promyelocytic Leukemia

APL is an AML in which abnormal promyelocytes predominate and is characterized by a recurring genetic abnormality, namely t(15;17)(q22;q12).

APL has two morphologic variants: the hypergranular variant and a hypogranular variant. The hypergranular variant is characterized by abnormal promyelocytes with markedly granular cytoplasm. Most cases of hypergranular APL also demonstrate Auer rods in the cytoplasm of some leukemic cells. In the hypogranular variant of APL, the leukemic cells have an apparent paucity or absence of granules in their cytoplasm. Nevertheless, both variants of APL have identical staining patterns by enzyme cytochemistry [i.e., strong reactivity with myeloperoxidase (MPO), Sudan Black B-SBB, and chloroacetate-CAE, and negativity (or weak reactivity) in 25% of cases with nonspecific esterases alpha-naphthyl acetate esterase (ANAE) and alpha-naphthyl butyrate esterase (ANBE)] and also by flow cytometric immunophenotyping (i.e., CD33+, CD13+, CD11b–, CD14–, CD34–, HLA-DR–, CD64dim, and CD117v). The above features are helpful in distinguishing the hypogranular variant of APL from other subtypes of AML, which may have overlapping morphologic features (i.e., AML, M5b).

Acute Monocytic Leukemia

AML may resemble the hypogranular variant of APL morphologically, but has a different immunophenotype and is not associated with a t(15;17)(q22;q12). It is important to distinguish these two types of AML, since they have different prognoses and different therapeutic regimens.

The leukemic cells of acute monocytic leukemia (AML, M5b) are composed of blasts and promonocytes (considered blast equivalents for diagnostic purposes). The blasts and promonocytes are often convoluted and do not contain apparent cytoplasmic granulation. This subtype of AML is characterized by the following enzyme cytochemical staining pattern and flow cytometric immunophenotype: ANBE++, ANAE++, MPO–/+, SBB–/+, CAE weakly+ and CD14–/+, CD64+, HLA-DR+, CD13+, CD33+, CD15+, CD11b–/+ CD34–, and CD117–/+.

Acute Myeloid Leukemia with Minimal Differentiation (AML, M0)

AML, M0 may be distinguished from ALL primarily by immunophenotyping. AML, M0 shows no evidence of myeloid differentiation by morphology or enzyme cytochemistry (MPO, SBB, ANAE, ANBE, and CAE are all negative or stain <3% of blasts). The myeloid lineage is recognized in this AML by immunophenotyping (primarily by flow cytometry) and shows the following immunophenotype: CD34+, HLA-DR+, CD117+/–, CD13+/–, CD33+/–, CD14–, CD11b–, CD15–, CD64–, cCD3–, CD79a–, and cCD22–; aberrant CD7+/–.

B Lymphoblastic Leukemia

B lymphoblastic leukemia (B-ALL) is a neoplasm of precursor B cells with the following immunophenotype: CD19+, cCD70a+, cCD22+, CD10+ (most), sCD22+ (most), CD24+ (most), Tdt+ (most), CD20v, CD34v, CD45dim/–, and sIg and light chain–. There may be aberrant expression of myelomonocytic antigens (i.e., CD13, CD33, CD15, or CD11b) and this aberrant expression does not exclude a diagnosis of B-ALL. The blasts are negative for MPO, SBB, ANAE, ANBE, and CAE by enzyme cytochemistry. B-ALL is classified primarily by cytogenetic and/or molecular findings (see Table 14-8), due to prognostic implications or unique

CASE STUDY: Acute Promyelocytic Leukemia

A 41-year-old female presents with pancytopenia.
  WBC count: 800/µL
  Hgb: 8.4 g/dL
  Platelet count: 51,000/µL

The BM aspirate smear reveals hypercellular (>90% cellular) marrow particles with the following 500-cell-differential count: 72% leukemic cells, 0% myelocytes, 3% maturing granulocytes, 1% erythroid, 21% lymphocytes, and 3% plasma cells. The leukemic cells are characterized by marked cytoplasmic granulation (**Figure 14-12A**).

The enzyme cytochemical stains performed on the BM aspirate smears demonstrate that MPO, SBB, and CAE stain virtually all of the leukemic cells (Figure 14-12B).

ANAE and ANBE stain less than 20% of the nonerythroid marrow cells. Flow cytometric analysis of the BM aspirate reveals a hypocellular specimen (7350/µL) with cells differentiated as indicated. A major population of 71% cells analyzed demonstrates moderate CD45 and moderate-to-high side scatter. This cell population expresses CD33, CD64, and dim /partial CD117 (Figure 14-12C–D). These cells do not express CD34, HLA-DR, CD11b, CD13, CD14, CD15, or the T-cell and B-cell antigens analyzed. This immunophenotype is characteristic of promyelocytes, Cytogenetic analysis reveals the following karyotype: 47,XX,+8,t(15;17)(q22;q12)[17]/46,XX[3].

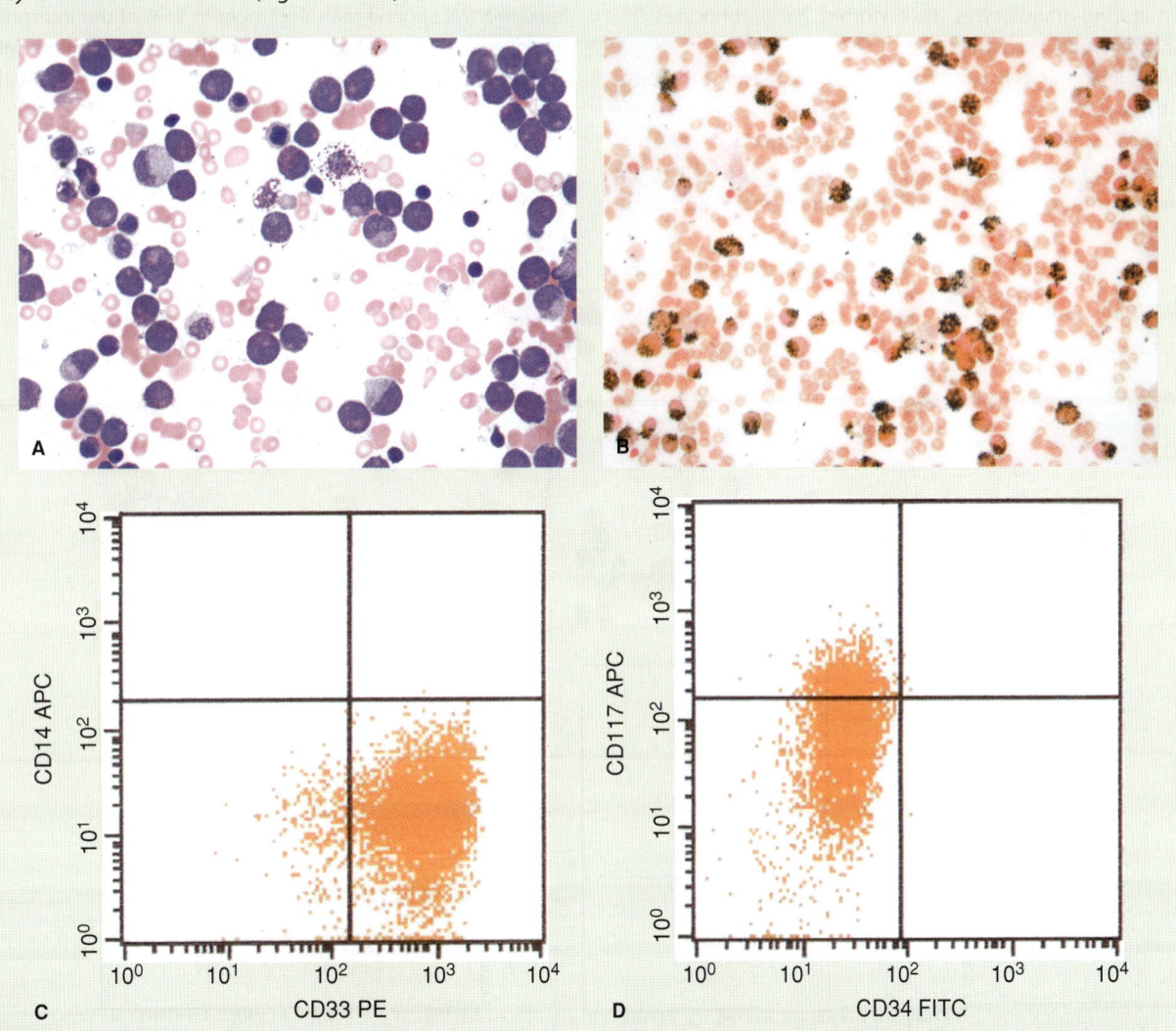

FIGURE 14-12 **Acute promyelocytic leukemia.** BM aspirate (**A**, Wright stain, ×600) in case of acute promyelocytic leukemia demonstrates an increase in abnormal promyelocytes with markedly increased cytoplasmic granulation. They show intense positivity for MPO (**B**, MPO stain, ×600). The corresponding flow cytograms of the BM aspirate demonstrate that the immature cells express CD33 and are negative for CD14 (**C**, lower right and upper left boxes, respectively. They dimly express CD117 and are negative for CD34 (**D**, upper left and lower right boxes, respectively).

CASE STUDY: Acute Monocytic Leukemia (AML, M5)

A 64-year-old male with a history of leukocytosis is evaluated for suspected leukemia.

CBC Data upon presentation
WBC count: 134,600/μL
Hgb: 11.5 g/dL
Platelet count: 30,000/μL
Monocyte count: 59,300/μL
Blasts: 54%

The PB smear reveals a leukocytosis with neutrophilia and monocytosis. There are numerous blasts and promonocytes (54% by manual differential count).

The BM aspirate reveals hypercellular marrow particles (>95%) with the following 500-cell differential count: 77% blasts, 3% maturing granulocytes, 3% erythroid, 7% lymphocytes, 9% monocytes, and 1% plasma cells.

The leukemic cells are characterized by blasts with abundant hypogranular cytoplasm containing occasional vacuoles and variably convoluted nuclear contours (Figure 14-13A).

The enzyme cytochemical stains performed on the BM aspirate smears demonstrate that ANAE and ANBE stain the great majority (>80%) of leukemic cells, MPO and SBB stain virtually all of the leukemic cells, and CAE shows faint granular punctate staining in >80% of leukemic cells (Figure 14-13B).

Flow cytometric analysis of the BM aspirate reveals a hypercellular specimen with 80% of cells found in the "monocytic" cell region. Cells within this region variably express CD11b, CD13, CD14, CD15, CD33, CD64, HLA-DR, and aberrant CD56. These cells do not express CD10, CD34, CD117, or the T- or B-cell antigens analyzed (Figures 14-13C–D). This immunophenotype is characteristic of aberrant monocytic cells.

Cytogenetic analysis reveals an abnormal karyotype: 46,XY,t(9;11)(p22;q23). A FISH assay detects a mixed lineage leukemia (MLL) gene rearrangement in 96% of the interphase nuclei examined. These findings are characteristic of the MLL/MLLT3 translocation often associated with a monocytic leukemia with an aggressive course.

The morphology combined with the ancillary study results supports a diagnosis of AML FAB subtype: AML, M5b; WHO classification: AML with t(9;11)(p22;q23)(MLLT3-MLL).

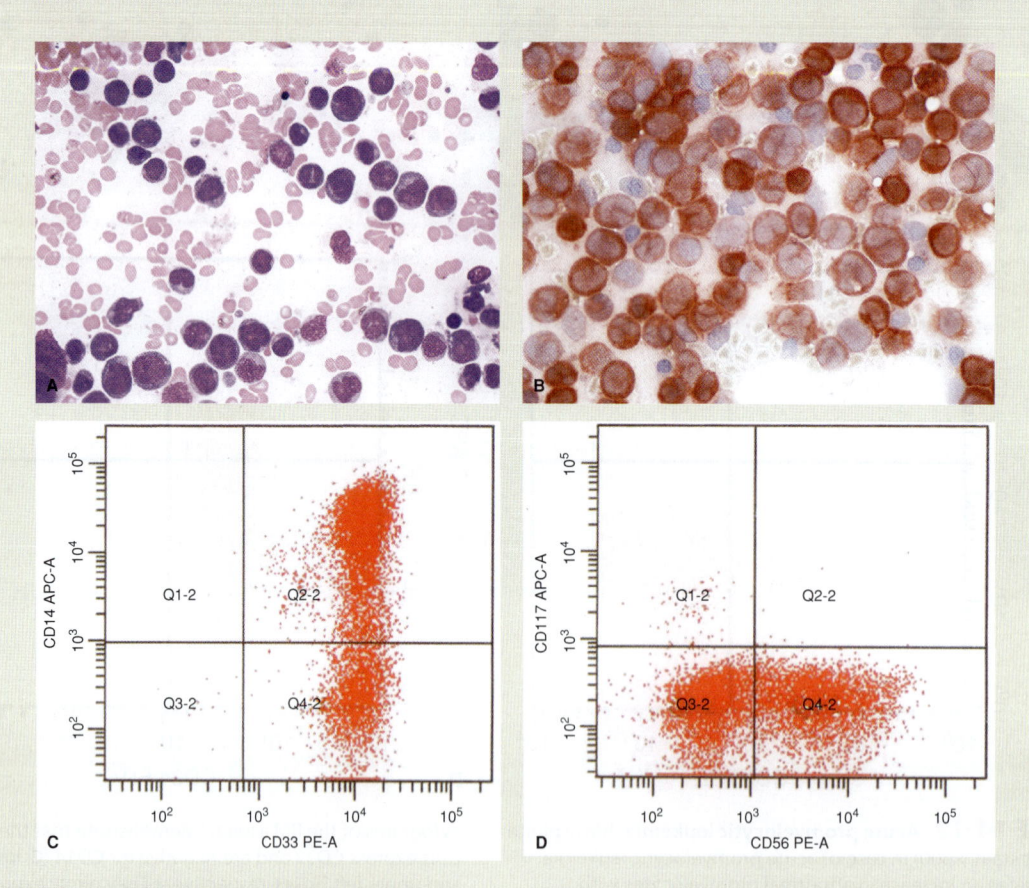

FIGURE 14-13 **Acute monocytic leukemia.** BM aspirate (**A**, Wright stain, ×600) in case of acute monocytic leukemia demonstrates an increase in blasts associated with abundant hypogranular cytoplasm containing occasional vacuoles and variably convoluted nuclear contours. They show intense positivity for one of nonspecific esterase stains—ANBE (**B**, ANBE stain, ×600). The corresponding flow cytograms of the BM aspirate demonstrate that the blasts variably express CD33 and CD14 (**C**, right boxes), as well as CD56 (**D**, lower right box). They are negative for CD117 (**D**, upper left box).

CASE STUDY: Acute Myeloid Leukemia, Minimally Differentiated (AML, M0)

AML, M0 is characterized by no evidence of myeloid differentiation by morphology or enzyme cytochemical staining. Myeloid differentiation is recognized by flow cytometric immunophenotyping.

A 69-year-old female is transferred from an outside hospital for further evaluation and treatment of suspected acute leukemia.

CBC Data upon presentation
WBC count: 23,500/μL
Hgb: 9.5 g/dL
Platelet count: 247,000/μL
Blasts: 89

Review of the PB smear reveals numerous blasts characterized by their relatively small size and small amounts of associated hypogranular cytoplasm (**Figure 14-14A**).

The bone marrow aspirate is hypercellular (80%) with the following differential: 75% blasts, 20% erythroid, and 5% lymphocytes.

The enzyme cytochemical stains performed on the BM aspirate smears demonstrate that MPO and SBB stain less than 3% of blasts. ANAE, ANBE, and CAE do not stain the blasts (Figure 14-14B).

Flow cytometric analysis of the PB reveals an elevated WBC count (23,500/ I) with 86% cells found in the blast cell region. Cells within the blast region express CD117, CD34, and HLA-DR (Figure 14-14C and D). These cells do not express CD56, CD10, T cell, B cell, or the other myelomonocytic markers analyzed. This immunophenotype is characteristic of myeloblasts.

Cytogenetic analysis reveals a normal karyotype: 46,XX.
This AML meets the criteria for a diagnosis of AML, M0.

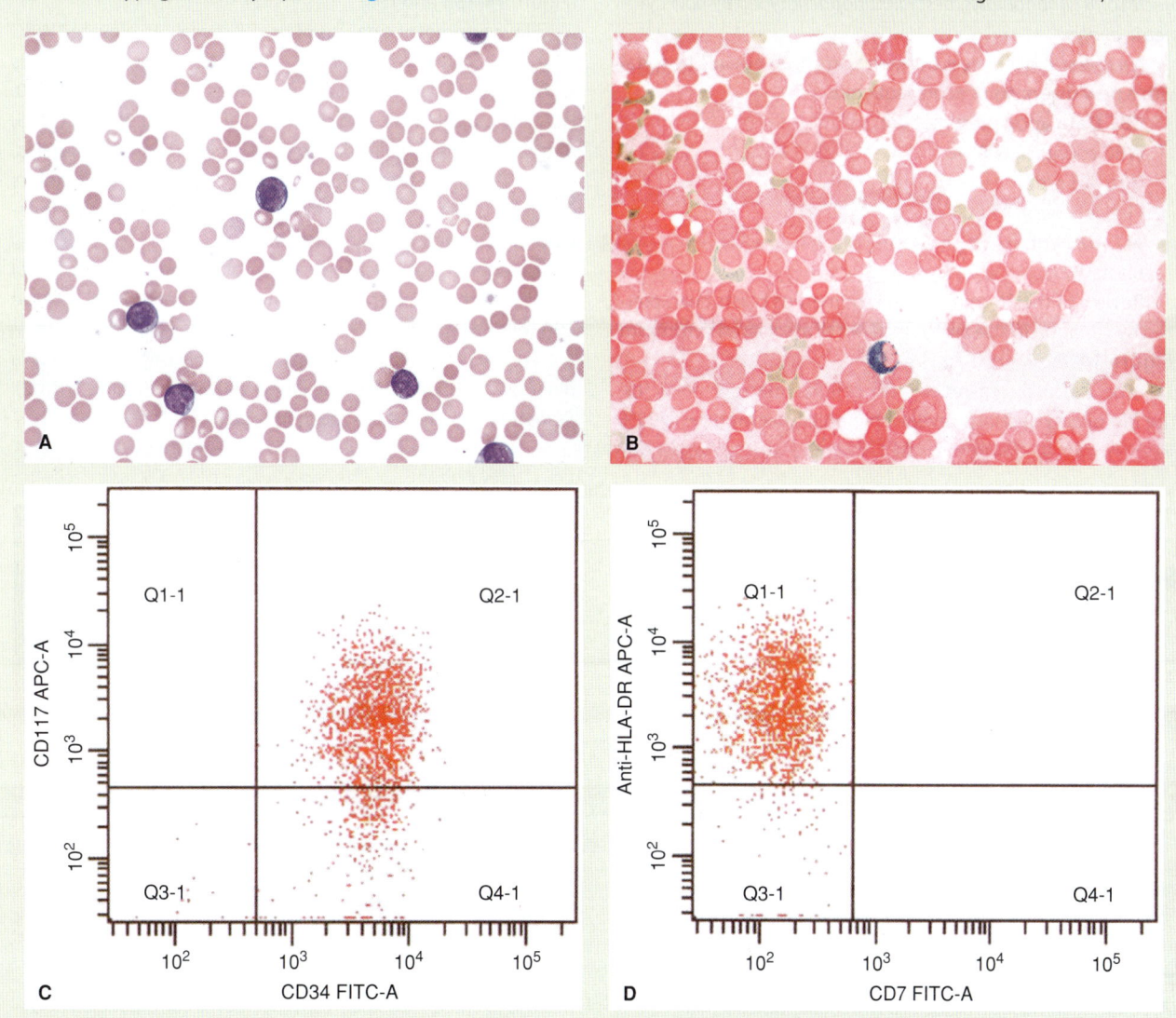

FIGURE 14-14 AML, M0. PB smear (**A**, Wright stain, ×600) in a case of AML, M0 demonstrates relatively small blasts with a small amount of hypogranular cytoplasm. The MPO stain of the BM aspirate reveals negativity of the blasts for MPO (**B**, MPO stain, ×600). The corresponding flow cytograms of the PB demonstrate that the blasts express CD117 and CD34 (**C**, upper right box) as well as HLA-DR (**D**, upper left box).

immunophenotypic and genetic features supporting a distinct entity. Those associated with hyperdiploidy or with t(12;21)(p13;q22); *TEL-AML1 (ETV6-RUNX1)* have a favorable prognosis. Those associated with hypodiplody, t(9;22)(q34;q11.2) (*BCR/ABL-1*), or a rearrangement of 11q23 (*MLL*) have an unfavorable prognosis.

T Lymphoblastic Leukemia

T lymphoblastic leukemia (T-ALL) is a neoplasm of precursor T-cells, which are usually TdT+ and variably express CD1a, CD2, CD3 (most often cCD3), CD4, CD5, CD7, and CD8. There may be aberrant expression of CD10 and myeloid antigens (i.e., CD13 or CD33) and this aberrant expression does not exclude a diagnosis of T-ALL. The blasts are negative for MPO, SBB, ANAE, ANBE, and CAE by enzyme cytochemistry.

Acute Leukemias of Ambiguous Lineage

Acute leukemias of ambiguous lineage include those leukemias that show no clear evidence of differentiation along a single lineage. In general, they are rare and have a poor prognosis.

CASE STUDY: B Lymphoblastic Leukemia (BLL)

B lymphoblastic leukemia is a group of neoplasms composed of precursor B lymphoblasts, best immunophenotyped by flow cytometric analysis.

A 47-year-old female is transferred from an outside hospital with a new diagnosis of acute leukemia.

CBC Data upon presentation:
WBC count: 36,600/μL
Hgb: 7.3 g/dL
Platelet count: 17,000/μL
ALC: 6200/μL
Blasts: 82%

Review of the PB smear reveals numerous blasts characterized by variation in size and a small rim of associated cytoplasm (**Figure 14-15A**).

The BM aspirate reveals no cellular marrow particles. The BM biopsy sections reveal a hypercellular marrow (>95% cellular) with sheets of immature cells and marked necrosis (Figure 14-15B and C).

Flow cytometric analysis of the PB reveals an elevated WBC count (36,600/ l) with 70% of cells in the blast region. Cells within the blast region variably express CD10, CD19, CD20, HLA-DR, partial CD34, and dim / partial aberrant CD11b, CD15, and CD33. These cells do not express surface light chains, CD56, T-cell, or the other myeloid or monocytic markers (Figure 14-15D and E). This immunophenotype is characteristic of precursor B lymphoblasts.

Cytogenetic analysis reveals an abnormal FISH (*BCR/ABL*) result with the (9;22) translocation demonstrated in 88% of the 100 cells examined.

This acute leukemia meets the diagnostic criteria for a diagnosis of B-lymphoblastic leukemia with t(9;22)(q34;q11.2); *BCR–ABL1*, which has a poor prognosis.

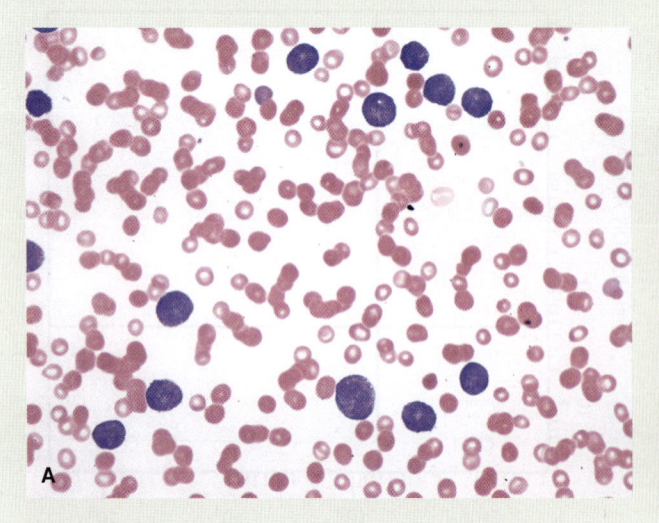

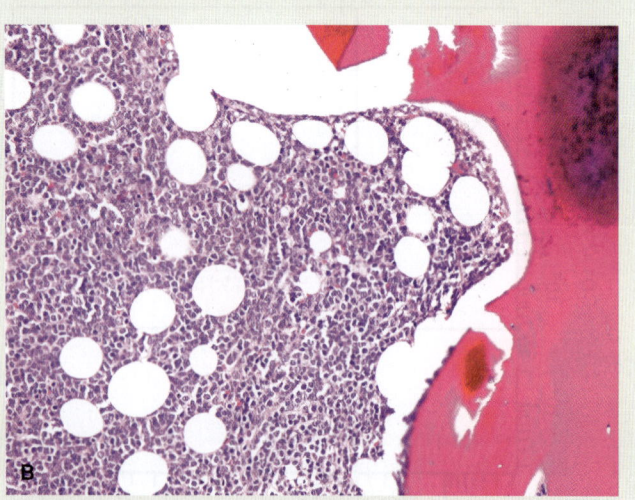

FIGURE 14-15 B-Lymphoblastic leukemia. PB smear (**A**, Wright stain, ×600) in a case of B-lymphoblastic leukemia demonstrates blasts characterized by their variation in cell size, blastic chromatin, and a small rim of associated cytoplasm. The BM biopsy demonstrates areas of hypercellularity and other areas of necrosis (**B** and **C**, H&E stain, respectively). The corresponding flow cytograms of the PB demonstrate that the blasts express CD19 and CD10 (**D**, upper right box), as well as partial CD34 (**E**, lower right).

FIGURE 14-15 *(Continued)*

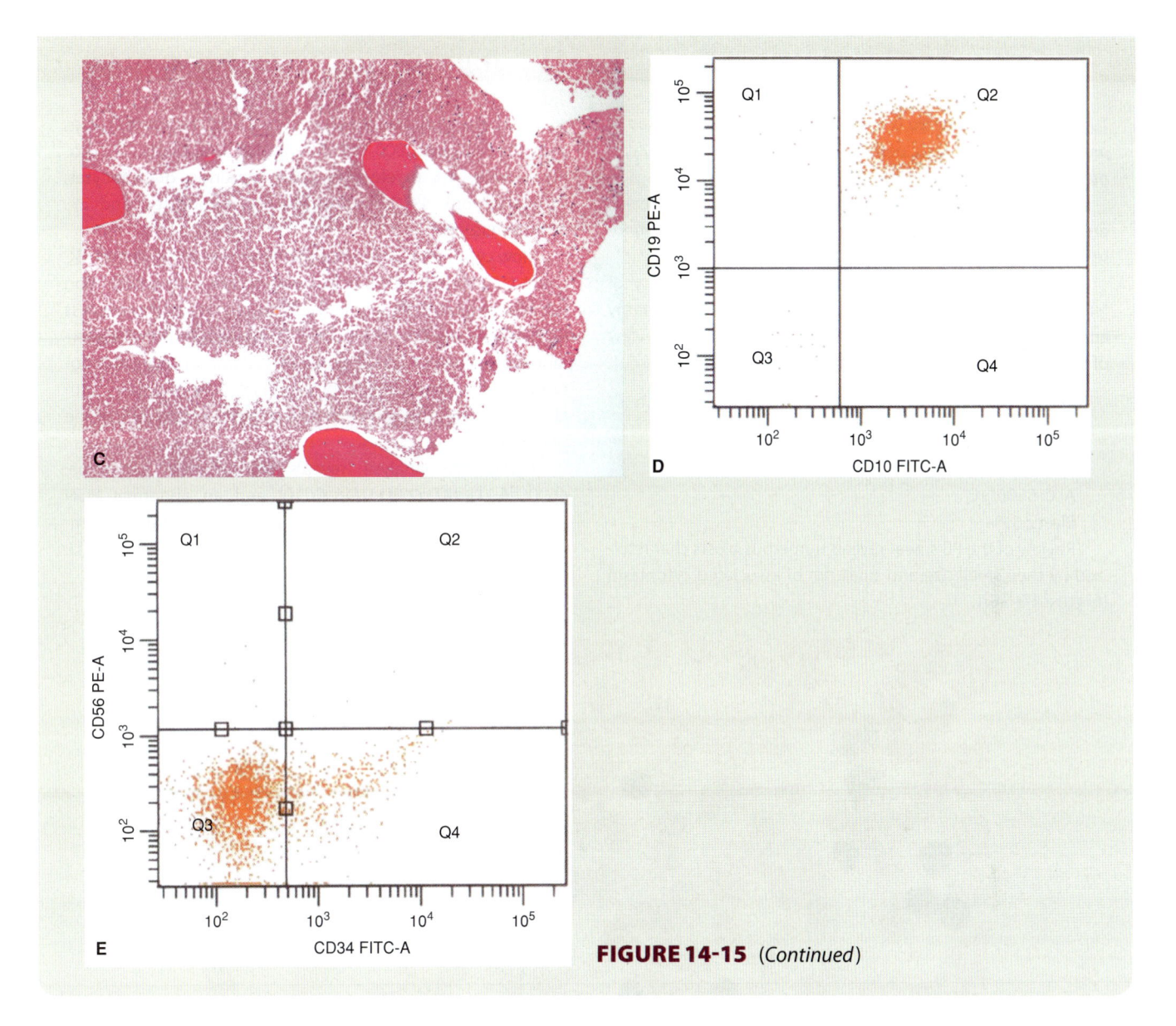

Plasma Cell Dyscrasias

PCDs are a group of neoplastic disorders of clonal plasma cell, typically secreting a single homogeneous (monoclonal) immunoglobulin (Ig) called a paraprotein or M protein. They must be differentiated from benign causes of plasmacytosis. The causes of BM plasmacytosis are listed in Table 14-9.

PCDs represent a heterogenous group of neoplastic disorders of terminally differentiated B cells, typically secreting a single homogeneous (monoclonal) Ig called a paraprotein or M protein. The most classic PCD, multiple myeloma, is a relatively common neoplasm, with approximately 20,000 new cases diagnosed annually. Clinical presentation is dependent on the degree to which the monoclonal Ig affects end-organ function, extent of associated immune suppression, and local tissue destruction or invasion. These tumors are diagnosed and classified based on clinical presentation, radiographic features, and laboratory data.

TABLE 14-9 Benign and malignant causes of bone marrow plasmacytosis.

Malignant	Benign
MGUS	MGUS
Smoldering myeloma	Autoimmune disease
Multiple myeloma	HIV infection
Plasmacytoma	Drug effect
POEMS syndrome	
Lymphomas associated with plasma cell differentiation:	
Lymphoplasmacytic lymphoma	
Marginal zone lymphoma	

MGUS, monoclonal gammopathy of undetermined significance; POEMS syndrome, *P*olyneuropathy, *O*rganomegaly, *E*ndocrinopathy, *M*onoclonal gammopathy, *S*kin changes; HIV, human immunodeficiency virus.

CASE STUDY: T Lymphoblastic Leukemia (TLL) with MLL Rearrangement

T lymphoblastic leukemia is a group of neoplasms composed of precursor T lymphoblasts, best immunophenotyped by flow cytometric analysis.

It is important to distinguish AML, B-lymphoblastic leukemia, and T-lymphoblastic leukemia, since they have different prognoses and therapeutic regimens.

A 25-month-old male presents with a recent history of "strep throat" 2 weeks ago with persistent lymphadenopathy and "blasts" reported on peripheral smear. Pathologist's review of the PB smear and flow cytometry are requested.

CBC Data upon presentation
WBC count: 15,800/μL
Hgb: 11.7 g/dL
Platelet count: 248,000/μL
ALC: 5500/μL
Blasts: 39%

Review of the PB smear reveals numerous blasts characterized by their small size and small rim of associated cytoplasm (**Figure 14-16A**).

The bone aspirate reveals cellular (70%) marrow particles with the following 800-cell differential: 48% blasts, 1% promyelocytes, 4% myelocytes, 20% maturing granulocytes, 17% erythroid, 4% lymphocytes, 4% monocytes, and 2% eosinophils.

Flow cytometric analysis of the PB reveals an elevated WBC count (15,800/μL) with a population of 39% cells gated upon the blast region. Cells within the blast region variably express CD2, CD3, CD4, CD5, CD7, CD10, CD34, and HLA-DR with aberrant expression of CD33 (Figures 14-16B and C). This immunophenotype is characteristic of precursor T-lymphoblasts with aberrant myeloid antigen expression, representing 39% of the peripheral WBCs.

Cytogenetic analysis reveals an abnormal karyotype: 46,XY,t(6;11)(q27;q23)[11]/46,XY[10] and an abnormal FISH (MLL) result with an MLL rearrangement in 29.5% nuclei examined. Translocations involving MLL may occur in 8% of T-ALL cases.

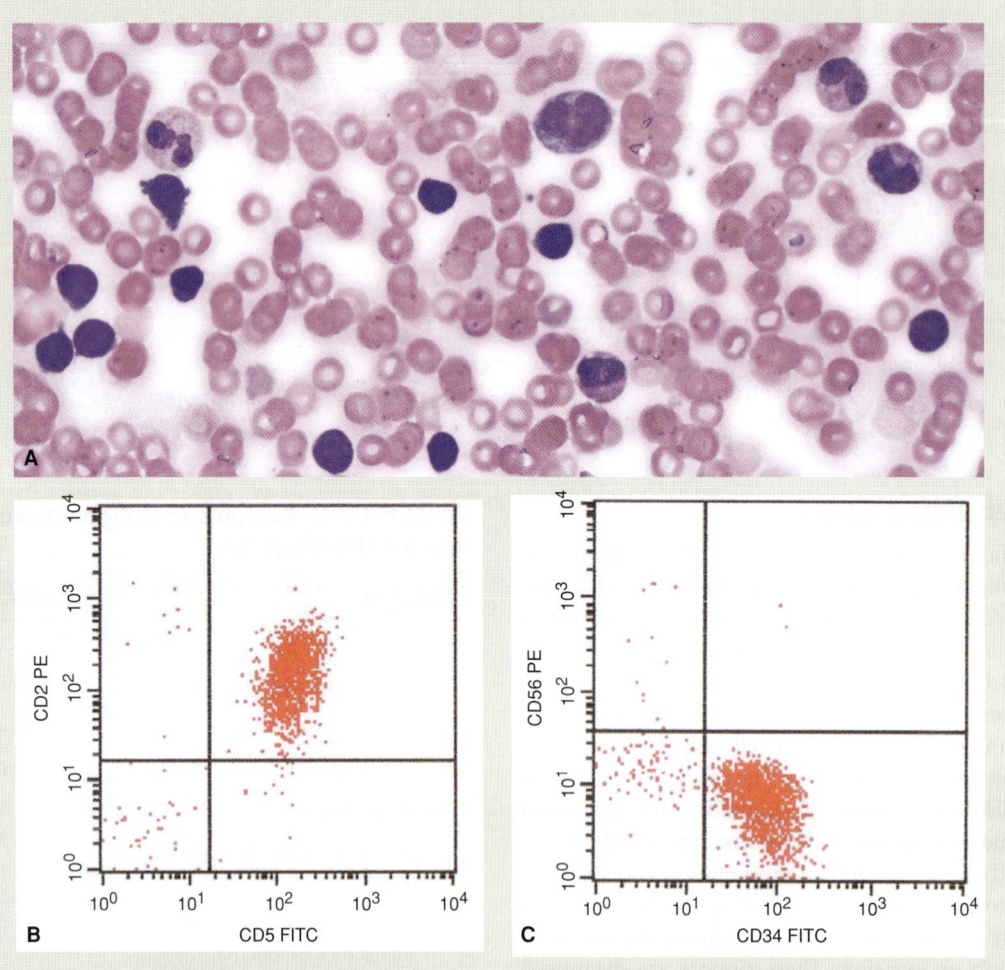

FIGURE 14-16 **T-Lymphoblastic leukemia.** PB smear (**A**, Wright stain, ×600) in a case of T-lymphoblastic leukemia demonstrates blasts characterized by their small size and small rim of associated cytoplasm. The corresponding flow cytograms of the PB demonstrate that the blasts express CD2 and CD5 (**B**, upper right box) as well as CD34 (**C**, lower right box).

> ### CASE STUDY: Monoclonal Gammopathy of Undetermined Significance (MGUS)
>
> MGUS is defined as the presence in the serum of an M protein <30 g/L, BM clonal plasma cells <10%, no end-organ damage [i.e., no hypercalcemia, renal insufficiency, anemia, bone lesions (CRAB)], and no evidence of B-cell lymphoma or other disease known to produce an M protein. Electrophoresis studies are the classic methods for evaluating distribution of proteins in the serum and urine. If an M spike is identified, immunofixation studies are performed to qualify the monoclonal protein.
>
> A 57-year-old man with a history of poorly controlled hypertension was previously found to have mild proteinuria. The PB evaluation was generally unremarkable, with the exception of low-normal Hgb concentration. Urine electrophoresis confirmed the proteinuria, but no monoclonal protein was identified. Serum protein electrophoresis, and associated immunofixation electrophoresis, demonstrated an IgM kappa monoclonal protein at a concentration of 5 g/L. The BM biopsy (Figure 14-17) demonstrates a normocellular BM with appropriate numbers of plasma cells in an appropriate distribution. Stains for kappa and lambda light chain reveal polyclonal staining of the plasma cell population. Some cases of MGUS, typically the non-IgM forms, can progress to myeloma. However, in many cases, there is no definitive underlying causative factor identified.
>
> **FIGURE 14-17 Monoclonal gammopathy of uncertain significance.** Immunohistochemical stain for CD138, a specific plasma cell marker in the BM, demonstrates no significant overall increase in plasma cells and occasionally physiologically expected plasma cell clusters along marrow vessels (arrow) (×400). Stains for kappa and lambda light chain (not shown) reveal polyclonal staining of the plasma cell fraction.

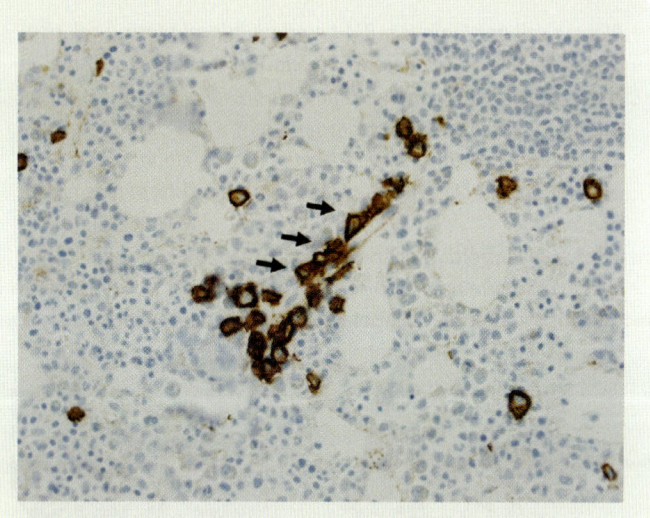

Polyneuropathy, organomegaly, endocrinopathy, monoclonal gammopathy, and skin changes (POEMS) syndrome may rarely occur in association with "osteosclerotic" myeloma. In this rare PCD, the focal plasma cell aggregates are surrounded by thickened bone (i.e., osteosclerosis). The systemic manifestations are variable and often nonspecific, complicating timely diagnosis of this entity.

PRIMARY LYMPH NODE DISORDERS

The major compartments of the lymph node include the cortex, paracortex, medullary cords, sinuses, and connective tissue framework. The cortex is the predominantly B-cell region of the lymph node. Scattered in the cortex are primary and secondary follicles.

The germinal centers are predominantly composed of follicle center B cells with some intermixed small T lymphocytes. The mantle zones are composed of a heterogeneous population of small B lymphocytes. In nonstimulated lymph node, most follicles are primary follicles (Figure 14-19). Secondary follicles are formed as a reaction to T-cell-dependent antigens. The germinal centers of the secondary follicles comprise a dark zone at the lower pole and a light zone toward the apical pole, where the mantle is thicker (corona) and faces the direction of antigen influx (marginal sinus).

The paracortex is the T zone of the lymph node. It is rich in high endothelial venules and composed predominantly of T cells (CD4 > CD8), which are represented by small lymphocytes with occasional intermixed immunoblasts. There may be scattered B lymphocytes, plasma cells, and Langerhans cells. Paracortical hyperplasia typically occurs in response to a viral infection, a hypersensitivity state, or regional tumor and may be observed in dermatopathic lymphadenopathy.

The medullary cords are composed of mature plasma cells and may be expanded in conditions with a B-cell reaction, such as reactive follicular hyperplasia (FH).

The sinuses receive the afferent lymphatics drainage that flows into the efferent lymphatic at the hilum of the lymph node. The sinuses often contain histiocytes and some lymphoid cells.

Primary lymph node disorders include reactive processes (i.e., FH) and neoplastic disorders (i.e., malignant lymphomas).

The major forms of reactive lymphadenopathies include (1) FH (to be differentiated from follicular lymphoma, FL), (2) an interfollicular or diffuse increase in large lymphoid cells (to be differentiated from a diffuse large cell lymphoma), (3) parenchymal histiocytic reaction (including granuloma formation), and (4) prominent necrosis. Malignant lymphomas are divided into non-Hodgkin lymphomas (NHLs) and Hodgkin lymphomas (HLs). The NHLs may be of B-or T-cell origin, and the HLs are further divided into nodular lymphocyte-predominant HL (NLPHL) and classical HL. The 2008 WHO classification of malignant lymphomas (see Table 14-1 for future reference) includes an exhaustive list and is beyond the scope of this book.

We will focus on the most common B-cell lymphomas (i.e., FL and diffuse large B-cell lymphoma, DLBCL), the most common group of T-cell lymphomas [i.e., peripheral T-cell lymphoma, not otherwise specified (PTCL, NOS)], and the HLs in

CASE STUDY: Plasma Cell Myeloma

Plasma cell myeloma is a BM-based multifocal plasma cell neoplasm associated with an M protein in serum and/or urine. In contrast to MGUS, clonal plasma cells are identified in the BM of myeloma patients and typically represent >10% of marrow cells. In combination with the identification of this clonal plasma cell population, clinical features of CRAB are diagnostic of plasma cell myeloma.

A 65-year-old African-American man presents with progressive fatigue and reports "foamy urine" for the past several months. A complete laboratory evaluation reveals anemia, hypercalcemia, and renal insufficiency. Skeletal radiographs demonstrate lytic lesions of the calvarium, ribs, and spine. Serum protein electrophoresis/immunofixation demonstrates an IgG kappa M spike, quantified at 37 g/L, and free kappa light chains are identified in the urine.

A BM biopsy is performed (Figure 14-18), demonstrating a massive expansion of the marrow space by predominantly mature appearing plasma cells, corroborated by immunohistochemistry for CD138 (i.e., a plasma cell specific marker in the BM). In situ hybridization studies confirm that the infiltrate of plasma cells expresses kappa light chain, in keeping with the serologic and urine studies.

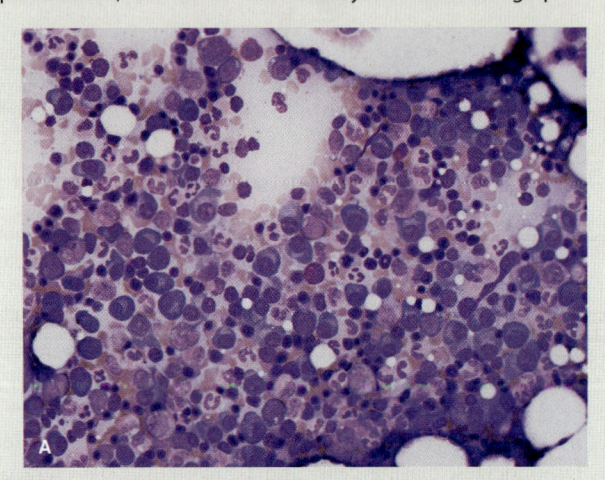

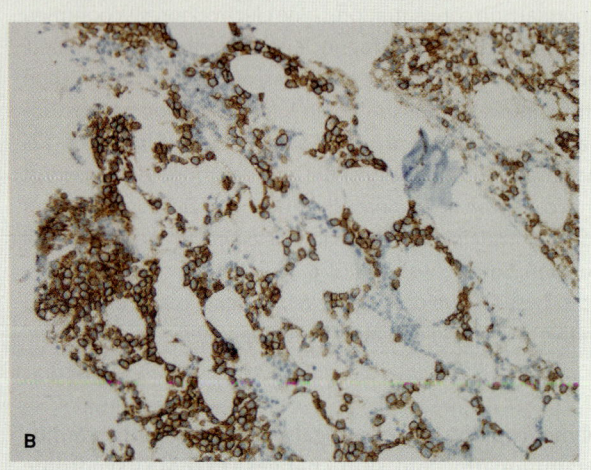

FIGURE 14-18 Multiple myeloma. The Wright-Giemsa-stained BM aspirate demonstrates a hypercellular marrow with marked increase in plasma cells (**A**, ×400). Typically, the plasma cells are morphologically normal, although occasionally lager and/or multinucleated forms may be identified. Immunohistochemistry reveals a marked increase in CD138 staining in the BM biopsy (**B**, ×200).

---

relation to their distinction from reactive processes and from each other. These lymphoma types are highlighted in Table 14-10.

FH is a reactive proliferation of lymphoid follicles (i.e., germinal centers) in the lymph node that may be difficult to distinguish from FL.

Distinguishing Follicular Hyperplasia from Follicular Lymphoma

> **QUICK REVIEW**
>
> It may be difficult to distinguish between florid reactive hyperplasia and FL. The most important criterion is the architectural arrangement of the follicles at low magnification. A pattern of "back-to-back" follicles disposed throughout the entire nodal parenchyma (with little-or no-interfollicular tissue) is characteristic of FL. In contrast, the follicles in FH have the following features (Figure 14-20A):
>
> - Discrete and well-separated follicles with at least some interfollicular tissue
> - Variably sized and shaped follicles
> - Well-defined mantle zones
> - Heterogeneous population of follicle center cells (large cells may outnumber small cells in large follicles that are mitotically active)
> - Numerous tangible-body macrophages
> - Cellular polarization seen in at least some follicles (i.e., due to centrocytes and centroblasts occupying different zones)
> - Very rare follicle formation in perinodal tissue
>
> In diagnostically challenging cases, morphological features may overlap. In such cases, ancillary studies (i.e., flow cytometric immunophenotyping, immunhistochemistry, and molecular studies) may be necessary. FH will display no evidence of a monoclonal B-cell population by flow cytometry (Figure 14-20B). By immunohistochemical staining, bcl-2 will be negative in the germinal centers of FH (and is generally positive in the malignant nodules of FL—see below). Genotypic studies will demonstrate lack of Ig gene and *bcl-2* gene rearrangements in FH (which should both be identified in FH—see below). *In patients less than 20 years of age, a diagnosis of FL should not be based on histologic features alone, but should be supported in such cases by ancillary techniques.*

HEMATOPATHOLOGY

Follicular Lymphoma

Nodular growth patterns may also be demonstrated in other types of NHLs of B-cell origin (i.e., mantle cell lymphoma, etc.), as well as in subclassifications of HLs, and may cause diagnostic confusion with FL.

Nodular Lymphocyte-Predominant Hodgkin Lymphoma

HLs (see below) are also of B-cell derivation and are composed of two disease entities: **NLPHL** and **classical Hodgkin lymphoma (cHL discussed below)**.

NLPHL is a monoclonal B-cell neoplasm characterized by a nodular and diffuse proliferation of scattered large neoplastic B cells. It shares the following features with cHL: usually arising in lymph nodes (preferentially in the cervical region), majority manifest clinically in young adults, neoplastic cells are scattered in a rich mixed inflammatory background, and the neoplastic T cells are often ringed by surrounding T cells. NLPHL may be confused diagnostically with FL, since it typically has at least a partial nodular growth pattern. It is classified under HL since it shares some features with cHL, discussed below.

Histologically, the lymph node architecture is effaced by at least a partially nodular proliferation composed predominantly of small lymphocytes, histiocytes, and intermingled neoplastic cells. The neoplastic cells (LP or "lymphocytic and histiocytic—LH" cells) are characterized by their large size, mononucleation, folded or "multilobated" nuclei, and scant cytoplasm. They are often referred to as "popcorn" cells, due to their nuclear appearance. The nucleoli are usually multiple basophilic, and smaller than the neoplastic

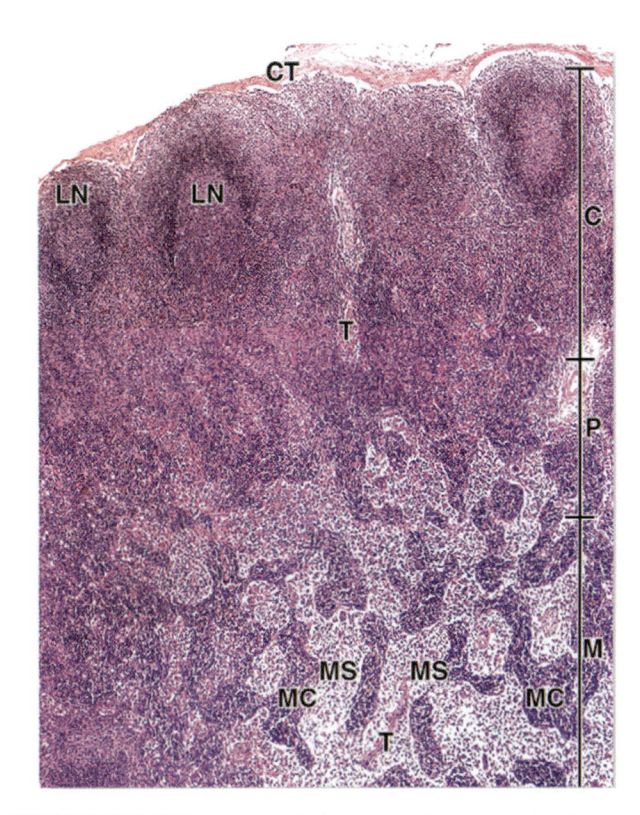

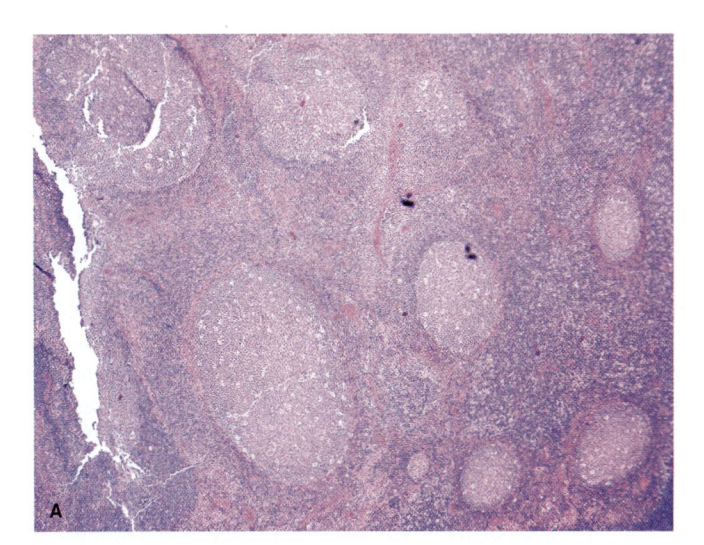

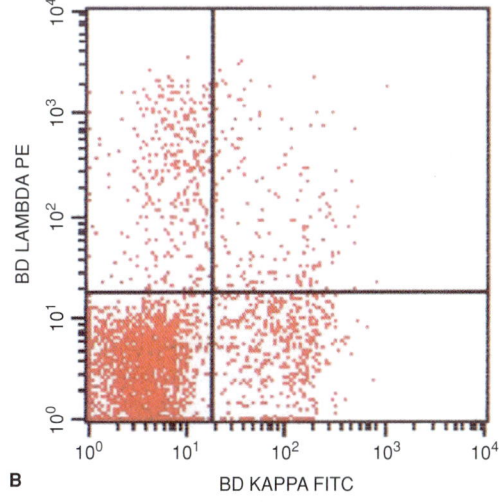

FIGURE 14-19 **Regions of a lymph node.** A low-magnification section of a lymph node showing the three functional regions: the cortex (C), the paracortex (P), and the medulla (M). Connective tissue of the capsule (CT) completely surrounds each lymph node and extends as several trabeculae (T) throughout the lymphoid tissue. Major spaces for lymph flow are present in this tissue under the capsule and along the trabeculae. A changing population of immune cells is suspended on reticular fibers throughout the cortex, paracortex, and medulla. Lymphoid nodules (LN) are normally restricted to the cortex and the medulla is characterized by sinuses (MS) and cords (MC) of lymphoid tissue. X40. H&E. (Reproduced with permission from Mescher AL. Junqueira's Basic Histology: Text and Atlas. 12th Edition, New York: McGraw Hill Lange, 2010:241 (Figure 14–18)).

FIGURE 14-20 **FH.** This section of lymph node in a case of FH demonstrates reactive germinal centers with polarization of the mantle zone and numerous tangible body macrophages (**A**, H&E stain, ×400). The corresponding flow cytogram of the lymph node demonstrates no evidence of monoclonal expression of either kappa or lambda on the **B**-cells analyzed (B, upper left and lower right boxes).

TABLE 14-10 WHO classification: Hodgkin and non-Hodgkin lymphomas.

Hodgkin Lymphoma
- Nodular lymphocyte-predominant Hodgkin lymphoma
- Classical Hodgkin lymphoma
  - Nodular sclerosis classical Hodgkin lymphoma
  - Lymphocyte-rich classical Hodgkin lymphoma
  - Mixed cellularity classical Hodgkin lymphoma
  - Lymphocyte-depleted classical Hodgkin lymphoma

Non-Hodgkin Lymphoma
Mature B-Cell Neoplasms
- Chronic lymphocytic leukemia/small lymphocytic lymphoma
- B-cell prolymphocytic leukemia
- Splenic marginal zone lymphoma
- Hairy cell leukemia
- Splenic lymphoma/leukemia, unclassifiable
  - Splenic diffuse red pulp small B-cell lymphoma
  - Hairy cell leukemia-variant
- Lymphoplasmacytic lymphoma
  - Waldenström macroglobulinemia
- Heavy chain diseases
  - Alpha heavy chain disease
  - Gamma heavy chain disease
  - Mu heavy chain disease
- Plasma cell myeloma
  - Monoclonal gammopathy of undetermined significance
  - Solitary plasmacytoma of bone
  - Extraosseous plasmacytoma
- Extranodal marginal zone B-cell lymphoma (MZL) of mucosa-associated lymphoid tissue (MALT lymphoma)
- Nodal MZL
  - Pediatric type nodal MZL
- Follicular lymphoma
  - Pediatric type follicular lymphoma
- Primary cutaneous follicle center lymphoma
- Mantle cell lymphoma
- Diffuse large B-cell lymphoma (DLBCL), not otherwise specified
  - T cell/histiocyte-rich large B-cell lymphoma
  - Primary DLBCL of the CNS
  - Primary cutaneous DLBCL, leg type
  - EBV positive DLBCL of the elderly
- DLBCL associated with chronic inflammation
- Lymphomatoid granulomatosis
- Primary mediastinal (thymic) large B-cell lymphoma
- Intravascular large B-cell lymphoma
- ALK+ large B-cell lymphoma
- Plasmablastic lymphoma
- Large B-cell lymphoma arising in HHV8-associated multicentric Castleman disease
- Primary effusion lymphoma
- Burkitt lymphoma
- B-cell lymphoma, unclassifiable, with features intermediate between diffuse large B-cell lymphoma and Burkitt lymphoma
- B-cell lymphoma, unclassifiable, with features intermediate between diffuse large B-cell lymphoma and classical Hodgkin lymphoma

Mature T-Cell Neoplasms
- T-cell prolymphocytic leukemia
- T-cell large granular lymphocytic leukemia
- Chronic lymphoproliferative disorder of NK cells
- Aggressive NK cell leukemia systemic
- EBV+ T-cell lymphoproliferative diseases of childhood
  - Systemic EBV+ T-cell lymphoproliferative disease of childhood
  - Hydroa vacciniforme-like lymphoma
- Adult T-cell leukemia/lymphoma
- Extranodal NK/T cell lymphoma, nasal type
- Enteropathy-associated T-cell lymphoma
- Hepatosplenic T-cell lymphoma
- Subcutaneous panniculitis-like T-cell lymphoma
- Mycosis fungoides
- Sezary syndrome
- Primary cutaneous CD30+ T-cell lymphoproliferative disorders
  - Lymphomatoid papulosis
  - Primary cutaneous anaplastic large-cell lymphoma
- Primary cutaneous peripheral T-cell lymphomas, rare subtypes
  - Primary cutaneous gamma-delta T-cell lymphoma
  - Primary cutaneous CD8+ aggressive epidermotropic cytotoxic T-cell lymphoma
  - Primary cutaneous CD4+ small/medium T-cell lymphoma
- Peripheral T-cell lymphoma, not otherwise specified
- Angioimmunoblastic T-cell lymphoma
- Anaplastic large cell lymphoma, ALK+
- Anaplastic large cell lymphoma, ALK−

CASE STUDY: Follicular Lymphoma

FL is a neoplastic proliferation of lymphoid follicles characterized by a back-to-back proliferation of clonal follicles.

A 48-year-old male presents with a history of a large left neck mass that is biopsied. The node demonstrates a tightly packed follicular pattern of cells that efface normal nodal architecture. The neoplastic follicles have a severely attenuated mantle zone and scant tingible body macrophages. Immunophenotyping indicates the cell to be of monoclonal B cell origin.

FL is a neoplasm composed of follicle center (i.e., germinal center) Bcells, composed of varying numbers of centrocytes and centroblasts/large transformed cells, with at least a partial follicular (i.e., nodular) growth pattern. *If diffuse areas of any size composed predominantly (or entirely) of blastic cells are present in any case of FL, a diagnosis of DLBCL is also made.*

FL accounts for about 20% of the lymphomas with the highest incidence in the United States and Western Europe. As mentioned previously, FL primarily affects adults and rarely occurs in individuals under the age of 20 years.

Most cases have a predominantly follicular pattern with closely packed follicles that efface the nodal architecture. In contrast to FH, the neoplastic follicles are closely packed without intervening interfollicular tissue, usually have attenuated or absent mantle zones, and lack polarization and tingible body macrophages (**Figure 14-21A** and **B**). The neoplastic cells of FL are monoclonal B-cells that have the following immunophenotype: CD19+, CD20+, CD79a+, CD10+ (80% of cases), CD5−, (Figures 14-21C and D) bcl-6+, and bcl-2+ (Figure 14-21E). Bcl-6 is a marker of germinal center derivation and will be seen in the follicles of FH and FL, whereas bcl-2 positivity is only demonstrated in FL and not in FH. FL is genetically characterized by the t(14;18)(q32;q21) and *BCL2* gene rearrangements. *BCL6* rearrangements are found infrequently in most typical cases of FL.

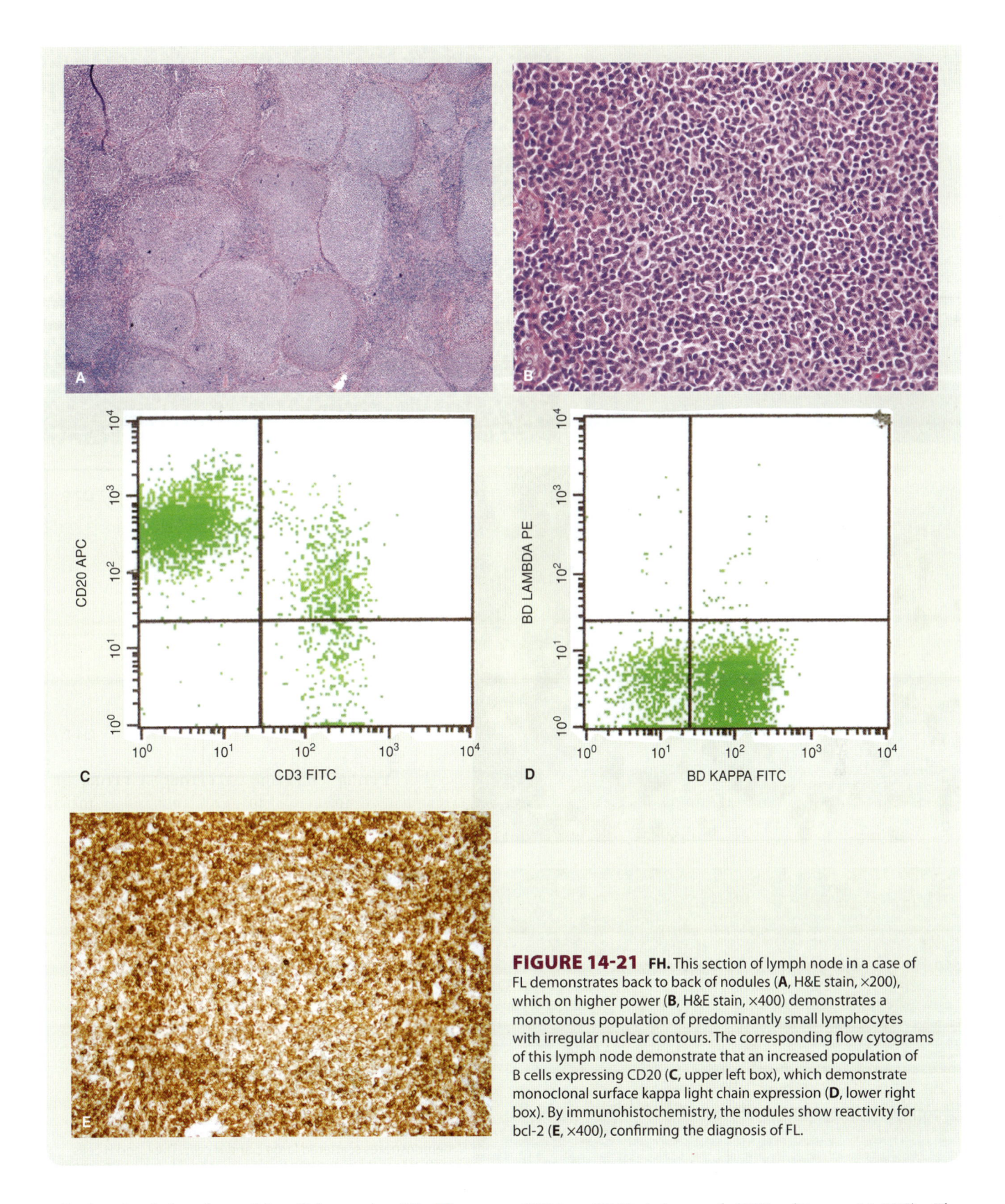

FIGURE 14-21 FH. This section of lymph node in a case of FL demonstrates back to back of nodules (**A**, H&E stain, ×200), which on higher power (**B**, H&E stain, ×400) demonstrates a monotonous population of predominantly small lymphocytes with irregular nuclear contours. The corresponding flow cytograms of this lymph node demonstrate that an increased population of B cells expressing CD20 (**C**, upper left box), which demonstrate monoclonal surface kappa light chain expression (**D**, lower right box). By immunohistochemistry, the nodules show reactivity for bcl-2 (**E**, ×400), confirming the diagnosis of FL.

cells (i.e. Reed–Sternberg, RS, cells) seen in cHL (Figure 14-22A and B).

The neoplastic cells of NLPHL are monoclonal B cells with the following immunophenotype: CD20+, CD79a+, bcl-6+, CD45 (i.e., leukocyte common antigen-LCA)+, CD15–, CD30–/wk+, and EBV– (Figure 14-22C). The architectural background of NLPHL is composed of large spherical meshworks of follicular dendritic cells, which are predominantly filled with small B cells and numerous CD3+/CD57+ cells. The small B-cells are not neoplastic (i.e.,

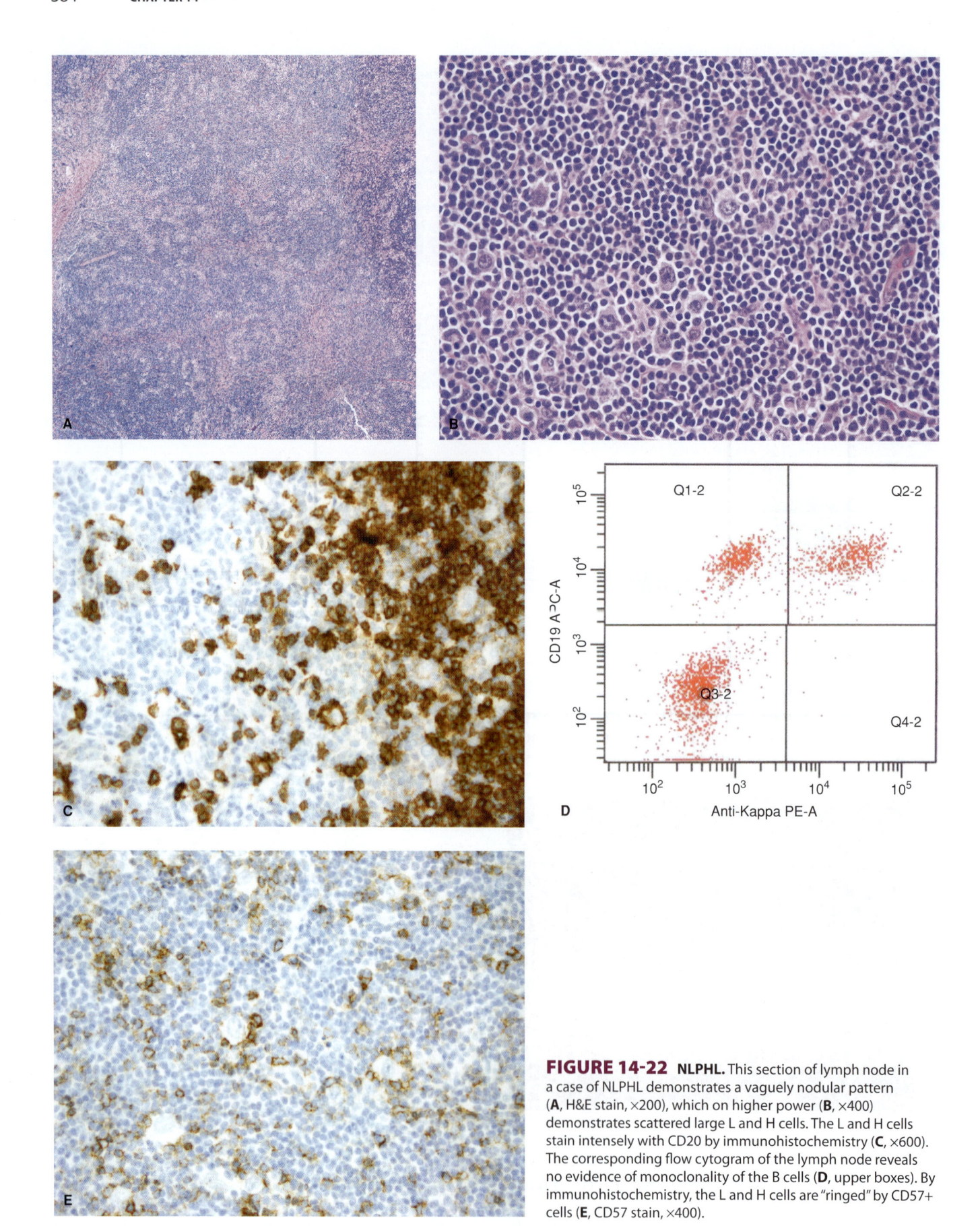

FIGURE 14-22 NLPHL. This section of lymph node in a case of NLPHL demonstrates a vaguely nodular pattern (**A**, H&E stain, ×200), which on higher power (**B**, ×400) demonstrates scattered large L and H cells. The L and H cells stain intensely with CD20 by immunohistochemistry (**C**, ×600). The corresponding flow cytogram of the lymph node reveals no evidence of monoclonality of the B cells (**D**, upper boxes). By immunohistochemistry, the L and H cells are "ringed" by CD57+ cells (**E**, CD57 stain, ×400).

polyclonal by flow cytometry—Figure 14-22D) and the neoplastic LP cells are often "ringed" by the numerous CD3/CD57+ cells (as demonstrated by immunohistochemistry—Figure 14-22E). LP cells have clonally rearranged *IG* genes, usually only detectable by single cell isolation of the LP cells. *BCL6* rearrangements are frequent in NLPHL.

> **QUICK REVIEW**
>
> Although the nodular pattern and predominance of small B cells may cause diagnostic confusion with FL, the following features of NLPHL allow distinction of these two entities:
>
> - Paucity of the neoplastic LP cells
> - Ringing of the LP cells by CD3 and/or CD57 by immunohistochemistry
> - Absence of a monoclonal B-cell population by flow cytometry
> - No evidence of t(14;18)(q32;q21) and *BCL2* gene rearrangements

Nodular growth patterns may also even be rarely demonstrated in NHLs of T-cell origin.

Diffuse Large B-Cell Lymphoma

NHLs and HLs may also grow in a diffuse pattern, as eluded to previously. The most common lymphoma growing in a diffuse pattern is DLBCL.

> **HUNTING FOR ZEBRAS**
> **Follicular Variant of T-Cell Lymphoma**
>
> This rare variant of T-cell lymphoma is characterized by replacement of the lymph node architecture by back-to-back nodules, superficially resembling FL. The nodules are composed of neoplastic T cells associated with remnants of normal germinal centers, including a variable number of germinal center B cells and follicular dendritic cells. The neoplastic cells show a spectrum of size and are often atypical with irregular nuclear contours, hyperchromatic nuclei, and abundant clear of pale cytoplasm. The residual germinal centers may be compressed to one side of the nodules, which may aid in distinguishing from FL. The perifollicular sinus surrounding the tumor nodules is often expanded by lymphoma cells, suggesting that spread may occur via this sinus.
>
> The neoplastic cells most often demonstrate a follicular T-helper cell immunophenotype: CD3+, CD4+, CD5+, Bcl-6+, and Bcl-2+ with variable positivity for CD10. Thus, similar to FL, the follicular variant of T-cell lymphoma may demonstrate positivity for CD10, bcl-6, and bcl-2 by immunophenotyping. *However, further immunophenotyping should demonstrate a B-cell origin in FL and a T helper cell origin in the follicular variant of T-cell lymphoma. Distinguishing FL from T-cell follicular variant is important because of differences in prognosis and therapy between the two.*

Distinguishing DLBCL from Reactive Proliferation

DLBCL may be distinguished from reactive immunoblastic proliferation, which demonstrates the following features:

- Presence of some residual normal lymph node architecture
- Lack of atypia of the large transformed cells
- Polymorphous appearance with the immunoblasts showing a range of sizes and cytoplasmic basophilia, as well as intermixed plasmablasts and plasma cells
- Immunoblastic proliferation merging imperceptibly with adjacent reactive follicles and paracortical zones
- Immunohistochemistry showing that the large lymphoid cells represent a mixture of B and T cells
- Flow cytometric immunophenotyping demonstrating a mixture of reactive T cells and polytypic B cells

These features usually aid in this differential diagnosis; however, as discussed previously, there are morphologic variants of DLBCL (i.e., T-cell rich DLBCL) that may cause diagnostic confusion. In such cases, molecular studies (i.e., analysis for a B-cell gene rearrangement) may be indicated and may aid in distinguishing these entities.

Distinguishing DLBCL from T-Cell Lymphoma

Although NHLs of mature T-cell origin (i.e., **PTCL**) typically grow in a diffuse pattern, DLBCL occurs much more commonly than PTCL. It is important to distinguish DLBCL from PTCL, since PTCL generally has a worse prognosis. The distinction is primarily done by immunophenotyping, as described above.

Peripheral T-Cell Lymphoma, Not Otherwise Specified (PTCL, NOS)

PTCL, NOS represents a heterogeneous category of nodal and extranodal mature T-cell lymphomas that do not correspond to any of the specifically defined entities of mature T-cell lymphoma in the current classification and may be confused with DLBCL.

PTCL, NOS accounts for 30% of PTCLs in Western countries. Histologically, they are characterized by effacement of lymph node architecture by neoplastic paracortical or diffuse infiltrates, which may show broad cytologic features. Most cases demonstrate numerous medium-sized and/or large cells with irregular, pleomorphic, hyperchromatic, or vesicular nuclei and prominent nucleoli, associated with numerous mitotic features (**Figure 14-24**). RS-like cells may be seen in some cases. In addition, rare cases may demonstrate a predominance of small lymphocytes with atypical, irregular nuclei. An inflammatory background (composed of small lymphocytes, eosinophils, plasma cells, large B-cells, and in some cases clusters of epithelioid histiocytes) is often present.

The neoplastic cells usually demonstrate an aberrant immunophenotype (i.e., CD3+), most frequently CD4+/CD8– and with frequent loss of expression of CD5 and CD7. CD30 may occasionally be expressed and CD15 is generally negative. T-cell receptor genes are clonally rearranged in most cases.

CASE STUDY: Diffuse Large B-Cell Lymphoma

DLBCL is a neoplasm of large B-cells growing in a diffuse growth pattern.

A 76-year-old male presents with a history of a left groin mass suspicious for lymphoma that is biopsied. The node demonstrates diffuse large cells of lymphocytic appearance but having abnormally large nuclei at least twice as large as that of normal lymphocytes. Immunophenotyping reveals the cells to be of monoclonal B-cell origin.

DLBCL is a neoplasm with a diffuse growth pattern composed of large B lymphocytes with a nuclear size equal to or exceeding the size of a normal tissue macrophage or more than twice the size of a normal lymphocyte (Figure 14-23A).

DLBCL may demonstrate several morphologic variants, the most common being a centroblastic variant, an immunoblastic variant, or an anaplastic variant. Some cases may have a mixture of medium-sized cells, may be rich in background reactive T cells (T-cell-rich variants), or may display RS-like cells (see below).

The neoplastic cells are monoclonal B-cells with the following immunophenotype: CD19+, CD20+, CD79a+, and CD22+, but may lack one or more of these (Figure 14-23B). There may be variable expressions of CD10, bcl-6, and MUM1.

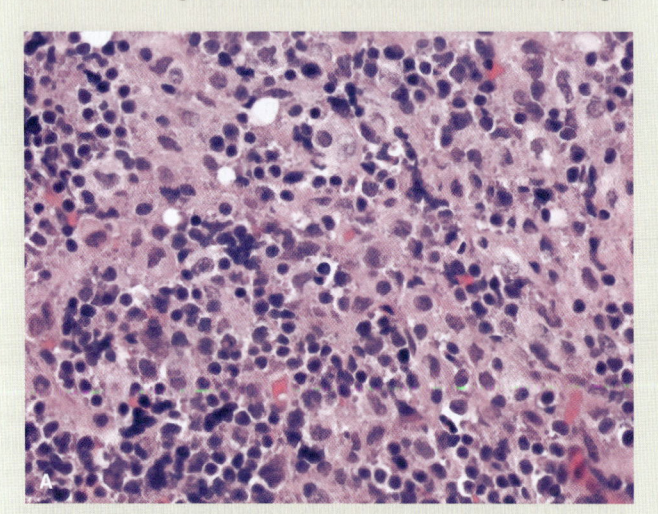

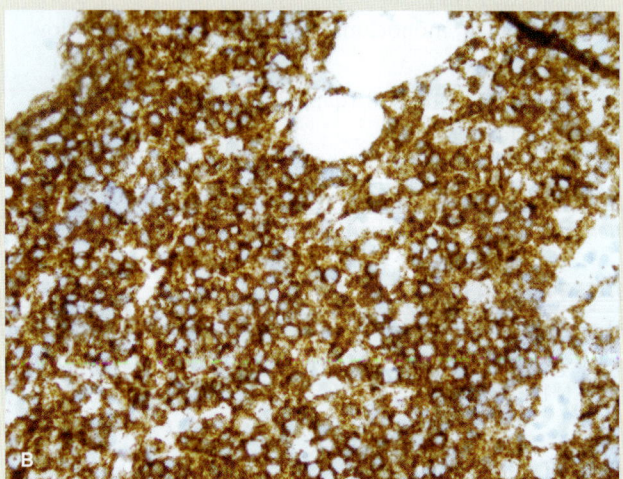

FIGURE 14-23 Diffuse large B-cell lymphoma. This section of lymph node demonstrates sheets of large cells infiltrating in a diffuse growth pattern (**A**, H&E stain, ×600). By immunohistochemistry, the large cells are intensely reactive with CD20 (**B**, CD20 stain, ×600), confirming a diagnosis of DLBCL.

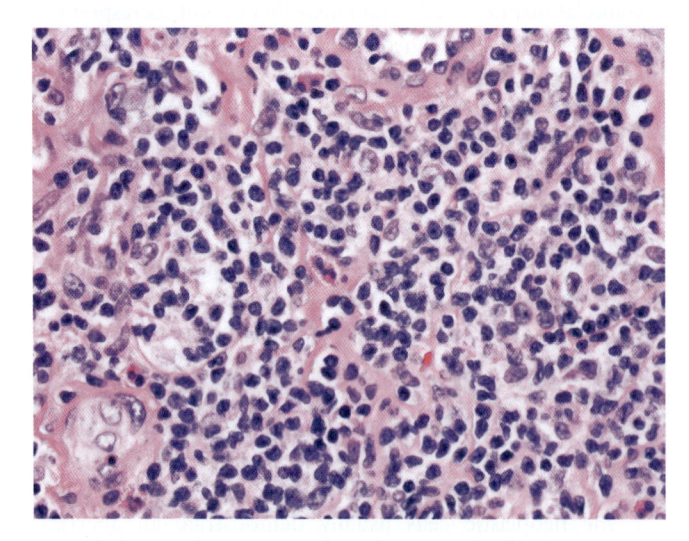

FIGURE 14-24 PTCL, NOS. This section of lymph node in a case of peripheral T-cell lymphoma, NOS demonstrates effacement of the lymph node architecture by a heterogenous population of lymphoid cells with irregular nuclear contours (H&E stain, ×600).

Due to the varying morphologic features, PTCL, NOS should be differentiated from reactive paracortical hyperplasia, as well as from other NHL (i.e., B-cell lymphomas, such as DLBCL) and cHLs (i.e., mixed cellularity type).

Morphologic features favoring reactive paracortical hyperplasia include the following:

- No erosion of the mantle zones or germinal centers of residual follicles
- Cellular composition of two distinct populations (not a continuous range of cell sizes): small lymphocytes and large activated cells lacking atypical features
- No clear cells identified

PTCL, NOS may be distinguished from DLBCL and cHL (see below) by immunophenotyping.

Classical Hodgkin Lymphoma

cHL is a monoclonal lymphoid neoplasm most often derived from B cells and composed of mononucleated or multinucleated neoplastic RS cells. There is typically an inflammatory

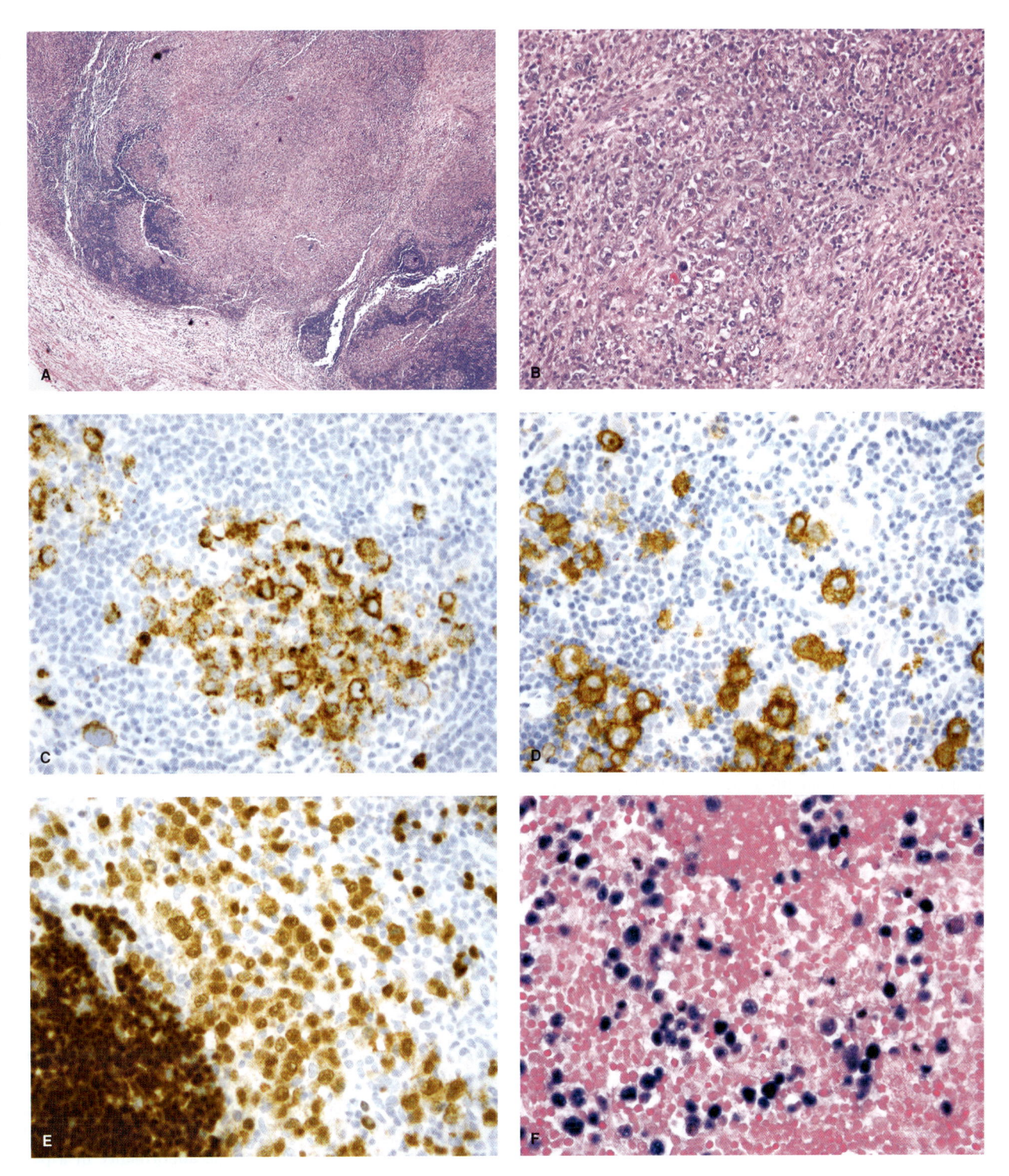

FIGURE 14-25 cHL. This section of lymph node in a case of the nodular sclerosing subtype of cHL demonstrates a thickened capsule and a nodular effacement of the lymph node at low power (**A**, H&E stain, ×200). On higher power (**B**, H&E stain, ×400), the sheets of RS cells and variants are seen. By immunohistochemistry or in situ hybridization (ISH), the RS cells and variants are reactive with CD15 (**C**, ×600), CD30 (**D**, ×600), PAX-5 (**E**, ×600), and EBV-ISH (**F**, ×600).

background composed of non-neoplastic small lymphocytes, eosinophils, neutrophils, histiocytes, plasma cells, and fibroblasts with or without collagen fibrosis. Based on the characteristics of the inflammatory background, there are four histological subtypes: lymphocyte-rich, nodular sclerosis, mixed cellularity, and lymphocyte-depleted (Figure 14-25A and B). In some cases, there may be an associated granulomatous component, which may be marked in a subset.

The neoplastic cells of all four subtypes have the following immunophenotype, representing a B cell with defective B-cell transcription: CD30+, CD15+ (75–80% of cases), PAX5+, CD20v+ (minority of neoplastic cells), CD45–, and EBVv+ (*EBNA-1+*) (75% of mixed cellularity cHL and 10-40% of nodular sclerosis cHL) (Figures 14-25C–F).

Due to the paucity of neoplastic cells relative to the inflammatory background, immunophenotyping is preferably performed by immunohistochemistry and the neoplastic cells are not typically identified by flow cytometric immunophenotyping. The neoplastic cells contain clonal *IG* gene rearrangements in more than 96% of cases and clonal T-cell receptor gene rearrangements in rare cases.

Since some case of cHL may have a marked granulomatous component, such cases should be distinguished from a granulomatous lymphadenitis. This may be accomplished by the lack of neoplastic cells by morphology and immunohistochemical immunophenotyping. Likewise, cHL may be distinguished from DLBCL (especially from those with a T cell or lymphohistiocytic-rich background or those with RS-like cells) and from PTCL, NOS (with RS-like cells) by careful attention to the immunophenotypic features.

B-Cell Lymphoma, Unclassifiable, with Features Intermediate Between DLBCL and Classical HL (DLBCL/cHL)

To complicate the situation even further, there are a group of lymphomas that have features intermediate between DLBCL and cHL. Such lymphomas *do not clearly have the morphology and immunophenotype to satisfy the diagnostic criteria as previously described for either DLBCL or for cHL.*

Features that would qualify a case as DLBCL/HL include

- Strong expression of CD15 in a case otherwise resembling DLBCL or
- Strong and diffuse expression of CD20 and/or other B-cell markers, such as CD79a in a case morphologically suggestive of cHL but very rich in large neoplastic cells

PRIMARY DISORDERS OF SPLEEN

Few diseases are primary to the spleen and any pathologic findings often represent disease processes that originate in other parts of the body. Commonly, the spleen is removed for therapeutic reasons and the role of the pathologist is to confirm a diagnosis that was suspected clinically (and possibly confirmed by other hematologic, microbiologic, and histologic studies of tissues from other organ systems) and to exclude any unsuspected pathology.

The division of the spleen into white and red pulp components forms the basis for pathologic evaluation. Conditions involving the spleen are divided into those disorders affecting the two main compartments.

Disorders of White Pulp

The evaluation of the spleen should begin at low power to determine which major compartment, the white pulp or the red pulp, is involved in the disease process. With white pulp involvement, the white pulp, or lymphoid areas, is typically expanded and often appear nodular.

Primary disorders of the splenic white pulp include reactive processes (i.e., FH), infectious processes [granulomatous disorders), and neoplastic disorders (i.e., malignant lymphomas—Hodgkin and non-Hodgkin)] (Table 14-11).

TABLE 14-11 Disorders predominating in splenic white pulp.

Reactive hyperplasia
Follicular
Rheumatoid arthritis (Felty syndrome)
Immune thrombocytopenic purpura
Thrombotic thrombocytopenic purpura
Acquired hemolytic anemia
AIDS
Nonfollicular
Acute infections
Graft rejection
Idiopathic antigenic stimulation
Malignant lymphomas and other lymphoproliferative disorders
Chronic lymphocytic leukemia/Small lymphocytic lymphoma
Lymphoplasmacytic lymphoma
Mantle cell lymphoma
Marginal zone lymphoma
Follicular lymphoma
Large B-cell lymphoma
T-cell lymphoma
Peripheral
Hepatosplenic
Angioimmunoblastic
Anaplastic large cell
Mycosis fungoides
Hodgkin lymphoma

Follicular Hyperplasia

Reactive FH (or the presence of secondary germinal centers) implies antigenic stimulation and may result from a number of infectious or immune-mediated causes (i.e., rheumatoid arthritis and immune thrombocytopenic purpura). Frequently, it is the major pathologic abnormality in a patient with splenomegaly or hypersplenism and no well-defined clinical condition, known as idiopathic reactive FH.

Morphologically, the reactive follicles are similar to those seen in lymph nodes with features including variation in size and shape, a mixed follicle-center cell population, tingible body macrophages, and polarized appearing mantle zones. Benign follicles may at times be difficult to distinguish from the neoplastic follicles of FH and additional testing to include immunohistochemical staining, flow cytometric analysis, and cytogenetic studies may be necessary to help determine a benign versus malignant process. Other lymphomas, such as marginal zone lymphoma, small lymphocytic lymphoma, and mantle cell lymphoma may present with a nodular pattern and may also need to be excluded. Importantly, most lymphomas are not primary to the spleen and represent more generalized disease.

Infectious processes may result in FH as described above or with granulomata that are often nodular and well circumscribed. The granulomata are composed of a loose collection of macrophages and may be surrounded by a rim of inflammatory cells, including lymphocytes, plasma cells, and acute inflammatory cells. Frequent infectious causes of splenic granulomas include viral, fungal, mycobacterial, bacterial, and parasitic/protozoal infections. Additionally, noninfectious causes of granulomata include systemic (sarcoidosis, vasculitis, rheumatoid arthritis), malignancy-associated (carcinoma, melanoma, lymphoma), immunodeficiency, foreign body, and idiopathic etiologies.

Primary Splenic Marginal Zone Lymphoma

Primary splenic marginal zone lymphoma is a B-cell neoplasm composed of small lymphocytes that surround and replace the

> ### CASE STUDY: Follicular Hyperplasia
>
> *FH may occur in the white pulp of the spleen and needs to be distinguished from malignant lymphoma.*
>
> A 38-year-old woman with chronic ITP has frequent nosebleeds, menorrhagia, and platelet count of 15,000 per mm. Because her disease is resistant to steroid therapy her spleen is removed.
>
> ITP is a process of autoimmune platelet destruction. The spleen may be removed in steroid refractory cases and the histologic findings are variable, but include reactive FH, as seen in this case (Figure 14-26). 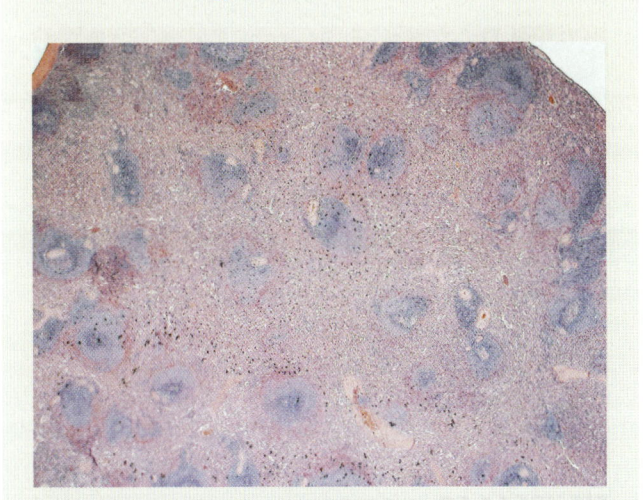
>
> **FIGURE 14-26** Spleen, FH. Prominent white pulp expansion with scattered germinal centers.

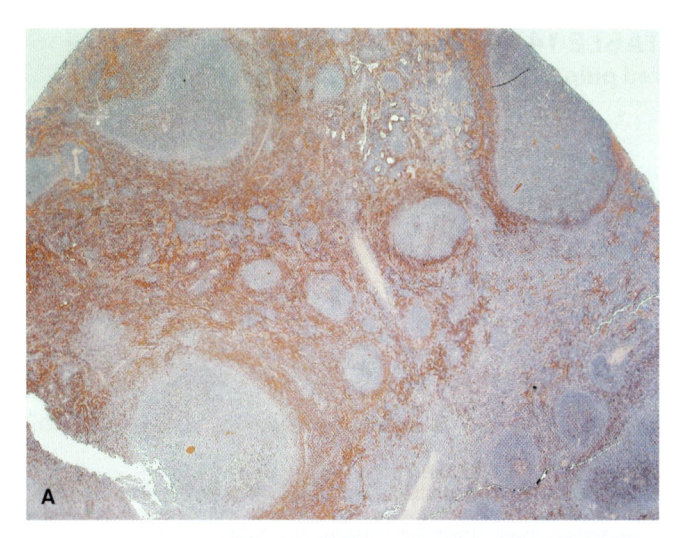

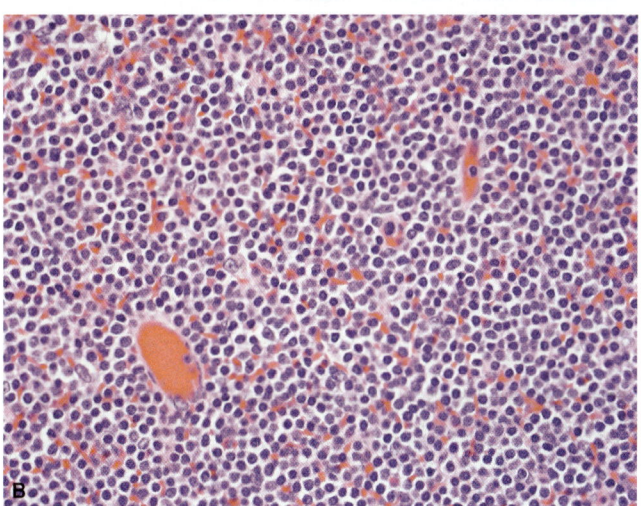

FIGURE 14-27 (A) Spleen, splenic marginal zone lymphoma, 2×. Nodular expansion of white pulp by a monotonous population of pale appearing cells. (B) Spleen, splenic marginal zone lymphoma, 40×. Monotonous population of small lymphocytes with pale cytoplasm.

splenic white pulp germinal centers, effacing the follicle mantle (see Figure 14-27A and B, for a case example).

Disorders of Red Pulp

Primary disorders of the splenic red pulp include non-neoplastic disorders of erythrocytes, granulocytes, and platelets; disorders of the monocyte-macrophage system; neoplastic hematolymphoid disorders (i.e., acute and chronic leukemias); non-neoplastic vascular lesions, and splenic cysts, nonhematolymphoid tumors, and tumorlike lesions (Table 14-12).

Again, in the disorders of the red pulp, the spleen is often removed for therapeutic, not diagnostic, reasons. Most of the above entities have associated or specific histologic findings that can be used to confirm a diagnosis that has already been established clinically. Importantly, metastatic disease to the spleen should always be considered when dealing with mass or tumorlike lesions.

TABLE 14-12 Disorders predominating in splenic red pulp.

- Congestion
    - Congenital and acquired hemolytic anemias
    - Fibrocongestive splenomegaly
- Infections
    - Infectious mononucleosis
    - Acute septic splenitis
    - Bacillary angiomatosis
- Histiocytic proliferations
    - Lipid histiocytoses
    - Ceroid histiocytosis
    - Gaucher disease
    - Hemophagocytic syndromes
    - Histiocytic and dendritic cell neoplasms
- Leukemias, myeloproliferative disease, and myelodysplastic syndrome
    - Chronic myelogenous leukemia
    - Myelodysplasia
    - Hairy cell leukemia
    - T-cell large granular lymphocytic leukemia
    - Systemic mastocytosis
- Nonhematopoietic tumors
    - Developmental
    - Cysts
    - Hamartomas
    - Vascular neoplasms
    - Hemangiomas
    - Lymphangiomas
    - Littoral cell angiomas
    - Angiosarcomas
    - Nonvascular sarcomas
    - Metastases
    - Inflammatory pseudotumor

Hairy Cell Leukemia

Hairy cell leukemia results in marked expansion of the red pulp with frequent red cell lakes. Hairy cell leukemia is named for the unique appearance of the cells observed on PB smear. The cells preferentially infiltrate the red pulp of the spleen and result in marked expansion of the red pulp with frequent red cell lakes and obliteration of white pulp (Figure 14-29A–C). Splenomegaly is often massive and may be the only abnormal physical finding. However, the spleen is rarely removed and the diagnosis is most often made by evaluation of the blood and BM.

Hepatosplenic T-Cell Lymphoma

Hepatosplenic T-cell lymphoma is a rare form of lymphoma, derived from cytotoxic T cells usually of gamma delta T-cell receptor type. It is usually composed of medium-sized lymphoid cells demonstrating sinusoidal infiltration of the spleen,

CASE STUDY: Hypersplenism Due to Sickle Cell Anemia

Sickle cell anemia, the most common of the hemoglobinopathies, is an inherited multisystem disorder due to the presence of mutant sickle cell hemoglobin (Hgb S). It is characterized by chronic hemolytic anemia and is associated with recurrent episodes of pain and other vaso-occlusive complications. Sickle cell anemia may result in marked expansion of the red pulp due to sequestration of the sickled erythrocytes. Splenic infarcts are often present and old fibrotic infarcts encrusted with iron and calcium (Gamna–Gandy bodies) may be seen. Because splenic sequestration recurs in about 50% of patients, most pathology specimens are from patients after the first acute sequestration crisis. In advanced stages, however, the spleen is small and extensively fibrotic, a process known as autosplenectomy.

A 2-year-old boy with a history of sickle cell anemia and splenic sequestration crisis has his spleen removed. It is enlarged and weighs 65 g. The microscopic sections are demonstrated in Figure 14-28A and B.

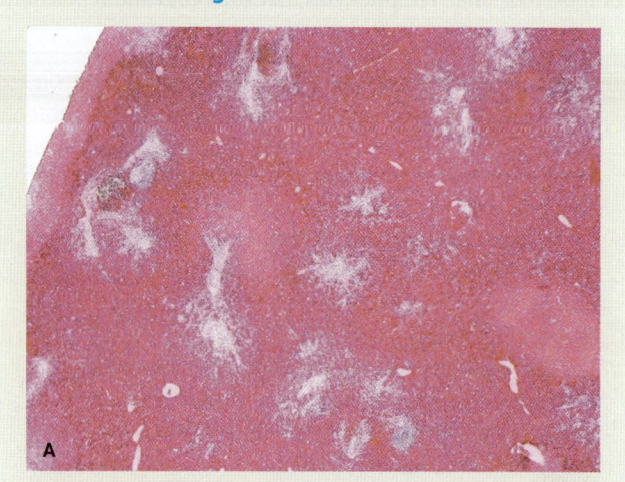

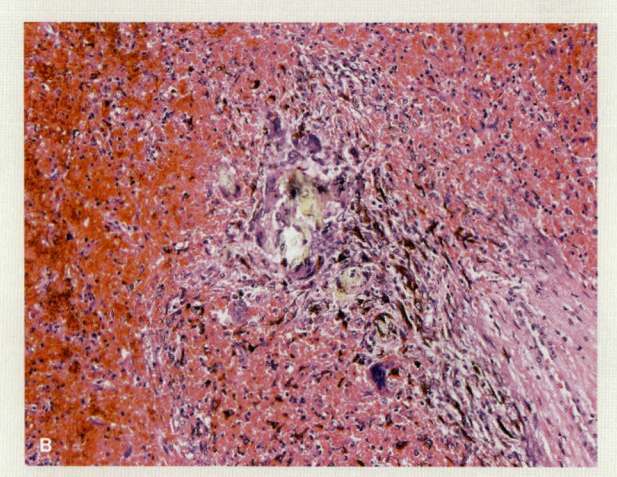

FIGURE 14-28 (A) Spleen, sickle cell anemia, 2 ×. Prominent red pulp congestion. (B) Spleen, sickle cell anemia, Gamna–Gandy body, 20×. Fibrotic infarct encrusted with iron and calcium.

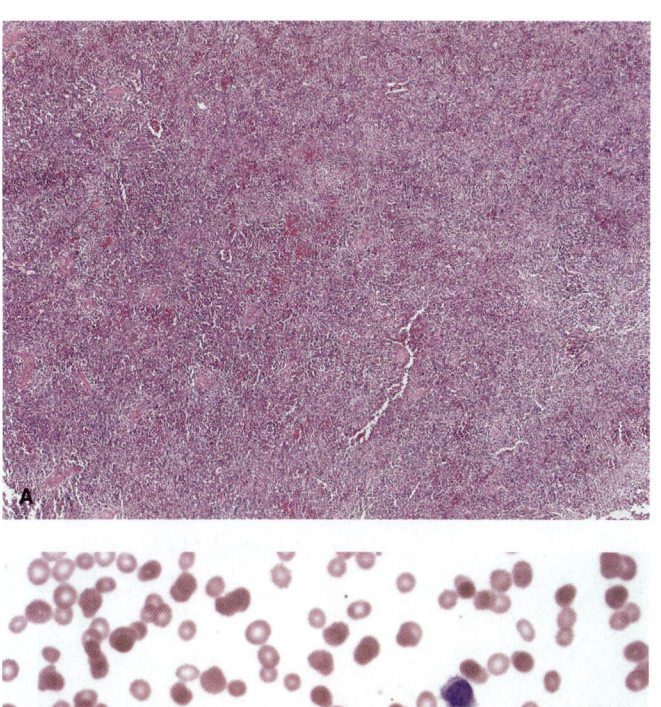

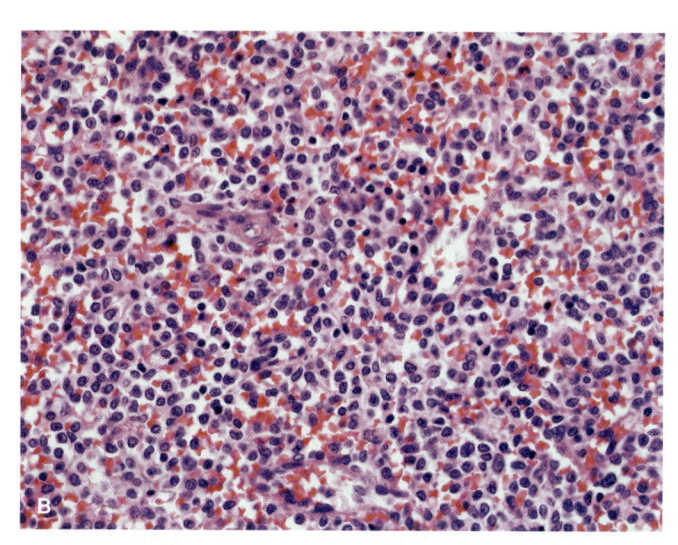

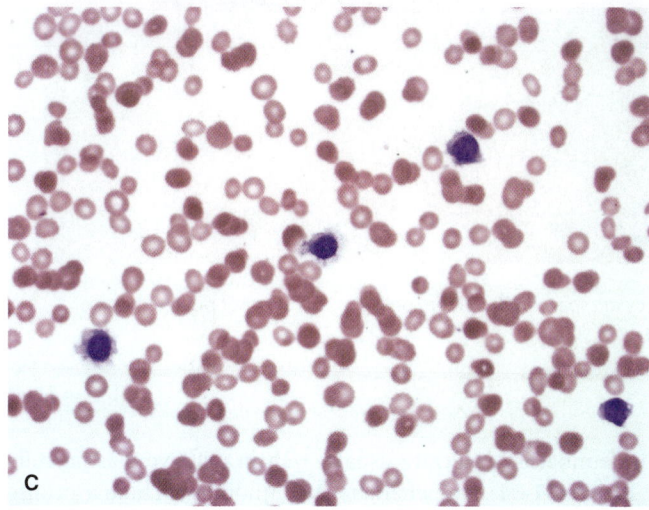

FIGURE 14-29 **(A) Spleen, hairy cell leukemia, 2 ×.** Effacement of splenic architecture and expansion of red pulp by a monotonous population of small lymphocytes. **(B)** Spleen, hairy cell leukemia, 40×. High-power image of a monotonous population of small lymphocytes with abundant pale pink cytoplasm. **(C)** Spleen, hairy cell leukemia, PB smear. Small lymphocytes with cytoplasmic projections imparting a "hairy" appearance.

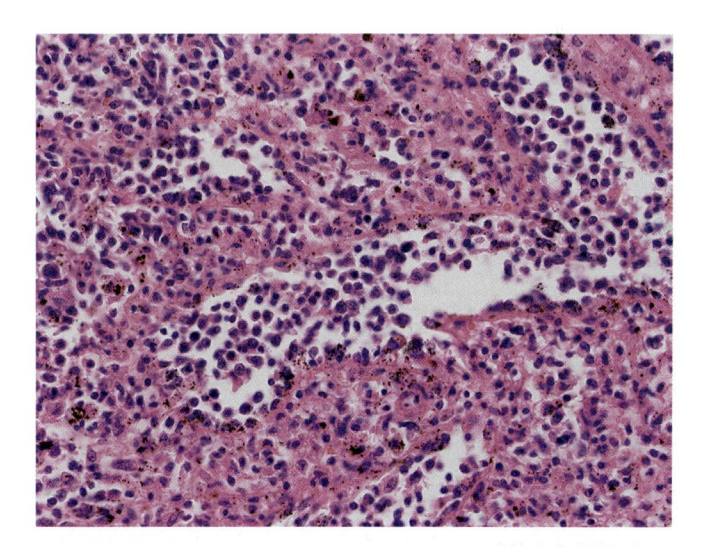

FIGURE 14-30 **Spleen, hepatosplenic T-cell lymphoma.** Diffuse infiltration of the red pulp and sinuses by small-to-medium lymphocytes.

liver, and BM (Figure 14-30). Patients usually present with hepatosplenomegaly. Microscopically, the neoplastic cells diffusely infiltrate the red pulp cords and conspicuously fill the sinuses. Features may be similar to those of hairy cell leukemia, but red cell lakes are not seen in hepatosplenic T-cell lymphoma.

Benign Vascular Tumor (Hemangioma)

Hemangiomas are the most common benign neoplasm of the spleen. They are usually solitary and well circumscribed. Two major subtypes occur in the spleen: capillary and cavernous. Microscopically, they are analogous to their counterparts at other sites. Capillary hemangiomas demonstrate lobulated, unencapsulated aggregates of thin-walled vessels lined by flattened endothelium. Cavernous hemangiomas are characterized by large, dilated vascular channels. In most cases, the lesion is an incidental finding, but may result in hemorrhage or hypersplenism.

CASE STUDY: Peliosis

Peliosis a non-neoplastic vascular lesion may involve the spleen, demonstrating cystic spaces with flattened sinus lining cells. Peliosis of the spleen is usually associated with peliosis hepatis and may result in splenic rupture or death. The pathogenesis is unknown, but it occurs in patients with wasting diseases such as tuberculosis or cancer. It is also commonly seen with anabolic and contraceptive steroids. Many other diseases, including hematologic malignancies, have been associated with this disorder.

A 73-year-old male with untreated chronic leukemia presents with splenic rupture. The features of splenic peliosis are demonstrated in **Figure 14-31A** and **B**.

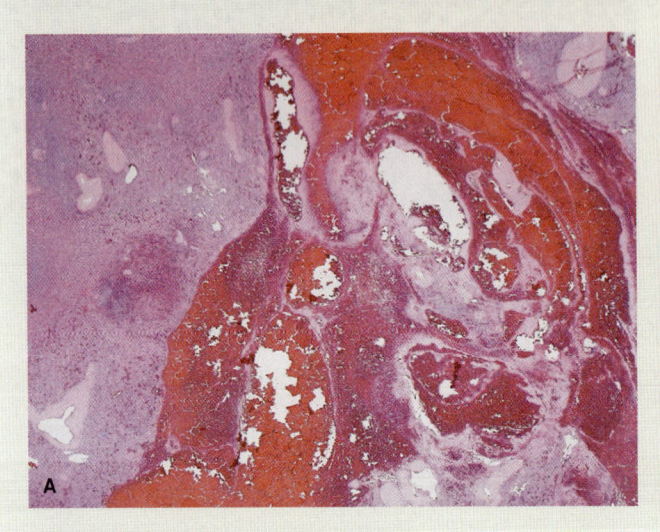

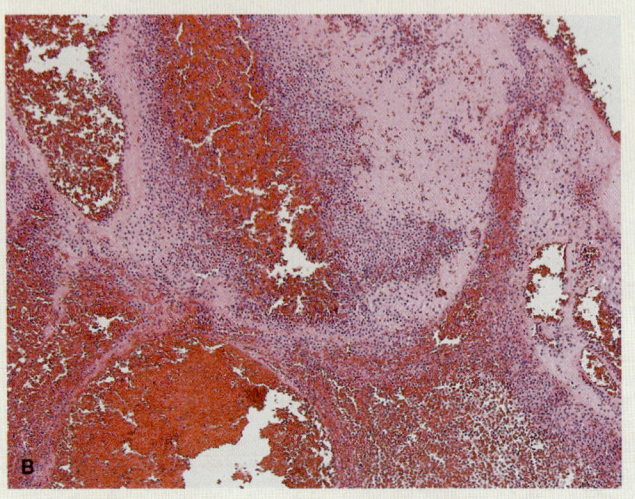

FIGURE 14-31 (A) Spleen, peliosis, 2 ×. Lesion with blood-filled cystic spaces. (B) Spleen, peliosis, 10 ×. Higher power image of cystic spaces with flattened sinus lining cells.

TUMORLIKE LESIONS

Inflammatory Pseudotumors

Inflammatory pseudotumor is a benign tumor-like lesion composed of proliferating spindle cells admixed with an inflammatory infiltrate usually rich in reactive plasma cells (**Figure 14-34**). The characteristic findings include a proliferation of bland-appearing spindle cells and a polymorphic background of monocytes, lymphocytes, granulocytes, and plasma cells.

HUNTING FOR ZEBRAS
Hemangioendothelioma Versus Angiosarcoma

Hemangioendothelioma is characterized by vascular lesions demonstrating well-formed vascular channels, mild atypia, absence of necrosis, a low mitotic rate, and borderline malignant potential. The histologic and clinical features are intermediate between the benign, well-differentiated hemangiomas and the frankly malignant angiosarcoma.

True angiosarcoma of the spleen is uncommon and is distinguished from hemangioendothelioma by dissecting growth, more significant cellular atypia, higher mitotic activity, and the presence of necrosis (**Figure 14-32**).

The microscopic features are quite variable and may be solid, papillary, or have freely anastomosing vascular channels. The cells are usually atypical and hyperchromatic with occasional intracytoplasmic hyaline globules.

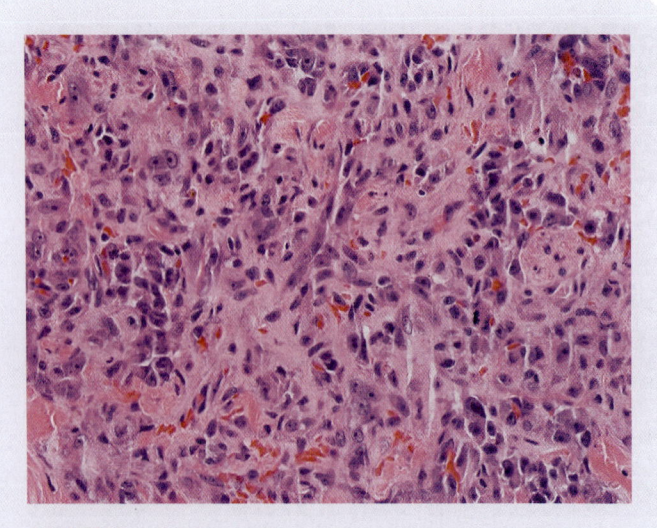

FIGURE 14-32 High-grade angiosarcoma. Vascular channels lined by highly atypical cells with hyperchromatic nuclei.

CASE STUDY: Hamartoma

Splenic hamartoma is a tumor-like lesion composed of structurally disorganized, mature splenic red pulp elements.

The endothelial-type cells that line the anastomotic channels express vascular antigens, including factor VIII and CD31, as well as CD8. Although hemangiomas may appear similar histologically, the cells in these tumors lack CD8. Hamartomas lack white pulp elements, but extramedullary hematopoiesis may be present.

A 68-year-old female presents with a splenic mass found incidentally by CT scan while being evaluated for diverticulitis. The histologic features of the "mass" are typical of a hamartoma (Figure 14-33).

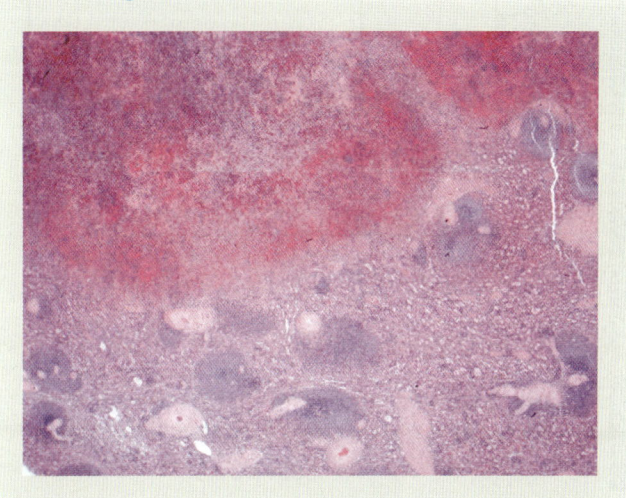

FIGURE 14-33 Spleen, hamartoma, 2 ×. Circumscribed lesion composed of disorganized red pulp elements.

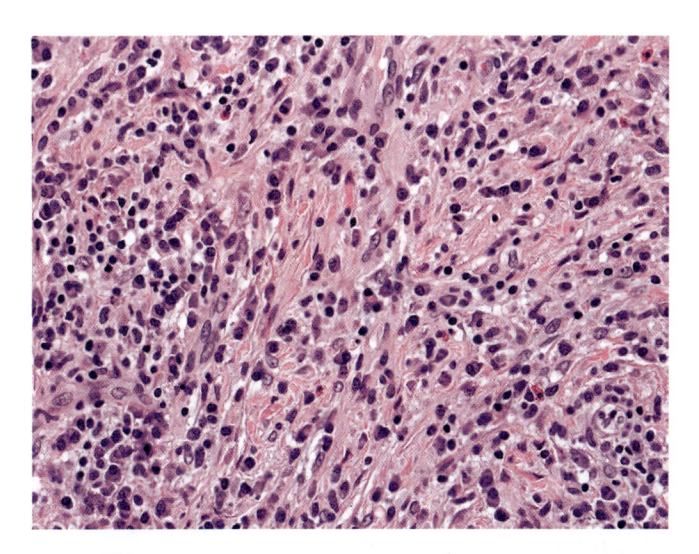

FIGURE 14-34 Inflammatory pseudotumor. Proliferation of bland-appearing spindle cells with an inflammatory infiltrate composed of plasma cells, small lymphocytes, and rare eosinophils.

Because of the inflammatory appearance of these lesions, stains for microorganisms including acid-fast bacillus (AFB), Gomori methenamine silver (GMS), and periodic acid-Schiff (PAS) may be necessary in some cases. Additionally, the lesion should be differentiated from splenic hamartomas and inflammatory myofibroblastic tumor, a true neoplasm of neoplasm of spindle cells of myofibroblastic lineage.

PRIMARY DISORDERS OF THYMUS

Primary disorders of the thymus include reactive conditions (thymic hyperplasia) as well as benign and malignant neoplasms derived from epithelial and lymphoid components. Thymic aplasia (or hypoplasia) may also occur and results in an immunodeficiency syndrome (i.e., DiGeorge syndrome). See Table 14-13.

Thymic Hyperplasia

True thymic hyperplasia is defined as an increase in the size and weight of the thymus and demonstrates a normal microscopic appearance. The weight of the normal thymus is mainly related to age: it is greatest in relation to body weight at the time of birth, weighing an average of 15 g. It continues to increase in size and weight until puberty to reach an average weight of 30–40 g. Subsequently, thymic weight declines during the process of aging involution and at 60 years of age is 10–15 g. Death from asphyxia (largely in young persons) and several cardiovascular conditions are associated with higher than normal thymic weight, including myocardial fibrosis; coronary thrombosis, myocardial infarction, and ruptured myocardium; cor pulmonale; hypertensive heart disease with congestive heart failure; and coronary occlusion due to atheroma. Thymic hyperplasia has been recognized in several instances as a complication of chemotherapy for HL and germ cell tumors, and has been interpreted as the expression of an immunologic "rebound" phenomenon. A similar enlargement of the thymus has been reported in children recovering from thermal burns and in infants following cessation of administration of corticosteroids.

Thymoma

Thymoma (and thymic carcinoma also derived from thymic epithelial cells) is an extremely heterogeneous group of neoplastic lesions with an exceedingly wide spectrum of morphologic appearances (Figures 14-36A–D).

Thymoma is defined as a benign or low-grade malignant tumor of the thymic epithelium with characteristic histologic features, frequently associated with a variable population of immature, but non-neoplastic T cells. Thymoma is divided into noninvasive (encapsulated or circumscribed) and invasive

TABLE 14-13 Primary disorders of the thymus.

Aplasia/hypoplasia (DiGeorge syndrome)
True thymic hyperplasia
Thymoma (benign or malignant)
Thymic carcinoma

CASE STUDY: Thymic Hyperplasia with Associated Pure Red Cell Aplasia

Thymic hyperplasia represents an enlargement of the thymus and is non-neoplastic. Lymphoid (i.e., follicular) hyperplasia of the thymus is characterized by the microscopic finding of FH, independent of size and weight. Lymphoid hyperplasia of the thymus is most commonly associated with myasthenia gravis, but has also been observed in a number of immunologically mediated disorders, including systemic lupus erythematosus (SLE), rheumatoid arthritis, scleroderma, allergic vasculitis, and thyrotoxicosis. Red cell aplasia has been noted to occur with several disease states involving the thymus (thymoma and myasthenia gravis) but is of unknown significance.

The patient, a 35-year-old female, was found to have an enlarged thymus on CT that was not evident on plain chest X-ray examination. Thymectomy for the enlarged thymus was performed and followed rapidly by a full hematologic recovery. See Figure 14-35A. By flow cytometric analysis, true thymic hyperplasia shows a population of cells with variable expression of T-cell markers as well as the common thymocyte antigen, as demonstrated in Figures 14-35B–D.

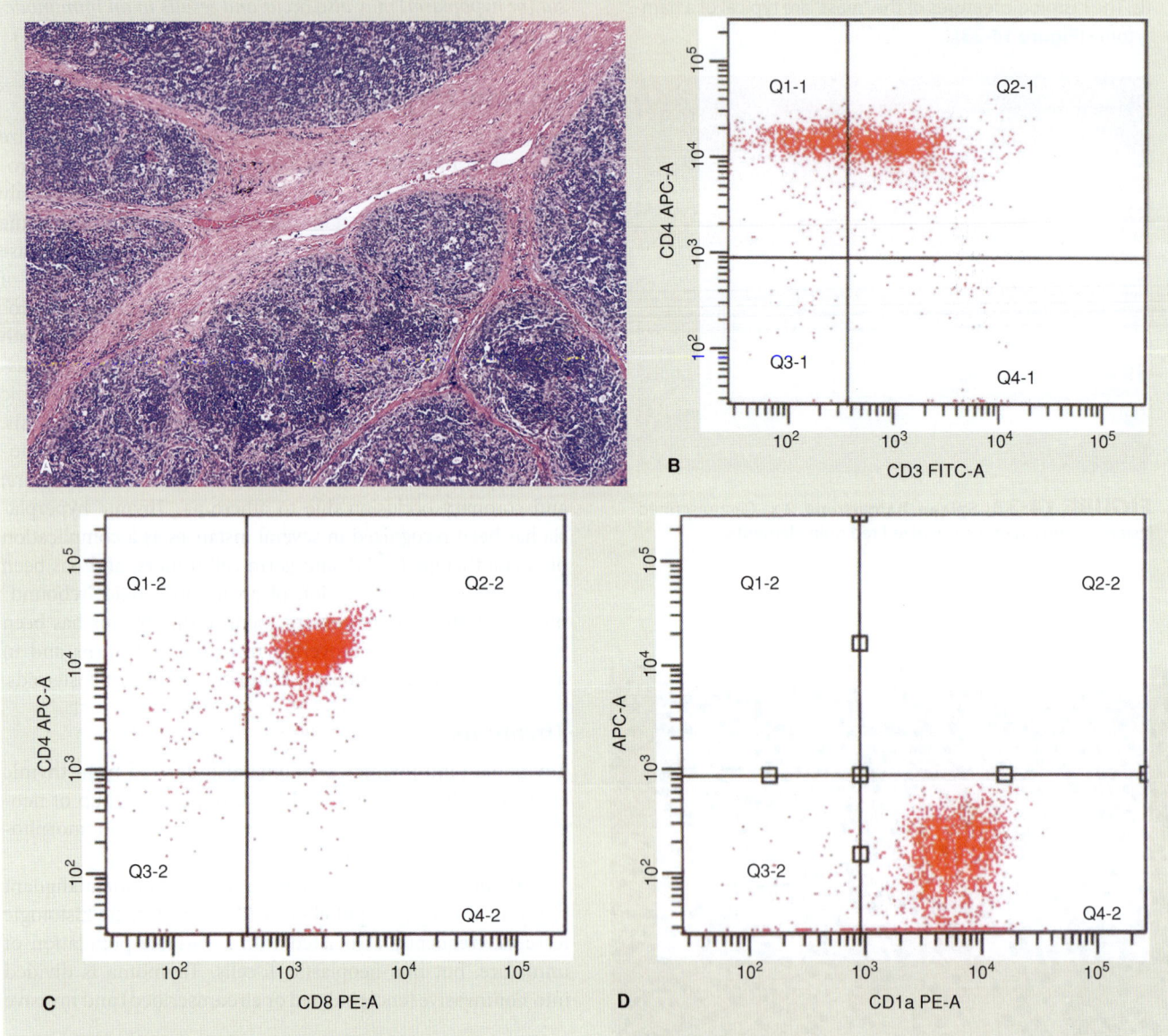

FIGURE 14-35 True thymic hyperplasia. This section of thymic tissue in a case of true thymic hyperplasia demonstrates a normal microscopic appearance (i.e., of normal thymus) (**A**, H&E stain, ×400). The corresponding flow cytograms of the thymic tissue demonstrate a smear pattern of CD3 and CD4 expression (**B**, upper boxes), coexpression of CD4 and CD8 (**C**, upper right box), as well as expression of the common thymocyte antigen, CD1a (**D**, lower right box).

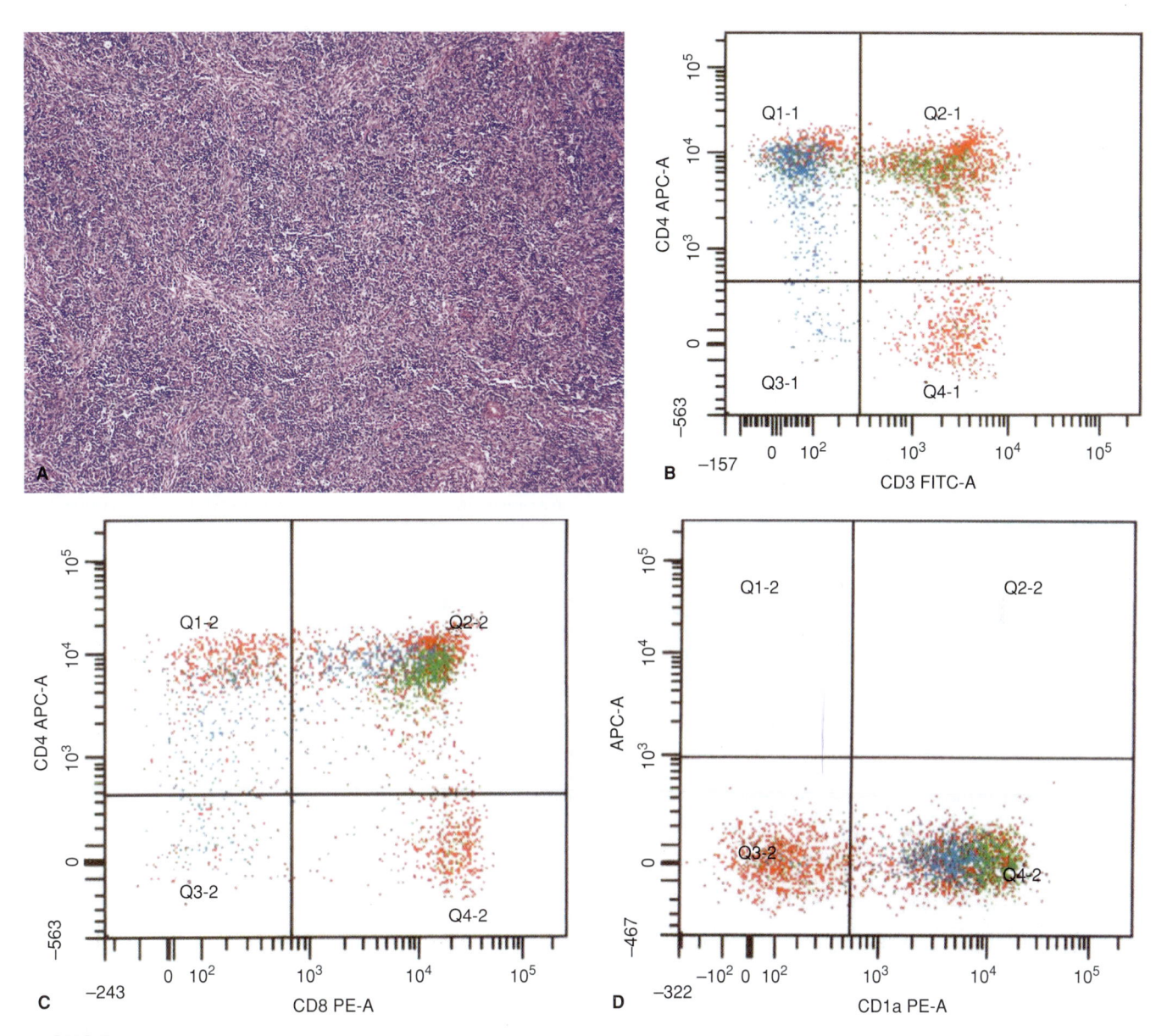

FIGURE 14-36 Thymoma. This section of thymic tissue in a case of thymoma demonstrates the typical histology with varying components of epithelioid, spindle, and lymphoid cells (**A**, H&E stain, ×400). The corresponding flow cytograms of the thymic tissue demonstrate that the lymphoid cells show a smear pattern of CD3 and CD4 (**B**), coexpression of CD4 and CD8 (**C**, upper right box), and expression of CD1a (**D**, lower right box).

HUNTING FOR ZEBRAS
Thymoma Versus Thymic Carcinoma

Thymic carcinoma is uncommon, representing only about 1.5% of all cancer cases. Previously classified as a type C thymoma, it is characterized by having the most aggressive morphology and clinical course.

Thymic carcinoma and thymoma may be distinguished histologically in most cases. The presence of immature T cells, even in implanted and distant metastatic foci of thymoma, indicates that the epithelial cells of thymoma are capable of attracting immature T cells from the BM; the presence of medullary differentiation in thymoma indicates that immature T cells have the ability to mature in the environment of the thymoma. These phenomena suggest that thymoma is a functional tumor with regard to T-cell maturation. In contrast, thymic carcinoma has lost this property.

types; the latter occasionally shows pleural implantation and rarely lymphatic and hematogenous metastases. Cytologically, thymoma is divided into spindle cell type, polygonal (round or oval) cell type, and mixed cell type. A distinction between noninvasive, invasive, and metastasizing types on the basis of the cytologic features is impossible.

Thymic Carcinoma

Thymic carcinoma is a cytologically malignant thymic epithelial tumor. It is defined as a tumor composed of nests and diffuse growth of obviously atypical cells of an invasive nature, as seen in carcinomas of other organs, although completely encapsulated in rare instances (Figure 14-37). There are no immature (or cortical) T cells. The phenotype of the infiltrating lymphocytes is similar to that of carcinomas of other organs.

T-Lymphoblastic Lymphoma

It is important to distinguish not only thymomas from thymic carcinoma (as described previously) but also from

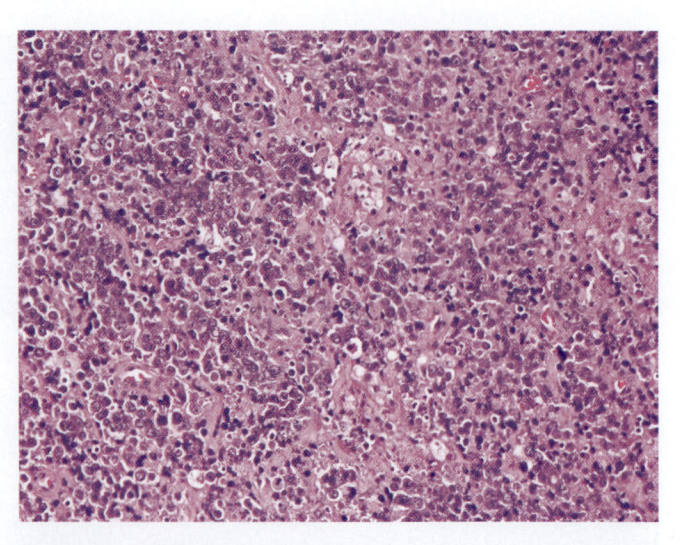

FIGURE 14-37 Thymic carcinoma. This section of thymic tissue in a case of thymic carcinoma demonstrates cytologically malignant cells infiltrating in a variably cohesive growth pattern (H&E stain, ×600).

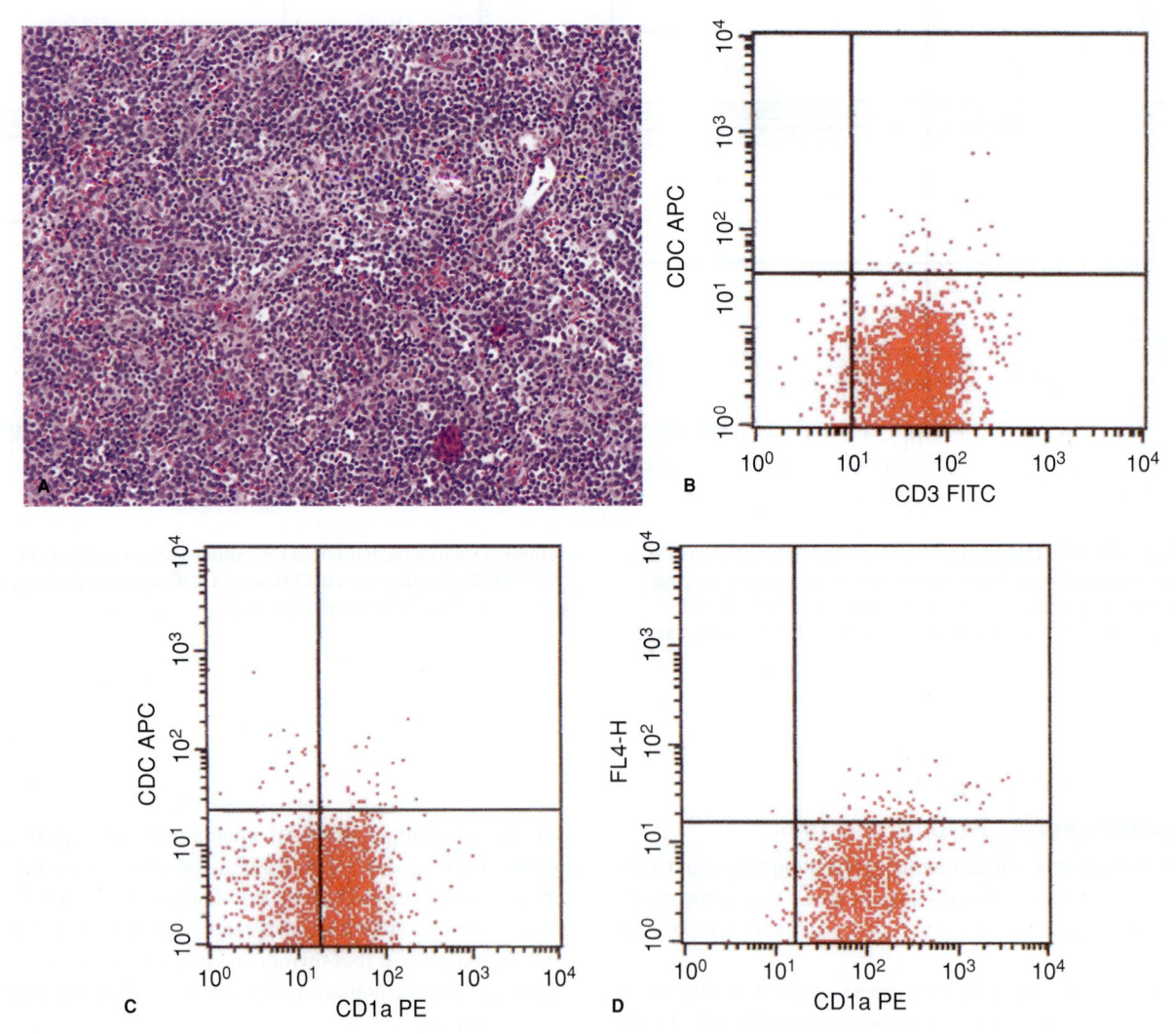

FIGURE 14-38 T-Lymphoblastic lymphoma. This section of a mediastinal tumor reveals sheets of immature cells with a focal starry-sky appearance (**A**, H&E stain, ×400). The corresponding flow cytograms of this tumor demonstrate expression of CD3 (**B**, lower right box) without expression of CD4 (**B**, upper boxes), but with expression of CD8 (**C**, lower right box) and CD1a (**D**, lower right box). This aberrant immunophenotype in correlation with the cytomorphology is diagnostic of involvement by T-lymphoblastic lymphoma.

T lymphoblastic lymphoma. The distinction between thymoma and T-lymphoblastic lymphoma may actually be more problematic, since they have similar immunophenotypes.

T-lymphoblastic lymphoma (the lymphomatous form of T lymphoblastic leukemia (previously discussed)) is composed of a neoplasm derived from thymic precursor T-cells forming a lymphomatous mass. There are various stages of differentiation that a T-lymphoblastic lymphoma may represent, including a common thymocyte stage—identical to the immunophenotype of thymoma. It must be differentiated from thymoma due to the marked difference in prognosis and treatment (Figures 14-38A–D).

The lymphoblasts in T lymphoblastic lymphoma are morphologically indistinguishable from those of Burkitt lymphoma (the other high-grade lymphoma) and are composed of sheets of lymphoblasts with a starry-sky appearance. Thus immunphenotyping is necessary to distinguish these entities.

Differential Diagnosis: Burkitt Lymphoma

Burkitt lymphoma is a high grade B-cell lymphoma composed of monomorphic medium-sized transformed cells, sometimes appearing cohesive with squared off borders, and typically demonstrating a starry-sky appearance (Figure 14-39 and Table 14-10). The neoplastic cells are typically CD10+ monoclonal B-cells, consistent with a follicle center cell origin. Genotypically, Burkitt lymphoma demonstrates a *MYC* translocation.

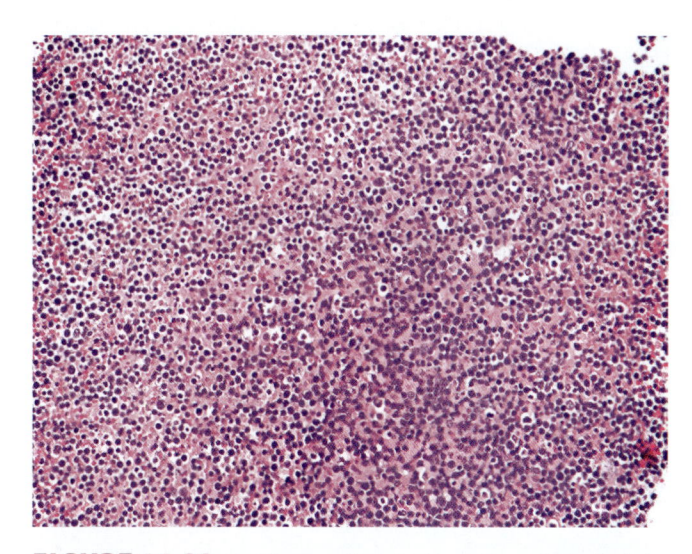

FIGURE 14-39 Burkitt lymphoma. This section of lymph node in a case of Burkitt lymphoma demonstrates typical histology with a diffuse growth pattern infiltrated by a monomorphic population of intermediate-sized cells with marked individual cell necrosis and a starry-sky appearance.

CHAPTER 15

Pathology of the Endocrine System

Catherine A. Hammett-Stabler and Susan J. Maygarden

Disorders stemming from the endocrine system are among the most frequently encountered patient problems. Currently, diabetes (discussed under Pancreas) and thyroid disorders rank within the top ten most encountered diagnoses. On a broader scale, endocrinopathies cross all ages and genders and often manifest as other clinical entities that make diagnosis challenging. Because multiple organ systems are usually involved, endocrinology can seem daunting in an organ-based approach. However, it can be divided into more manageable sections by approaching the topic first by the gland involved, that is, pituitary, adrenal, or thyroid, and then from the clinical perspective of hyperfunction or hypofunction, based on the concentrations of the respective hormones or peptides secreted into the circulation. This chapter will thus be divided by system or gland and subdivided by functional defect. Diagnosis of endocrine disorders makes heavy use of clinical laboratory testing and that emphasis is reflected in this chapter.

QUICK REVIEW
Basic Principles of Clinical Endocrinology
Glands, Hormones, and Receptors

The key glands of the endocrine system include the hypothalamus, pituitary, thyroid, parathyroids, adrenals, pancreas, and gonads. These organs synthesize and secrete specific biochemical messengers, known as hormones, into the blood in a synchronized collaboration with the central nervous system (CNS) and the immune system to regulate metabolism, growth, development, and reproduction (Figure 15-1). *Other tissues, such as adipose and gut, are also metabolically active and involved in these activities as well. The term hormone, derived from the Greek* hormon *meaning to set in motion, was chosen because these compounds act on cells some distance from their site of origin (hence the derivation of the word* **endocrine**, *from the Greek krino, to separate). Now we know that many hormones also act locally on neighboring cells at the* **paracrine** *level, and even on the very cell from which they originate in an* **autocrine** *manner.*

Several classification schemes of hormones are recognized, but the simplest consists of three broad groups: peptides, steroids, and amino acid derivatives. The *peptide* hormones represent the largest and most diverse hormone class and include examples such as growth hormone (GH), adrenocorticotropic hormone (ACTH), and insulin. These are typically synthesized and stored for quick release into the circulation when needed, either as specific gene products or through post-translational modification of precursors and are usually water-soluble. All *steroid* hormones are derived from cholesterol, and as such, are lipophilic. Compounds in this class are not stored, so the rate of synthesis regulates secretion. Examples of steroid hormones include cortisol, aldosterone, and the androgens. The last group, *amines,* is derived from the amino acid tyrosine and includes the thyroid hormones (thyroxine (T4) and triiodothyronine (T3)) and the catecholamines (epinephrine, norepinephrine, and dopamine). Each of these compounds is stored as granules in the cytoplasm until needed.

Hormone Transport—The Role of Proteins

Upon release by the respective endocrine gland, a hormone is transported through the circulation to various tissues. En route to the target tissue the hormone is exposed to degradation by numerous proteolytic enzymes. Hormones circulate either as free (i.e., not protein bound) forms, or bound to one or more proteins. Free hormones are readily available for receptor interaction and thus exhibit the greatest biological activity, but they are most susceptible to degradation. Protein binding serves as a means of transporting hormones safely through the circulation to the target tissue and as a way of assuring sufficient hormone is available should the amount of bioavailable hormone decline. Examples of hormones and their related binding proteins are seen in Table 15-1. How tightly the hormone is bound to a protein is important since this affects the hormone's potential to interact at the receptor, that is, its biological activity. *Those that are found in the free state, along with those hormones that are weakly protein bound, are considered to have the greatest bioavailability; while hormones bound to proteins with high affinity have the least.*

Peptide hormones typically circulate in an unprotected free form. They must reach their destination and act within

Hypothalamus
Antidiuretic hormone (ADH)
Oxytocin (OT)
Regulatory hormones

Pituitary gland
Anterior pituitary secretes:
  Adrenocorticotropic hormone (ACTH)
  Follicle-stimulating hormone (FSH)
  Growth hormone (GH)
  Luteinizing hormone (LH)
  Melanocyte-stimulating hormone (MSH)
  Prolactin (PRL)
  Thyroid-stimulating hormone (TSH)
Posterior pituitary releases:
  Antidiuretic hormone (ADH)
  Oxytocin (OT)

Pineal gland
Melatonin

Thyroid gland
Calcitonin (CT)
Thyroid hormone (TH)

Parathyroid glands
(located on posterior surface of thyroid)
Parathyroid hormone (PTH)

Thymus
Thymopoietin
Thymosins

Heart
Atriopeptin

Adrenal glands
Cortex:
  Corticosteroids
Medulla:
  Epinephrine (E)
  Norepinephrine (NE)

Gastrointestinal (GI) tract
Cholecystokinin (CCK)
Gastric inhibitory peptide (GIP)
Gastrin
Secretin
Vasoactive intestinal peptide (VIP)

Kidney
Calcitriol
Erythropoietin (EPO)
Renin

Pancreatic islets
Glucagon
Insulin
Somatostatin
Pancreatic polypeptide

Testes (male)
Androgens
Inhibin

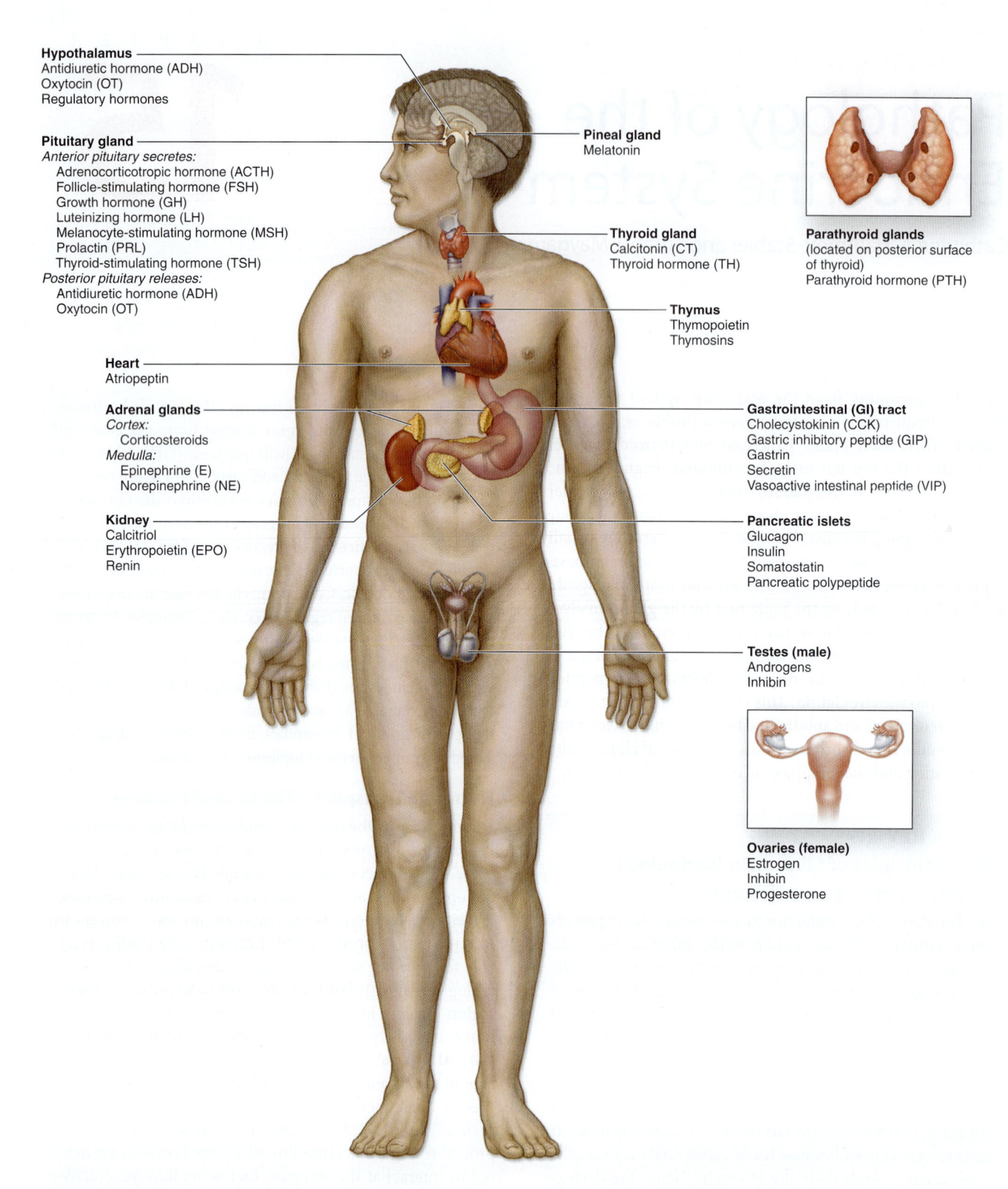

Ovaries (female)
Estrogen
Inhibin
Progesterone

FIGURE 15-1 Endocrine system. The endocrine glands and major hormones they secrete are listed with their locations. In parentheses are shown other organs, including the heart, kidney, thymus, gut, and gonads, which contain endocrine cells and have important endocrine functions. In addition, many widely distributed tissues and cells throughout the body have endocrine functions but are not shown here. These include adipose cells, which secrete the hormone leptin, and vascular endothelial cells, which produce polypeptides called endothelins, which promote vasoconstriction. (Reproduced with permission from McKinley M, O'Loughlin V.D. Human Anatomy. 2nd ed. New York: McGraw-Hill, 2004 (Figure 20-1).)

TABLE 15-1 Hormone transport proteins.

Protein	Hormone
Albumin	All
Thyroid-binding globulin (TBG)	T3, T4
Thyroid-binding prealbumin (TBPA, transthyretin)	T4
Cortisol-binding globulin (CBG)	Cortisol
Sex hormone-binding globulin (SHBG)	Estradiol, testosterone
Vitamin D-binding globulin (VDBG)	Vitamin D

minutes before being degraded. At the target cell surface, these compounds bind to specific receptors and in doing so activate intermediate messengers that cause a downstream response. *Steroid hormones circulate in combination with a protein. As a result, they have longer half-lives (on the order of hours). Their lipophilic nature facilitates entry into the target cell in order to bind to specific intracellular receptors.* The steroid–receptor complex interacts with the nucleus to elicit an alteration in gene expression and protein synthesis. Although steroids typically travel some distance from the site of origin, the importance of their actions at the local level is now recognized. Additionally, the local metabolism of hormone precursors also contributes to many of the biological effects observed. *Amines circulate both free and protein bound and act via cell surface receptors (catecholamines) and through nuclear receptors (thyroid hormones).*

Regulation and Rhythms

A recurring theme in the following sections is the pattern of secretion observed for many hormones. Two observations must be considered when using hormone measurements in patient care. First, many display a distinctive circadian or diurnal pattern characterized by a gradual rise and subsequent fall in concentrations over the 24-hour period. The circadian pattern observed is tied to the individual's biological clock, which in turn is synchronized to a combination of events including retinal response to light-dark, hormonal signals from sleep, awakening, and feeding, and is subject to neuronal and humoral signals originating from the suprachiasmatic nucleus as well as peripheral tissues (heart, gut, muscle). Second, although one may observe rapid rises, or pulses, in concentration to allow the body to respond quickly to changing needs, the concentrations quoted in reference ranges result from more long-term effects on the pattern of hormone secretion.

One of the most important features of the endocrine system is its ability to self-regulate by either positive or negative feedback control. Positive feedback control is stimulatory resulting in rapid changes. An example is the release of oxytocin to stimulate uterine contractions, which, in turn, stimulates the release of more oxytocin. In contrast, the overall effect in negative feedback control is inhibition. Negative feedback mechanisms exist throughout the endocrine system, and the hypothalamic–pituitary–thyroid axis is often used as an illustration. In response to the circulating levels of the key secretory hormones (thyroxin, T4 and triiodothyronine, T3) released by the thyroid, the hypothalamus and pituitary alter production of their own hormonal products, in this example, thyrotropin releasing factor (TRH) and thyroid stimulating hormone (TSH), respectively. In the case of decreased thyroid function, less T4 and T3 are released into the circulation and the hypothalamus and pituitary respond by increasing their appropriate hormones in an attempt to stimulate the thyroid. Conversely, should the thyroid become over active as in hyperthyroid states, the hypothalamus and pituitary sense the elevated T4 and T3 concentrations, and in turn, decrease production of their hormones, TRH and TSH. These events are collectively known as negative feedback and help to maintain the secretory hormone within a narrow range.

Hormonal control is further defined by the individual's set point that some consider one's personal reference range. The set point typically falls within the expected population reference range but is unlikely to be at the mean or median of that range. *The concept is important to remember when a change in a patient's hormone concentration is observed along with clinical signs and symptoms even if the concentration remains within the reference range.*

HYPOTHALAMIC–PITUITARY AXIS

The hypothalamus serves as a link between the CNS and the endocrine system. The pituitary gland, also known as the **hypophysis**, is located beneath the hypothalamus in the bony sella turcica. Structurally, the pituitary can be divided into the **anterior** (**adenohypophysis**) and **posterior** (**neurohypophysis**) sections. The anterior pituitary is further subdivided into the **pars distalis** (accounting for the bulk of the region), **pars tuberalis, and pars intermedia** (Figure 15-2). Within the hypothalamus, hypophysiotropic neurons secrete specific factors that travel via the adenohypophyseal portal system to the anterior pituitary where they bind to receptors to either stimulate or inhibit the secretion of the five major anterior pituitary hormones. In addition, neurons located primarily in the supraoptic and paraventricular nuclei of the hypothalamus secrete vasopressin and oxytocin from axons extending into the neurohypophysis.

QUICK REVIEW

Histologically, the pars distalis of the anterior lobe is composed of cords of secretory cells, that is, the somatotrophs, lactotrophs, thyrotrophs, corticotrophs, and gonadotrophs (Table 15-2). By the names alone, one can surmise that they are responsible for the synthesis and release of specific hormones: growth hormone (GH), prolactin (PRL), thyroid-stimulating hormone (TSH), adrenocorticotropin,

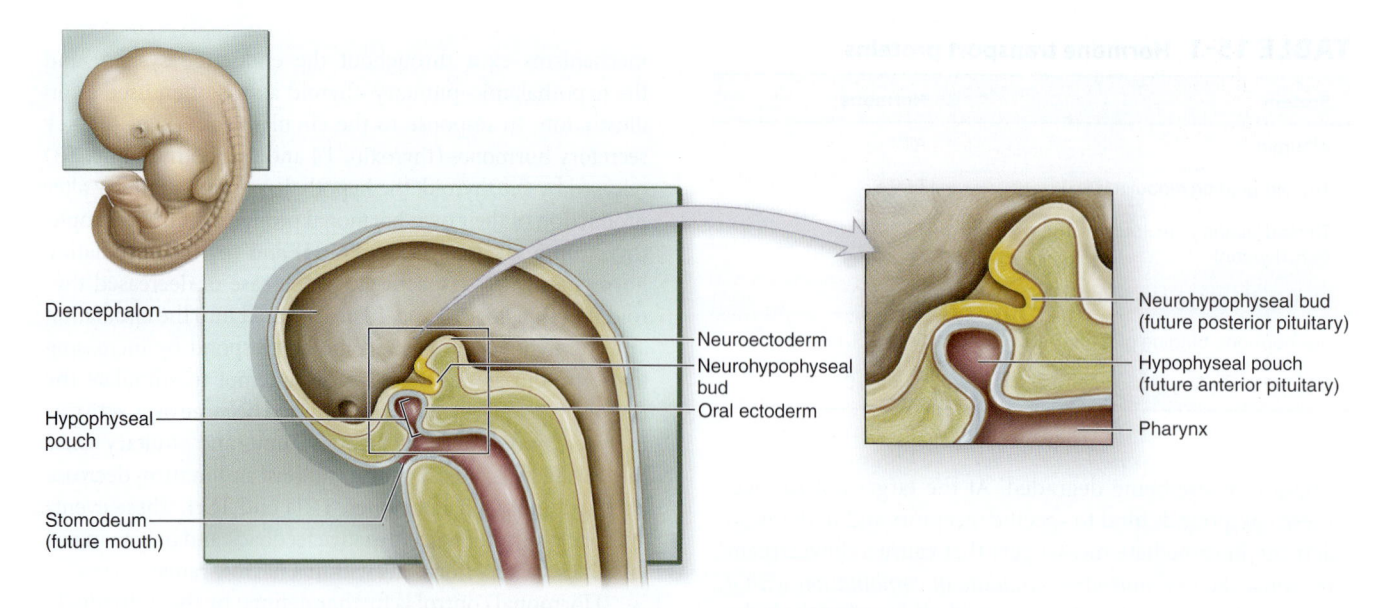

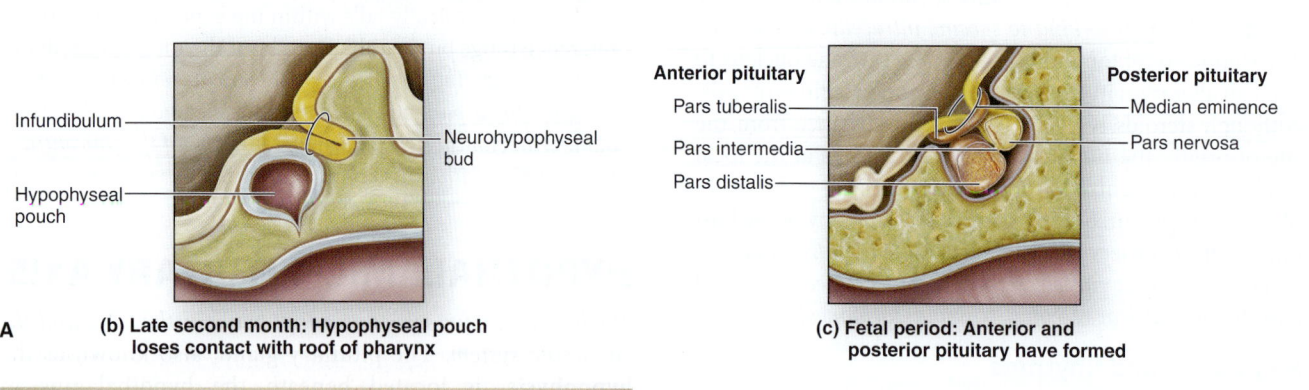

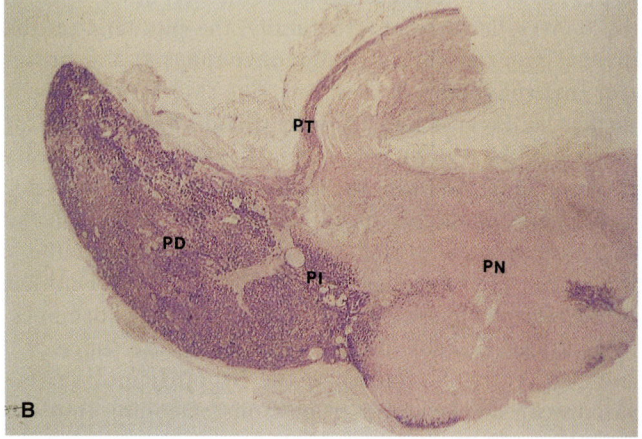

FIGURE 15-2 **(A) Formation of the pituitary gland.** The pituitary gland is formed from two separate embryonic structures. (a) During the third week of development, a hypophyseal pouch (or Rathke pouch, the future anterior pituitary) grows from the roof of the pharynx, while a neurohypophyseal bud (future posterior pituitary) is formed from the diencephalon. (b) By late in the second month, the hypophyseal pouch detaches from the roof of the pharynx and merges with the neurohypophyseal bud. (c) During the fetal period, the anterior and posterior parts of the pituitary complete development. (Reproduced with permission from McKinley M, O'Loughlin VD Human Anatomy. 2nd ed. New York: McGraw-Hill, 2004 (Figure 20-15).) **(B)** Histology of the pituitary gland. Histologically, the two parts of the pituitary gland reflect their origins, as seen in this low-magnification section of an entire gland. The infundibular stalk (IS) and pars nervosa (PN) of the neurohypophysis resemble CNS tissue, while the adenohypophysis' pars distalis (PD), pars intermedia (PI), and pars tuberalis (PT) are typically glandular in their level of staining. X15. Hematoxylin and eosin (H&E). (Reproduced with permission from Berman B. Color Atlas of Basic Histology. 3rd ed. New York: McGraw-Hill, 2003 (Figure 17-1).)

TABLE 15-2 Summary of pituitary hormones.

Pituitary Hormone	Cells Responsible for Synthesis	Hypothalamus Releasing Hormones	Inhibiting Factors	Target Gland or Tissue	Function
Adrenocorticotropin hormone (ACTH)	Corticotrophs	Corticotropin-releasing hormone (CRH); Arginine vasopressin (AVP)		Adrenal	Stimulation of corticosteroids and adrenal androgens
Growth hormone (GH)	Somatotrophs	GH-releasing hormone (GHRH)	Somatostatin (somatotropin-release inhibiting hormone, SRIF)[c]	Peripheral tissue, liver	Direct and indirect (insulin-like growth factor 1, IGF-1) stimulation of growth, metabolism, homeostasis
Prolactin (PRL)	Lactotrophs	Oxytocin, thyrotropin-releasing hormone (TRH)	Dopamine[d]	Mammary gland	Stimulation of lactation
Thyrotropin or thyroid-stimulating hormone (TSH)[a]	Thyrotrophs	TRH	Somatostatin	Thyroid	Stimulation of thyroid hormone release
Luteinizing hormone (LH)[a]	Gonadotrophs	Gonadotropin-releasing hormone (GnRH)[b]		Ovary, testis	Stimulation of estrogen and testosterone production
Follicle-stimulating hormone (FSH)[a]	Gonadotrophs	GnRH[b]		Ovary, testis	Regulation of theca and Sertoli cell function
Human chorionic gonadotropin (hCG)[a]	Gonadotrophs	GnRH	unknown	unknown	Differs from placental and trophoblastic isoforms. The role of pituitary hCG is unknown—it may serve to facilitate some of the LH functions

[a]TSH, LH, FSH and hCG belong to the glycoprotein hormone family.
[b]GnRH is also known as luteinizing hormone-releasing hormone, LHRH.
[c]SRIF is also known as somatostatin and growth hormone inhibitory hormone (GHIF or GHIH).
[d]Other PRL-release inhibiting factors are known.

and luteinizing hormone (LH) and follicle-stimulating hormone (FSH), respectively. Although one can use traditional histological staining methods to distinguish between the cell types, these methods cannot be used to identify the specific hormonal products. In general, however, the somatotrophs and lactotrophs exhibit acidophilic staining, while the corticotrophs, thyrotrophs, and gonadotrophs exhibit basophilic staining (Figure 15-3). The posterior lobe is nervous tissue composed of axons whose neuronal cell bodies are in the hypothalamus and modified glial cells (also known as pituicytes).

TROPIC HORMONES OF THE ANTERIOR PITUITARY

The hormones of the anterior pituitary include GH, PRL, ACTH, TSH, LH, and FSH. *Abnormalities associated with GH and PRL are of particular significance in terms of anterior pituitary pathology.*

Growth Hormone

GH is the most abundant hormone produced by the anterior pituitary. The hormone is a relatively small, single-chain peptide that circulates in both free and protein-bound forms in about a 50-50 ratio. Hypothalamic **growth hormone releasing hormone** (GHRH) stimulates release, while **somatotropin-release inhibiting factor** (SRIF, somatostatin) inhibits release. The actions of GHRH, that is, release, are now thought to dominate since disruption of the pathway leads to GH deficiency. Negative feedback through a short feedback loop also plays a role as GH itself stimulates the hypothalamus to produce SRIF.

Hypopituitarism and Deficiency of Growth Hormone

GH deficiency is a problem encountered in children who have not achieved their normal stature. This excludes children who are genetically predisposed to being short statured, who are malnourished, or who have an underlying systemic illness.

The terms hypopituitarism and GH deficiency are often used interchangeably because pituitary dysfunction rarely occurs without GH deficiency. Hypopituitarism has many causes, as seen in Table 15-3, and the presentation varies depending on the age of the patient. Disorders of the hypothalamus may cause GH deficiency by impairing GHRH secretion, whereas lesions of the pituitary or the pituitary stalk may directly cause GH deficiency. Unfortunately, "idiopathic hypopituitarism" is the most frequent cause of GH deficiency in children and may occur as a result of trauma during birth or in the perinatal period. For others, as yet unrecognized genetic mutations are

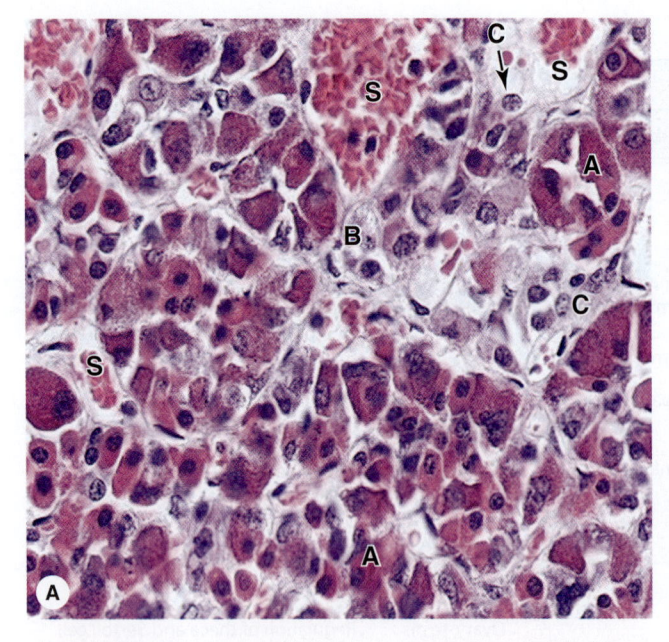

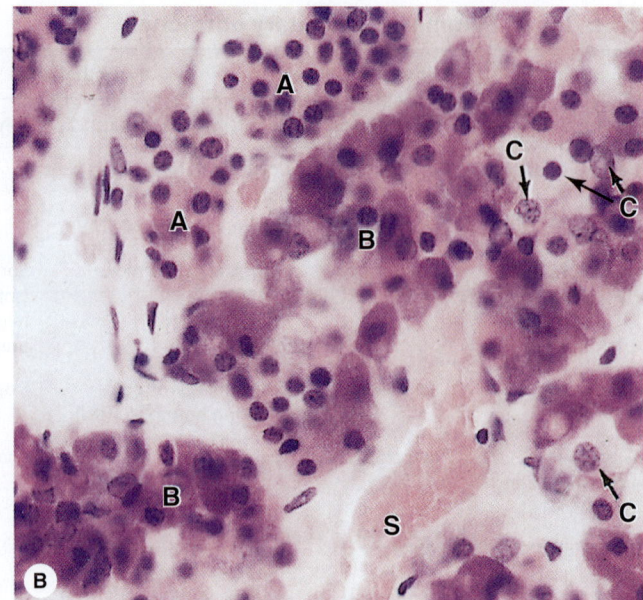

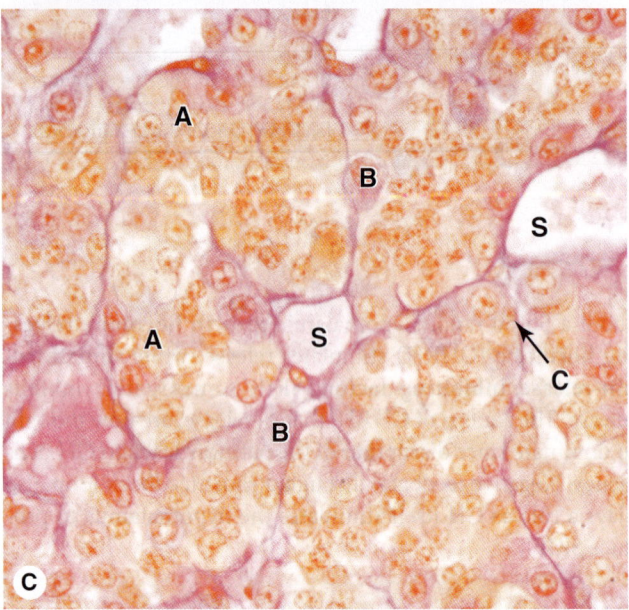

FIGURE 15-3 **Pars distalis:** Acidophils, basophils, and chromophobes. **(A,B).** Most general staining methods simply allow the parenchymal cells of the pars distalis to be subdivided into acidophil cells (A), basophils (B), and chromophobes (C) in which the cytoplasm is poorly stained. ×400. H&E. **(B)** Gomori trichrome provides similar information. ×400. Cords of acidophils and basophils vary in distribution and number in different regions of the pars distalis, but are always closely associated with capillaries and sinusoids (S) in the second capillary plexus of the portal system. The vascular plexus carries off secreted hormones into the general circulation. Specific acidophil or basophil cells can be identified immunohistologically with antibodies against their hormone products. Chromophobes are less numerous and represent various undifferentiated parenchymal cells. Their number and density also vary in different regions. (Reproduced with permission from Mescher AL. Junqueira's Basic Histology: Text and Atlas. 12th ed. New York: McGraw Hill Lange, 2010:353 (Figure 20-6).)

likely. In many cases, nutritional, psychological, or pharmacological causes are suspected.

Most defects in multiple pituitary hormone secretion are related to compressive or other tissue destructive causes including CNS tumors (craniopharyngioma being a notable example), neurological insults, and cranial radiotherapy. In such cases the cells responsible for the hormone synthesis will usually cease, functioning in a specific order. Loss of GH typically occurs first followed by loss of LH/FSH, then loss of TSH, and finally ACTH.

Congenital deficiencies of pituitary hormones are uncommon (1 in 50,000 births). They may affect pituitary gland development and be associated with hyposecretion of multiple pituitary hormones (**combined pituitary hormone deficiency CPHD** or **panhypopituitarism**). Congenital CPHD results from mutations in genes for developmental factors necessary for pituitary gland maturation. Most of these genes affect the anterior pituitary. Mutations in two transcription factors (POUF-1/PIT-1 and PROP1) are associated with CHPD (the latter accounting for about 30% of cases) in which GH as well as PRL and TSH are deficient.

Isolated growth hormone deficiency (IGHD) is associated with mutations in the growth hormone gene (GH1) and in the GHRH receptor gene. The most severe form (Type 1A) is associated with deletion of the GH1 gene. Most cases of IGHD are idiopathic (not currently associated with a known genetic defect). Genetic defects in hypothalamic factors have also been associated with congenital pituitary defects. Therapy relies on recombinant human GH. Patients with Type 1A disease may become refractory to therapy as a result of developing neutralizing antibodies to the recombinant protein.

TABLE 15-3 Causes of hypopituitarism.

Pituitary Diseases	
Genetic etiologies	Aplasia and hypoplasia due to mutations in a pituitary transcription factors, such as Prop-1 and Pit-1. Isolated GH deficiency due to mutation in the GH-N gene
Intrasellar tumors	Craniopharyngiomas, adenomas, and metastatic tumors
Nontumorous destruction	Infarction associated with trauma, infection, head irradiation, postpartum necrosis (Sheehan syndrome)
Disorders of the Hypothalamus	
Idiopathic	Often associated with birth trauma and other forms of perinatal injury
Familial forms	Midline central nervous system (CNS) and facial development defects: septo-optic dysplasia, holoprosencephaly, cleft lip or palate, single upper central incisor
Infections and inflammatory diseases	Tuberculosis, sarcoidosis
Histiocytosis	
Hypothalamic tumors	Craniopharyngiomas, neurofibromas, gliomas, germinomas, metastatic tumors to the hypothalamus
Functional disorders	Psychosocial dwarfism, anorexia nervosa
Disorders of Growth Hormone (GH) Responsiveness (GH high, IGF-I low)	
Receptor abnormalities	Laron dwarfism (GH receptors mutations), pygmies
Biologically inactive GH	
Protein-calorie malnutrition	

WHAT WE DO

Diagnosis of Hypopituitarism and GH Deficiency in Children

In the newborn or neonatal period, IGHD and even panhypopituitarism may be difficult to identify. Growth is usually not affected during this period and there may be few, if any, symptoms with IGHD. A significant clue of panhypopituitarism during this period, however, is the occurrence of episodes of hypoglycemia due to the combined deficiency of cortisol and GH. In childhood, a decrease in linear growth velocity is a hallmark feature of both IGHD and panhypopituitarism. This is often apparent after 6 months of life, but can occur at any age. These children are often modestly overweight and look younger than their age due to immature facial bone structure. *Without treatment, those with panhypopituitarism will not progress through puberty and will eventually exhibit signs and symptoms of TSH and/or ACTH deficiency as the disease progresses.*

A single GH measurement is not an optimal measure to assess deficiency. In children, it is better to assess the response of the pituitary to a stimulus such as the tests shown in **Table 15-4** (GH stimulation tests). IGF-1 contributes to GH regulation by directly stimulating the hypothalamus to release SRIF. Because IGF-1 has a much longer half-life compared with GH, it is useful as a substitute for GH testing when evaluating patients. Although GH-deficient patients will usually have corresponding low IGF-1 concentrations, a low IGF-1 is not specific for GH deficiency but may be related to poor nutrition, renal disease, hypothyroidism, or psychological disorders.

Diagnosis of Hypopituitarism in Adults

The presentation of hypopituitarism in an adult depends on the hormone(s) that are deficient, the magnitude of the deficiency, and the rapidity of occurrence. For example, symptoms, including those of ACTH deficiency, may occur quite rapidly following infarction or postpartum necrosis (**Sheehan syndrome**).

Progression of hypopituitarism may be insidious following cranial irradiation and symptoms may be subtle for many years. Adults typically are diagnosed after they encounter symptoms related to secondary hypogonadism (amenorrhea for women and impotence for men). With progression or involvement of the thyrotrophs, signs and symptoms of secondary hypothyroidism may develop. In some cases, the patient is diagnosed when symptoms of secondary hypoadrenalism develop and they are unable to handle a stress—in severe cases, a life-threatening adrenal crisis may ensue causing vascular collapse.

Testing will show low tropic hormones from the pituitary and low secretory hormones from the endocrine gland, for example, a low TSH with a low thyroxine. Additional provocative testing may be needed to sort through apparent mild or subtle deficiencies. These include the use of GnRH to test FSH and LH reserve, ACTH to test adrenal reserve, TRH to distinguish pituitary from hypothalamic causes of abnormal thyroid function, and so on.

CASE 15-1

A 21-year-old female is found unresponsive at home. In the emergency room, she is found to have altered metal status, is afebrile with a pulse rate of 50 beats per minute, respiration 12 per minute, and blood pressure is 100/60 mmHg. Stat laboratory results (with reference ranges) include sodium 134 mmol/L (135–145), potassium 4.0 mmol/L (3.5–5.0), chloride 110 mmol/L (98–107), and a whole blood glucose (point of care) 40 mg/dL (65–179). (Quick review of these laboratory values: the most significant result is the critically low glucose, consistent with hypoglycemia. The sodium is mildly decreased and the chloride is mildly increased. As part of the exercise, you may want to stop and think about the causes of these changes.)

She became responsive with emergent treatment that included intravenous administration of 50% dextrose. Her family reports that she gave birth to her third child 4 months earlier. Since that time she has complained of fatigue, malaise, and weakness, which was attributed to postpartum depression and the care of three children plus full-time employment. They also note, however, that she has had episodes of vomiting, abdominal pain, and diarrhea. She does not use alcohol or drugs, is not diabetic, and until the delivery was in good health and active.

The patient's hypoglycemia may be a life-threatening event. Many times its occurrence is related to the effect of a medication or alcohol use, but other causes include liver disease, uremia, neoplasms (insulinoma, for example), metabolic disorders such as glycogen storage diseases, and endocrinopathies such as hypoadrenalism, hypopituitarism, and glucagon deficiency. Additional testing reveals a TSH of <0.1 μIU/mL (0.4–4.5), cortisol less than 1.5 μg/dL (5–20), FSH 1.0 μIU/mL (1.5–12), PRL 1.3 ng/mL (3–20).

With these results, panhypopituitarism resulting from postpartum infarction of the anterior pituitary, also known as **Sheehan syndrome***, is suspected.* This condition was first described in 1937 by a British pathologist. Improved obstetrical care has reduced the frequency in developed countries, but it still occurs. The blood flow to and within the anterior pituitary is among the highest of any other organ. During pregnancy, the pituitary enlarges and becomes vulnerable to ischemia. In the event of severe postpartum hemorrhage, the resulting systemic hypotension may lead to vasospasm and pituitary infarction.

GH Excess and Pituitary Adenomas

Excessive GH production leads to **acromegaly** *in adults and* **gigantism** *when it occurs in children. At least 90% of all cases of acromegaly are associated with pituitary adenomas.* Neoplasms of the pituitary are almost invariably benign and common. Autopsy and radiographic studies suggest that between 15% and 20% of normal persons have unapparent tumors; symptomatic tumors are much less common (0.1% in community-based studies). Although benign, pituitary adenomas may have serious clinical consequences involving mass effects (such as headache, cranial nerve palsies, bitemporal hemianopia, and visual defect in the temporal half of each eye's visual field), panhypopituitarism and ultimately destruction of the sella as a result of pressure-related damage. Symptoms relating to mass effects are usually associated with **macroadenomas** (larger than 1cm in diameter). Rapid expansion of a macroadenoma as a result of infarction and/or hemorrhage may result in **pituitary apoplexy**, the acute onset of symptoms related to mass effects requiring prompt surgical intervention. Hyperfunction of the pituitary, and in particular excess of a single hormone, is (as noted above) most often the result of a functional (hormone secreting) adenoma, which comprises about 80% of pituitary adenomas.

Most adenomas are derived from the anterior pituitary and are monoclonal, demonstrating sheets or cords of uniformly stained cells (Figure 15-4). Twenty-five percent of pituitary adenomas are lactotrophs (**prolactinomas**) and are the most common type. Somatotropic (GH secreting) adenomas are relatively uncommon (5–15% of adenomas). Twenty-five percent of GH secreting adenomas also secrete PRL. A proportion of such multiple hormone secreting tumors is polyclonal. Monoclonal, pluripotent primitive stem cell-derived tumors occur, are aggressive, and are associated with gigantism in teenagers. Pituitary adenomas may be sporadic or familial and details of the molecular pathology of such are available.

The patient who has acromegaly has a distinctive physical appearance due to acral growth of flat bone that leads to large, broad features of the hands, feet, and nose. The skin becomes thickened due to excess collagen. Physical examination will reveal a generalized enlargement of the organs. These disorders can progress slowly and not be recognized for some time. These patients usually have elevated GH concentrations that do not suppress (see below). *Because (as noted above) IGF-I concentrations are directly influenced by GH and are not subject*

TABLE 15-4 Examples of growth hormone stimulating tests.

Stimulus	Time of Peak GH Release
20–30 minutes of vigorous exercise	20 minutes after beginning
Arginine	60–120 minutes
Glucagon	120–180 minutes
L-dopa	30–120 minutes
Clonidine	90 minutes

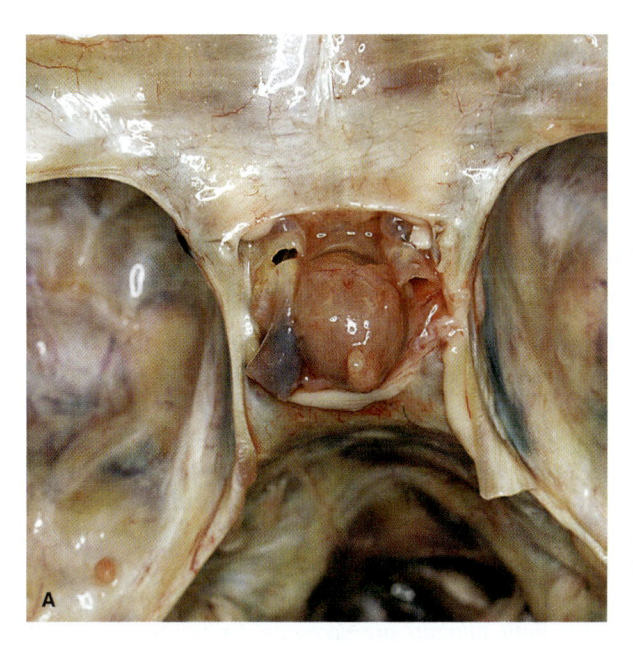

FIGURE 15-4 Pituitary adenoma. **(A)** Gross photograph of organ exposed in sella turcica of sphenoid. **(B)** Photomicrograph of pituitary pars dorsalis demonstrating adenoma in upper half of image. Note uniform population of acidophilic cells in contrast to mixed population in the normal area (bottom half of the image). ((4a) Contributed with permission of Clay Nichols, MD NC Medical Examiners Office.)

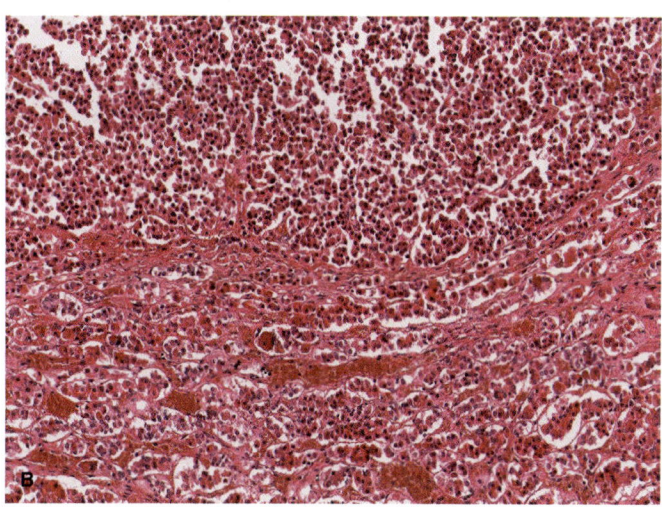

to rapid fluctuations, they are now used in the diagnosis of these patient suspected to have excess GH production. IGF-I concentrations also correlate well with clinical severity of the disease. Treatment is complex and includes radiosurgical approaches or the use of pharmacological agents including somatostatin receptor ligands (somatostatin analogues) and GH receptor antagonists.

Prolactin

PRL is a 198 amino acid protein produced by the lactotrophs. As the name of these cells suggest, PRL controls initiation and maintenance of lactation providing the breast tissue has been primed by estrogens, progestins, corticosteroids, thyroid hormone, and insulin. Regulation of PRL is unique in that primary control is inhibitory rather than stimulatory. Dopamine appears to be the main PRL inhibitory factor, but there may be others. Several PRL releasing factors have been identified including thyrotropin-releasing hormone (TRH), vasoactive intestinal peptide, and estrogen. PRL deficiency is important during the postpartum period because it is necessary for lactation. In such cases the PRL deficiency may be related to Sheehan syndrome (see Case 15-1). Outside of this period and in males, the impact is not well defined.

The diagnosis of hyperprolactinemia, the most common hypothalamic–pituitary disorder, can be quite challenging as there are multiple etiologies for the disorder. Mild elevations in PRL may be seen in chronic renal failure, following breast stimulation, in primary hypothyroidism, in empty sella syndrome, and in response to many drugs (antihypertensives, phenothiazines, morphine, methyldopa, and some antidepressants). Even mild hyperprolactinemia can inhibit ovulation

WHAT WE DO

The diagnosis of acromegaly is confirmed by performing an oral glucose tolerance test and noting the failure of the GH concentration to suppress as seen in **Figure 15-5**. A normal response (diamonds) is a suppressed serum GH to <1 ng/mL. In contrast, all acromegaly patients respond abnormally showing either (1) a lack of suppression, (squares) or (2) a paradoxical increase (triangles), a response seen in ~20% of cases for unknown reasons.

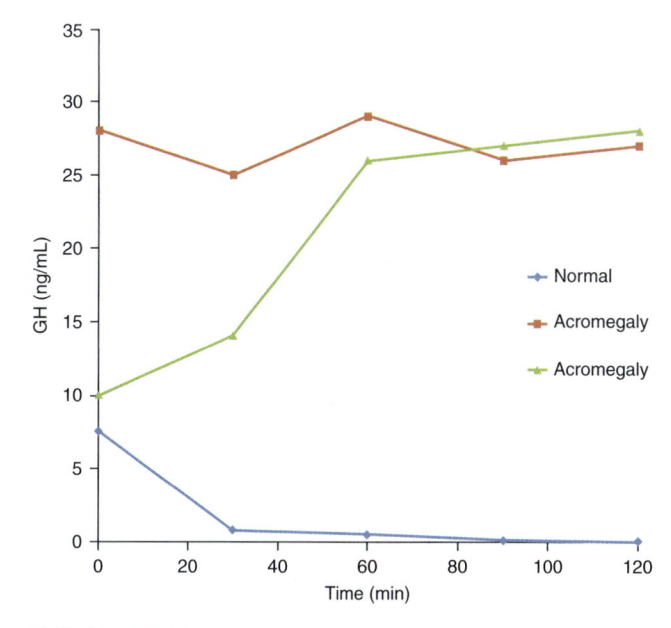

FIGURE 15-5 Serum growth hormone response to oral glucose.

> **CASE 15-2**
>
> ED is a 42-year-old female who begins to experience frequent headaches that she thinks are related to a need for new glasses. On a routine examination by her optometrist, she is found to have a visual field defect and was immediately referred for workup. He immediately refers ED to you. During her history and physical, she reports she has had irregular menses for a number of years but few other complaints or problems. MRI reveals a tumor of approximately 1.2 cm in size within the sella. Laboratory testing is within normal limits with the exception of PRL, which is elevated at 1152 ng/mL. In the absence of PRL-stimulating drugs or a recent pregnancy, the increased PRL concentration suggests the tumor is a prolactinoma.

and lead to infertility. Patients who are found to have a macroprolactinoma can have very elevated PRL concentrations. Tumors of the lactotrophs vary considerably in size and in their production of PRL. However, many prolactinomas are less than 1 cm in diameter and grow slowly thus permitting careful monitoring if detected. The elevated PRL inhibits the secretion of gonadotropin releasing hormone (GnRH) that leads to ovarian dysfunction, amenorrhea, and galactorrhea. This syndrome is the most common presentation of patients with functioning pituitary adenomas. Nonsurgical treatment involves the use of dopamine D2 receptor agonists such as bromocriptine and cabergoline, which directly inhibit hormone secretion.

Besides PRL and other hormones discussed earlier, additional tropic hormones secreted by the anterior pituitary include ACTH, TSH, LH, and FSH and are discussed as follows.

Adrenocorticotropin Hormone

ACTH is a product of the corticotrophs. This 39 amino acid polypeptide fragment originates from a larger precursor molecule, **proopiomelanocortin** (POMC) that also gives rise to β-lipotropin. **Corticotropin-releasing hormone** (CRH) and proinflammatory cytokines stimulate release of the peptide in response to biorhythms and various stimuli. ACTH synthesis can also be stimulated by high concentrations of **antidiuretic hormone** (ADH) interacting with the vasopressin type 3 receptors on the corticotrophs. ACTH exerts a number of effects on the adrenal cortex including the incorporation of lipoprotein-bound cholesterol into the gland, stimulation of RNA and protein synthesis, and promotion of cell differentiation. *Most importantly, it is the primary regulator of the secretion of cortisol and androgenic steroids by the adrenal cortex.*

Because of this close relationship, ACTH and cortisol follow very similar patterns of release. During a 24-hour period, maximal (peak) concentrations are achieved between 0400 and 0800 with the lowest (trough) concentrations seen approximately 12 hours later in response to sleep-wake cycles. Individuals who have altered hours of sleep and wakefulness such as those who work the midnight shift, for example, have a shift, even a reversal, in their diurnal rhythm. In addition to the characteristic diurnal pattern, episodic increases in concentrations are associated with various stressors.

Luteinizing Hormone and Follicle-Stimulating Hormone

LH and **FSH** are synthesized and released from gonadotrophs located in the anterior pituitary in response to GnRH. GnRH is secreted by the hypothalamus in a pulsatile manner in response to estrogen in the female and testosterone in the male. Biochemically, LH and FSH are glycoproteins consisting of an α- and β-subunit. The α-subunit that is involved in receptor binding is identical in structure to the α-subunit of both TSH and human chorionic gonadotropin (hCG). The unique β-subunit of each provides immunospecificity and hormonal activity. Both subunits are necessary for full biological activity. Once released from the gonadotrophs, LH and FSH travel through the circulation to the gonads. In the female, FSH stimulates the growth and maturation of ovarian follicles, stimulates estrogen secretion, and promotes endometrial changes of the proliferative phase of the menstrual cycle. LH acts with FSH to promote ovulation and secretion of androgens and progesterone. LH also initiates and maintains the secretory phase of the menstrual cycle and contributes to the formation of the corpus luteum. For each hormone, serum concentrations in women vary with the menstrual cycle and increase postmenopause. In the male, FSH stimulates spermatogenesis through its actions on the Sertoli cells, while LH stimulates development and function of Leydig cells in the testes.

Because of the actions of LH and FSH on gonadal function, gonadal failure is often the earliest symptom of pituitary insufficiency. The most direct approach to ruling out primary gonadal insufficiency from pituitary insufficiency is to measure the pituitary gonadotropins. In these cases, depressed LH and FSH concentrations are suggestive of pituitary insufficiency, while elevated concentrations rule out pituitary deficiency.

Thyroid-Stimulating Hormone (Thyrotropin) and Human Chorionic Gonadotropin

TSH (thyrotropin) stimulates growth and vascularity of the thyroid gland, growth of the follicular cells, and promotes most of the steps in thyroid hormone synthesis. TSH release is regulated by hypothalamic TRH and the thyroid hormones, T3 and T4. TSH is a 31-kDa glycoprotein composed of two subunits: the α-subunit shared with other glycoproteins (LH, FSH, and hCG) and a unique β-subunit that confers specificity. TSH will be discussed in greater detail in the thyroid section of the chapter.

hCG is not typically thought of as a pituitary hormone, but in fact, small amounts of this hormone can be produced by the gonadotrophs, most often during the peri- and postmenopausal periods. The pituitary-derived hCG concentrations found in the serum and urine are low (usually <15 IU/L), but may raise concerns of pregnancy or gestational trophoblastic disease. An elevated FSH is helpful in the immediate assessment of a patient to rule out pregnancy prior to an urgent procedure. hCG of pituitary origin should suppress with 2 weeks of estrogen replacement. If the low hCG levels persist, trophoblastic disease must be considered.

TUMORS AFFECTING PITUITARY FUNCTION

Pituitary Adenomas

Adenomas are by far the most common tumors of the pituitary. These have already been discussed in the section "GH Excess and Pituitary Adenomas."

Craniopharyngioma

Craniopharyngiomas are among the more common causes of panhypopituitarism in children. Adamantinomatous (demonstrating areas of calcification) craniopharyngiomas are most common in youth. Such tumors are commonly associated with mutations in the β-catenin gene, an activator of the Wnt signaling pathway. Squamous papillary tumors are more common in adults and are not associated with a known genetic lesion (Figure 15-6). In either case, craniopharyngiomas are composed of epithelial cells that proliferate and occupy space in and above the sella turcica, encroaching on adjacent pituitary and hypothalamic tissue. Although the tumors are defined as benign by histology, they grow slowly in an invasive pattern and tend to recur, particularly when complete surgical removal is problematic. The tumors proliferate such that symptoms manifest in the first few years of life, though there are cases in which the lesion is not apparent clinically until late in life.

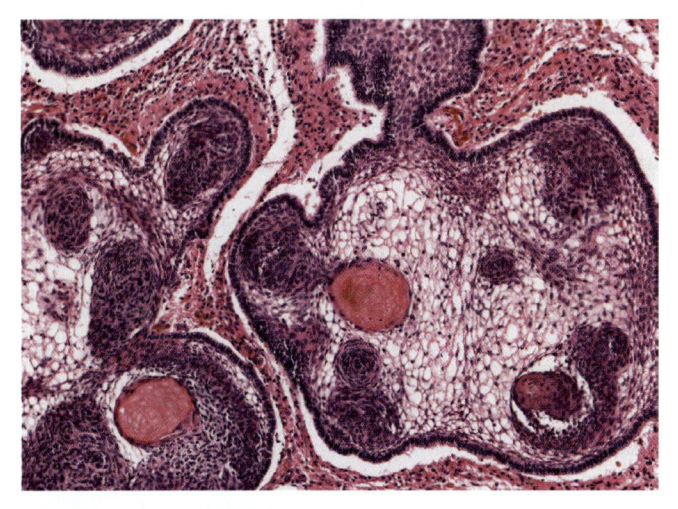

FIGURE 15-6 **Suprasellar craniopharyngioma.** Photomicrograph demonstrates epithelial islands that are surrounded by a layer of palisading cells. The islands contain amorphous pink areas of keratinization.

Pathogenesis of Pituitary Adenomas

IN TRANSLATION

Forty percent of sporadic GH secreting tumors have an activating mutation in the G protein subunit α-gene (GNAS or gsp) that results in constitutively elevated levels of cAMP. Somatic mosaicism for such activating GNAS mutations result in **McCune–Albright syndrome** (MAS), which is characterized by bone abnormalities (polyostotic fibrous dysplasia), dermal café-au-lait spots, and a spectrum of endocrine disorders notably including acromegaly. Although MAS is rare, somatic activating mutations for GNAS are common in sporadic pituitary adenomas (as noted above). Hence, such mutations are likely to play a role in adenoma generation. A number of familial inherited disorders are also associated with pituitary adenomas. The most important of which is **multiple endocrine neoplasia syndrome type 1 (MEN1)**. MEN1 is an autosomal dominant disorder associated with mutation in the *MEN1* gene, which encodes the nuclear protein **menin**. *MEN1* functions as a tumor suppressor and tumors are associated with loss of heterozygosity (LOH) at the locus. MEN1 is characterized by the formation of adenomas in multiple endocrine organs (including the parathyroid gland in 90% of patients and the pituitary gland in 10–60% of patients). In addition, endocrine tumors of the thyroid gland, adrenal cortex, and pancreas are common. Nonendocrine tumors include lipomas, meningiomas, facial angiofibromas, and carcinoids at various sites. MEN1 is responsible for 3% of pituitary adenomas, which when functional, most often secrete GH and PRL. Progression to malignancy, although uncommon, has been reported to occur.

Malignant Pituitary Tumors

Pituitary carcinomas *are exceedingly rare constituting no more than 0.2% of all pituitary tumors.* They are defined by their ability to metastasize beyond the pituitary to the cerebrospinal space or extracranial regions. Most pituitary carcinomas are functional with nearly half the tumors secreting ACTH, which is rarely secreted by adenomas.

POSTERIOR PITUITARY

The posterior pituitary is predominantly neural tissue derived from downward evagination of the neural tube. Most, but not all cells, are located in the supraoptic and paraventricular nuclei and are responsible for the synthesis of **oxytocin** and ADH (also referred to as vasopressin, arginine vasopressin, AVP). As with other hormones, oxytocin and ADH originate from two precursor proteins, that is, prooxyphysin and propressophysin.

Oxytocin is released in response to vaginal and lower uterine distention during labor. Upon release, oxytocin stimulates contractions of the uterine smooth muscle. In addition, oxytocin is released in response to suckling in order to stimulate the myoepithelial cells of the mammary alveoli thus causing milk ejection and efficient emptying of the breasts.

The release of ADH is mediated by osmoreceptors in the hypothalamus that respond to plasma osmolality. A decrease in plasma volume, stress, nicotine, morphine, and barbiturates can also stimulate release. The primary role of ADH is to reduce water excretion by concentrating urine through its actions on the distal tubules and medullary collecting ducts. Disorders of ADH can be divided into hypofunction (**polyuric states** and **diabetes insipidus, DI**) and hyperfunction (**syndrome of inappropriate ADH secretion**, SIADH).

Polyuria and Diabetes Insipidus

While "normal" urine output is not definable, any patient who excretes more than 2.5–3.5 L/day warrants investigation for polyuria. When there is insufficient ADH, the renal cells become impermeable to water and reabsorb little of the dilute filtrate entering from the proximal nephron. As a result, large volumes of very dilute urine are excreted. The range of impairment is extremely variable—in some, the effect is so intense that the person excretes 5–10 L/day. Usually, the urine-specific gravity is close to that of water (approximately 1.000) and the osmolality is also decreased to less than 300 mOsm/kg. **Hypothalamic diabetes insipidus** (HDI) occurs when there is insufficient ADH produced (also called neurohypophyseal or central DI). This is most commonly caused by trauma to the pituitary resulting from tumors or surgery. DI may also be related to renal disease or behavioral disturbances. The latter is associated with excessive fluid consumption (psychogenic polydipsia).

Syndrome of Inappropriate Antidiuretic Hormone Secretion

The syndrome represents the autonomous, sustained production of ADH in the absence of known stimuli. SIADH is associated with a broad range of potential etiologies including ectopic hormone production by neoplasias (including carcinomas and carcinoids), drug effects, pulmonary disease, and a host of neurological/psychiatric disorders. The diagnosis is mainly one of exclusion after investigating other causes that stimulate ADH production, for example, cardiac, hepatic, renal, thyroid, and adrenal failure, or medications. ADH levels increase disproportionately to (low) serum osmolality and to a normal or increased plasma volume. Water retention results in hyponatremia and serum hypo-osmolality without edema.

THE ADRENAL GLANDS AND THEIR HORMONES

The two adrenal glands are situated retroperitoneally at the upper pole of each kidney. Each gland consists of a reddish-brown medulla surrounded by a yellow to yellow-brown cortex. The lipid and steroid contents of the cortex can be judged macroscopically by this yellow color, with brown indicating lipid and therefore steroid depletion. In the healthy adult, each gland weighs approximately 4 g. With associated pathological conditions, adrenal size may vary considerably. For example, gland weights are usually somewhat less in conditions of deficiency, while weights may be increased as much as fourfold in conditions of excess (**Figure 15-7**).

The Adrenal Cortex

Each adrenal gland is 90% cortex that is histologically divided into three distinct zones: the outer **zona glomerulosa** *lying just beneath the capsule, the middle* **zona fasciculata**, *and the inner* **zona reticularis**. The zona glomerulosa consists of clusters of small cells and is responsible for the synthesis of the salt retaining hormone, **aldosterone**. The widest of the three, the zona fasciculata, is composed of larger lipid-laden cells arranged in parallel cords and is responsible for the majority of the **glucocorticoids**. A small portion of the androgens is also produced in this region. Finally, the innermost cells of the zona reticularis are important in the synthesis of the **C18 and C19 steroids and thus sex steroids hormones**. They also produce **glucocorticoids**.

All adrenocortical steroids are derived from cholesterol. While over 30 steroids are synthesized within the cortex, only a few with significant biological activity are released into the circulation. *Based on their predominant biological activity, the hormones produced are classified as glucocorticoids, mineralocorticoids, and androgens* (**Table 15-5**). All share the same nucleus, but other structural differences give rise to their biological activity. The glucocorticoids control intermediary metabolism. The mineralocorticoids have a predominant effect on the regulation of water and electrolyte metabolism. The androgenic steroids are important in maintaining secondary sex characteristics in both genders.

WHAT WE DO

Laboratory studies for polyuria include a random serum and urine osmolality, urine glucose, fasting serum glucose, and serum sodium. A 24-hour urine collection is necessary to measure and document urine volume. Most healthy individuals will excrete less than 2.5 L/day. If serum osmolality ≥295 mOsm/kg, serum sodium ≥145 mmol/L, or glucose is >100 mg/dL the polyuria is most likely due to a condition other than diabetes insipidus-diabetes mellitus, for example. The combination of a urine osmolality less than 300 mOsm/kg with a serum osmolality above 300 mOsm/kg or with hypernatremia suggests DI is likely. If both serum and urine osmolality are decreased, psychogenic polydipsia should be considered.

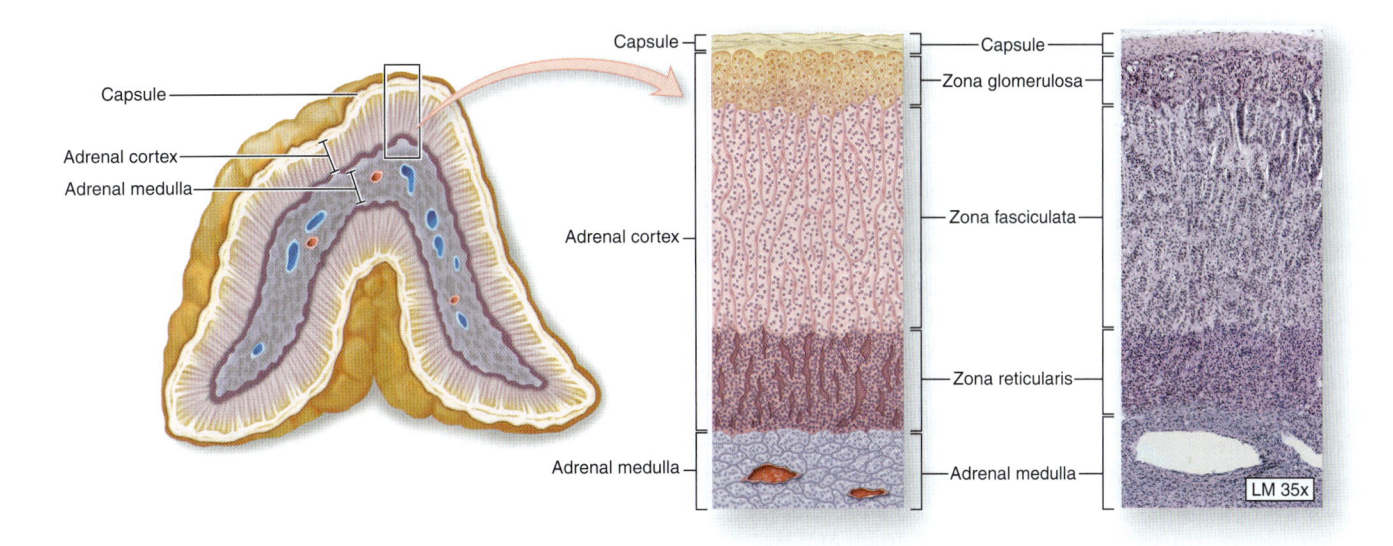

FIGURE 15-7 Adrenal gland. Inside the capsule of each adrenal gland is an adrenal cortex, formed from embryonic mesodermal cells, which completely surrounds an innermost adrenal medulla derived embryologically from neural crest cells. Both regions are very well vascularized with fenestrated sinusoidal capillaries. Cortical cells are arranged as three layers: the zona glomerulosa near the capsule, the zona fasciculata (the thickest layer), and the zona reticularis. (Reproduced with permission from McKinley M, O'Loughlin VD. Human Anatomy. 2nd ed. New York: McGraw-Hill, 2004 (Figure 20-13C,D).)

Regulation of the Adrenal Hormones

QUICK REVIEW

Three systems contribute to the regulation of adrenal function (Table 15-5). As with other endocrine systems, the hypothalamic–pituitary axis plays an integral role, but the immune system and the renin-angiotensin system also contribute.

The hypothalamic–pituitary–adrenal (HPA) axis: CRH from the hypothalamus is secreted into the portal venous nexus of the pituitary stalk to stimulate the synthesis and release of ACTH that, in turn, is carried to the adrenal where it binds to specific cortical cell membrane receptors. Through a series of steps involving adenylate cyclase and protein kinase, the adrenal cortex responds to synthesize corticosteroids. The rising cortisol concentration is sensed by the pituitary and hypothalamus and ACTH and CRH release are decreased via negative feedback. Androgen synthesis is regulated by both ACTH and androgen-stimulating hormone (also from the pituitary). Glucocorticoid and androgen synthesis usually parallel each other because of the coinfluence of ACTH, but occasionally, androgen synthesis is maintained when glucocorticoid production is decreased most likely due to the influence of androgen-

TABLE 15-5 Summary of adrenal hormones and their roles.

Class	Major Steroid	Site of Synthesis	Biological Activity and Physiological Function

Glucocorticoids	Cortisol	Zona fasciculata
		Zona reticularis
			1. Carbohydrate metabolism
			  a. Promotion of gluconeogenesis
			  b. Deposition of liver glycogen
			  c. Reduction in glucose utilization
			2. Inhibition of amino acid uptake and protein synthesis in peripheral tissues
			3. Fat distribution
			4. Anti-inflammatory and immunosuppressive effects

Mineralocorticoids	Aldosterone	Zona glomerulosa	1. Regulation of salt homeostasis
			  a. Sodium conservation
			  b. "waste" potassium
			2. Regulation of extracellular fluid volume

Adrenal Androgens	Dehydroepiandrosterone (DHEA) and DHEA-S	Zona reticularis Zona fasciculata	Indirect via peripheral conversion to testosterone
Catecholamines	Epinephrine Norepinephrine Dopamine	Chromaffin cells	1. Neurotransmitters 2. (epi) Increases metabolism in response to stress

stimulating hormone. In contrast, the HPA axis has minimal influence on aldosterone regulation.

The immune system: Proinflammatory cytokines such as IL-6, IL-1, and TNF-α also act through ACTH to stimulate the synthesis of cortisol. In turn, cortisol has many effects on immunity and hematopoiesis. The hormone stimulates erythropoiesis and causes functional leukocytosis by decreasing the adherence of polymorphonuclear leukocytes to endothelial cells and increasing their level in the circulation. In addition, increased levels of cortisol result in lymphocytopenia, monocytopenia, and eosinopenia. Negative feedback by the glucocorticoids dampen production of the cytokines.

Renin-angiotensin: Within the zona glomerulosa, the regulation of aldosterone involves potassium and the renin-angiotensin system with a minor influence from ACTH. Thus, while exhibiting a diurnal pattern, the concentrations measured in the circulation reflect the system's response to changes in dietary sodium and potassium, body position (recumbent to upright), and conditions of abnormal blood volume and/or blood pressure. In this region of the adrenal, potassium causes a membrane depolarization effect that opens calcium channels to activate cell-signaling mechanisms. Regulation via the **renin-angiotensin system** involves a series of events, the first of which is the release of renin, a proteolytic enzyme, by the renal juxtaglomerular epithelial cells. These cells release renin in response to four interdependent factors: (1) decreased renal arteriolar pressure, (2) decreased oncotic pressure, (3) increased sympathetic drive to the macula densa of the juxtaglomerular apparatus, and (4) a negative sodium balance. In the circulation, renin hydrolyzes its substrate, angiotensinogen, a hepatically produced glycoprotein, to yield angiotensin I that is metabolized in the lung via angiotensin-converting enzyme to angiotensin II. Angiotensin II directly stimulates aldosterone secretion in the zona glomerulosa by increasing CYP11B2 transcription, the gene responsible for aldosterone synthase.

ADRENAL HORMONES

Cortisol

Cortisol is released into the circulation in a circadian pattern with highest concentrations observed about 0800 and lowest in the late evening, approximately 2000 hours. Between 90% and 97% of circulating cortisol is bound to **cortisol-binding globulin (CBG)**, a hepatically produced α-1-globulin, with smaller amounts bound to albumin and sex hormone-binding globulin. The 3-10% of circulating cortisol that is not protein bound is known as "free cortisol" and represents the biologically available and active form of the steroid. It is free cortisol that promotes gluconeogenesis, acts on peripheral tissues to inhibit protein uptake, and feeds back on the pituitary and hypothalamus. Usually, measurements of total cortisol are sufficient as changes in the total concentration parallel those in the free hormone. An exception to this occurs when the patient has a physiological condition or is taking a medication that alters CBG concentrations (Table 15-6) and thus impacts the concentration of total serum cortisol. Conditions or drugs that increase CBG will cause the total cortisol to increase; and conversely those that decrease CBG will decrease total cortisol. *Even though these conditions alter the total cortisol concentration, the amount of free cortisol remains unaffected emphasizing the fact that it is free cortisol that is biologically active and involved in negative feedback.*

WHAT WE DO

Currently, there are very few analytical methods that can accurately measure cortisol in the range expected for the unbound portion. Fortunately, an alternative means of estimating the amount of circulating free cortisol is possible through the measurement of urinary cortisol, since cortisol excreted in the urine is reflective of the amount of circulating free hormone. A 24-hour sample is optimal but a timed sample may suffice in some cases. Another, relatively new option is the measurement of the hormone in saliva as free cortisol readily diffuses into that fluid. Because of the circadian pattern of cortisol, it is important to note the time of day to interpret serum and salivary concentrations.

Aldosterone

Aldosterone is produced at a rate of about 1/100th of that of cortisol. The hormone is weakly bound to CBG and transported primarily by albumin to a variety of tissues where its actions are mediated through a high-affinity mineralocorticoid receptor. Its major functions include regulation of the extracellular fluid volume and regulation of potassium metabolism. In the renal distal convoluted tubule and the cortical collecting duct, aldosterone promotes reabsorption of sodium in exchange for potassium excretion. As discussed above, the primary regulators of aldosterone are the renin–angiotensin system and potassium. *When interpreting aldosterone test results, it is important to document position since serum concentrations are higher on standing compared with recumbent and sodium intake by collecting 24-hour urine for Na (urinary aldosterone concentrations inversely correlate with urinary Na excretion).*

TABLE 15-6 Drugs and conditions that affect cortisol-binding-globulin (CBG) and cortisol concentrations.

Increase CBG	Decrease CBG
Estrogens	Malnutrition
Hyperthyroidism	Chronic liver disease
Diabetes	Androgens Hypothyroidism

Dehydroepiandrosterone and Androstenedione

Dehydroepiandrosterone (DHEA) and androstenedione are normally released in tandem with cortisol. The production of adrenal sex hormones is age dependent. Release begins in late childhood, peaks in the twenties, and declines slowly thereafter. This age-related decline does not happen with cortisol. DHEA has a short half-life and a circadian pattern. *The sulfated precursor (DHEA-S) has little androgenic activity and is useful when assessing adrenal androgen production because little of it is formed in the gonads, it has a longer half-life, and concentrations are relatively constant throughout the day.*

ADRENAL CORTICAL INSUFFICIENCY

Thomas Addison's description of patients presenting with primary adrenal insufficiency remains quite relevant: "The leading and characteristic features of the morbid state to which I would direct attention are anemia, general languor, and debility, remarkable feebleness of the heart's action, irritability of the stomach, and a peculiar change in the color of the skin." Additional signs and symptoms may include weight loss, salt craving, hypotension, anorexia, syncope, and/or vertigo.

Etiology of Adrenal Insufficiency

Several of Addison's original cases were caused by tuberculosis and metastatic disease; others had no identifiable etiology. For many years, tuberculosis was the most common cause of primary adrenal insufficiency; and it remains so today worldwide, particularly in underdeveloped countries. *However, in the USA and other developed areas, up to 90% of primary adrenal insufficiency is caused by an autoimmune destruction of the cortex.* The process is gradual, and while patients may be identified before complete destruction, eventually, all cortical adrenal steroids become deficient. When examined either post-adrenalectomy or on autopsy, both adrenal glands are usually atrophied, sometimes severely. The capsule is fibrous and the cortical zones may be completely destroyed so that the medulla is separated from the capsule by only a collapsed stroma and a few cells. A diffuse lymphocytic infiltration also occurs that in severe cases may cause the adrenals to appear of normal size. Most cases of autoimmune adrenal insufficiency are isolated and have no defined genetic component. The medulla usually remains intact but may show some lymphocytic infiltration (Figure 15-8).

> ### HUNTING FOR ZEBRAS
> Two uncommon familial **polyglandular autoimmune syndromes** (**APS 1** and **APS 2**) are associated with adrenal insufficiency and other autoimmune endocrine (and non-endocrine) disease. The more common **APS 2** (alternately PGA 2) has a female predominance and generally is recognized in the third to fourth decade of life. It is associated with the combination of autoimmune adrenal and thyroid disease and/or type 1 diabetes. The disease is associated with certain HLA-DR types, but other, as yet undefined, environmental or intrinsic factors are important in triggering the autoimmune response. **APS 1** (alternately PGA 1) is an extremely uncommon syndrome associated with adrenal insufficiency, hypoparathyroidism, and mucocutaneous candidiasis. The disease is usually diagnosed in childhood and demonstrates a near equal sex ratio. As a rare autosomal recessive trait, it almost always occurs in familial/ethnic clusters. The defect is in the *AIRE* gene, a transcription factor important in the elimination of self-reactive clones in the thymus during immune development (see also section "Hypoparathyroidism").

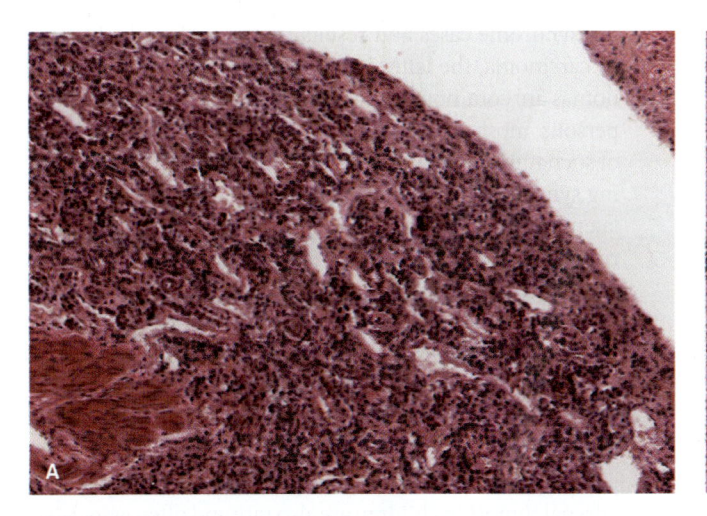

FIGURE 15-8 Adrenal insufficiency. **(A)** Photomicrograph of an adrenal gland from patient with long-standing adrenal insufficiency believed to be of autoimmune etiology. There is no residual cortex. The gland is hypoplastic and consists solely of the medullary region.

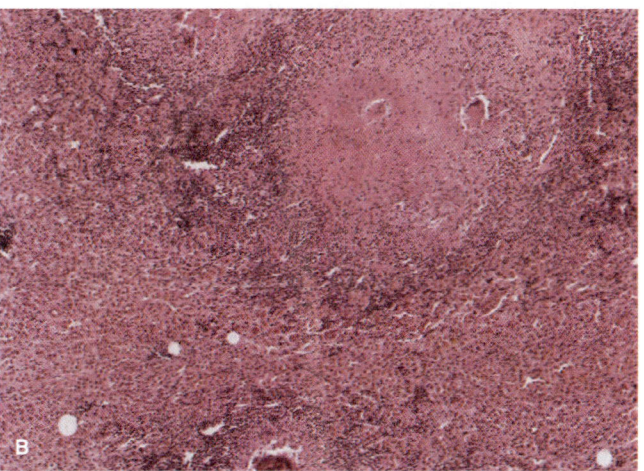

(B) Photomicrograph demonstrtaing adrenal tuberculosis. A characteristic caseating granuloma with giants cells is present in the upper part of the field.

Most cases of adrenal insufficiency are iatrogenic in origin and associated with glucocorticoid usage. **Secondary adrenal insufficiency** may be related to pituitary or hypothalamic defects resulting in defects in either the synthesis or release of ACTH. Rare congenital defects in the ACTH receptor of glucocorticoid secreting cells have also been characterized in many individuals with **familial glucocorticoid deficiency,** an autosomal recessive condition.

Diagnosis of Adrenal Insufficiency

Patients presenting in the early stages of adrenal insufficiency in the absence of stress may be difficult to diagnose because of unremarkable laboratory data. Steroid levels may be within normal limits and stimulation studies may be within normal limits or only slightly suppressed. If the disease is not associated with infection or neoplasm, adrenal antibodies may be detected in the patient's serum. Laboratory studies of patients presenting in later stages usually demonstrate hyponatremia, hyperkalemia, metabolic acidosis, increased urea nitrogen, and mild normocytic anemia, eosinophilia, and lymphocytosis.

CASE 15-3

GL is a 17-year-old male referred to the pediatric endocrine clinic for the evaluation of "underdevelopment and shortness of stature." He has had a long history with multiple hospitalizations for infections. He says he does not do much after school, does poorly in physical education classes (tires after just a few minutes), and tends to stay indoors. His mother confirms that he rarely played outside as a child, and even today comes home after school and falls asleep until dinner. She also confides that he struggles with his school work, a change seen since he entered high school. Physical examination reveals an underdeveloped, thin youth, well tanned, with mild orthostatic hypotension.

Weakness, anorexia, easy fatigability, and a mild decrease in blood pressure on standing are common findings in many disorders. But in this case, the patient's tanned appearance despite his history suggested a possible pituitary or adrenal cause.

Laboratory results (with reference ranges) include hemoglobin 9.4 g/dL (11.7–15.5), WBC 7.5×10^9/L (4.8–10.8), Na 136 mmol/L (135–145), K = 4.4 mmol/L (3.5–5), fasting glucose 99 mg/dL (60–110), cortisol (AM) <2 μg/dL (AM, 7–25), aldosterone 3.2 ng/dL (recumbent 1–16), renin 9.4 ng/mL/h 0.5–1.5 ng/mL/h), ACTH 840 pg/mL (10–50). Urine chemistries: Na 142 mmol/24 h (40–220), K = 58 mmol/24 h (25–125), glucose nondetected, aldosterone 3.6 μg/24 h (2–20), cortisol <2 μg/dL (20–90). In addition, serum cortisol remained <2 μg/dL after ACTH stimulation. This patient was diagnosed with primary adrenal insufficiency – the finding of adrenal autoantibodies confirmed an autoimmune process as the cause.

Hypoglycemia and hypercalcemia may also be present. *Depending on the amount of destruction, serum cortisol concentrations are quite low, even nondetectable, throughout the day. Most importantly, the hormone does not respond to ACTH stimulation or stressors.* In parallel, urine-free cortisol levels are also quite low. Serum and urine aldosterone levels are low and remain so even on stimulation with postural changes and spontaneous or induced sodium deprivation.

ADRENAL CORTICAL HYPERFUNCTION

Hyperfunction of the cortex is usually classified according to the clinical syndromes resulting from excessive exposure to the dominating hormone:

- Glucocorticoid excess results in **Cushing syndrome**
- Mineralocorticoid excess is associated with **Conn syndrome**
- Androgen excess is associated with **congenital adrenal hyperplasia (CAH)**

Corticosteroid Excess (Cushing Syndrome)

Cushing syndrome is a generic term used to describe the finding of hypercortisolism and the resulting pathophysiological changes. However, the eponym does not describe the underlying causes of the hypercortisolism. Four etiological categories can be described:

1. **Cushing disease** is the most common cause of Cushing syndrome (approximately 70–80% of patients). In these cases, the primary defect is not in the adrenal but rather the pituitary, usually in the form of a benign microadenoma. The tumor-produced ACTH stimulates both adrenals leading to bilateral hyperplasia and greatly increased serum and urinary cortisol concentrations.
2. **Adrenal Cushing syndrome** is responsible for 8% of Cushing syndrome cases and results from an adrenal adenoma or carcinoma, the latter being rare. Although adrenal adenomas are common, being found in 1–2% of asymptomatic persons, most are considered incidental findings since 80% of such tumors are nonfunctional. Generally, adrenal Cushing syndrome occurs more commonly in females and unilaterally, with the left adrenal most commonly affected. The remaining normal adrenal tissue often atrophies (**Figure 15-9**). Adrenal adenomas are more likely to develop in children, while pituitary adenomas (Cushings disease) occur more frequently in adults. Several rare inherited conditions (including MEN1—see above) are associated with adrenal adenomas. As noted, adrenal carcinomas are uncommon comprising less than 1% of all incidentally discovered presumptive adrenal adenomas (**Figure 15-10**). Malignant adrenal tumors in children are also rare and often associated with mutations in tp53 and the Li–Fraumeni syndrome.
3. **Ectopic Cushing syndrome** accounts for 10–15% of Cushing syndrome cases and is due to overproduction of

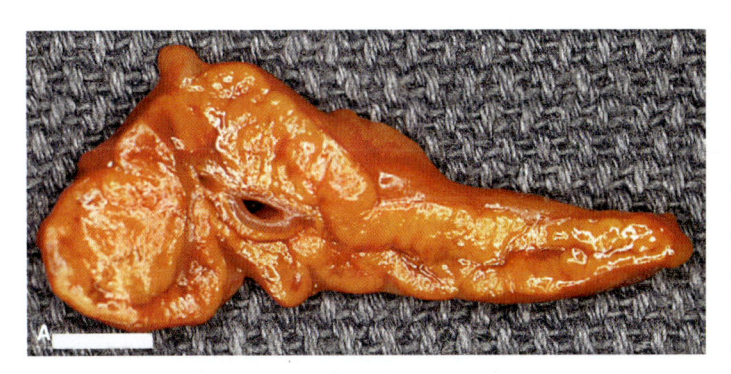

FIGURE 15-9 Adrenal cortical adenoma. **(A)** Gross image, adenoma is on left side of gland (bar 1 cm). **(B)** Photomicrograph of adrenal adenoma. Cells are uniform and similar to those in the fasciculata layer of gland. ((9a) Contributed with permission of Clay Nichols, MD NC Medical Examiners Office.)

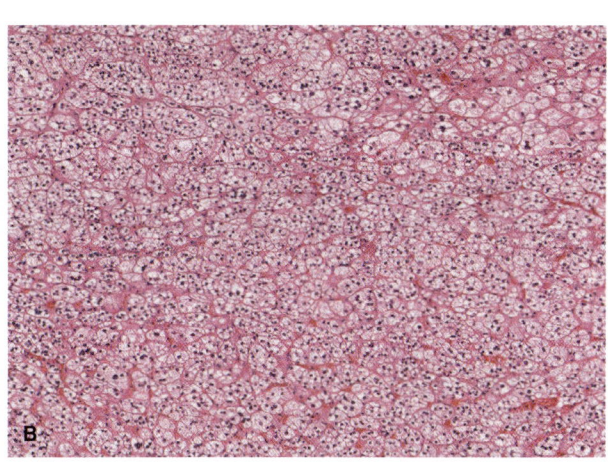

biologically active ACTH by nonendocrine tumors. Most often, these tumors are small cell carcinomas of the lung, but thymomas, islet cell tumors, carcinoid tumors, or paragangliomas originating. As in Cushing disease, bilateral adrenal hyperplasia results.

4. **Exogenous or iatrogenic Cushing syndrome** usually results from excessive steroid therapy or factitious use over extended periods of time. The exogenous steroids suppress pituitary production of ACTH, and in turn, adrenal synthesis of cortisol. Once the exogenous exposure is removed, the adrenals may need time to return cortisol synthesis to pre-suppression levels and during this time patients are at risk of adrenal insufficiency. This is why prescribed doses of steroids are tapered and not stopped abruptly.

Categories 1, 3, and 4 are sometimes considered as secondary hypercortisolism; category 2 as primary disease.

Regardless of the etiology, any prolonged increase in cortisol concentrations leads to a similar clinical presentation in patients with Cushing syndrome. Fat accumulates in the face (this is often referred to as "moon facies") and often around the neck and upper body in the supraclavicular and dorsocervical areas (hence, these patients are described as having a "buffalo hump"). As the epidermis and underlying connective tissue atrophies, the skin becomes thin and may appear transparent. This also accounts for the **plethora** (the ruddy complexion noted in the patient) and frequent bruising. The loss of connective tissue in the truncal area may result in pronounced striae. Because of the interrelation between cortisol, the immune system and repair, these patients often report frequent fungal infections and poor wound healing. Since the zona fasciculata is also responsible for the synthesis of androgens, many female patients who have Cushing syndromes have hirsutism and acne. Muscle weakness, fatigue, and back pain are commonly reported, as is osteopenia. Other common features include edema and glucosuria along with neurological changes such as irritability and depression.

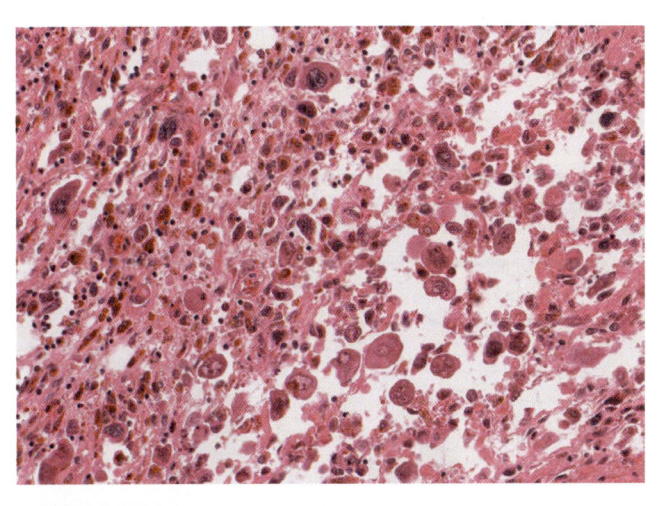

Diagnosis of Cushing Syndrome

Laboratory testing includes timed serum cortisol, urine-free cortisol (preferably as a 24-hour collection), and plasma ACTH. Because these hormones may be elevated, even significantly, in non-Cushing disorders, a **suppression test** (Table 15-7) is usually necessary to assess the integrity of the negative feedback mechanism of the HPA axis and to distinguish between the various causes of Cushing syndrome. Dexamethasone is the steroid of choice for these studies.

Mineralocorticoid Excess or Hyperaldosteronism

Primary hyperaldosteronism (PH) accounts for up to 13% of cases of hypertension. The condition is most usually a sporadic occurrence in adults and is more common in females. Primary disease is uncommon in children. Adrenal adenomas (Conn

FIGURE 15-10 Adrenal cortical carcinoma. Photomicrograph of an anaplastic variant of adrenal carcinoma. Neoplastic giant cells have bizarre hyperchromatic nuclei, which are sometimes multiple.

CASE 15-4

TP is a 26-year-old female who is seen as the first appointment in a primary care clinic for a checkup. She is concerned about increasing hirsutism and irregular menstrual cycles over the past 2 years. She notes that she feels exhausted at the end of her workday – her job requires standing and some light lifting. She has a history of mild hypertension and mild glucose intolerance. Her blood pressure is 146/110 mmHg. She has acne on the chest and back. Although she has little acne on her face, it is puffy and hirsute with a ruddy color. She is moderately obese, but there is no evidence of localized fat pads.

Blood is collected for several laboratory tests. She is asked to complete a 24-hour urine collection and to return to the clinic the following afternoon for an additional test. Laboratory results (and reference ranges) from the early morning visit include Na 144 mmol/L (135–145), K = 3.4 mmol/L (3.5–5.0), fasting glucose 115 mg/dL (65–100), hematocrit 46% (37–44), hemoglobin 13.6 g/dL (12–16), cortisol 44 µg/dL (5–20), LH, mid follicular 6 mU/mL (5–20), FSH 10 mU/mL (2.6–16), DHEA-S 4.5 µg/mL (0.8–3.2), testosterone 500 ng/dL (20–80). Urinary free cortisol 160 µg/24 h (20–90). A serum cortisol collected at 4 pm is 37 µg/dL (2–14). Plasma ACTH was 135 pg/mL (20–70).

The elevated serum (with loss of diurnal pattern) and urine cortisols suggest *Cushing syndrome*. The etiology of the hypercortisolism is distinguished by reassessing the suppressibility of cortisol following administration of dexamethasone: first overnight and then at a higher dose. For this particular patient, the morning cortisol following a low dose of dexamethasone remained elevated at 21 µg/dL. Following a higher dose, the cortisol concentration declined to less than 1.5 µg/dL suggesting Cushing disease. Additional studies revealed a pituitary tumor confirming the diagnosis (Table 15-7).

Syndrome) and idiopathic hyperaldosteronism (IHA) account for nearly all cases of PHA, the latter accounting for 60% or more of PHA. Rare adrenocortical carcinomas and three uncommon inherited conditions account for less than 1% of cases. IHA is characterized by bilateral micro or macronodular adrenocortical hyperplasia and is variable in severity. The cause of IHA remains unknown.

Laboratory testing (Table 15-8) reveals hypokalemia, hypernatremia, alkalosis, hypochloremia, elevated plasma, and urine aldosterone with suppressed renin. Failure of aldosterone to suppress following salt loading confirms the diagnosis. **Secondary hyperaldosteronism** develops in response to enhanced production and release of renin from the kidneys, as it occurs in hyponatremia, decreased renal perfusion, renal artery stenosis, or depletion of the vascular volume.

HUNTING FOR ZEBRAS

Familial hyperaldosteronism (FH) Type I. FH Type I is associated with hyperaldosteronism in response to normal levels of ACTH and is associated with a dominant mutation resulting in a chimeric gene linking *CYP11B1* (the 11 β-hydroxylase gene) and *CYP11B2* (the aldosterone synthase gene). This results in ACTH dependent regulation of the gene and production of aldosterone in the zona fasciculata and hyperplasia of this region. The mutation is reported to be rare but may be under-diagnosed. FH type II is an autosomal dominant mutation occasionally associated with adrenocortical adenomas that remain poorly characterized.

TABLE 15-7 Summary of expected laboratory results in corticosteroid excess (Cushing syndrome).

	Reference Range	Cushing Disease	Ectopic ACTH Syndrome	Adrenal Tumor
Serum cortisol (0800 h)	4.5–23 µg/dL	↑, Loss of circadian pattern	N to ↑	N to ↑
Urinary free cortisol (random)	<100 µg/dL	>120 µg/dL	>120 µg/dL	>120 µg/dL
Plasma ACTH (0800 h)	10–60 pg/mL	wnl to ↑↑	wnl to ↑↑↑	<10 pg/mL
Overnight Dexamethasone Suppression Test				
Serum cortisol (0800 h)	<3 µg/dL	>10 µg/dL No suppression	>10 µg/dL	>10 µg/dL
High-dose Dexamethasone Suppression Test				
Serum cortisol (0800 h)		Suppression	Fails to suppress	Fails to suppress

TABLE 15-8 Summary of test results in mineralocorticoid excess (hyperaldosteronism).

Expected responses: low-Na diet or upright posture or diuretic use increases plasma aldosterone, while a high-Na diet or supine position decreases aldosterone secretion

Document position at time of blood collection
Collect urine to assess Na intake
Remember plasma aldosterone and renin activity are inversely proportional to urine Na

	Plasma Renin	Plasma Aldosterone	Serum K
Primary aldosteronism	↓	↑	↓
Secondary aldosteronism			
Malignant hypertension	↑	↑	↓
Renin-secreting tumors	↑	↑	N or ↓

Congenital Adrenal Hyperplasia (Excess Androgen Synthesis)

Androgen excess occurs in response to disorders of both the adrenals and the ovaries. Adrenal causes include Cushing syndrome, adrenal carcinoma, and CAH. Androgen-secreting adrenal tumors are the most common cause in adults, while CAH, premature adrenarche (increased adrenal activity associated with puberty), or adrenal carcinoma are the most common causes in children.

CAH is a group of autosomal recessive disorders that result from loss of function mutations in a variety of enzymes active in the biochemical pathway of cortisol synthesis. The most common mutations that are responsible for over 90% of cases are in the *CYP21A* 21 hydroxylase gene. The case frequency is about 1 per 15,000 individuals but is much higher in selected populations where carrier frequency may be 1 in 5. Hence, screening for CAH is common in most newborn screening programs. CAH is most often recognized at birth or early childhood because of the occurrence of ambiguous genitalia, early virilization, or salt wasting. Clinical presentation is complex and, as expected, differs in males and females. In the newborn period, the patient may present with mixed findings of both adrenal deficiency and hyperfunction: Cortisol synthesis is decreased, yet androgen synthesis is increased. Both adrenals become hyperplastic due to the resulting increase in ACTH. Since the enzymatic block is usually partial, the patient may be able to maintain cortisol and aldosterone concentrations within the reference range when not stressed.

Adrenal Medulla

The medulla is composed of catecholamine secreting **chromaffin** *cells. Catecholamines are derived from tyrosine and include dopamine, norepinephrine, and epinephrine that* are also produced in the axon terminals of sympathetic postganglionic neurons, the CNS, and in scattered groups of chromaffin cells found in the abdomen and neck. Which compounds are produced depends on the tissue. Neurons within the CNS release all three. The majority of norepinephrine originates from the postganglionic neurons, whereas only a small amount is synthesized by the adrenal medulla. The opposite is true for epinephrine with most of it being synthesized in the adrenal medulla.

> ### QUICK REVIEW
> The catecholamines are responsible for the physiological responses summarized by the well-known phrase "fright, fight, or flight." The physiological effects observed in response to catecholamine release are related to the interaction of each with receptors on the cellular membranes. Dopamine interacts with specific dopaminergic receptors that stimulate or inhibit adenylate cyclase. Norepinephrine and epinephrine bind to either α- or β-adrenergic receptors. The two can interact with either receptor, but the affinity varies. Metabolic effects occur as a result of direct receptor interaction at the target tissue or through an indirect route involving other hormones or peptides. Direct actions include stimulation of hepatic glucose production, stimulation of tissues to glycogenolysis and glycolysis with increased lactate and pyruvate production, stimulation of lipolysis, stimulation of hepatic ketogenesis, stimulation of potassium and phosphate intracellular transport, and stimulation of thermogenesis. Indirect actions are observed as catecholamines alter the secretion of hormones or peptides that in turn elicit a specific effect. The major indirect actions involve the suppression of insulin and stimulation of GH and glucagon secretion. Catecholamines are stable within the storage granules of the adrenal medullary cells, but once released, the compounds are rapidly degraded by the enzymes catechol-O-methyltransferase and monoamine oxidase. Less than 2% of the released products are excreted into the urine as free catecholamines. Most is excreted metabolic products, namely metanephrines or vanillylmandelic acid.

Neoplastic Disease of the Adrenal Medulla: Pheochromocytoma

Neoplasia is the primary cause of disease in the adrenal medulla with pheochromocytoma being the most common. Tumors of neuronal origin such as **neuroblastoma** *and* **ganglioneuroma** *also occur and are of particular note in children where they are the most common childhood cancer.* **Pheochromocytomas**, tumors of neural crest origin, can occur at any location along the primitive chromaffin system. Approximately 90% of these tumors originate in the adrenal medulla, but 5–10% are extra-adrenal (and often termed **paraganglioma**) and appear anywhere along the sympathetic ganglia of the abdominal aorta. Many students find the mnemonic "rule of 10" useful in remembering the characteristics of pheochromocytomas:

- 10% are outside the extra-adrenal
- 10% occur in children
- 10% are multiple or bilateral
- 10% are malignant
- 10% recur after surgical removal
- 10% are familial

Pheochromocytomas in children tend to be familial. The frequency of bilateral tumors is higher than in adults (about 30%) and malignant disease frequency is half than that of seen in adults. Familial pheochromocytomas account for up to 30% of cases and have been associated with several syndromes including the most common of which are MEN, von Hippel–Lindau (VHL) syndrome, and neurofibromatosis type 1 (NF1).

MEN2A (Sipple syndrome) and 2B are autosomal dominant syndromes both associated with different mutations in the *RET* oncogene. Both subtypes are associated with a 50% or greater risk of pheochromocytoma, most commonly bilateral and benign. The MEN2 subtypes differ in phenotype, 2A is characterized by the development of medullary thyroid carcinoma (MTC) and primary hyperparathyroidism, 2B patients also express MTC but also develop mucosal neuromas and have a Marfanoid habitus. In both MEN syndromes, MCT often develops before the pheochromocytoma. Thus patients who develop MTC are monitored for the occurrence of a pheochromocytoma.

VHL syndrome, resulting from mutations of the tumor suppressor *VHL*, is characterized by benign cerebellar hemangioblastomas, retinal angiomas, multiple pancreatic and renal cysts, and pheochromocytomas that are often extra-adrenal. The risk of pheochromocytoma in VHL depends on the nature of the mutation and ranges from 10% (VHL type I) to 50% (in VHL type II).

Pheochromocytomas occur in about 10% of **NF1 (Von Recklinghausen syndrome)** cases, an autosomal dominant disorder inactivating the tumor suppressor *NF1 gene* and characterized by formation of multiple neurofibromas.

Pheochromocytomas often show necrosis and hemorrhage and tend to encompass the adrenal. The enlarged medullary region may be striking, reducing the adrenal cortex to a thin layer. Tumor cells characteristically form nests of tumor cells termed *zellballen* (German for cell balls) surrounded by a fibrovascular stroma (Figure 15-11). Intracellular enzymatic activities of the enzymes involved in catecholamine synthesis are enhanced, whereas the actions of enzymes involved in metabolism are reduced. As a result, tumors usually produce higher concentrations of parent compounds than that of metabolites. The patient's signs and symptoms relate to the pharmacologic actions of the specific catecholamines secreted, and the severity of the symptoms relates both to the amount of catecholamine secreted and the duration of secretion. Hypertension, often labile and resistant to pharmacotherapy, is the most common symptom. The symptomatic triad consists of sweating, tachycardia/palpitations, and headache. At least one of this set of symptoms occurs in a paroxysmal manner in essentially all patients.

Testing has recently favored the measurement of the metabolites in plasma or urine as the parent compounds have very short half-lives and are easily degraded, thus requiring extremely careful patient preparation, sample collection, and handling. Furthermore, since tumor secretion may be episodic or sporadic rather than continuous, testing of a single, random urine, or plasma may show only modestly elevated or even normal levels of catecholamines. The best sensitivity is obtained using a 24-hour urine or plasma metanephrine determination. Follow-up care includes repeat measurement of urinary metabolites approximately 1 week postoperatively and periodically thereafter.

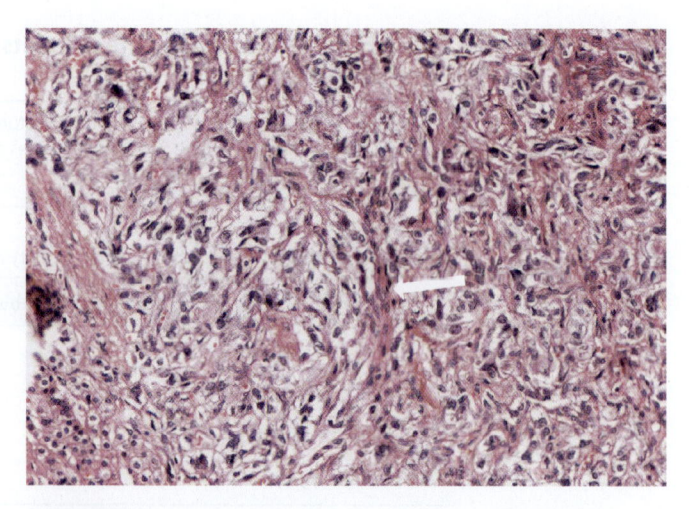

FIGURE 15-11 Pheochromocytoma. Photomicrograph demonstrates formation of cell nests separated by fibrovascular stromal elements (not prominent in this example arrow). Cells are pleomorphic with nuclei that appear to have inclusion-like structures.

THYROID

The thyroid gland, often described as butterfly in appearance, is found as two lobes connected by the isthmus lying anterior and lateral to the trachea. It originates during the 4th week of development from an out-pouching of pharyngeal epithelium that descends in front of the pharyngeal gut into the anterior midline of the neck as the **thyroglossal duct**. *Developmental transcription factors, notably thyroid transcription factors 1 and 2 (TTF-1, TTF-2) and paired homeobox-8 (PAX-8) synchronize*

CASE 15-5

PW is a 59-year-old male admitted with hypertension, chest pain, and respiratory distress. Blood pressure is 238/150 mmHg. Troponin is mildly elevated but does not increase over the next 8 hours. Random drug tests are negative for stimulants such as cocaine and amphetamines. Myocardial infarction is ruled out and the patient is discharged. Over the next few months he experiences several 5–10-minute episodes of palpitations, sweating, and light-headedness; he describes as "spells during which he thinks he is going to die." His last episode was approximately 1 week ago.

Plasma and a random urine are collected during the office visit while he is asymptomatic. Given the episodic nature of the events, he is given a urine container and instructions to collect a sample following his next episode and to either come to the clinic or to the emergency room. The catecholamines and metanephrines profiles reported for the samples collected during office visit were, as expected, within the reference ranges.

Two weeks later, he presents to the office with a sample and reports an episode that occurred within the past 30 minutes. During the examination, he reports having another episode. A plasma sample is collected.

The following laboratory results are obtained: urinary metanephrine 86 μg/dL (30–180) and normetanephrine 4256 μg/dL (111–419), plasma metanephrine 62 pg/mL (<100), and normetanephrine 2703 pg/mL (<167).

A unique opportunity arose when this patient became symptomatic during the visit. Since he was symptomatic, one would expect both parent catecholamines and the metabolites to be elevated. The primary care provider ordered only the metanephrine metabolites since she was not prepared to properly collect and handle the more labile parent compounds. The elevated metanephrines reflect increased catecholamine production and are consistent with the pheochromocytoma later removed surgically.

---

development at the cellular level and induce the genes involved in key proteins such as thyroglobulin (Tg), thyroid peroxidase (TPO), the sodium iodide symporter (NIS), and the thyroid-stimulating hormone receptor (TSH-R). By adulthood, the gland normally weighs about 20 g. (**Figure 15-12**).

Histological features include well-defined **follicles** (acini) lined by **epithelial follicular cells** surrounding **colloid**. The follicles are responsible for the synthesis and release of T4 and **T3**, two hormones key to development and overall metabolism. Smaller populations of **parafollicular** or C cells derived from the neural crest are located between the follicles. Parafollicular cells are characterized by their secretion of **calcitonin**, a hormone involved in regulating calcium levels (**Figure 15-13**).

T4 and G3 are unique in that they contain iodine. They exhibit multiple actions within most cells of the body and are integral to development and overall metabolism.

TSH stimulates the growth and vascularity of the thyroid gland, and promotes the uptake and processing of iodine, the synthesis of the thyroid hormone precursors, and the proteolytic release of thyroid hormones from Tg. Upon binding to its receptor on the follicle basal membrane, TSH activates several signaling systems (including a cyclic adenosine monophosphate pathway), and in doing so stimulates iodine metabolism, along with the initiation of thyroid hormone synthesis and release. As might be expected, based upon concepts learned in the previous sections, rising concentrations of T4 and T3 in the circulation exert negative feedback actions at the pituitary suppressing the release of TSH.

QUICK REVIEW

An in-depth discussion of the synthesis and release of thyroid hormones is beyond the scope of this text, but is found in most biochemistry texts. Briefly, the process includes the active uptake of iodine from the circulation, the oxidation and incorporation of iodine into the tyrosine residues of Tg through a process known as organification, the coupling of iodotyrosine molecules within Tg forming T4 and T3, and proteolysis of Tg with release of free iodothyronines and iodotyrosines. Excess iodine is removed from the non-T4 or T3 tyrosine residues for reuse. Much of the T4 released into the circulation undergoes peripheral conversion to either T3 or to a metabolically inactive form. In fact about 85% of T3 is derived from this process. T3 is three to eight times more potent than T4.

Upon release into the circulation, more than 99% of each hormone is quickly bound by thyroxine-binding globulin (TBG), transthyretin (thyroxine-binding prealbumin), and albumin. It is the remaining unbound, or free, portions of each hormone that is responsible for the hormone's biologic effects. Hence, changes in the circulating concentrations of the binding proteins in response to disease (hepatic or renal dysfunction), drugs (estrogens, anabolic steroids, etc.), or normal physiologic events (pregnancy) are clinically relevant. Changes in free hormone concentration resulting from altered binding protein levels respond rapidly to return to normal so the patient remains euthyroid. This differs from the situations to be discussed shortly in which thyroid dysfunction leads to under production (hypothyroidism) or overproduction (hyperthyroidism) of thyroid hormone.

T4 and T3 are involved in numerous functions from exerting a calorigenic effect on tissues to growth, development, and sexual maturation. They also stimulate heart rate and contraction, stimulate protein synthesis and carbohydrate metabolism, increase lipid synthesis and degradation, increase vitamin requirements, and enhance the sensitivity of β-adrenergic receptors to catecholamines.

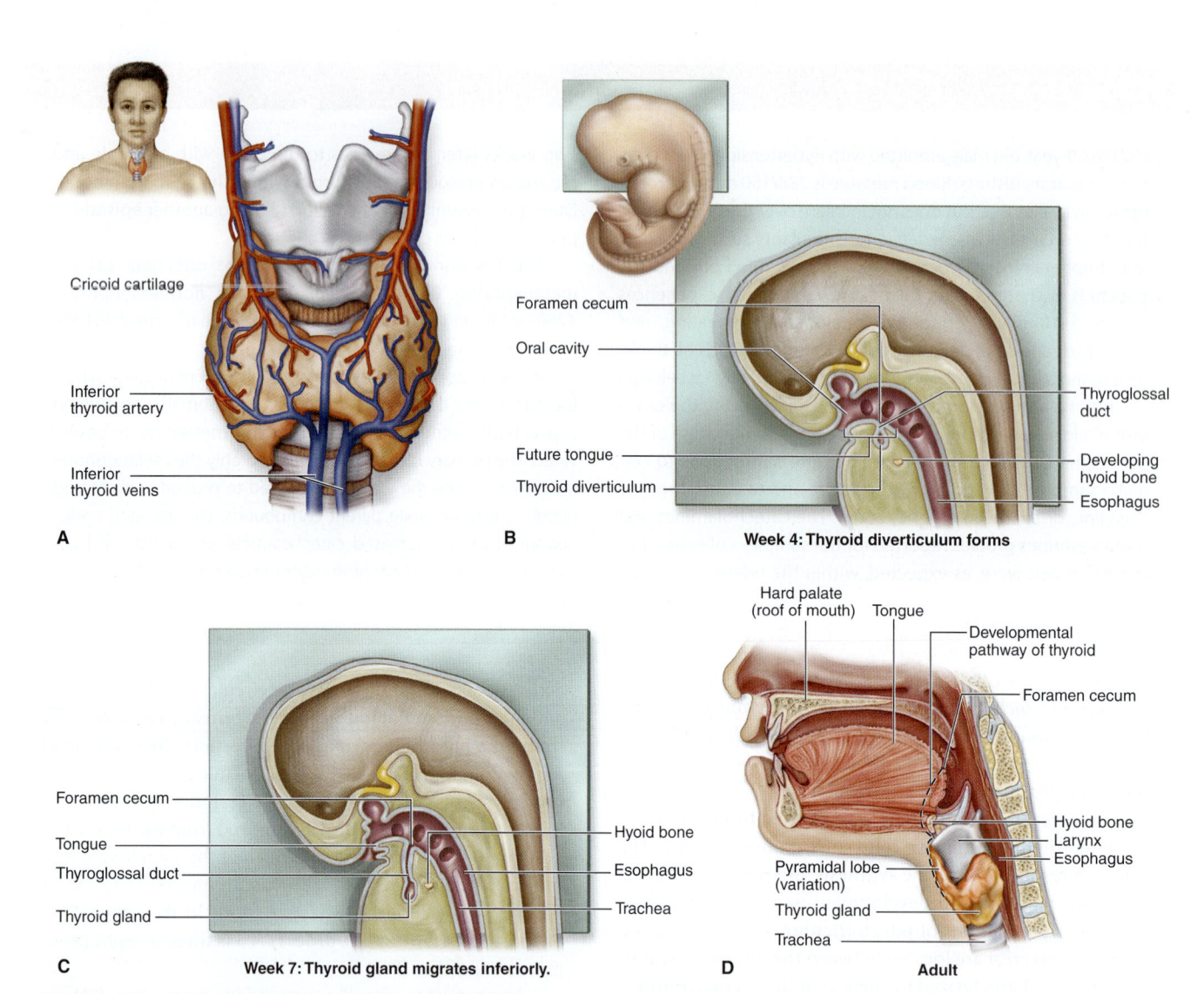

FIGURE 15-12 Thyroid gland and its development. (A) The thyroid is a highly vascular, butterfly-shaped gland, approximately 5 cm × 5 cm and weighing 20–30 g in adults, surrounding the anterior surface of the trachea just below the larynx. Immigrating neural crest cells infiltrate the epithelium as precursors to the thyroid's parafollicular C cells. **(B)** Thyroid development begins in the fourth week as an epithelial diverticulum growing down from the endodermal lining of the foregut. **(C)** The thyroid diverticulum continues to grow in an inferior direction and its connection to the developing pharynx, the thyroglossal duct, later regresses. **(D)** By fetal stages, the thyroid has attained its normal adult position. (Reproduced with permission from McKinley M, O'Loughlin VD. Human Anatomy. 2nd ed. New York: McGraw-Hill, 2004 (Figures 20-9A, 20-16B to D).)

Thyroid Function Testing

Assessment of thyroid function begins with the measurement of TSH and T4, and for some cases includes T3 and selected thyroid antibodies. Methods, most commonly immunoassays, are readily available for the measurement of TSH, total T4, total T3, free T4 (FT4), and free T3 (FT3). Current TSH immunoassays are very sensitive and have changed the way in which patients are tested. When hypothalamic–pituitary function is normal, the amount of TSH measured in the serum reflects the combined action of FT4 and FT3 on the pituitary. The response of the pituitary is so sensitive to circulating thyroid hormone levels that a 2-fold change in FT4 results in a 100-fold change in serum TSH. This response plus the analytical sensitivity and precision of the current methods makes TSH the best test in terms of clinical sensitivity for detecting thyroid dysfunction and forms the basis for using TSH as the primary test of organ function.

A number of algorithms have been designed to screen various populations for thyroid disease that start with a sensitive TSH assay and then proceed to FT4. All of these schemas are designed for use in otherwise healthy, ambulatory patients and should not be used when assessing hospitalized or chronically ill patients.

Abnormal thyroid function studies are often encountered when performed on nonambulatory patients who are acutely or chronically ill, a condition known as the sick-euthyroid syndrome. These patients are found to have

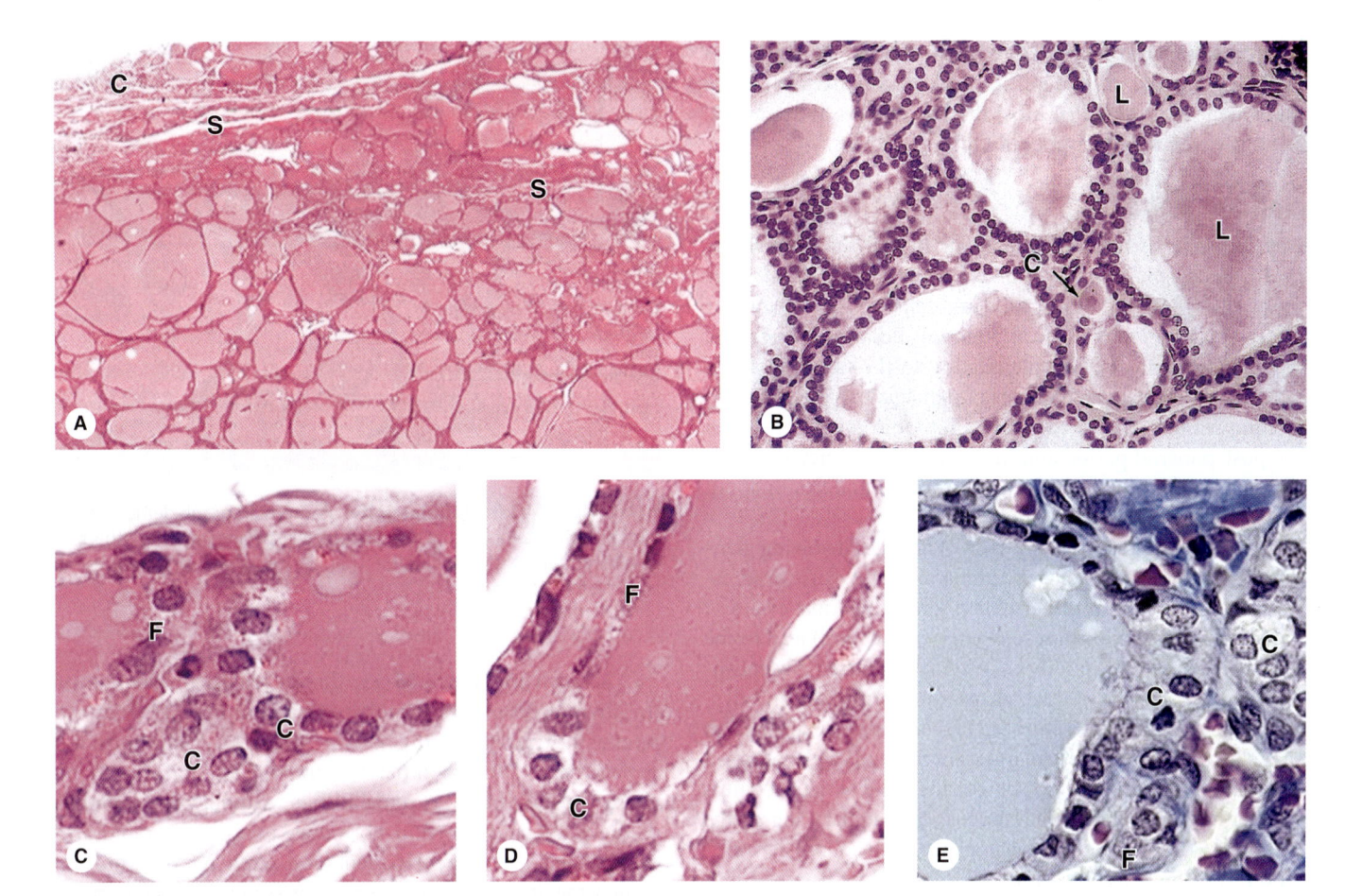

FIGURE 15-13 Thyroid follicular cells and parafollicular cells. **(A)** A low-power micrograph of thyroid gland shows the thin capsule (C), from which septa (S) with the larger blood vessels, lymphatics, and nerves enter the gland. The parenchyma of the organ is distinctive, consisting of colloid-filled epithelial follicles of many sizes. The lumen of each follicle is filled with a lightly staining colloid of a large gelatinous protein called thyroglobulin. ×12. H&E. **(B)** The lumen (L) of each follicle is surrounded by a simple epithelium in which the cell height ranges from squamous to low columnar. Also present are large pale-staining parafollicular or C cells (C) that secrete calcitonin, a polypeptide involved with calcium metabolism. ×200. H&E. **(C,D,E)** C cells may be part of the follicular epithelium or present singly or in groups outside of follicles. Follicular cells (F) can usually be distinguished from C cells (C) by the smaller size and darker staining properties. Unlike follicular cells, C cells seldom vary in their size or pale staining characteristics. C cells are somewhat easier to locate in or between small follicles. (C and D) ×400. H&E; e: ×400. Mallory trichrome. (Reproduced with permission from Mescher AL. Junqueira's Basic Histology: Text and Atlas. 12th ed. New York: McGraw Hill Lange, 2010:367 (Figure 20-19).)

- A decreased peripheral conversion of T4 to T3,
- Increased synthesis of biologically inactive thyroid hormones,
- Decreased synthesis of binding proteins,
- Increased presence of binding protein inhibitors,
- Decreased T3/T4 receptors, and
- Decreased cellular activity of T3.

In addition, many of the drugs often administered to ill patients, such as heparin, dopamine, and glucocorticoids, alter TSH secretion or thyroid hormone protein binding. If testing is necessary, a combination of TSH and FT4 may help determine if the patient has a thyroid disorder.

Congenital Abnormalities

Ectopic thyroid tissue, which may be functional, is occasionally present in abnormal locations along the line of fetal migration, most commonly within the tongue. There is a sevenfold preponderance in females. Ectopic thyroid tissue is generally asymptomatic, although occasionally it can cause problems because of interference with swallowing and breathing. Failure of the thyroglossal duct to involute may result in thyroglossal duct cysts, the most common congenital anomaly of the neck. They present as cystic masses with thyroid tissue found in the walls. The cysts occur along the midline between the location of the adult thyroid and tongue and are often attached to the hyoid bone. In some cases, the cysts and ectopic thyroid may represent the only functional thyroid tissue in a person, a finding that should be considered prior to surgical intervention.

Benign Diseases of the Thyroid

Abnormalities of the thyroid relating to function and structure are common. *Thyroid hyperplasia, which may be either diffuse or nodular, is referred to as* **goiter** *(a term generally used to* refer to non-neoplastic processes). Most thyroid abnormalities are benign; however, nodules in children is more likely to be malignant than in adults. Most thyroid cancers are indolent, but there are a small number of aggressive forms.

Nodular Goiter

Nodular goiter is most often nontoxic in that the hyperplastic gland does not produce symptoms related to abnormal endocrine thyroid function, neoplastic, or inflammatory disease. Nodular goiters may come to medical attention because of cosmetic or other concerns of patients relating to the neck mass. On occasion, such masses may cause dysphagia or stridor related to compression of neck structures. Sporadic goiter appears in the post-pubertal period and increases in frequency with age. Autopsy studies demonstrate small thyroid nodules in about half of the post 60 years old population.

Goiters encompass a spectrum of changes involving glandular hyperplasia, colloid accumulation, and with progression, the formation of discernible nodules. Multiple cycles of hyperplasia and **involution** (colloid accumulation) lead to the formation of multiple poorly circumscribed or partially encapsulated areas. Fibrosis, hemorrhage, cyst formation, and dystropic calcification are common. Hyperplasia is expressed at the cellular level as diffuse enlargement of glands with collapsed follicles decreased in colloid content and lined with tall columnar epithelium. Follicles may have focal papillary ingrowths **(Figure 15-14)**. Involution is associated with colloid accumulation in distended follicles, which are lined by flattened epithelium. Large nodules may require sampling by **fine-needle aspiration** (FNA) to exclude cancer. Treatment most often involves drug suppression; surgery is rarely necessary.

Hypothyroidism

Hypofunction of the thyroid results from loss or atrophy of the thyroid tissue, impaired hormone synthesis, or, rarely, insufficient stimulation of the gland (secondary or tertiary hypothyroidism). Clinical signs and symptoms include cold intolerance, slowing of physical and mental activity, hoarse voice, constipation, mild weight gain, and muscle weakness.

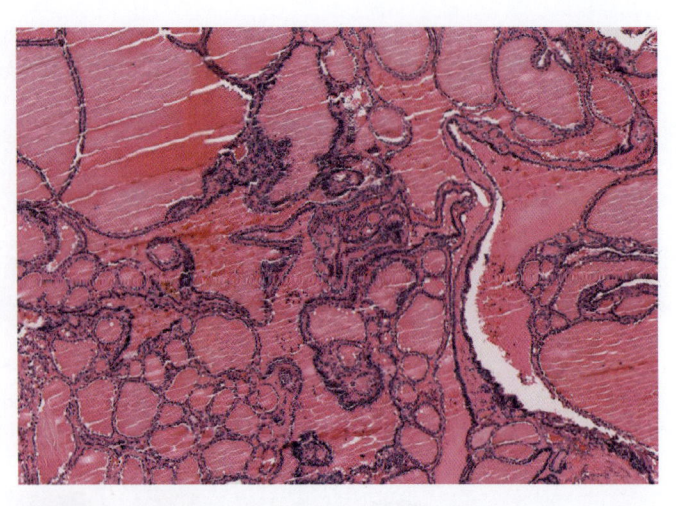

FIGURE 15-14 Nodular goiter. Photomicrograph demonstrates variability in size of thyroid follicles, some large and inactive, others smaller and hyperplastic. Complex papillary invaginations are present in some follicles.

As seen in **Figure 15-15**, the decreased production of the thyroid hormones stimulates secretion of TSH from the pituitary. Primary hypothyroidism is treated by daily hormone replacement. During initial treatment, FT4 concentrations change quickly, but TSH remains high. Although the response of the pituitary to thyroid hormones is normally rapid and exaggerated, since these patients are often hypothyroid for some time, it may take 4–8 weeks for serum TSH concentration to reach a new steady state (this is sometimes called the pituitary lag). In these first few weeks, FT4 is usually the best test to monitor replacement. Once the set point is re-established, TSH becomes the best monitor.

Congenital hypothyroidism is a serious finding and requires immediate treatment to prevent neurological and skeletal consequences (cretinism) (see below). Screening programs to detect neonatal hypothyroidism exist in almost every developed country. A combination of TSH and FT4 is used to monitor therapy.

Hypothyroidism occasionally occurs as a result of pituitary (secondary) or hypothalamic (tertiary) diseases that produce a

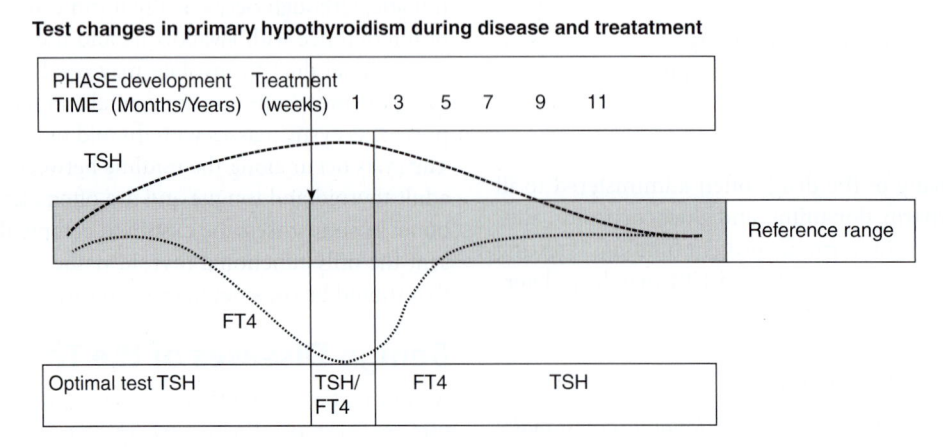

FIGURE 15-15 Changes in hormone pattern in hypothyroidism.

deficiency in TSH, TRH, or both. Isolated TSH deficiency is very rare and most patients have deficiencies in other pituitary hormones. Without stimulation from TSH, thyroid hormone production declines. In this situation, T4 and/or T3 concentrations are low and TSH concentrations are low or within the reference range.

Endemic and Other Hypofunctioning Goiters

Historically, nodular goiter was endemic in populations with low dietary iodine and associated with **cretinism** (physical and mental developmental defects relating to neonatal hypothyroidism that result from congenital iodine deficiency). Supplementation of table salt ("iodized salt") has prevented endemic goiter in developed countries, but the consequences of iodine deficiency are still seen in some areas of the world where diets are low in natural iodine and iodized salt is either expensive or unavailable. A number of foodstuffs such as cassava and drugs including lithium interfere with iodine uptake and are **goitrogenic**, associated with sporadic goiter (either nontoxic or associated with thyroid hormone suppression and presenting as hypothyroid goiter). Genetic defects in a number of metabolic pathways including mutations affecting the synthesis or release of thyroglobulin result in neonatal congenital hypothyroidism and goiter. *Where sufficient iodine is available, the most common cause of hypothyroidism after age 6 years is* **Hashimoto thyroiditis***, a condition characterized by the gradual, autoimmune-based destruction of the thyroid, which will be discussed below under thyroiditis.*

Toxic Multinodular Goiter

Patients with asymptomatic multinodular goiter can develop functioning (toxic) nodules. The disease is 10-fold more common in women over the age of 60 and is more frequent in areas with an endemic lack of iodine in the diet. Overall toxic multinodular goiter is the second most common cause of hyperthyroidism after **Graves disease** (see below) in developed countries. In toxic multinodular goiter, nodules function autonomously. Such lack of central control of thyroid hormone synthesis is frequently associated with somatic mutations of the TSH receptor or less commonly, the α-subunit of guanyl nucleotide stimulatory protein receptor of the TSH signal transduction pathway. Some nodules are monoclonal in origin and represent benign functional thyroid adenomas. The risk of finding neoplastic disease in multinodular goiter is low. About 5% of surgically removed nodules had evidence of thyroid cancer.

Hyperthyroidism

Primary hyperfunction of the thyroid has a number of causes, but the majority of cases, 60–80%, are related to **Graves disease** *(see below).* Excessive thyroid hormone concentrations lead to the classic symptoms of nervousness, fatigue, palpitations, heat intolerance, and weight loss. Complications of hyperthyroidism, if untreated, are far reaching and include stroke, congestive heart failure, and osteopenia.

Graves Disease

Graves disease and **Hashimoto thyroiditis** (discussed below under section "Thyroiditis" and clinically associated with hypothyroidism) are the most common members of the clinical spectrum of **autoimmune thyroid diseases (AITD)**. Graves disease (also known as **toxic diffuse goiter**) is the most common cause of hyperthyroidism in the United States. The disease is autoimmune in origin and results from the binding of antibodies (thyroid-stimulating immunoglobulins) to the TSH receptor of follicular cells resulting in dysregulated hypersecretion. About 10% of patients with Graves disease have additional autoimmune disease with rheumatoid arthritis being the most common. The disease is also associated with ophthalmopathy (affecting the orbital and periorbital tissue) characterized by eyelid retraction, proptosis, and edema of the periorbital area. In Graves disease, the thyroid gland becomes diffusely enlarged. Colloid is depleted, epithelial cells are tall, and hyperplastic and lymphocytic infiltration occurs (**Figure 15-16**).

Thyroid Autoantibody Detection in AITD

Thyroid-related autoantibodies are directed to a number of thyroid-specific targets such as the TSH-R TPO, Tg, and even T3 and T4. The antibodies are diagnostically useful because they may be present in patients who have mild biochemical changes and mild clinical symptoms. They are not, however, diagnostic as they are often present in low concentrations in 10–15% of the clinically euthyroid population.

TSH receptor antibodies are a group of related immunoglobulins that bind to thyroid cell membranes at, or near, the TSH receptor site and are frequently associated with Graves disease. This group of autoantibodies can be confusing as some stimulate the thyroid, while others decrease the gland's activity by blocking the action of TSH, and others have no effect. Stimulatory antibodies (sometimes termed LATS or long-acting

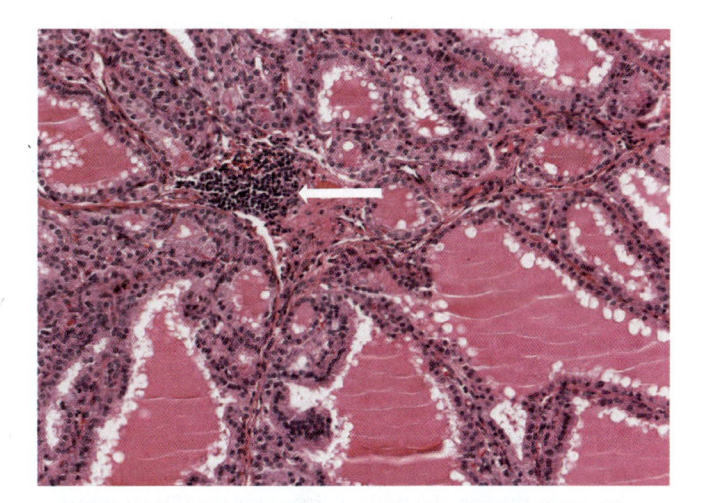

FIGURE 15-16 Graves disease (diffuse toxic goiter). Extensive hyperplastic small follicles lined by tall active follicular cells showing scalloping of colloid are present. A nest of lymphocytes is evident (arrow).

thyroid stimulator) are primarily responsible for the hyperfunction of the gland in *Antithyroid peroxidase antibodies (TPOAb)* a component of thyroid microsomes, titers are usually elevated in both Graves disease and HT. Low levels of these antibodies are known to precede thyroid dysfunction in euthyroid patients. Monitoring of such patients is useful as a rise in titer is associated with an increased risk of developing overt disease. However, the role of TPOAb in disease pathogenesis is unclear.

Thyroiditis

Inflammatory disorders of the thyroid may be caused by infectious agents and autoimmune mechanisms. Thyroiditis may be further subdivided into acute, subacute, and chronic forms differing in their etiology.

Acute Suppurative Thyroiditis

Acute suppurative thyroiditis is an uncommon childhood bacterial infection of the gland most often associated with *Staphylococcus aureus*, and *Streptococcus pyogenes*. The thyroid is highly resistant to bacterial infections. Hence, most cases are associated with congenital malformations such as a pyriform sinus, a fistulous connection between the pharynx and (generally) the left side of the thyroid capsule. Thyroglossal duct remnants may also be a route of infection.

> **IN TRANSLATION**
>
> As is the case with other autoimmune diseases, both environmental and genetic factors play a role in the etiology and pathogenesis of **AITD** including Graves disease and **Hashimoto thyroiditis** (discussed below). Environmental agents including increased iodine intake, certain drugs, infectious agents (notably hepatitis C, related in part to interferon α-therapy), stress, and ionizing radiation have been associated with autoimmune disease of the thyroid, but the relative importance of each in triggering AITD is unknown. Induction of HLA class II antigen expression on thyroid follicular cells as a result of environmentally induced epithelial cell injury is likely to play a role by allowing these cells to play a role in thyroid-specific antigen presentation.
>
> Multiple loci are involved in genetic susceptibility to AITD with each locus playing a small but additive role. A number of genes and chromosomal regions including variants of HLA-class II region are associated with susceptibility to Graves disease. HLA-D3 (and more specifically DRb1 Arg74 rather than Ala or Gln) is a strong risk factor for Graves disease. A similar association is found with Hashimoto thyroiditis. Variation in the CD40 molecule (important in terminal B cell differentiation), *PTPN22*, a lymphoid tyrosine phosphokinase, the gene for thyroglobulin, and the TSH receptor gene (*TSHR*) are all associated with increased risk of Graves (and other autoimmune thyroid) disease.

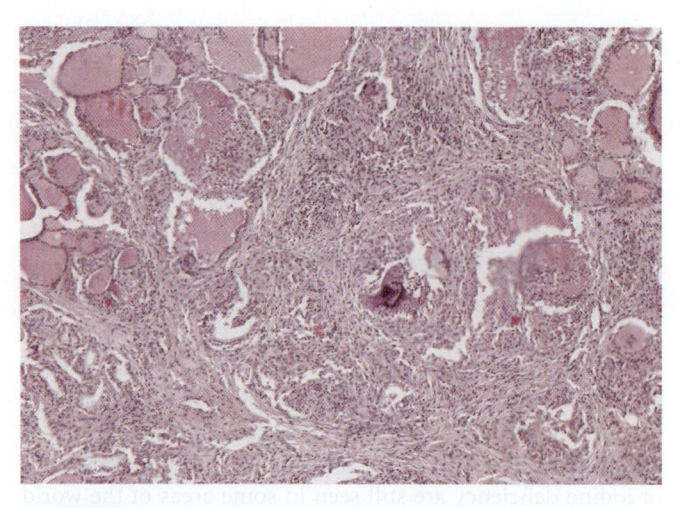

FIGURE 15-17 DeQuervain thyroiditis (granulomatous thyroiditis). Photomicrograph shows granuloma surrounding a giant cell. Residual follicles are present peripherally.

Subacute Thyroiditis

The most common form of **subacute thyroiditis** (also referred to as *granulomatous thyroiditis* or *DeQuervain thyroiditis*) is likely to have a viral etiology based on occurrence of the disease post-upper respiratory tract infections. The list of associated viremias is long and includes mumps, measles, influenza, and many others. The disease is fivefold more prevalent in women and is associated with positivity for the HLA-Bw35 antigen. The disease is self-limited and is characterized by a hyperthyroid periods associated with follicular destruction and release of thyroid hormone in the absence of accelerated synthesis. Hypothyroidism then occurs as a result of glandular depletion followed by a slow return to a euthyroid state in almost all patients. The disease is characterized by neck pain and an enlarged asymmetric, fibrotic appearing thyroid. There is an initial acute inflammation of the gland followed by granulomatous inflammation with replacement of follicles by histiocytes and giant cells. Patchy fibrosis is common **(Figure 15-17)**.

Chronic Autoimmune Thyroiditis (Hashimoto Thyroiditis)

Hashimoto thyroiditis and Graves disease (discussed above under section "Hyperthyroidism") are the most common members of the clinical spectrum of AITD. After age 6 years, Hashimoto thyroiditis is the most common cause of hypothyroidism in the United States and other areas of the world with adequate iodine intake. The disease shows a 7- to 10-fold female preponderance and is predominantly a disease of middle age. The disease is characterized by extensive infiltration of the thyroid by lymphocytes and plasma cells, often accompanied by germinal center formation. Enlarged follicular oncocytic cells (Hürthle cells, as mentioned above) are a common finding **(Figure 15-18)**. T cells are predominantly Th1 CD4 in phenotype and play a role in the destruction of thyrocytes by

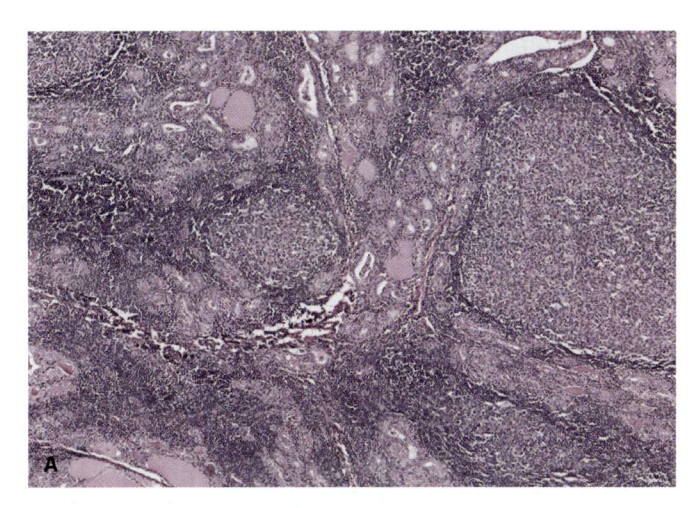

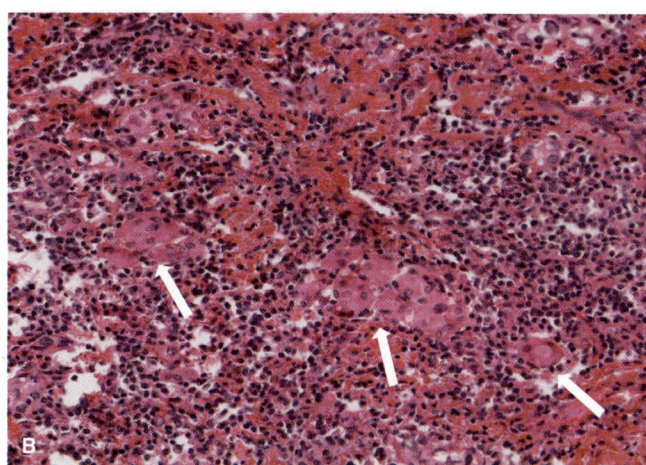

FIGURE 15-18 **Hashimoto thyroiditis (A)** Low-power photomicrograph demonstrates extensive lymphoid infiltration and the presence of germinal centers surrounding residual follicles. **(B)** Hürthle cells surrounding small residual follicles (arrow).

mediating cytotoxic T-cell-induced apoptosis. Intrathyroid B cells produce antibodies directed against a variety of thyroid-specific antigens, predominantly thyroglobulin and TPO, a diagnostic hallmark of the disease. Occasionally antibodies to the TSH receptor occur, but unlike those found in Graves disease, such antibodies block rather than stimulate the receptor. Antithyroid antibodies in Hashimoto thyroiditis have the potential to be cytotoxic (through complement mediated and other mechanisms). Antibody secreting cells may also play a role in antigen presentation to T cells. Additional information on the etiology of AITD is noted above.

Fibrosis may be present both in late stage disease and as a distinct variant associated with high levels of IgG 4. This variant is a member of the group of **IgG4-related systemic diseases (IgG4-RSD)**, which includes autoimmune pancreatitis. These hyper-IgG4 diseases are characterized by the increased level of this normally trace immunoglobulin subtype combined with lymphoplasmacytic infiltration by IgG4-positive plasma cells and diffuse fibrosis. Patients are most often initially euthyroid but become hypothyroid in late stage disease. The initial presentation may be that of hyperthyroidism and Graves disease, which may precede the occurrence of Hashimoto thyroiditis. Hashimoto thyroiditis is associated with an increased incidence of papillary carcinoma of the thyroid and primary thyroid lymphoma (especially extranodal marginal zone B cell lymphomas).

Neoplasms of the Thyroid

Benign Neoplasms—Follicular Adenoma

Thyroid nodules are extremely common. About 5% of the population has thyroid nodules on palpation, but up to 60% have nodules at autopsy or when imaging of the neck is performed for reasons unrelated to the thyroid gland. Most nodules are non-neoplastic (related to functional thyroid disease such as multinodular goiter), but 5–20% are neoplasms. Of these neoplastic nodules the majority are benign, termed follicular adenomas. Follicular adenomas are much more likely to be solitary nodules and are usually cold (nonfunctional) on thyroid scans. Solitary, solid (non cystic) cold nodules are usually investigated by FNA. However, the diagnosis of follicular adenoma is difficult to make by FNA, and is often indistinguishable from cellular nodules in a goiter or follicular carcinoma (see What We Do box, page 419).

Follicular adenomas are defined as completely encapsulated nodules that show a different pattern inside the nodule than in the surrounding thyroid gland (Figure 15-19). The adenoma may show a variety of patterns (microfollicular, macrofollicular, trabecular) and may be composed of normal appearing follicular cells or oncocytic (Hurthle) cells (Hurthle cell adenoma). By definition, adenomas do not breach the capsule and do not invade into blood vessels. Pathologists must examine the entire capsule of an encapsulated nodule to exclude capsular or vascular invasion before making a diagnosis of follicular adenoma.

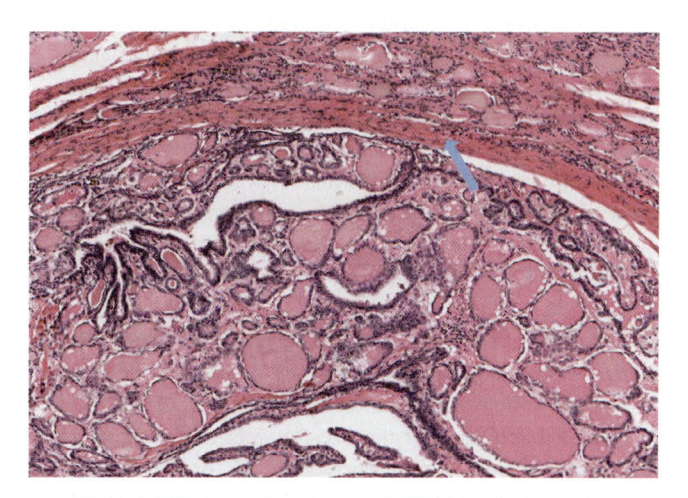

FIGURE 15-19 **Follicular adenoma of thyroid.** Follicular adenoma (bottom of field) shows no sign of having breached the intact capsule (arrow).

Malignant Neoplasms

Follicular Cell-Derived Thyroid Carcinoma

Thyroid cancer is relatively rare, comprising 1% of all new cancers in the United States each year. The great majority arise from follicular cells. These tumors span a spectrum from well-differentiated to undifferentiated, and their biologic behavior can be very indolent to extremely aggressive. Fortunately, the majority are on the well-differentiated end. Tumors occur over a wide age range with young individuals having a more benign course in most instances. Risk factors for the development of thyroid cancer include radiation exposure, particularly in children (as documented by the Chernobyl nuclear disaster). Other risk factors include mutational events such as somatic mutations in familial polyposis tumor suppressor gene and of the RET proto-oncogene.

The principal thyroid cancers that arise from follicular thyroid cells are as follows:

- Papillary thyroid carcinoma
- Follicular thyroid carcinoma
- Poorly differentiated thyroid carcinoma
- Anaplastic thyroid carcinoma

Papillary thyroid carcinoma (PTC) represents about 80% of all thyroid cancers in the United States. PTC has a strong association with radiation exposure, either for therapeutic purposes or as a result of environmental exposure. PTC is about threefold more common in females. The average age of presentation is between 35 and 40, but PTC may occur in young children. The prognosis is excellent in young people (25 year survival rate >95%) even with lymph node metastases), but aggressive disease may occur in particularly in males and older patients and in the case of some unusual histologic variants of PTC. The tumor spreads by lymphatic invasion; regional lymph node metastases are common and may be the presenting sign. Distant blood-borne metastatic disease is uncommon.

PTCs have a white invasive appearance on gross examination and show indistinct margins. Tumor may invade locally and extend beyond the thyroid. On microscopic evaluation, tumors are most often unencapsulated. Papillae consist of a neoplastic epithelium surrounding vascular stalks. Papillary architecture is not required for diagnosis, which is based on cytologic features of the neoplastic cells. Cytologic features of PTC are characteristic and diagnostic. Such features include crowded cells, nuclei with finely dispersed chromatin and nuclei showing irregular contour, grooves, and intranuclear pseudoinclusions. Psammoma bodies (calcific concretions) are present in about half of cases (Figure 15-20). Such features may be easier to appreciate using cytology (as with FNA) than in histology material. **Papillary microcarcinomas** are small (1 cm or less), incidentally detected carcinomas. They are the most common form of papillary carcinoma. *Up to a quarter of thyroidectomies for benign disease and up to a third of autopsies harbor papillary microcarcinomas. These usually have an excellent prognosis, though rarely may spread to cervical lymph nodes.*

Nuclear changes characteristic of PTC may occur in tumor areas showing follicular (rather than papillary) architecture and such tumors are classified as a **follicular variant of papillary thyroid carcinoma (FVPTC)** and have similar behavior to "conventional" PTC. Several additional variants of PTC are defined including **encapsulated PTC**, which has a better prognosis than conventional PTC and **tall-cell variant PTC** (characterized by the presence of tall, columnar malignant cells that are about twice as tall as wide) having an aggressive behavior. *BRAF* gene mutations (discussed above) are particularly common in this variant.

IN TRANSLATION

Activation of two receptor tyrosine kinases as a result of chromosomal rearrangements is detected in about half of all sporadic cases of PTC. The majority of cases demonstrate fusion of the 3' tyrosine kinase portion of the *RET* gene to the 5' portion of a number of different genes, which (unlike *RET*) are normally expressed in follicular thyroid cells. This results in a constitutively activated *RET* gene (termed *RET-PTC*) in follicular cells. Fifteen percent of cases show rearrangement of the *NTRK1* tyrosine kinase gene by a similar mechanism resulting in a constitutively active *TRK* gene in follicular cells. Activation of the serine/threonine kinase *BRAF* gene either by fusion gene formation or (much more commonly) by point mutations is a common finding in sporadic PTC and results in activation of the RAS-RAF-MEK-MAPK signaling pathway as does the presence of *RET-PTC* or *TRK*. A single point mutation at residue 600 (val600glu) in *BRAF* accounts for over 98% of all such mutations.

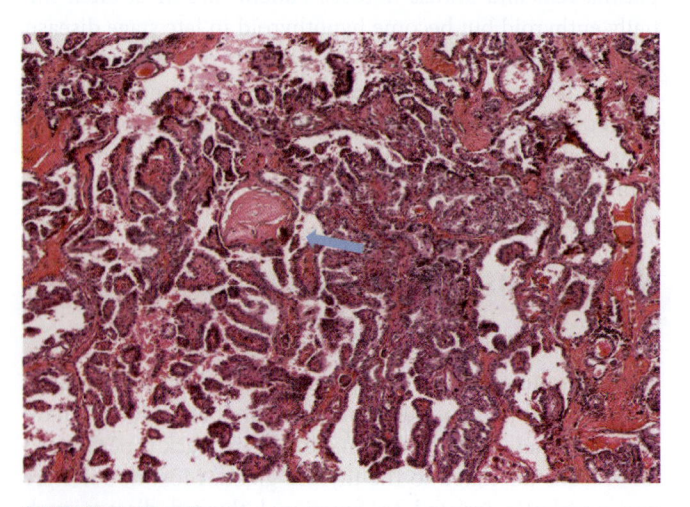

FIGURE 15-20 Papillary carcinoma of the thyroid. Photomicrograph demonstrates the complex papillary structure characteristic of this lesion. A psammoma body is present (arrow).

Poorly Differentiated Thyroid Carcinoma

A small subset of follicularly derived thyroid carcinomas are intermediate between the well differentiated papillary and follicular carcinomas and undifferentiated anaplastic thyroid carcinoma discussed below. These are termed poorly differentiated thyroid carcinoma. Most have a solid or insular (nested) architecture. These are thought to be de-differentiations of well differentiated thyroid cancer, and often transitions are seen between the well-differentiated and poorly differentiated portions of the tumor. The mean 5-year survival is about 50%.

Undifferentiated (Anaplastic) thyroid carcinoma (ATC): ATC is a rare and highly malignant disease, which although responsible for only 2% of all thyroid cancer results in 40% of deaths. It is found predominantly in elderly female patients in their seventh to ninth decade. Metastatic disease (usually to the lung) is often present at diagnosis. Five-year survival is less than 10% and most patients are dead within 1 year of diagnosis, often as a result of invasion of vital structures of the neck leading to impairment of respiration. A number of anaplastic cellular variants are described including squamoid, spindle cell, and giant cell types. Most cases are diagnosed by FNA, since patients typically are not surgical

> **HUNTING FOR ZEBRAS**
>
> A small percentage of PTC is associated with familial syndromes that increase the risk of cancer in multiple organ systems; an example being Gardner syndrome (**familial adenomatous polyposis, FAP**). In this autosomal dominant syndrome in which the *APC* tumor suppressor gene is inactivated, there is a 2–12% incidence of PTC, roughly a 10-fold excess over that expected in this population. Young women with FAP show an extraordinary 160-fold excess of thyroid cancer. Familial disease (unlike sporadic PTC) tends to be multicentric, bilateral, and has a propensity for invasion and metastasis.

Follicular thyroid carcinoma (FTC): FTC usually presents as a solitary cold thyroid nodule in the fifth and sixth decade developing about three times more often in females. Hürthle cell carcinomas (FTC-like tumors composed of oncocytic Hürthle cells) are considered as a subtype of FTC, although they demonstrate a higher percentage of invasive disease. FTC may present with distant metastatic disease, most frequently to the bone and lung. Unlike PTC, FTC is spread via a blood born route. FTC may present as an encapsulated tumor or as disseminated disease in which tumor has spread throughout the thyroid and invaded perithyroid tissues. There is a 70-100% 10-year survival if the lesion has an intact capsule. However, 10-year survival falls to 15–45% for disseminated disease. *Recurrent disease occurs in half of patients showing any sign of angioinvasion in vessels either within or beyond the tumor capsule, even in the absence of tumor spread to the thyroid parenchyma (grossly encapsulated angioinvasive FTC)* (Figure 15-21).

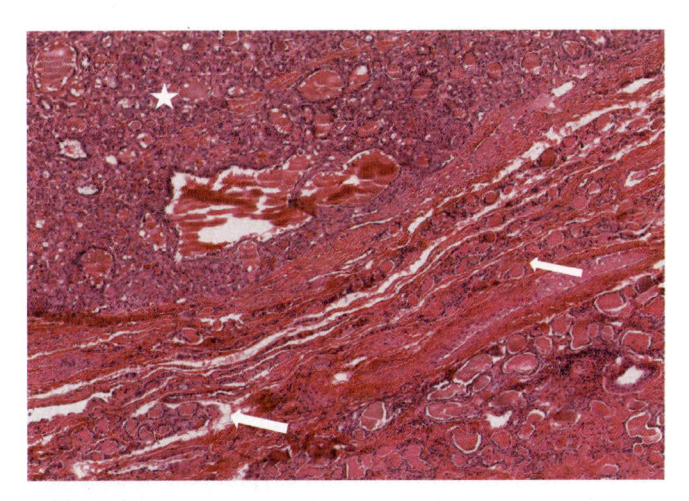

FIGURE 15-21 Follicular carcinoma of the thyroid. Invasion of the neoplastic cell population (★) through the tumor capsule is evident (arrow).

> **WHAT WE DO**
>
> The mainstay of diagnosis of solid thyroid masses is FNA. These are usually done on nodules that are cold on thyroid scan. FNA is excellent for tumors that have characteristic cytology, such as papillary, medullary, and undifferentiated (anaplastic) thyroid carcinoma. Likewise, cytology is very dependable for benign goiters, especially those that contain a large amount of colloid. Colloid can be easily seen in FNA slides and reliably indicates that the lesion is benign. The problem with thyroid FNA is with lesions that show crowded follicular cells in an acinar architecture, since this pattern can be seen in hyperplastic nodules in benign goiters, follicular adenomas, and follicular carcinomas. Distinction between these depends on architectural features such as encapsulation and invasion, which cannot be done by a small sample from the center of the lesion. Thus, cytology cannot reliably distinguish between these entities, and needle aspirates from all three types of cases are usually signed out in a nondefinitive, atypical way. To help refine this heterogeneous group of cytology diagnoses, several commercial molecular-based tests exist that look either the proprietary genetic signature of benign thyroid tissue (Afirma Gene Expression Classifier) or known gene mutations and rearrangements that have been associated with thyroid cancer (such as RET, BRAF, KRAS, PAX8, the miRInform Thyroid Test). These tests, while expensive, may add additional information to that obtained by cytology, and may help decide between a likely benign or likely malignant diagnosis for planning further care.

candidates. Undifferentiated thyroid carcinoma is readily recognized as malignant by cytology, and yield highly cellular samples with bizarre tumor cells. Similar BRAF and RAS mutations to those found in FTC and PTC are also found in ATC suggesting a progression of pro-neoplastic genetic alterations. ATC also demonstrates frequent additional mutation in the TP53 gene (for p53) CTNNB1 (encoding a β-catenin), which may be involved in tumor dedifferentiation.

Neuroendocrine Cell-Derived Thyroid Carcinoma: Medullary Thyroid Carcinoma (MTC)

MTC is a neuroendocrine tumor arising from the parafollicular C cells responsible for calcitonin production. The tumor is responsible for about 5% of thyroid cancer and about 80% of cases are sporadic. However, 20% of cases are associated with the autosomal dominant disease **MEN2** so familial clusters occur. Because the malignant C cells secrete calcitonin, increased serum levels of this hormone in the presence of a thyroid nodule are virtually diagnostic for MTC. The overall prognosis for MTC is worse than for patients with well-differentiated follicular cell-derived tumors. The 10-year survival rate is 65% combining sporadic and familial forms. Prognosis varies with MEN2 variants but is generally better in the young. Cervical lymph node metastases are common at diagnosis. Multicentric bilateral disease occurs in familial disease (but not sporadic) disease.

> ### IN TRANSLATION
> MTC is strongly associated with gain of function mutations in the *RET* receptor tyrosine kinase proto-oncogene in both sporadic and familial disease. Three subtypes of familial MEN are recognized all of which are associated with specific mutational events in *RET* and all with a near 100% lifetime risk of MTC.
>
> **MEN2A (Sipple syndrome)** is the most common form of MEN2 accounting for up to 80% of cases. As many as 95% of MEN2A patients develop MTC often with lymph node involvement before 35 years of age. The syndrome is also associated with development of pheochromocytomas and hyperparathyroidism. **MEN2B** is the least common variant comprising 5% of cases and is associated with aggressive MTC occurring at an early age in the absence of thyroidectomy prior to 1 year. The disease is also associated with pheochromocytomas, mucosal neuromas, and a Marfanoid habitus. **Familial MTC** accounts for up to 20% of MEN2. This variant of MEN2 is solely associated with MTC and a later age of disease onset and lower penetrance than MEN2A and B. The disease is most commonly diagnosed in families showing late onset MTC with *RET* mutations. Sporadic MTC is associated with *RET* mutations in 50% of cases and with *RAS* mutations in about 25% of cases.

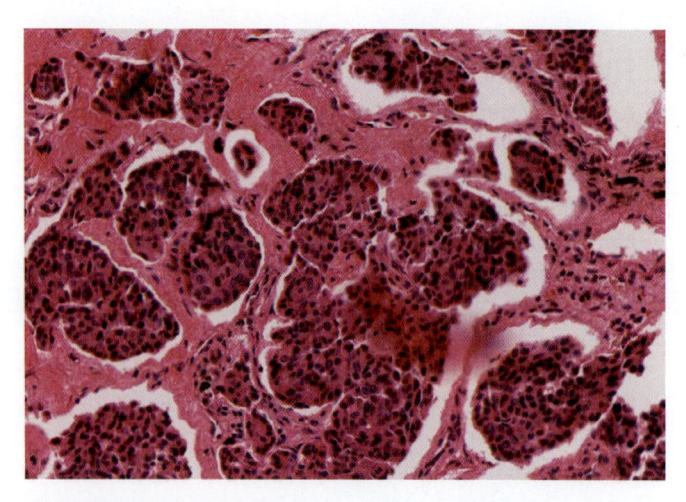

FIGURE 15-22 Medullary carcinoma of the thyroid. High-power photomicrograph from a metastasis to a lymph node demonstrates islands of medullary cells surrounded by amorphous amyloid deposition.

Grossly, MTCs are unencapsulated and found in the middle and upper thyroid lobes, the location of thyroid parafollicular cells. Focal calcifications may be observed. C cell hyperplasia is associated with inherited disease prior to onset of MTC in MEM 2 and is a likely precursor lesion. The neoplastic C cells infiltrate and destroy thyroid follicles and have a typical neuroendocrine appearance, demonstrating packets of uniform round, oval, or spindle-shaped cells (Figure 15-22). The stroma in MTC may show deposition of amyloid with green birefringence upon Congo red staining.

PARATHYROID

Parathyroid glands (PT) are derived from branchial clefts III and IV. Four glands are most commonly found, but the number can vary between 1 and 12. Glands are small (about 3×6 mm weighing less than 50 mg each) and are most commonly found embedded in the posterior thyroid capsular surface with one gland on the anterior and posterior pole of each thyroid lobe (Figure 15-23). Embryonic migration is variable and parathyroid tissue may reside in the mediastinum, pericardium, near the recurrent laryngeal nerve, and attached to the thymus in 10% of individuals. The frequent association with thymic tissue relates to the development of the inferior parathyroid, which originates from a combined thymus–parathyroid primordia derived from the third pharyngeal pouch. Separation of the primordia into inferior parathyroid and thymus is not complete in some individuals.

The parathyroid glands are encapsulated and septate containing clusters of secretory cell. Approximately 75% of the gland is composed of small polygonal **chief cells**, which secrete **parathyroid hormone (PTH)** and **oxyphil** cells of uncertain function. The chief cells form cords clustered around capillaries. Oxyphil cells are larger, have a distinctive pink cytoplasm, are arrayed in small clusters and are increased in number in

PATHOLOGY OF THE ENDOCRINE SYSTEM 429

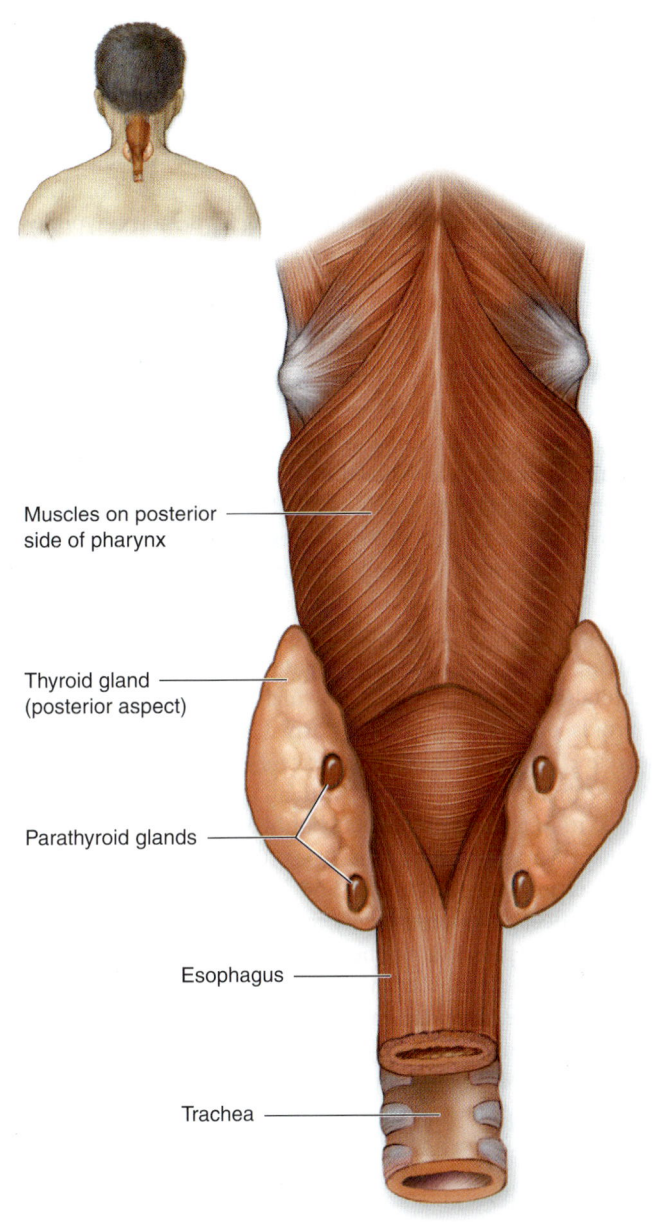

FIGURE 15-23 Parathyroid glands. The parathyroid glands are four small nodules normally embedded in the capsule on the posterior surface of the thyroid gland. They arise embryologically from the third and fourth pharyngeal pouches and migrate to the developing thyroid, a process that frequently leads to ectopic or additional parathyroid glands, often associated with the thymus. (Reproduced with permission from Mescher AL. Junqueira's Basic Histology: Text and Atlas. 12th ed. New York: McGraw Hill Lange, 2010:369 (Figure 20-22).)

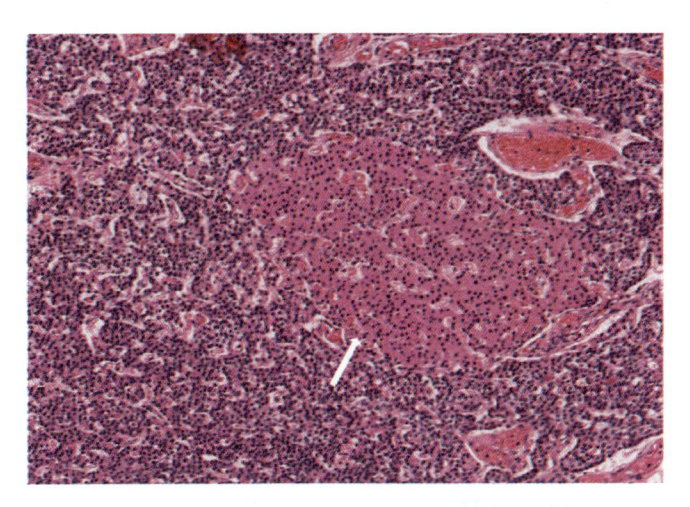

FIGURE 15-24 Parathyroid gland normal histology. Chief cells are predominant. An island of oxyphil is present (arrow).

glands from the elderly The balance of the parathyroid gland is composed of adipocytes, amounts of which also increase with age (Figure 15-24).

PTH is secreted into the circulation as an 84 amino acid protein hormone derived from a 115 amino acid preproparathyroid hormone. The bioactivity of the hormone is mediated via binding of the amino terminal 34 amino acids to the type 1 PTH receptor (PTHR1). The intact molecule has a very short plasma half-life and represents no more than 30% of circulating hormone being rapidly degraded into carboxy-terminal fragments missing the PTHR1 receptor-binding region. Certain of these fragments (confusingly called nonparathyroid hormone 1-84), lacking in canonical Ca^{2+} regulating activity, may inhibit the bone resorption activities of osteoclasts and hence have hypocalcemic activity. For this reason, the exact epitope specificity of the immunoassay used to measure PTH may be of clinical significance. This is of particular concern in chronic renal disease where "nonparathyroid hormone" peptides may be clinically significant.

QUICK REVIEW

PTH has a number of critical physiological functions mediated via its action on its major end organs: bone, kidneys, and intestine.

- PTH increases the level of circulating Ca^{2+} by increasing levels of osteoclast stimulating factor production by osteoblasts thereby serving to increase bone resorption with subsequent release of Ca^2. The increased level of ion suppresses PTH production in a negative feedback loop. Calcitonin serves an opposing function by inhibiting osteoclast activation and promoting bone growth.
- PTH stimulates the synthesis of active vitamin D (1,25 dihydroxyvitamin D3) from its precursor by activating a 1-hydroxylase in the renal tubules. 1,25 dihydroxyvitamin D3 promotes Ca^2 uptake by intestinal epithelial cells.
- PTH inhibits the resorption of phosphorus by renal tubular cells and increases uptake of Ca^{2+} thereby reducing blood phosphate and increasing blood Ca^{2+} levels.
- In **hyperparathyroidism** blood Ca^{2+} levels are increased and blood phosphate levels are decreased while the opposite (low blood Ca^{2+}, high blood phosphate) occurs in **hypoparathyroidism**.

Hypoparathyroidism

Primary hypoparathyroidism (HypoPT) results from decreased or absent of PTH secretion and is characterized by hypocalcemia and hyperphosphatemia. The most common cause of primary HypoPT is iatrogenic, resulting from surgical removal of all parathyroid glands. Such removal may be the result of surgery for thyroid or neck malignancies, in an attempt to treat MEN2A-related disease (see above) or other forms of parathyroid hyperplasia. In **secondary hypoparathyroidism**, there is low PTH combined with an elevated level of serum calcium. Processes external to the parathyroid glands, most commonly associated with malignancy or an osteolytic process, are responsible for the hypercalcemia.

Autoimmune Hypoparathyroidism

Autoimmune disease (either restricted to the parathyroids and often idiopathic in nature, or as part of **autoimmune polyglandular syndrome 1 [APS 1] alternately [PGA 1]**) is an uncommon cause of primary HypoPT and is also discussed above under adrenal hypofunction. Antibodies directed toward **parathyroid calcium sensing receptor (CaSR)** are found in both APS 1 and idiopathic autoimmune parathyroid disease. Activating antibodies directed toward CaSR (as well as congenital activating mutations in the protein) lead to HypoPT, while inactivating antibodies (and mutations) lead to **hyperparathyroidism (HyperPT)**. Antibodies to an additional parathyroid antigen (NALP5) occur in half of APS 1 patients and are also associated with autoimmune HypoPT.

Congenital Hypoparathyroidism

*A number of congenital syndromes involving PT maldevelopment are associated with HypoPT. The most common of these is **DiGeorge syndrome (DGS)**, which occurs in about 1 in 4000 live births.* The syndrome is associated with conotruncal cardiac defects, characteristic craniofacial defects, and thymic and parathyroid hypoplasia or absence, resulting in T-cell-associated immunodeficiency disease and neonatal hypocalcemia (in 20–60% of patients). DGS is best understood as a "field defect" involving development of structures dependent on third and fourth pharyngeal pouches and associated neural crest derived tissue, which is found in patients with deletions of the 22q11.2 chromosomal region. This region subtends 30–50 genes, but the critical gene is TBX1 a T-box transcription factor whose function is required in early patterning and development of the pharyngeal pouch derivative structures. DGS occurs sporadically in 85% of cases, but 7% of cases are inherited and point mutations have been detected solely in TBX1 in inherited disease.

Pseudohypoparathyroidism

Pseudohypoparathyroidism (PHP) is a result of end-organ insensitivity to the effect of PTH, which results in hypocalcemia, hyperphosphatemia, and *increased* PTH levels. The best understood form of PHP, **Albright hereditary osteodystrophy (AHO)** now classified as **PHP type 1a**, is the result of a dominant mutation in the *GNAS1 gene* responsible for the α-subunit of a stimulatory G protein that couples receptor peptide-hormone binding to adenylate cyclase activation. In addition to PHP and resistance to PHA administration, patients have a variety of skeletal defects, a stocky habitus, and short stature. Lack of sensitivity to other peptide hormones (and in particular thyrotropin resulting in primary hypothyroidism) occurs in many patients with PHP type 1a.

Hyperparathyroidism

Primary hyperparathyroidism (HyperPT) relates to overproduction of PTH by the parathyroid gland with resultant high serum calcium and low serum phosphate. **Secondary (renal) HyperPT** is associated with chronic renal disease and presents with extreme levels of PTH combined with normal to low serum calcium and bone demineralization related to renal osteodystrophy. Rising calcium and falling phosphate levels provide the stimulus for excess PTH production. **Tertiary HyperPT** refers to long-standing chronic renal disease patients treated by renal transplantation (and in some cases subtotal parathyroidectomy) in which the hyperplastic parathyroids do not return to a normal state and continue to secrete PTH autonomously and excessively.

Primary HyperPT occurs with an age-adjusted frequency of two to four cases per 10,000, but in elderly populations the frequency may be higher than 1 per 1000. The disease is three times as frequent in females and is generally diagnosed in the fifth decade or later. Eighty to ninety percent of cases are related to the presence of a benign solitary adenoma generally involving one gland. Carcinomas of the parathyroid gland are extremely rare. They are most often active in secreting PTH and constitute 1% or less of cases of primary HyperPT. Hyperplasia and/or multiple adenomas are responsible for the balance of cases. Most cases of primary HyperPT are sporadic; a few are associated with inherited syndromes (Figure 15-25).

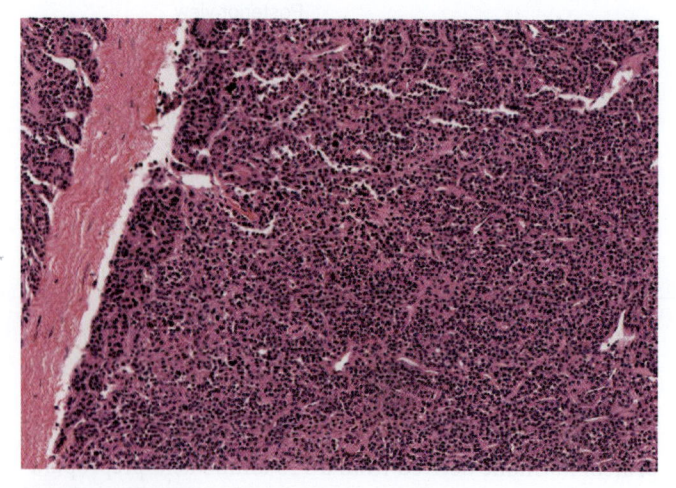

FIGURE 15-25 Hyperplastic parathyroid gland. Marked chief cell hyperplasia in a multinodular pattern is demonstrated. A connective tissue septum is present vertically on the left of the field.

Treatment of primary HyperPT requires surgical removal of the adenoma(s). In the hands of an experienced surgeon, the success rate is excellent with low morbidity and recurrence. The finding of persistent or recurrent hypercalcemia is consistent with either incomplete resection of hyperplastic parathyroid tissue or a missed adenoma. The extremely short half-life of PTH and the availability of reasonably rapid methods (<20 minutes) allow for the evaluation of surgical success, that is, an intraoperative PTH. The protocol establishes patient's baseline PTH level prior to surgery for comparison to a second sample collected 5–10 minutes post-gland excision. If all hypersecreting tissue has been removed, the PTH level will drop by at least 50% with the second sample.

Familial Hyperparathyroidism

Familial hypoparathyroidism is responsible for about 5% of patients with HyperPT. Defects in several genes are responsible disease in kindreds and also in some cases of sporadic disease. MEN1 (Werner syndrome—also discussed above) is an autosomal dominant disorder characterized by parathyroid, pancreatic islet and pituitary hyperplasia and tumor formation. HyperPT is most characteristic of the disease with a 50% or greater penetrance by the age of 50. Hyperplasia occurs in multiple glands and has a very high postoperative recurrence rate. The syndrome is associated with germ line mutations in *MEN1 locus*. LOH is required for tumor formation. LOH and somatic mutations at the MEN1 locus have also been detected in a significant number of sporadic parathyroid adenomas. MEN2A (Sipple disease—also discussed under section "Medullary thyroid carcinoma") is most associated with MTC, but parathyroid gland hyperplasia and hyperPT occur in about 20% of cases.

Osteitis Fibrosa Cystica

Osteitis fibrosa cystica (OFC) also known as **brown tumor of hyperparathyroidism** is a now uncommon complication of poorly treated hyperPT. *OFC is not a neoplasm but rather a spectrum of PTH driven bone changes that result in increased osteoclast activity, fibrosis, cyst formation, and concurrent hemorrhage (hence the brown coloration)* (Figure 15-26). OFC is associated with bone pain, swelling, and pathologic fractures and can mimic "true" bone neoplasms in radiographs.

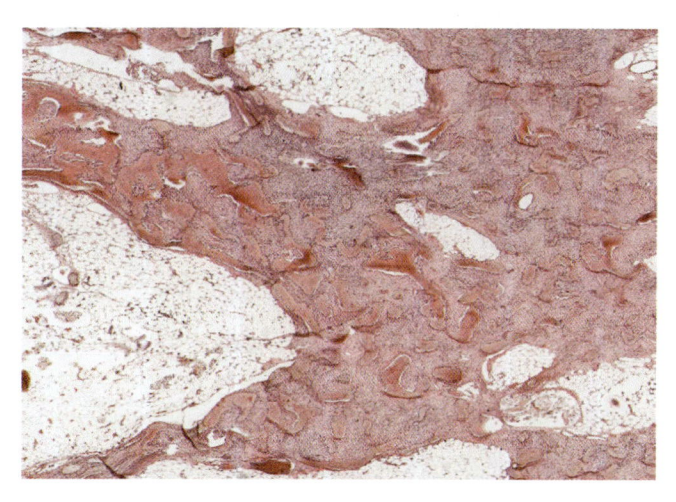

FIGURE 15-26 Osteitis fibrosa cystica. Extensive cyst formation and osteoclastic activity occurs. Brown areas result from hemosiderin accumulation.

CHAPTER 16

Breast Pathology

Chad A. Livasy, M.D.

INTRODUCTION

CASE 16-1

A 32-year-old G4P4 woman presents with complaints of a new lump in her left breast. Her past medical history is negative for a family history of breast carcinoma. Physical examination reveals a 3 cm firm, ill-defined mass that is tender to palpation. Ultrasound studies demonstrate a 4 cm solid-appearing mass with ill-defined borders. Due to the solid-appearing nature of the lesion and ill-defined borders, the lesion is categorized as suspicious and biopsy is recommended. Ultrasound-guided core biopsy is performed yielding the histology demonstrated in **Figure 16-1**.
    Pathologic diagnosis: Granulomatous mastitis.

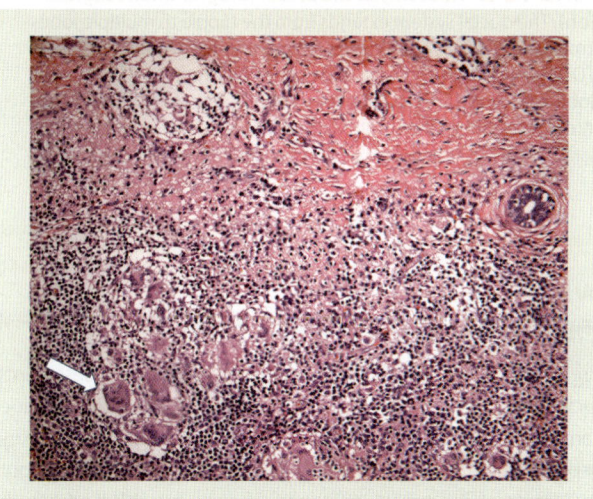

FIGURE 16-1 Granulomatous mastitis. The breast stroma is involved by a dense inflammatory process consisting of dense aggregates of histiocytes (arrow) and a background of lymphocytes.

Normal Anatomy and Histology

The breast lies anterior to the chest wall over the pectoralis major muscle and typically extends from the second to the sixth rib in the vertical axis and from the sternal edge to the midaxillary line in the horizontal axis. Bundles of dense fibrous connective tissue, the suspensory ligaments of Cooper, extend from the skin to the pectoral fascia and provide support for the breast. At puberty, estradiol and progesterone levels increase to initiate breast development. The adult female breast consists of a series of branching ducts that terminate in lobules. The arrangement of these structures resembles a branching tree with 5–10 primary milk ducts in the nipple, 20–40 segmental ducts, and 10–100 subsegmental ducts that end in glandular units called terminal-duct lobular units (TDLU) **(Figure 16-2)**. The TDLU represents the functional unit of the breast **(Figure 16-3)**. During lactation, there is a dramatic increase in the number of lobules, and the epithelial cells in the TDLU undergo secretory changes consisting of cytoplasmic vacuoles **(Figure 16-4)**. The accumulated secretions are then transported via the ductal system to the nipple. When lactation ceases, the lobules involute and return to their normal resting appearance. The mammary ducts and lobules are embedded within a stroma composed of varying amounts of fibrous and adipose tissue. The stromal component comprises the major portion of the nonlactating adult breast, consisting of lobular stroma and interlobular stroma. The proportions of fibrous and adipose tissue vary with age and among individuals and may affect the sensitivity and specificity of mammographic studies. During menopause, as a result of reduction in estrogen and progesterone, there is involution and atrophy of the TDLUs associated with loss of the specialized intralobular stroma. The postmenopausal breast is characterized by marked reduction

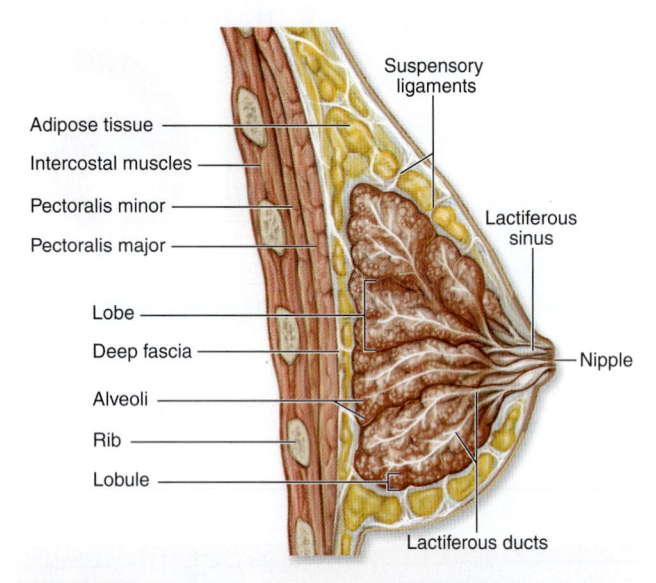

FIGURE 16-2 **Anatomy of the breast (diagrammatic sagittal section).** The ductal system extends from the nipple to multiple lobes of terminal-duct lobular units (TDLUs) branching in a treelike fashion. The TDLU is the site of origin for most breast carcinomas. The ducts and lobular acini are lined by two layers of cells: the inner luminal cells and outer myoepithelial cells. (Reproduced with permission from McKinley M, O'Loughlin VD. Human Anatomy, 2nd ed. New York: McGraw-Hill; 2008.)

in the glandular and fibrous stroma components, typically with concomitant increase in stromal adipose tissue.

The cells lining the ductal-lobular system are bilayered. The inner luminal cell layer is cuboidal to columnar in shape and typically shows relatively uniform round nuclei. Most pathologic epithelial lesions of the breast, including carcinoma, arise from the luminal cell layer. The outer myoepithelial (basal) cell layer is typically comprised of flattened-appearing cells with compressed nuclei and scant cytoplasm. It is critical to understand this concept as preservation or loss of this bilayered arrangement is used to distinguish benign from malignant epithelial lesions of the breast (Figure 16-5).

Clinical Symptoms of Breast Disease

The various presenting clinical symptoms of breast disease are summarized in Table 16-1. These symptoms include breast mass/lump, breast pain, nipple-related problems, and skin changes. Breast mass/lump is the most common presenting symptom. Each symptom should bring to mind a differential diagnosis depending on the clinical context. Benign conditions predominate in younger patients and breast cancer becomes increasingly more prevalent with advancing age. Breast cancer does not have specific signs and symptoms that allow reliable

WHAT WE DO
Clinical Evaluation of Breast Disease

Breast abnormalities are usually evaluated with "triple assessment" including physical examination, imaging studies, and tissue sampling for suspicious or indeterminate breast lesions. Key aspects of physical examination include palpation of the four quadrants of the breast, palpation of axilla for enlarged lymph nodes, examination of breast skin/areola/nipple, and evaluation of nipple discharge. Most mass lesions in women >35 years of age are evaluated with mammography, often in conjunction with ultrasound studies. The advantage of mammography as an imaging modality is that it is quick to perform and interpret its images essentially the whole breast and has a reasonably high sensitivity to detect invasive carcinoma (identified as density, architecture distortion or asymmetry) and ductal carcinoma in situ (DCIS) (calcifications). It is important to understand that not all cancers are seen using mammography and that palpable masses not identified on imagines studies still require further investigation. Approximately 10% of breast cancers are mammographically occult. Ultrasound may assist in the identification of palpable masses and densities detected by mammography. Ultrasound is particularly useful in determining whether a lesion is solid or cystic. Magnetic resonance imaging (MRI) is useful in certain clinical situations in the detection of breast cancer. These include patients at high risk of the development of breast cancer and dense breast tissue, local staging of breast cancer prior to breast conserving therapy, and identification of occult breast cancers in patients presenting with metastatic carcinoma within axillary lymph nodes.

While MRI demonstrates high sensitivity, a drawback of MRI is lower specificity. Several benign lesions may have a worrisome appearance by MRI evaluation. The optimal utilization of MRI studies is a source of controversy and ongoing research.

Breast lesions that are indeterminate or suspicious by imaging studies typically undergo biopsy evaluation in which a small piece of the lesion is removed and evaluated in surgical pathology for definitive classification of the lesion. A list of the various types of breast biopsies is provided in Table 16-2. Solid lesions are usually biopsied under ultrasound guidance using a large cutting needle with a spring-loaded, automated biopsy instrument to obtain tissue specimens for histologic evaluation. Biopsies taken in this manner are called core biopsies. Ultrasound cores are typically 1–2 cm in length and 1–2 mm in thickness depending on the gauge of needle used. Biopsy of calcifications requires the use of stereotactic guidance to ensure sampling of the calcifications in the core biopsy tissue. Most of the stereotactic biopsies are performed with vacuum-assisted systems using a 14, 11, or 8 gauge needle, allowing multiple core samples to be taken to help ensure thorough sampling of the breast tissue in the region of concern. The core biopsy tissues are then evaluated in the pathology lab using light microscopy and a report is generated listing the pathologic diagnoses. Lastly, fine-needle aspiration technique using a 22–25 gauge needle may also be used in certain clinical situations, such as cyst evaluation. Fine-needle aspirations remove individual cells that are then smeared on a slide to be evaluated by a pathologist. Cyst aspirations yielding bloody fluid are one example in which pathologic evaluation of the fluid is recommended to exclude malignancy.

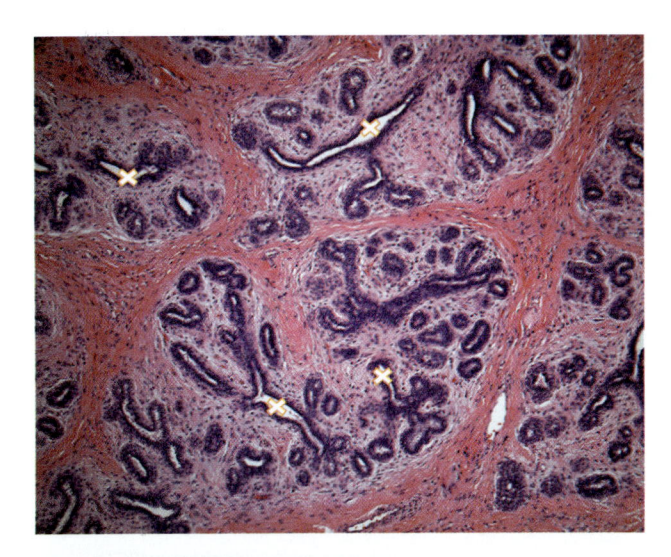

FIGURE 16-3 Terminal-duct lobular units (TDLUs). Multiple TDLUs are displayed with terminal ducts designated by X and surrounded by numerous smaller lobular acini. The TDLU represents the functional unit of the breast.

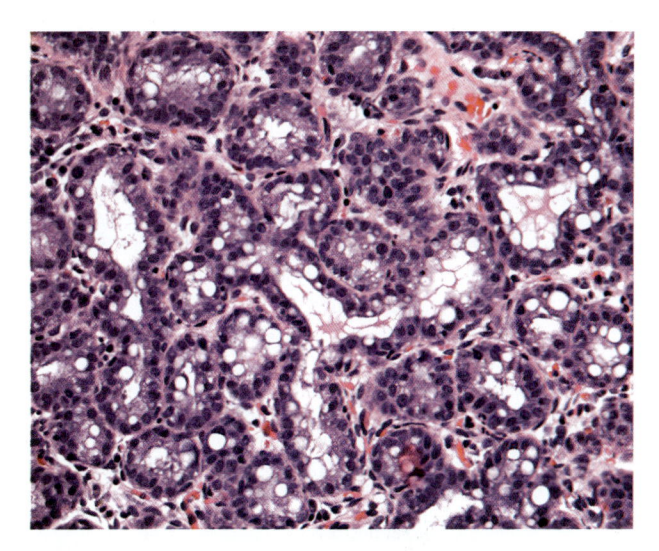

FIGURE 16-4 Lactational change. Lactational changes include increased density of lobular acini with the luminal cells containing abundant clear secretory-type vacuoles with production of pink secretory material seen with the lobular acini and terminal duct lumens.

distinction from the various benign breast conditions. Breast abnormalities often require thorough clinical examination, imaging studies, and tissue sampling (biopsy) for definitive classification of disease. In asymptomatic women, abnormal findings on screening breast imaging are a common cause of referral to breast clinic and tissue biopsy for diagnosis.

It is essential that all pathologic diagnoses are correlated with the imaging findings to ensure adequate sampling of the lesion of concern. In some cases, such as a particularly small or poorly defined nodule, the core biopsy may miss the target resulting in a false negative study. Pathologic–radiographic correlation helps identify these rare cases such that repeat tissue sampling can be performed.

BENIGN BREAST DISEASE

Inflammatory Lesions

Granulomatous Mastitis (Case 16-1)

Most cases of granulomatous mastitis represent an idiopathic granulomatous inflammatory process, typically occurring in parous women between the ages of 20 and 40. The idiopathic form has been designated granulomatous lobular mastitis. Systemic diseases such as sarcoidosis and Wegener granulomatosis and atypical infections from fungi and mycobacteria may also rarely cause granulomatous mastitis and should be clinically excluded. Women with granulomatous lobular mastitis may present with

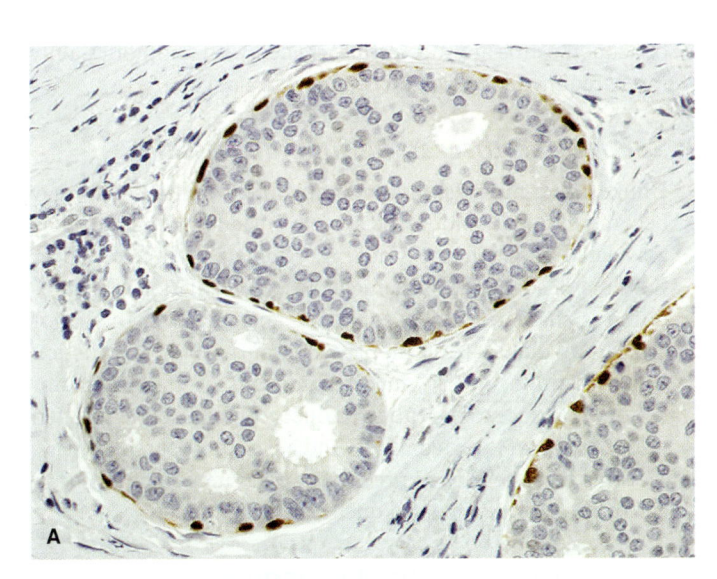

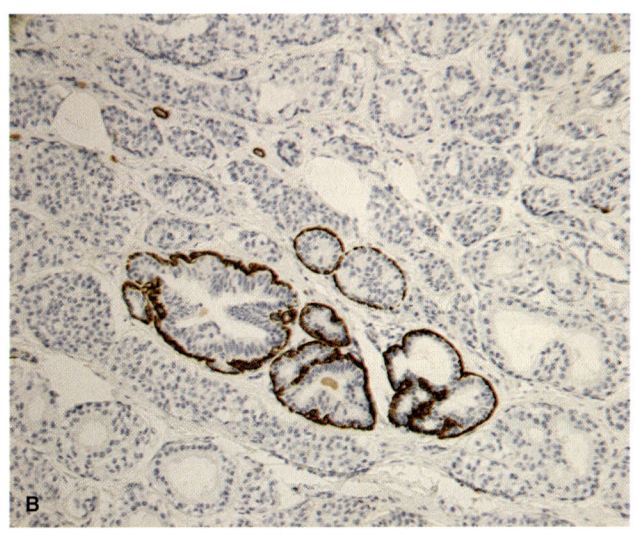

FIGURE 16-5 Myoepithelial cells. Myoepithelial cells surround all of the ducts and lobules of the breast and are preserved in cases of ductal carcinoma in situ (DCIS) (**A**) as highlighted here by an immunohistochemical stain for p63. The myoepithelial cell nuclei stain brown. In contrast, invasive carcinomas show infiltration into the breast stroma with loss of the myoepithelial cell layer (**B**). A small focus of normal breast tissue with surrounding myoepithelial cells highlighted by smooth muscle actin immunostain is present in the center of the image.

TABLE 16-1 Symptoms and causes of breast disorders.

Symptom or Finding	Differential Diagnosis
Discrete lump	
Age <30	Fibroadenoma
	Cyst (fibrocystic change)
	Intramammary lymph node
	Inflammatory lesions
	Fat necrosis
	Inflammatory lesions
	Hereditary breast carcinoma (rare)
Age 30–50	Cyst (fibrocystic change)
	Fibroadenoma
	Carcinoma
	Inflammatory lesions
	Fat necrosis
Age >50	Carcinoma
	Cyst (fibrocystic change)
	Fat necrosis
	Fibroadenoma
Other rare	Phyllodes tumor
	Fibrous mastopathy
	Pseudoangiomatous stromal hyperplasia
Diffuse lumpiness	Fibrocystic change
Indiscrete lump	Fibrocystic change (fibrosis)
	Normal breast tissue
	Inflammatory lesions
	Carcinoma (especially lobular)
Breast pain	
Cyclic	Hormone related
Noncyclic	Inflammatory conditions
	Fat necrosis related to trauma
	Cyst (fibrocystic change)
	Carcinoma
Nipple discharge	
Galactorrhea	Hyperprolactinemia, hypothyroidism, drugs
Single duct (bloody)	Intraductal papilloma
	Carcinoma
Single duct (nonbloody)	Fibrocystic change
	Duct ectasia
Nipple changes	
Erythema/scaling	Dermatitis
	Paget disease
Skin changes	
Erythema	Inflammatory dermatologic condition
	Inflammatory breast carcinoma
Induration/dimpling	Inflammatory conditions
	Carcinoma
	Fat necrosis

TABLE 16-2 Breast specimen types and indications.

Specimen Type	Indications
Core biopsy	Standard biopsy used to evaluate most breast abnormalities
Ultrasound core	Solid masses/nodules/densities
Stereotactic core	Calcifications, tiny nodules, architecture distortion
Fine-needle aspiration	Cysts
	Some inflammatory lesions
Excisional biopsy	Complete excision of lesion/region of concern
	Used in breast conserving therapy (BCT)
	Discordance between imaging and core biopsy results
Lumpectomy	Complete excision of a mass lesion
	Used in breast conserving therapy (BCT)
Mastectomy	Failure to achieve negative margins with BCT
	Large/multicentric malignancy not amendable to BCT
	Hereditary breast cancer
	Patient preference

a breast mass that is suspicious for malignancy by imaging studies. The characteristic non-necrotizing granulomas are typically centered on the lobules and associated with few background neutrophils and lymphocytes.

Acute Mastitis

Acute mastitis is an inflammatory condition characterized by a neutrophilic response to bacteria, often *Staphylococcus aureus* or streptococci. Most cases are associated with breast-feeding secondary to the development of cracks and fissures in the nipple allowing bacteria to enter the breast tissue. Patients typically present with breast pain and erythema. Most cases of acute mastitis are successfully treated with antibiotics, only rarely requiring surgical incision and drainage.

Subareolar Abscess (Periductal Mastitis)

Unlike acute mastitis, this inflammatory condition that may become chronic is not associated with lactation, but strongly associated with tobacco smoking. Nipple piercing complications may also result in subareolar abscess formation. This condition is characterized by squamous metaplasia of the major lactiferous ducts of the nipple resulting in duct obstruction from keratinous debris, duct rupture, and an intense inflammatory response to the ruptured ducts contents. Patients often present with an inverted nipple and a painful subareolar mass. A fistula tract develops in recurrent cases necessitating surgical excision of the involved ducts and fistula tract.

Lymphocytic/Fibrous Mastopathy

This condition is often identified in patients with a history of type 1 diabetes mellitus or autoimmune disease, suggesting

CASE 16-2

A 45-year-old woman presents with complaints of a firm breast lump present over the last 4 months. Her past medical history is significant for type 1 diabetes mellitus, hypertension, and Hashimoto's thyroiditis. Physical examination reveals a fairly discrete, very firm mass in the right breast. The mass is not tender on palpation. Mammographic and ultrasound studies reveal a dense solid mass with focally ill-defined borders. The lesion is categorized as suspicious and biopsy is recommended. Ultrasound-guided core biopsy is performed yielding the histology demonstrated in **Figure 16-6**.

Pathologic diagnosis: Dense stromal fibrosis with periductal and perivascular chronic inflammation, consistent with fibrous mastopathy.

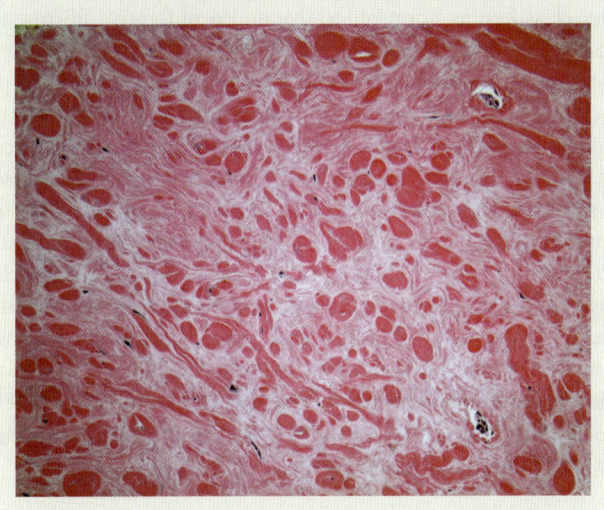

FIGURE 16-6 **Fibrous mastopathy.** The breast stroma shows a dense region of bland stromal fibrosis. In this case, the stromal cells show a keloid-like fibrosis.

CASE 16-3

A 48-year-old woman presents with a 1 cm ill-defined breast lump located in the subareolar region of the left breast. The patient also reports a history of thick proteinaceous nipple secretions without blood from the left breast. Her past medical history is unremarkable. Ultrasound evaluation reveals a cystically dilated duct with thick walls favoring a benign process. The patient desires to have the lesion excised and an excisional biopsy of the lesion is performed yielding the histology demonstrated in **Figure 16-7**.

Pathologic diagnosis: Duct ectasia.

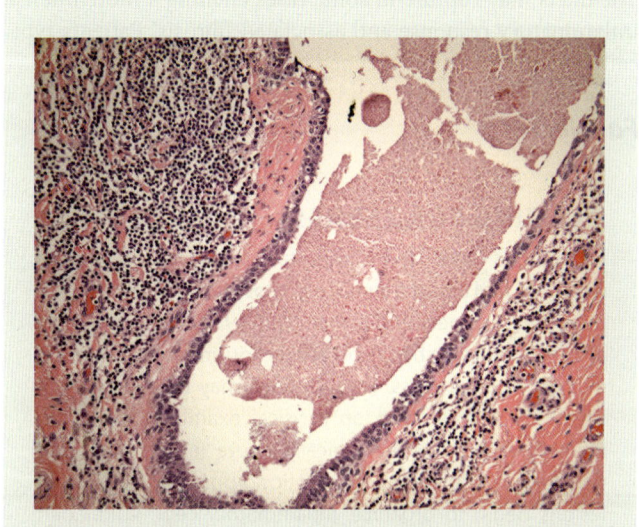

FIGURE 16-7 **Duct ectasia.** The central duct is dilated and filled with thick secretions and there is a surrounding cuff of chronic inflammation in the periductal stroma.

CASE 16-4

A 64-year-old woman presents with complaints of a new 5 cm firm breast mass. The patient's past medical history is remarkable only for hypertension with no family history of breast cancer. Physical examination reveals a large firm mass measuring at least 5 cm. Mammographic and ultrasound imaging reveals a solid density with irregular margins categorized as highly suspicious for malignancy. Ultrasound-guided core biopsy is performed yielding the histology demonstrated in **Figure 16-8**. After obtaining the diagnosis, further questioning reveals that the patient was in a motor vehicle accident 3 months earlier resulting in trauma to her chest region.

Pathologic diagnosis: Fat necrosis.

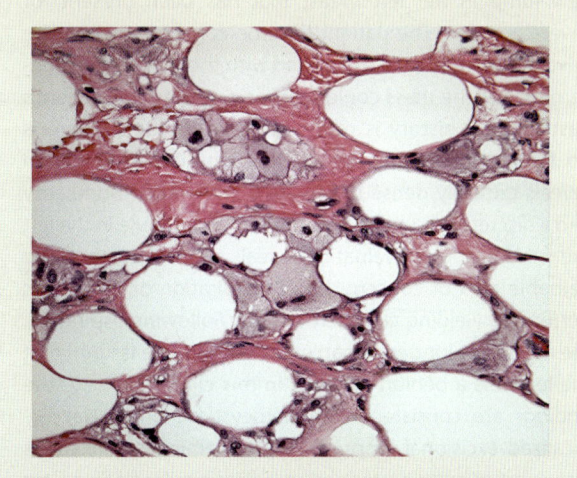

FIGURE 16-8 **Fat necrosis.** The adipose tissue contains multiple clear cystic spaces that are surrounded by foamy histiocytes.

an underlying autoimmune etiology Case 16-2. The lesions, which may be multiple, are characterized by dense collagenous stroma associated with mild periductal and perivascular chronic inflammation. Patients present with a firm breast mass or masses. Imaging studies often reveal an indeterminate mass requiring biopsy evaluation.

Duct Ectasia

Duct ectasia Case 16-3 is characterized by dilated ducts filled with thick proteinaceous material and numerous lipid-laden macrophages. The periductal stromal often contains a mild infiltrate of lymphocytes surrounding the involved ducts. The ducts may rupture in some cases eliciting a more intense inflammatory response and associated fibrosis. Patients typically present with an ill-defined breast mass.

Fat Necrosis

> **HUNTING FOR ZEBRAS**
>
> Fat necrosis Case 16-4 is important to consider in women who have had breast trauma (e.g., motor vehicle accident) or prior breast surgery and present with a breast mass. History of breast trauma should be elicited during the evaluation of a new breast mass. These lesions may closely mimic a breast carcinoma, both on physical examination and on imaging studies. Microscopically, acute lesions are often paucicellular consisting of necrotic adipose tissue. As these lesions begin to organize, inflammatory cells, lipid-laden macrophages, and fibrosis become apparent. Dystrophic calcifications may form in older lesions.

Benign Epithelial Lesions

Fibrocystic Change

Fibrocystic change Case 16-5 is extremely common, with more than one-third of females between the ages of 20 and 45 years of age showing some evidence of this condition on physical examination. Fibrocystic change of the breast includes a wide variety of changes of the breast ducts and stroma resulting in "lumpy" change of the breasts on physical examination. Gross examination of breast tissue involved by fibrocystic change reveals dense white stromal tissue admixed with variably sized cysts that may have a brown or blue (blue-dome cyst) discoloration (Figure 16-9). Microscopically these changes entail fibrosis of the breast stroma, cystic dilation of ducts, apocrine metaplasia, adenosis, and variable degrees of usual-type ductal epithelial hyperplasia (Figure 16-10). These changes are further classified as nonproliferative and proliferative fibrocystic change depending on the degree of ductal hyperplasia present. Nonproliferative fibrocystic change is not associated with increased risk of breast cancer, while proliferative fibrocystic change is associated with slight increased risk of breast cancer (1.5–2.0× increased relative risk). Cases of proliferative fibrocystic change typically show an intraductal proliferation of luminal and myoepithelial cells that may fill and distend the duct lumen. The cysts and nodular areas of dense stromal sclerosis presenting as breast masses in patients may require further evaluation to exclude breast cancer. Microcalcifications are often associated with fibrocystic change, observed in association with apocrine metaplasia, adenosis, and cysts. These microcalcifications may require sampling if their appearance on mammogram is suspicious.

CASE 16-5

A 28-year-old woman presents with complaints of a new lump in her left breast that has been present for several months. The patient became concerned when she developed breast pain associated with the mass. She is concerned that the mass could be breast cancer. The patient's past medical history is otherwise unremarkable. There is no family history of breast cancer. Physical examination reveals diffusely dense firm breasts with vague nodularity and a discrete, circumscribed, tender 1 cm nodule in the left breast. Ultrasound evaluation reveals a cystic lesion in the palpable area of concern. Needle aspiration of the cyst is performed yielding clear serous fluid. Following aspiration, the mass is no longer palpable. The patient is reassured that the lesion is a benign cyst and in this clinical context, the findings are consistent with fibrocystic change. Needle-localized excisional biopsy of the remaining calcifications was subsequently performed revealing similar findings. No carcinoma was identified.

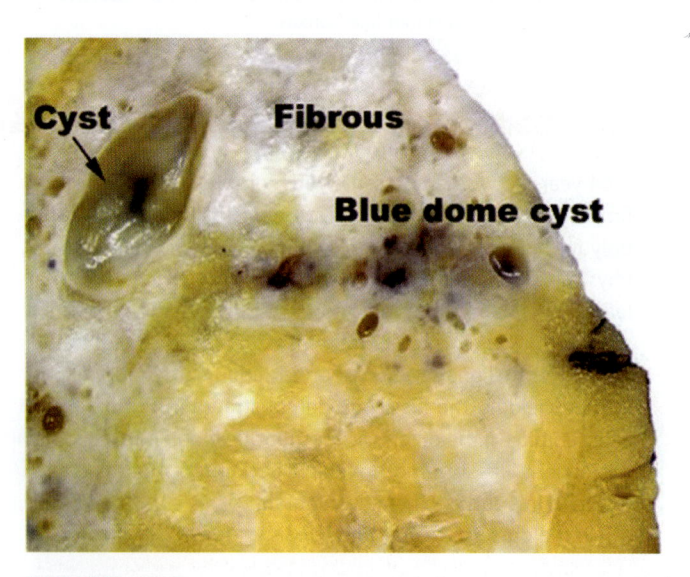

FIGURE 16-9 Fibrocystic change. The cut surface of this breast specimen contains variably sized cysts in a background of dense white fibrous tissue. Blue-dome cysts have a vaguely blue appearance on gross examination. (Image from Internet: doctorsgates.blogspot.com-atlas-of-pathology-images)

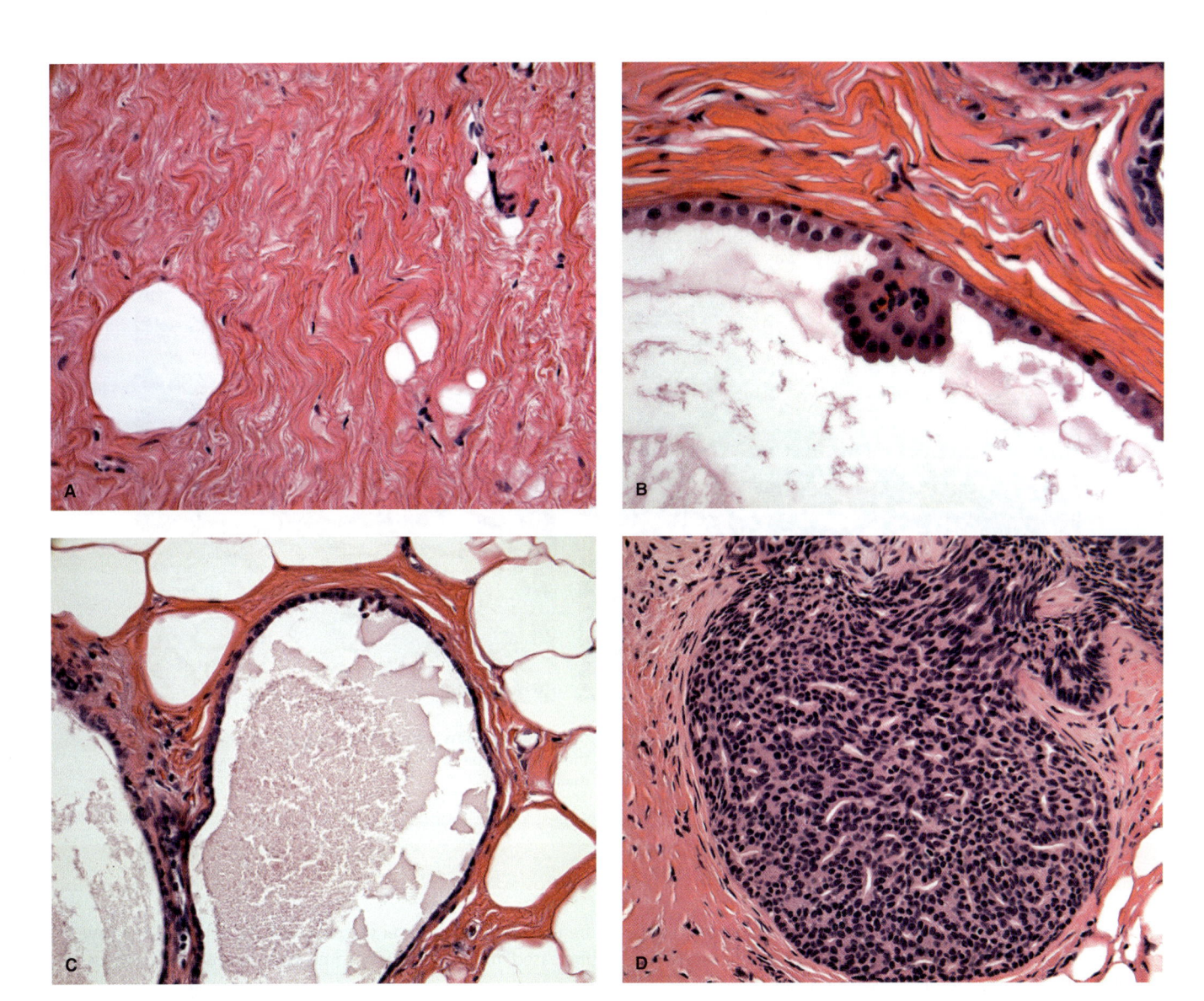

FIGURE 16-10 Components of fibrocystic change. Fibrocystic change consists of regions of stromal fibrosis (**A**), apocrine metaplasia characterized by abundant pink granular cytoplasm (**B**), cystically dilated ducts (**C**), and in cases of proliferative fibrocystic change, ductal epithelial hyperplasia (**D**).

Sclerosing Adenosis

Sclerosing adenosis Case 16-6 is the most common form of adenosis, and arises in the TDLU. Sclerosing adenosis is often an incidental finding in breast biopsies; however, it may present as a mammographic abnormality either due to associated calcifications or nodularity. Microscopically, sclerosing adenosis is characterized by lobulocentric proliferation of acini with preservation of the luminal epithelial and peripheral myoepithelial cell layers, accompanied by stromal sclerosis. Due to the complexity of some lesions, sclerosing adenosis may mimic the histology of an invasive carcinoma and is a recognized pitfall for pathologists. Special immunohistochemical stains may be used by pathologist to highlight the myoepithelial cells within the lesion.

Columnar Cell Lesions

Columnar cell lesions typically occur in premenopausal women 35–50 years of age. Columnar cell lesions come to clinical detection due to the mammographic detection of the calcifications frequently associated with these lesions. Columnar cell lesions are a frequent finding in stereotactic core biopsies performed for indeterminate calcifications. The spectrum of columnar cell lesions includes columnar cell change, columnar cell hyperplasia, and flat epithelial atypia (Case 16-7). Columnar cell change and columnar cell hyperplasia (>2 cell layer thick proliferation) are characterized by the presence of columnar cells lining the TDLU, often with associated expansion of the lobule acini. Cytologic nuclear atypia and architectural atypia (loss of polarity) may be observed in columnar cell lesions and this finding has been designated flat epithelial atypia. There is mounting evidence that flat epithelia atypia

CASE 16-6

A 46-year-old woman was recalled from screening mammography with the detection of an ill-defined breast mass with associated calcifications. Ultrasound revealed a 5 mm nodule with irregular margins. Biopsy was recommended. The patient's past medical history was unremarkable. Ultrasound-guided core biopsy yielded the histology demonstrated in Figure 16-11. Special stains for myoepithelial cells were ordered by the pathologist to help exclude invasive carcinoma.

Pathologic diagnosis: Nodular sclerosing adenosis.

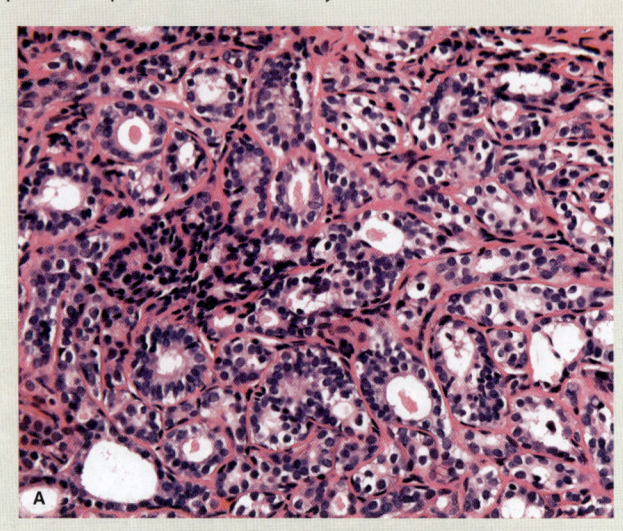

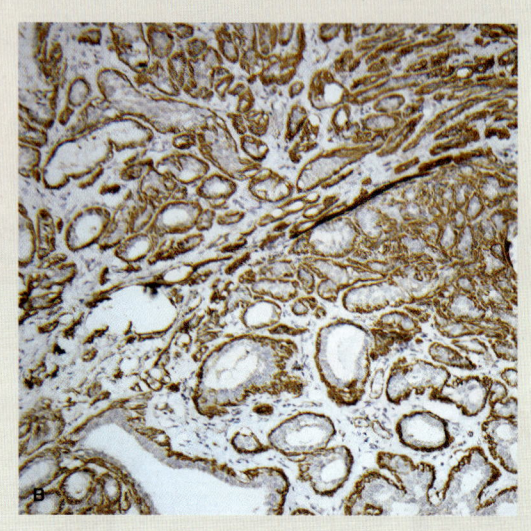

FIGURE 16-11 Sclerosing adenosis. High-power image shows densely packed acini in a pattern that may mimic some invasive carcinomas **(A)**. Immunohistochemical stain for smooth muscle actin stains the myoepithelial cells brown **(B)**, confirming the preservation of myoepithelial cells and benign nature of the lesion.

CASE 16-7

A 50-year-old woman was recalled from screening mammography due to a finding of suspicious calcifications. The calcifications were present 1 year ago but demonstrated a benign appearance. Over the past year, the calcifications have increased in number and become more irregular. Stereotactic core biopsy of the calcifications was recommended. The patient

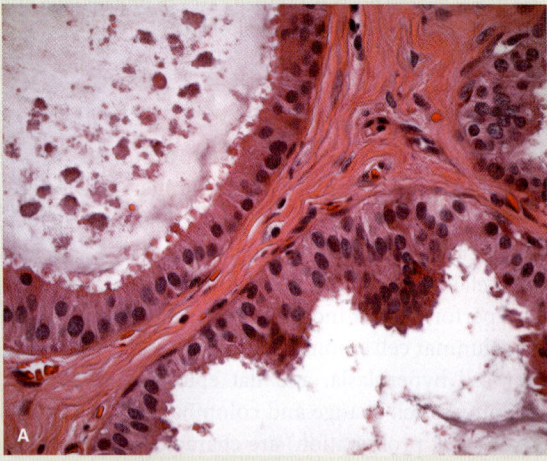

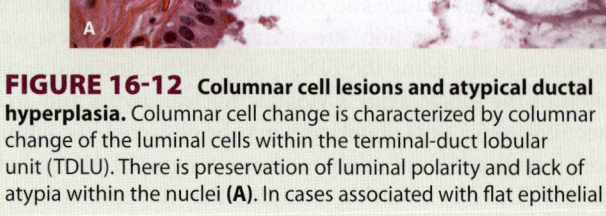

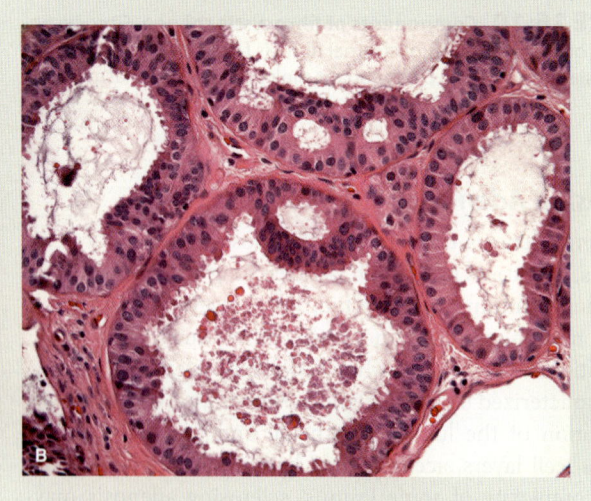

FIGURE 16-12 Columnar cell lesions and atypical ductal hyperplasia. Columnar cell change is characterized by columnar change of the luminal cells within the terminal-duct lobular unit (TDLU). There is preservation of luminal polarity and lack of atypia within the nuclei **(A)**. In cases associated with flat epithelial atypia and atypical ductal hyperplasia **(B, C)**, there is focal loss of polarity within the proliferation associated with cellular stratification and monomorphism (flat epithelial atypia), and rigid epithelial arcades and micropapillary tufts (atypical ductal hyperplasia).

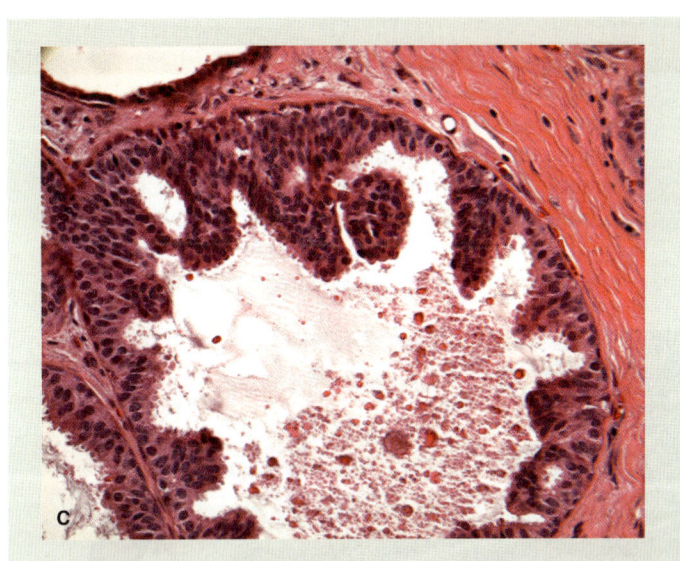

FIGURE 16-12 *(Continued)*

IN TRANSLATION

Molecular analysis has demonstrated that the majority of columnar cell lesions are clonal and neoplastic rather than hyperplastic, showing similar chromosomal alterations to those found in adjacent ADH and low-grade DCIS. Epidemiologic studies of flat epithelial atypia have shown a 1.5–2-fold increased risk of the development of breast cancer. Flat epithelial atypia identified in a core biopsy is typically followed by needle-localized excisional biopsy to rule out a more serious lesion.

represents an early precursor lesion for ADH and low-grade DCIS. There is also an association between flat epithelial atypia and lobular neoplasia.

Radial Scar/Complex Sclerosing Lesion

A variety of breast lesions are characterized by benign tubules entrapped and distorted by fibrous or fibroelastotic stromal tissue, often with accompanying adenosis and epithelial hyperplasia architecturally arranged in a radial fashion from the central scar Case 16-8. The terms radial scar and complex sclerosing lesion (for larger lesions >1 cm) have been used for the majority of these lesions. The mammographic appearance of radial scar/complex sclerosing lesion may closely mimic that of an invasive carcinoma. These lesions have been reported to be associated with increased risk of carcinoma and atypical hyperplasia; consequently, surgical excision of the entire lesion is recommended.

Papillary Lesions

The spectrum of papillary neoplasms includes benign intraductal papillomas (vast majority of papillary lesions), atypical papillomas, and papillary carcinomas. Benign intraductal

has no family history of breast cancer and has received no prior breast biopsies. Stereotactic core biopsies are performed yielding the histology demonstrated in Figure 16-12.

Pathologic diagnosis: Atypical ductal hyperplasia (ADH) arising in a background of flat epithelial atypia and columnar cell change, with associated microcalcifications.

CASE 16-8

A 57-year-old woman is recalled from screening mammography due to the detection of a 7 mm region of architectural distortion with faintly visible associated calcifications. Based on the radiographic findings, the differential diagnosis includes a small invasive carcinoma and radial scar. Ultrasound core biopsy followed by needle-localized excisional biopsy is performed yielding the histology in Figure 16-13.

Pathologic diagnosis: Radial scar.

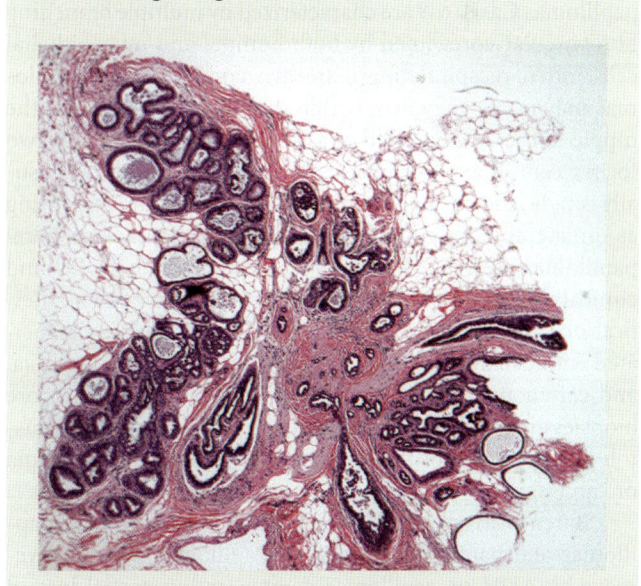

FIGURE 16-13 **Radial scar.** There is an irregular radial arrangement of the architecture with the central region containing fibroelastotic change of the stroma. When the lesion is large enough, the architectural distortion may be appreciated on imaging studies.

CASE 16-9

A 45-year-old woman presents with new onset bloody nipple discharge from the left nipple. The patient's family history is remarkable for a sister who developed breast cancer at the age of 52. The patient reports that her sister's breast cancer presented with bloody nipple discharge. Physical examination reveals a vague 1.0 cm subareolar mass. The left nipple is negative for redness, scaling, ulceration, or retraction. Mammographic studies confirm a 1.0 intraductal mass in the subareolar region of the left breast. The patient undergoes ultrasound-guided core biopsy of the lesion followed by major duct excision yielding the histology in Figure 16-14.

Pathologic diagnosis: Benign intraductal papilloma.

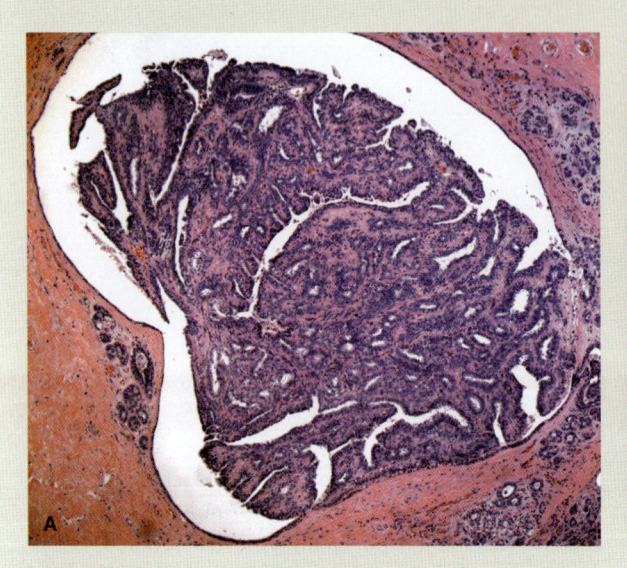

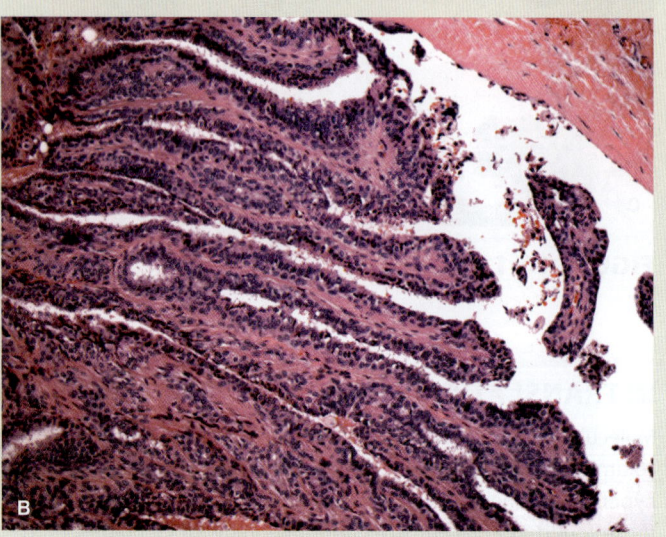

FIGURE 16-14 **Intraductal papilloma.** There is an intraductal proliferation characterized by the presence of papillae (A), often with a treelike configuration. On higher magnification (B), the papillae are lined by luminal and myoepithelial cells and contain a central fibrovascular core.

papillomas Case 16-9 are characterized by multiple branching fibrovascular cores lined by both luminal and myoepithelial cells, often recapitulating a treelike configuration. Papillomas may occur anywhere within the ductal system from the nipple to the TDLU. Papillomas are broadly divided into two forms: central and peripheral. The central papilloma is usually single and located in the subareolar region presenting as unilateral bloody nipple discharge in patients. Peripheral papillomas are typically multiple, located in the TDLU and clinically occult or identified in biopsy specimens for calcifications. Peripheral papillomas are more frequently associated with usual-type ductal hyperplasia, atypical hyperplasia, and carcinoma. Mass-forming papillomas identified in core biopsies are typically surgically excised to allow complete histologic evaluation of the lesion and exclusion of focal atypia or carcinoma.

Rarer forms of papillary neoplasms include atypical papillomas and papillary carcinomas. Papillomas with involvement by ADH or papillomas demonstrating partial loss of myoepithelial cells have been designated atypical papillomas. Papillary carcinomas are more common in elderly women and male breast cancers. The detailed classification of papillary carcinomas is complex and beyond the scope of this review.

Atypical Hyperplasias

Atypical hyperplasias of breast are categorized as either ADH or atypical lobular hyperplasia (ALH) and are associated with moderate increased risk of the development of breast cancer. Atypical hyperplasias share some of the same features as carcinoma in situ but are not sufficiently developed to meet criteria as a carcinoma. ADH typically comes to detection through biopsy of screen-detected calcifications Case 16-10. ALH is often an incidental finding in biopsies performed for other reasons and not associated with calcifications.

ADH is a neoplastic intraductal proliferation possessing some of the features of low-grade DCIS, but lacking sufficient quantitative or qualitative features for a diagnosis of DCIS. Foci of ADH are typically small in size (<2 mm). ADH is characterized microscopically by a monomorphic intraductal cell population with solid, micropapillary or cribriform architecture.

ALH is a neoplastic lobular proliferation of cells resembling those of lobular carcinoma in situ (LCIS), but lacking the quantitative extent of the lobular proliferation for a diagnosis of LCIS. The neoplastic lobular cells do not fill or distend more than 50% of the acini within the involved lobules as is seen with LCIS.

CASE 16-10

A 51-year-old woman was recalled from screening mammography due to a 9 mm cluster of indeterminate calcifications. Physical examination of the breast was negative for findings. The patient reports a family history of breast cancer. Her mother was diagnosed with breast cancer at the age of 55. Stereotactic core biopsies of the calcifications are performed yielding the histology demonstrated in Figure 16-15.

Pathologic diagnosis: ADH with associated microcalcifications. Due to patient's family history of breast cancer and diagnosis of ADH, the patient was referred to high-risk breast clinic to further discuss radiographic surveillance measures and possible chemoprevention with tamoxifen.

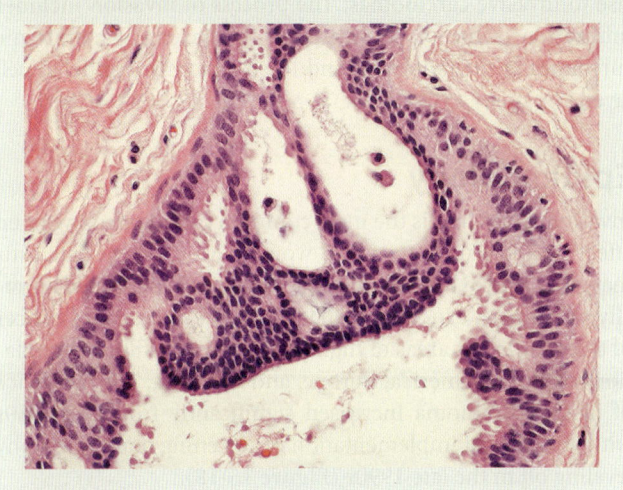

FIGURE 16-15 Atypical ductal hyperplasia. The key histologic features of the intraductal proliferation include cellular monomorphism with formation of rigid epithelial arcades and cribriform architecture. Unlike DCIS, only a portion of the duct is involved in this proliferation.

Fibroepithelial Lesions

Fibroadenoma

Fibroepithelial tumors are categorized into the very common fibroadenoma Case 16-11 and the very rare phyllodes tumor. Fibroadenomas are the most common benign tumor of the female breast and arise from intralobular breast stroma. Fibroadenoma occurs most frequently in women of childbearing age and juvenile forms exist in teenagers. These benign tumors present as painless, firm, slow growing, circumscribed, mobile nodules. Fibroadenomas are usually solitary but may be multiple in some patients. These tumors may increase in size during pregnancy due to hormonally responsive epithelium. On gross examination, the masses are circumscribed and lobulated with a tan cut surface. Fibroadenomas are a benign biphasic tumor comprised of benign stroma and epithelium with an intracanalicular or pericanalicular growth pattern. The appearance of

CASE 16-11

A 23-year-old woman presents with complaint of a breast mass present for over a year. The patient is currently pregnant (1st trimester) and has noted that the mass is increasing in size. Physical examination reveals a 2 cm mobile mass in the upper outer quadrant of the right breast. The patient's past medical history is otherwise unremarkable. Core biopsy of the mass is performed yielding the histology in Figure 16-16.

Pathologic diagnosis: Fibroadenoma.

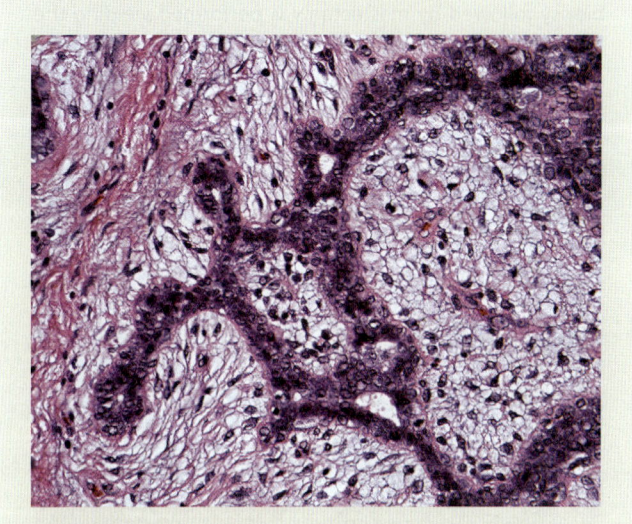

FIGURE 16-16 Fibroadenoma. This benign fibroepithelial lesion is characterized by a proliferation of the intralobular stroma resulting in distortion and compression of the glandular elements (intracanalicular pattern). Some cases such as this one may show myxoid change of the stromal proliferation.

the stromal component is highly variable ranging from hypocellular to hypercellular and hyalinized to myxoid. The cellular variant of fibroadenoma may raise concern for a phyllodes tumor, particularly when sampling of the lesion is limited in a core biopsy. In these cases, excision of the entire mass is recommended to definitively exclude a phyllodes tumor.

Phyllodes Tumor

Phyllodes tumors are rare fibroepithelial tumors that are thought to also arise from breast intralobular stroma. These tumors are present in an older age group than fibroadenomas. The clinical presentation is variable depending on the biology of the tumor. Patients with malignant phyllodes tumors may present with a rapidly enlarging breast mass. The physical examination and radiographic findings often resemble a fibroadenoma with the exception that most phyllodes tumors are typically larger (>4 cm) at the time of detection. The majority of phyllodes tumors are benign but show a propensity for local recurrence if not completely excised. The recurrent tumors may demonstrate more aggressive biology than the primary tumor

CASE 16-12

A 57-year-old woman presents with complaint of an enlarging breast mass over the last several months. Physical examination reveals an 8 cm breast mass with well-defined margins. No skin changes are observed. Mammography and ultrasound show a large, 8 cm circumscribed mass with central lobulations. The findings are concerning for malignancy with the differential diagnosis including phyllodes tumor and carcinoma. Ultrasound-guided core biopsy followed by mastectomy is performed yielding the histology in Figure 16-17.

Pathologic diagnosis: Malignant phyllodes tumor with liposarcomatous differentiation.

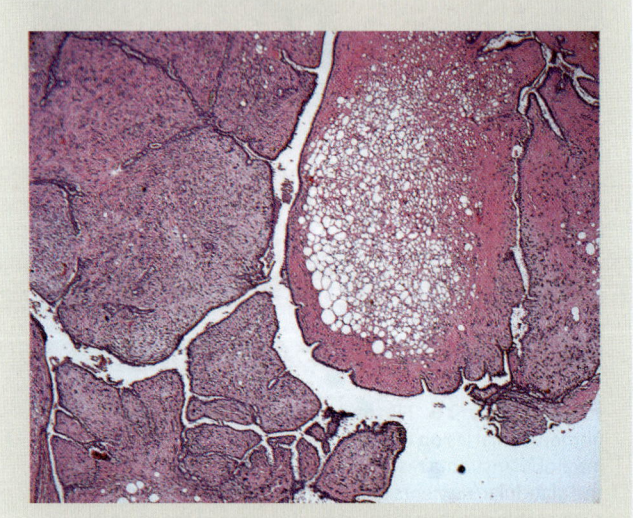

FIGURE 16-17 **Phyllodes tumor.** The histologic appearance of phyllodes tumor is highly variable. This tumor demonstrates characteristic leaflike projections of hypercellular stroma. In some cases, the distinction of phyllodes tumor from fibroadenoma may be particularly difficult, especially in small biopsy specimens.

and show stromal overgrowth, a condition where the epithelial component of the tumor is markedly diminished or absent. The term "phyllodes" means leaf-like that is the characteristic architectural pattern of this tumor. Phyllodes tumors show higher stromal cellularity than fibroadenomas and are typically associated with at least some degree of cytologic atypia and mitotic activity. Phyllodes tumors are divided into three groups: benign, borderline, and malignant depending on the constellation of histologic findings including number of mitoses, cytologic atypia, stromal cellularity, and tumor border Case 16-12. Malignant and some borderline phyllodes tumors may metastasize in a hematogenous fashion to distant sites such as lungs.

Gynecomastia

A benign enlargement of the male breast tissue. Patients present with unilateral or bilateral subareolar enlargement. The mass effect is due to a proliferation of breast stromal connective tissue and duct epithelium. Causes include hyperestrogen states secondary to cirrhosis or increased production of adrenal estrogens, drugs (e.g. marijuana), and alcohol.

CARCINOMA OF THE BREAST

Definitions

It is essential to understand the difference between in situ and invasive mammary carcinoma. Invasive carcinomas are comprised of malignant epithelial cells that infiltrate the breast stromal tissues associated with a tendency for tumor metastasis to regional and distant sites. In situ carcinomas are confined inside the ductal-lobular system and are not capable of producing metastatic disease. In situ carcinomas give rise to invasive carcinomas. The process of invasion includes infiltration of tumor cells through the basement membrane surrounding ducts/lobules and loss of the myoepithelial cell layer.

Epidemiology

Invasive carcinoma is the most common carcinoma in women affecting approximately 1 in 8 women. Most recent data estimate that approximately 207,000 women are diagnosed annually with breast cancer and 40,000 will die annually of cancer of the breast. The areas of highest risk are the affluent populations of North America, Europe, and Australia. The incidence of in situ carcinoma increased significantly from the 1980s with widespread implementation of screening mammography leveling off in the late 1990s (Figure 16-18).

Risk Factors

There is extensive information published on the risk factors associated with breast carcinoma. These risk factors are summarized in Table 16-3. The etiology of breast cancer is multifactorial and involves complex interactions between genes, hormonal, and environmental factors. Hormone-related risk factors such as young age at menarche, older age at first term birth, nulliparity, older age at menopause, and postmenopausal hormone replacement therapy (estrogen + progesterone) underscore the importance of hormones in the development of breast cancer. It is imperative to assess patient risk of breast cancer by taking a thorough clinical history. Statistical models exist to estimate breast cancer risk using a patient's medical history. The Gail model has been tested in large populations of white women and has been shown to provide accurate estimates of breast cancer risk.

Breast Cancer Predisposition Syndromes

Mutations in BRCA1/BRCA2, TP53, CHEK2, PTEN, LKBI/STK11, and ATM genes are associated with hereditary breast and ovarian cancer syndrome, Li–Fraumeni

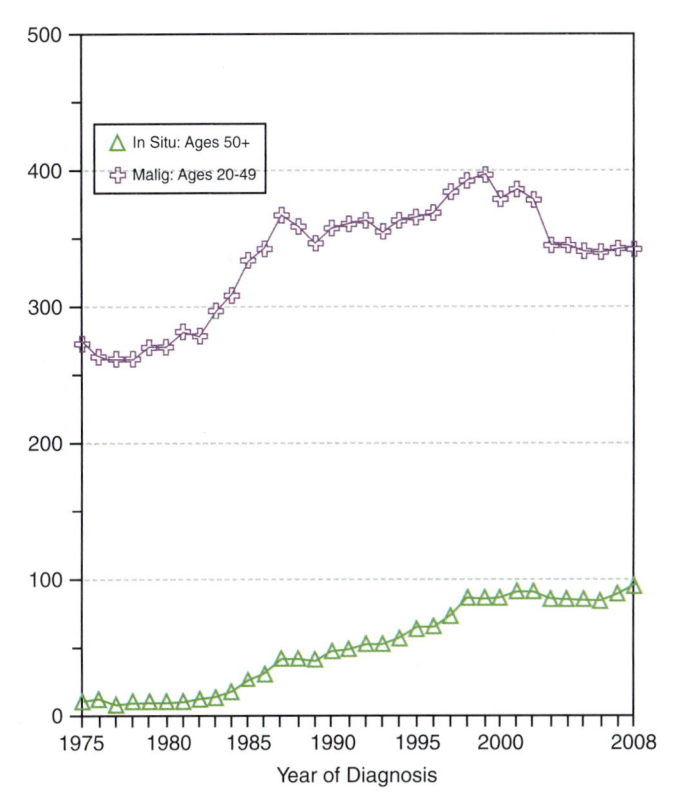

FIGURE 16-18 **Epidemiologic trends in breast cancer.** SEER data from 1975 to 2008 demonstrates increased incidence of in situ carcinoma from the 1980s with widespread implementation of screening mammography leveling off in the late 1990s. In 2003, there was an abrupt decrease of 6.7% in the incidence of invasive breast cancer in women >50 years of age. It is hypothesized that this change was due in large part to discontinuation of hormone replacement therapy among postmenopausal women.

TABLE 16-3 Risk factors for breast cancer.

Strong Risk Factors
Age
Female
BRCA1 or BRCA2 mutation
Family history of breast cancer
>1 immediate family member
1 family member with early age at detection
Atypical hyperplasia (4–6 times increase in relative risk)
Radiation therapy during youth
Personal history of cancer
High breast density
Weak/Moderate Risk Factors
Family history of breast cancer (advanced age at detection)
High levels of blood estrogens or androgens
Age at first period <12 years
Age at menopause >55 years
Nulliparity
Late age at first child birth (age >35)
Hormone replacement therapy (estrogen plus progesterone)
Postmenopausal weight gain
Proliferative benign breast conditions (1.5–2 times increase in relative risk)
Columnar cell lesions/flat epithelial atypia
Radial scar
Usual-type ductal hyperplasia
Sclerosing adenosis
Alcohol intake
Westernized diet
Environmental toxins

syndrome, Li–Fraumeni variant syndrome, Cowden syndrome, Peutz–Jeghers syndrome, and ataxia telangiectasia, respectively. The deleterious mutations in these genes are autosomal dominant and highly penetrant. The inheritance of a susceptibility gene is the primary cause of approximately 10–12% of breast cancers. The known high-risk breast cancer genes account for only about 25% of familial breast cancers.

BRCA1 (17q21)/BRCA2 (13q12-13) genes are involved in DNA repair. Female BRCA1 mutation carriers have a lifetime risk of developing breast cancer of approximately 40–80%, while female BRCA2 mutation carriers have a lifetime risk of developing breast cancer of approximately 30–60%. These patients are also at high risk of developing high-grade serous carcinomas of the fallopian tube fimbria and ovary. The frequency of BRCA1/BRCA2 mutations is rare in the general population, 0.1% or 0.2%. Some population groups such as those of Ashkenazi Jewish descent have higher risk (2–3%) of carrying certain mutations in the BRCA1/BRCA2 genes. Patients with a personal history of breast cancer plus one or more of the following may be candidates of genetic counseling and testing: diagnosis before age 45, diagnosis before age 50 with close relatives diagnosed before 50 or one close relative with ovarian cancer, two breast cancers with at least one diagnosed before age 50, at least two close relatives with breast cancer, close male relative with breast cancer, personal history of ovarian cancer, and ethnicity associated with higher mutation frequency.

Breast cancers developing in patients with germ line BRCA1 mutations are typically high-grade tumors with tumor infiltrating lymphocytes, a hormone receptor-negative and HER2-negative phenotype (triple negative), and basal-like gene expression pattern (discussed later). BRCA2 tumors do not show such characteristic features; the majority are high-grade, hormone receptor-positive and HER2-negative tumors.

IN TRANSLATION
Molecular Evolution of Breast Cancer

The molecular mechanisms underlying the development of breast cancer are far from being completely understood. Like other cancers, these tumors arise from the acquisition of somatic, genetic, and epigenetic alterations leading to changes in gene sequence, copy number, and expression. Historically, breast cancer progression was seen as a linear multistep process similar to colon carcinogenesis encompassing progressive changes from hyperplasia, atypical hyperplasia, carcinoma in situ, and invasive carcinoma. No longer is breast cancer carcinogenesis perceived as a single pathway, but a complex series of stochastic genetic events leading to distinct and divergent pathways toward invasive breast cancer. The complexity of these pathways correlates with the tremendous biologic diversity observed in breast cancers and further support that breast cancer is not a single disease, but instead a collection of multiple diseases.

The genetics of low and high-grade breast cancers is segregated by the type of genetics aberrations. Low-grade, hormone receptor-positive tumors show a low number of genomic alterations with highly recurrent losses of 16q. High-grade carcinomas, particularly hormone receptor negative tumors, show complex genotypes frequently harboring loss of 11q, 14q, 8p, 13q; gain of 17q, 8q, 5p; and amplifications on 17q12, 17q22–24, 6q22, 8q22, 11q13, and 20q13. The marked differences in these molecular profiles indicate that progression from low-grade carcinoma to high-grade carcinoma is

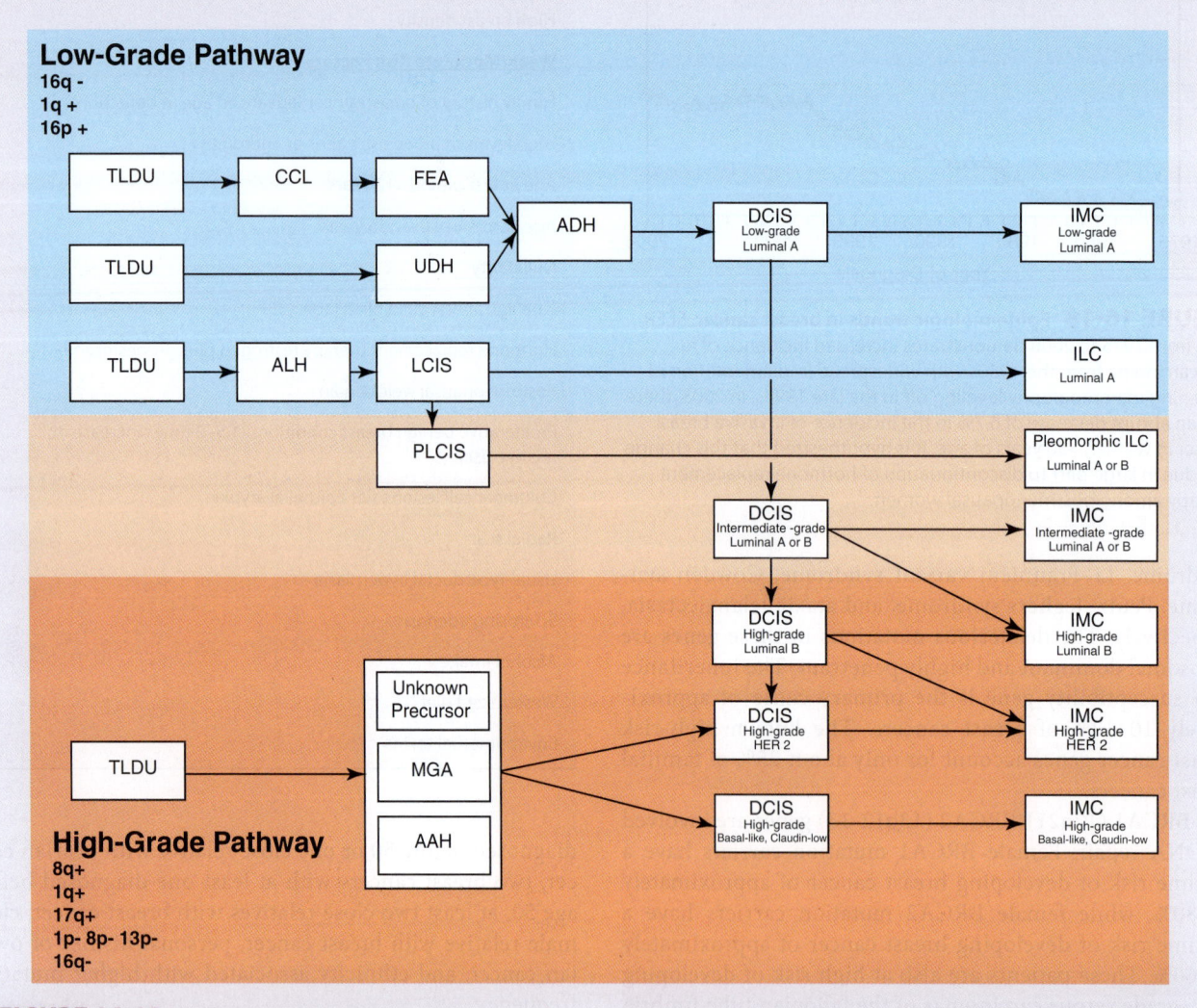

FIGURE 16-19 Multistep model of breast cancer progression. There are two distinct pathways of progression: low- and high-grade pathways. The low-grade precursor lesions include usual-type ductal hyperplasia (UDH), columnar cell lesions (CCL), flat epithelial atypia (FEA), atypical ductal hyperplasia (ADH), atypical lobular hyperplasia (ALH), well-differentiated ductal carcinoma in situ (DCIS), and lobular carcinoma in situ (LCIS). The low-grade pathway typically gives rise to hormone receptor-positive, HER2-negative invasive mammary carcinomas (IMC) with a low proliferation rate. The early precursor lesions for most of invasive carcinomas in the high-grade pathway are unclear. Microglandular adenosis (MGA) and atypical apocrine hyperplasia (AAH) are likely candidates for some of these tumors. High-grade DCIS and pleomorphic LCIS may give rise to high-grade tumors. While diverse in their gene expression patterns, the high-grade tumors fall into three broad groups: (1) hormone receptor-positive, HER2-negative with high proliferation rate (luminal B), (2) triple-negative (basal like/claudin-low), and (3) HER2 positive. In general, invasive mammary carcinomas show tremendous biologic diversity including tumors that do not fit into the low- or high-grade pathway, showing intermediate-grade biology.

infrequent. Precursor lesions for the low-grade pathway include columnar cell change, flat epithelia atypia, ADH, lobular neoplasia, and low-grade DCIS. The entire constellation of these lesions may be identified in excisional biopsies for low-grade invasive mammary carcinoma, such as tubular carcinoma. The high-grade pathway is less well understood. The precursor lesions for high-grade DCIS are not known in many cases. In some cases, low-grade ductal carcinoma may progress to high-grade ductal carcinoma. Other potential precursor lesions for high-grade carcinoma include atypical apocrine proliferations and microglandular adenosis. A schematic drawing of the multistep model of breast cancer progression is demonstrated in **Figure 16-19**.

Much more detailed molecular genetic information from breast cancers is now being obtained through the use of next-generation sequencing technologies that reveal the entire sequence of tumor genomes. In the breast cancer cases studied to date, most rearrangements in breast cancer are intrachromosomal. Tandem duplications seem to be the most common subclass. The high prevalence of tandem duplications in a subset of cancers suggests the presence of a defect in DNA maintenance that generates this particular class of rearrangement. Breast cancers with many tandem duplications are usually hormone receptor negative and classified by expression profile as basal like. Cancers with few rearrangements are usually hormone receptor positive and classified as luminal A or luminal B.

CASE 16-13

A 53-year-old woman presents with complaints of scaling, redness, and itching of her right nipple. Physical examination reveals a red ulcerated region involving the nipple. The patient's past medical history is otherwise unremarkable. Mammographic examination of the breast is performed demonstrating extensive pleomorphic linear branching calcifications involving multiple quadrants of the breast, extending from the chest wall to the nipple. Stereotactic core biopsies of calcifications from two different quadrants of the breast are performed, followed by total mastectomy, yielding the pathology results in **Figure 16-20**.

Pathologic diagnosis: High-grade multicentric DCIS associated with Paget disease. No invasive carcinoma is identified.

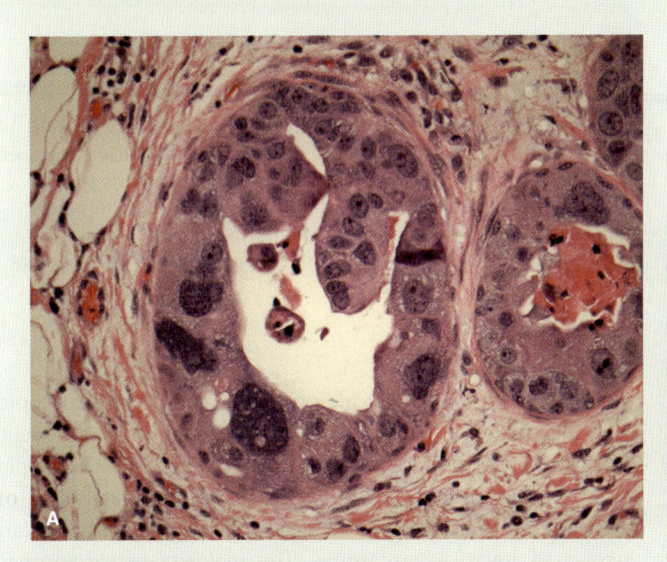

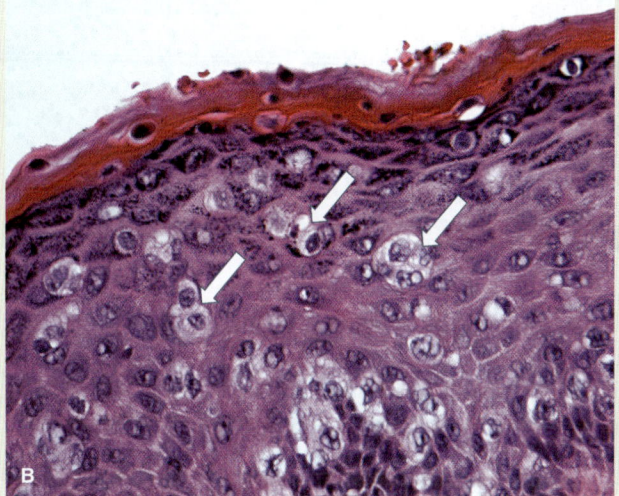

FIGURE 16-20 High-grade ductal carcinoma in situ (DCIS) and Paget disease. The marked nuclear pleomorphism seen here is characteristic for high-grade DCIS **(A)**. The central necrosis identified in the right duct is often present in these lesions. The skin from this case shows nests and single cells of carcinoma infiltrating the epidermis diagnostic of Paget disease **(B)**. The carcinoma cells (arrows) show nuclear atypia and pale cytoplasm allowing their distinction from the adjacent squamous cells in the epidermis.

Ductal Carcinoma In Situ

DCIS is defined as a neoplastic intraductal lesion characterized by increased epithelial proliferation, mild-to-severe nuclear atypia, and an inherent but not obligate tendency to progress to invasive carcinoma **Case 16-13**. Most cases of DCIS are detected as a result of calcifications; however, DCIS may also present as a vague nodular mass or a discrete mass lesion (mass-forming DCIS). DCIS lesions are highly heterogeneous in their phenotype. The degree of nuclear pleomorphism is minimal in low-grade DCIS and prominent in cases of high-grade DCIS. Central necrosis is a common finding in intermediate and high-grade DCIS. DCIS architecture demonstrates a variety of patterns including cribriform, micropapillary, and solid **(Figure 16-21)**. Because we are currently unable to determine

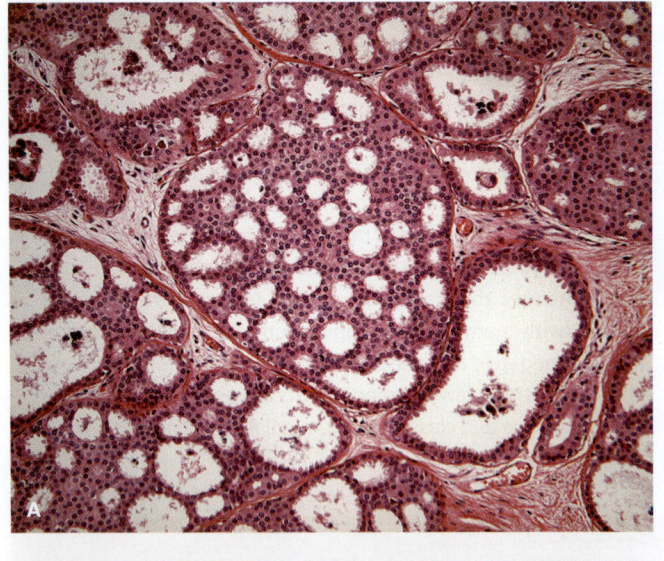

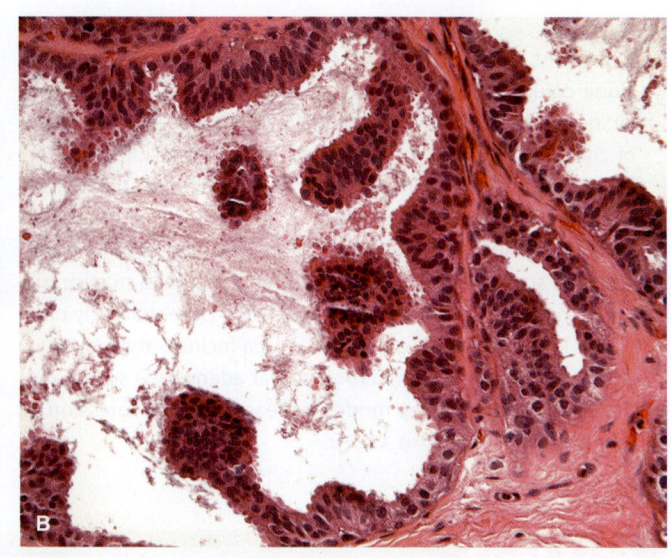

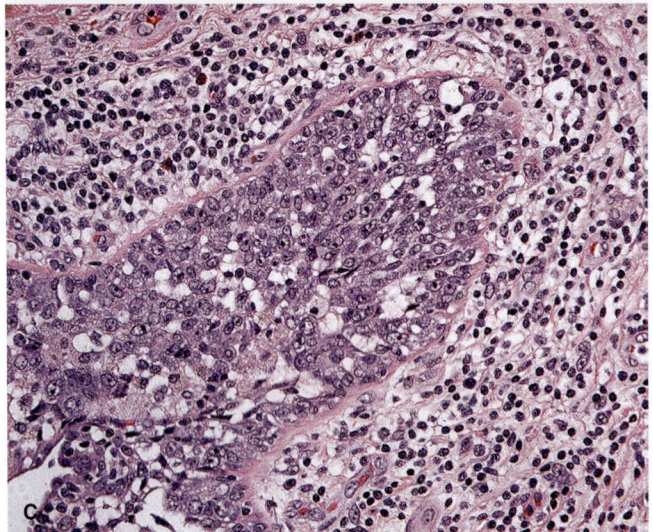

FIGURE 16-21 Patterns of ductal carcinoma in situ (DCIS). There is tremendous diversity of the architectural and nuclear features of DCIS. Common patterns include cribriform **(A)** where the tumor cells form sieve-like architecture and micropapillary **(B)** where the tumor cells form micropapillae without fibrovascular cores. High-grade solid DCIS **(C)** is also demonstrated showing solid arrangement of tumor cells within the duct.

which DCIS cases will progress to invasive carcinoma, all cases of DCIS are treated with surgical excision, often followed by radiation therapy and tamoxifen (for estrogen receptor [ER]-positive DCIS cases). Risk factors for recurrence of DCIS after treatment include high-grade histology, large size of DCIS, and positive or close surgical margins. Pathology reports for DCIS lesion include information on tumor grade (nuclear grade), presence or absence of necrosis, size of lesion, and margins status. Positive margins for DCIS are re-excised in an effort to obtain clear margins. DCIS involving multiple quadrants of the breast (multicentric) often requires a total mastectomy. All cases of DCIS are tested for ER expression by immunohistochemistry. The benefit of tamoxifen therapy appears confined to patients with ER-positive DCIS.

Paget Disease

Paget disease of the nipple is an uncommon presentation of breast cancer. Patients with Paget disease present with nipple abnormalities including scale crust and itching. Microscopic sections of Paget disease demonstrate nests of tumor cells extending from DCIS within the ductal system into the nipple skin. An underlying mass is present in approximately half of the patients presenting with Paget disease, indicative of an associated invasive carcinoma. The majority of carcinomas associated with Paget disease are high grade and show HER2 overexpression (discussed later).

Lobular Carcinoma In Situ

Classic LCIS is typically an incidental finding identified in breast specimens Case 16-14. Occasionally, LCIS is identified in biopsies for calcifications where the calcifications are present within the LCIS. Microscopy shows a monomorphic population of loosely cohesive cells with low nuclear grade filling and expanding the majority of acini within lobules. LCIS, like all forms of lobular neoplasia, demonstrate loss of expression of E-cadherin, a cell adhesion protein that contributes to the cohesion

CASE 16-14

A 31-year-old woman with macromastia undergoes reduction mammoplasty. A total 715 g of tissue is removed from the left breast and 890 g of tissue is removed from the right breast. Gross inspection of breast tissue reveals no abnormalities. Preoperative imaging studies of the breast revealed no abnormalities. Random representative sections of the breast tissue are submitted for microscopic evaluation yielding the histology in **Figure 16-22**.
Pathologic diagnosis: LCIS.

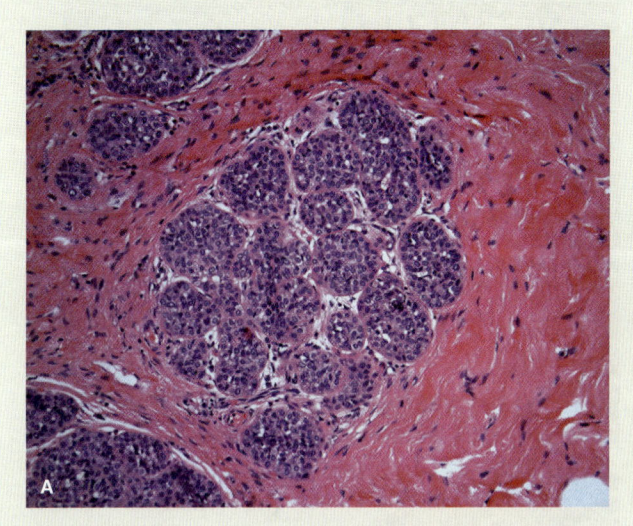

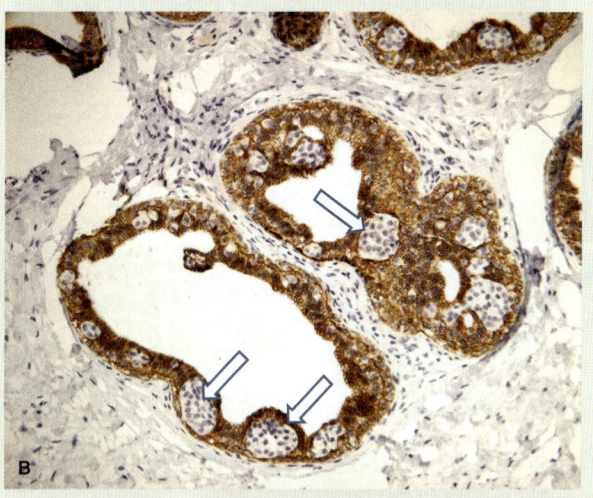

FIGURE 16-22 **Lobular carcinoma in situ (LCIS).** The lobule acini are filled and distended by a monomorphic population of cells with low-grade cytology **(A)**. LCIS may show pagetoid extension into the ducts that are demonstrated by E-cadherin immunostain **(B)**. The nests of LCIS involving the duct wall are negative for staining (arrows), while the duct cells show brown membranous immunoreactivity.

of normal breast epithelial cells. Unlike DCIS, most forms of LCIS are not managed as a direct precursor lesion for invasive carcinoma. Surgical margins positive for LCIS in biopsy specimens are not re-excised in an effort to obtain negative margins. An exception to this rule is in cases showing variant pleomorphic histology with comedo necrosis, so-called pleomorphic LCIS. There is mounting evidence that such lesions act as direct precursors for invasive pleomorphic lobular carcinoma and these cases should be managed similarly to DCIS.

Microinvasive Carcinoma

In some cases, stromal invasion is detected at a very early stage such that the extent of stromal invasion measures no more than 1 mm. These lesions are designated "DCIS with microinvasion" and represent the earliest form of invasive mammary carcinoma. If only one or a few foci of microinvasion are identified, the long-term prognosis for the patient is excellent, similar to that of pure DCIS.

Invasive Mammary Carcinoma

Invasive mammary carcinomas Case 16-15 are identified microscopically by the infiltration of breast stroma by tumor cells that have broken through the basement membrane that typically surrounds the breast ducts and lobules. The invasive process is associated with loss of myoepithelial cells as the tumor invades. The infiltrating tumor cells incite a host desmoplastic response in most cases characterized by fibroblastic/myofibroblastic proliferation and inflammation, resulting in a mass lesion that can be palpated or detected in mammographic images as areas of increased density. Gross examination of invasive carcinomas typically reveals a spiculated to rounded mass that is significantly firmer than the adjacent benign breast tissue (**Figure 16-24**). Invasive carcinomas may gain access to lymph-vascular channels and metastasize to regional (axillary lymph nodes) and distant sites (e.g., bone, brain, lung, skin, and liver). Unusual sites of metastasis include peritoneal surfaces, GI tract, and reproductive organs.

Traditionally, invasive carcinomas have been classified into histologic subtypes based on their appearance under the microscope (Figure 16-23). Invasive ductal carcinoma (no special type) comprises the largest group of invasive breast cancers. This is a heterogeneous group of tumors that fail to exhibit sufficient characteristics to be classified as a special histologic type (Figures 23A–C). A list of the most common histologic subtypes along with key histologic features is provided in Table 16-4. Some histologic subtypes are generally associated with a favorable prognosis such as tubular and mucinous carcinoma, while other subtypes such as metaplastic are associated with poor prognosis.

450   CHAPTER 16

CASE 16-15

A 36-year-old woman presents with complaints of a change in her breast examination. She has noted a mass in the upper outer quadrant of the left breast. The mass has increased in size over the last few months. Physical examination reveals a firm, ill-defined breast tethered to the skin. The patient's past medical history is unremarkable, but there is a significant

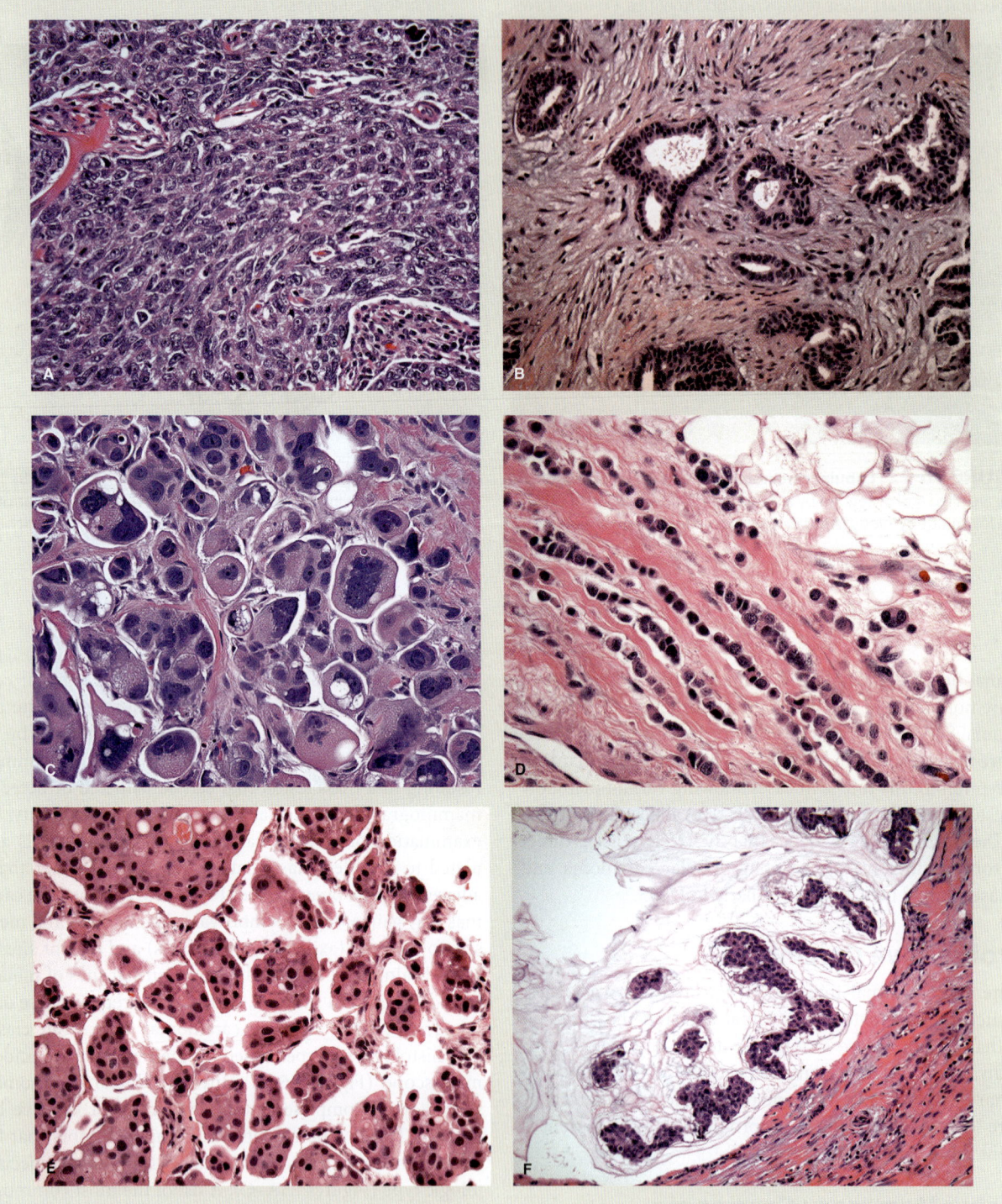

FIGURE 16-23 Histologic diversity of invasive mammary carcinoma. Invasive carcinomas of the breast show diverse histology correlating with the biologic diversity of these tumors. High-grade tumors are characterized by solid architecture, nuclear pleomorphism, and a high mitotic rate (**A, C**). In contrast, low-grade tumors show well-formed tubules, uniform nuclear cytology, and a low mitotic rate (**B**). Special types of invasive mammary carcinoma include lobular (**D**), micropapillary (**E**), mucinous (**F**) and metaplastic (**G**).

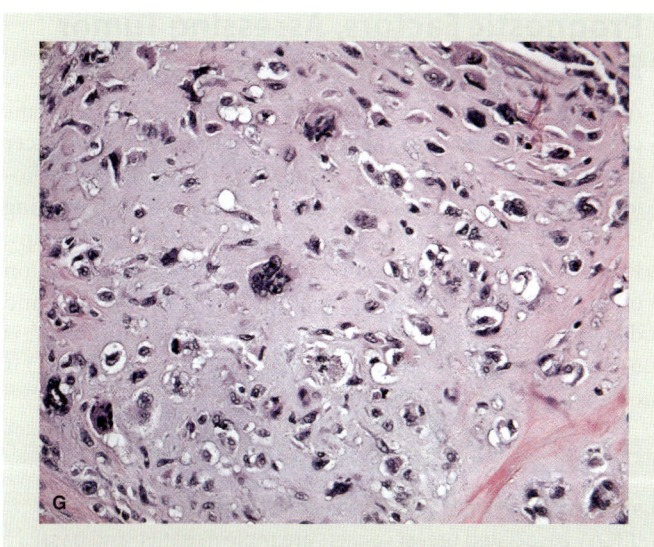

FIGURE 16-23 (Continued)

family history for breast cancer. The patient's mother and only sister were both diagnosed with premenopausal breast cancer. One maternal aunt has a history of ovarian carcinoma. Bilateral mammograms and ultrasound studies are performed. Interpretation of the mammographic images is limited by high breast density. A vague 2 cm ill-defined density is identified in the upper outer quadrant of the left breast corresponding to clinically detected mass. MRI studies are performed revealing two additional enhancing lesions, each <1 cm, in the lower outer quadrant of the breast. Second look ultrasound identifies both lesions and all three breast masses undergo core biopsy evaluation yielding the pathology in Figure 16-23A.

Pathologic diagnosis: Invasive mammary carcinoma, no special type, Nottingham grade 3, involving all three core biopsy sites. Hormone receptor and HER2 studies performed on all three tumors show a triple negative phenotype (ER/PR negative, HER2 negative). Prior to definitive surgery the patient undergoes genetic counseling with BRCA testing. The results return as positive for a deleterious mutation of BRCA1. Bilateral total mastectomies are performed with bilateral sentinel lymph node evaluation. Three separate invasive carcinomas are identified in the left breast, the largest measuring 1.9 cm, showing similar high-grade histology. All of the sentinel lymph nodes are negative for metastatic tumor.

Invasive lobular carcinomas are the second most common histologic subtype of mammary carcinoma Case 16-16. Invasive lobular carcinomas frequently present as irregular and poorly delimited tumors that can be difficult to define on physical examination and radiographic studies. As a result, it is not uncommon that the extent of tumor involvement in the breast is larger than clinically appreciated. Invasive lobular carcinomas may demonstrate unique patterns of distant metastasis involving GI tract, reproductive organs, and serosal lining. A defining trait of lobular carcinomas is loss of expression of E-cadherin,

CASE 16-16

A 62-year-old woman presents with complaints of a change in breast examination. Over the last few years, she has noted an enlarging area of skin thickening in her left breast. Physical examination reveals no discrete mass lesion, but a broad region of skin thickening is appreciated in the left breast. Mammographic and ultrasound studies performed a couple of years earlier were reported as negative. Repeat radiographic studies are performed and identify a vague region of asymmetry in the left breast. A corresponding lesion is identified on ultrasound and a core biopsy is performed yielding the histology in Figure 16-23D.

Pathologic diagnosis: Invasive lobular carcinoma, Nottingham grade 1. The tumor is strongly positive for hormone receptors and negative for HER2 amplification. MRI study reveals multinodular enhancement throughout the entire left breast. Total mastectomy with sentinel lymph node evaluation is performed. Approximately 8 cm of invasive lobular carcinoma is identified. The tumor focally infiltrates the dermis of the skin. One of four sentinel lymph nodes is positive for metastatic carcinoma, measuring 5 mm in greatest dimension.

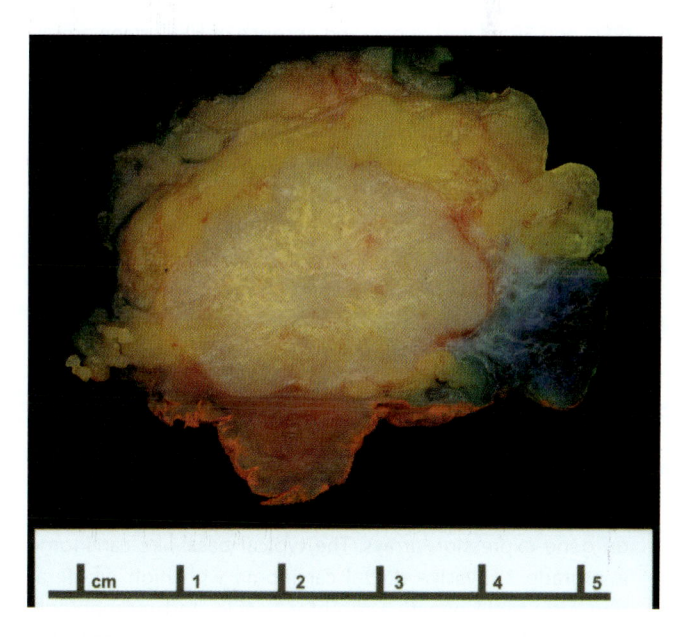

FIGURE 16-24 Gross specimen of invasive mammary carcinoma. This triple-negative breast carcinoma shows a pushing margin of invasion and a tan-yellow cut surface. The foci of yellow discoloration within the tumor represent geographic zones of necrosis.

a cell adhesion molecule that functions as a tumor suppressor, which may be demonstrated by immunohistochemistry. This finding is due to loss of expression of the CDH1 gene, due to deletions, mutations, or epigenetic inactivation.

Inflammatory carcinoma is a particular form of invasive mammary carcinoma with a distinct clinical presentation and poor prognosis. Patients present with diffuse breast skin erythema, edema, induration, and tenderness. An underlying mass may or may not be identified. The histopathologic correlation to inflammatory carcinoma is the presence of tumor emboli within the dermal lymphatics of the skin. In some cases, a punch biopsy of the breast skin may be warranted to confirm the diagnosis.

Prognostic Factors, Assessing Tumor Biology, and Predictive Factors

A summary of important prognostic factors in breast cancer is summarized in Table 16-5. Staging of breast cancer has tremendous prognostic value. Both clinical and pathologic staging is used for breast carcinomas. Clinical staging is based on information gathered before definitive therapy. Pathologic staging is based on the pathologic examination of the resected primary tumor, regional lymph nodes, and distant metastasis when relevant. The TNM classification is used to stage breast cancers. The pathologic tumor size (T) is

IN TRANSLATION

Gene expression profiling is another way to classify the biology of breast cancers. Microarray chips, which can measure the relative quantities of mRNA for thousands of gene simultaneously, have resulted in the development of a molecular classification system for breast cancer. Each of the intrinsic subtypes is defined by the expression of a characteristic set of genes, providing a distinct molecular portrait of the tumor. The molecular subtypes do not account for all the biologic diversity observed in breast cancers, but do provide significant prognostic and predictive information on tumors. The most common molecular subtypes include luminal A, luminal B, basal like, HER2, and claudin-low.

Luminal A tumors comprise the largest group, approximately 50% of invasive ductal carcinomas. The typical luminal A tumor is a grade 1 invasive carcinoma with a low proliferative rate, high expression of estrogen and progesterone receptors (PRs) and ER-related genes, and absence of HER2 gene amplification. These tumors are associated with favorable prognosis, likely to respond to endocrine therapy and unlikely to show significant response to chemotherapy.

Luminal B tumors comprise approximately 15–20% of invasive ductal carcinomas. The typical luminal B tumor is a grade 3 invasive carcinoma with high proliferative rate and positive expression of hormone receptors, although the quantitative levels may be low. Some of these tumors may show HER2 gene amplification. These tumors are associated with poorer prognosis than luminal A tumors and are more likely to show significant response to chemotherapy.

Basal-like tumors comprise approximately 15–20% of invasive ductal carcinomas and are associated with a poor prognosis. Although not synonymous, the majority of triple negative breast cancers carry the basal-like molecular profile on gene expression arrays. The typical basal-like carcinoma is a grade 3 invasive ductal carcinoma with high proliferation rate, triple negative receptor profile, and morphologic features showing pushing border of invasion, geographic tumor necrosis, solid/sheet-like growth pattern, lymphocytic infiltrate, and large central acellular zone. The majority of BRCA1-associated breast cancers are triple negative and basal like. Epidemiologic studies illustrate a higher prevalence of basal-like breast cancers among younger women and women of African descent. Increasing evidence suggests that the risk factor profile for development of basal-like tumors is different than those associated with the more common luminal subtypes. While basal-like carcinomas appear to be more sensitive to chemotherapy than luminal tumors, higher relapse rates are observed among tumors not completely eradicated by chemotherapy. Early relapse is common and a predilection for visceral metastasis, including brain metastasis, is seen.

The HER2-positive subtype comprises approximately 10% of invasive ductal carcinomas and is associated with aggressive biology. The typical HER2-positive subtype carcinoma is a grade 3 invasive ductal carcinoma showing loss of hormone receptor expression and HER2 gene amplification. HER2-positive tumors are further discussed below.

The rare claudin-low subtype shows low-to-absent luminal differentiation and high enrichment for epithelial-to-mesenchymal markers and immune response genes. This subtype is associated with poor prognosis. The typical claudin-low carcinoma is a grade 3 invasive metaplastic carcinoma with a triple negative receptor profile. These tumors have a response rate to chemotherapy that is intermediate between that of basal like and luminal tumors.

Reverse transcriptase polymerase chain reaction (RT-PCR)-based assays are currently the main methodology used for gene expression profiling of clinical breast cancer cases in the United States. The advantage of these assays is that they can be performed on formalin fixed, paraffin embedded tissue blocks, and do not require fresh tissue. The Genomic Health Oncotype DX Recurrence Score is widely used to help determine the clinical benefit of adjuvant chemotherapy for patients with hormone receptor-positive, lymph node-negative breast cancer. This assay further exemplifies the importance of understanding the tumor biology for optimizing individual patient therapy.

TABLE 16-4 Histologic subtypes of invasive breast cancer.

Subtype	Percentage	Characteristic Histologic Features
Ductal, no special type	75%	No special histologic features
Lobular	5–15%	Linear/single cell infiltration, discohesion
Tubular	2%	Well-formed tubules with apocrine snouts
Mucinous	2%	Abundant extracellular mucin
Papillary	1%	Fibrovascular cores, pushing margin
Micropapillary	1%	Micropapillary nests with surrounding cleft
Metaplastic	<1%	Squamous, sarcomatoid, matrix production
Other rare subtypes	<1%	Depends on subtype

TABLE 16-5 Prognostic factors in breast cancer.

Prognostic Factor	Comment
Tumor stage	
Tumor size	Measured from the primary resection specimen
Regional lymph nodes	Most important prognostic factor in patients without distant disease
Distant metastasis	Cure unlikely once distant metastases develop
Histologic grade	Nottingham grade ranges from 1 to 3 Grade 1 favorable Grade 3 unfavorable
Hormone receptors	Positive hormone receptor expression is favorable Loss of hormone receptor expression is unfavorable
HER2 status	HER2 gene amplification associated with aggressive tumor biology (unfavorable)
Proliferation rate	Measured by counting mitotic figures or Ki-67 index using immunohistochemistry High proliferation rate is unfavorable
Lymph-vascular invasion	Poor prognosis finding in the lymph node negative patients Associated with increased risk of local recurrence
Gene expression profiling	
Recurrence score	21-gene assay Used for ER-positive, lymph node negative tumors High recurrence score associated with high risk of developing distant metastasis over the next 10 years if treated with tamoxifen only Low recurrence score associated with low risk (<10%) of developing distant metastasis over the next 10 years if treated with tamoxifen only
MammaPrint	70-gene assay Used for lymph node negative tumors Classifies tumor as low or high risk of development of distant metastasis
Molecular subtype	Subtypes include luminal A, luminal B, basal like, HER2-positive and claudin-low

based on the measurement of the invasive component. The pathologic nodal status (N) is based on histologic examination of lymph nodes and requires detailed quantitation of the tumor burden within the lymph nodes. Axillary lymph node status is the most important prognostic factor for invasive carcinoma in the absence of distant metastasis. Axillary lymph node staging is now accomplished with sentinel lymph node biopsy. If the sentinel lymph nodes are negative for tumor, it is highly unlikely that any of the remaining axillary lymph nodes contain tumor, and the patient can be spared the morbidity (e.g., lymphedema) associated with a complete axillary lymph node dissection. The (M) designation is for distant metastasis.

Multiple methods are used to predict the biology of invasive mammary carcinomas including tumor histologic grade, receptor profile and gene expression profile. Numerous studies have documented the prognostic value of tumor histologic grade. The histologic grade is reported by pathologists for all invasive breast carcinomas. The Nottingham grade ranges from 1 to 3 and is based on tumor glandular differentiation, nuclear pleomorphism, and mitotic rate. Grade 1 tumors are associated with more favorable prognosis and hormone receptor positivity. Grade 3 tumors are associated with poorer prognosis and are more likely to be ER-negative than grade 1 or 2 tumors.

WHAT WE DO

All invasive breast carcinomas are tested for ER, PR and HER2 overexpression/amplification. The main utility of these studies is to guide therapy for patients. Hormone receptor-positive status, particularly when strong, is associated with response to hormonal therapy such as tamoxifen and aromatase inhibitors. Hormone receptor testing is currently evaluated using immunohistochemistry where nuclear staining is classified as positive (Figure 16-25A). Hormone receptor status may also be evaluated using quantitative RT-PCR assays to quantify mRNA levels. There is strong correlation between the results of immunohistochemical and RT-PCR-based assays.

Approximately 15–20% of breast cancer harbor amplifications involving the HER2 (also called ERBB2) gene locus located on chromosome 17. HER2 gene amplification results in a marked increase in the number of HER2 molecules at the membrane of tumor cells. The overexpression of HER2 promotes dimerization with members of the HER-receptor family and activation of intracellular signaling cascades that drive cellular proliferation, promote angiogenesis, and enhance cell survival pathways, resulting in aggressive tumor biology and clinical behavior. Even small HER2-positive breast cancers (<1 cm) may metastasize and cause mortality. Identification of HER2 driven tumors has become extremely important with the evolution of highly efficacious therapies that target HER2. These therapies target HER2-positive tumor cells using humanized monoclonal antibody (trastuzumab) against HER2 or tyrosine kinase inhibitors that interrupt the HER2 growth receptor pathway. Trastuzumab induces antibody-mediated cellular toxicity, inhibits HER2-mediated signaling, and prevents cleavage of the extracellular domain of HER2. In HER2-positive breast cancer, trastuzumab has shown a survival advantage in early and metastatic disease and is now the standard of care. Assessment for HER2-positive disease can be performed using immunohistochemistry to detect the markedly increased copies of HER2 receptors in cell membranes (Figure 16-25B) or in situ hybridization to detect HER2 gene amplification (HER2/CEP17 ratio >2.0).

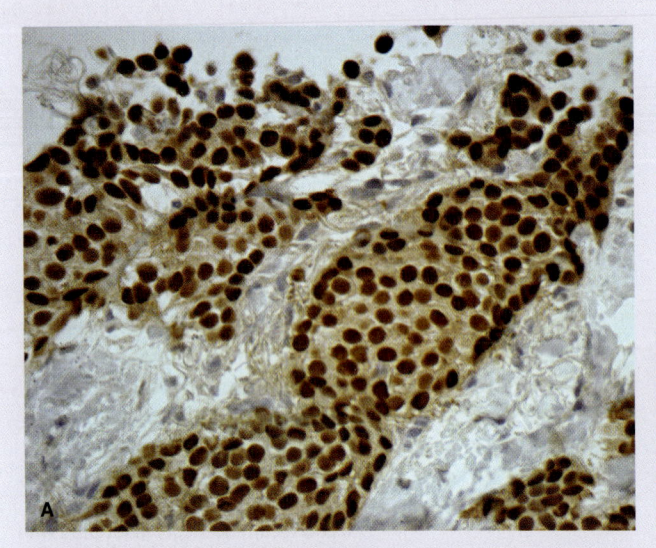

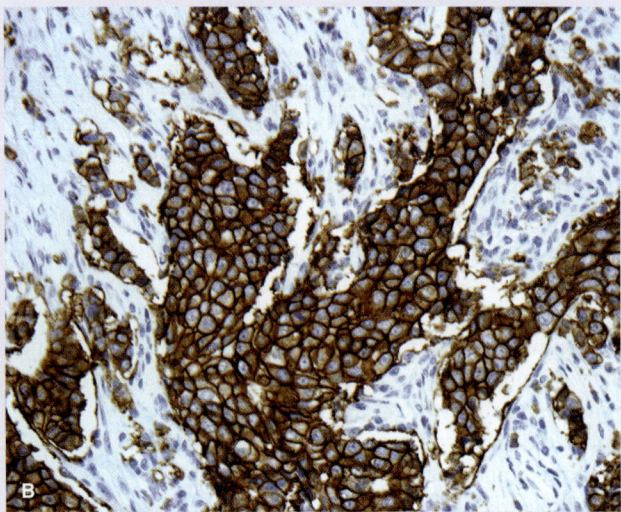

FIGURE 16-25 Receptor studies. Immunohistochemical stain for estrogen receptor shows strong positive staining in the nuclei of the invasive mammary carcinoma (A). Immunohistochemical stain for HER2 protein shows diffuse strong membranous overexpression typical for a HER2-amplified tumor (B).

CHAPTER 17

The Female Reproductive Tract

Natalie Banet, M.D. and Ruth A. Lininger, M.D., M.P.H.

INTRODUCTION

The role of the pathologist in diagnosing gynecologic disease includes a broad range of conditions from infectious to congenital and from benign to malignant neoplasms in all parts of the female reproductive tract. The following two cases are typical of those seen in the practice of gynecologic pathology.

CASE 17-1

A 57-year-old woman presents to her gynecologist with the complaint of postmenopausal bleeding. During her workup, a CT scan of her abdomen shows a 12-cm right ovarian mass. Clinical lab values drawn prior to removal of the mass include a markedly elevated inhibin level. Photos of the tumor are shown below (Figure 17-1). What is your diagnosis? What is the significance of her postmenopausal bleeding?

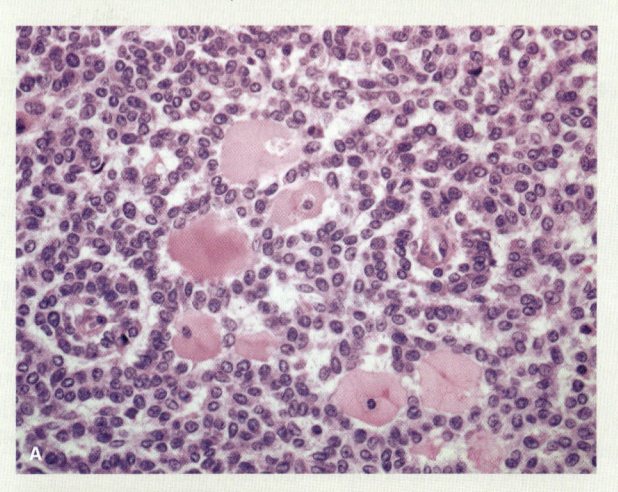

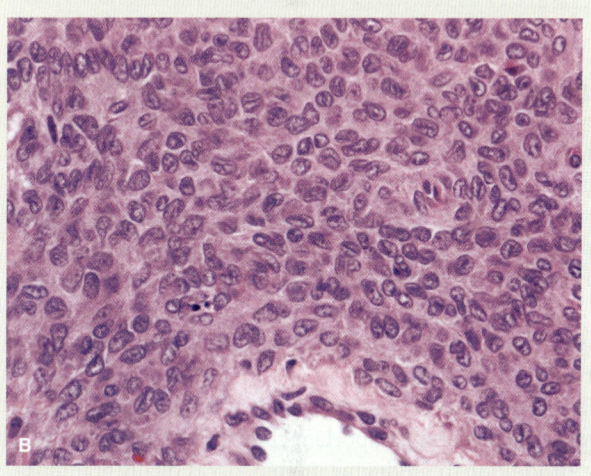

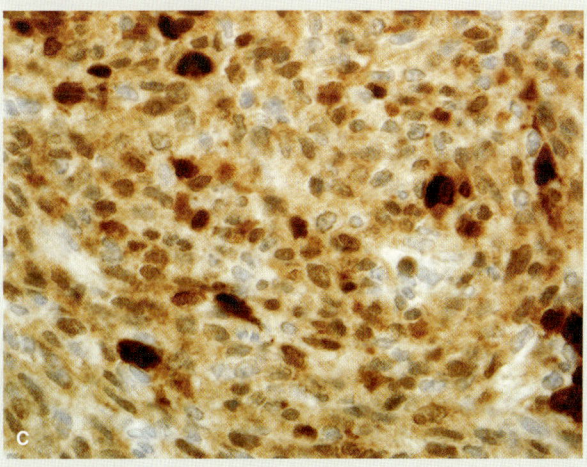

FIGURE 17-1 Granulosa cell tumor of the ovary.
(A) Ovarian gonadal stromal cells resembling the granulosa cell layer of the developing ovarian follicle are shown here forming Call-Exner bodies (microfollicular spaces filled with pale, eosinophilic material). (B) Nuclear grooves ("coffee bean nuclei") are characteristic (high-power view). (C) Immunohistochemical expression of inhibin.

CASE 17-2

A 30-year-old woman presents to the emergency department with left-lower quadrant abdominal pain. She admits to being sexually active, but has an intrauterine device. A urinary human chorionic gonadotropin (hCG) test is positive, and an ultrasound shows a mass in the left fallopian tube. A section from the intratubal mass is shown (**Figure 17-2**). What is your diagnosis? What about this patient's history made you suspect this condition? What are the clinical implications?

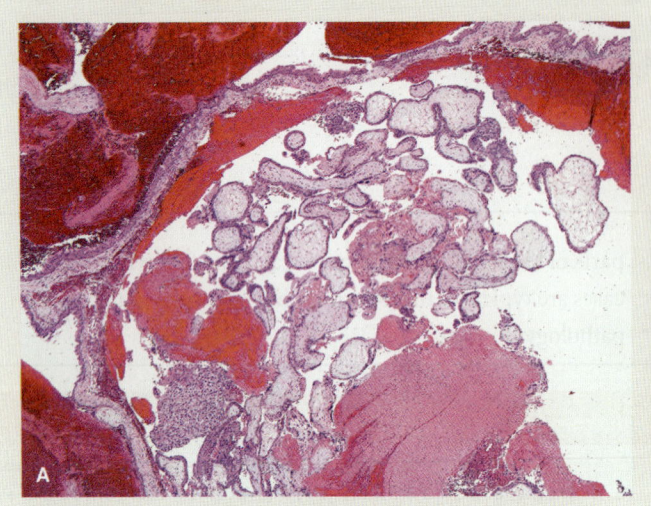

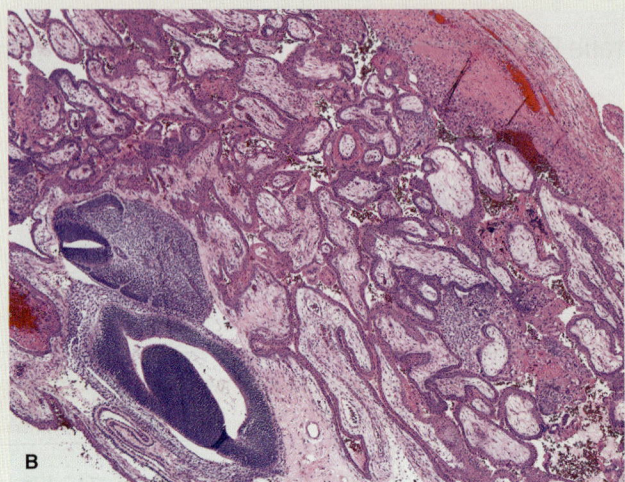

FIGURE 17-2 Tubal ectopic pregnancy. (A) Products of conception and blood are noted within this dilated segment of fallopian tube (low-power view). **(B)** At high power view fetal parts are seen, evidenced by embryonic neural tube and embryonic mesenchyme (lower left); the immature chorionic villi are shown in the top right.

The diagnosis for **Case 17-1** is adult granulosa cell tumor. Figure 17-1 depicts classic histology: neoplastic cells arranged in sheets with characteristic focal gland-like structures arranged around acellular pink material, known as Call-Exner bodies. The positive immunohistochemical staining confirms via immunofixation that this tumor overexpresses inhibin, which corresponds to the elevated blood level. The granulosa cell is a normal component of the ovarian follicle, which supports the follicle. Their classification will be discussed under tumors of the ovary.

The presentation of this patient with postmenopausal bleeding highlights one of the important clinical implications of this tumor. In addition to producing inhibin, occasionally granulosa cell tumors also produce estrogen. In a postmenopausal woman, unopposed estrogen stimulation can lead to a proliferation of the endometrial lining which can be premalignant or malignant (see section on "Endometrial Hyperplasia"), which can present with abnormal bleeding. Before operating on this patient's ovarian mass, an endometrial biopsy would be obtained to rule out a concurrent malignancy of the endometrium.

Figure 17-2 shows an ectopic pregnancy, with placental tissue composed of immature chorionic villi, syncytiotrophoblast, and the neural tube of the fetus. This condition arises when a fetus implants at any location other than inside the uterus, with the fallopian tube being the most common site. The incidence increases the most in women who have a history of pelvic inflammatory disease (PID), although women with an intrauterine device also have an increased risk.

Most patients with this condition usually present with severe abdominal pain, which can be a sign that the ectopic pregnancy has ruptured. This can be a life-threatening condition, requiring urgent surgical intervention to prevent excessive blood loss.

EMBRYOLOGY/ADULT ANATOMY

A basic knowledge of the development of the female genital tract can be extremely beneficial in the understanding of the pathogenic processes that affect these organs. Of particular importance is that fact that the ovary develops from a different cell type than the fallopian tube and uterus.

QUICK REVIEW
Embryology

The germ cells that give rise to the follicles of the ovary begin in the wall of the yolk sac, and are endodermal origin. Three weeks after fertilization, these cells migrate to the urogenital ridge, where they join a proliferating group of cells, which form the supporting stroma of the ovary.

The lining of the uterus (endometrium) and muscular wall of the uterus (myometrium) are of mesodermal origin. They are formed from the fusion of the Mullerian ducts, as is the vagina. The precise origin of the cervix is still the subject of debate, but it is likely that it is also derived from Mullerian remnants.

Adult Anatomy

The adult ovaries are located on either side of the uterus and are approximately 30 times the size of the newborn ovaries. They are divided into a cortex, which contains connective tissue that invests follicles at varying stages of development, and a medulla, which contains blood vessels, loosely arranged mesenchymal tissue, and remnants of ovarian development called hilar cells.

In the prepubertal female, the majority of the uterus is composed of cervix. The size and proportions of the adult uterus vary with size and the number of pregnancies (parity). The uterus is divided into three sections. The isthmus begins just above the cervix and is contiguous with the corpus (body). The fundus is the portion of the uterus above the fallopian tubes. The uterus is located between the bladder (anteriorly) and the rectum (posteriorly). It is supported by the round ligaments and the utero-ovarian ligaments, and is invested in a layer of pelvic peritoneum.

The fallopian tubes are hollow epithelial-lined muscular tubes that merge with the uterine cavity on one end and terminate into a patent end, which empties into the peritoneum. The portion closest to, and contiguous with, the uterus, is called the isthmus. The distal portion, termed ampulla, merges with the dilated end, termed fimbriae.

The anatomy of the external genital tract will be discussed in the appropriate sections below (Figures 17-3 and 17-4).

INFECTIONS

The presentation of the patient in Case 17-3 is common, as the majority of Chlamydial infections are asymptomatic. Routine screening for this disease in sexually active women is important due to the potentially grave complications of untreated infections. While some patients have only mild side effects, like urethritis and cervicitis, others may go on to develop PID. PID represents spread of an infection from the lower to the upper reproductive tract, and can lead to life-threatening illness, scarring, and infertility.

CASE 17-3

A 20-year-old sexually active woman presents to her family physician for a refill of her oral contraceptive pills (OCPs). She has had two sexual partners in the past year, and has used condoms inconsistently. Her physical exam is unremarkable. As part of her annual exam, testing for *Neisseria gonorrhoeae* and *Chlamydia trachomatis* are performed, the latter of which returns a positive result. Is it common for this disease to present in this way? What are the implications of this infection for the patient?

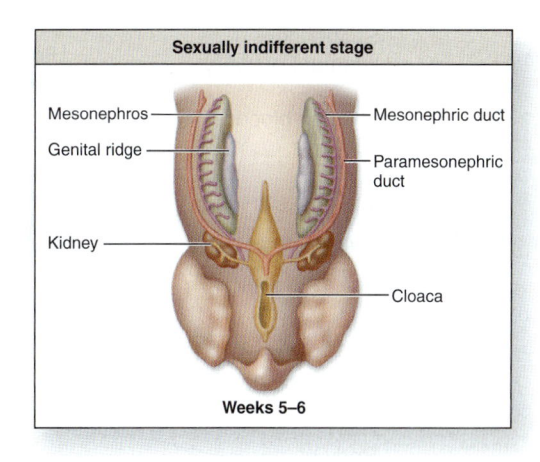

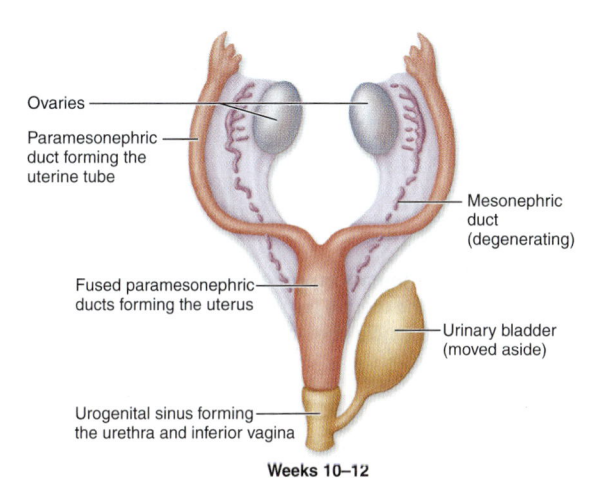

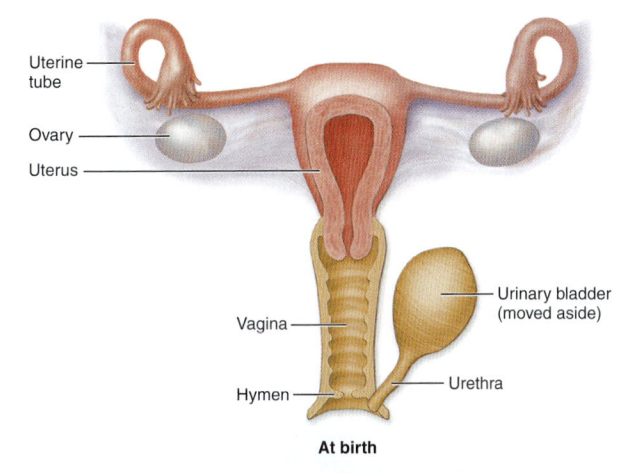

FIGURE 17-3 Embryonic development of the female reproductive tract. (Modified as shown from McKinley & O'loughlin. Human Anatomy. 2nd edn. McGraw Hill: New York, 2007, Figure 28.18.)

Fitz-Hugh–Curtis syndrome is a less common sequela of PID. This syndrome represents spread of the infection to the space around the liver and to the liver capsule (Glisson's capsule; perihepatitis), which may result in perihepatic adhesions. Perihepatic inflammation will present in women as right-upper quadrant pain, and may be confused with more common causes of pain in that location like cholecystitis.

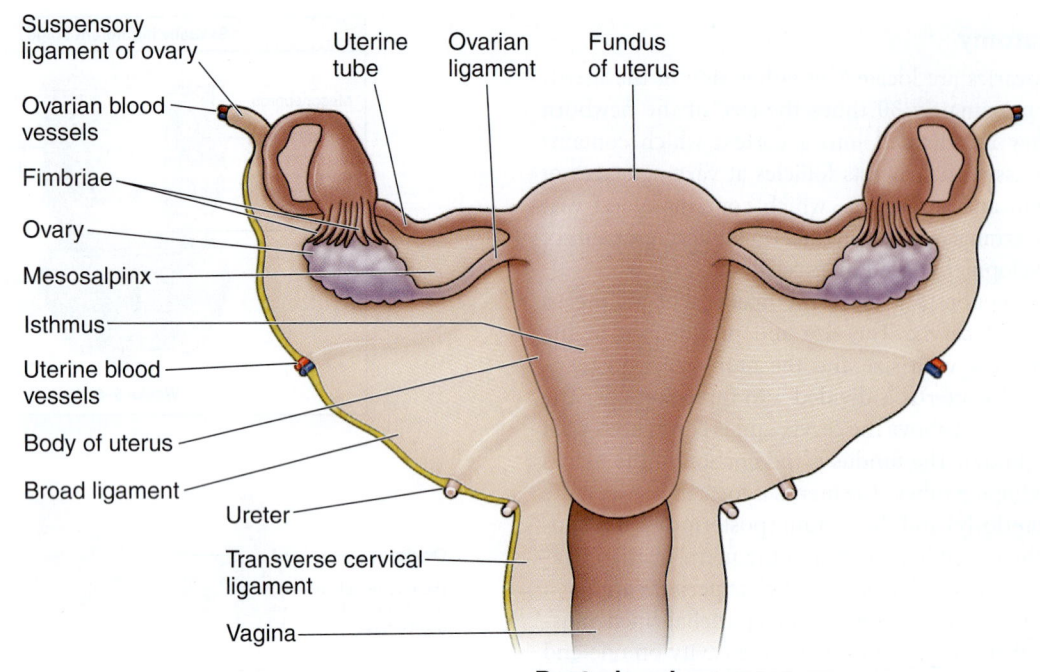

FIGURE 17-4 The female reproductive system. The relationship between the uterine tube and the uterus is shown in a posterior view (left) and a partially cut-away diagram (right).

Modified as shown from McKinley & O'loughlin. Human Anatomy. 2nd edn. McGraw Hill:New York, 2007, Figure 28.7.)

CASE 17-4

A 30-year-old woman calls her gynecologist complaining of intense vaginal itching and whitish discharge of 2 days duration. She has been on antibiotic therapy for 10 days for recent bronchitis. A pap smear, collected the day before she called the office, showed the organism pictured below (Figure 17-5). What is your diagnosis?

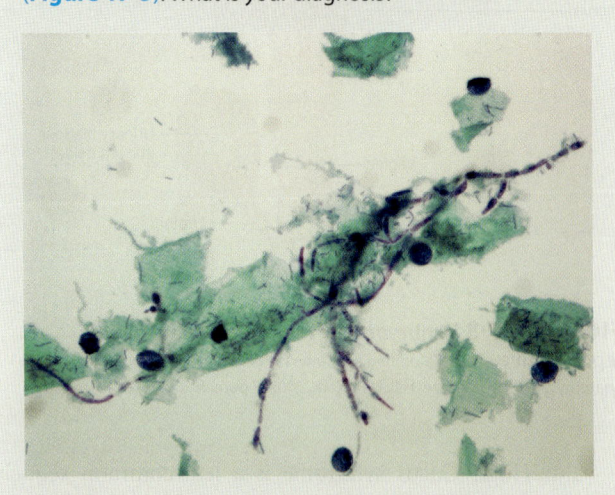

FIGURE 17-5 Candida fungal hyphae in Pap smear. Candida fungal pseudohyphae are noted here (staining purple), associated with benign squames (staining green). Normal bacterial vaginal flora (bacterial rods consistent with lactobacilli) are also present in the background (Pap smear, Thin Prep).

The organism in Figure 17-5 is *Candida albicans*, a yeast which is a normal part of the vaginal milieu. Symptomatic candidiasis results when a disturbance of the normal flora permits the overgrowth of this yeast, resulting in vaginal and vulvar redness, itching, and inflammation. A few conditions associated with increased incidence of yeast infection are: diabetes, recent antibiotic therapy, and pregnancy.

> **QUICK REVIEW**
> For a summary of other common sexually transmitted and genital infections, see Table 17-1.

VULVA

Anatomy

The external female genitalia consists superiorly of the mons pubis and clitoris, laterally of the labia majora and more medially of the labia minora. The posterior aspect, referred to as the posterior fourchette, abuts the perineum. The opening to the vagina is termed the vestibule. Bilateral and named glands in the area consist of Skene glands (also known as periurethral glands), which open just lateral to the urethral meatus, and Bartholin glands, present laterally, which empty via ducts that drain into the posterior aspect of the vestibule.

Developmental Anomalies

Clitoromegaly at birth suggests an abnormality of testosterone production, which may be caused by a number of conditions,

TABLE 17-1 Common sexually transmitted and genital infections.

Infectious Organism	Characteristics	Presentation	Diagnosis
Calymmatobacterium granulomatis	Gram-negative coccobacillus that causes granuloma inguinale. Rarely seen in United States, more common in tropical climates	Genital papules that develop into ulcers, heal with scarring	Identification of Donovan bodies (macrophages that have ingested the organism) on tissue section, also PCR assays now available
Candida albicans	Yeasts and pseudohyphae that are part of the normal vaginal flora. Common infectious agent, especially in diabetics and those on antibiotic therapy	Pruritic vaginitis with white discharge and erythematous mucosa	Direct visualization from a clinical sample, occasionally empirically treated based on symptoms
Chlamydia trachomatis	Most common sexually transmitted infection in women and men	Urethritis, cervicitis, pelvic inflammatory disease, FHC syndrome	Preferred method: detection of Chlamydia-specific DNA in urine or from a swab of affected area
Gardnerella vaginalis	Gram-negative rod causes bacterial vaginosis. "clue cell"—squamous cell covered in organisms	Malodorous vaginal discharge, rise in vaginal pH (>5.5)	Direct visualization from a clinical sample, occasionally empirically treated based on symptoms
Haemophilus ducreyi	Gram-negative rod that causes chancroid	Painful ulcers in the genital and perianal areas, enlarged inguinal lymph nodes	Clinical symptoms, culture is available
Herpes simplex virus	Sexually transmitted virus that infects and then remains latent in sensory ganglia, can cause recurrent outbreaks	Vesicles that ulcerate on the vulva, cervix, or perianal area. If during pregnancy, delivery by cesarean to prevent infection of fetus	PCR of a swab from the center of the ulcer. Can also screen for past infection with blood antibodies
Human Papilloma virus	Sexually transmitted virus that can lead to genital warts, or dysplasia and cancer of the cervix	Low-risk types—genital warts. High-risk types—cervical dysplasia, cancer (see section on "Cervix" below)	Clinical symptoms, on Pap smear by changes in the cellular appearance, or by PCR on Pap specimen
Neisseria gonorrhoeae	Common gram-negative diplococci, sexually transmitted	Pelvic inflammatory disease with involvement of tubes (salpingitis) and ovaries, scarring that can lead to infertility, FHC syndrome	Preferred method: detection of Chlamydia-specific DNA in urine or from a swab of affected area
Treponema pallidum	Sexually transmitted spirochete that causes syphilis, progresses when left untreated	Primary—solitary, painless chancre. Secondary—maculopapular rash on palms, soles, and trunk. Tertiary—neurosyphilis, gummas, and aortitis	First test: nonspecific (VDRL, RPR). Second test: confirmatory (FTA-ABS)
Trichomonas vaginalis	Sexually transmitted flagellated protozoan with tumbling motility	Vaginitis, urethritis, "strawberry-colored" cervix, greenish vaginal discharge	Direct visualization from a clinical sample, occasionally empirically treated based on symptoms

including adrenogenital syndrome and exogenous maternal ingestion.

Dermatologic Diseases/Benign Tumors

A common benign lesion in this part of the body, the Bartholin cyst, actually represents the accumulation of secretions from the corresponding glands due to plugging of duct outflow, and characteristically presents with a palpable mass located in the lateral aspect of the vestibular orifice. Although they may recur, these cysts are benign, and may require excision when draining alone is not curative. A common cause of infection in a Bartholin gland cyst is N. gonorrhoeae.

The diagnosis associated with Figure 17-6 is lichen sclerosus et atrophicus. This is an inflammatory skin disorder that is more common in postmenopausal women. It is characterized by all of the physical exam findings present in this patient. Microscopically, the epidermis is thinned by almost complete loss of the basal layer, with loss of rete pegs, and superficial hyperkeratosis (Figure 17-6). The superficial dermis is characterized by homogenization and edema, often with a band of pink, subepithelial collagen. There may be chronic

CASE 17-5

A 72-year-old woman presents to her gynecologist with a long-standing history of itching and discomfort of the labia majora and minora. Physical exam shows the affected areas of the vulva to be pale, with white plaque-like areas, thinned "parchment-like" skin, and focally, ulcerated patches. A skin biopsy is performed (Figure 17-6). What is your diagnosis? What are the implications for the patient?

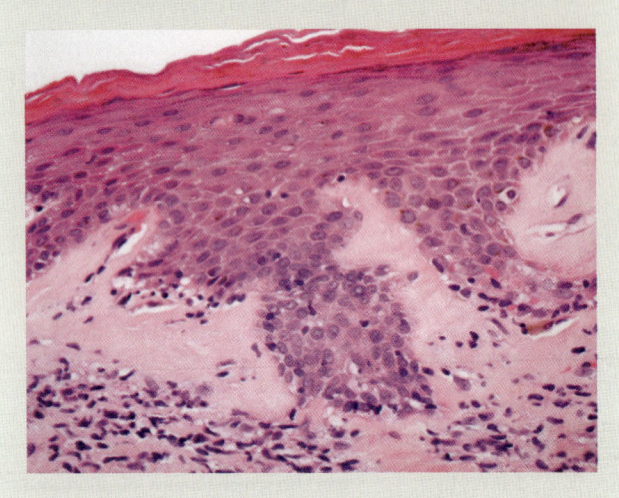

FIGURE 17-6 Lichen sclerosus et atrophicus (LSEA) of the vulva. Skin of the vulva shows a collagenized stroma underlying epidermis which is thinned, with hyperkeratosis.

inflammatory cells at the junction of the dermis and epidermis. Although it is not considered a premalignant lesion, patients with lichen sclerosus have a slightly increased risk of developing squamous cell carcinoma.

Inflammatory skin disorders that affect other areas of the body can also affect the vulva, including lichen planus, psoriasis, seborrheic dermatitis, and spongiotic dermatitis. For a more thorough discussion of these diseases, please see Chapter 20.

Premalignant and Malignant Tumors

The diagnosis of the biopsy illustrated in Figure 17-7 is vulvar intraepithelial neoplasia (VIN), which represents a spectrum of dysplasia from low grade (VIN1) to high grade (VIN3). Changes in the squamous cells include: increased nuclear to cytoplasmic ratios, nuclear pleomorphism, and a lack of maturation as the cells move toward the surface. Because the nuclear abnormalities are confined to the lower third in this patient's epithelium, this represents VIN1. The diagnosis of VIN2 is used when the abnormalities are confined to the lower two thirds, and when they are fully thick, VIN3.

There are three types of VIN. The first two: warty and basaloid, are associated with high-risk human papillomavirus (HPV) infection, most commonly HPV 16. This is the type of VIN present in this patient (pictured in Figure 17-7). Many women with these types of VIN have concurrent neoplasia of the genital tract, making this patient's history of cervical dysplasia (also caused by infection with high-risk HPV) not surprising.

CASE 17-6

A 45-year-old woman presents to her gynecologist with the chief complaint of vulvar irritation and pruritus. She has a past medical history significant for cervical dysplasia. Physical exam shows white papules on the labia majora. A biopsy of these lesions is performed (Figure 17-7). What is your diagnosis? What are the risk factors for this condition? What serious conditions can follow as a consequence?

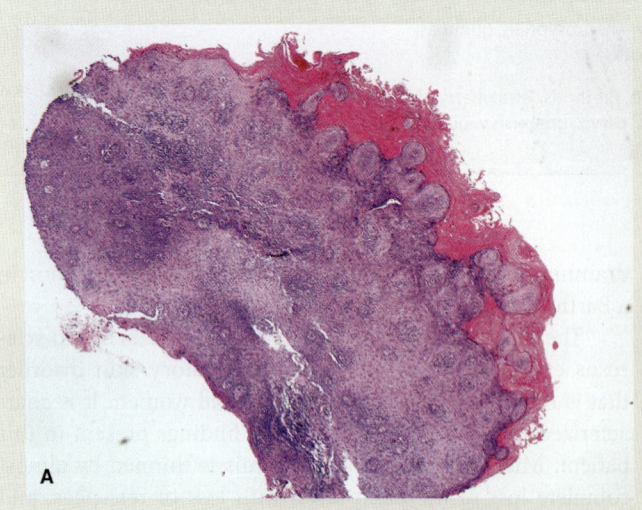

FIGURE 17-7 Vulvar condyloma. Warty vulvar squamous epithelial proliferation showing papillary projections with overlying mounds of hyperkeratosis and hypergranulosis as well as koilocytotic atypia (HPV viral cytopathic effect) **(A)** low- and **(B)** high-power view.

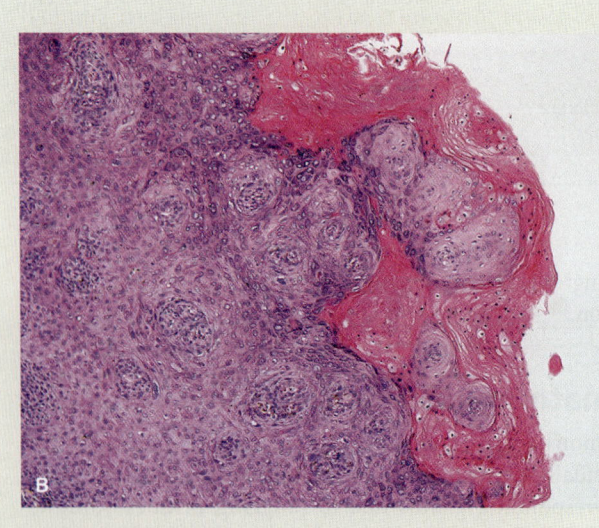

CASE 17-7

A 70-year-old woman presents to her gynecologist with the chief complaint of vulvar pruritus and erythema which had existed for some time, and which did not resolve with a variety of topical medications. She has no significant past medical history. Physical exam shows an eczematous, slightly raised erythematous area of the labia majora with focal whitish areas. A biopsy is performed (Figure 17-8). Immunohistochemical staining is performed to confirm the origin of the neoplastic cells. What is your diagnosis? For what other conditions must you screen this patient?

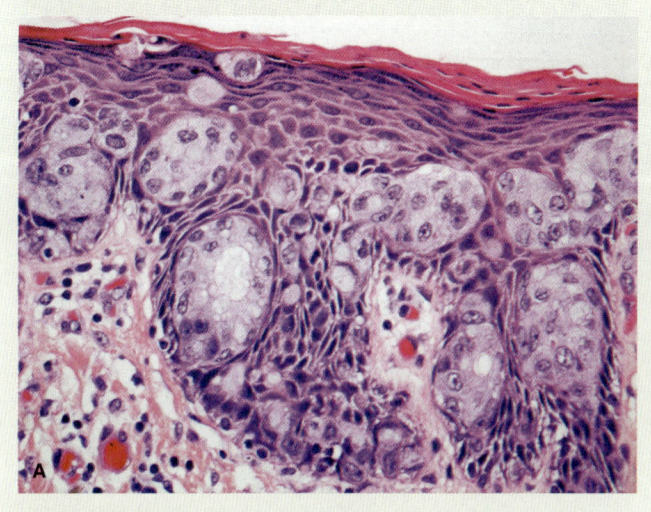

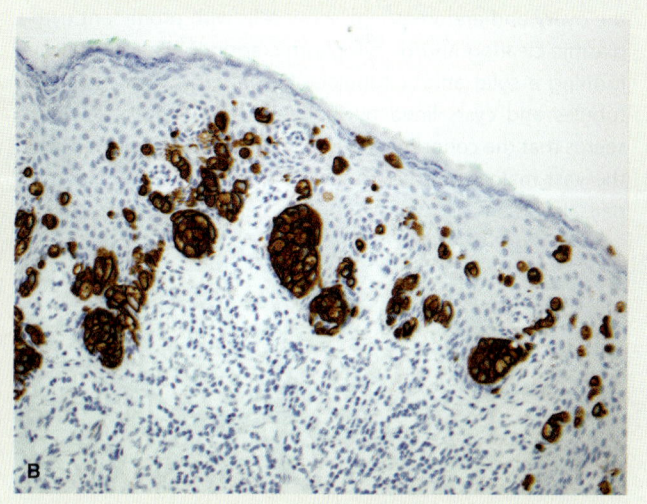

FIGURE 17-8 **Paget disease of the vulva. (A)** Intraepidermal extension of clusters of tumor cells and rare glands are noted here. **(B)** Immunostain for cytokeratin highlights the intraepidermal tumor, confirming it is an adenocarcinoma, and not a melanoma.

The third type of VIN is termed differentiated VIN (or VIN, simplex type), and while not associated with HPV infections, its incidence is increased in women with inflammatory dermatitis of the vulva, most notable lichen sclerosus. Though their causative agents are not the same, all three subtypes of VIN represent precursor lesions for vulvar squamous cell carcinoma.

The biopsy illustrated in Figure 17-8 demonstrates extramammary Paget disease. The Paget cells are distinct from surrounding epithelium, with paler cytoplasm and more prominent nuclei. They are present in large numbers at the junction of the epidermis and dermis, sometimes in nests and rarely small glands, and other times as single cells. Paget disease can present as a solitary finding of primary cutaneous origin (primary cutaneous Paget disease), or may be a manifestation of an underlying malignancy of the surrounding skin, the anal–rectal region, or the bladder (secondary Paget disease or Paget disease of noncutaneous origin).

Microscopically, the cells of Paget disease mimic those of a cutaneous malignancy, which can present in this part of the body, malignant melanoma. Immunohistochemistry can help to differentiate between these two entities. As shown in Figure 17-6, the neoplastic cells are epithelial in origin, staining positively with low molecular weight cytokeratins CK7 and CAM5.2, and do not stain for the melanoma markers, S100, HMB-45, and MART-1.

VAGINA

Benign Lesions and Malformations

Developmental abnormalities include a septate (doubled) vagina, which is often accompanied by a duplicate uterus (uterus didelphys).

Infectious organism of the external genitalia often affects the vagina. For details, see Table 17-1. In addition, systemic inflammatory diseases, such as Crohn disease and Stevens–Johnson syndrome, may also affect the vagina.

Premalignant and Malignant Neoplasms

The most common malignant tumor of the vagina is metastatic cervical carcinoma. Although primary squamous cell carcinoma of the vagina is rare when compared to cervical and vulvar carcinoma, it does occur. Like vulvar carcinoma, it is preceded by three levels of dysplasia, and uses the same criteria to differentiate between the grades of vaginal intraepithelial neoplasia. Risk factors include HPV infection, immunosuppression, and a history of ionizing radiation.

HUNTING FOR ZEBRAS

Clear Cell Carcinoma of the Vagina: Originally, a rare diagnosis made in postmenopausal women, from 1970 to 1990, it was noted that cases of clear cell carcinoma were being diagnosed in much younger women (mean age of 19). The cause was linked to intrauterine exposure to diethylstilbestrol, a drug used by many pregnant women from 1940 to 1970 to prevent miscarriage. These tumors, identical to their counterparts in the ovary and endometrium, show cells with prominent cytoplasmic clearing and/or cytoplasmic eosinophilic cell change forming a solid and/or tubulocystic patterns, with the small tubules and cysts lined by "hobnail" cells (Figure 17-9). It seems that the cohort of exposed females have now aged, and the vast majority of new cases are once again in postmenopausal women.

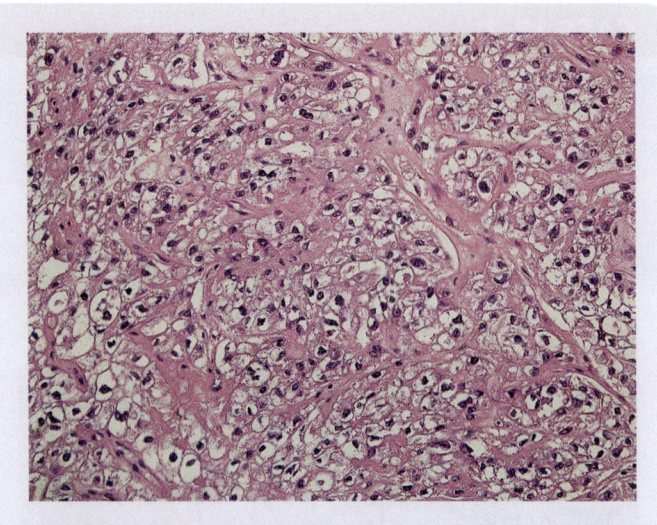

FIGURE 17-9 Clear cell carcinoma of the endometrium. This tumor demonstrates solid sheets of atypical cells with eosinophilic cytoplasm and prominent intracytoplasmic clearing.

IN TRANSLATION

Embryonal Rhabdomyosarcoma: Representing the most common primary vaginal neoplasm in infants and children, the malignant cell of origin in this tumor is skeletal muscle. The most common subtype, called sarcoma botyroides, is characterized by a "cambium layer" of condensed rhabdomyoblasts beneath the epithelium (Figure 17-10). When the tumor mass is large, some patients will present with the classic "cluster of grapes" protruding from the vaginal orifice.

Embryonal rhabdomyosarcoma is frequently associated with loss of heterozygosity in a region of the short arm of chromosome 11 (11p15.5), which is rich in imprinted genes. This could potentially lead to inactivation of a tumor suppressor gene or activation of a proto-oncogene resulting in neoplastic progression. Defects

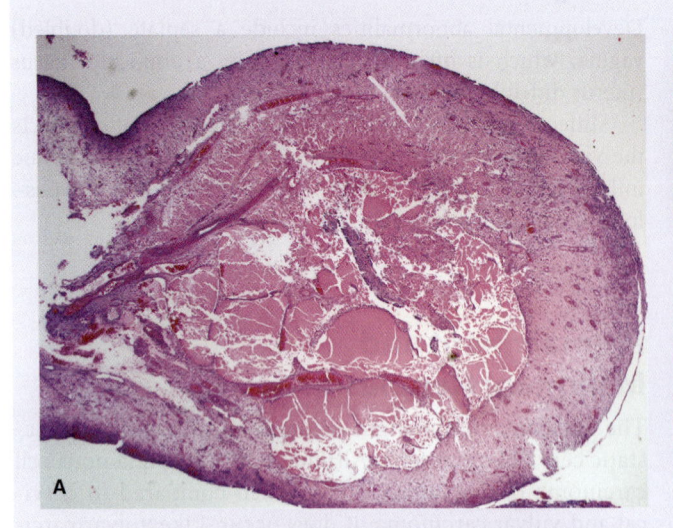

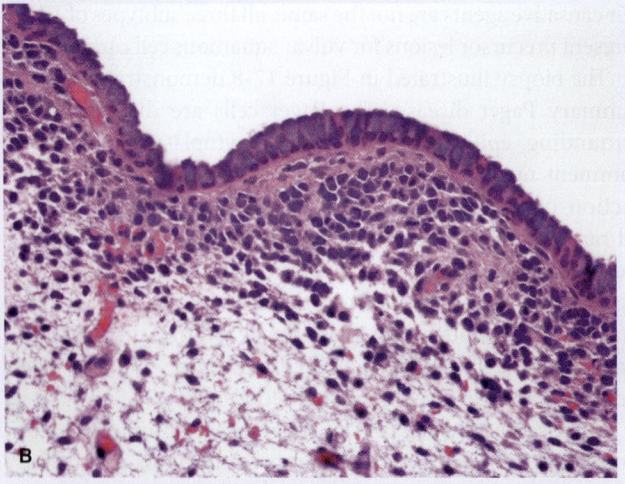

FIGURE 17-10 Sarcoma botryoides (embryonal rhabdomyosarcoma, botryoid type). (A) An edematous, grape-like structure is noted in this tumor (low-power view). **(B)** At high-power view, the surface of the tumor shows benign glandular epithelium with periglandular stromal condensation by the malignant mesenchymal component (the so-called "cambium layer").

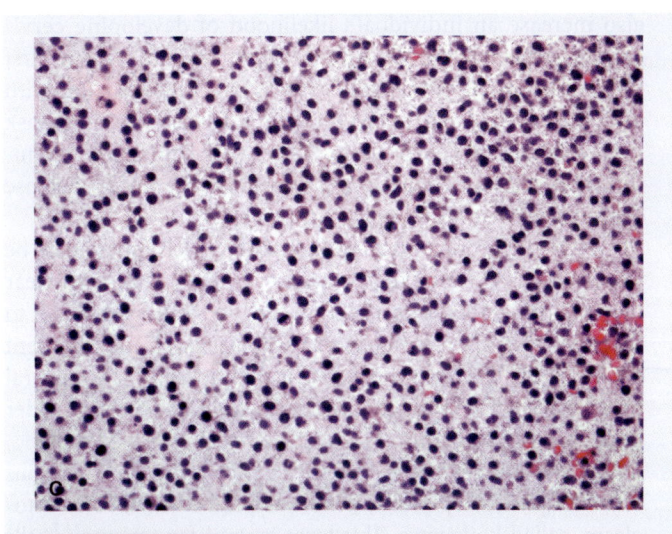

FIGURE 17-10 *(Continued)* **(C)** This field is entirely represented by sheets of embryonal rhabdomyosarcoma with a very undifferentiated appearance.

in this chromosomal region are also associated with Beckwith–Wiedemann syndrome (BWS). Children with BWS have an over 500-fold risk for developing several embryonal tumors, such as Wilms tumor and hepatoblastoma.

CERVIX

Anatomy

The uterine cervix consists of the endocervix, which is contiguous with the uterus, and the outer portion that opens into the vagina, the exocervix. The patent center of the cervix is called the os. The endocervix is lined by mucous-secreting cells, while the exocervix is lined by squamous epithelium. The area where these two meet is called the transformation zone. This zone is pathologically important, as it is the preferred locale for infection by HPV, a known precursor of cervical dysplasia and carcinoma. The transformation zone migrates throughout life as the cervix elongates (Figures 17-4 and 17-11).

Benign Findings of the Cervix

Inflammation: The normal flora of the vagina is dominated by Lactobacilli, which produce acid and maintain the vaginal pH below 4.5. This environment curbs the growth of other organisms, like yeast. However, normal physiologic events, like menstruation, can alter the vaginal pH and result in shifts in vaginal flora. These normal changes lead most women to show signs of inflammation in the cervix. Marked or destructive inflammation, however, must be noted on cervical biopsies, as it may be the harbinger of a more serious upper tract infection like *Chlamydia*, Herpes Simplex Virus, or gonococcus (see Table 17-1).

Benign Lesions of Cervix: Two benign lesions of the cervix are noted here due to their potential confusion for a malignant condition. Leiomyomas are benign, circumscribed tumors of smooth muscle. Although they occur most frequently in the uterus, cervical leiomyomas can cause reactive atypia of the overlying epithelium. Cervical polyps are relatively common exophytic growths that occur in adult women. Because they can present with vaginal bleeding and a mass, they occasionally cause clinical concern. However, simple excision shows them to be benign fibrous tissue covered by columnar epithelium.

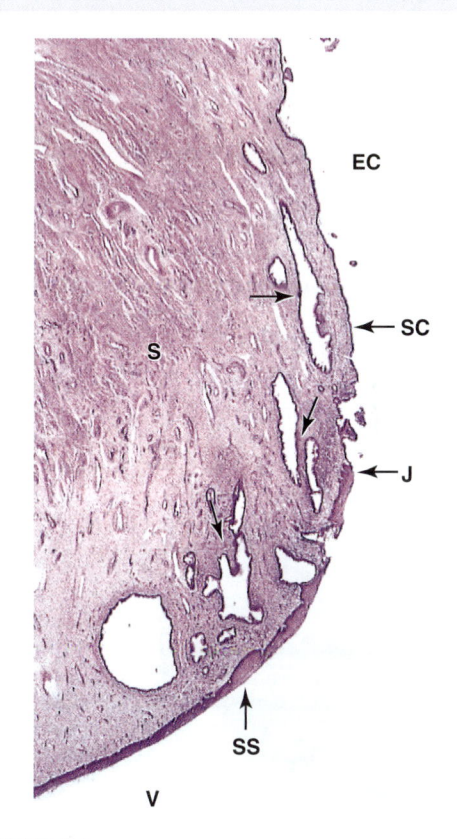

FIGURE 17-11 Cervix. The cervix is the lower part of the uterus, which extends into the upper vagina. Micrograph shows that the mucosa of the endocervical canal (EC) is continuous with the endometrium and like that tissue is lined by simple columnar epithelium (SC). The endocervical mucosa has folds and many large branched cervical glands (arrows) secreting mucus under the influence of the ovarian hormones and often becoming quite dilated. At the external os, the point at which this canal opens into the vagina (V), there is an abrupt junction (J) between this simple epithelium and the stratified squamous epithelium (SS) covering the exocervix and vagina. The junctional region defines the transformation zone ×15. H&E. (Modified from Mescher AL, Junqueira's Basic Histology Text and Atlas. 12th edn. McGraw Hill Lange New York, Figure 22-21.)

Occasionally, entrapped mucous-filled spaces, termed, Nabothian cysts, may present as a cervical polyp as well.

Premalignant and Malignant Neoplasms

Squamous Cell Lesions: The implementation of screening for squamous cell carcinoma of the cervix is an important success story in the history of medicine. Early detection of precursor lesions by Pap smear (named after its creator, Papanicolaou), allows for clinical intervention before carcinoma develops in the vast majority of cases. Once a relatively common condition, invasive squamous cell carcinoma has been decreasing in incidence in the West for some time as a result, although it continues to be a major public health problem in less developed countries throughout the world.

The pathogenesis of cervical carcinoma has been linked to infection with HPV, a DNA virus that has many subtypes. There are known types that are "high risk" for causing cervical carcinoma, namely, HPV 16 and 18, and others that are "low risk," and tend to cause lesions like genital warts, namely, HPV 6 and 11. Risk factors that increase exposure to HPV infections also increase an individual's likelihood of developing cervical dysplasia and cancer. Among these are: early age at first intercourse, multiple sexual partners or a male partner with multiple previous partners, persistent infection with high-risk HPV subtypes, and high parity. Other risk factors, like immunosuppression and smoking, compromise the body's defense against the infecting virus.

HPV infection, even with high-risk serotypes, can be transient. It is known that younger women more often clear the virus. It is, therefore, essential for the treating clinician to take into account a woman's age when making management decisions for patients with cervical dysplasia. The general trend is to manage younger patients less aggressively, and older patients more vigilantly.

The Pap smear in Figure 17-12 shows benign squamous cells with pink cytoplasm and more atypical cells with blue cytoplasm, called koilocytes. This term is used for squamous cells that show changes due to HPV infection. In addition to the perinuclear halo (seen above as a clear space around the nucleus), nuclear changes present in the koilocytes include enlargement, irregular borders, and clumping of chromatin. The diagnosis in this patient is low-grade squamous intraepithelial lesion.

CASE 17-8

A 26-year-old woman with no past medical history presents to her gynecologist for her annual exam. She has had six lifetime sexual partners. Her Pap smear is shown in **Figure 17-12**. What is your diagnosis?

The results of her Pap smear prompts cervical biopsies, one of which is pictured in **Figure 17-13**. What is your diagnosis? Why was a biopsy performed?

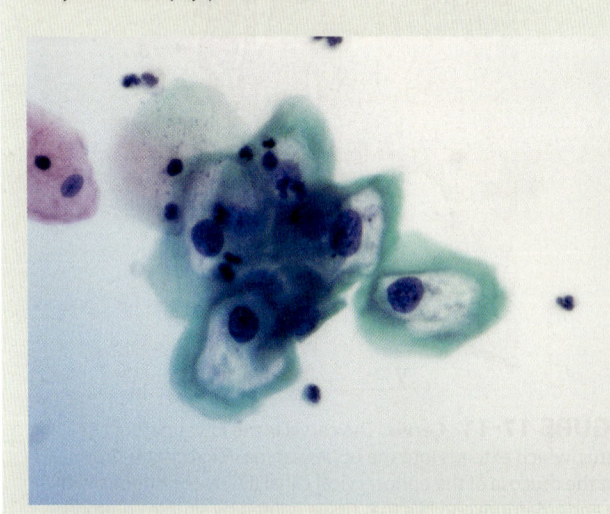

FIGURE 17-12 Low-grade squamous intraepithelial lesion (LGSIL) of the cervix. Dysplastic squamous epithelial cells (located centrally) show twofold nuclear enlargement compared to the small nuclei of normal squames (present at top left); perinuclear haloes present in the dysplastic cells signify accompanying koilocytosis (HPV viral cytopathic effect).

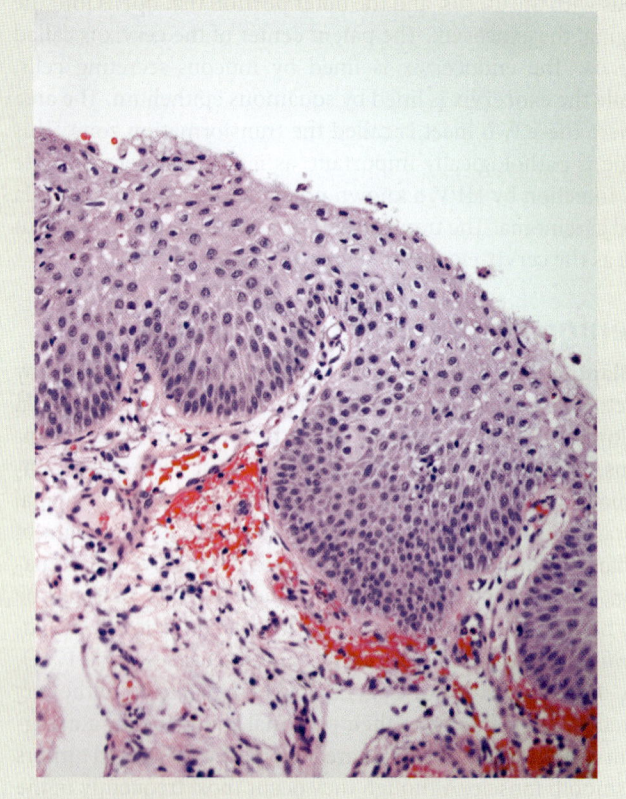

FIGURE 17-13 Cervical intraepithelial neoplasia 1 (CIN 1). CIN1 demonstrated here is characterized by mild koilocytotic atypia, and proliferation of the basal layer with some nuclear enlargement and nuclear irregularity.

THE FEMALE REPRODUCTIVE TRACT   465

TABLE 17-2 Abnormal cytologic diagnosis for squamous cell lesions of the cervix on Pap smear.

Diagnosis	Features
Atypical cells of uncertain significance (ASCUS)	Many appearances, mature squamous cells with some abnormality which makes them suspicious for LSIL
Low-grade squamous intraepithelial lesion (LSIL)	Intermediate-sized cells Koilocytes—nuclear enlargement with irregular borders, coarse chromatin, and perinuclear halo
High-grade squamous intraepithelial lesion (HSIL)	Smaller cells Single cells or groups with high nuclear to cytoplasmic ratios, markedly coarse chromatin
Squamous cell carcinoma	Features of HSIL with large nucleoli, tumor diathesis (necrotic debris in background), and "tadpole" cells with abnormal cytoplasmic outlines

QUICK REVIEW

For a summary of Pap smear diagnostic criteria, please see Table 17-2. A Pap smear showing high-grade squamous intraepithelial lesion (HSIL) is shown for comparison (see Figure 17-14).

The histologic images presented show cervical intraepithelial neoplasia 1 (CIN1). It is the first on a three-tiered scale of dysplasia from mild to severe. In the lower third of the epithelium above are multiple koilocytes, which have similar features to their counterparts in the Pap smear, but are pictured here in tissue sections. The progression to CIN2 (Figure 17-15) requires these dysplastic cells to extend into the upper two thirds of the epithelium, while full thickness dysplasia warrants a diagnosis of CIN3 (Figure 17-16). The diagnosis of invasive squamous cell carcinoma of the cervix is made when the neoplastic cells invade into the underlying stroma. Often there is a paradoxical redifferentiation with invasion, with the invasive squamous cells acquiring more abundant cytoplasm and often keratinization, sometimes manifesting as keratin "pearls."

Biopsies were performed in this patient for several reasons. It is known that not all patients' dysplasia of the cervix will inevitably proceed to high-grade dysplasia or develop invasive carcinoma. An example of invasive squamous cell carcinoma on a Pap smear and a surgical biopsy specimen are available in Figures 17-17 and 17-18, respectively.

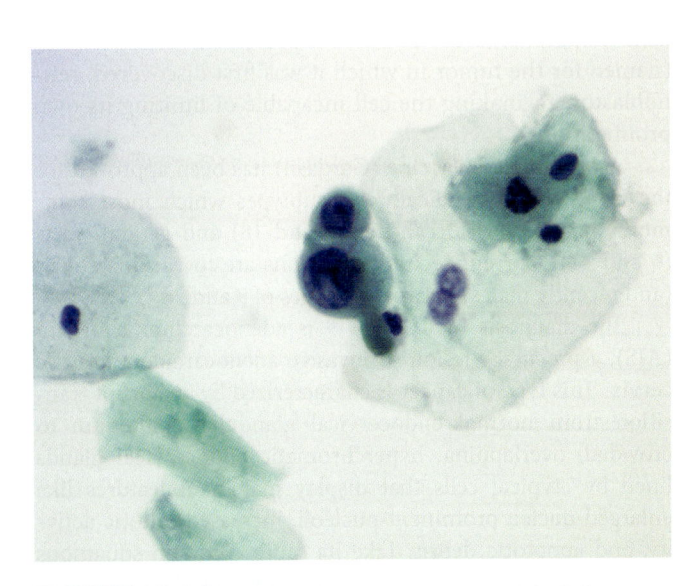

FIGURE 17-14 High-grade squamous intraepithelial lesion (HSIL) of the cervix. Squamous epithelial cells in the center of the image show a high nuclear: cytoplasmic ratio, nuclear hyperchromasia, an irregular nuclear membrane representing HSIL.

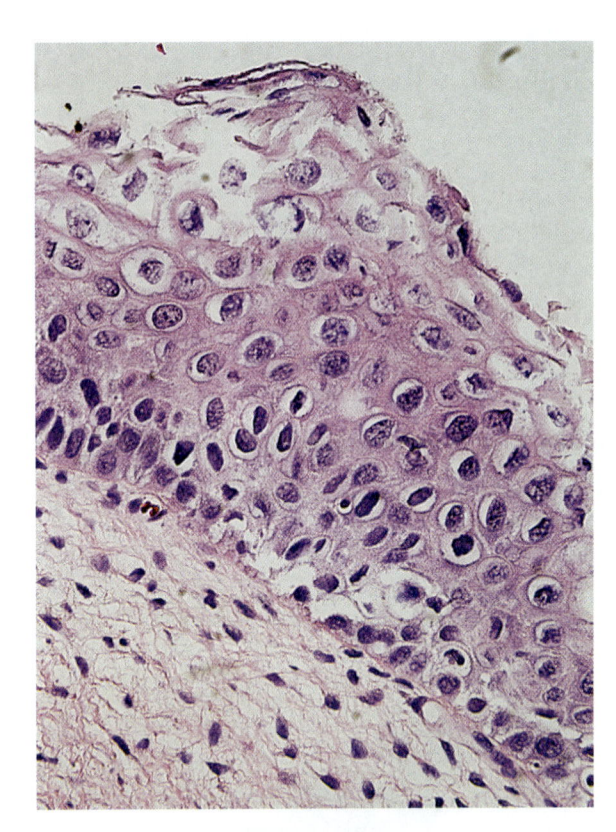

FIGURE 17-15 Cervical intraepithelial neoplasia 2 (CIN 2). CIN2 shows dysplastic changes extending into the mid-zone with increased koilocytotic atypia.

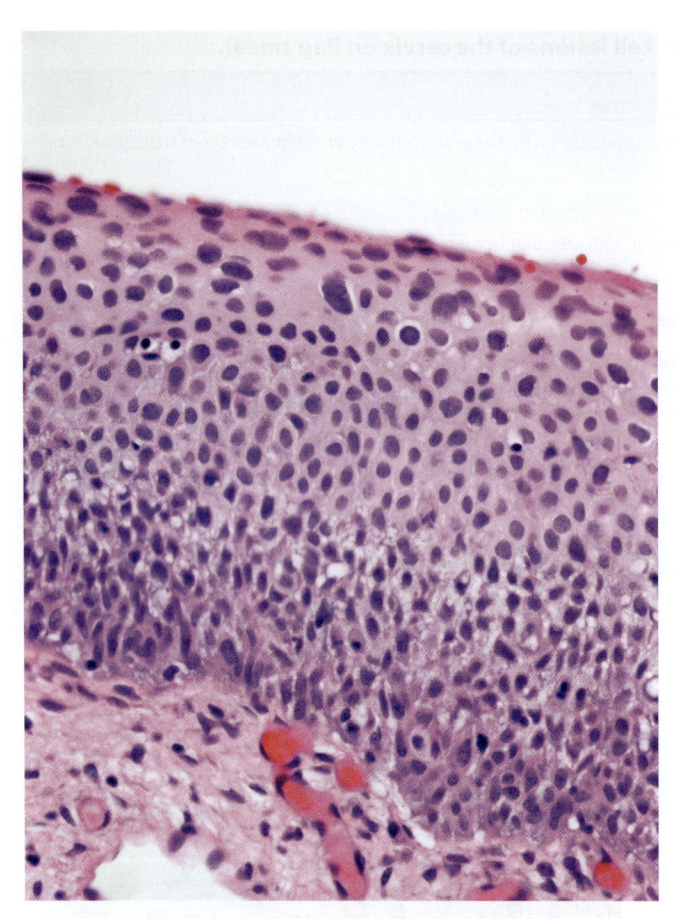

FIGURE 17-16 Cervical intraepithelial neoplasia 3 (CIN 3). CIN3 shows a full thickness proliferation of dysplastic cells with homogenization of the nuclear chromatin.

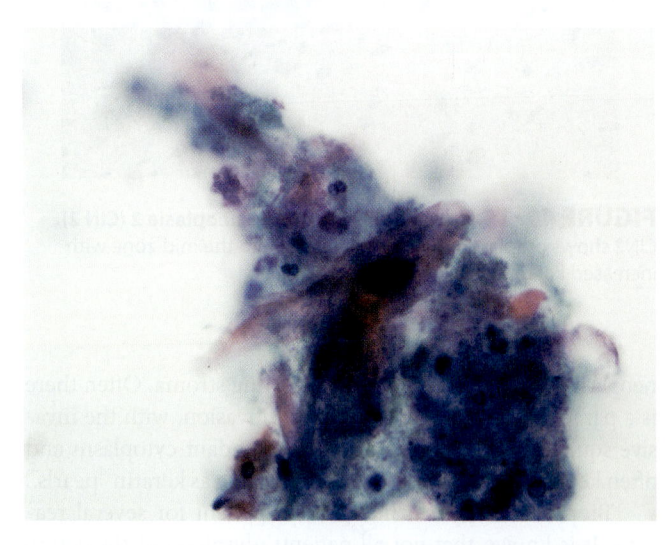

FIGURE 17-17 Squamous cell carcinoma of the cervix, Pap smear. Within the three-dimensional cell cluster in the center of this image is an enlarged, pink–red, amphophilic, elongated atypical squamous epithelial cell ("tadpole cell") with nuclear enlargement, irregularity, and hyperchromasia.

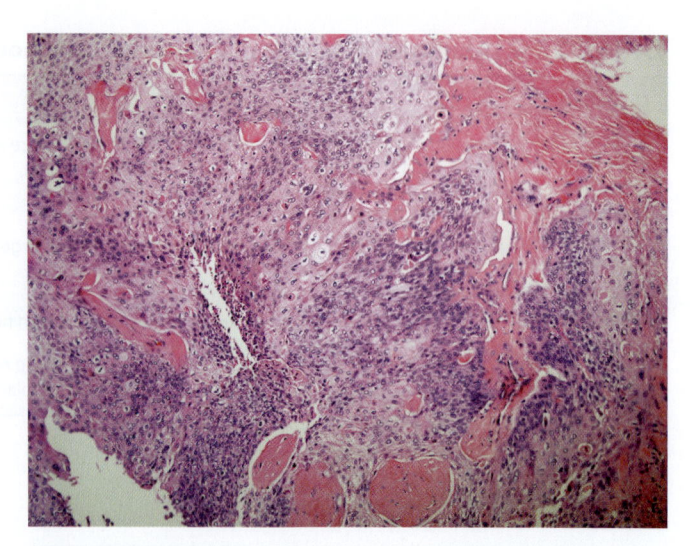

FIGURE 17-18 Invasive squamous cell carcinoma of the cervix. Infiltrating malignant squamous epithelium showing keratinization manifested by extracellular areas of pink acellular, keratinaceous debris, and intracellularly as cells showing hard pink cytoplasm.

Molecular Biology of HPV-Related Cervical Carcinogenesis

HPV belongs to the Papillomavirus family, a group of double-stranded DNA viruses. The pathogenesis of cervical infection begins when HPV infects the cervical epithelium during sexual intercourse, which affords the virus a chance to infect the cervical epithelium and maintain low copy numbers within the cells. Progression to invasive cervical carcinoma is characterized by integration of viral DNA into the host genome, which can destabilize the host DNA and make the keratinocytes immortal. One of the best characterized changes occurs when a viral protein E7 binds to pRB (named for the tumor in which it was first discovered, retinoblastoma), making the cell incapable of limiting its own proliferation.

A preventative vaccine (Gardasil) has been approved for the HPV virus, specifically the subtypes which most commonly cause cervical cancer (16 and 18) and genital warts (6 and 11). Current recommendations are to vaccinate girls (and recently males) between the ages of 9 and 26.

The diagnosis in **Case 17-9** is adenocarcinoma in situ (AIS), a precursor lesion to invasive adenocarcinoma of the cervix. This type of cancer is characterized by an abrupt transition from normal endocervical glandular epithelium to crowded, overlapping, hyperchromatic endocervical glands lined by atypical cells that display malignant features like enlarged nuclei, prominent nucleoli, increased mitotic activity, and apoptotic debris. Like its more common squamous counterpart, AIS is caused by infection with HPV, most commonly high-risk HPV types 16 and 18. Cervical cancer screening is extremely effective at detecting precancerous squamous lesions, but relatively poor at detecting glandular ones.

IN TRANSLATION
HPV Testing in Cervical Specimens

In certain patient groups, it is now routine to test for HPV in the cervical cells that are submitted for cytologic evaluation (Pap smear). The general trend is to test only those patients who have a decreased chance of clearing the virus (age >30) or those patients with an equivocal result [atypical squamous cells of undetermined significance (ASCUS) on Pap smear], and whose treatment algorithm would be affected by the result. Various testing platforms have been approved for use, all of which detect specific serotypes of HPV viral nucleic acids (DNA, RNA) in clinical samples. DNA detection methods include in situ hybridization using a DNA probe, hybridization using an RNA probe followed by signal amplification, and DNA amplification by PCR. RNA detection methods target high-risk viral E6/E7 mRNA.

CASE 17-9

A 35-year-old woman visited her family physician for her annual exam. Her Pap smear was read as ASCUS (Table 17-2). HPV testing was performed on the Pap smear and was positive for a high-risk subtype (HPV 18). A subsequent biopsy is available (Figure 17-19). What is your diagnosis?

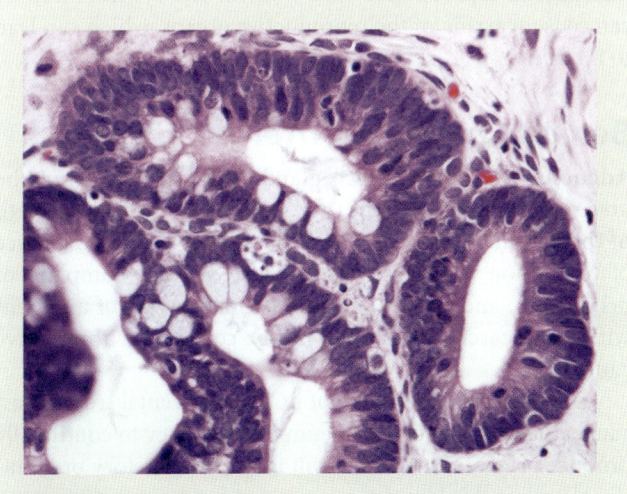

FIGURE 17-19 Adenocarcinoma in situ of the cervix. The endocervical glands show nuclear stratification, atypia, nuclear enlargement, increased mitotic activity, intestinal (goblet cell) metaplasia, and focally an intraglandular cribriform pattern, qualifying for endocervical adenocarcinoma in situ (AIS; H&E stain).

UTERINE CORPUS

Menstrual Cycle

The uterine lining undergoes a cyclic change approximately every 30 days in response to hormonal changes. The proliferative (follicular) phase of the endometrium is mediated by increases in estrogen produced by the developing ovarian follicle, corresponding to an increase in follicle stimulating hormone produced by the anterior pituitary gland. Proliferative endometrium is characterized by regularly spaced tubular endometrial glands with nuclear stratification and scattered mitotic figures (Figure 17-20). Ovulation occurs at the end of the proliferative phase in response to a surge in luteinizing hormone (LH). After ovulation, and in the setting of elevated estrogen and progesterone levels produced by the corpus luteum, the endometrium progresses through the secretory (luteal) phase, characterized by irregularly shaped, coiled endometrial glands with characteristic subnuclear and supranuclear vacuoles and stromal edema (Figure 17-21). In the absence of embryo implantation, the corpus luteum involutes and all the hormone levels fall, resulting in breakdown of endometrial glands, chronic inflammation, and stromal hemorrhage, the final step in the cycle (the menstrual phase; Figures 17-22 and 17-23).

Effects of Hormone Therapy/Dysregulation

OCPs generally contain some mixture of estrogen, which prevents the midcycle estrogen surge, and therefore ovulation, and progesterone, which arrests the proliferative phase and causes gland atrophy. Also beneficial in preventing pregnancy, OCPs render cervical mucous hostile to sperm, and alter fallopian tube motility.

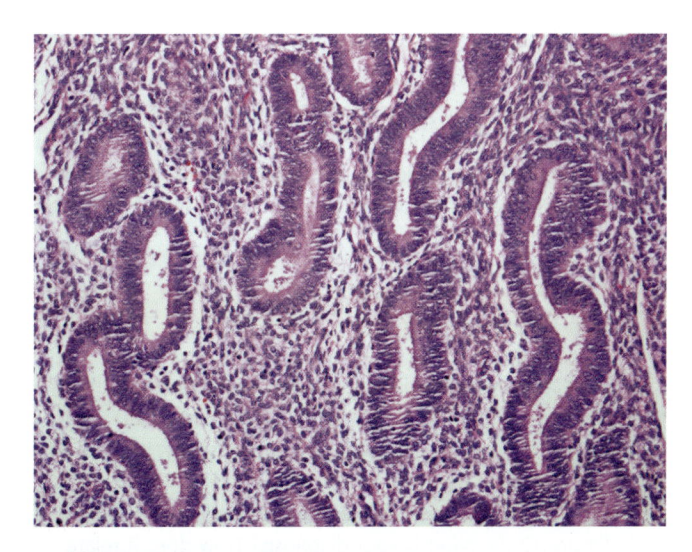

FIGURE 17-20 Proliferative endometrium. Seen here are benign tubular endometrial glands with nuclear stratification and often showing mitotic figures.

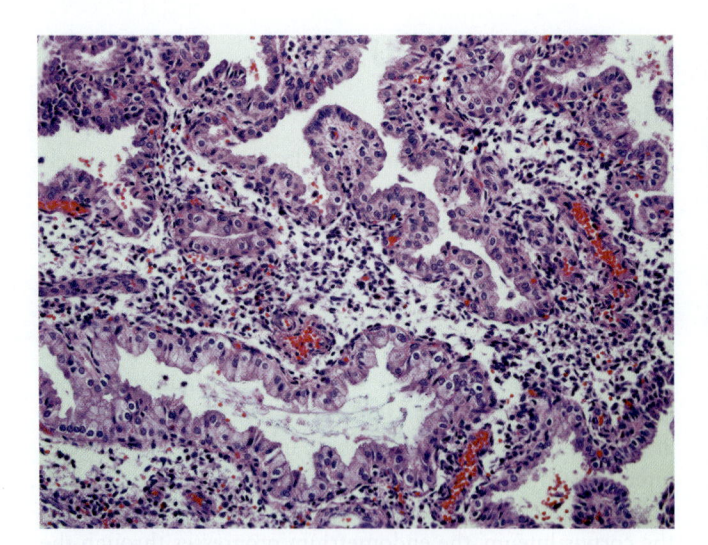

FIGURE 17-21 Secretory endometrium. Coiled, S-shaped endometrial glands showing intraglandular secretions as seen here are characteristic of secretory endometrium.

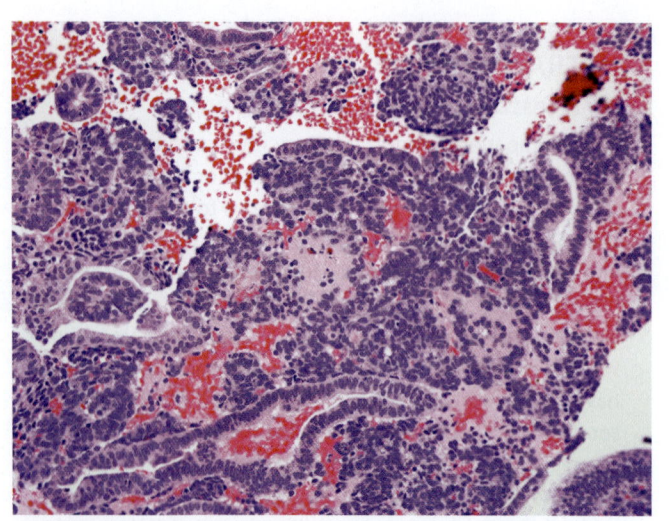

FIGURE 17-22 Menstrual endometrium. Endometrial glandular and stromal breakdown with stromal collapse and abundant blood are present. Eosinophilic surface syncytial metaplasia of the overlying endometrial epithelium may also be seen.

Many women seek treatment for disturbances in the menstrual cycle. Examples include menorrhagia (heavy bleeding at the time of a patient's menstrual period), and metrorrhagia (irregular bleeding between her menstrual period). These conditions may be the result of an anatomic lesion like a polyp, leiomyoma, or even neoplastic proliferations like endometrial hyperplasia (see "Hyperplasia and Carcinoma of the Uterus").

Dysfunctional uterine bleeding refers to bleeding apart from normal menses in the absence of an organic lesion. Usually caused by an imbalance of hormones, this is a common complaint that affects women of all ages, but especially those who are perimenopausal.

Endometriosis

Figure 17-24 shows endometrial glands and stroma in abnormal locations, confirming the diagnosis of endometriosis. Because these ectopic glands respond to the cyclic hormones of the menstrual cycle, they bleed and, therefore, appear brown on gross examination. Indeed, the "chocolate cyst" classically grossly described in the ovary is an endometriotic focus filled with aged blood, and their laparoscopic appearance has been described as "burn marks."

The most common site for endometriosis is the ovary, followed by the uterine serosa. It is not impossible, however, to see foci distant from the uterus (e.g., lung and lymph nodes). There are two widely accepted theories as to the origin of endometriosis. The first is retrograde flow through the fallopian tubes, the most likely cause in this patient. The second is spread of the glands through the bloodstream or lymphatics, which can explain lesions in the lung and lymph nodes.

Endometriosis is a common cause of pelvic pain and infertility in reproductive-aged women. The cyclical bleeding can cause scarring of the reproductive organs, which can lead to infertility.

Benign Changes of Uterus

Adenomyosis: Referring to glands and stroma within the uterine wall (Figure 17-25), it represents a downward growth of the endometrium into the myometrium. The importance of this lesion is twofold. First, these patients complain of pelvic pain, and second, glands within the wall of a patient with adenocarcinoma should not be confused with invasive cancer.

Pregnancy: Production of hCG by placental trophoblast causes the ovarian corpus luteum of pregnancy to continually produce progesterone. The result is a hypersecretory or gestational endometrial lining.

Infections: Acute endometritis is not a common condition, and almost always follows a normal pregnancy or miscarriage. Causative agents are bacterial. Chronic endometritis is diagnosed when plasma cells are present in the endometrial stroma. It may result from chronic PID, an intrauterine device, or retained products of conception after delivery.

> **CASE 17-10**
>
> A 32-year-old woman visits her gynecologist with the chief complaint of pain during menses (dysmenorrhea) and difficulty becoming pregnant. On laparoscopy, multiple brown, smudgy areas are noted on the exterior surface of the uterus and ovaries. Biopsies are taken, which are shown in Figure 17-24. What is your diagnosis? How does it relate to her infertility?

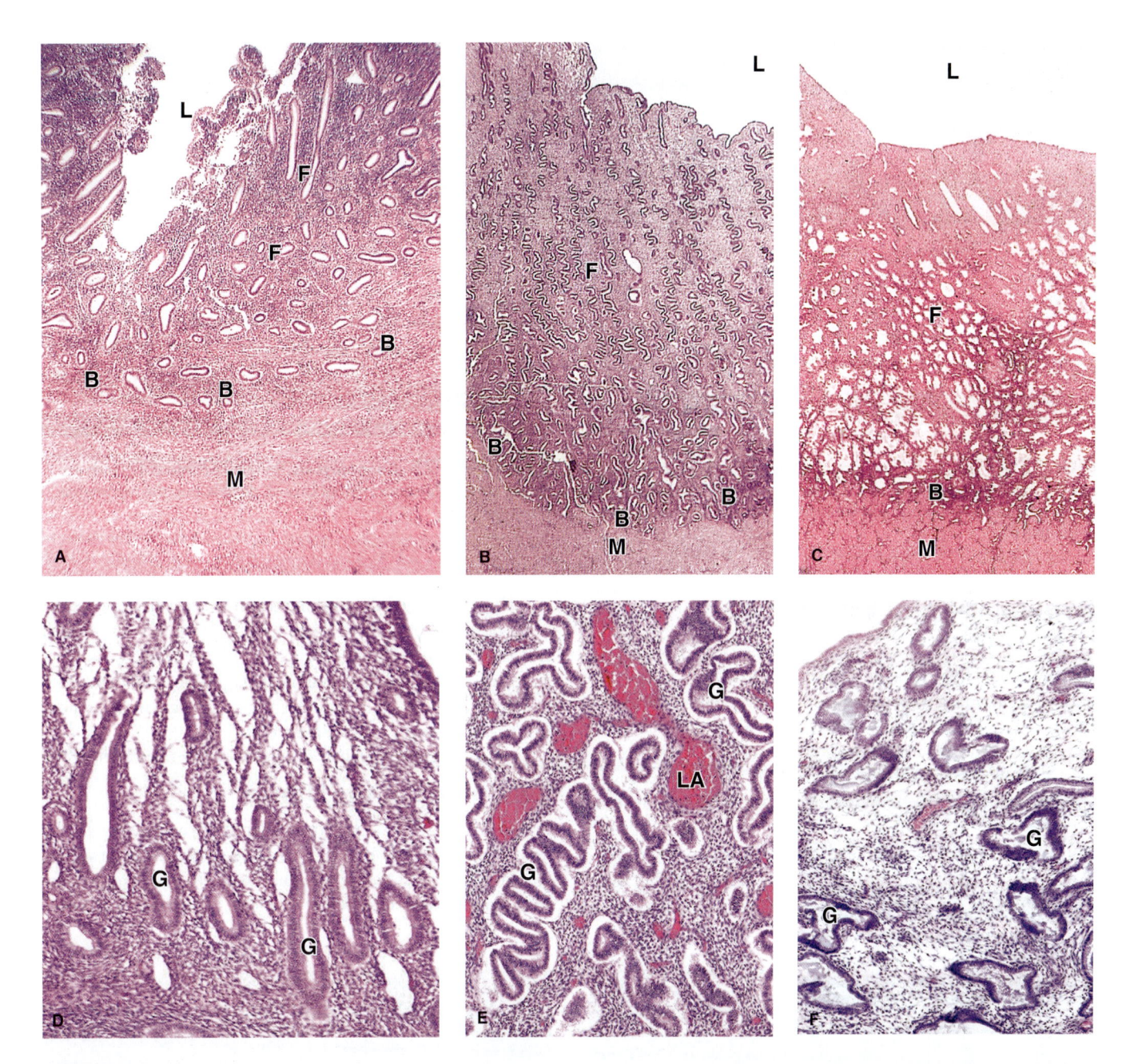

FIGURE 17-23 Proliferative, secretory, and premenstrual phases in the uterus. The major phases of the uterine cycle overlap, but produce distinctly different and characteristic changes in the functional layer (F) closest to the lumen (L) with little effect on the basal layer (B) and myometrium (M). Characteristic features of each phase include the following. During most of the proliferative phase (**A** and **D**) the functional layer is still relatively thin, the stroma is more cellular and the glands (G) are relatively straight, narrow, and empty. In the secretory phase (**B** and **E**) the functional layer is less heavily cellular and perhaps four times thicker than the basal layer. The tubular glands have wider lumens containing secretory product and coil tightly up through the stroma, giving a zigzag or folded appearance histologically. Superficially in the functional layer, lacunae (La) are widespread and filled with blood. The short premenstrual phase (**C** and **F**) begins with constriction of the spiral arteries, which produces hypoxia that causes swelling and dissolution of the glands (G). The stroma of the peripheral functionalis is more compact and that near the basal layer typically appears more sponge-like during this time of blood stasis, apoptosis, and breakdown of the stromal matrix. (**A**) ×20; (**B** and **C**) ×12; (**D**, **E**, and **F**) ×50. All H&E. (Modified from Mescher AL, Junqueira's Basic Histology Text and Atlas. 12th edn. McGraw Hill:New York, Figure 22-17.)

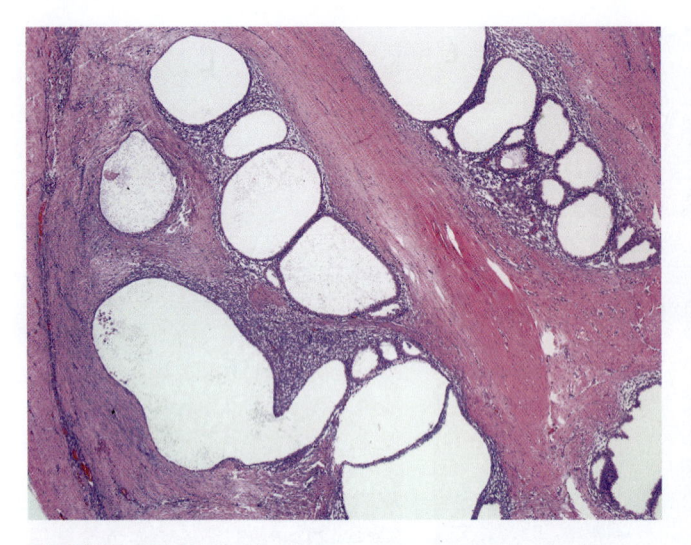

FIGURE 17-24 **Endometriosis.** This view shows deposits of benign endometrial-type glands associated with endometrial stroma, which may contain hemosiderin-laden macrophages, in a site outside of the uterus.

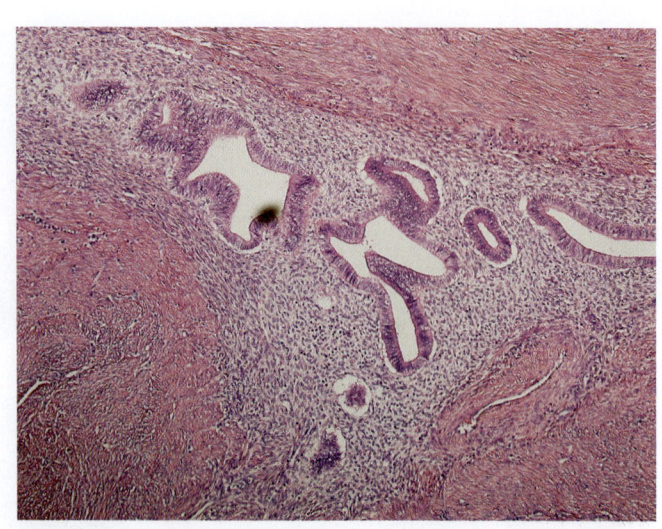

FIGURE 17-25 **Adenomyosis.** Benign endometrial glands are shown here within endometrial stroma, deep within the myometrial wall (H&E stain).

Hyperplasia and Carcinoma of the Uterus

Endometrial hyperplasia: Because estrogen causes the endometrial lining to proliferate in the first half of the menstrual cycle, an excess of estrogen can lead to unchecked growth of glands that can lead to an increased risk of cancer. A variety of conditions can lead an excess of estrogen stimulation, including anovulatory cycles (common around menopause), exogenous administration of estrogen, obesity (due to peripheral conversion of estrogen), or estrogen-producing ovarian conditions, like polycystic ovarian syndrome (PCOS).

Hyperplasia of the endometrium is classified by examining both the pattern of gland growth (simple vs. complex) and the cytologic features (atypical or not) of the cells. This gives rise to a four-tiered system that stratifies a patient's risk of cancer and can assist in determining clinical management (Figures 17-26 to 17-28; Table 17-3).

Carcinoma of the Uterus

Endometrial cancer is the most common malignancy of the female genital tract. Although all types of these cancers more commonly occur in postmenopausal women, there are two distinct groups that show different histologic features and prognosis.

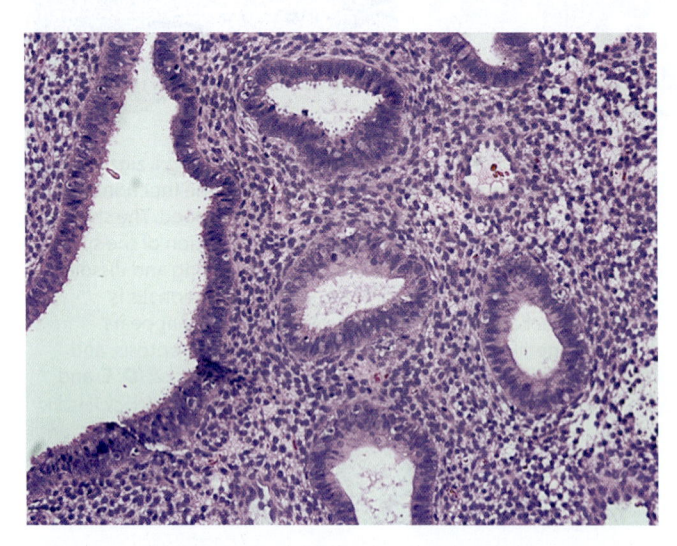

FIGURE 17-26 **Simple hyperplasia of the endometrium/ anovulatory pattern.** Generally, tubular proliferative phase endometrial glands are seen here showing ciliated cell (tubal) metaplasia and a cystically dilated gland (to the left) which suggests anovulation and which some pathologists may consider simple hyperplasia.

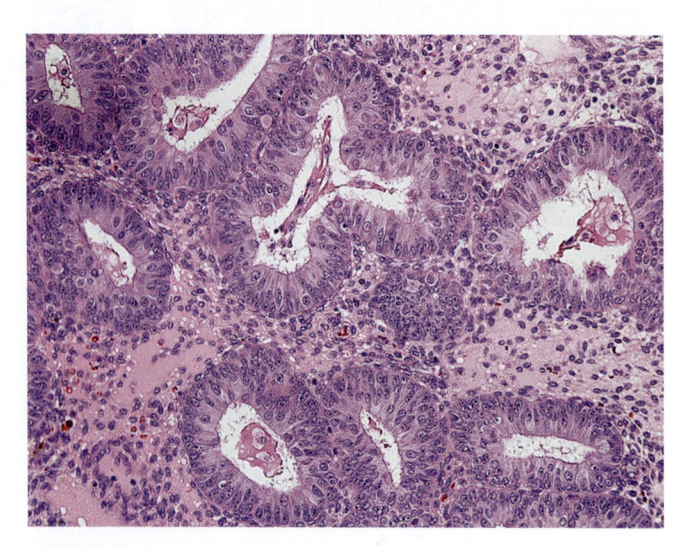

FIGURE 17-27 **Complex hyperplasia of the endometrium.** This slide shows crowded endometrial glands that show a somewhat thickened hyperplastic layer of endometrial epithelium with some nuclear enlargement and nuclear hyperchromasia, but no cytologic atypia.

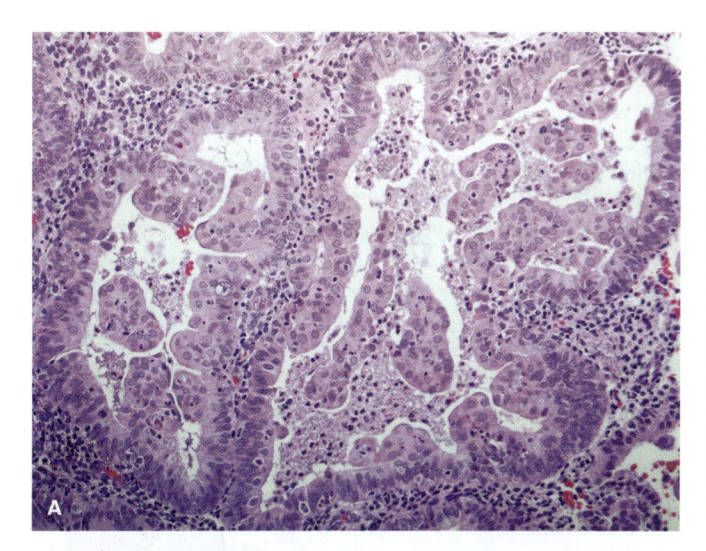

FIGURE 17-28 Complex atypical hyperplasia of the endometrium. (A) This image shows two crowded and complex endometrial glands showing atypical architectural features consisting of intraglandular papillary projections as well as cytologic atypia. Note there is still intervening stroma between the glands. **(B)** This focus shows an architecturally atypical endometrial gland with an intraglandular cribriform pattern.

Type I Endometrial Carcinoma

The most common types of endometrial carcinoma fit into this group, including those that follow endometrial hyperplasia, as discussed above. As in hyperplasia, the greatest risk factor is exposure to unopposed estrogen. Distinct from the other type of endometrial cancer, these tumors tend to share molecular alterations like mutations in *PTEN*, *PIK3CA*, *KRAS*, and occasionally, show microsatellite instability.

Grade 1 endometrioid adenocarcinoma (Figure 17-29) is characterized by back-to-back endometrial glands lined by cytologically malignant cells. Because the glands

TABLE 17-3 Common types of hyperplasia of the endometrium.

Type of Hyperplasia	Picture	Microscopic Findings	Association with Endometrial Cancer
Simple hyperplasia without atypia[a]		Cystically dilated glands with little architectural complexity Cell nuclei show no atypia	1% of patient progress to carcinoma
Complex hyperplasia without atypia		The number and size of glands increases, so glands appear crowded No cytologic atypia	3% of patients progress to carcinoma
Complex hyperplasia with atypia		The number and size of glands are increased, with marked glandular crowding and little remaining stroma Nuclei are irregularly shaped, with open chromatin and nucleoli	Statistics differ, anywhere from 25% to 48% progress to carcinoma

[a]Simple hyperplasia with atypia is not common, but does occur.

CASE 17-11

An obese 58-year-old woman with postmenopausal bleeding presents to her physician. An endometrial biopsy is performed (**Figure 17-29**). What is your diagnosis?

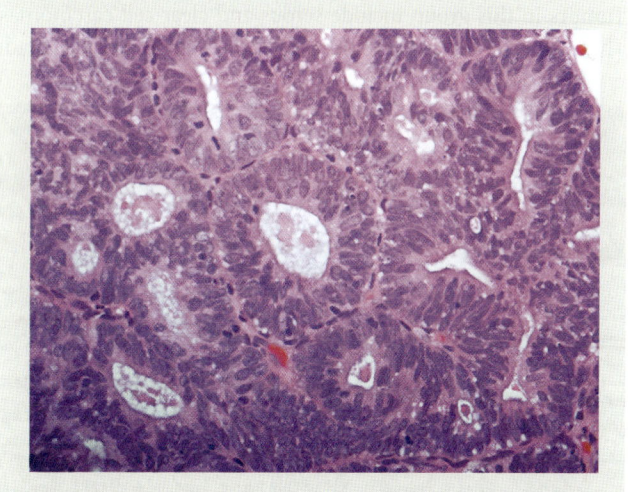

FIGURE 17-29 Endometrioid adenocarcinoma, well differentiated. This tumor shows atypical endometrial glands with a back-to-back glandular arrangement devoid of intervening endometrial stroma. The presence of glandular differentiation and absence of a solid pattern or tumor cells showing marked cytologic atypia makes this a well-differentiated tumor.

WHAT TO DO
Each endometrial adenocarcinoma is stained for estrogen and progesterone antibodies by the pathologist. Overexpression of these hormone receptors help predict whether the patient will benefit from treatment with progestins.

IN TRANSLATION
Two inherited genetic syndromes carry an increased risk of endometrial carcinoma. Hereditary nonpolyposis colon cancer syndrome is characterized by a defect in a DNA mismatch repair gene. Inactivation of these genes leads to carcinomas with microsatellite instability, most commonly of colon. The second most common tumor in these patients is endometrial carcinoma. Cowden syndrome is characterized by mutations in the PTEN gene, which normally acts as a tumor suppressor. This leads to an increased risk of carcinoma of the breast, thyroid, and endometrium.

resemble those of normal endometrium, they are called *endometrioid*. Other histologic patterns, including mucinous adenocarcinoma, are included in type I tumors. The gland architecture is preserved; hence, this is a Grade 1 tumor. Grade 2 tumors show some glands and some solid areas, while Grade 3 (Figure 17-30) tumors often show little resemblance to normal endometrial glands and have a significant solid architecture.

Type II Endometrial Carcinoma
Tumors in this group include serous and clear cell carcinomas. These tumors characteristically are of a high histologic grade

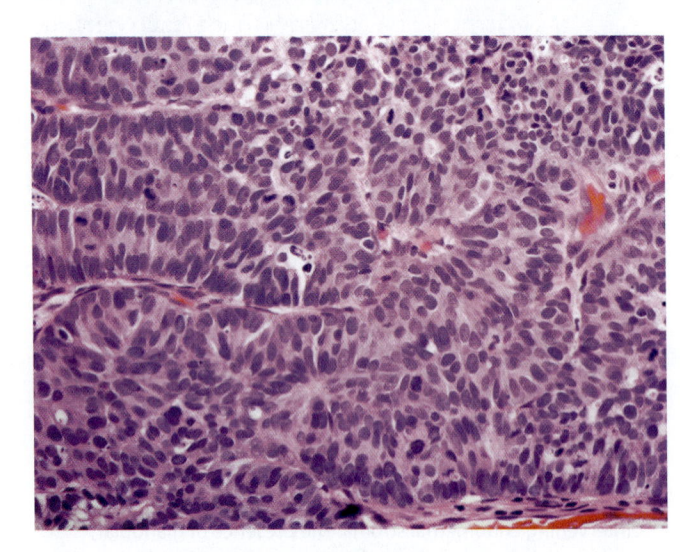

FIGURE 17-30 Endometrioid adenocarcinoma, poorly differentiated. This image shows tumor with back-to-back endometrial glands showing a significant solid pattern and high-grade nuclear atypia.

CASE 17-12
A 70-year-old woman presents to her gynecologist with postmenopausal bleeding. She has no significant past medical history. An endometrial biopsy is performed which shows a malignant epithelial proliferation that prompts a hysterectomy (Figure 17-31). Sections of the tumor with respect to the myometrium are shown below. What is your diagnosis? How does this affect the patient?

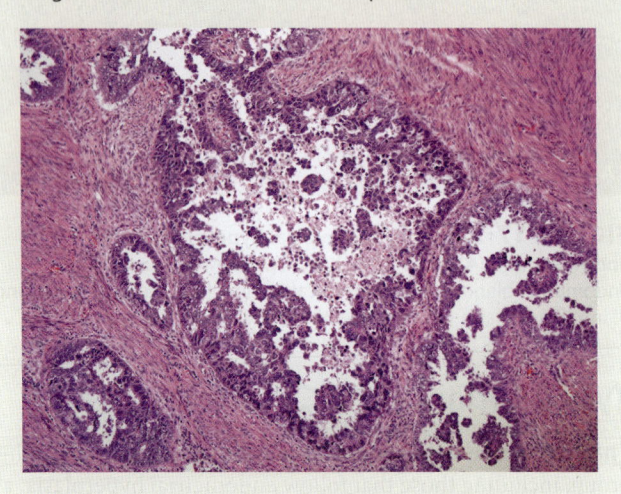

FIGURE 17-31 Serous carcinoma invading the myometrium. The tumor shows infiltrating glands with slit-like spaces, lined by atypical cells with high-grade cytologic atypia showing detached single cells and minute papillary cell clusters.

(Grade 3), commonly present at a more advanced stage, and have a worse prognosis. They tend to develop in women who are on average one decade older than type I tumors, and do not typically arise in a background of endometrial hyperplasia. In general, these cancers have mutations in the tumor suppressor gene *TP53*.

These sections in Figure 17-31 show the tumor infiltrating into the outer half of the wall of the uterus. The overtly malignant cells above are characteristic of serous carcinoma of the uterus, with papillary stalks lined by cells with enlarged and irregularly shaped nuclei, mitotic figures, and nucleoli. The dark purple calcified lamellar structures, psammoma bodies, are also characteristic findings.

Together with other information from the specimen, this influences the stage of the tumor. The percentage of invasion into the myometrium (greater than or less than one half of the myometrial wall) is an important prognostic factor for type I and II endometrial cancers.

Another member of the type II endometrial cancer is malignant mixed Mullerian tumor, also called carcinosarcoma. It is notable for showing both malignant carcinomatous and sarcomatous components. These tumors most commonly arise via progressive malignant transformation of the epithelial component, although a minority may arise from adenosarcomas where the benign glandular component then becomes malignant. They also characteristically harbor mutations in the *TP53* gene and have a poor prognosis.

THE FEMALE REPRODUCTIVE TRACT

CASE 17-13

A 43-year-old woman who has no significant past medical history presents to her gynecologist complaining of menorrhagia and dysmenorrhea. An ultrasound shows a 3 cm submucosal mass within the wall of the uterus. As the patient no longer desires fertility, a hysterectomy is performed. Sections of the mass are shown below (**Figure 17-32**). What is your diagnosis? How does this relate to her symptoms?

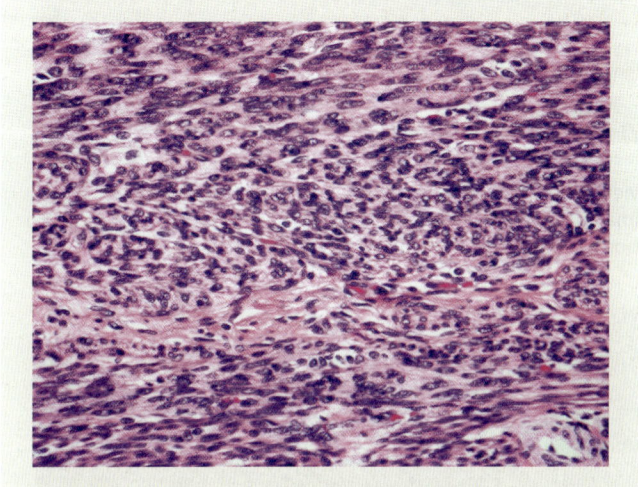

FIGURE 17-32 **Uterine leiomyoma.** Benign appearing spindled smooth muscle cells form intersecting fascicles.

HUNTING FOR ZEBRAS

Intravenous leiomyomatosis is a rare condition in which benign smooth muscle, either from a preexisting leiomyoma or from the surrounding vein, grows into veins of the uterus and pelvic region. Although this would normally be interpreted as malignant behavior, these tumors do not metastasize, although they may spread to distant sites via embolization. Grossly they resemble "worm-like" plugs, and treatment consists of hysterectomy and removal of the intravenous tumor (**Figure 17-33**).

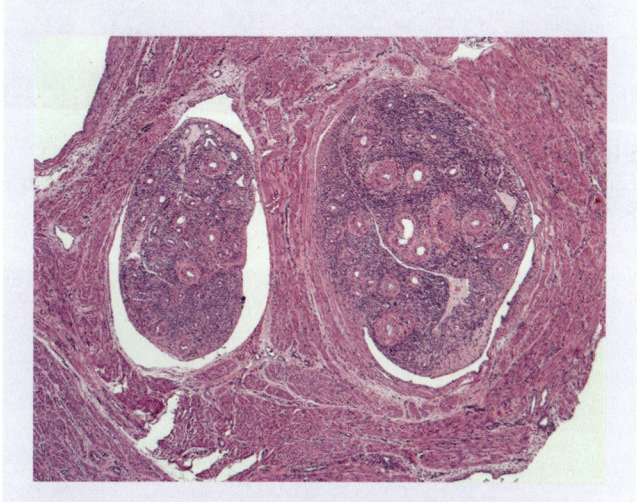

FIGURE 17-33 **Intravenous leiomyomatosis (IVL).** Within this myometrial vessel is a plug of benign appearing smooth muscle, representing intravenous extension from an adjacent uterine leiomyoma.

Mesenchymal (Stromal) Lesions of the Uterus

Smooth Muscle Tumors of Uterus

Leiomyomas (Figure 17-32) are common benign tumors derived from the smooth muscle in the uterine wall. Grossly, they are sharply circumscribed masses with firm, white, whorled cut surfaces. Histologically they show intersecting fascicles of smooth muscle with bland, spindle-shaped nuclei and no tumor cell necrosis. Mitotic figures are rare. Commonly referred to as fibroids, these lesions can cause pain and heavy flow during the menstrual cycle.

Leiomyosarcoma is a malignant tumor that arises from smooth muscle. Although these tumors are rare when compared to carcinoma of the endometrium, they are notable for their dismal prognosis. They are distinct tumors from their benign counterparts, and do not arise from leiomyomas. Their typical presentation is of a large, solitary mass that either protrudes into the endometrial cavity or invades the uterine wall. Large areas of necrosis are common. Histologic sections show markedly atypical cells, increased mitotic activity, and tumor necrosis (**Figure 17-34**).

Endometrial Stromal Tumors

The endometrial stroma may undergo malignant transformation giving rise to endometrial stromal tumors and endometrial stromal sarcomas, the latter of which is defined by the presence of stromal invasion. These tumors are composed of a solid proliferation of atypical cells that morphologically resemble endometrial stroma but form a mass. Formerly termed "endolymphatic stromal myosis," endometrial stromal sarcomas often spread to myometrial vessels. These tumors are characteristically estrogen receptor and progesterone receptor positive (**Figure 17-35**).

FALLOPIAN TUBES

- **Inflammation:** The most common abnormality of the fallopian tubes is acute salpingitis (**Figure 17-36**). This is most likely due to ascending infection from a lower genital tract infection. *N. gonorrhoeae*, *Escherichia coli*, and *Chlamydia* are commonly involved, though most infections are polymicrobial.
- **Ectopic Pregnancy:** Defined as implantation that develops outside the endometrium, over 95% occur in the fallopian tube. See the Case Study in the Introduction for further information.
- **Neoplasms:** The most common neoplasm of the fallopian tube is a metastatic focus from another site. Primary malignancies are uncommon. Benign lesions include adenomatoid

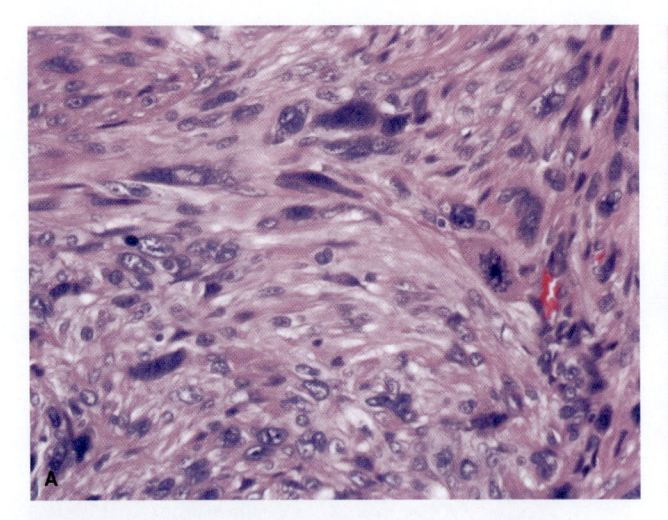

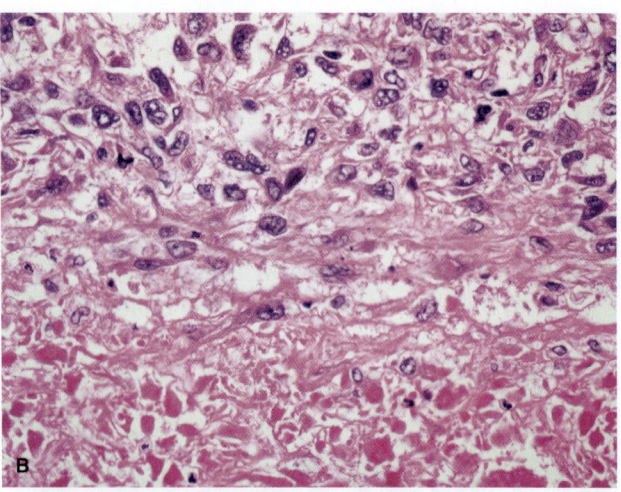

FIGURE 17-34 **Leiomyosarcoma. (A)** Malignant tumor composed of smooth muscle cells showing significant (moderate to severe) cytologic atypia and increased mitotic activity (high-power view). **(B)** Coagulative tumor cell necrosis (present in lower half of image) is present within this leiomyosarcoma, which shows a sharp border with the viable tumor (present at top of image).

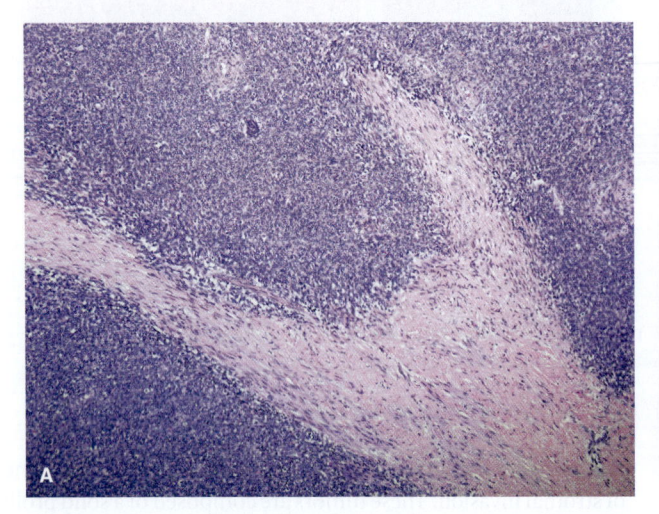

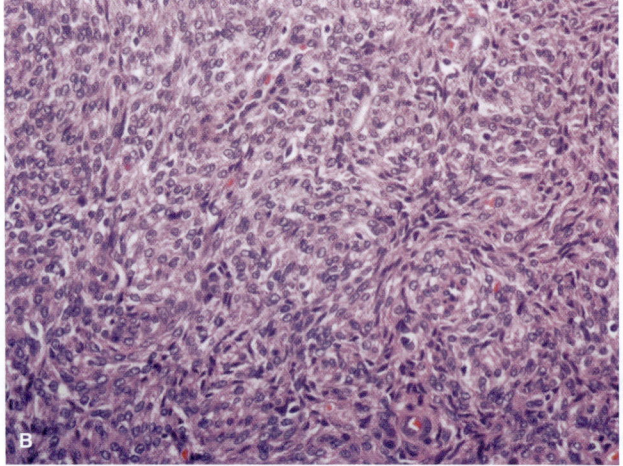

FIGURE 17-35 **Endometrial stromal sarcoma.** Infiltrating solid nests of spindle cells resembling endometrial stroma are seen here at low- **(A)** and high-power view **(B)**.

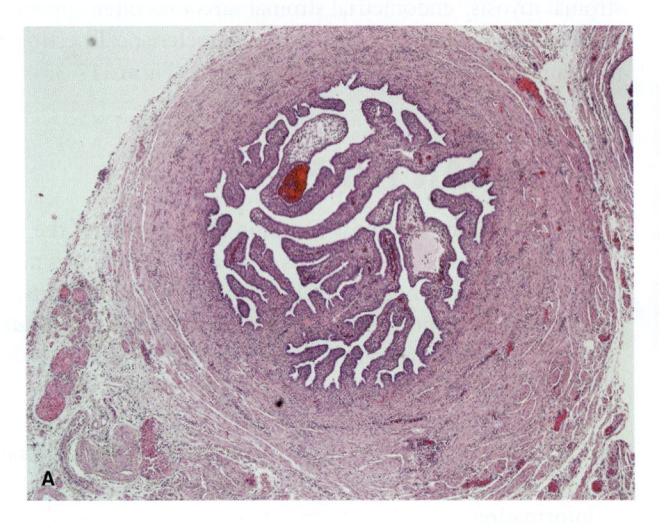

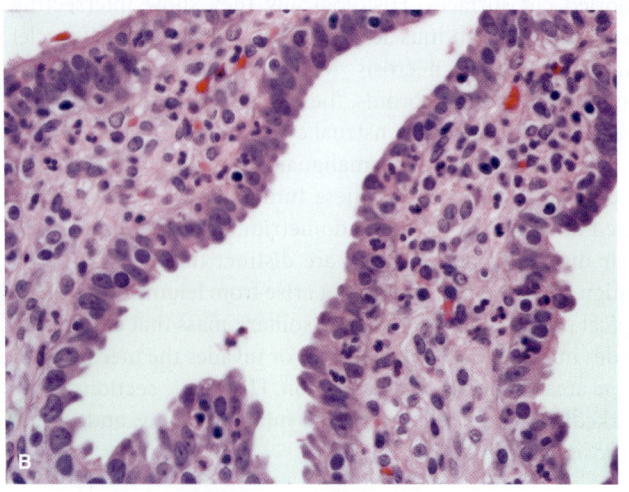

FIGURE 17-36 **Acute salpingitis. (A)** At low-power view, a cross-section of fallopian tube showing increased stromal cellularity is noted. **(B)** At high-power view, the increased cellularity in the fallopian tube fimbria is noted to be due to an infiltration of neutrophils and occasional lymphocytes within the tubal epithelium and in underlying stroma (H&E stain).

tumors, which resemble mesothelioma, and resemble their counterparts in the testis. Primary malignant tumors of the tube may be of serous or endometrioid subtypes. Recently, there has also been evidence that some ovarian cancers may originate from the fallopian tube (discussed below).

OVARY

Nonneoplastic Lesions of the Ovary

Several benign cystic lesions may present clinically, which are a consequence of normal ovulation. Follicular and luteal cysts represent the site of prior ovulation that has since sealed off. They are common near the surface of the ovary. They are normally small, but can become enlarged up to 5 cm and may clinically present with pelvic pain.

PCOS (previously known as Stein–Leventhal syndrome) is characterized clinically by infertility, obesity, and hirsutism. It is a common cause of infertility in reproductive-aged women. The ovaries in these patients are enlarged, often doubled in size, and show multiple follicular cysts within the ovarian cortex (Figure 17-37). Symptoms arise from an excess of androgen and LH and a paucity of follicle-stimulating

CASE 17-14

A 28-year-old woman presents to her physician with the chief complaint of difficulty in becoming pregnant. Physical exam shows an obese female with hirsutism. Ultrasound of the ovaries shows multiple cysts just beneath the surface of the ovary bilaterally. A representative section of an ovary from a patient with the same condition is shown below (Figure 17-37).
What is your diagnosis?

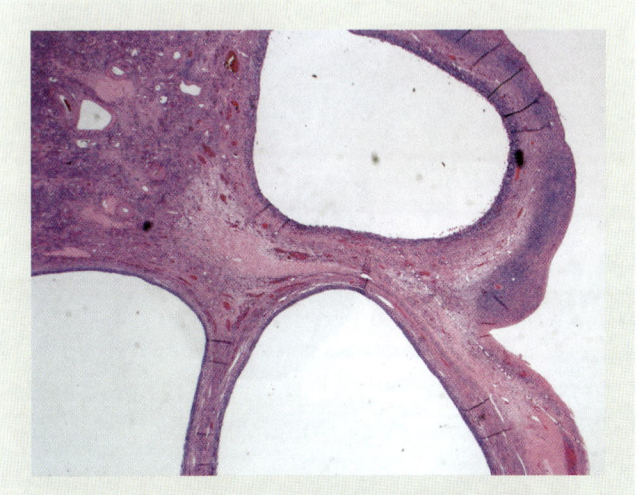

FIGURE 17-37 Polycystic ovarian syndrome (PCOS). This ovary at low-power view shows multiple, enlarged follicular cysts in the ovarian cortex, associated with cortical fibrosis. Numerous corpus albicans (not seen in this view) are often seen, which represent follicular cysts that have involuted.

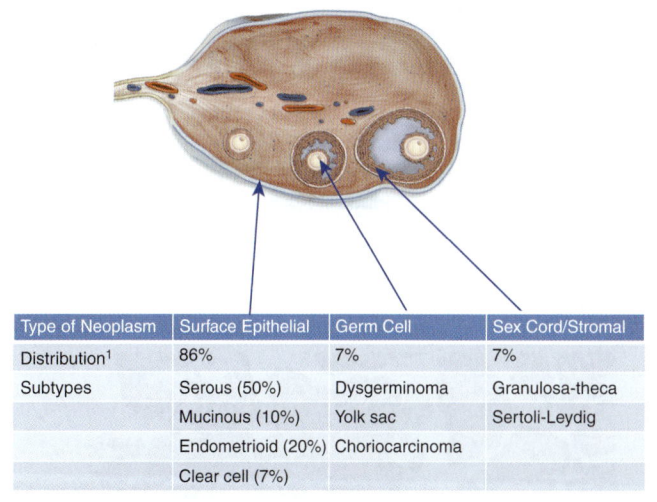

Type of Neoplasm	Surface Epithelial	Germ Cell	Sex Cord/Stromal
Distribution[1]	86%	7%	7%
Subtypes	Serous (50%)	Dysgerminoma	Granulosa-theca
	Mucinous (10%)	Yolk sac	Sertoli-Leydig
	Endometrioid (20%)	Choriocarcinoma	
	Clear cell (7%)		

[1]% of primary ovarian neoplasms (approximate)
[2]% of epithelial ovarian neoplasms (approximate)

FIGURE 17-38 Cellular origin of ovarian tumors. Data on frequency are approximate. (Modified from Mescher AL, Junqueira's Basic Histology Text and Atlas. 12th edn. McGraw Hill Lange New York, Figure 22-11 (inset B).)

hormone secretion by the ovaries. Women with PCOS are at an increased risk of endometrial hyperplasia and malignancy.

Tumors of the Ovary

Although ovarian cancer is not the most common malignancy of the female genital tract, it is the most lethal. Because these tumors can arise from multiple cell types (the ovarian surface epithelium, germ cells, or the gonadal stroma), ovarian tumors are also very diverse in appearance, presentation, and behavior. An overview of the origin of different ovarian tumors is shown below, and each respective tumor is discussed in the appropriate section (Figure 17-38).

Epithelial Tumors

The so-called "surface epithelial tumors" of the ovary are the most common subtype by far. Their origin is the subject of ongoing research, with two competing theories. One suggests that they are derived from the cells that line the surface of the ovary, while others maintain they result from small pieces of fallopian tube that are implanted on the surface of the ovary. Regardless of their origin, this category of tumor accounts for most of the deaths caused by ovarian cancer.

Figure 17-39 demonstrates a serous tumor of low malignant potential (serous borderline tumor), with papillary structures lined by cuboidal to columnar cells with generally mild atypia. Ovarian surface epithelial tumors are classified first by the cell type, with serous and mucinous being the most common, and second by architectural complexity and cytologic atypia. Lesions that have only one cell layer, no papillary areas, and no cytologic atypia are cystadenomas, while those with some architectural complexity and generally mild cytologic atypia represent tumors of low malignant potential. Regardless

CASE 17-15

A 45-year-old woman undergoes abdominal imaging after being involved in a motor vehicle accident. It shows a unilateral ovarian mass that measures 15 cm. It is removed and sent to pathology. Gross exam shows a multiloculated tumor with a smooth, glistening external surface. Representative sections all resemble those below (Figure 17-39). What is your diagnosis?

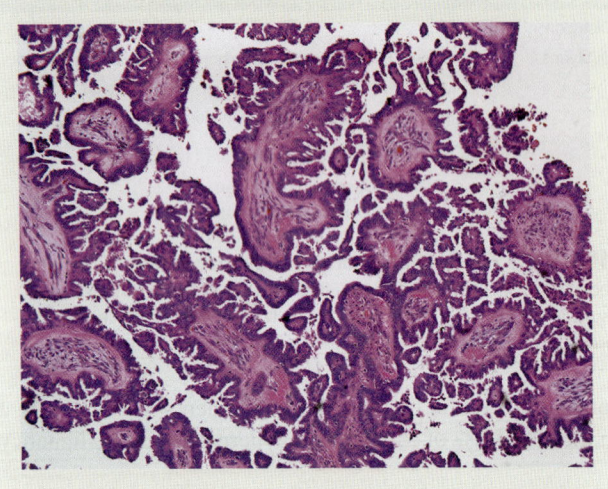

FIGURE 17-39 Serous tumor of low malignant potential (LMP) of the ovary. Papillary projections that are progressively branching with terminally located detached papillary clusters lined by serous (tubal type) epithelium with low-grade nuclear atypia are present. Psammoma bodies may be associated with these tumors (not demonstrated in this field).

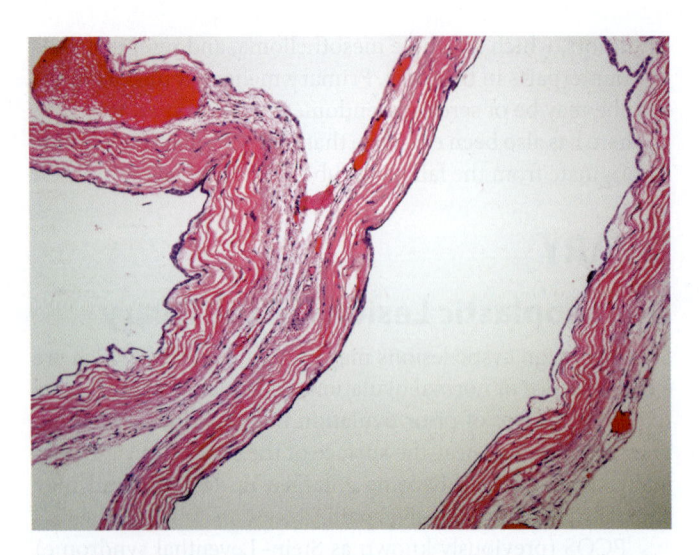

FIGURE 17-40 Ovarian serous cystadenoma. A section of the cyst wall showing a single, simple layer of benign serous epithelium (atrophic appearing in this section).

of architectural features, tumors with marked cytological atypia are classified as carcinoma. The spectrum of serous neoplasms of the ovary includes serous cystadenoma (Figure 17-40) and serous carcinoma (Figure 17-41).

For further characterization and list of other surface epithelial tumors, see Table 17-4.

Germ Cell Tumors

Case 17-6 shows structures not normally found in the ovary, like skin and sweat glands, making this a mature cystic teratoma (dermoid tumor). These tumors originate from pluripotent germ cells present in the ovary, and can form structures from

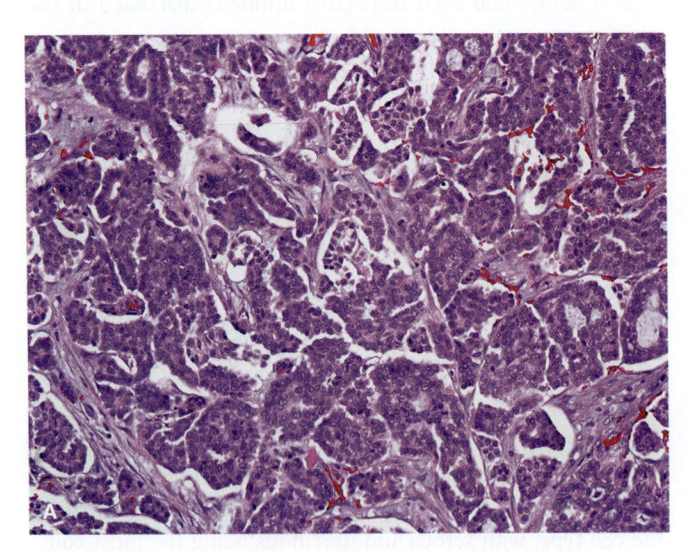

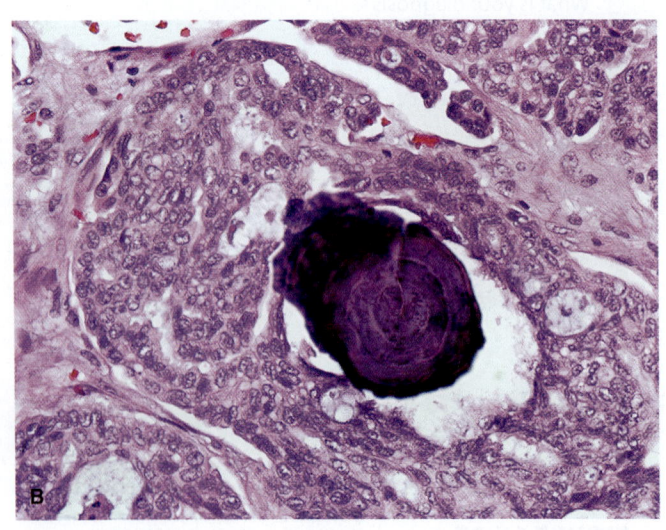

FIGURE 17-41 Papillary serous carcinoma of the ovary. **(A)** Tumor forming papillary formations, some of which show fibrovascular cores, as well as slit-like spaces, and some solid areas, invading the ovarian stroma (low-power view). **(B)** At high-power view, the tumor here shows significant cytologic atypia and a psammoma body (focus of dystrophic calcification forming concentric rings).

TABLE 17-4 Surface epithelial neoplasms.

Tumor Lining	Tumor Type	Histology	Age at Presentation	Molecular Alterations	General Facts
Serous	Cystadenoma	Single layer of tall columnar epithelium	20–45	–	Serous tumors bilateral 25%
	LMP	Papillary structures with little to no cytologic atypia	20–45	Mutations in *KRAS* and *BRAF*	Most common ovarian neoplasm
	Carcinoma	Overtly atypical cells, usually arranged in papillary groups	45–65	Vast majority harbor mutations in *TP53* gene	Carcinoma accounts for 30% of serous tumors
Mucinous[a]	Cystadenoma is most common (80%), LMP and carcinoma (10% each)	Lining of mucinous cells that most commonly resemble the endocervix, carcinoma shows atypia and/or invasion into stroma	Mean = 50	*KRAS* mutations	Bilateral less frequently (5% in benign, 20% in carcinoma)
					Less likely to be malignant (carcinoma = 15%)
Brenner tumor[a]	Most common is benign form	Nests of transitional-type epithelium (like urothelium) encased in a fibrous stroma	All ages	–	May coexist within the wall of a mucinous tumor
Endometrioid[a]	Most common is carcinoma	Tubular glands that resemble those of the endometrium, may be well differentiated or high grade	55–58 years (Carcinoma)	Mutations in *PTEN* tumor suppressor gene, *KRAS*, and *Beta-Catenin*, microsatellite instability	15–20% coexist with endometriosis (probable origin)
					40% bilateral, may have concurrent tumor of endometrium
Clear cell[a]	Most common is carcinoma	Large cells with abundant clear cytoplasm and bizarrely shaped nuclei	Mean = 50–53	Limited studies, however, overexpression of HNF1-β noted	Also frequently coexists with endometriosis

LMP = low malignant potential, also known as "borderline tumor."
[a] These tumors can also be present in all three tumor types (cystadenoma, LMP, and carcinoma, but are abbreviated for simplicity).

CASE 17-16

A 20-year-old woman presents to her physician with pelvic pain. A physical exam reveals a palpable left adnexal mass, which on abdominal imaging measures 7 cm and reveals multiple cysts with calcification (Figure 17-42) What is your diagnosis? What is the prognosis?

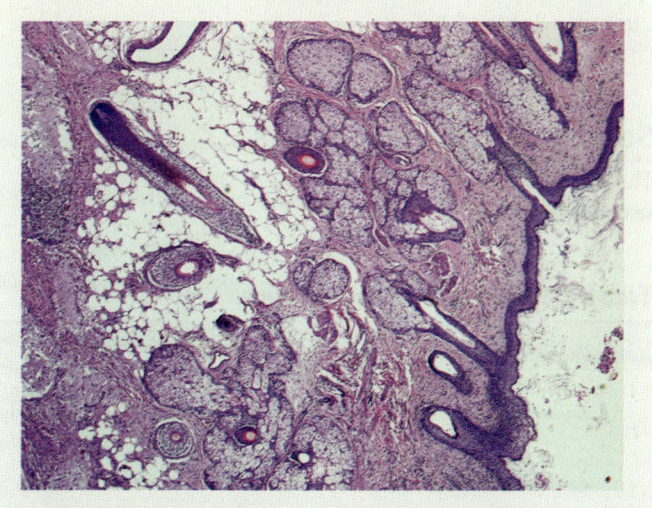

FIGURE 17-42 Mature cystic teratoma of the ovary.
A section of the cyst wall of this ovarian teratoma shows skin, sebaceous glands, hair follicles, and mature adipose tissue. Grossly hair is often noted.

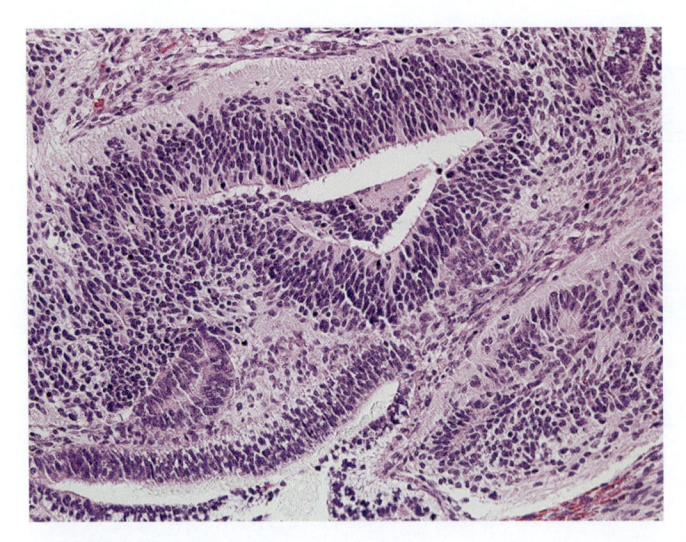

FIGURE 17-43 **Immature teratoma.** Note the neuroectodermal tubules and surrounding immature mesenchyme.

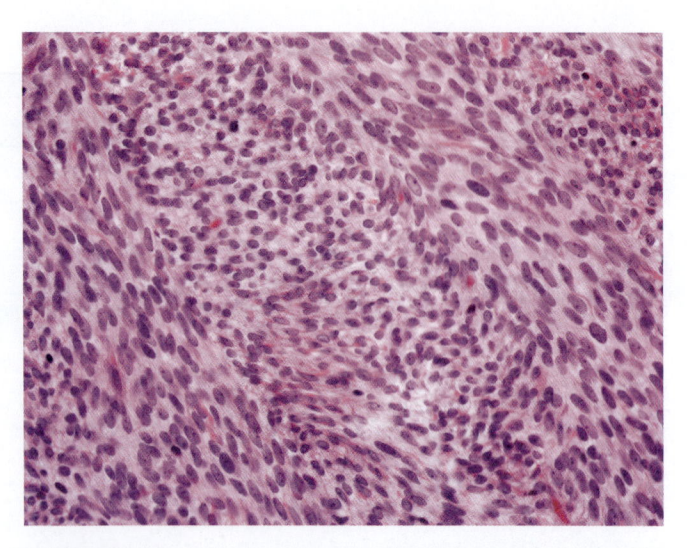

FIGURE 17-44 **Ovarian fibroma.** This section shows bland spindle cells forming fascicles with no cytologic atypia or increased mitotic activity.

all three germ layers. It is not uncommon to see teeth (which accounts for the calcification seen on imaging), respiratory epithelium, and even neural tissue. A unique type of teratoma composed of only thyroid tissue is known as struma ovarii.

The prognosis for this patient is excellent. Mature teratomas only rarely harbor a high-grade malignancy, and the most common type to arise here is squamous cell carcinoma. Immature teratomas are usually larger masses with mostly solid areas. They are characterized by the presence of immature embryonic tissue, such as neuroectodermal tubules and immature mesenchyme (Figure 17-43). The prognosis for these patients is not as favorable.

> **QUICK REVIEW**
>
> A summary of the remaining germ cell tumors can be found in Table 17-5.

Sex Cord/Stromal Tumors

The least common ovarian tumors arise from the supporting sex cord (gonadal) stroma.

Fibroma/Thecoma: These lesions either show spindled cells resembling fibroblasts (fibroma; Figure 17-44) or plump, lipid-filled cells (thecoma). The pure fibroma is the most common tumor, but a mixture of the two elements is not uncommon, which is termed a fibrothecoma. When present as a pure fibroma, these tumors are hormonally inactive, however, some secrete estrogens. For unknown reasons, some of these tumors present as bilateral ovarian tumors with ascites and right-sided hydrothorax, a condition known as Meigs syndrome.

Sertoli–Leydig cell tumor: Because these tumors differentiate toward male structures, it is not uncommon for them to produce masculinization. A minority, however, have estrogenic effects. Microscopically, well-differentiated tumors show tubules composed of Sertoli cells and interspersed Leydig cells in the stroma, while less differentiated tumors have these elements present in less recognizable forms (Figure 17-45).

Granulosa Cell Tumor: This tumor is notable for being the most common malignant member of this group. More common in postmenopausal women, secretion of estrogens by these neoplasms is not uncommon. Inhibin levels in the blood are frequently elevated. For further information, see the introduction case at the start of the chapter (Figure 17-1).

TABLE 17-5 Germ cell neoplasms.

Tumor Type	Photo	Microscopic Features	Clinical Characteristics
Dysgerminoma		Counterpart of seminoma of the testicle, shows polygonal cells, clear cytoplasm, centrally placed nuclei, and surrounding chronic inflammation	Low-stage tumors (do not extend beyond the ovary) have excellent prognosis, all tumors respond well to chemotherapy
Endodermal sinus (yolk sac) tumor		Glomerulus-like structures called Schiller–Duval bodies (see picture, left) with a blood vessel lined by papillae protruding into a space lined by tumor cells	Elevated levels of α-fetoprotein in blood, respond well to chemotherapy
Choriocarcinoma		Mostly these occur as part of a germ cell tumor of the ovary, pure choriocarcinoma is rare. Show cells present in placental villi (cytotrophoblasts and syncytiotrophoblasts)	Elevated levels of human chorionic gonadotropin, present in prepubertal girls (after this, metastasis from intrauterine site or origin in an ovarian primary must be excluded)

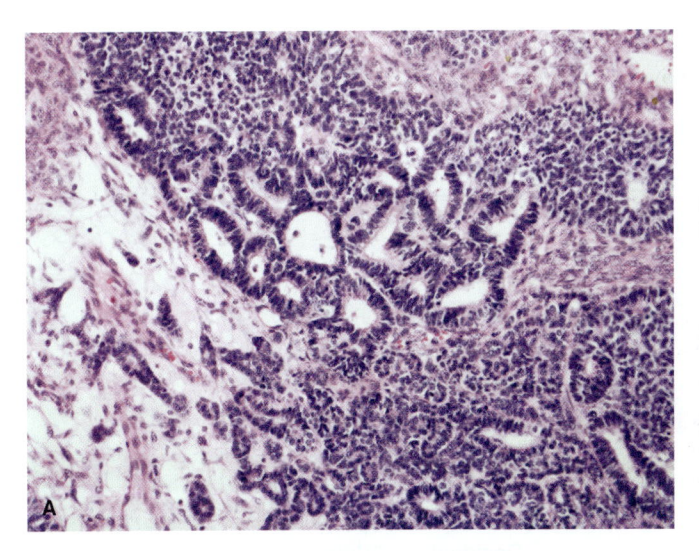

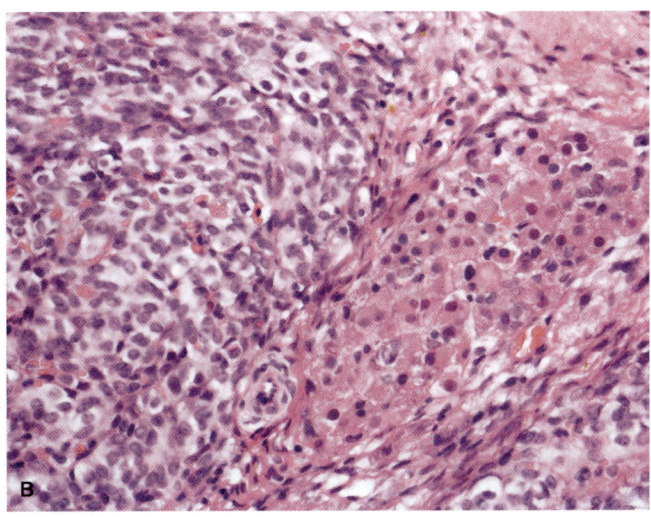

FIGURE 17-45 Sertoli–Leydig cell tumor. (A) Area showing the Sertoli cell tumor component forming sertoliform tubules merging with solid areas of tumor. **(B)** High-power view of the poorly differentiated, solid Sertoli cell tumor component (on the left) and the Leydig cell component showing prominent eosinophilic cytoplasm (on the right); the Leydig cell component is often sparse.

Yolk Sac Tumor: These tumors arise from primitive gonadal stroma that resembles the embryologic yolk sac. They express α-fetoprotein, which can be detected as elevated serum levels in the blood, or detected immunohistochemically within sections of the tumor **(Figure 17-46)**. This tumor can have many patterns. Although more common in the younger patient, it may occur in older women as well.

Metastatic Tumors to the Ovary

Strictly speaking, the most common metastatic tumor to the ovaries originates from within the lower genital tract (uterus, fallopian tubes, cervix, or contralateral ovary). Metastasis from an extra-Mullerian site should be suspected when ovarian tumors are bilateral, or the implants of tumor are present only on the ovarian surface. The most common offenders are carcinomas of the breast and gastrointestinal tract (stomach, intestine, and pancreas).

The much-discussed Krukenberg tumor represents bilateral metastases to the ovaries of a signet-ring cell adenocarcinoma, most commonly of gastric origin.

PLACENTAL AND GESTATIONAL DISEASE

Development and Anatomy: The placenta exchanges gas and nutrients from maternal to fetal circulation through specialized structures of fetal origin called chorionic villi. These provide a large surface area where the maternal blood can surround the villi in the intervillous spaces, communicating with the fetal blood, which is present within the villi. A schematic diagram is pictured in **Figure 17-47**.

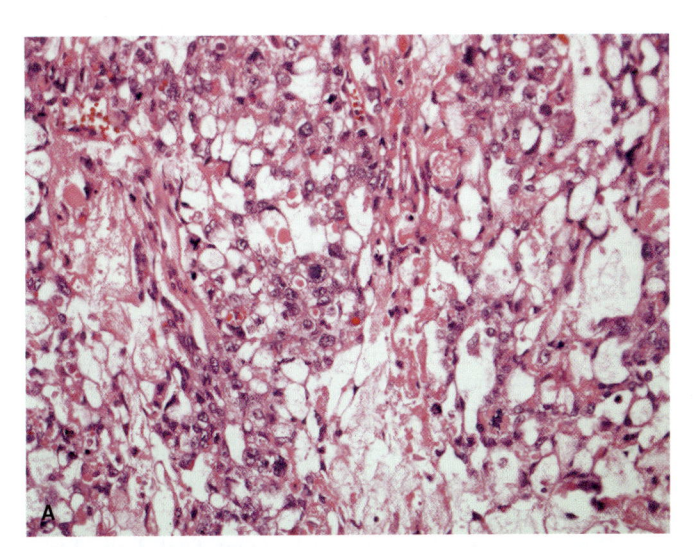

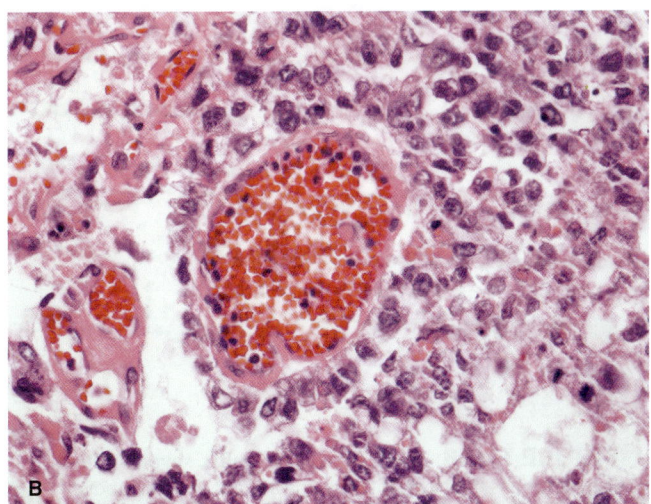

FIGURE 17-46 Yolk sac tumor of the ovary. (A) Solid sheets of tumor cells showing vacuolization, eosinophilic hyaline globules (low-power view) and **(B)** Schiller–Duval bodies (perivascular bodies), structures resembling the rat endodermal sinus (high-power view).

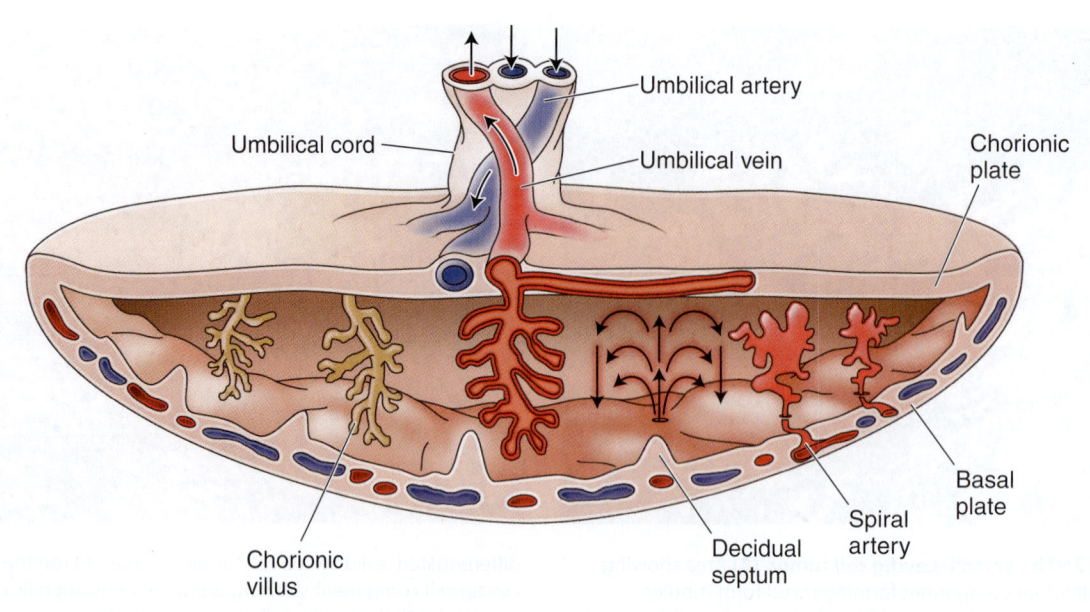

FIGURE 17-47 **Drawing of a section through a full-term placenta.** Maternal blood flows into the intervillous spaces in funnel-shaped spurts. Exchange occurs with fetal blood as maternal blood flows around the villi. Inflowing arterial blood pushes venous blood into the endometrial veins, which are scattered over the entire surface of the decidua basalis. Note also that the umbilical arteries carry deoxygenated fetal blood to the placenta and that the umbilical vein carries oxygenated blood to the fetus. Placental lobes are separated from each other by the placental (decidual) septa. (Cunningham F. et al. 2010. Williams Obstetrics, 23rd edn. McGraw Hill Medical New York, Figure 3-24.)

CASE 17-17

A 21-year-old woman presents to the emergency department in labor at 36 weeks gestation. Her membranes ruptured the day prior to arrival. Over the next few hours, she delivers and her placenta is sent to pathology. Gross examination shows "cloudy" placental membranes. Sections of the amnionic membranes are shown in **Figure 17-48**. What is your diagnosis? How does it relate to this patient's presentation? What are the most common causes?

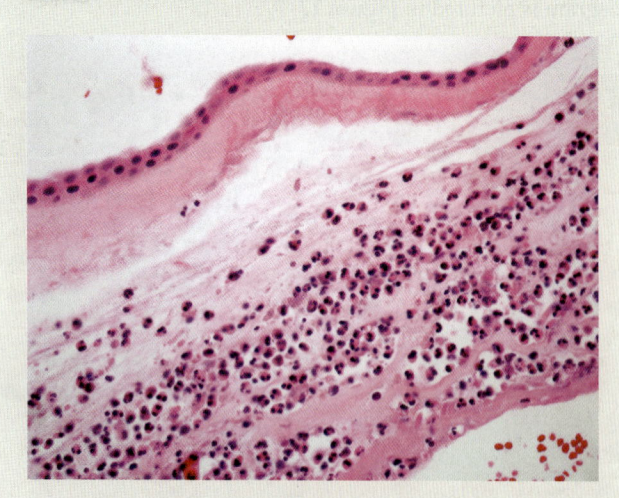

FIGURE 17-48 **Acute chorioamnionitis, severe.** Note the numerous neutrophils within the amnion, located above the chorionic plate (H&E stain).

Infections

Figure 17-48 show dense, acute inflammation of the placental membranes, both at the fetal surface (amnion) and maternal surface (chorion). Chorioamnionitis is a condition that results due to infection in the placenta. Most commonly, these infections arrive via the ascending route, passing upward through the vagina, or less commonly, through spread from the bloodstream of the mother.

Most of the common infectious etiologies for placental infections arising via the ascending route are normal components of vaginal flora. Offenders include: group B *Streptococcus sp.*, *E. coli*, *Enterococcus*, *Staphylococcus*, *Bacteroides*, and *Mycoplasma hominis*. Infections may also be caused by Candida species. Hematogenous infectious agents have been given the moniker "TORCH" (Toxoplasma, Others, Rubella, Cytomegalovirus, and Herpes simplex), and typically cause more severe inflammation around the chorionic villi and may also cause developmental fetal damage as a result of infection.

Preeclampsia/Eclampsia

Preeclampsia is a condition that occurs during pregnancy characterized by the clinical symptoms of hypertension, proteinuria, and edema. It is a relatively common condition, occurring in approximately 5% of pregnancies, and is more common in primigravidas. Eclampsia develops in those who have seizures. The etiology of preeclampsia is still unclear, but it is evident that the placenta plays a key role, as the symptoms resolve soon after delivery.

During normal placental development, fetal-derived trophoblasts invade the maternal arteries of the uterus and form hybrid vessels. In preeclampsia, this process is underdeveloped, and can lead to ischemia of the placenta late in gestation. Additional systemic coagulation abnormalities are likely caused by factors secreted into maternal circulation by the placenta, although this is still under investigation.

The placenta may show various signs of ischemia in preeclampsia including infarcts, which are evident by the presence of dead villi. The villi can be abnormally mature in response to decreased oxygen, and will be decreased in size and have an increase in blood vessels. Vasculitic changes in this setting, termed acute atherosis, are manifested as fibrinoid necrosis of the vessel's wall with accumulation of lipid-laden macrophages.

Placental Attachment Disorders

Improperly attached placentas can compromise the well-being of the infant. Placenta previa occurs when implantation is too low, as in the lower uterine segment or cervix, and can cause severe third trimester bleeding. If the implantation is directly into the myometrium and has little or no intervening maternal decidua, the result is placenta accreta. Following delivery, the placenta may not detach normally, and this placenta accreta can cause significant postpartum bleeding.

Multiple Gestations

Twin gestations are the result of the fertilization of two eggs (dizygotic) or the division of one egg after fertilization (monozygotic). This results in different divisions of the chorion and amnion. Specifically, the presence of only one chorion implies a monozygotic gestation. This is an important distinction, as a condition called twin–twin transfusion system can only occur in a monochorionic twin gestation. A vascular anastomosis connects the circulation of the twins, shunting blood disproportionately to one twin. This can result in the death of potentially both fetuses (Figure 17-49).

Gestational Trophoblastic Disease

Gestational trophoblastic disease is a spectrum of diseases from relatively benign to highly malignant. A unifying characteristic of these lesions is production of hCG, though the amounts differ.

Hydatidiform moles are abnormal proliferations of trophoblastic tissue, and are divided into complete and partial subtypes (Figures 17-50 and 17-51, respectively). Distinction between the various types is very important, as each carries a different risk of subsequent malignancy. Contrast the abnormal placental villi in molar gestations with that from a normal placenta (Figure 17-52). In cases that lack defining characteristics, staining for the p57 protein can be helpful. Because it is paternally imprinted, it is only expressed in maternal tissues. See Table 17-6 for details.

The multinucleated cells above are syncytiotrophoblasts, while the single cells are cytotrophoblasts. Together, they are characteristic of choriocarcinoma, a malignant neoplasm derived from the trophoblasts of the placenta. It most

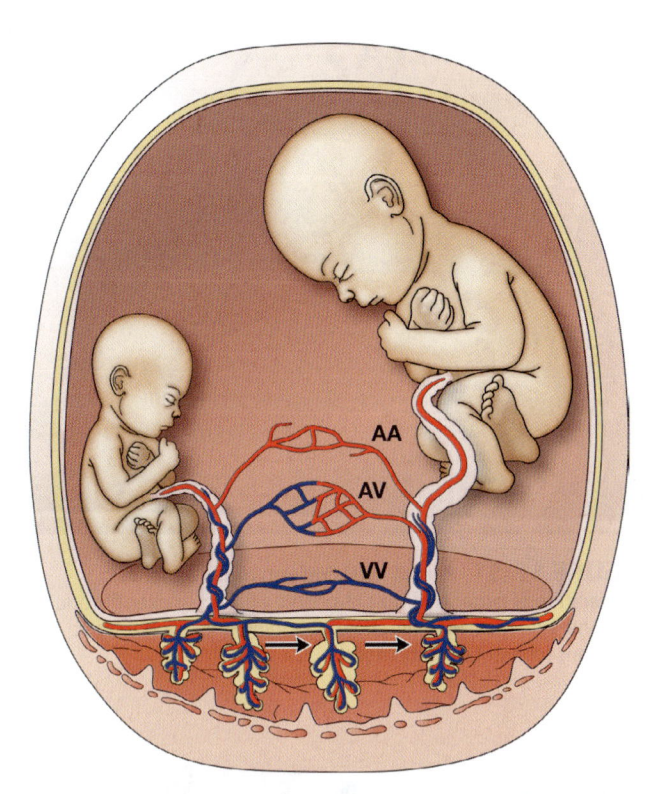

FIGURE 17-49 Anastomoses between twins may be artery to venous (AV), artery to artery (AA), or vein to vein (VV). Schematic representation of an AV anastomosis in twin–twin transfusion syndrome that forms a "common villous region" deep within the villous tissue. Blood from a donor twin may be transferred to a recipient twin through this shared circulation. This transfer leads to a growth-restricted discordant donor twin with markedly reduced amniotic fluid. (Cunningham F. et al. 2010. Williams Obstetrics, 23rd edn. McGraw Hill Medical New York, Figure 39-18.)

commonly follows a hydatidiform mole (50%), but may also follow a miscarriage (25%) or a normal pregnancy (22%). The remaining few cases originate from ectopic pregnancies, or rarely, from pluripotent cells within the gonads.

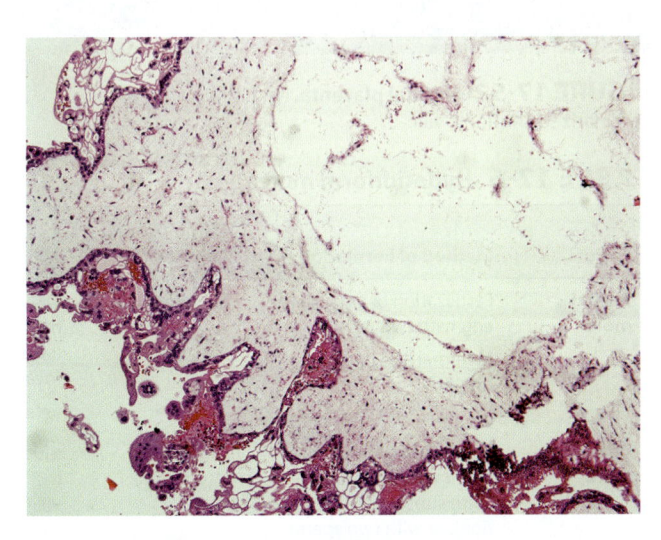

FIGURE 17-50 Complete mole. This image shows an enlarged, hydropic chorionic villous with trophoblastic hyperplasia and atypia (at the bottom) and a central cistern (top right).

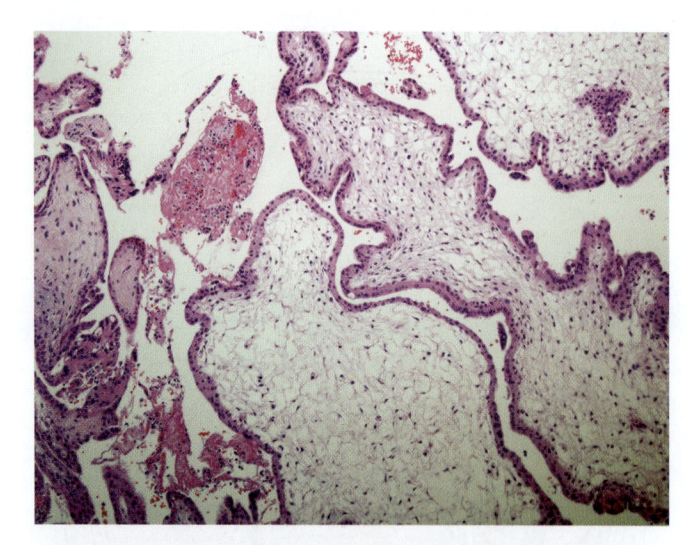

FIGURE 17-51 **Partial hydatidiform mole.** A biphasic proliferation of larger, hydropic chorionic villi and smaller, fibrotic chorionic villi. The larger villi show scalloping and trophoblastic inclusions (one noted at top right).

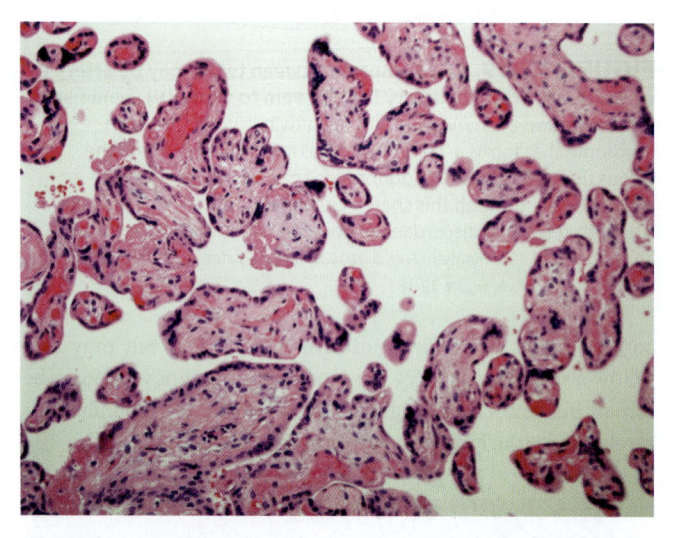

FIGURE 17-52 **Normal placenta.** Note the mature small, vascularized chorionic villi.

CASE 17-18

Choriocarcinoma

A 28-year-old woman who recently experienced a miscarriage presents to her gynecologist complaining of vaginal bleeding. A urine pregnancy test is positive, but a quantitative confirmatory test is elevated well outside the normal range for pregnancy. A CT scan of the chest, abdomen, and pelvis shows a small intrauterine mass and multiple nodules in the parenchyma of the lungs. A uterine curettage is performed **(Figure 17-53)**. What is your diagnosis? Is this a common presentation of this illness?

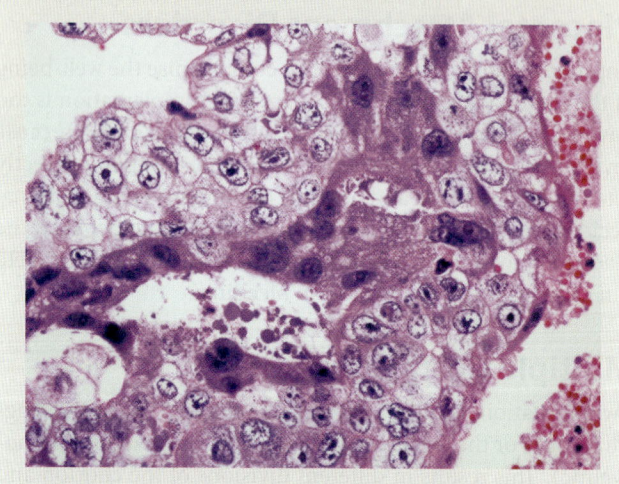

FIGURE 17-53 **Choriocarcinoma.** This image shows the classical "biphasic" pattern of choriocarcinoma, consisting of syncytiotrophoblast (in the center) directly apposed to cytotrophoblast (located above and below; H&E stain).

It is not uncommon for these tumors to present with vaginal bleeding and distant metastasis (the likely cause of the lung nodules in this patient). Other common sites of metastasis include the vagina, brain, liver, and kidney. The elevated hCG is a result of production by the syncytiotrophoblasts. Once extremely lethal, these tumors have an extremely good prognosis due to their response to chemotherapy.

TABLE 17-6 Hydatidiform moles.

Lesion	Method of Formation	Chromosomal Composition	Microscopic Features	p57 Expression	Risk of Choriocarcinoma
Partial mole	Fertilization of a normal egg with two sperm. Maternal and paternal in origin	Triploid 69, XXY	Only a fraction of villi show abnormalities, with hydropic changes (swelling), trophoblastic rimming focal. Fetal parts present	Positive (maternal tissue present)	Rare
Complete mole	Fertilization of an empty ovum with one sperm (with subsequent duplication), or with two sperm. Entirely paternal in origin	Diploid 46XX, 46XY	Clusters of swollen villi are seen, resembling bunches of grapes. All villi are abnormally formed with circumferential growth of abnormal trophoblasts. No fetal parts	Negative (no maternal tissue present)	2% risk

Soft Tissue and Bone Pathology

CHAPTER 18

Karen J. Fritchie, M.D.

INTRODUCTION

WHAT WE DO

Although malignant neoplasms of soft tissue are relatively uncommon, accounting for about 0.6% of all cancer deaths in the United States in 2010, soft tissue pathology is often considered as an overwhelming and intimidating area. Soft tissue pathology includes a wide spectrum of tumors from several supportive nonepithelial tissue types mostly of mesodermal origin (adipose tissue, smooth muscle, skeletal muscle, etc.) and the peripheral nervous tissue of neuroectodermal origin. Additionally, there are a significant proportion of tumors that cannot be classified beyond the generic term "sarcoma" despite the use of immunohistochemical tools, cytogenetic techniques, and molecular studies. The simplest way to approach soft tissue pathology is to divide the tumors into groups based on the line of differentiation of the neoplastic population. Therefore, this chapter will systematically explore the different types of soft tissue neoplasms based on lineage. Within each subset of tumors (lipomatous, smooth muscle, nerve sheath, etc.), there is a certain set of rules or principles that provide an approach to diagnostic workup. An understanding of these rules helps the pathologist to navigate through each group of tumors. The overall approach to the analysis of soft tissue masses will start with imaging studies most often using CT or MRI technology to define the location and extent of tumor and assay for the presence of potential metastatic lesions. Early biopsy using fine-needle aspiration, core needle, or open incisional biopsy will provide tissue to allow classification, histological grading, and often cytogenetic or molecular analysis. The study of chromosomal abnormalities is of particular importance in the classification of certain soft tissue tumors. For example, about 95% of Ewing sarcomas (ES) (see below) have a translocation involving the *EWS* gene on 22q12.

LIPOMATOUS TUMORS

Normal Adipose Tissue Histology

Adipose tissue can be divided in to white fat and brown fat. White fat consists of spherical adipocytes containing a single lipid vacuole that compresses a crescent-shaped nucleus at the periphery of the cell (Figure 18-1A). White fat provides several key functions such as thermal insulation, mechanical protection, and storage and release of lipid/free fatty acids in response to physiologic stimuli. Brown fat has the primary function of heat production and is typically found during the neonatal period in areas such as the axilla, perirenal region, and posterior neck. The abundant mitochondria in brown fat cells along with tissue vascularity are responsible for the red-brown coloration of this tissue. Microscopically, brown fat consists of a mixture of multivacuoloated, granular cells with centrally placed nuclei and univacuolated cells that appear similar to cells of white fat (Figure 18-1B).

Lipoblasts are embryonic mesenchymal cells that are the center of much controversy in the topic of lipomatous neoplasms. Morphologically, these cells have a hyperchromatic-scalloped nucleus that is multiply indented by numerous fat vacuoles or indented by a single large fat vacuole. It is critical to appreciate that lipoblasts can be seen in both benign and malignant fatty tumors and the identification of lipoblasts is not always requisite for the diagnosis of liposarcoma (Figure 18-2).

QUICK REVIEW
Rules for Lipomatous Neoplasms

1. Location, location, and location. Superficial (dermal, subcutaneous) lipomatous tumors are usually benign, while deep-seated (subfacial, intramuscular, retroperitoneal) fatty lesions are worrisome.
2. The three morphologic cell types/patterns that you should be able to recognize are fat necrosis (Figure 18-3), atypical hyperchromatic stromal cells (Figure 18-7), and lipoblasts (Figure 18-2B).

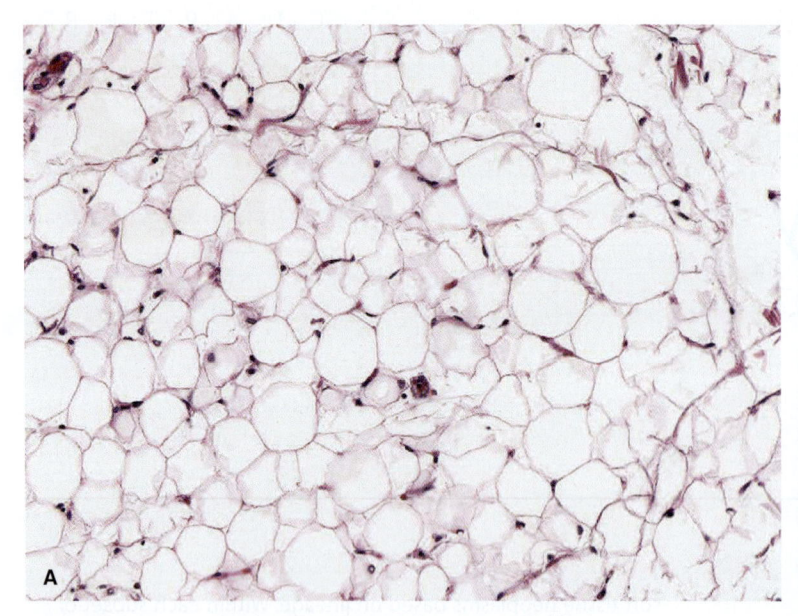

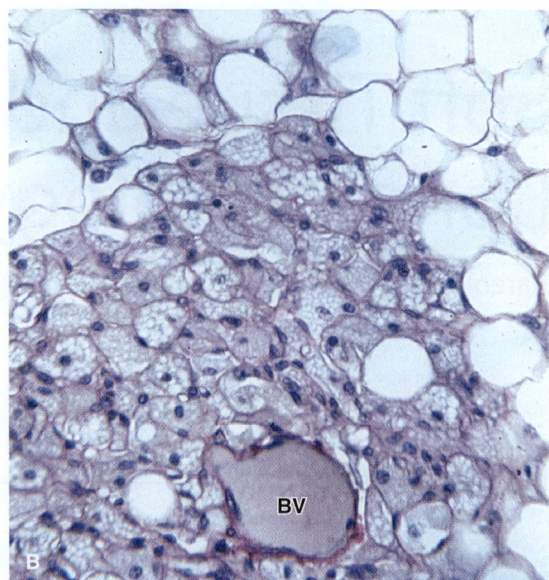

FIGURE 18-1 **(A) White fat.** Note single lipid vesicles and peripheral nuclei. **(B) Brown fat.** Note the multivacuolated nature of the cells and the centrally placed nuclei. BV indicates a small blood vessel. (Modified from Mescher AL, Junqueira's Basic Histology Text and Atlas 12th edn. McGraw Hill Lange New York 2010, Figure 6-4A, page 113).

3. Almost all fatty neoplasms have described cytogenetic abnormalities. Fluorescence in situ hybridization for *MDM2* gene amplification in atypical lipomatous tumors/well-differentiated liposarcoma (ALTs/WDL) and rearrangements of *CHOP (DDIT3)* in myxoid liposarcoma are often critical in the workup of these entities.

The most common soft tissue tumors are of lipomatous differentiation. Lipomatous tumors occur in both superficial and deep soft tissue. Location (subcutaneous, intramuscular, retroperitoneal) is often helpful in making the correct diagnosis. While immunohistochemistry is frequently used to elucidate a line of differentiation in other soft tissue tumors, the use of immunohistochemistry is limited in

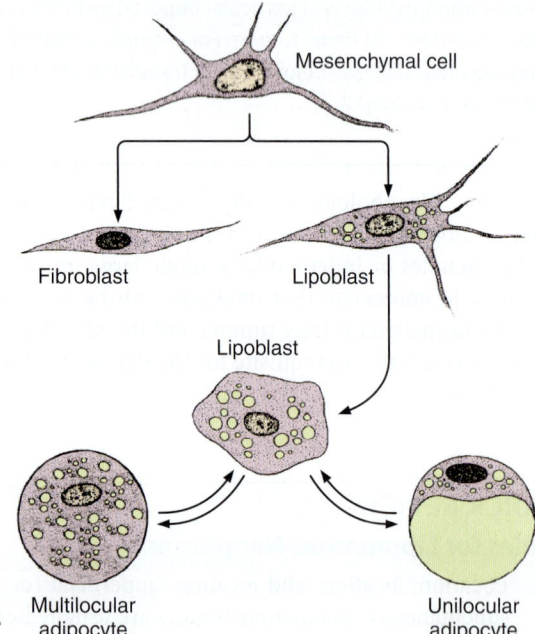

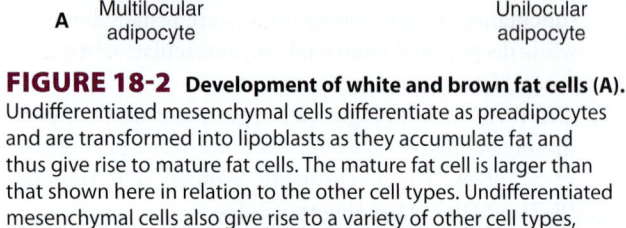

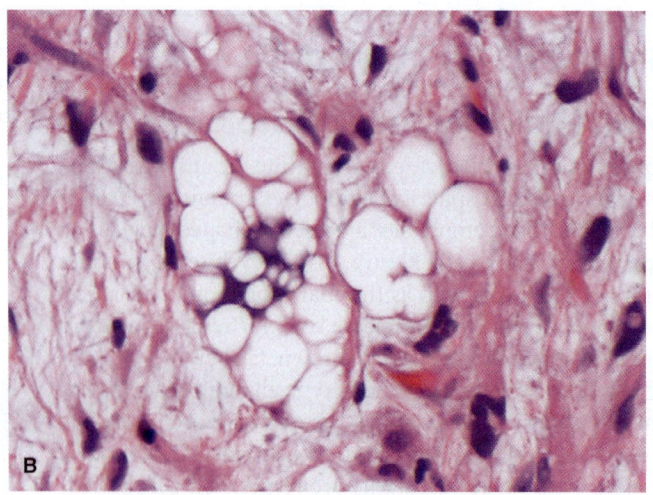

FIGURE 18-2 **Development of white and brown fat cells (A).** Undifferentiated mesenchymal cells differentiate as preadipocytes and are transformed into lipoblasts as they accumulate fat and thus give rise to mature fat cells. The mature fat cell is larger than that shown here in relation to the other cell types. Undifferentiated mesenchymal cells also give rise to a variety of other cell types, including fibroblasts. When a large amount of lipid is mobilized by the body, mature unilocular fat cells may return to the lipoblast stage. **(B) Lipoblast** demonstrating central scalloped nucleus and numerous fat vesicles. (Figure 2a source from Mescher AL, Junqueira's Basic Histology Text and Atlas 12th edn. McGraw Hill Lange New York 2010, Figure 6-3, page 112.)

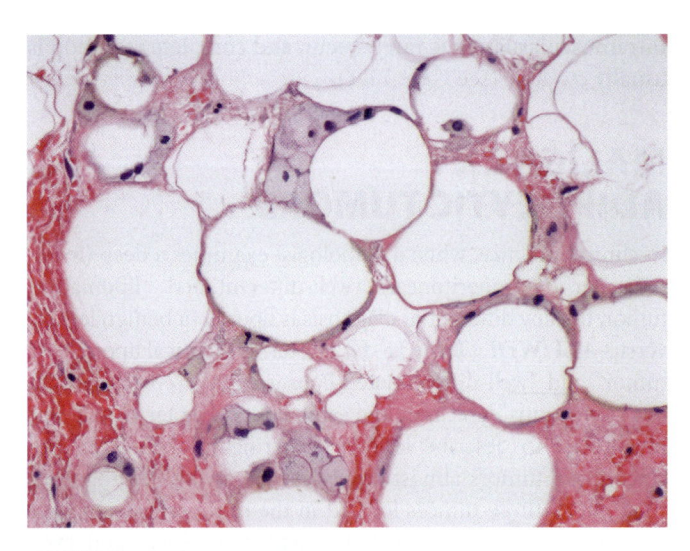

FIGURE 18-3 Fat necrosis.

fatty neoplasms. Instead, ancillary studies such as cytogenetics and molecular techniques are invaluable in the categorization and diagnosis of some of these lesions. Distinct cytogenetic aberrations have been described in almost all fatty tumors.

> ### CASE 18-1
>
> A 40 year-old male presents with a 15 cm thigh mass.
>
> Cytogenetic studies revealed a translocation involving chromosome 3 and 12. No supernumerary ring or giant marker chromosomes were identified. Morphologic features, coupled with the cytogenetic findings, support the diagnosis of intramuscular lipoma. The case demonstrates the importance of cytogenetic analysis in differentiating between benign, and malignant lesions of adipocytic lineage (Figure 18-4).

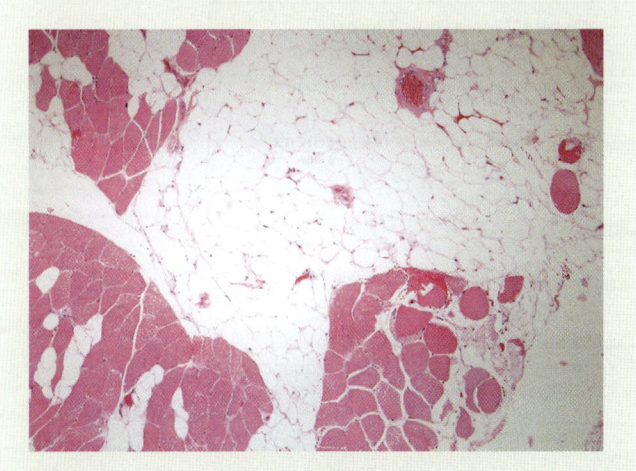

FIGURE 18-4 **Intramuscular lipoma.** Note the infiltrative nature of the neoplasm and the lack of atypical stromal cells.

BENIGN ADIPOCYTIC TUMORS

Lipomas are the most common soft tissue tumor and rarely are clinically significant. They typically present as a slowly growing painless subcutaneous mass in anatomic locations such as the back, shoulder, neck, abdomen, or proximal extremities. They may become large but average 3 cm in size. When superficial they are generally well circumscribed, but lipomas can have a diffuse pattern of growth if deep seated. Morphologically, lipomas consist of mature adipose tissue and have the gross yellow appearance of fat. Although these lesions are well vascularized, the blood vessels are usually compressed by the adipocytes and relatively inconspicuous. While thin fibrous bands may be identified, these septae are hypocellular without atypical cells. Up to two-thirds of lipomatous tumors show cytogenetic abnormalities, with aberrations involving 12q13-15 being most common. Lipomas only rarely recur after excision.

Variant forms of benign lipomas include angiolipomas, spindle cell/pleomorphic lipoma, and intramuscular lipomas. **Angiolipomas** are benign lipomatous neoplasms with unique clinical and morphologic features. The classic clinical presentation is a young adult male with multiple tender subcutaneous nodules. Morphologically, these tumors are composed of mature adipose tissue and clusters of capillary-sized vessels most easily recognized at the periphery of the lesion. Thrombi are seen in the lumens of the intralesional vessels (Figure 18-5). This type of lipomatous tumor is unusual because although familial cases have been reported, no distinct cytogenetic aberration has been characterized to date.

Spindle cell/pleomorphic lipoma is another benign lesion with a characteristic clinical history: an older male with posterior neck/back mass. In fact, with that clinical history, spindle cell lipoma should always be the first thing on the differential diagnosis. These tumors are well-circumscribed

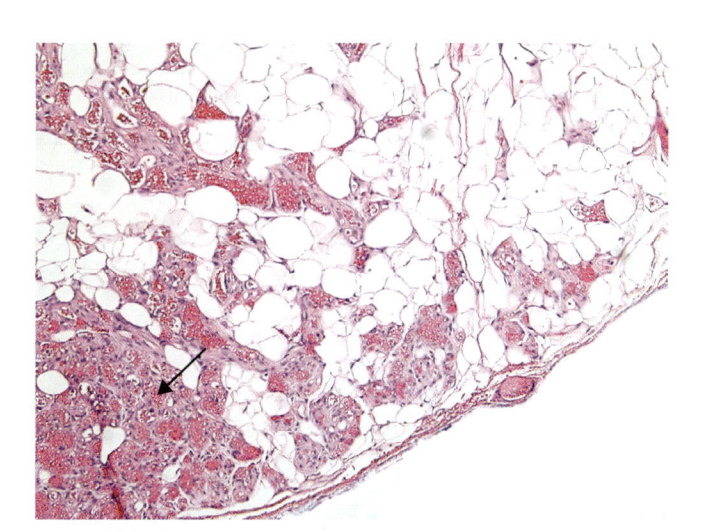

FIGURE 18-5 **Angiolipoma.** Thrombosed capillary-sized vessels are prominent at the periphery of the tumor (arrow).

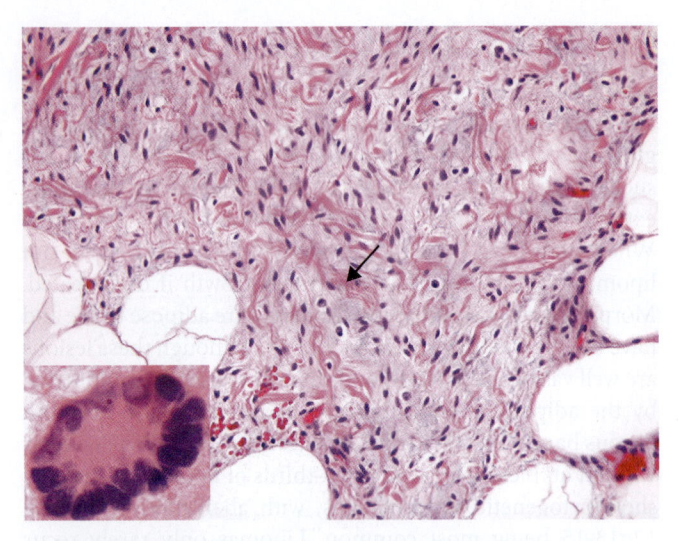

FIGURE 18-6 Spindle cell/pleomorphic lipoma. The specimen shows the three components of the tumor; bland spindle cells, mature adipose tissue, and ropey collagen fibers (arrow). Inset shows a multinucleated floret-like giant cell.

subcutaneous lesions that are composed of three elements: mature adipose tissue, bland spindle cells, and ropey collagen. Occasionally, multinucleated floret-like giant cells may be a component of these tumors (Figure 18-6). The spindled cells of spindle cell/pleomorphic lipoma are strongly CD34 positive, the one exception to the teaching that immunohistochemistry is not useful in fatty tumors.

Intramuscular lipomas are benign fatty tumors that occur within skeletal muscle of the extremities. Therefore, these tumors are deep-seated and are of clinical concern. Intramuscular lipomas rarely recur, and complete resection is usually curative (see Case 18-1).

MALIGNANT ADIPOCYTIC TUMORS

In clinical practice, when a pathologist examines a deep (intramuscular, retroperitoneal) well-differentiated lipomatous tumor, the key differential diagnosis is lipoma (a benign lesion) versus **ALT/WDL** (Table 18-1). The terms "atypical lipomatous tumor" and "well-differentiated liposarcoma" are best thought of as synonyms describing the same entity. The term ALT was introduced to describe lesions occurring in the extremities since those tumors almost always have a favorable prognosis. In contrast, those tumors located in the retroperitoneum have a worse clinical course with frequent recurrences and even death. There are several gross, microscopic, and cytogenetic/molecular features that can be helpful in making the distinction between lipoma and ALT/WDL. First, lipomas are typically grossly homogeneous, whereas examination of ALT/WDL may reveal fibrous bands. Second, ALT/WDL is characterized histologically by atypical hyperchromatic stromal cells that exhibit large, hyperchromatic smudgy nuclei. Such cells are often found in fibrous septae and vessel walls (Figure 18-7). It is the identification of these cells, not lipoblasts, which solidify the diagnosis of ALT/WDL. As alluded to earlier, ALT/WDL can recur and cause death. Those tumors located on the extremity recur in approximately 40% of cases, while retroperitoneal lesions have a recurrence rate of over 90%. ALT/WDL can recur but do not metastasize. However, with time, these tumors are at risk of dedifferentiation, and dedifferentiation occurs

TABLE 18-1 Comparison of lipoma and atypical lipomatous tumor (ALT)/well-differentiated liposarcoma.

	Lipoma	Atypical Lipomatous Tumor/Well-Differentiated Liposarcoma
Age	40–60 years of age	Middle-aged to elderly
Site	Superficial (subcutaneous), occasionally intramuscular	Deep (intramuscular or retroperitoneal including groin)
Morphology	Mature adipose tissue No atypical hyperchromatic stromal cells	Mature adipose Fibrous septae Atypical hyperchromatic stromal cells (can be focal)
Cytogenetics	Translocation involving 12q13–15	Supernumerary ring and giant marker chromosomes with amplified sequences of 12q14-15 region
Molecular	No amplification of MDM2	MDM2 amplification
Behavior	Benign, only rarely recur	Extremities: recur, rarely dedifferentiate Retroperitoneum: frequently recur; up to 20% dedifferentiate

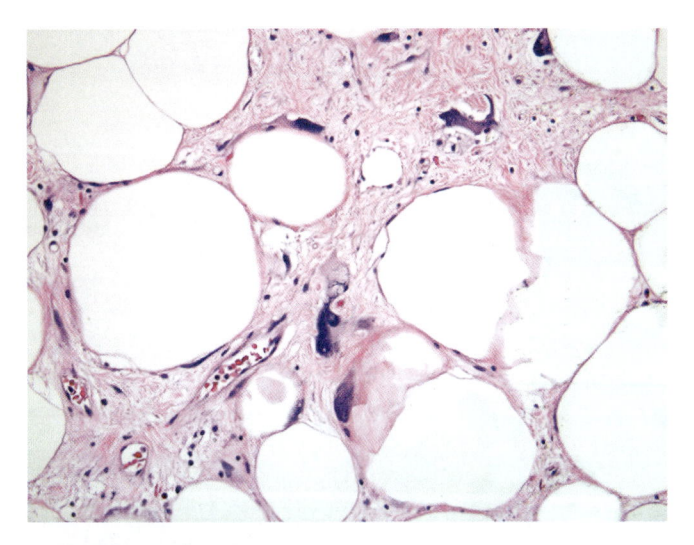

FIGURE 18-7 Atypical lipomatous tumor/well-differentiated liposarcoma. Atypical hyperchromatic stromal cells with smudged nuclei are prominent in this specimen that also contains numerous fibrous bands.

more frequently with retroperitoneal lesions than with those tumors involving the extremities. Morphologically, **dedifferentiated liposarcoma** is characterized by well-differentiated liposarcoma immediately adjacent to a high-grade nonlipogenic sarcoma, usually with an abrupt transition (Figure 18-8) Cytogenetic analysis has shown that these tumors contain the same abnormalities as well-differentiated liposarcoma (giant marker and ring chromosomes) but also usually have additional abnormalities.

Myxoid liposarcoma is another malignant lipomatous neoplasm. This tumor commonly presents in young to middle-aged adults in deep soft tissue of the extremities. Histologically, myxoid liposarcoma is characterized by round to stellate-shaped cells in a myxoid background with a prominent plexiform capillary network. Signet ring and less commonly multi-vacuolated lipoblasts can be identified in these tumors. Additionally, foci of "round cell differentiation" can be seen. These areas are composed of sheets of virtually back-to-back round cells with vascularity that is obscured by cellularity (Figure 18-9).

IN TRANSLATION

Fusion between the *CHOP (DDIT3)* gene on chromosome 12 and the *FUS* gene on chromosome 16 is sensitive and specific for the diagnosis of myxoid liposarcoma, and this finding can be helpful on small biopsy specimens when the diagnosis is in doubt. Myxoid liposarcoma can recur and metastasize, and tumors with >5% round cell differentiation have a worse prognosis.

WHAT WE DO

Current Trends: Fluorescence in Situ Hybridization (FISH) for *MDM2* Gene Amplification

Ancillary techniques utilizing cytogenetic and molecular tools can be critical in arriving at the correct diagnosis (Table 18-2). Frequently, atypical hyperchromatic cells are only found focally, and they may be missed due to chance or poor sampling. Therefore, the finding of supernumerary ring or marker chromosomes with cytogenetic studies or *MDM2* gene amplification with fluorescence in situ hybridization is virtually diagnostic of ALT/WDL. In deep-seated lesions that are clinically worrisome but where histologic review fails to reveal cytologic atypia or in small biopsy samplings, cytogenetic and molecular tools are invaluable.

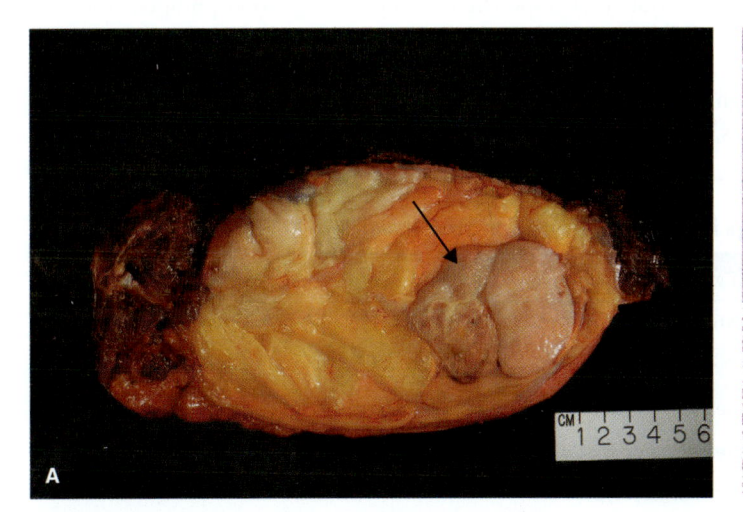

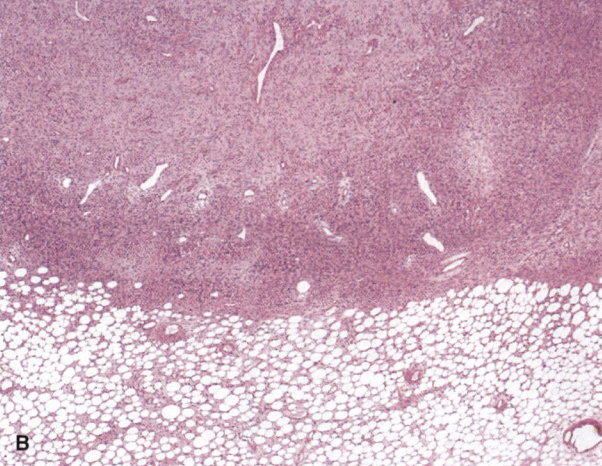

FIGURE 18-8 High-grade nonlipogenic sarcoma within a well-differentiated liposarcoma. (A) Gross surgical specimen showing tan area of "dedifferentiation" within the yellow lipogenic tumor (arrow). **(B)** Histology specimen shows abrupt transition between lipogenic well-differentiated area of tumor (lower third) and "dedifferentiated" high-grade nonlipogenic sarcoma (upper two thirds).

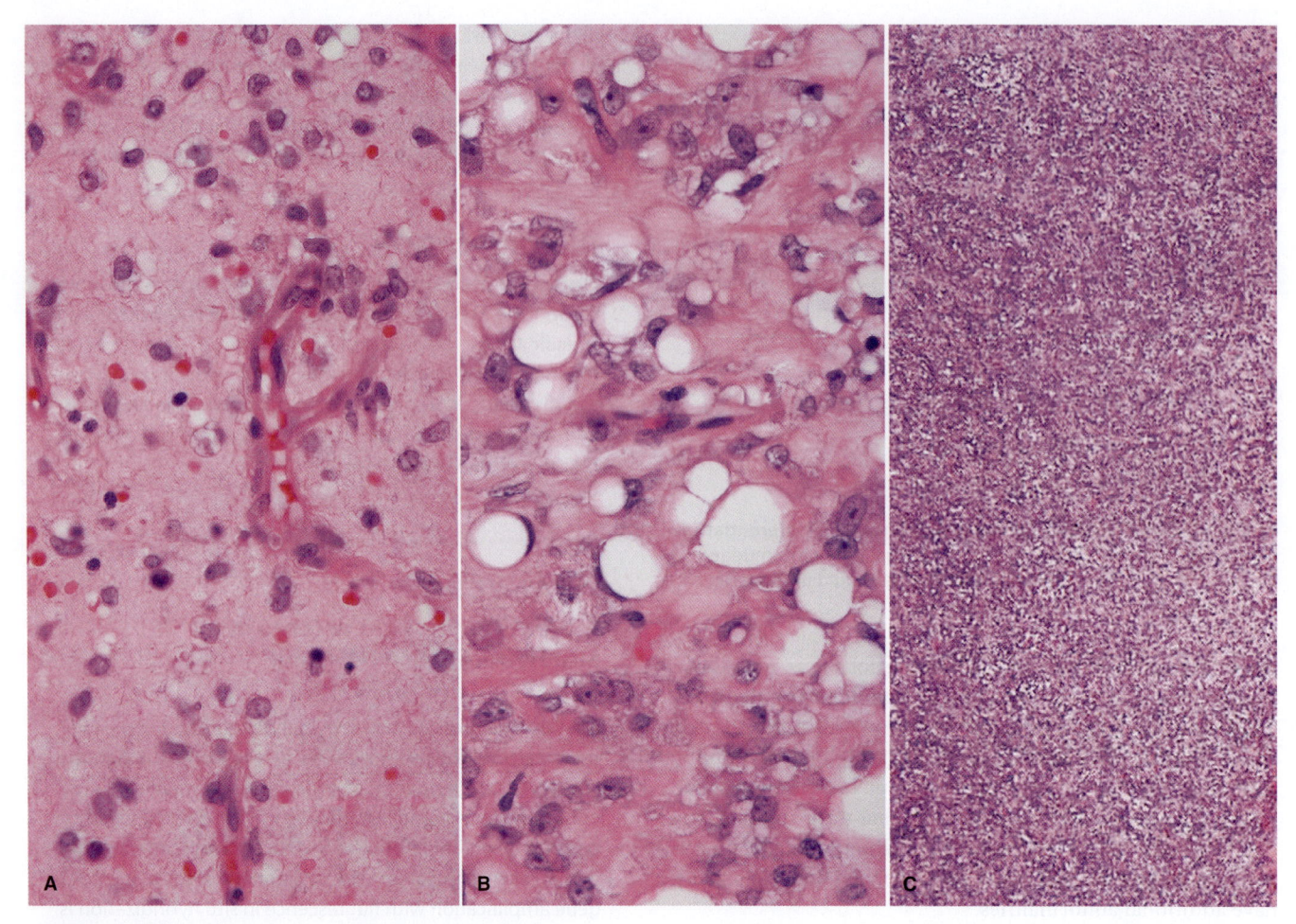

FIGURE 18-9 Myxoid liposarcoma. **(A)** typical stellate cells in a myxoid background and a prominent plexiform pattern of capillaries. **(B)** area with prominent signet ring lipoblasts. **(C)** demonstrates "round cell dedifferentiation."

VASCULAR TUMORS

Normal Histology

The vascular system consists of a series of vessels through which blood flows and can be divided into arterial (arteries, arterioles) and venous (veins, venules) systems. The arterial system is responsible for delivering blood pumped from the heart to capillary beds that are the site of gas exchange. Blood is returned to the heart via the venous system. Most vessels in the vascular system have the same basic structure: tunica intima, tunica media, and tunica adventitia. The tunica intima

TABLE 18-2 Cytogenetic findings in lipomatous neoplasms.

Tumor	Cytogenetic Finding
Lipoma	Aberration of 12q13-15
Spindle cell/pleomorphic lipoma	Deletion of 16q and 13q
Hibernoma	Rearrangement of 11q13-21 in several cases
Lipoblastoma	Rearrangement of 8q11-13
Angiolipoma	Normal karyotype
Atypical lipomatous tumor/well-differentiated liposarcoma	Supernumerary ring and giant marker chromosomes with amplified sequences of 12q14-15 region
Myxoid liposarcoma	t(12;16)(q13;p11)

consists of a flattened endothelial layer surrounded by a basement membrane. The tunica media is an intermediate muscular layer and exhibits the most variation in arterial and venous components. The outer supporting layer is called the tunica adventitia. Capillaries consist only of a single layer of endothelial cells without muscular or advential components. Besides serving as a conduit for blood delivery, blood vessels play a role in coagulation and immune function (Figure 18-10).

The lymphatics are a unidirectional system of vessels and transport excess fluid from the interstitium to regional lymph nodes and finally to the venous system. Lymphatic vessels are found in almost all tissues, and the structures of lymphatics are similar to that of vessels of the venous system. In fact, it is often not possible to distinguish between veins and lymphatics on hematoxylin and eosin (H&E) sections.

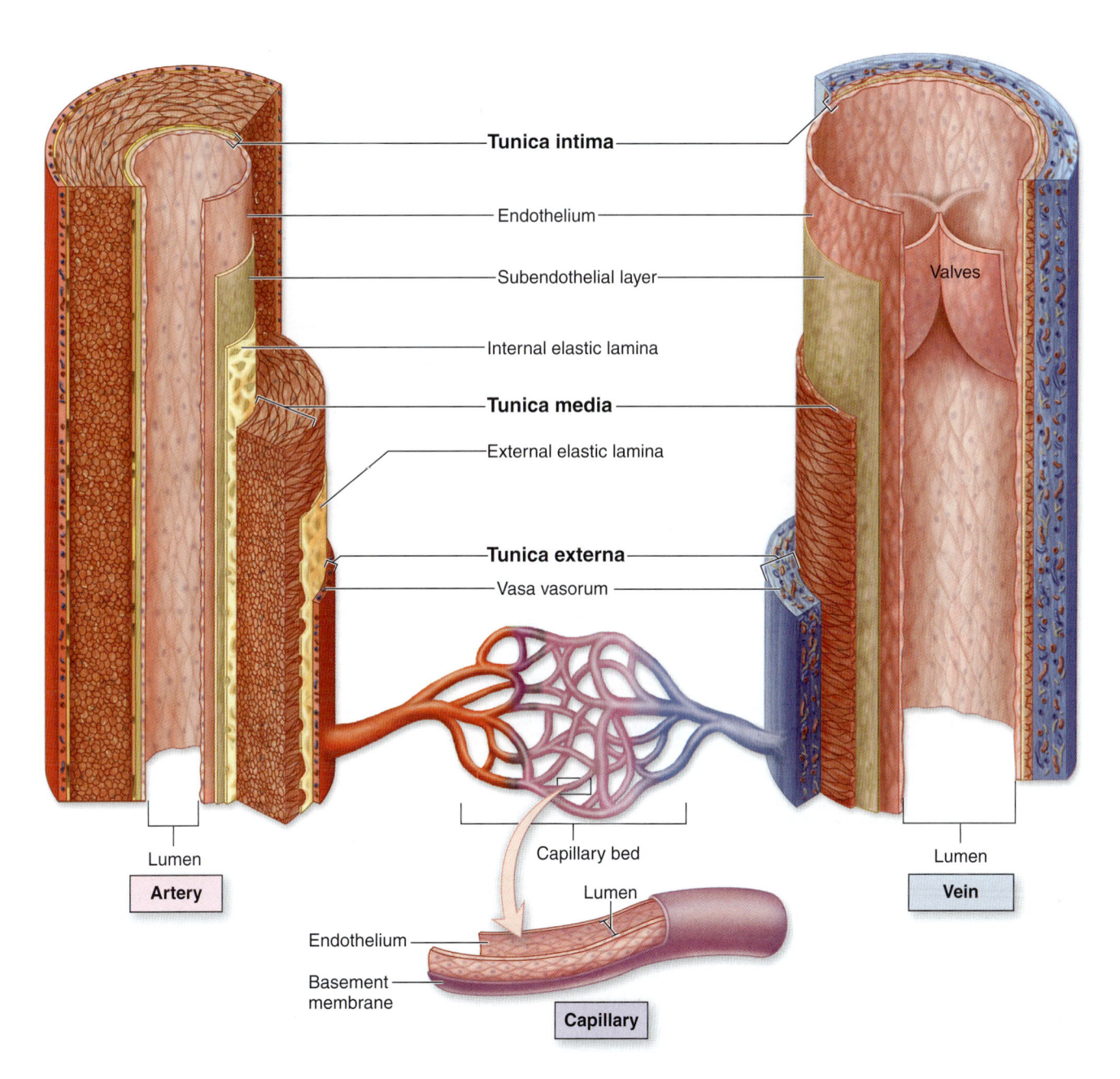

FIGURE 18-10 Walls of arteries, veins, and capillaries.
Walls of both arteries and veins have a tunica intima, tunica media, and tunica externa (or adventitia), which correspond roughly to the heart's endocardium, myocardium, and epicardium. An artery has a thicker tunica media and relatively narrow lumen. A vein has a larger lumen and its tunica externa is the thickest layer. The tunica intima of veins is often folded to form valves. Capillaries have only an endothelium, with no subendothelial layer or other tunics.
(From Mescher AL, Junqueira's Basic Histology Text and Atlas 12th edn. McGraw Hill Lange New York 2010, Figure 11-7, page 190.)

CASE 18-2

A 10-year-old male presents with forehead lesion.

Histologic examination reveals a well-circumscribed dermal-based proliferation with a lobular low-power appearance. At a higher power, well-formed capillary-sized vessels can be identified. The nuclei of the endothelial cells are uniform with significant atypia. These findings are consistent with **hemangioma** (Figure 18-11).

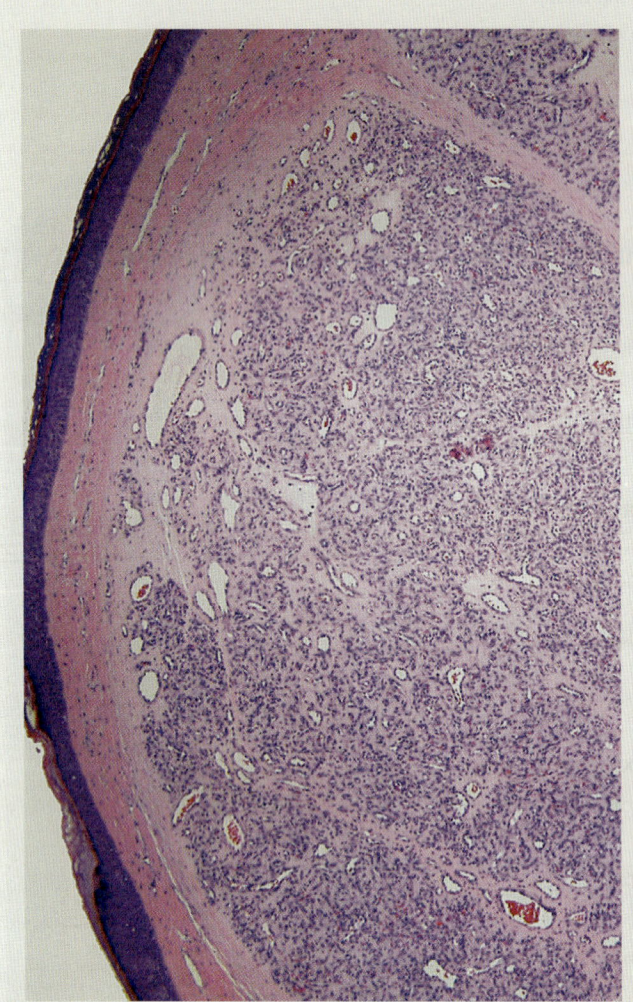

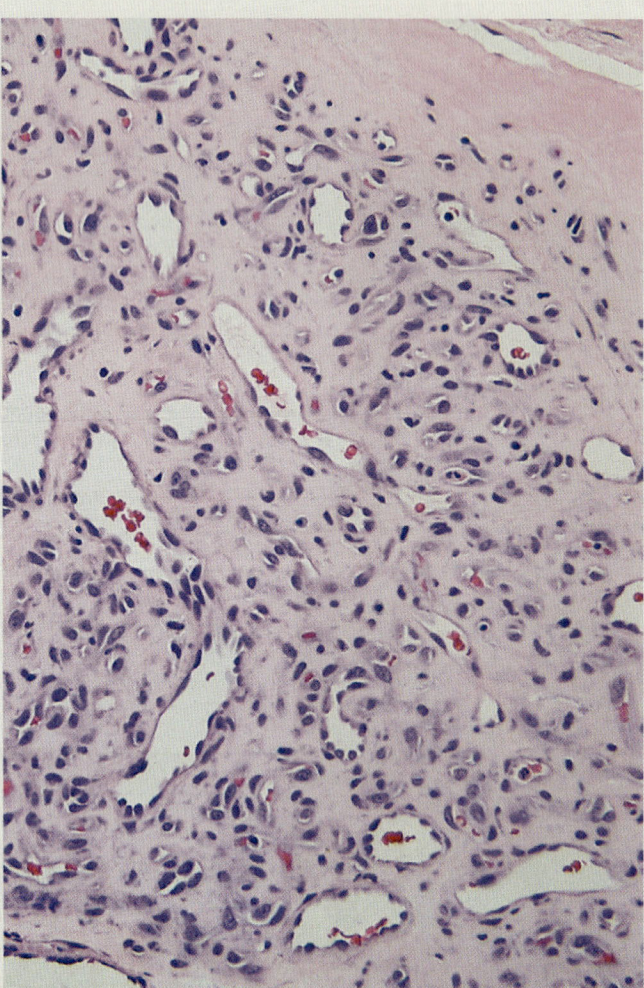

FIGURE 18-11 Hemangioma. Left (low-power view) demonstrates well-circumscribed, dermal nature of the lesion. Right (high-power view) shows well-formed capillary vessels lined with uniform, endothelial cells whose nuclei show no significant atypia.

QUICK REVIEW
Rules for Vascular Lesions

1. Low-power architecture is critical. Reactive and benign vascular lesions have a well-circumscribed, lobular low-power appearance. Diffuse, infiltrative vascular proliferations are worrisome. Once you have assessed the lesion at low power, features at high power that can be worrisome include nuclear atypia, nuclear stratification, and poorly formed vessels (Figure 18-12) (see Table 18-3).

2. Vascular differentiation is a spectrum and may be difficult to recognize. Well-differentiated vascular lesions contain recognizable vessels with lumen formation. In some cases, vascular differentiation is in the form of cells with a single intracytoplasmic lumen. Rarely, vascular differentiation is so primitive that the lesion shows no morphologic evidence of endothelial lineage. In this situation, immunohistochemistry is needed to prove vascular differentiation. Helpful immunostains are CD31 and CD34.

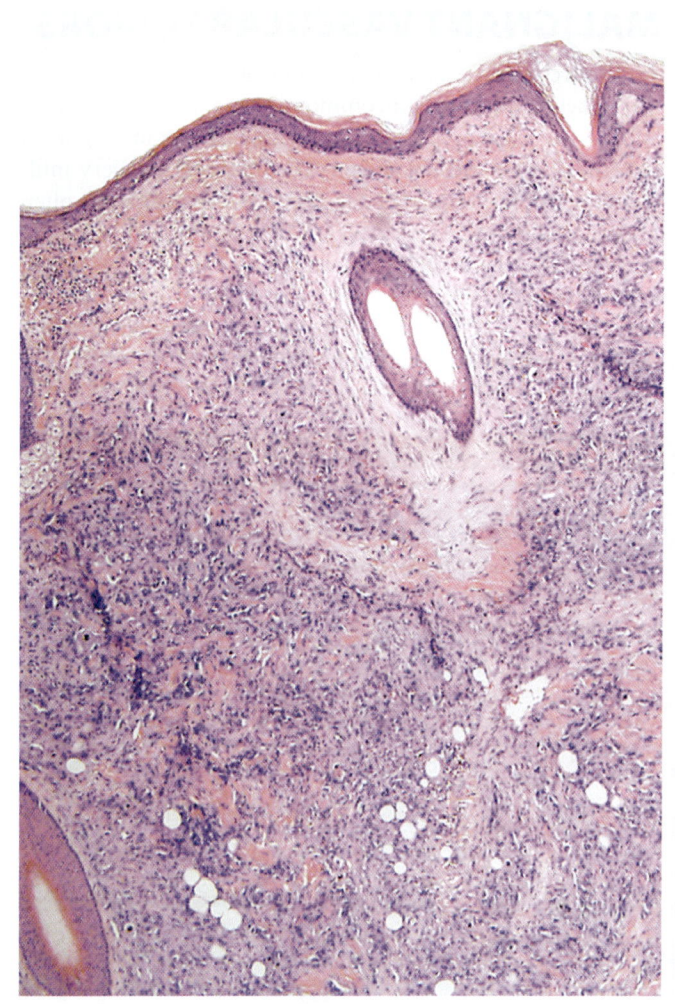

FIGURE 18-12 Angiosarcoma. Left (low-power view) compares this diffuse, infiltrative lesion with Figure 18-11left. Right (high-power view) notes the poorly defined vascular structures. Neoplastic endothelial cells demonstrate hyperchromatic, pleomorphic nuclei that show stratification.

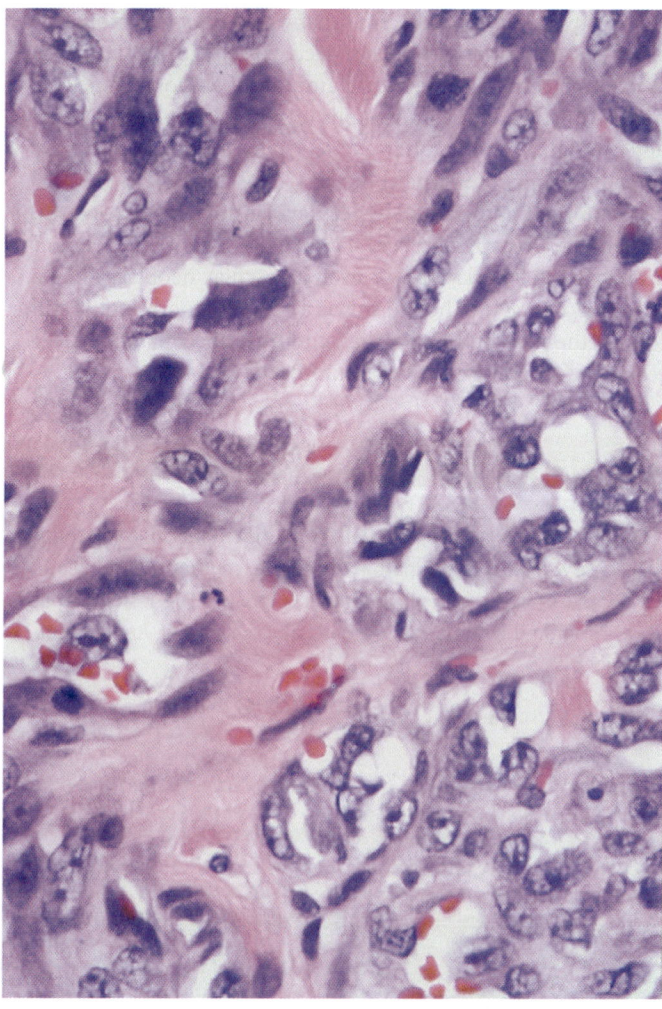

BENIGN VASCULAR TUMORS

Hemangiomas are benign neoplasms of endothelial cells. These lesions are relatively common and occur most frequently in the head and neck region of infants and children. It is often difficult if not impossible to distinguish hemangiomas from arteriovenous malformation. Some regress over time, and others reach a relative stable size. Hemangiomas do not undergo malignant transformation.

Variants: There are several types of hemangioma including lobular capillary hemangioma, pyogenic granuloma, and cherry angioma. While these lesions have varying clinical presentations, they share a common morphologic appearance.

Lobular capillary hemangiomas (see Case 18-2) are characterized by a circumscribed nodular arrangement of small capillary size vessels with a larger feeder-type vessel.

Pyogenic granulomas are polypoid hemangiomas that occur on mucosal surfaces and skin with a granulation tissue appearance. Some are associated with trauma or pregnancy.

Cherry angiomas typically present in adults, usually occur on the trunk or extremities, and have a ruby red appearance.

Some vascular lesions occur in deep soft tissue. Although most of these are benign and do not metastasize, they may recur and even be locally aggressive. **Intramuscular hemangioma** usually presents as a deep soft tissue mass in the lower

TABLE 18-3 Comparison of benign and malignant vascular lesions.

	Benign	Malignant
Low-power architecture	Circumscribed, lobular	Infiltrative, dissection through collagen
Nuclear features	Uniform nuclei	Nuclear atypia and hyperchromasia
Nuclear stratification	No	Yes
Degree of vascular differentiation	Well-formed vessels	Poorly formed vessels

extremity of young adults. They many contain small capillary-sized vessels, larger cavernous-sized vessels, or a mix of the two. Some contain a significant amount of adipose tissue and may be mistaken for a lipomatous tumor. Intramuscular hemangiomas may be difficult to excise. Up to 20% recur; they may be challenging to manage clinically.

Papillary endothelial hyperplasia is not a true neoplasm; rather it is a reactive process that usually involves the wall of a preexisting blood vessel or even a vascular neoplasm like a hemangioma. Even though this is a reactive condition, it still follows the rules outlined earlier: circumscribed, bland nuclear features. Complete excision is curative.

MALIGNANT VASCULAR TUMORS

Angiosarcoma is a malignant tumor of vascular differentiation. These tumors are uncommon lesions that usually affect adults. The classic clinical presentation is a skin lesion on head/neck of an elderly person. These tumors are very infiltrative (poorly circumscribed) and gross examination often underestimates the true extent of the lesion. For this reason, surgeons may have difficulty completely excising the lesion, and the surgical margins may be positive. Microscopically, these tumors are composed of an intricate network of poorly defined vascular structures diffusely infiltrating the dermis or

CASE 18-3

A 70-year-old man presents with large subcutaneous thigh mass. Low-power examination reveals a multinodular myxoid neoplasm centered in subcutaneous tissue. The lesional cells are spindled with hyperchromatic atypical nuclei. Arching curvilinear blood vessels are visible. In some areas, the neoplastic cells are more closely packed and exhibit fascicular growth with little intervening myxoid stroma. These features are consistent with **myxofibrosarcoma (Figure 18-13)**.

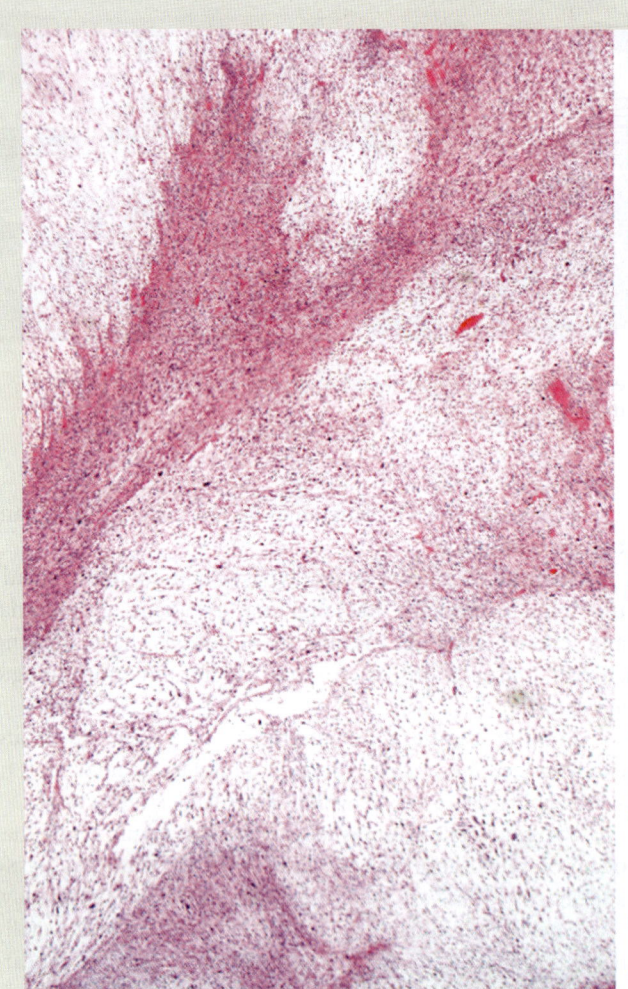

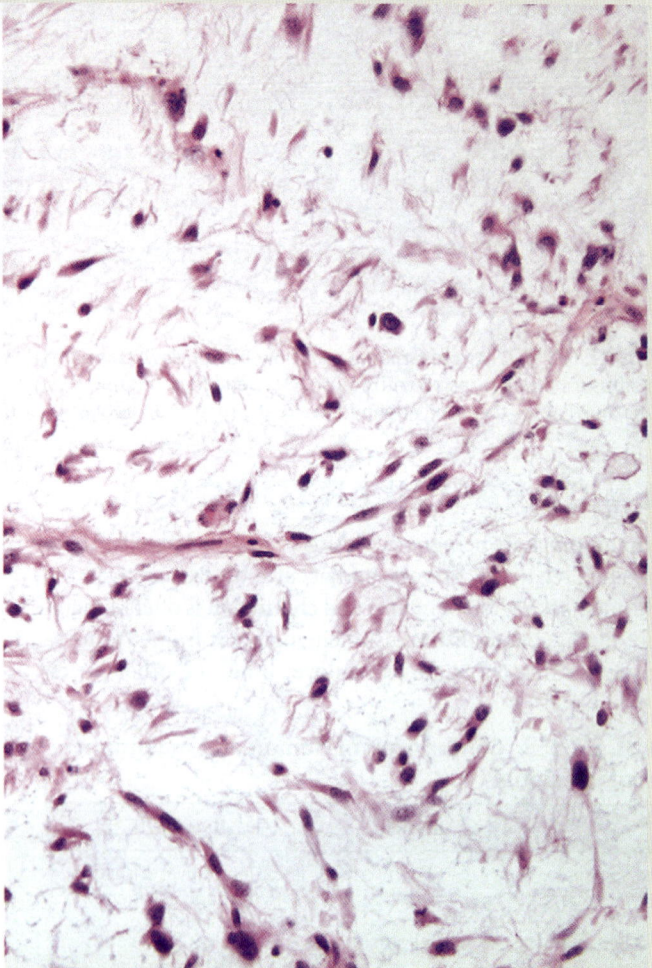

FIGURE 18-13 **Myxofibrosarcoma.** Left (low-power view) demonstrates a multinodular myxoid neoplasm in the subcutis. Both myxoid and close-packed fascicular areas of growth are evident. Right (high-power view) shows neoplastic cells with pleomorphic, hyperchromatic nuclei in a myxoid background.

other tissue. In some cases, primitive vessels may be identified, but in other lesions the neoplastic cells show no evidence of endothelial differentiation (Figure 18-12). The neoplastic cells have hyperchromatic and pleomorphic nuclei and nuclear stratification. Even though mitotic figures should not be used to distinguish between reactive/benign and malignant vascular lesions since reactive/benign lesions can have brisk mitotic activity, the mitotic rate in angiosarcomas is usually high. In cases where the pathologist cannot be confident of endothelial differentiation by H&E morphology, immunohistochemical stains such as CD31 and CD34 can be used. Angiosarcoma is an aggressive tumor, and the overall long-term survival is poor.

Angiosarcoma can occur in several clinical scenarios. Although the most common clinical scenario involves the head/neck of the elderly, angiosarcoma may also arise with chronic lymphedema, following radiation treatment or with exposure to certain chemicals like Thorotrast or vinyl chloride. Despite the clinical differences, the morphologic features are similar, and prognosis is dismal in all types.

FIBROBLASTIC AND MYOFIBROBLASTIC LESIONS

Normal Histology

Fibroblasts are slender spindled cells with pale cytoplasm, indistinct cell borders, uniform nuclei, and pinpoint nucleoli. They are responsible for the production of extracellular matrix of fibrous connective tissue including collagen, elastin, and glycosaminoglycans. Myofibroblasts are the most important cell type in tissue repair, and they have overlapping features of fibroblasts and smooth muscle. Microscopically, they are also spindled cells with lightly eosinophilic cytoplasm and bland nuclei, but unlike fibroblasts they contain bundles of intracytoplasmic microfilaments that provide a mechanism of cell contraction.

> **QUICK REVIEW**
> **Rules for Fibroblastic and Myofibroblastic Lesions**
> Fibroblastic and myofibroblastic lesions can be divided into reactive and neoplastic conditions, and often it is difficult to distinguish the two. Frequently reactive lesions will be more heterogeneous in cellular composition, while fibroblastic/myofibroblastic neoplasms will have a more organized appearance with a regular distribution of blood vessels. While marked cytologic atypia favors a malignant process, some reactive lesions may have some cellular pleomorphism while neoplasms may appear deceptively bland. Similarly, atypical mitotic figures are a worrisome finding, but the mere presence of mitotic activity is generally not helpful diagnostically. Finally, fibroblasts and myofibroblasts variably express smooth muscle markers, but typically immunohistochemical stains are most useful in excluding other entities in the differential diagnosis.

Fibroblastic and myofibroblastic lesions can be characterized as reactive, benign and malignant lesions including nodular fasciitis, fibromatosis, and myxofibrosarcoma.

REACTIVE FIBROBLASTIC LESIONS

Nodular fasciitis is a self-limited fibroblastic and myofibroblastic proliferation that is often clinically concerning because patients present with a rapidly growing mass. These lesions most commonly affect young adults, in areas such as upper extremity. In children, nodular fasciitis has a predilection for the head and neck. Histologic examination shows bland spindle cells without significant cytologic atypia. Mitotic figures are usually easily found, but no atypical mitotic figures are present (Figure 18-14). These lesions are benign , and they should not recur after excision. *Nodular fasciitis is an important entity to be aware of because it is the most common reactive/benign lesion that is misdiagnosed as a sarcoma.* Recent work has shown most cases of nodular fasciitis harbor rearrangements of the *USP6* gene, supporting the notion that this entity ia a "transient neoplasia".

BENIGN FIBROBLASTIC TUMORS (FIBROMATOSIS)

Fibromatoses are a group of locally aggressive but nonmetastasizing tumors composed of fibroblasts and myofibroblasts. There are two main types of fibromatosis: superficial and deep. Both superficial and deep groups share are characterized by a bland but infiltrative spindle cell proliferation of fibroblasts and myofibroblasts in long sweeping fascicles with a regular distribution of thin-walled blood vessels. Although these superficial and deep fibromatosis are impossible to distinguish by microscopic examination, they differ in clinical presentation and behavior.

Superficial fibromatosis includes plantar and palmar subtypes. Palmar fibromatosis, also known as Dupuytren contracture, affects up to 20% of people over 65 and presents as a single nodule or multiple small nodules. Plantar fibromatosis also occur in adults but occasionally occur in children and young adults. Although superficial fibromatosis has the same morphologic features as the deep type, they have a much better clinical outcome with surgery reserved for symptomatic cases.

Deep fibromatosis can be divided into abdominal, intra-abdominal, and extra-abdominal subtypes. The abdominal type arises from the musculoaponeurotic structures of the abdominal wall and usually occurs in women of childbearing age. Intra-abdominal fibromatosis includes mesenteric and pelvic fibromatosis. Extra-abdominal fibromatosis mainly affects muscles and overlying fascia of the pelvic and shoulder girdle of young adults. Even though the clinical features of these subtypes are variable, all forms of deep fibromatosis have similar morphologic features. While deep fibromatoses do not metastasize, they can cause significant morbidity

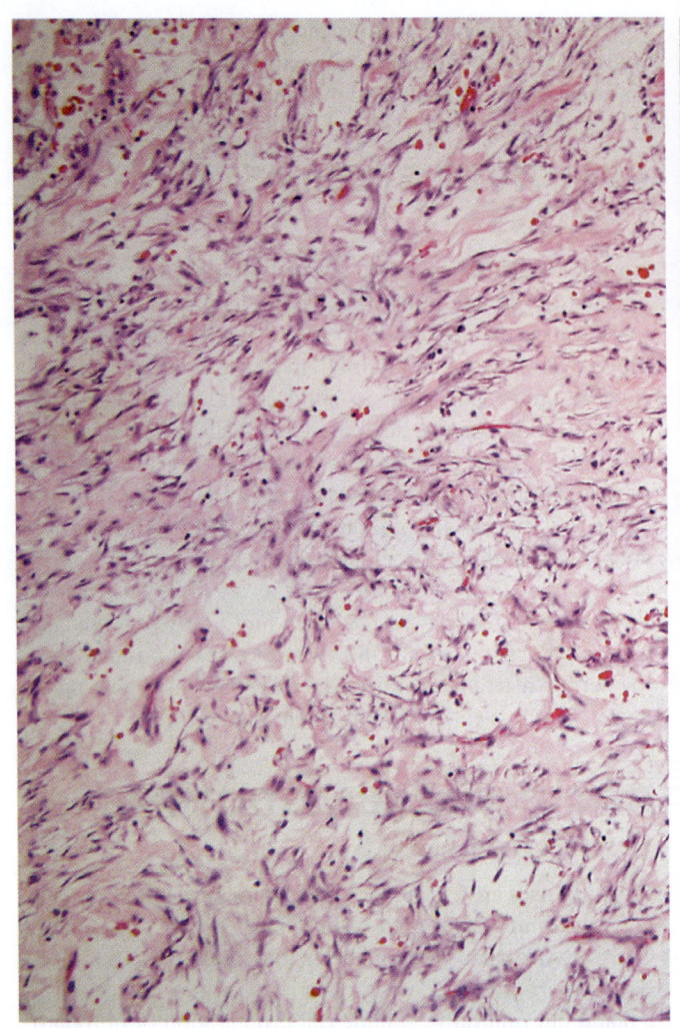

FIGURE 18-14 Nodular fasciitis. Two high-power views of a bland circumscribed lesion. Left shows a relatively open area with some extravasated red cells present. Right shows a denser area. The spindle cells are bland and lack significant atypia.

and mortality from aggressive local behavior. Recurrence rates following excision vary, but reach almost 80% in some series.

> **IN TRANSLATION**
>
> Almost all deep fibromatosis have mutations in the β-catenin or APC gene causing intranuclear accumulation of β-catenin that results in diffuse staining with β-catenin immunohistochemical stain. Conversely, reactive fibroblastic and myofibroblastic proliferations will be negative for β-catenin. Therefore, immunohistochemistry can be a useful tool in distinguishing fibromatosis from reactive proliferations on small biopsy specimens. Since Gardner syndrome is an autosomal dominant disease caused by germline mutation in the APC gene, affected patients are at a substantially higher risk of deep fibromatosis than the general population. Patients with Gardner syndrome also may present with intestinal polyposis, osteomas, and skin cysts.

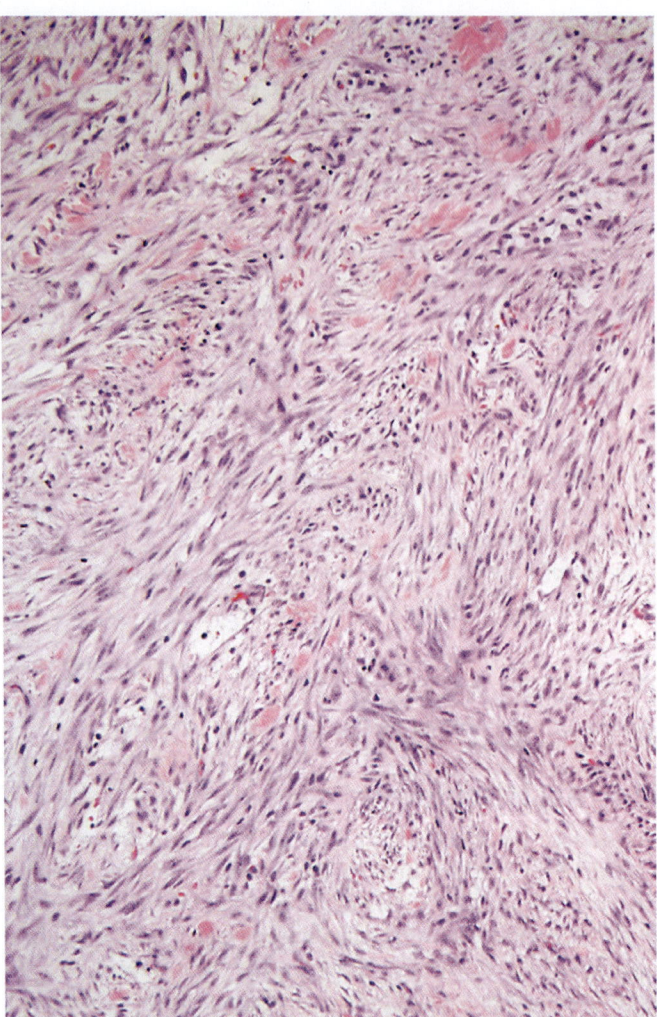

MALIGNANT FIBROBLASTIC TUMORS

Myxofibrosarcoma is a malignant fibroblastic lesion that classically presents as a superficial mass in the lower extremity of the elderly. Grossly these tumors are lobular and have a gelatinous cut surface. Microscopically, the amount of myxoid stroma varies by case and correlates with less aggressive course (see Figure 18-13). Conversely, those tumors with increased cellularity are high grade and are at risk of more aggressive behavior including more frequent local recurrence and potential for distant metastasis (see Case 18-13).

FIBROHISTIOCYTIC LESIONS

Lesional Histology

Fibrohistiocytic lesions are a group of entities that contain a mixture of histiocytes and fibroblasts. Histiocytes are cells derived from monocyte–macrophage lineage. They have eosinophilic cytoplasm containing lysosomes that are

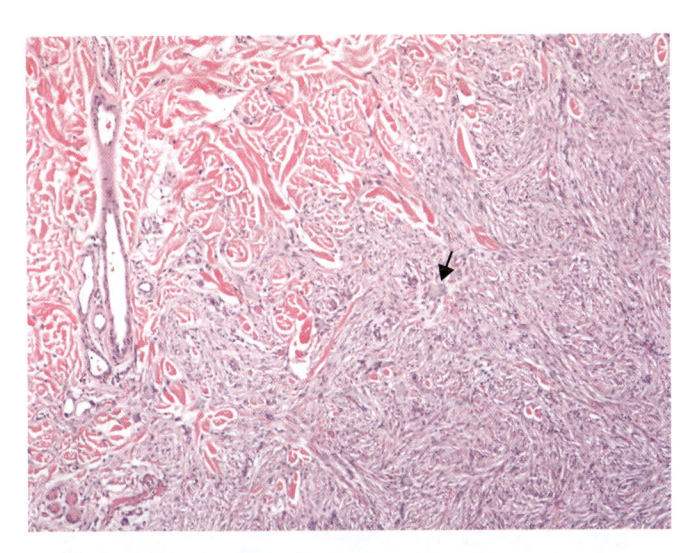

FIGURE 18-15 **Benign fibrous histiocytoma.** Medium-power view from margin of lesion shows both spindle-shaped and rounded histiocyte-like cells. Occasional giant cells are evident (arrow). Cells appear to surround ("trap") collagen fibers.

enzyme-containing organelles used to break down cellular waste material.

BENIGN FIBROHISTIOCYTIC TUMORS

Benign fibrous histiocytoma is a benign lesion that usually present as a solitary slowly growing nodule in adults in the dermis. Microscopically, this lesion consists of a mixed cellular population including spindle cells, xanthoma cells, multinucleated giant cells, inflammatory cells, and hemosiderin-laden macrophages. Epidermal hyperplasia and peripheral collagen trapping are helpful clues to the diagnosis (Figure 18-15). Simple excision is curative as these lesions rarely recur.

Numerous variants of fibrous histiocytoma are recognized and vary in morphology and clinical behavior. For example, **atypical fibrous histiocytoma** exhibits cytologic atypia and mitotic activity in a background that resembles classic benign fibrous histiocytoma. These variants have a higher recurrence rate than benign fibrous histiocytoma.

QUICK REVIEW
Current Trends: Fibrosarcoma And Malignant Fibrous Histiocytoma

It was not long ago that the diagnoses of fibrosarcoma and malignant fibrous histiocytoma (MFH) were two of the most common diagnoses in soft tissue pathology. Fibrosarcoma was described as a malignant spindle cell sarcoma of fibroblasts and typically exhibited a "herringbone" growth pattern. MFH was a pleomorphic sarcoma subdivided into five subtypes: pleomorphic, giant cell, inflammatory, angiomatoid, and myxoid. However, with the advent of improved immunohistochemical and molecular techniques, current thinking about these two entities has changed dramatically. While over 65% of sarcomas were diagnosed as fibrosarcoma in the early 1900s, the diagnosis is virtually extinct. We now realize that many things that were labeled as fibrosarcoma were actually monophasic synovial sarcoma, malignant peripheral nerve sheath tumor (MPNST), and fibrosarcomatous dermatofibrosarcoma protuberans. Similarly, with further investigation we now know that "MFH" is not a reproducible diagnosis, and there is no evidence that tumors with this label are histiocytic in derivation. In fact, many lesions called "MFH" in previous years can now be classified as lymphoma, poorly differentiated carcinoma, dedifferentiated liposarcomas, and various other malignancies. The history of "fibrosarcoma" and "MFH" illustrates the fluidity of the field of pathology and shows how much our understanding of tumors has grown over the past hundred years.

SMOOTH MUSCLE

Normal Histology

Smooth muscle is found throughout the body in organs such as the genitourinary tract, gastrointestinal tract, and respiratory tract and provides relatively continuous contractions of low force in a rhythmic or wavelike pattern. The activity of smooth muscle is influenced by the autonomic nervous system, hormones, and local metabolites.

Smooth muscle cells have distinct histologic features and usually can be identified by H&E morphology. One of the characteristic properties of a smooth muscle cell is its brightly eosinophilic cytoplasm. The cells are elongated and spindled, and the nuclei have blunt ends that give them a "cigar-like" appearance. Smooth muscle cells are bound together into fascicles (Figure 18-16). Ultrastructurally,

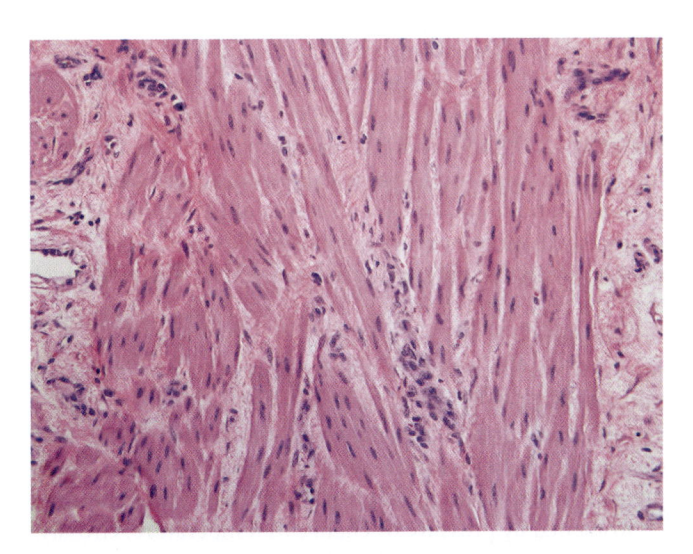

FIGURE 18-16 **Normal smooth muscle cells.** Fascicles of normal smooth muscle cells. The cells have an elongate spindle shape and bright, eosinophilic cytoplasm. The elongate nuclei are centrally located at the cells maximum width.

smooth muscle cells have three types of filaments: myosin, actin, and intermediate. Oftentimes when the lineage of spindle cells is in question, immunohistochemistry can help to prove muscle origin by positive staining for actin, desmin, or H-caldesmon.

> ## QUICK REVIEW
> ### Rules for Distinguishing Smooth Muscle Neoplasms
> Having decided that a tumor is derived from smooth muscle, there are three histologic features to look for: atypia, mitotic figures, and coagulative tumor necrosis. Mitotic figures are the most objective criteria for malignancy, and as a general rule, any mitotic activity in a soft tissue smooth muscle tumor is a worrisome finding. Atypia includes nuclear hyperchromasia or pleomorphism. Atypia is usually subjectively stratified in to mild, moderate, and severe grades. However, any more than mild atypia may be indicative of a malignant tumor. Necrosis in smooth muscle tumors may be of the hyalinized or coagulative-tumor type. In hyalinized-type necrosis, there is a gradual transition between viable and necrotic tissue. In contrast, the demarcation between viable and nonviable tissue is typically sharp in coagulative tumor necrosis and the nuclei in the necrotic cells retain their hematoxyphilia. While hyalinized-type necrosis can be seen in benign smooth muscle neoplasms, coagulative tumor necrosis is a concerning finding.

Benign Smooth Muscle Tumors

Superficial or cutaneous leiomyoma can be divided into two types: those arising from pilar arrector muscles and the genital form. Leiomyoma of pilar arrector origin may be solitary or multiple and present as small 1–2 cm brown-red papules that may coalesce. These lesions typically arise during early adulthood and, like angiomyomas, may be painful. Genital leiomyomas are usually solitary and affect sites such as the scrotum, vulva, and areola of the nipple. Microscopically these tumors are composed of bundles of smooth muscle. Genital leiomyomas are usually more circumscribed than the pilar arrector type. Close examination is necessary to make sure that the lesion does not contain worrisome features such as nondegenerative atypia, necrosis, or increased mitotic activity.

Angiomyoma is a benign smooth muscle tumor that classically affects middle-aged women. Patients usually present with a slowly enlarging and painful mass that may be worsened by pressure or change in temperature. Grossly, the mass is circumscribed with a white-gray cut surface. Microscopically, these lesions are composed of smooth muscle concentrically arranged around thick-walled blood vessels. Myxoid change, calcification, and hyalinization may be seen. While degenerative atypia may be seen, these lesions should not have mitotic activity or necrosis. Simple excision is curative.

Leiomyomatosis peritonealis disseminata may be clinically alarming because patients present with multiple small subperitoneal nodules throughout the abdominal cavity. The clinical presentation is often worrisome for a metastatic process. However, histologic examination reveals nodules of smooth muscle. The etiology of this condition is unclear but evidence points to a hormonal factor since this lesion almost exclusively occurs in females and most are patients of childbearing age. No treatment is necessary, and some of these nodules regress following pregnancy or removal of the estrogenic source.

Malignant Smooth Muscle Tumors

Leiomyosarcoma is a malignant tumor of smooth muscle (see **Case 18-4**). While the retroperitoneum is a common

> ### CASE 18-4
> A 65-year-old woman presents with a large retroperitoneal mass.
>
> Histologic sections show an atypical spindle cell proliferation composed of cells with brightly eosinophilic cytoplasm and organized in a fascicular growth pattern. These morphologic features are suggestive of smooth muscle origin. Smooth muscle actin and desmin immunohistochemical stains are strongly positive in the neoplastic population. Examination at higher power reveals significant cytologic atypia and frequent mitotic figures. These findings are consistent with **leiomyosarcoma (Figure 18-17)**.
>
> **FIGURE 18-17 Leiomyosarcoma.** High-power view shows elongate eosinophilic cells arranged in a fascicular pattern. There is marked nuclear atypia with frequent mitotic figures visible.

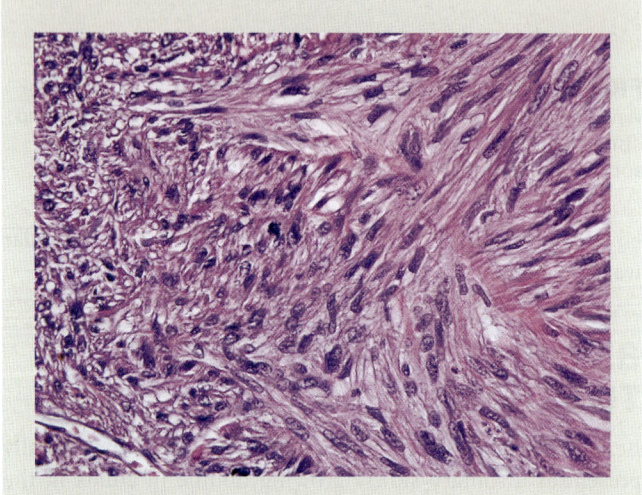

site, they also may occur in places like the skin, deep soft tissue, bone, and visceral organs. Middle aged and older adults are most commonly affected. Although there is no gender preference overall, retroperitoneal lesions are more common in women. Key morphologic features include perpendicularly oriented bundles of spindle cell with brightly eosinophilic cytoplasm. The neoplastic nuclei have blunt ends and exhibit atypia. Mitotic figures are typically easy to find (Figure 18-17). Some lesions may have myxoid or epithelioid change. Usually, smooth muscle derivation is evident by H&E morphology, but immunohistochemical markers for smooth muscle actin, desmin, and H-caldesmon can be also be used. Prognosis depends on site. Leiomyosarcomas limited to the dermis almost never metastasize, while those arising in the retroperitoneum have a much worse outcome.

Leiomyosarcoma variants may arise from large veins such as the vena cava. Inferior vena cava leiomyosarcoma classically affects older female patients. Presentation varies depending on which portion of the vena cava is involved. Those tumors arising in the inferior portion of the inferior vena cava cause

HUNTING FOR ZEBRAS

A 5-year-old patient presents with multiple liver lesions. The patient has a history of liver transplant for alpha-one-antitrypsin deficiency.

Histologic review demonstrates a spindle cell proliferation of relatively uniform cells in interlacing fascicles. Only minimal cytologic atypia is identified, and the mitotic rate is low. A smooth muscle actin stain is diffusely positive in the lesional cells, supporting smooth muscle origin. Numerous lymphocytes are admixed with the spindle cell population as highlighted by a CD3 immunohistochemical stain. The clinical and morphologic findings are suggestive of EBVSMT. To confirm the diagnosis, in situ hybridization for EBER (Epstein–Barr virus early RNA) is performed and is positive (Figure 18-18).

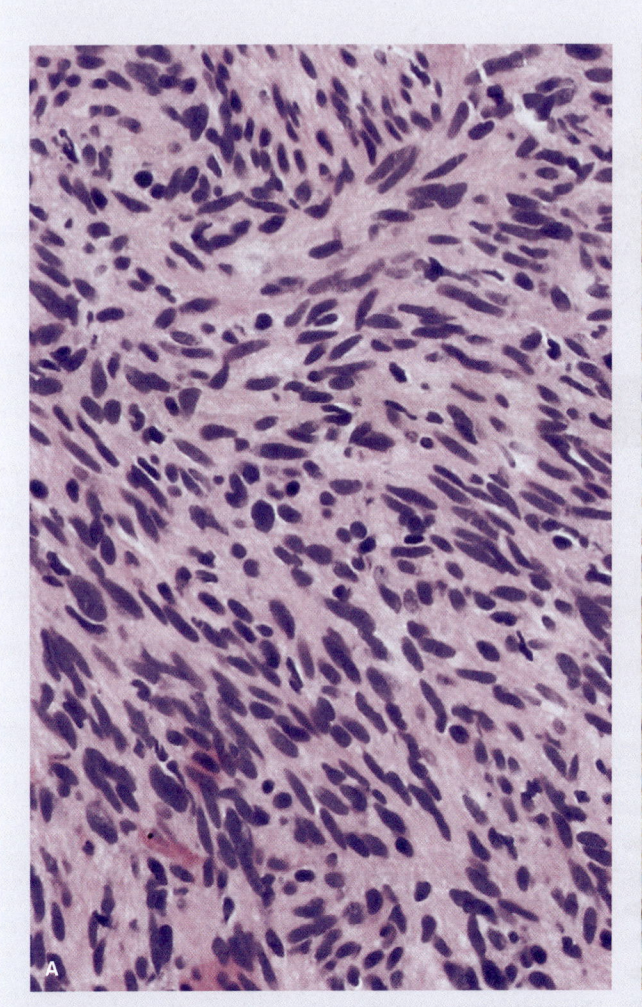

FIGURE 18-18 Epstein–Barr virus-associated smooth muscle tumor (EBVSMT). **(A)** A tumor composed of spindle-shaped cells arranged in fascicles. **(B)** Immunostaining for smooth muscle actin is positive. **(C)** Infiltrating lymphocytes are highlighted by CD3 immunostaining. **(D)** Positive in situ staining for EBV early viral RNA confirms the diagnosis.

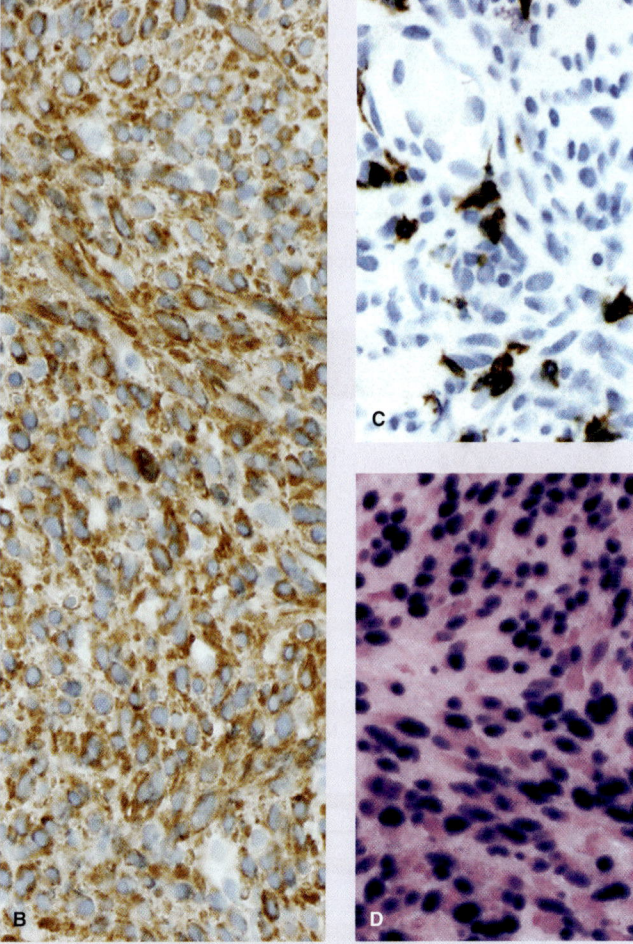

lower extremity edema, while those patients with a tumor in the superior portion present with Budd–Chiari syndrome (hepatomegaly, jaundice and ascites). Tumors in the lower inferior vena cava may be treated surgically, whereas those in the upper portion are usually unresectable. Overall, the long-term outcome is poor.

Epstein-Barr Virus associated smooth muscle tumor (**EBVSMT**) is a rare entity. Although it has been known for some time that smooth muscle tumors are more common in immunocompromised individuals, the link between EBV infection and these tumors was first described in 1995. EBVSMTs usually develop in children in sites such as soft tissue, liver, lung, spleen, and dura. Morphologically, these tumors are less pleomorphic than traditional leiomyosarcoma. Studies suggest that multifocal lesions are the result of multiple infections rather than metastases. Even with multiple lesions, EBVSMT has a better prognosis than leiomyosarcoma.

SKELETAL MUSCLE
Normal Histology

One of the key roles of skeletal muscle is locomotion. Skeletal muscle cells are specialized for the function of movement. Myoblasts are the most immature skeletal muscle cell. These are small mononuclear cells with granular cytoplasm but no microscopically detectable filaments. Myoblasts fuse to form myotubes that contain multiple centrally placed nuclei and cytoplasmic filaments including desmin and vimentin. During development, myofibrils enlarge and become more numerous, and eventually cross-striations can be seen. Myotubes eventually differentiate into muscle fibers, syncytial-like units with a cylindrical shape, peripheral nuclei and filaments arranged in sarcomeres. Sarcomeres are the contractile unit of skeletal muscle they are composed of parallel arrays of two types of myofilaments: actin (thin, 50–70 nm in diameter) and myosin (thick 140–160 nm in diameter) (Figure 18-19).

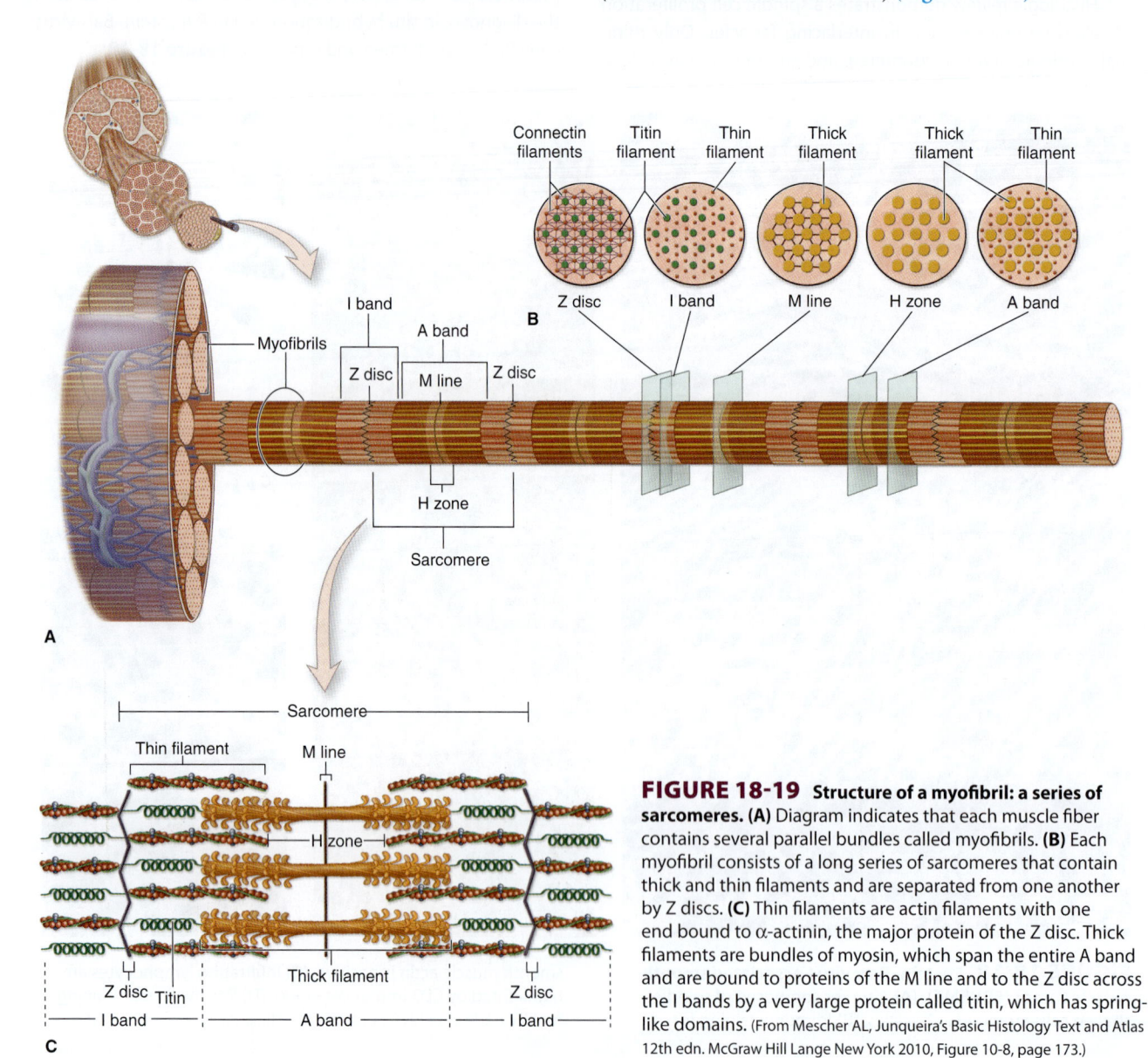

FIGURE 18-19 Structure of a myofibril: a series of sarcomeres. (A) Diagram indicates that each muscle fiber contains several parallel bundles called myofibrils. **(B)** Each myofibril consists of a long series of sarcomeres that contain thick and thin filaments and are separated from one another by Z discs. **(C)** Thin filaments are actin filaments with one end bound to α-actinin, the major protein of the Z disc. Thick filaments are bundles of myosin, which span the entire A band and are bound to proteins of the M line and to the Z disc across the I bands by a very large protein called titin, which has spring-like domains. (From Mescher AL, Junqueira's Basic Histology Text and Atlas 12th edn. McGraw Hill Lange New York 2010, Figure 10-8, page 173.)

SOFT TISSUE AND BONE PATHOLOGY   499

CASE 18-5

A 3-year-old male presents with a paratesticular mass.

Histologic sections show a cellular neoplasm adjacent to seminal vesicle. Alternating cellular and myxoid areas are evident at low power. The neoplastic cells have high N:C ratios and exhibit marked cytologic atypia. A myogenin stain highlights a proportion of the lesional nuclei. These findings are consistent with **embryonal rhabdomyosarcoma** (Figure 18-20).

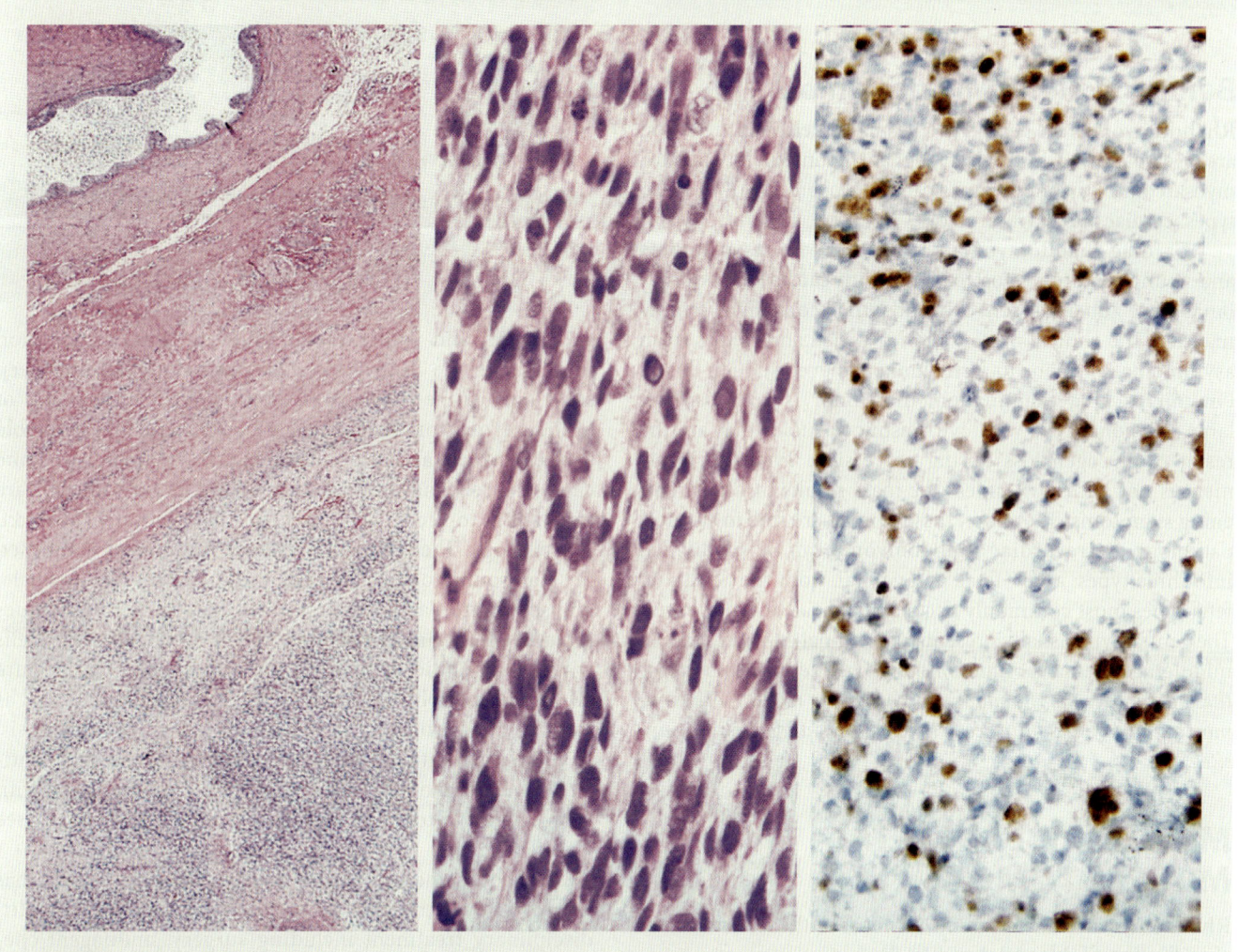

FIGURE 18-20 Embryonal rhabdomyosarcoma. Left (low-power view) shows tumor mass with cellular and myxoid areas adjacent to a seminal vesicle (upper part of image). Middle (high-power view) shows neoplastic cells with marked cellular atypia and a high N:C ratio. Right shows positive myogenin immunostain supporting the diagnosis.

QUICK REVIEW

Rules for Skeletal Muscle Neoplasms

1. Unlike other categories of soft tissue tumors, malignant skeletal muscle tumors outnumber benign ones.
2. Common sites for rhabdomyosarcomas are genitourinary tract and head/neck. Rhabdomyosarcoma is the most common soft tissue sarcoma in children under 15 years of age and should be included in the differential diagnosis of a mass at one of those sites in an infant or young child.
3. Microscopic clues to skeletal muscle differentiation in poorly differentiated tumors include eosinophilic cytoplasm, cross-striations, and immunohistochemical staining for myogenic markers. Immunohistochemical tools can be helpful in proving skeletal muscle differentiation. Desmin is an intermediate filament protein found in both smooth and skeletal muscle. Desmin is the most sensitive marker for skeletal muscle differentiation but it is not specific as smooth muscle cells as well as different types of nonmuscle cells may be positive. Myogenin and MyoD1 are nuclear

transcription factors and are more specific but less sensitive for skeletal muscle tumors. It is important to remember that myogenin and MyoD1 are nuclear stains, and only nuclear positivity should be considered as evidence of skeletal muscle differentiation (Figure 18-20).

Benign Skeletal Muscle Tumors

Rhabdomyomas are benign neoplasms of skeletal muscle, and are overshadowed by their malignant counterpart, rhabdomyosarcoma. Rhabdomyomas can be broken down into two types: cardiac and extracardiac.

Cardiac rhabdomyoma occurs in the hearts of infants and young children. Most patients with cardiac rhabdomyomas have tuberous sclerosis and other congenital abnormalities. The clinical presentation is varied and ranges from asymptomatic lesions to arrhythmia and even sudden death. On microscopic examination, the tumor is composed of large polygonal cells with cytoplasmic vacuoles that are the result of glycogen loss during processing. Typically, treatment is not necessary unless the mass results in life-threatening symptoms. Therefore, these tumors are rare in surgical pathology. **Extracardiac rhabdomyoma** can be subdivided into three types: adult, fetal, and genital. Both the adult and fetal types most commonly occur in the head and neck area. The genital type usually presents as a vaginal or vulva mass in middle-aged females. *Caution should be exercised in making these diagnoses, as rhabdomyosarcomas are much more common and also frequently occur in head/neck and genitourinary sites.*

MALIGNANT SKELETAL MUSCLE TUMORS

Rhabdomyosarcoma accounts for most of the lesions in this classification (Tables 18-4 and 18-5).

Embryonal rhabdomyosarcoma is most common in children younger than 10 year of age but may also affect

TABLE 18-4 Classification of rhabdomyosarcoma.

Rhabdomyosarcoma
Embryonal rhabdomyosarcoma
Botryoid rhabdomyosarcoma
Spindle cell/Sclerosing rhabdomyosarcoma
Anaplastic rhabdomyosarcoma
Alveolar rhabdomyosarcoma
Pleomorphic rhabdomyosarcoma

TABLE 18-5 Characteristics of embryonal and alveolar rhabdomyosarcoma.

	Embryonal RMS	Alveolar RMS
Age	Young children (0–15 years)	Adolescents
Site	Head/neck, GU tract	Extremities
Morphology	Small round blue cell	Small round blue cells
IHC	Desmin, myogenin and myoD1 positive	Desmin, myogenin and myoD1 positive
Cytogenetics	No recurrent abnormalities	t(1;13) and t(2;13)
Prognosis	Better prognosis	Worse prognosis

adolescents and young adults. These tumors are common in sites like the head/neck, genitourinary tract, and deep soft tissue of the extremities. The histologic appearance of rhabdomyosarcoma is extremely variable and may resemble skeletal muscle at any point during development. In some cases, the cells may be so poorly differentiated that they are impossible to recognize as skeletal muscle based on H&E morphology. The least differentiated tumors are composed of small round to spindled cells with hyperchromatic nuclei and scant cytoplasm. In these cases, helpful histologic clues include alternating densely packed and myxoid areas, cells with eosinophilic cytoplasm, and cross-striations (Figure 18-20). Immunohistochemistry can be an invaluable tool as staining for myogenin or MyoD1 confirms the diagnosis. In more differentiated tumors, rhabdomyoblasts are identified. Rhabdomyoblasts are larger round to ovoid cells with eosinophilic cytoplasm with a granular appearance (see Case 18-5).

The outcome of patients with rhabdomyosarcoma has improved over the past several decades because of multi-disciplinary treatment including surgery, multiagent chemotherapy, and radiotherapy. Prognosis is often dependent on many factors such as anatomic site, extent of disease (metastasis, lymph node involvement), and histologic subtype.

Botryoid-type rhabdomyosarcoma is a subtype of embryonal rhabdomyosarcoma with some unique features. It presents as a polypoid "grape-like" mass and affects mucosa-lined hollow organs such as the urinary bladder, vagina, and nasal cavity.

Alveolar rhabdomyosarcomas account for approximately one-third of rhabdomyosarcoma. They typically occur in a slightly older age group (adolescents) than those affected by embryonal rhabdomyosarcoma. Alveolar rhabdomyosarcomas frequently occur in deep soft tissue of the extremities as well as in the head/neck and genitourinary tracts. They are characterized by nests and loosely cohesive aggregates of small round blue cells separated by fibrous bands. The cells usually cling to the fibrous septa at the edge of the nests and become discohesive toward the center, mimicking the morphology of alveolar spaces (Figure 18-21 left). Another interesting difference between alveolar and embryonal subtypes is that alveolar rhabdomyosarcoma frequently has distinctive cytogenetic abnormalities.

Pleomorphic rhabdomyosarcoma is an uncommon tumor that usually affects adults with peak incidence in the fifth decade. The most sites include deep soft tissue, abdomen, chest wall, and retroperitoneum. These tumors are usually large with hemorrhage and necrosis. Microscopic examination reveals large atypical cells with hyperchromatic nuclei and brightly eosinophilic cytoplasm. Cytoplasmic eosinophilia is often the most helpful clue to the diagnosis that can be confirmed by staining for myoD1 or myogenin. Desmin staining alone is not confirmative since leiomyosarcoma may be positive for this marker. These tumors are clinically aggressive with patients often developing early metastases (Figure 18-21 right).

Spindle cell/Sclerosing rhabdomyosarcoma is an evolving subtype. The pediatric population seems to have a favorable outcome while cases in adults behave more aggressively.

> **IN TRANSLATION**
>
> Most alveolar rhabdomyosarcomas are characterized by a t(2;13)(q35;q14) translocation resulting in a PAX3-FKHR fusion gene. A smaller percentage of tumors have a t(1;13)(p36;q14) translocation creating a PAX7-FKHR fusion. Therefore, cytogenetics can be a helpful ancillary tool when the diagnosis is in doubt.

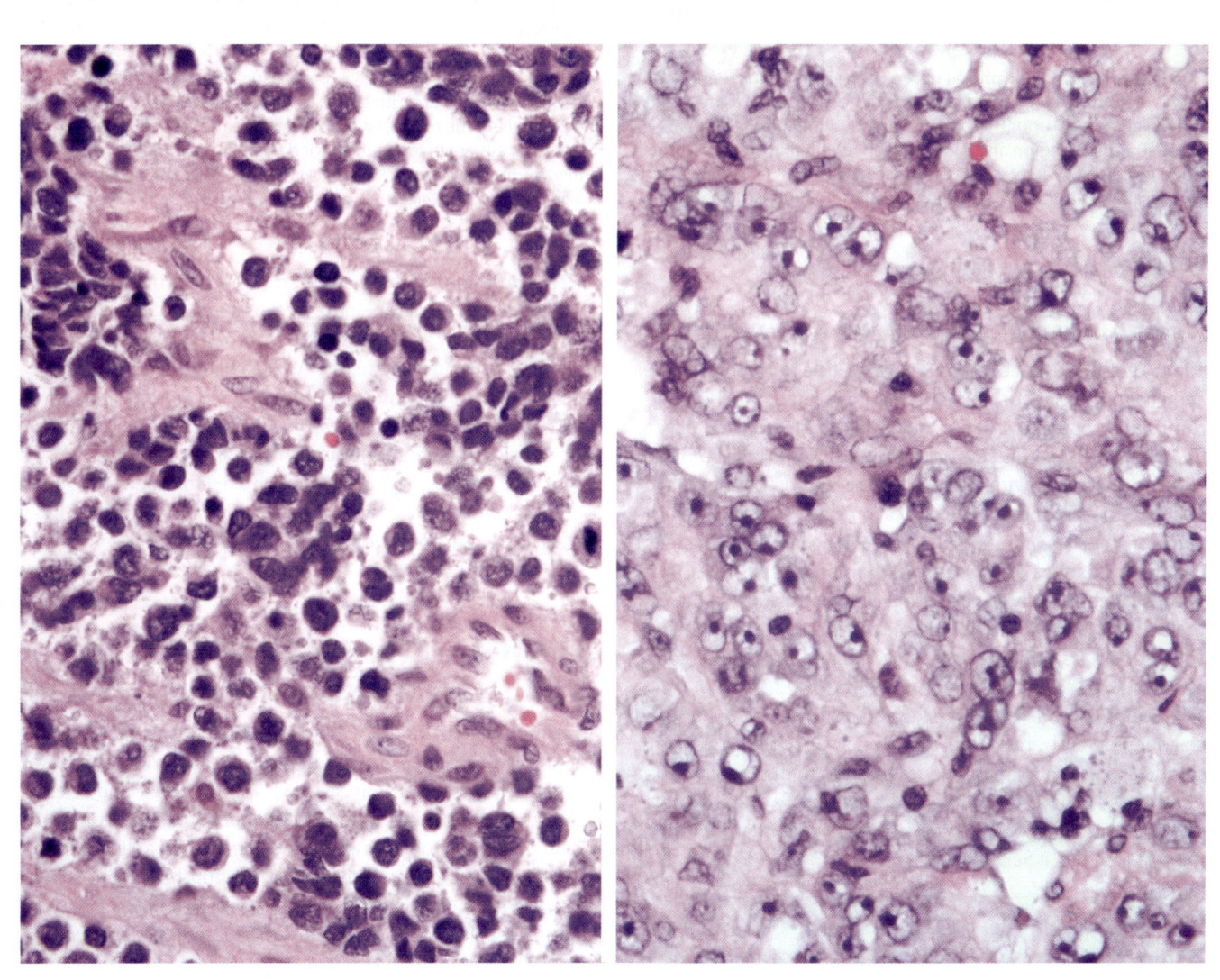

FIGURE 18-21 Variants of rhabdomyosarcomas. Alveolar rhabdomyosarcoma (left): Nests of loosely cohesive small round blue cells appear to cluster to septae at the edge of nests giving an "alveolar" appearance. Pleomorphic rhabdomyosarcoma (right): Malignant cells are large, polygonal in shape and tend to have marked eosinophilic cytoplasm. Atypical nuclei are prominent, vesicular, and may have prominent nucleoli.

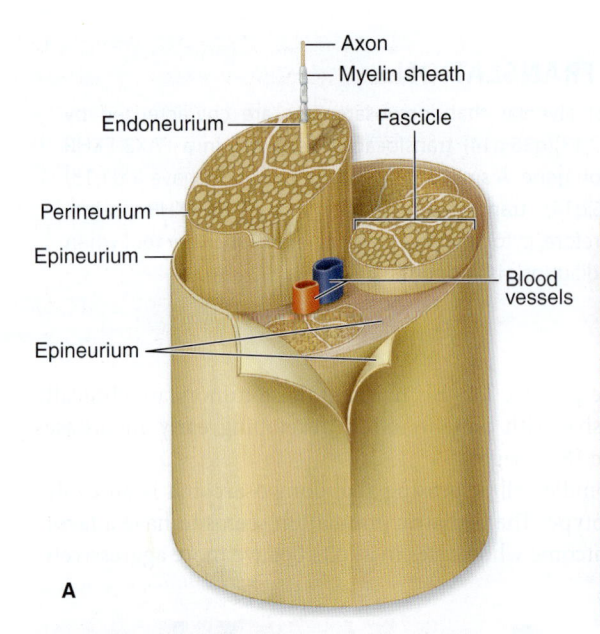

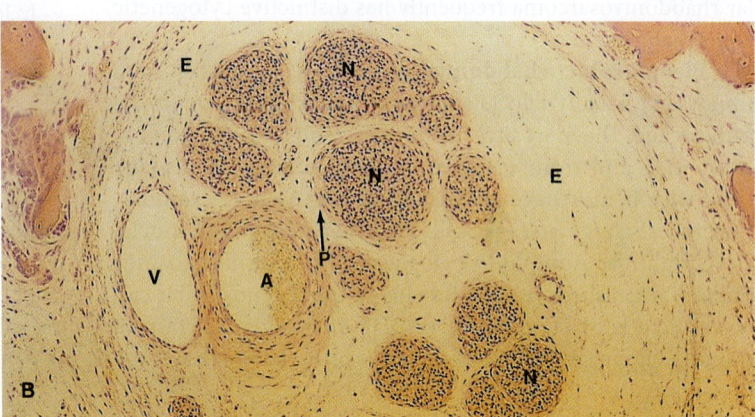

FIGURE 18-22 **Peripheral nerve connective tissue.** Peripheral nerves are protected by three layers of connective tissue, as depicted in the diagrams **(A)** and **(B)**: The outer epineurium (E) consists of a dense superficial region and a looser deep region that contains large blood vessels (A,V) and fascicles in which nerve fibers (N) are bundled. Each fascicle is surrounded by the perineurium (P), consisting of a few layers of unusual epithelial-like fibroblastic cells that are all joined at the peripheries by tight junctions to form a blood–nerve barrier that helps regulate the microenvironment inside the fascicle. Axons and Schwann cells are in turn surrounded by a thin layer of endoneurium. (From Mescher AL, Junqueira's Basic Histology Text and Atlas 12th edn. McGraw Hill Lange New York 2010, Figure 9-26, page 162.)

PERIPHERAL NERVE

Normal Histology

There are three main components of mature peripheral nerve: epineurium, perineurium, and endoneurium. The epineurium is the outermost layer and consists of collagen, elastic fibers, mast cells, and several nerve fascicles. The size of the epineurium varies with location of the nerve. The next layer is the perineurium that envelops each nerve fascicle. The perineurium consists of multiple layers of concentrically arranged flattened cells that are thought to be fibroblastic. By immunohistochemistry, these perineural cells express EMA. Finally, the smallest unit of the peripheral nerve is the endoneurium which encircles individual nerve fibers and is made of collagen, blood vessels, and fibroblasts (Figure 18-22).

Axons are encased by Schwann cells that provide crucial support and protection for the nerve. Schwann cells are spindled cells that sometimes are difficult to distinguish from fibroblasts on H&E morphology. Schwann cells are S100 positive, and this feature is very helpful in proving that the cell of interest is in fact a Schwann cell.

> ### QUICK REVIEW
> **Rules for Peripheral Nerve Diagnosis**
> 1. Tumor of peripheral nerve can mirror any element of the peripheral nerve (Schwann cells, fibroblasts, perineural cells, mixture of elements).
> 2. Immunohistochemistry can be helpful in confirming the derivation of the tumor. For example, a spindle cell lesion may be composed of fibroblasts, smooth muscle, or neural elements. An S100 stain would support Schwannian differentiation in the appropriate morphologic context, and would help make the diagnosis of a peripheral nerve sheath tumor.
> 3. Benign nerve sheath tumors are one of the few groups of benign soft tissue tumors that may undergo malignant transformation.

BENIGN PERIPHERAL NERVE TUMORS

Traumatic neuroma is a nonneoplastic but exuberant proliferation of nerve elements in response to prior trauma or surgery. When a nerve is severed, the proximal end tries to re-establish continuity with the distal portion. However, if the distal portion is too far away or does not exist, a disorganized proliferation of axons, Schwann cells, fibroblasts, and blood vessels results. Occasionally these lesions are painful, but the main clinical concern is usually to rule out recurrence of a neoplasm when these occur at the site of a previous cancer resection.

Schwannomas are one of the two main types of peripheral nerve sheath tumors (neurofibroma is the second). These

CASE 18-6

A 25-year-old woman presents with a 5 cm neck mass.

The gross specimen consisted of a well-encapsulated mass with a partially solid and partially cystic cut surface. Histologic review showed a spindle cell neoplasm surrounded by a thick fibrous capsule. Hypercellular areas (Antoni A) are composed of uniform spindle cells with hyperchromatic, wavy nuclei alternating with less cellular regions. Thick-walled, hyalinized vessels were scattered throughout the tumor. An immunohistochemical stain for S100 was strongly and diffusely positive. The clinical, morphologic, and immunophenotypic features are classic for **schwannoma** (Figure 18-23).

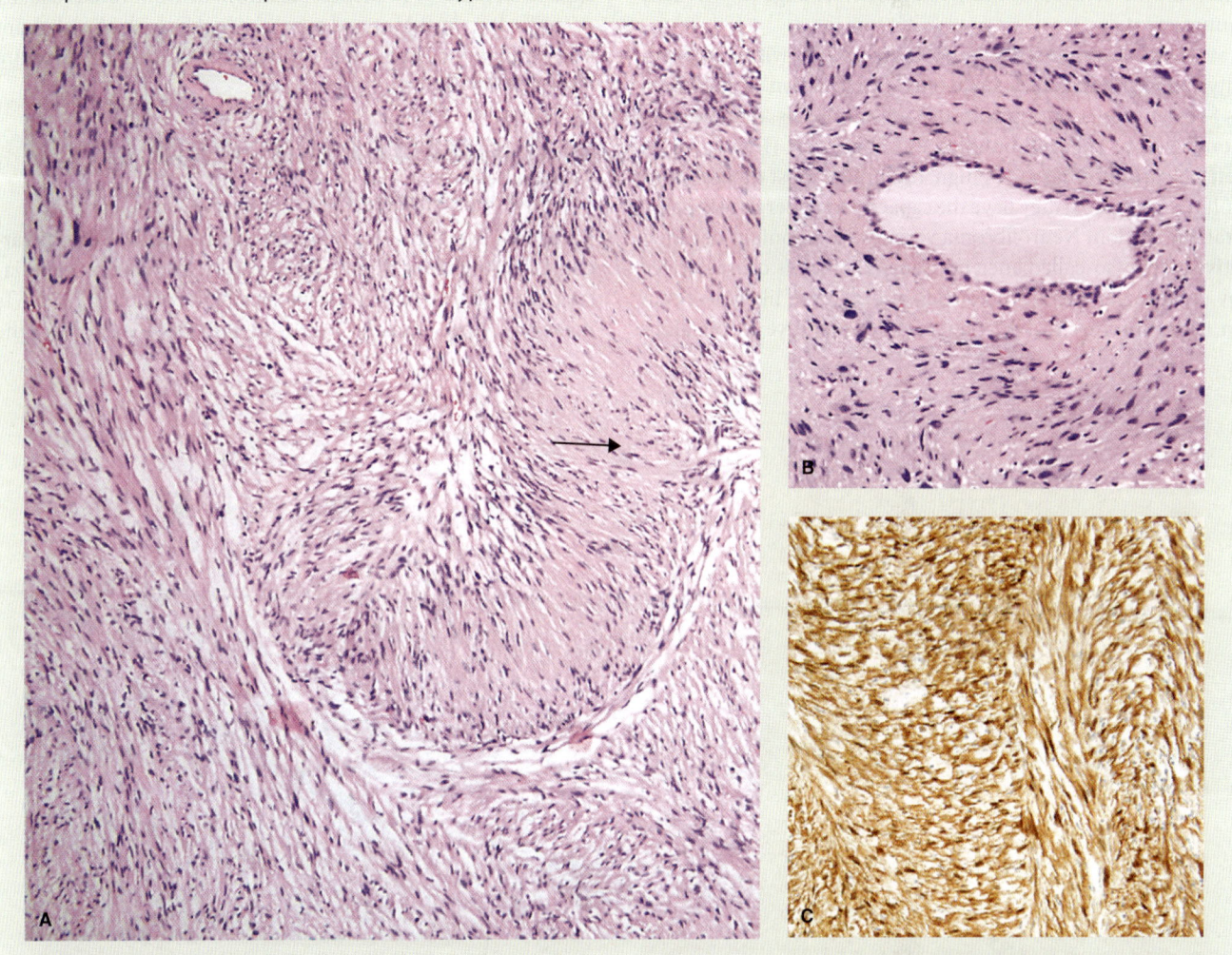

FIGURE 18-23 Schwannoma. **(A)** Spindle cell neoplasm demonstrating a hypercellular pattern of growth (Antoni A pattern) and a characteristic Verocay body consisting of two palisading columns of nuclei separating an amorphous area of fibrillary cell processes (arrow). **(B)** Characteristic hyalinized vessel within tumor. **(C)** S100 immunostaining characteristic of Schwann cells.

tumors are composed entirely of Schwann cells. Schwannomas occur most commonly in early to middle-aged adults. Head, neck, and flexor surfaces of the extremities are favored sites, although these tumors may also arise at other sites including the retroperitoneum and mediastinum. These tumors are slowly growing and usually do not cause any clinical symptoms unless they become large. Grossly, schwannomas are surrounded by epineurium, so they are truly encapsulated. Sectioning reveals a solid pink-tan cut surface with areas of cystic degeneration and calcification possible in older or larger lesions. Microscopically, the classic findings of this neoplasm are an alternating pattern of Antoni A and Antoni B areas. Antoni A areas are cellular and composed of spindled cells with nuclear palisading and Verocay bodies (two compact columns of nuclei separated by fibrillary cell processes). Antoni B areas consist of a disorganized arrangement of spindled cells in a background of collagen and inflammatory cells. Cystic change may be evident in these areas. Additionally, gaping thick-walled hyalinized vessels are a characteristic feature of schwannoma and often can provide a clue to the diagnosis in small biopsy specimens. Since these tumors are composed of Schwann cells, they are diffusely S100 positive (Figure 18-23). Schwannomas are benign tumors and simple excision is curative. Recurrences are very infrequent and, unlike neurofibromas, malignant change is virtually nonexistent.

Neurofibromas stain for S100 but usually with less intensity than schwannomas since only a proportion of the lesion is Schwann cells. Along with the Schwann cells, this tumor is composed of collagen bundles and fibroblasts (Figure 18-24 left). Neurofibromas are benign, but unlike most other benign soft tissue tumors, they have the capacity to undergo malignant transformation. Neurofibroma variants may contain degenerative atypia (so-called ancient change), which is characterized by enlarged, pleomorphic nuclei, and is more likely to occur in neurofibromas in NF1 patients. Degenerative atypia alone does not equate with malignancy, but should prompt a more extensive examination (Figure 18-24 right).

Plexiform neurofibroma is a unique type of neurofibroma because it is pathognomonic of Neurofibromatosis I (NF1). Therefore, the diagnosis should be made cautiously because of clinical implications. This form of neurofibroma is characterized by a gross appearance often referred to as "a bag of worms." Microscopically these lesions consist of tortuous expansion of nerve branches. Plexiform neurofibromas usually occur in deep locations and are at the highest risk of malignant transformation. Occasionally, these tumors can affect an entire limb causing marked disfigurement.

MALIGNANT PERIPHERAL NERVE TUMORS

Malignant peripheral nerve sheath tumors (MPNSTs) are sarcomas arising from peripheral nerves or showing differentiation of any element of the nerve sheath. Even though MPNSTs make up approximately 5–10% of soft tissue sarcomas, the

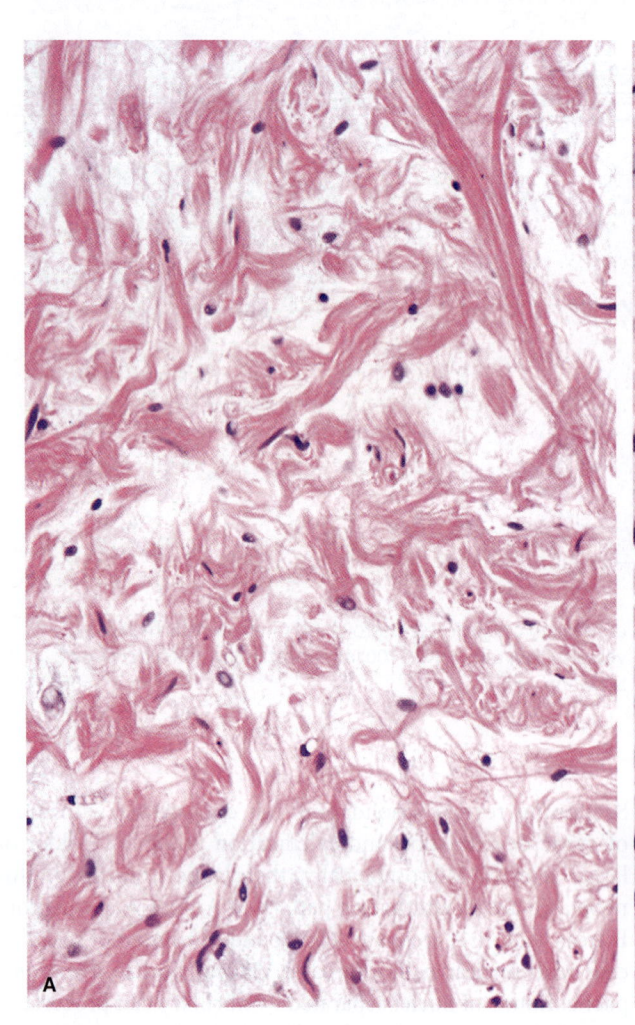

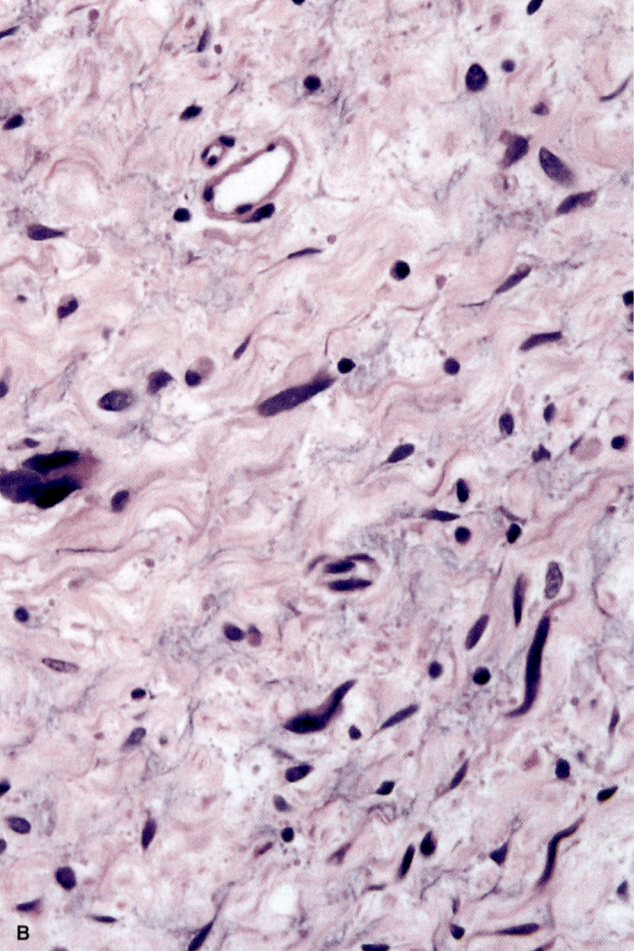

FIGURE 18-24 Neurofibroma. **(A)** Characteristic spindle cells with wavy hyperchromatic nuclei are scattered in a background of collagen bundles. **(B)** Neurofibroma shows degenerative atypia ("ancient change"). The myxoid background contains degenerating cells with enlarged hyperchromatic nuclei.

diagnosis of MPNST is often one of exclusion because there is no specific, reproducible morphologic, immunohistochemical, or molecular marker for this tumor. However, when a spindle cell sarcoma arises from a peripheral nerve or arises from a preexisting neurofibroma, one can usually be confident of the diagnosis. About one quarter to one half of MPNST arise in patients with NF1. Hence, enlargement or pain of a mass in a patient with NF1 should cause clinical concern for an MPNST. Grossly, these tumors are large and fleshy with frequent hemorrhage and necrosis. Microscopically MPNST is usually a high

HUNTING FOR ZEBRAS

A 45-year-old woman recently noted a small painless nodule on her tongue.

Sections show a submucosal lesion composed of nests of lightly eosinophilic cells with granular cytoplasm. The overlying epithelium appears acanthotic (thickened) without atypia. The clinical and morphologic features are consistent with **granular cell tumor** (Figure 18-25).

Initially granular cell tumors were thought to be of muscular differentiation. However, immunophenotypic and ultrastructural examination revealed that they are neural in origin. These benign tumors are common in middle adulthood and are more common in females than males. They may present in virtually any location including dermis, subcutis, submucosa, within muscle, or within visceral organs. Most are solitary and painless. Gross examination reveals a poorly circumscribed mass. Histologic review demonstrates a proliferation of polygonal cells with granular eosinophilic cytoplasm. The granular nature of the cytoplasm is the result of PAS-positive phagolysosomes. These tumors stain for S100 protein and other neural markers. These tumors are benign, and simple excision is the treatment of choice. It is not uncommon to see epithelial hyperplasia overlying these lesions. This may be so striking that the lesion may be mistaken for squamous cell carcinoma in the absence of recognition of the associated granular cell tumor.

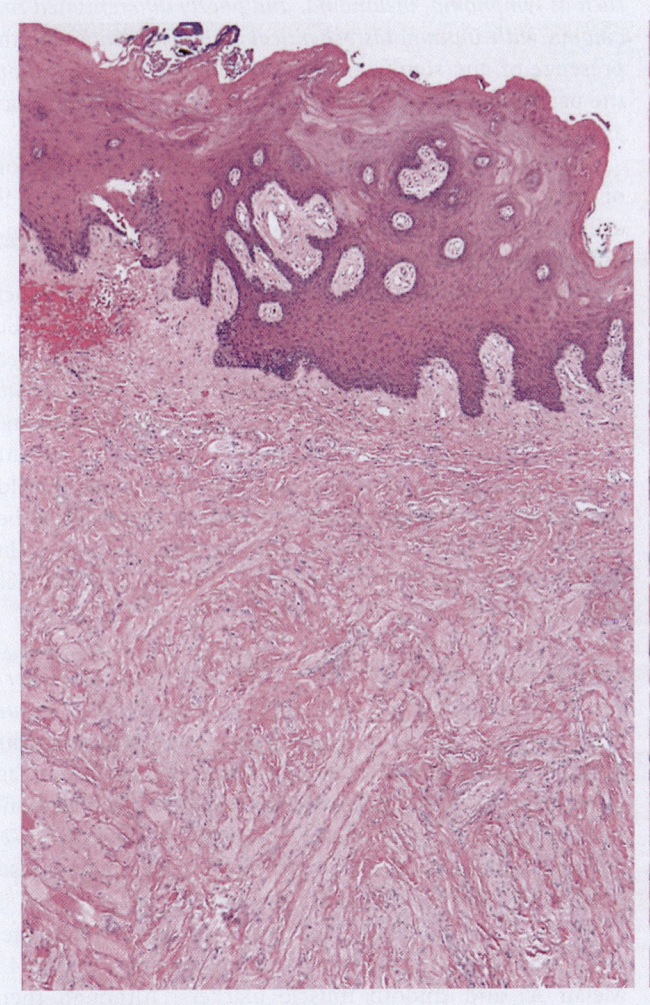

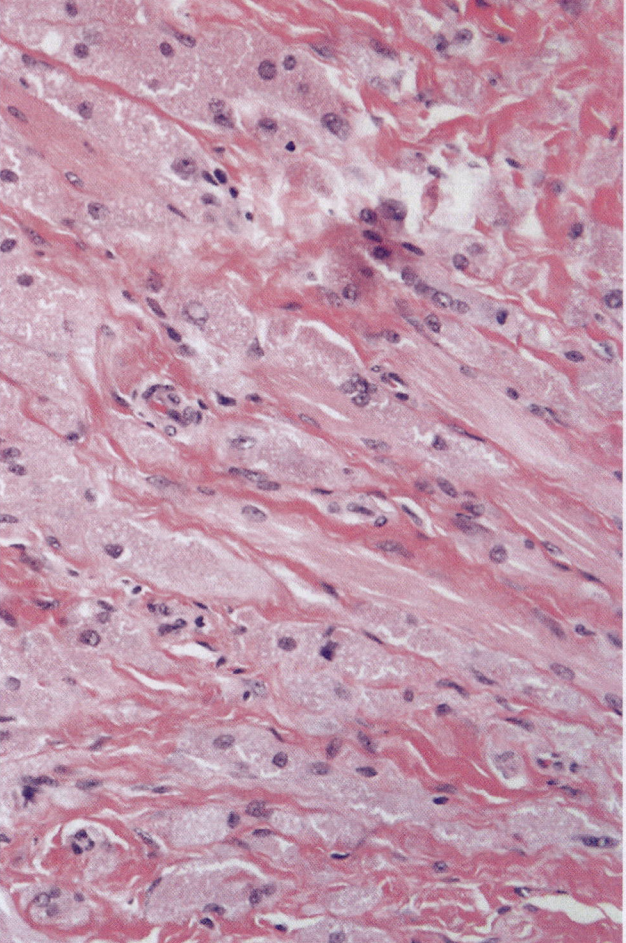

FIGURE 18-25 Granular cell tumor. Left (low-power view) shows a submucosal lesion with a thickened (acanthotic) overlying epithelium that shows no atypia. The neoplasm appears as cellular nests separated by collagen fibers. Right (high-power view) demonstrates nests of polygonal cells that have the granular eosinophilic cytoplasm characteristic of this neoplasm.

grade spindle cell tumor with fascicular growth. The neoplastic cells are typically spindled to fusiform in shape with high N:C ratios. Some lesions exhibit a marbled low-power appearance with alternating cellular and myxoid areas. Other tumors display increased cellularity in subendothelial zones. However, morphologic features are nonspecific and overlap with other spindle cell sarcomas. S100 is usually only weakly positive focally but may be entirely negative. Without the correct clinical context (arising from a nerve or preexisting neurofibroma), electron microscopy is the only way to prove nerve sheath differentiation. In the absence of such, MPNST becomes a diagnosis of exclusion. These tumors are highly aggressive sarcomas with the ability recur locally and metastasize.

SOFT TISSUE TUMORS OF UNCERTAIN DIFFERENTIATION

Introduction

Despite advances in immunohistochemical, cytogenetic, and molecular techniques, as well as, a better understanding of many soft tissue tumors, there are many entities in which the lineage remains unclear. Nevertheless, such tumors can be reproducibly diagnosed and sometimes a prognosis is determined. These "uncertain" tumors have distinct morphologic or molecular findings that aide in the diagnostic process.

Variants: This classification includes intramuscular myxoma, acral myxoinflammatory fibroblastic sarcoma, solitary fibrous tumor (SFT), perivascular epithelioid cell tumor (PEComa), synovial sarcoma, and desmoplastic small round cell tumor.

Intramuscular myxoma is a benign neoplasm that usually occurs in mid-to-late adult life and is more common in females than in males. Patients usually present with a painless mass at sites such as the proximal extremities, buttocks, and shoulder. Grossly these tumors have a glistening gray-white appearance and sectioning reveals gelatinous material. Although appearing circumscribed at low power, they typically infiltrate adjacent muscle. Histologic examination reveals an intramuscular mass composed of spindled to stellate-shaped cells with small but dark, pyknotic nuclei in a mucoid or myxoid stroma. Occasional thin-walled blood vessels are observed. These tumors are benign and rarely recur after resection. The lesional cells seem to be fibroblastic in origin but lineage remains uncertain.

Some patients may present with multiple intramuscular myxomas in the same region of the body. Almost all of these patients will have Mazabraud syndrome that includes a constellation of intramuscular myxomas and fibrous dysplasia most commonly of the femur and pelvis. Usually, the fibrous dysplasia is detected years before the intramuscular myxomas are evident. The intramuscular myxomas in Mazabraud syndrome are histologically identical to the sporadic forms.

Acral myxoinflammatory fibroblastic sarcoma (inflammatory myxohyaline tumor of the distal extremities with virocyte or Reed-Sternberg-like cells) frequently present in middle-to-late adulthood, usually in the distal extremities. Grossly the tumor is poorly circumscribed with a gelatinous cut surface. They usually are between 1 and 8 cm. These neoplasms have a variety of histologic patterns. Myxoid and hyalinized zones alternate with areas of marked chronic inflammation. Sometimes germinal centers are present. In cellular areas, bizarre, strikingly atypical cells are found. These worrisome cells have large nuclei and prominent nucleoli and bear resemblance to Reed-Sternberg cells. Sometimes the macronucleoli are sufficiently large so as to raise suspicion for a viral infection. Occasionally, vacuolated cells morphologically similar to lipoblasts are noted. Despite the alarming cytologic features of this lesion, the mitotic rate is low (Figure 18-26). These lesions appear to be capable of local recurrence. Wide local excision without chemotherapy or radiotherapy is the treatment of choice. *When one encounters a lesion like this, it is important to rule out entities such as lymphoma, melanoma, and poorly differentiated carcinoma with immunohistochemical stains. Additionally, the presence of any significant mitotic activity should prompt the pathologist to consider a fully malignant sarcoma such as myxofibrosarcoma* (Figure 18-13 right).

Solitary fibroma tumors (SFT) are mesenchymal tumors of uncertain differentiation composed of ovoid to spindle cells surrounding a branching vasculature. Variable stromal hyalinization is present.

The behavior of the SFT family of tumors is unpredictable. Approximately 10–15% will behave aggressively, but such behavior does not correlate with morphologic features. *Because the criteria for malignancy are not well established, the diagnosis of "benign SFT" is never made.* Although even bland-appearing tumors may metastasize, a mitotic count of greater than or equal to 4 per 10 high-power fields is suggestive of the potential for malignant behavior. Other findings including large tumor size, necrosis, increase cellularity, and cytologic atypia should also prompt closer clinical follow-up.

Perivascular cell tumors (PEComas) are a group of neoplasms composed of perivascular epithelioid cells. *Perivascular epithelioid cells (PECs) have no known counterpart in nonneoplastic tissue and are recognized only in tumors.* This group of cells is characterized by a typically radial perivascular location. PECs have pale eosinophilic cytoplasm and may be spindled or epithelioid in morphology (Figure 18-27 left). Occasionally, PECs may acquire lipid in their cytoplasm and mimic adipocytic cells. The immunophenotype of PECs is also unusual: myelomelanocytic in that they often stain for a combination of melanocytic (HMB-45, Melan A) and smooth muscle markers. Although there are several theories as to the derivation of PECs including neural crest lineage, the true origin of these cells remains uncertain.

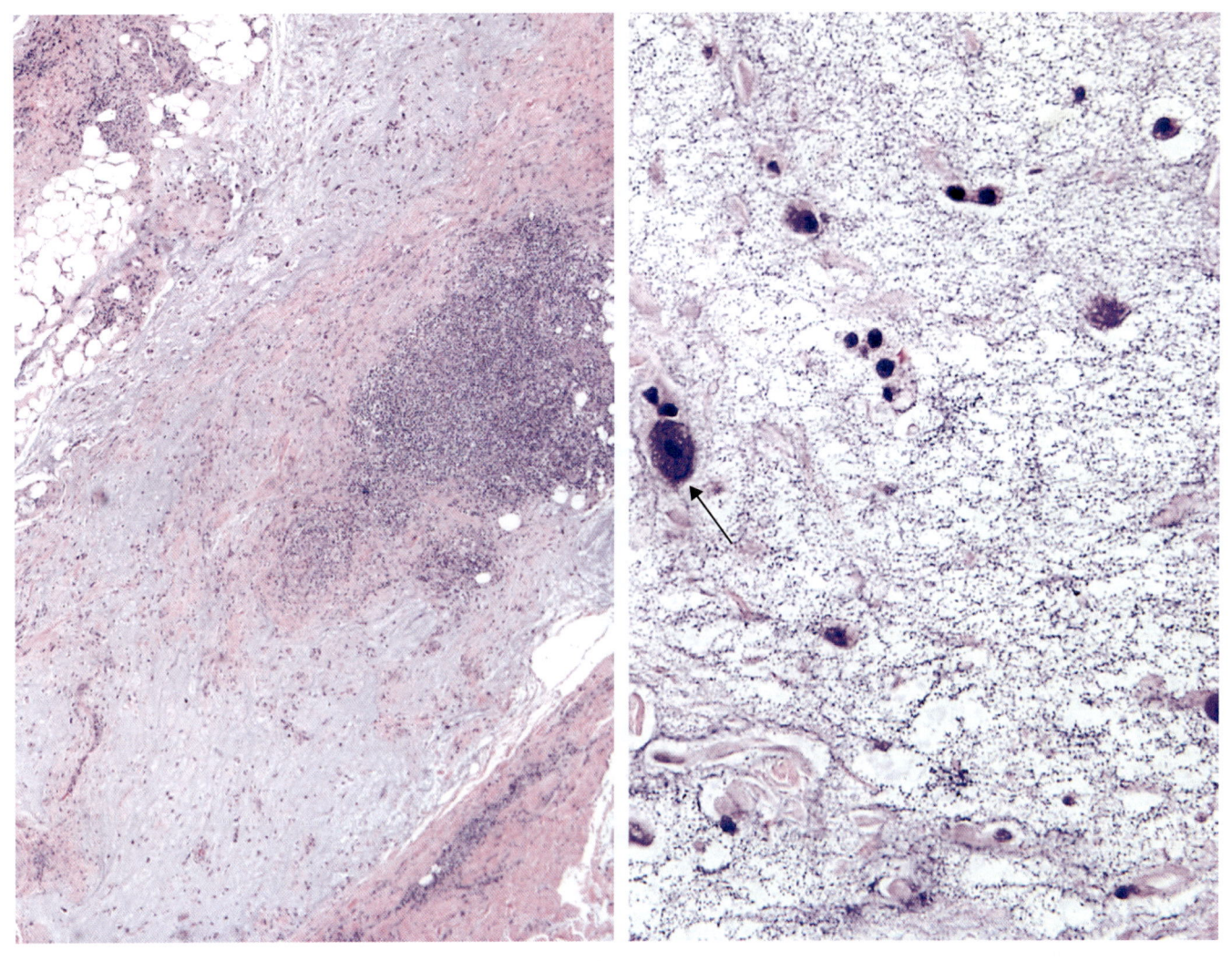

FIGURE 18-26 Acral myxoinflammatory fibroblastic sarcoma (inflammatory myxohyaline tumor of the distal extremities with virocytes or Reed-Sternberg-like cells). Left (low-power view) shows a nodular myxoid tumor with areas of intense inflammation. Right (high-power view) demonstrates a bizarre tumor cell in a myxoid area (arrow). The cell has a vesicular nucleus with a large prominent nucleolus.

Synovial sarcoma is a malignant soft tissue tumor that, despite its name, *does not* arise from synovium but rather is of unknown origin. This tumor typically affects young adults and tends to arise in deep soft tissue sites near joints. Common sites include knee, ankle, and foot. The mass may be present for several years before the patient presents for clinical workup, often after noting rapid growth. Sometimes, the lesion is misdiagnosed as a chronic inflammatory condition for a period of time before the correct diagnosis is made. The gross appearance of the tumor depends on the rate of growth. Slowly growing tumors tend to be more circumscribed than rapidly growing lesions. Cyst formation, hemorrhage, necrosis, and calcification may present. The latter provides a diagnostic clue in radiographic studies. Synovial sarcoma may be monophasic (having only a spindle cell population) or biphasic (also forming epithelial structures). The epithelial cells are characterized by cuboidal to columnar cells organized in cords, nests, or glands. The spindle cells have plump, hyperchromatic nuclei, scant cytoplasm and are arranged in a fascicular (herringbone) growth pattern. Mast cells, branching blood vessels, and areas of stromal hyalinization may be noted. Immunohistochemical stains may be helpful as these tumors typically stain for cytokeratins focally and are negative for CD34. MPNST (almost always the other main consideration in the diagnosis) can be differentiated from synovial sarcomas using cytogenetic and molecular techniques. Synovial sarcomas consistently have a balanced reciprocal translocation between the *SYT* gene on chromosome 18 and either the *SSX1* or *SSX2* gene on the X chromosome. This abnormality can be detected with cytogenetic studies or with fluorescence in situ hybridization or RT-PCR techniques on paraffin embedded tissue. The prognosis for patients with synovial sarcoma is variable, and there are numerous clinical and morphologic variables that affect

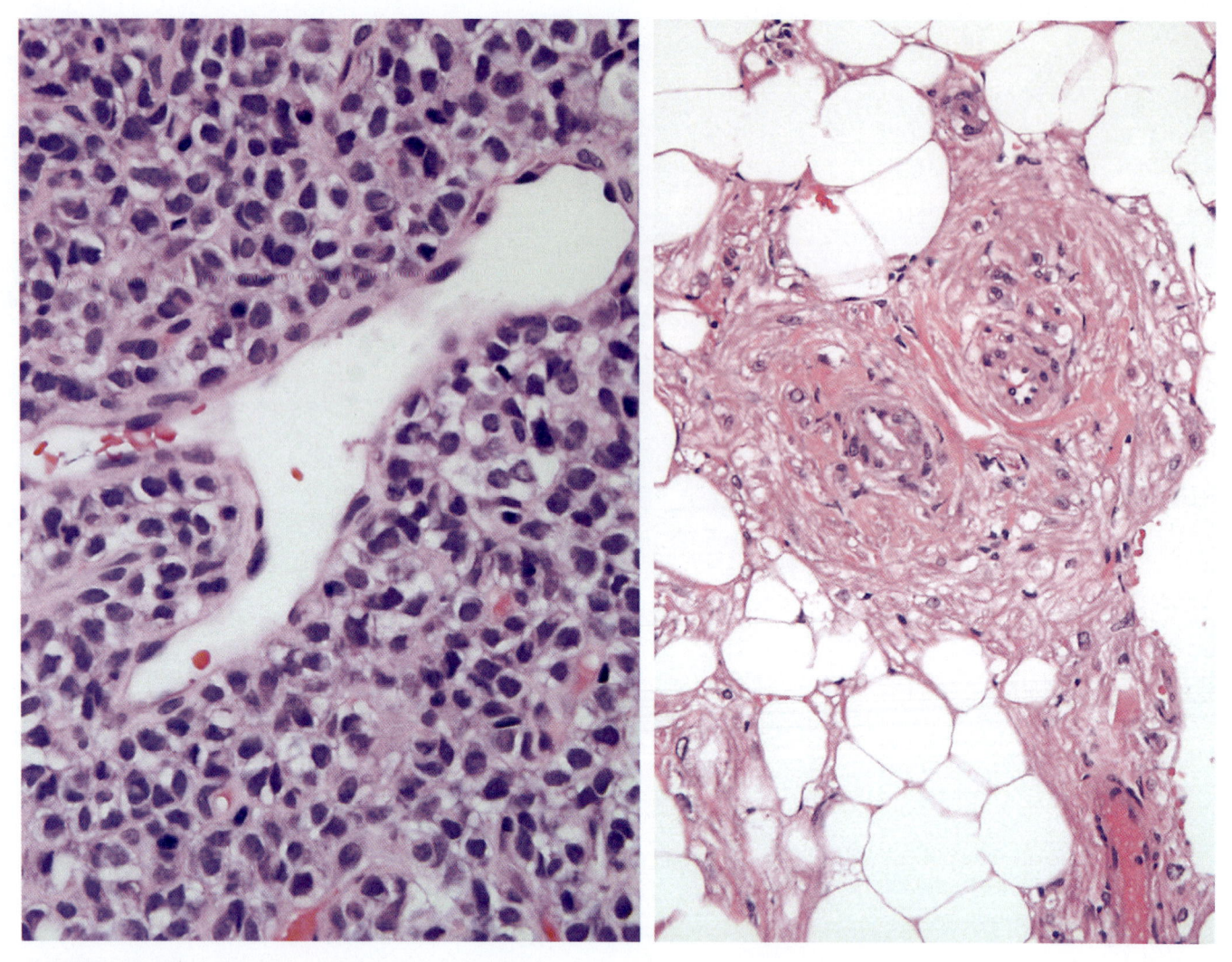

FIGURE 18-27 **Solitary fibrous tumor (left).** A patternless proliferation of round to ovoid neoplastic cells with a characteristic ectatic staghorn-shaped vessel. Perivascular cell tumor (PEComa) (right) showing a proliferation of spindle to epithelioid-shaped cells arranged around blood vessels.

survival such as age, location, size, amount of calcification, and poorly differentiated areas.

Desmoplastic small round cell tumor (DSRCT) most commonly affects male patients between the ages of 15 and 35. Most patients present with a large pelvic/abdominal mass with extensive peritoneal involvement that causes abdominal distention and constipation. Microscopic examination reveals well-demarcated nests of neoplastic cells with central necrosis embedded in a fibrotic or desmoplastic stroma (Figure 18-28). The lesional cells have high nuclear:cytoplasmic ratios, hyperchromatic nuclei, and eosinophilic cytoplasm. One of the unique features of this tumor is its immunoprofile. The neoplastic cells frequently stain for markers from multiple lines of differentiation including epithelial, mesenchymal, and neural markers. Desmoplastic small round cell tumor is a very aggressive neoplasm, and often the prognosis is poor. Although some studies have suggested mesothelial origin to the tumor, ultrastructural and immunohistochemical techniques have failed to support that theory. Currently, the origin of the neoplastic cells of this tumor is unknown.

IN TRANSLATION

Usually the diagnosis of DSRCT is not a dilemma because of its unique clinical and morphologic features. However, occasionally, the diagnosis may be attempted on a smaller biopsy specimen in which the characteristic desmoplastic stroma is not evident. In such cases, cytogenetic and molecular techniques can be helpful. Desmoplastic small round cell tumor has a unique cytogenetic abnormality t(11;22)(p13;q12), which results in a fusion of the *EWS* gene on 22q12 to the *WT1* gene on 11p13. This aberration can be detected by cytogenetic, reverse transcription polymerase chain reaction (RT-PCR), or FISH studies.

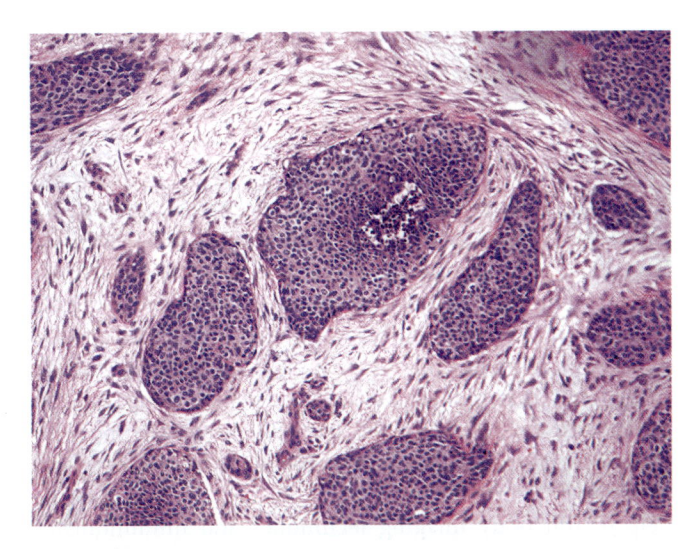

FIGURE 18-28 Desmoplastic small round cell tumor. The nests of lesional cells show hyperchromatic nuclei and scant cytoplasm and are surrounded by desmoplastic stroma.

BONE AND JOINT PATHOLOGY

Bone Organization

Bones are the main component of the human skeleton and are composed of osteoid, cartilage, fat, nerves, vessels, and bone marrow. The major functions of bone include metabolic, mechanical, and hematopoietic.

There are numerous organization schemes for the bones. The first major scheme divides the skeleton into two main regions: the axial skeleton (skull, vertebrae, ribs, pelvis) and appendicular skeleton (limbs, hands, feet, digits). This division is especially important in cartilaginous tumors. Long bones can be divided into different anatomic regions: epiphysis (end region near joint), diaphysis (central shaft), and metaphyseal (connecting region). Knowledge of clinical history and location of a bone lesion is critical because many tumors and tumor-like conditions have distinct predilection for certain anatomic sites.

Radiology and clinical history play an essential role in orthopedic pathology. In many situations, it is impossible to make an accurate diagnosis without knowledge of the radiologic features and clinical history. As a general rule, one should never sign out a bone case without review of the imaging.

Normal Histology

Bone is composed of a fibrous matrix, predominantly type I collagen, and mineral, hydroxyapatite. Bone can be divided into compact bone and cancellous bone based on gross and microscopic appearance. Compact bone makes up the cortex, while cancellous bone occupies the central region. Bone can also be classified by the organization pattern of its collagen into woven and lamellar bone. Woven bone is best thought of as temporary bone and typically is found in areas of rapid growth such as fracture callus and tumor. Woven bone consists of an irregular arrangement of collagen that forms randomly organized trabeculae of bone. Osteocytes are unevenly distributed within lacunae and osteoblasts are seen lining the trabeculae. In contrast, lamellar bone has a more orderly arrangement and is found in areas of slow growth. The collagen fibers are arranged in parallel sheets/bundles. In cortical bone, the fibers are circumferentially arranged, while the organization is longitudinal in cancellous bone (Figure 18-29).

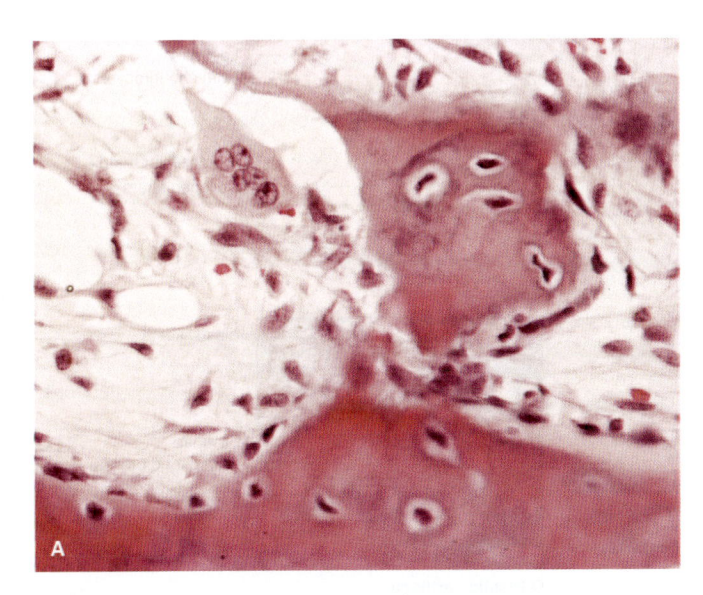

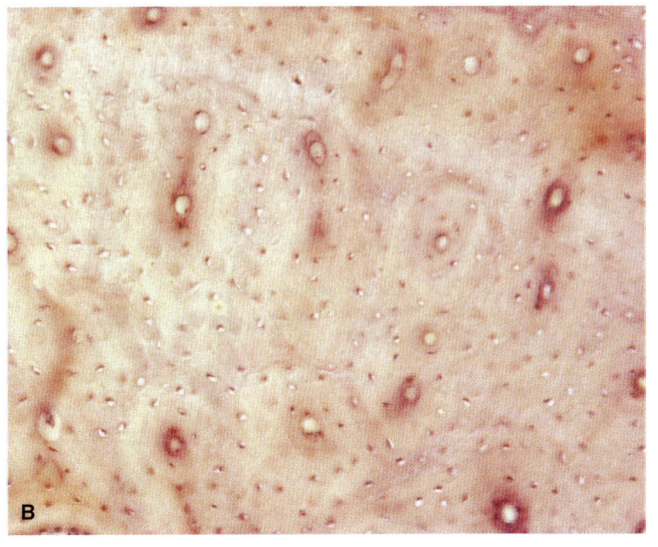

FIGURE 18-29 Primary (woven) bone and secondary (lamellar) bone. (A) Micrograph of a fractured bone undergoing repair. Primary bone is newly formed, immature bone, rich in osteocytes, with randomly arranged bundles of calcified collagen. Osteoclasts and osteoblasts are numerous in the surrounding endosteum. ×200. H&E. **(B)** Secondary or mature bone shows matrix organized as lamellae, seen faintly here as concentric lines surrounding osteonic canals. (From Mescher AL, Junqueira's Basic Histology Text and Atlas 12th edn. McGraw Hill Lange New York 2010, Figure 8-8, page127.)

Cartilage is another specialized type of connective tissue and is composed of chondrocytes and an extracellular matrix of collagen fibers in a proteoglycan matrix. Cartilage can be subdivided into three types based on morphologic features and composition of the extracellular matrix. The most common type of cartilage is hyaline cartilage that forms the model for the axial and appendicular skeleton. Hyaline cartilage is also found at the end of ribs, in tracheal and bronchial rings, and at articular surfaces. Histologically, hyaline cartilage is composed of chondrocytes with small, hyperchromatic nuclei embedded in pink-gray-pale blue extracellular matrix. Elastic cartilage is found in the sites such as the pinna of the external ear and epiglottis and is composed of chondrocytes in a matrix of elastin fibers. Fibrocartilage is primarily found in the intervertebral discs and symphysis pubis and consists of chondrocytes in a matrix of thick bundles of collagen (Figure 18-30).

Lesions of Bone

Lesions in this classification include metastatic tumors, osteoid osteoma, osteosarcoma, cartilaginous neoplasms, fibro-osseous lesions, fibrous and fibrohistiocytic lesions, and other tumors of bone such as Ewing sarcoma (**ES**).

METASTATIC DISEASE

The most common malignancy that a surgical pathologist will encounter in bone is metastatic disease and not a primary bone neoplasm. The skeleton is a common site for metastases, and autopsy series have shown up to 30% of patients who died of carcinoma had skeletal metastases documented with only gross examination or limited sampling. Common carcinomas that metastasize to bone include lung, kidney, breast, prostate, and thyroid. For patients presenting with metastatic disease without an undocumented primary, lung and kidney primaries are most likely. Fortunately, with the help of full body imaging techniques and immunohistochemical studies, the primary sites of most skeletal metastases can be identified. In children, rhabdomyosarcoma, neuroblastoma, and clear cell sarcoma of the kidney are three pediatric malignancies that have a high rate of bony metastases.

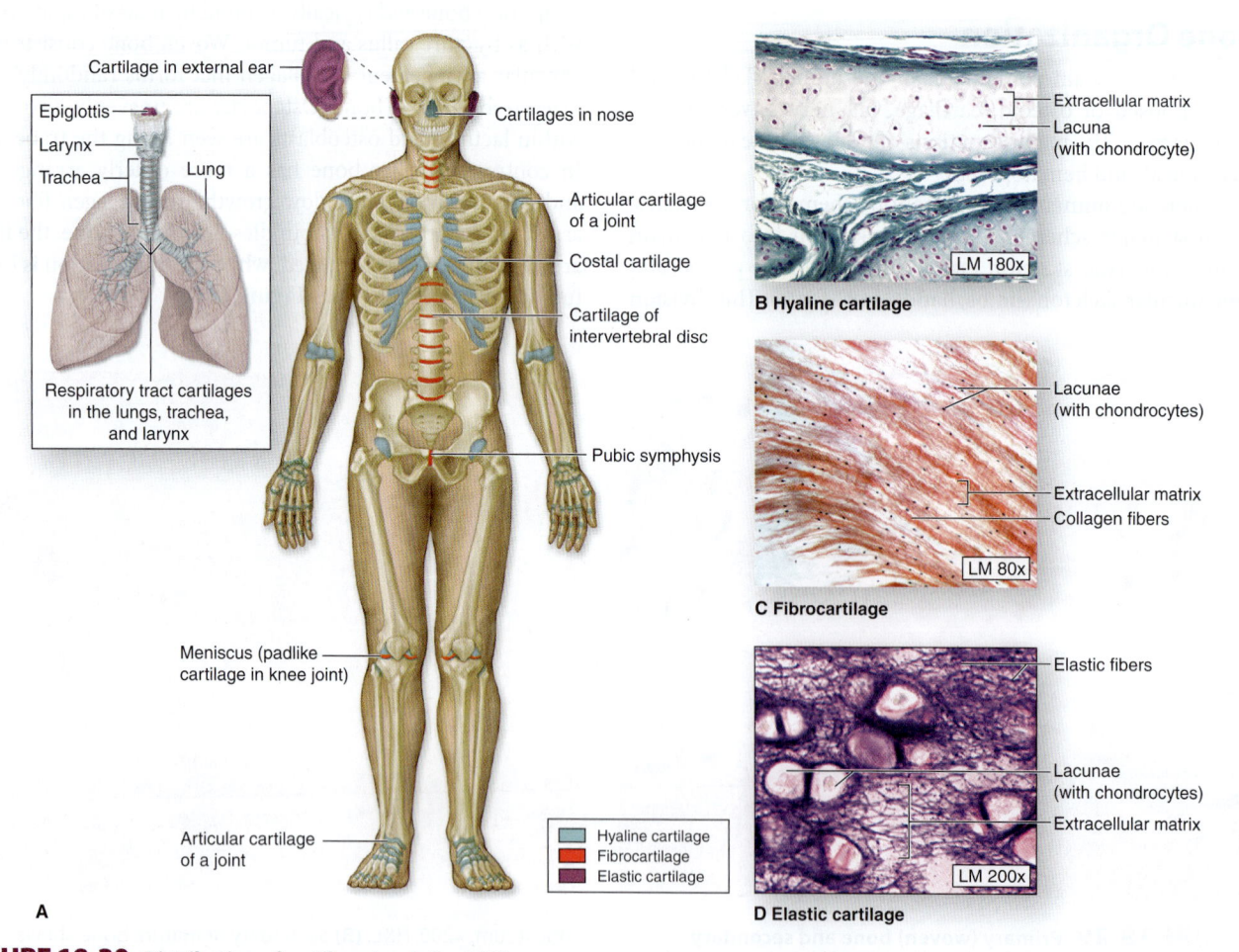

FIGURE 18-30 Distribution of cartilage in adults. (A) There are three types of adult cartilage distributed in many areas of the skeleton, particularly in joints and where pliable support is useful, as in the ribs, ears, and nose. Cartilage support of other tissues throughout the respiratory system is also prominent. The photomicrographs show the main features of **(B)** hyaline cartilage, **(C)** fibrocartilage, and **(D)** elastic cartilage. (Mescher AL, Junqueira's Basic Histology Text and Atlas 12th edn. McGraw Hill Lange New York 2010, Figure 7-1, page 115.)

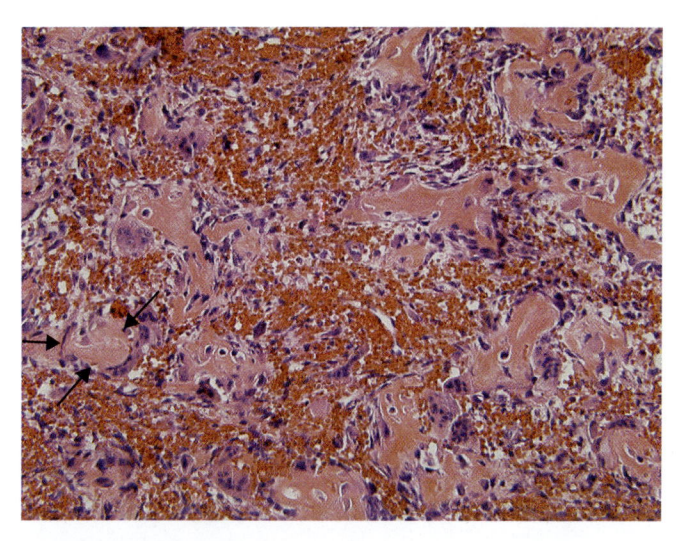

FIGURE 18-31 **Osteoid osteoma.** Irregular trabeculae of bone with prominent osteoblastic rimming is shown (arrow). The intervening stroma shows rich vascular connective tissue. No cytologic atypia is appreciated.

BENIGN BONE-FORMING TUMORS

Osteoid osteoma is a benign bone-forming tumor with a distinct clinical presentation. Patients are usually teenagers or young adults who report pain that is worse at night and alleviated by aspirin or other NSAIDs. The most common site for this lesion is the femoral neck, but these tumors also frequently occur in other long bones. Imaging is often diagnostic and shows a nidus (well-demarcated lytic lesion) surrounded by sclerosis. Gross examination typically reveals nidus tissue that is reddish and distinct from the surrounding sclerotic bone. Histologic examination reveals an interlacing network of bony trabeculae with varying degrees of mineralization. The trabeculae are lined by a prominent layer of osteoblasts. The surrounding stroma is often highly vascular. No cytologic atypia is identified (Figure 18-31).

Osteoblastoma is another benign osteoblastic tumor that is closely related to osteoid osteoma, and it is often impossible to distinguish these two entities based solely on morphologic grounds. Osteoblastoma typically occurs in the axial skeleton with more than 40% occurring in the vertebral column and sacrum. While osteoid osteoma rarely exceeds 1.5 cm in diameter, osteoblastoma has higher growth potential.

Complete surgical removal of osteoid osteoma and osteoblastoma is recommended. Radiofrequency ablation may be used as an alternative approach in the treatment of osteoid osteoma. Removal of the nidus tissue usually results in relief of symptoms.

MALIGNANT BONE-FORMING TUMORS

Osteosarcoma is the most common primary malignancy of bone. It can be divided into different subgroups based on histologic appearance and anatomic location. Histologic subgroups include in osteoblastic, chondroblastic, and fibroblastic, although there is no evidence that these subtypes have any prognostic value. Osteosarcoma can also be subdivided by location into intramedullary and surface osteosarcoma.

Intramedullary osteosarcoma usually presents in adolescence, although there is also a smaller peak in later adulthood (see Case 18-7). Patients typically report pain and sometimes swelling. The most common anatomic locations are the distal femur and proximal tibia. Even though the radiologic appearance of these tumors may vary from lytic to sclerotic, the destructive growth pattern of the lesion usually allows for a high degree of preoperative suspicion as to the diagnosis. In most cases, the tumor destroys the cortex and may extend into adjacent soft tissue. As the tumor penetrates the cortex, it can elevate the periosteum (termed Codman triangle by the radiologist) or produce a prominent periosteal reaction.

Gross examination yields a poorly circumscribed heterogeneous mass with variable amounts of ossification. Hemorrhage and necrosis are not unusual. The morphologic spectrum of osteosarcoma can be diverse, but the consistent histologic feature of this tumor is malignant cells producing osteoid matrix (Figure 18-32 left). Some osteosarcomas have an osteoblastic appearance with large pleomorphic cells with pronounced atypia admixed with an abundance of tumor bone. Other tumors show zones of chondroid-type matrix, and in some cases there may be very little osteoid formation. These lesions typically have high mitotic rates with numerous atypical mitotic figures.

Although conventional osteosarcoma is a highly aggressive neoplasm, the prognosis has improved with the advent of neoadjuvant chemotherapy. The use of preoperative chemotherapy regimens currently allows for limb-sparing surgery in many cases. Despite improved outcomes, osteosarcomas still frequently metastasize to sites such as lungs.

CARTILAGINOUS TUMORS

The two main types of neoplasms in this category are **enchondroma** (benign) and **chondrosarcoma** (malignant). Tumors in this group are interesting and complicated neoplasms presently not well understood. There are several important principles that must be observed when evaluating a cartilaginous tumor. Knowledge of the clinical presentation, radiologic findings, and morphologic features must be combined in order to arrive at the correct diagnosis.

Clinical characteristics are very important. Location is one of the most important factors in determining whether a cartilaginous neoplasm is benign or malignant. A pathologist must know the location of the tumor because criteria and thresholds for benign versus malignant depend on location. *Appendicular (hands/feet) cartilaginous lesions are almost always benign, whereas axial (ribs, scapula, pelvis) tumors are almost always malignant.* This is a critical fact because even the most bland looking midline cartilaginous lesions behave aggressively, while very worrisome-appearing lesions

CASE 18-7

A 18-year-old male presents with right leg pain. Imaging showed large distal femur mass with cortical destruction (**Figure 18-32**).

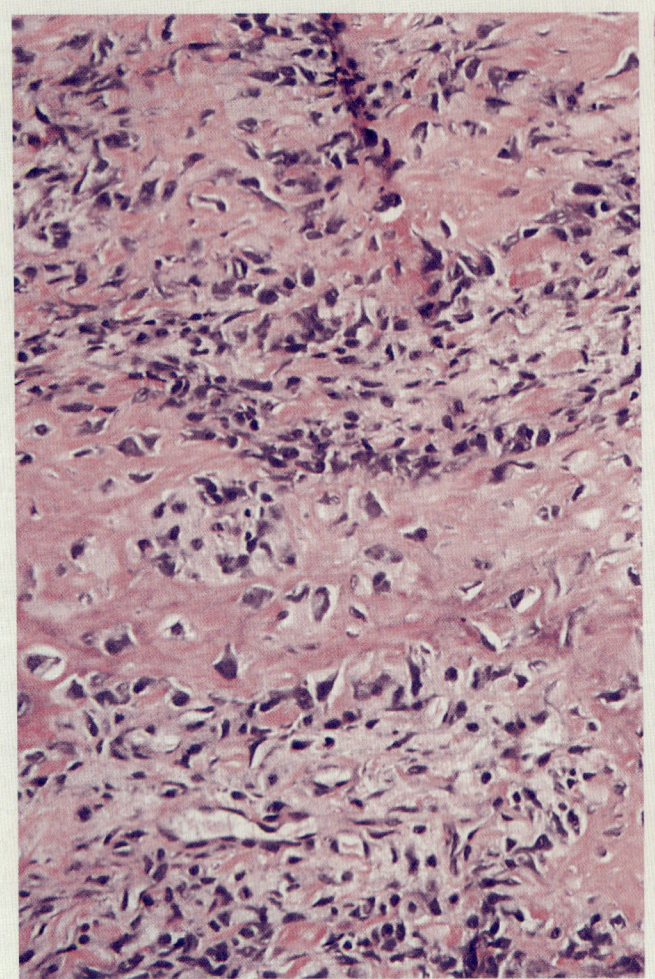

Histologic sections show sarcomatous cells producing osteoid. By definition, this is consistent with **osteosarcoma**. In some areas, the tumor has a chondroblastic morphology.

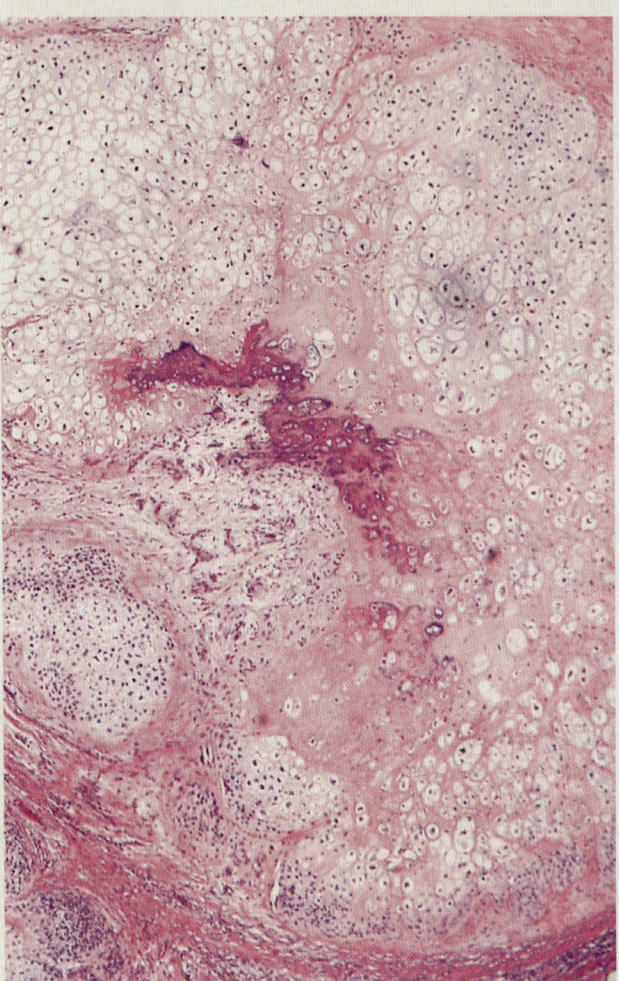

FIGURE 18-32 Osteosarcoma (left, high-power view). Atypical sarcoma cells producing amorphous pink osteoid. Other areas of tumor demonstrate a chondroblastic morphology (right).

in the small bones of the hands and feet usually pursue a benign course. Pain is also an important clinical feature. Benign cartilaginous lesions are frequently asymptomatic. **Chondrosarcoma**, however, often causes pain. An incidentally discovered well-differentiated cartilaginous mass in the proximal femur is much less worrisome than one that is causing pain.

Radiologists often recognize cartilaginous lesions by their appearance on imaging: radiolucent defect with punctuate or stippled calcifications. **Enchondromas** may expand the cortex but do not disrupt it. Cortical disruption and soft tissue extension are usual evidence of malignancy.

Histologic appearance is also of importance. Features that should be evaluated include cellularity, host bone engulfment, mucoid matrix change, and cytologic features. *Mucoid matrix degeneration and host bone engulfment are the two most helpful features in terms of classifying central cartilaginous tumors as benign or malignant* (**Table 18-6**).

Enchondroma is a common benign intramedullary cartilaginous neoplasm. It occurs in all age groups and most commonly develops in the small bones of the hands and feet. The second most common site of involvement is the long tubular bone. Histologically, as alluded to earlier, enchondroma usually has low cellularity without host bone engulfment. The

CASE 18-8

A 70-year-old man presents with a destructive lesion of the iliac crest (Figure 18-33 A and B). These sections show a cartilaginous proliferation, but there are major differences when comparing this case to a benign cartilaginous lesion (enchondroma—Figure 18-33 C and D). First, the overall cellularity in the patient's lesion is much higher. Second, the tumor is engulfing preexisting bone. Finally, the clinical setting is also important in that the tumor is axial (pelvis). Taken together, the clinical and morphologic features of this tumor are consistent with a malignancy, **chondrosarcoma**.

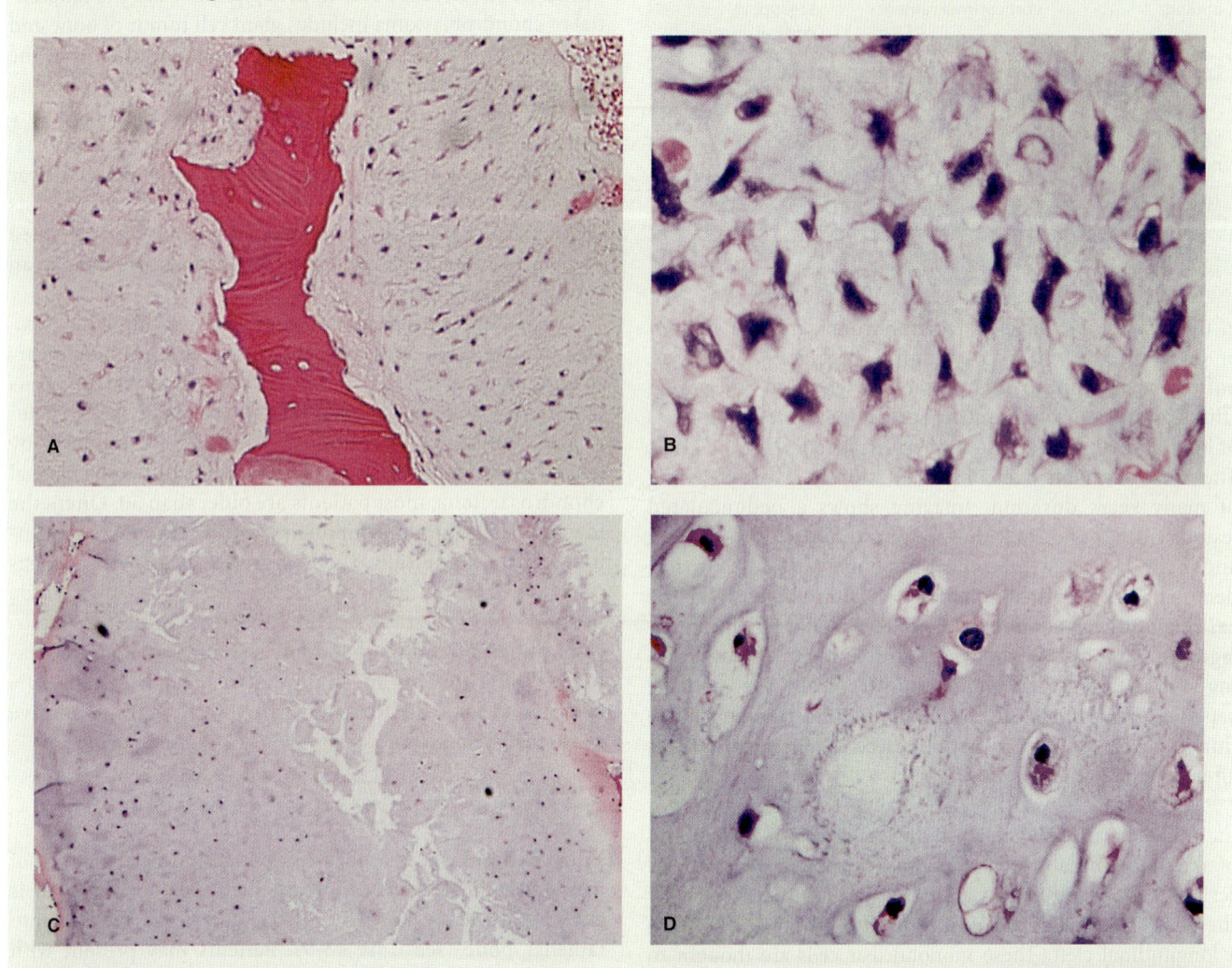

FIGURE 18-33 Comparison of enchondroma (benign) and chondrosarcoma (malignant) lesions. Enchondroma [(C) low-power view, (D) high-power view)] shows a well-differentiated cartilaginous proliferation of low cellularity. At high-power view, the neoplastic cell nuclei are pyknotic. Chondrosarcoma [(A) low-power view, (B) high-power view] shows a lesion with much greater cellularity. At low-power view, the tumor is engulfing preexisting bone. At high-power view, the neoplastic cells exhibit marked atypia.

chondrocytes have small pyknotic nuclei. Myxoid change is typically not found (Figure 18-33 C and D).

Chondrosarcoma is usually a tumor of mid-to-late adulthood with the majority of patients being older than 50 (see Case above and Figure 18-33 A and B). These tumors commonly involve midline bones such as the ribs, spine, sternum, and pelvic bones. Imaging reveals aggressive features such as endosteal scalloping, cortical destruction, or soft tissue extension. Histologically, these lesions are hypercellular. Neoplastic cartilage will permeate the marrow space and engulf preexisting cancellous bone trabeculae. The nuclei often show an open chromatin pattern with atypia. Mitotic figures may be seen but are not required for the diagnosis.

Other chondroid lesions include osteochondroma, chondroblastoma, and dedifferentiated chondrosarcoma. **Osteochondroma** is a cartilage capped bony projection that presents as an exophytic growth on the bone surface. The etiology of these lesions is thought to be due to displacement

TABLE 18-6 Comparison of benign and malignant cartilaginous tumors.

	Enchondroma	Chondrosarcoma
Pain	No	Yes
Location	Appendicular	Axial
Radiologic findings	Circumscribed without cortical involvement	Endosteal scalloping, cortical disruption
Cellularity	Low (but can be higher in appendicular sites)	Usually high
Bone engulfment/permeation	No	Yes
Myxoid change	No	Yes

of the physeal cartilage. Osteochondromas may be solitary or occur in the setting of multiple hereditary exostoses. **Solitary osteochondroma** presents in children and young adults as an outgrowth on the surface near the metaphysis of long tubular bones. About one-third occur near the knee. The most common clinical presentation is a hard swelling of many years duration. Imaging shows a pedunculated lesion with a bone stalk that is continuous with the cortex and medullary cavity of underlying bone. Histologic review demonstrates a cartilaginous cap overlying a bony stalk. The cartilaginous cap contains moderately cellular hyaline cartilage that mimics the epiphyseal growth plate. The underlying stalk contains cancellous bone. Typically the cartilage cap measures from 0.2 cm to 1 cm. In adults, the cap may be thin or absent because growth of these lesions usually stops after skeletal maturation.

Chondroblastoma is a rare benign cartilaginous tumor that characteristically involves the epiphyses of long bones of skeletally immature patients. Images show a well-circumscribed lytic lesion with a sclerotic margin. Microscopically these lesions are composed of round to polygonal cells with a longitudinal cleft. These mononuclear cells are thought to represent chondroblasts. Scattered multinucleated giant cells are typically present. Distinct cartilaginous matrix can usually be found, although level of cartilaginous differentiated varies. Calcification is a helpful diagnostic feature and usually is found as a fine linear deposition between mononuclear cells (so-called "chicken-wire" pattern) (Figure 18-34 left). Chondroblastomas are benign lesions, and can usually be treated with curettage and bone grafting. Rarely, they may recur. Few primary bone lesions occur in the epiphyses, and the differential of chondroblastoma includes giant cell tumor of bone and clear cell chondrosarcoma. Age of the patient can aid in the diagnosis. Chondroblastoma occurs in skeletally immature patients, while the other two tumors affect skeletally mature patients. Giant cell tumor of bone is composed of an even distribution of multinucleated giant cells in a sea of mononuclear cells (Figure 18-34 right). Clear cell chondrosarcoma consists of neoplastic cells with abundant clear cytoplasm embedded in a cartilaginous matrix. Clear cell chondrosarcoma is an extremely rare entity.

Dedifferentiated chondrosarcoma is a highly aggressive cartilaginous neoplasm composed of a low-grade cartilaginous proliferation and a high-grade sarcomatous component and an abrupt transition between the two elements. The femur is the most common site followed by pelvis, humerus, ribs, and scapula. Similar to conventional chondrosarcoma, most patients are older than 50. Often, the low- and high-grade components can be recognized radiologically. Histologically, the low-grade component consists of a well-differentiated chondroid lesion. The high-grade portion is a high-grade sarcoma that may exhibit heterologous differentiation (rhabdomyosarcoma, osteosarcomatous). These tumors are highly lethal, and less than 10% of patients with dedifferentiated chondrosarcoma survive more than year.

FIBRO-OSSEOUS LESIONS

Fibrous dysplasia is a fibro-osseous lesion best thought of as a defect in bone development such that bone growth is arrested at the level of woven bone and never matures into lamellar bone (see Case 18-9). Patients may present with solitary or multifocal disease in a variety of clinical settings. Most patients present with involvement of a single focus of a single bone (monostotic). Occasionally, multiple foci involving several bones will be identified (polyostotic). Associated extraskeletal manifestations such as skin hyperpigmentation and endocrine abnormalities may be observed and are more commonly seen with polyostotic disease. The most common sites of involvement are the ribs, craniofacial bones, proximal femur, and tibia. Patients usually present in the first three decades. Some lesions are discovered as an incidental finding on radiographs, while other patients report pain and swelling.

Imaging reveals a well-circumscribed medullary lesion with a ground-glass appearance. Often a thick rim of sclerotic bone is identified around the lesion. Gross examination shows a centrally located, sharply circumscribed mass with a variably

> **IN TRANSLATION**
>
> **Multiple hereditary exostosis** (multiple osteochondromas) is an autosomal dominant disorder characterized by inactivating mutations in exostosin 1 (*EXT1*) at 8q24 or *EXT2* at 11p11-13. Both loci are involved in the synthesis and cellular display of heparan sulfate. Patients usually present with multiple osteochondromas and other bone deformities. Osteochondromas in this disorder are usually larger than solitary lesions. Rarely, osteochondromas may undergo malignant transformation.

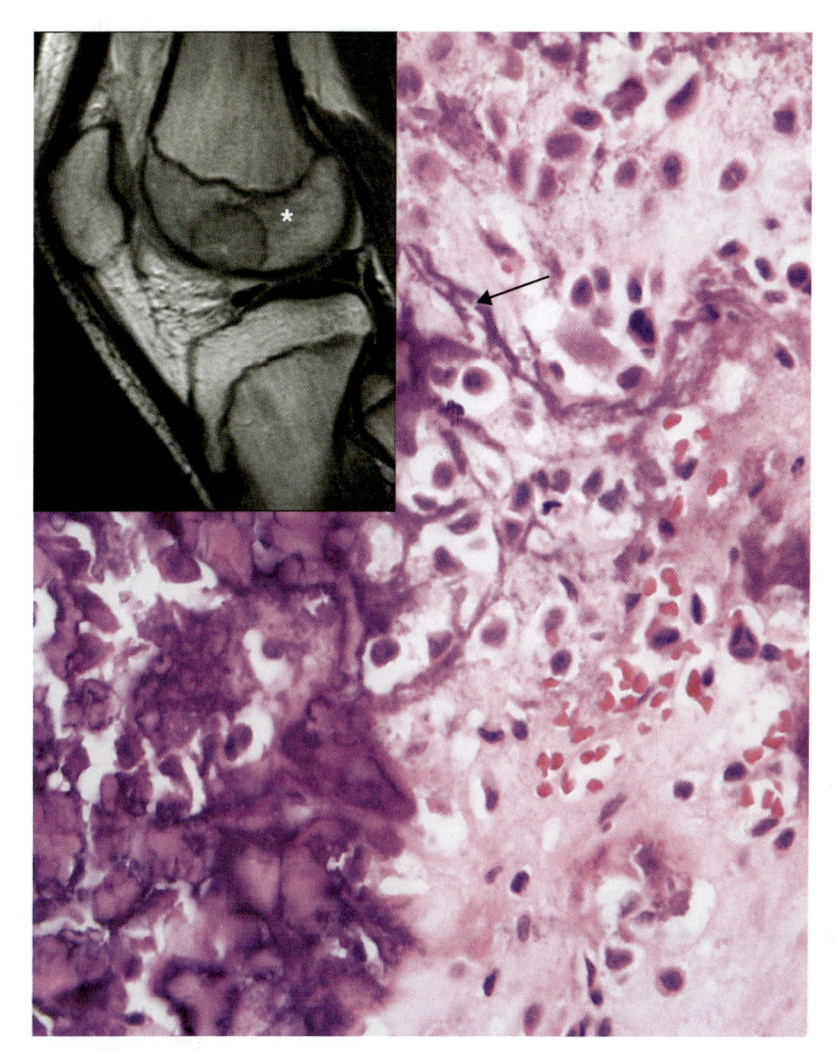

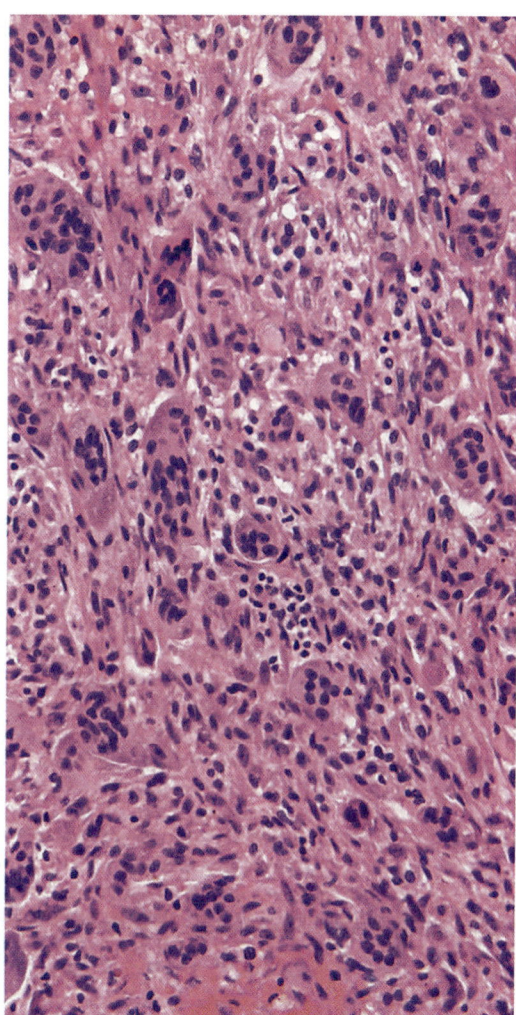

FIGURE 18-34 Chondroblastoma (left) and giant cell tumor (right). Chondroblastoma (left inset) radiograph shows circumscribed lytic lesion with sclerotic margin (*). Left (high-power view) shows pink cartilaginous matrix, chondroblastoma cells (often with a nuclear cleft), and a "chicken-wire" pattern of calcification surrounding individual cells (arrow). Occasional giant cells are also present. Giant cell tumor of bone (right) shows a striking even distribution of multinucleated giant cells surrounded by mononuclear cells.

tan to gray to white cut surface. Microscopic examination shows numerous irregularly shaped trabeculae of immature woven bone surrounded by bland spindle cells. Little or no osteoblastic rimming of the trabeculae is usually appreciated. Some lesions may be heavily ossified, while others show areas of cartilaginous differentiation or xanthomatous change. Importantly, the intervening spindle cell population is uniform without atypia (Figure 18-35 left).

Although the lesions of fibrous dysplasia may enlarge over time, they usually stabilize after puberty. If a solitary focus is at risk of pathologic fracture, curettage may be performed with bone grafting. Occasionally lesions in expendable bones such as the ribs are segmentally resected.

Osteofibrous dysplasia is a rare fibro-osseous lesion that occurs predominantly in the tibia but also occasionally in the fibula. Like fibrous dysplasia, osteofibrous dysplasia is composed of bony trabeculae and fibrous tissue. However, in osteofibrous dysplasia, the trabeculae are lined by osteoblasts (Figure 18-35 right). This lesion usually presents during the first two decades as a multiloculated radiolucent expansion of the anterolateral cortex of the tibia. Some have speculated that osteofibrous dysplasia is related to adamantinoma given their overlapping clinical, radiologic, and morphologic features.

Nonossifying fibroma is a relatively common nonneoplastic lesion that affects long tubular bones of skeletally immature patients. Current thinking suggests that the underlying pathogenesis may be related to incomplete ossification. Studies have estimated up to 30% of children may have nonossifying fibroma. Most of these are small, asymptomatic and typically resolve spontaneously by adulthood. Occasionally, these lesions may become large and undergo secondary pathologic fracture, bringing the individual to clinical attention. Histologic sections show a proliferation of uniform spindle cells in a storiform (whorled) pattern. Variable amounts of multinucleated giant cells, hemosiderin-laden macrophages,

CASE 18-9

A 30-year-old patient presents male with well-circumscribed medullary lesion in proximal femur. Radiology shows ground-glass appearance (Figure 18-35).

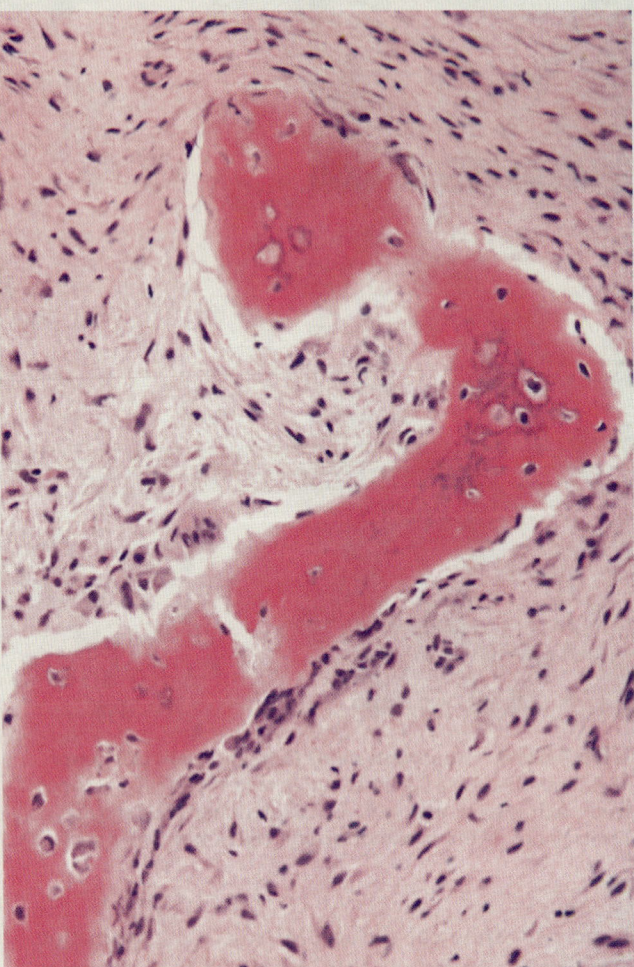

Histologic sections show a fibro-osseous lesion composed of irregular trabeculae of bone surrounded by a spindle cell proliferation. No osteoblastic rimming of the trabeculae is noted. The radiologic and morphologic features are consistent with **fibrous dysplasia**.

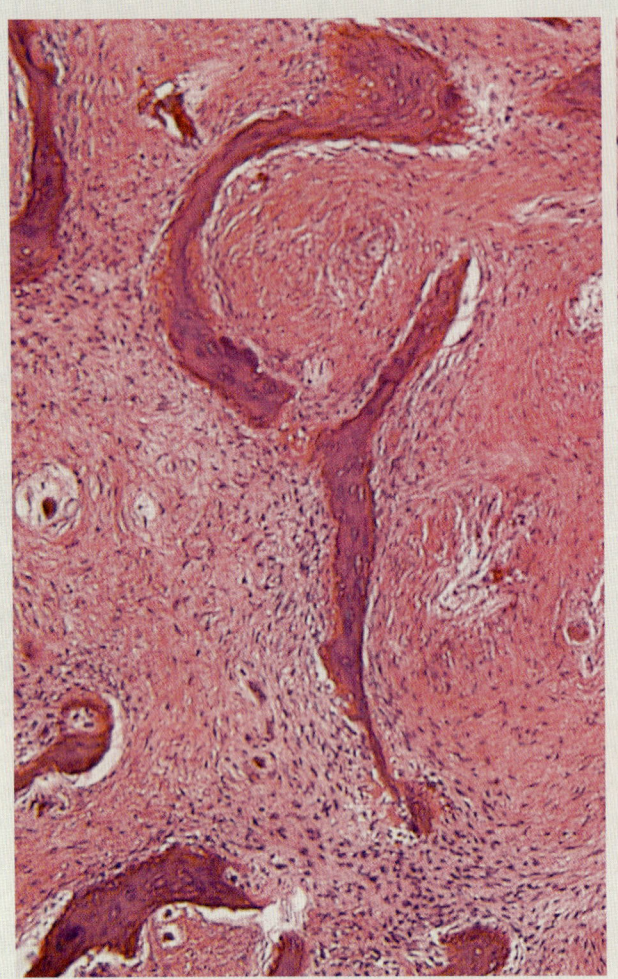

FIGURE 18-35 Fibro-Osseous lesions: **Fibrous dysplasia** (left) is composed of irregular trabeculae of bone surrounded by a spindle cell proliferation. No osteoblastic rimming of the trabeculae is noted. **Osteofibrous dysplasia** (right). Histologic sections show a fibro-osseous lesion composed of irregular trabeculae of bone surrounded by a spindle cell proliferation. Osteoblasts rimming of the trabeculae is noted.

and foamy histiocytes may be present. Sometimes the lesion may be complicated by secondary aneurysmal bone cyst (ABC) or pathologic fracture.

Other Tumors of Bone

This section includes Ewing sarcoma (ES), Langerhans cell histiocytosis (LCH), chordoma, and aneurysmal bone cyst (ABC).

ES usually affects adolescents and young adults, and is much more common in Caucasians than non-Caucasians. ES may arise at virtually any site, but is more common in soft tissue and bone. In bone, the ribs and long bones are common sites. Radiologic studies show a destructive, permeative lesion that typically affects the diaphysis of a long bone. It is not uncommon to see a soft tissue component to the mass. A characteristic radiologic finding is a

CASE 18-10

A 15-year-old patient presents with proximal femur mass. Imaging showed an ill-defined permeative destructive intramedullary lesion with prominent multilayered periosteal reaction.

Histologic sections show a small round blue cell neoplasm composed of uniform cells with a fine powdery chromatin pattern. Focal rosette formation is identified. A battery of immunohistochemical stains was performed and showed the tumor cells to exhibit strong membranous staining for CD99. The lesional cells were negative for cytokeratins, S100, and lymphoid markers. Cytogenetic studies showed a translocation involving chromosomes 11 and 22 (t(11;22)(24;q12)). The clinical, morphologic, immunophenotypic, and molecular findings are consistent with **ES** (Figure 18-36).

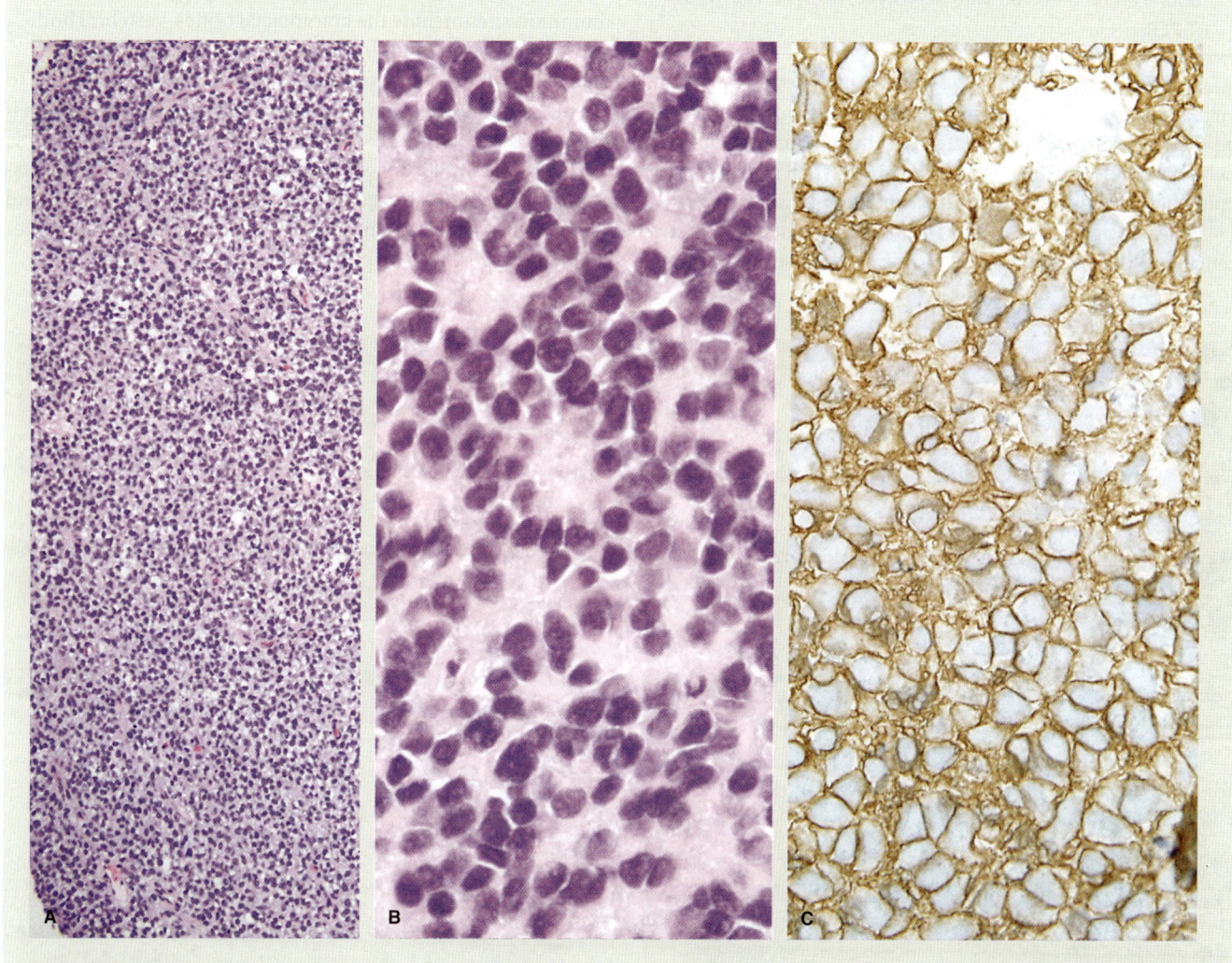

FIGURE 18-36 ES. Low-power view (**A**) shows a small round blue cell neoplasm composed of uniform cells. High-power view (**B**) demonstrates fine powdery nuclear chromatin pattern and focal rosette formation. (**C**) Immunostaining with CD 99 (MIC2) shows a positive membranous pattern consistent with ES.

significant multilayered periosteal reaction (onion skin). While this feature is not specific, it suggests consideration of ES.

Microscopic examination shows a lobular arrangement of relatively uniform round blue cells with round nuclei, powdery chromatin, and small nucleoli. Cytoplasm is scant but may be pale or vacuolated. The mitotic rate may be variable, but it is not uncommon to find areas of degeneration and necrosis. While not a prerequisite for diagnosis, rosettes may be identified (see Case 18-10 and Figure 18-36).

Ancillary studies are critical to the diagnosis since many tumors including lymphoma, melanoma, neuroblastoma, and other sarcomas may have the same morphologic features. Immunohistochemical stains are often the first line of the diagnostic workup. ES will show a strong membranous staining pattern for CD99. Although not specific, as

> **IN TRANSLATION**
>
> Cytogenetics and molecular studies are often used to confirm the diagnosis. The defining feature of this family of tumors is the translocation involving the *EWS* gene on 22q12 with a member of the ETS family of transcription factors. The most frequent translocation is t(11;22)(q24;q12) that fuses the *FLI-1* gene on 11q24 with the *EWS* gene on 22q12, which is found in about 90% of tumors. This translocation can be detected with karyotypic analysis, FISH, and RT-PCR.

virtually every other tumor in the differential diagnosis may be CD99 positive, it is a relatively sensitive marker and can help to exclude the diagnosis. In most cases, ES is negative for epithelial, melanocytic, myogenic, and lymphoid markers.

ES is an aggressive tumor with a high incidence of recurrence and distant metastases. However, the use of multimodality treatment including radiation and chemotherapy has significantly increased survival rates.

LCH is a clonal proliferation of cells with features of Langerhans cells, mononuclear cells with oval characteristically grooved nuclei and abundant eosinophilic cytoplasm. LCH includes eosinophilic granuloma (solitary focus), Hand–Schuller–Christian disease (multifocal skeletal), and Letterer–Siwe (multifocal skeletal and extraskeletal) diseases. LCH usually affects children and young adults, and disseminated forms of the disease usually present by age two. The most common sites include the craniofacial bones, vertebral bodies, ribs, pelvis, and femur. Imaging shows a lytic and well-demarcated "punched-out" intramedullary lesion ranging from 1 to 2 cm. Larger lesions may appear more aggressive and can even disrupt the cortex and extend into soft tissue. Microscopic features are similar for solitary and diffuse forms of the disease and include a mixed population of Langerhans cells and eosinophils. Other inflammatory cells, including multinucleated giant cells, may be present (Figure 18-37 left).

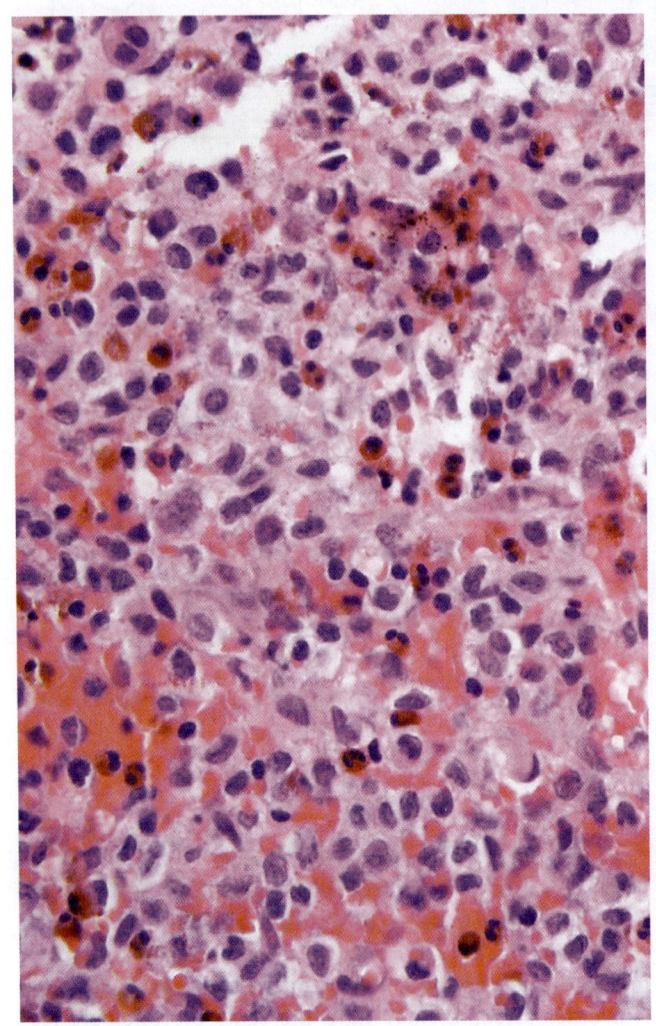

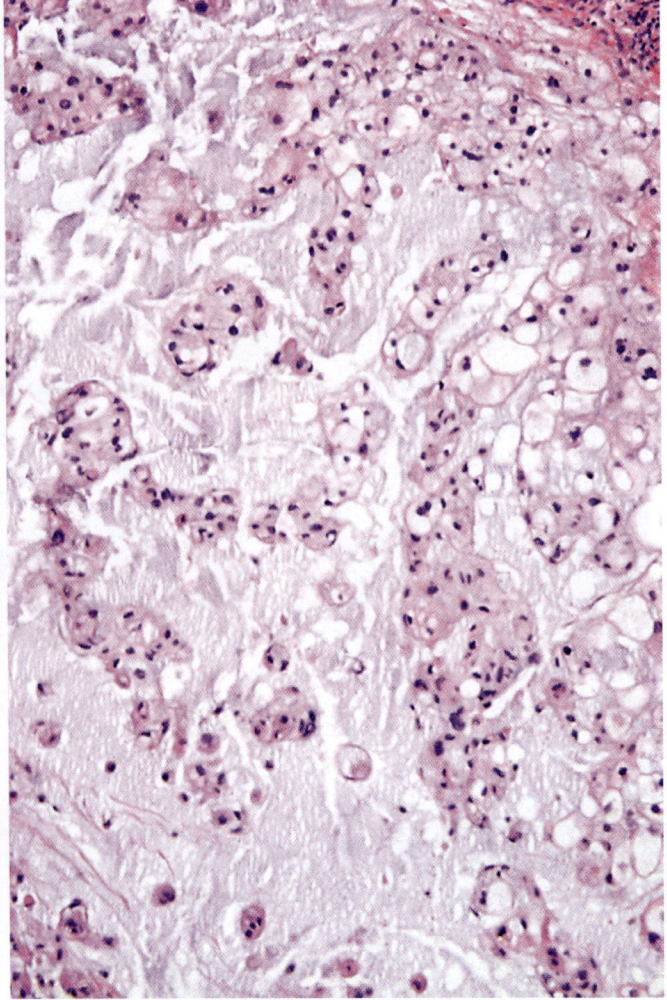

FIGURE 18-37 Langerhans cell histiocytosis (left) and chordoma (right). Left Langerhans cell histiocytosis demonstrates a mixed population of mononuclear cells and inflammatory cells. Most of the inflammatory cells are eosinophils. (Right) Chordoma section also showed a multilobulated neoplasm composed of chains and cords of ovoid cells with bubbly eosinophilic cytoplasm.

Immunohistochemical stains for S100 and CD1a will highlight these cells, while ultrastructural examination will reveal characteristic Birbeck granules. Clinical outcome depends on the form and extent of disease. Eosinophilic granuloma is usually benign and can be treated by curettage. When the disease affects multiple organs or organ systems, the outlook is less favorable.

Chordoma is a primary bone neoplasm that arises in midline locations such as the sacrococcygeal and sphenooccipital regions. Evidence suggests that these tumors arise from intraosseous remnants of the notochord. The incidence peaks during the fifth and sixth decades. Patients usually report pain secondary to compression of nerves in the sacrococcygeal region. On imaging, chordomas appear as a lytic lesion that expands and destroys normal bony structures. The microscopic appearance of chordomas is somewhat distinct. These tumors have a multilobular low-power appearance. Each lobule is composed of nests and cords of neoplastic cells in a myxoid matrix. The lesional cells have round nuclei and prominent nucleoli. The characteristic feature of these neoplasms is the physaliphorous (bubbly) cell that exhibits striking cytoplasmic vacuolization (Figure 18-37 right). Chordomas are notoriously difficult to treat because of their high propensity for local recurrence and location near vital structures. Complete surgical excision, if feasible, is the treatment of choice.

Aneurysmal bone cyst (**ABC**) is a benign cystic bone lesion that can involve any part of the skeleton. Patients are usually less than 20 years old and may present with pain and swelling from weeks to years duration. Radiologic features are usually characteristic and include a ballooned distention of the periosteum with a lytic, multilocular lesion. CT and MRI studies can show fluid-fluid levels, confirming the cystic nature of the lesion. Although it is rare to receive an intact specimen, these lesions would appear as a spongy, multiloculated mass containing blood. Microscopic examination reveals collapsed fibrous septa outlining cystic spaces filled with blood. The septa vary in thickness and some lesions may appear solid. A mixture of inflammatory cells, loose fibrous stroma, blood vessels, multinucleated giant cells, and thin seams of osteoid are found within the septa. Importantly, no cytologic atypia is found. *ABC must be distinguished from variants of osteosarcoma that are malignant and do demonstrate marked cytologic atypia.* Although they may be locally destructive, the overall prognosis is good. Most ABCs are treated with curettage and bone graft.

TRAUMATIC AND INFLAMMATORY CONDITIONS OF BONE

Fracture

Fracture can be defined as any discontinuity of one structure that was caused by stress on the involved bone. The terminology used to describe different types of fractures is more or less standardized. Open (or compound) fractures communicate through the skin, leading to contamination of the fracture site and an increased risk of infection. Closed fractures do not communicate with the outside environment. Simple fractures are those lesions where the bone is split into two fragments, whereas comminuted fractures result in more than two fragments. Intra-articular fractures pass through a joint. Pathologic fractures occur at sites where the bone has been weakened by another process.

The clinical signs and symptoms of a fracture include pain, swelling, and deformity. The usual radiologic appearance of a fracture of a long bone includes progressive calcification of the callus repair tissue followed by bridging of the fracture gap with new bone and disappearance of the fracture line.

The morphology of a fracture site depends on the time between injury and examination. Fractures typically interrupt the bony trabeculae and disrupt small blood vessels in the bone marrow causing hemorrhage. Fibroblasts and inflammatory cells invade the organizing hematoma. There is also a proliferation of capillary-sized blood vessels around the fracture site. Within a week, an osteoblastic response occurs along the fracture line and new osteoblasts produce osteoid that eventually mineralizes and unites the osseous callus. Variable amounts of cartilaginous tissue may form as part of the remodeling process. Union is complete when the fibrous tissue is replaced by bone. The persistence of fibrous tissue is referred to as nonunion (**Figure 18-38**).

Avascular Necrosis

Avascular necrosis may be caused by any condition that limits or impairs blood flow to the affected bone including corticosteroid use, alcohol abuse, trauma, and sickle cell disease. Clinical symptoms include sudden onset of pain. The femoral head is the most commonly affected bone. Imaging findings include collapse of the affected bone in the subchondral region. Gross examination reveals yellow-tan, soft necrotic bone that is detached from the overlying articular cartilage. Microscopic examination shows a triangular-shaped region of dead bone with empty lacunae and necrotic bone marrow.

Osteomyelitis

Osteomyelitis is inflammation of the bone marrow and is almost always associated with infection. It may be caused by all types of organisms, but is typically the result of infection with pyogenic bacteria or mycobacteria. The organisms may infect the bone through hematogenous spread or become directly implanted at the site through an open wound. Most cases of osteomyelitis are seen in elderly debilitated patients, immunocompromised patients, or as a direct result of surgery or open fracture. The morbidity and mortality rates due to osteomyelitis have decreased dramatically with the use of antibiotics, but osteomyelitis still remains a significant clinical problem.

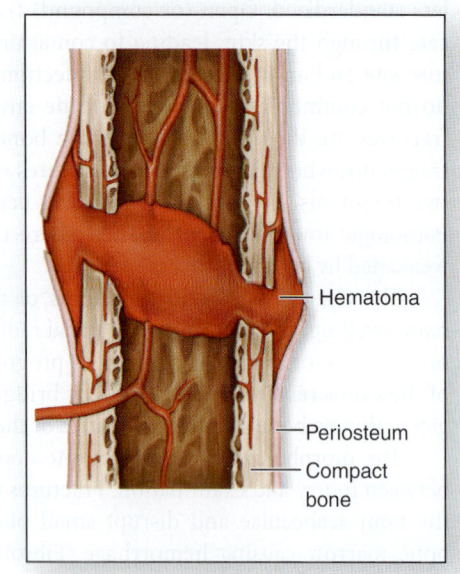

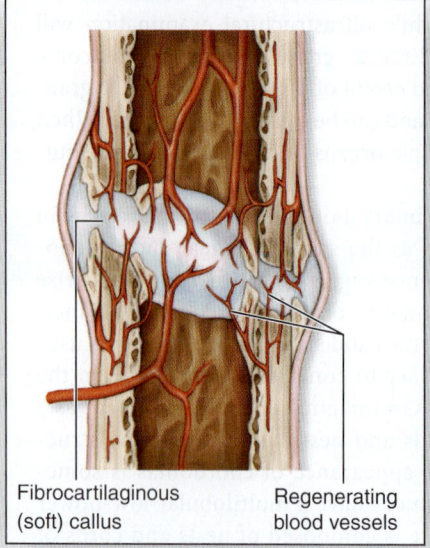

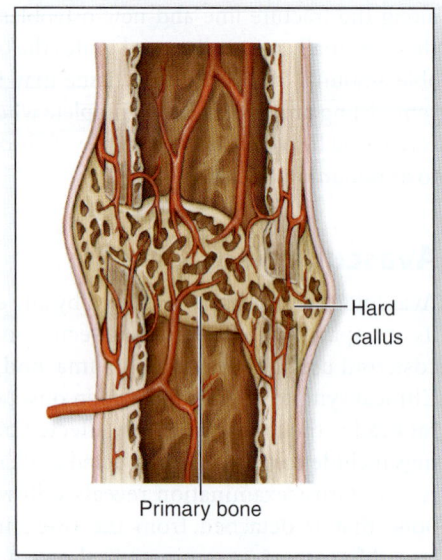

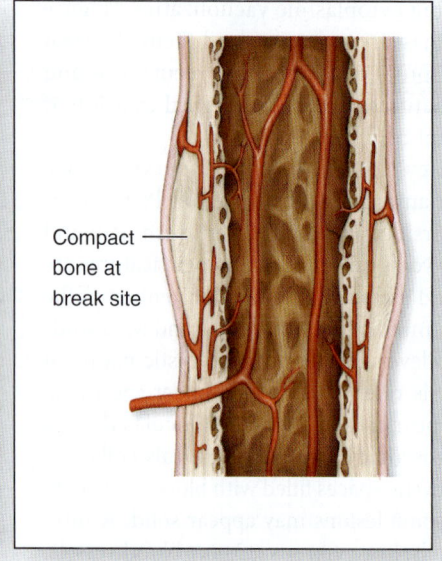

FIGURE 18-38 **Main features of bone fracture repair.** Repair of a fractured bone occurs through several stages, but utilizes mechanisms already in place for bone remodeling. **(1)** Blood vessels torn within the fracture release blood that clots to produce a large fracture hematoma. **(2)** This is gradually removed by macrophages and replaced by a soft fibrocartilage-like mass of procallus tissue rich in collagen and fibroblasts. If broken, the periosteum re-establishes continuity over this tissue. **(3):** This soft procallus is invaded by regrowing blood vessels and osteoblasts. In the next few weeks, the fibrocartilage is gradually replaced by trabeculae of primary bone, forming a hard callus throughout the original area of fracture. **(4)** The primary bone is then remodeled as compact and cancellous bone in continuity with the adjacent uninjured areas and fully functional vasculature is re-established. (From Mescher AL, Junqueira's Basic Histology Text and Atlas 12th edn. McGraw Hill Lange New York 2010, Figure 8-18, page 135.)

Acute hematogenous osteomyelitis results from a blood-borne infection that gains access to vascular channels in bone. *Staphylococcus aureus* is the most common organism responsible for hematogenous osteomyelitis in children over 3 years of age. This usually occurs in large venous channels in the metaphysis of children after mechanical trauma. Healthy adults are usually not at risk, but it is not uncommon to see acute osteomyelitis in older debilitated patients with chronic disease (diabetes, peripheral vascular disease). Genitourinary infections are also a risk factor in the elderly. Organisms such as *Pseudomonas aeruginosa* can gain access to the spine via the Batson venous plexus. While children may present with high fever and pain, symptoms in adults may be much more subtle.

Osteomyelitis resulting from direct inoculation may occur following puncture wounds, accidents, or surgery. Infections resulting from accidents may be polymicrobial (staphylococcus, streptococcus, gram-negative organisms) due to the diversity of foreign material that may be introduced to the wound. Iatrogenic infections may follow fracture fixation or prosthetic joint replacement. Infection after joint replacement may be acute or present years later.

Approximately 15–30% with acute osteomyelitis develop chronic osteomyelitis, frequently following inadequate antibiotic therapy or surgical debridement. Necrotic bone (sequestrum) prevents antimicrobial agents from reaching the microorganisms. Squamous cell carcinoma has been reported to be a late sequela of chronic osteomyelitis in approximately 1% of patients and typically is reported up to 30 or 40 years following the original infection.

Histologically, acute osteomyelitis is characterized by a neutrophilic infiltration actively destroying bone. Edges of bony trabeculae are eroded by bacterial enzymatic digestion. The morphologic appearance of chronic osteomyelitis is much more subtle, and changes may only include bony sclerosis, fibrosis, and marrow edema. In cases of chronic osteomyelitis, the histologic image is nonspecific and clinical correlation is often required.

DEVELOPMENTAL AND METABOLIC CONDITIONS OF BONE

A wide variety of developmental and metabolic conditions may affect the skeleton. Most of these conditions are rare, but their diversity speaks to the complex and intricate pathways of skeletal development. Achondroplasia, osteogenesis Imperfecta, osteopetrosis, rickets/osteomalacia, Paget disease, and osteoporosis fall into this classification.

Achondroplasia is an autosomal dominant disease caused by a defect in paracrine cell signaling, resulting in reduction in chondrocyte proliferation in the growth plate and shortened proximal extremities. Abnormalities in the components of bone matrix can also have variable effects from disability to death. **Osteogenesis imperfecta** is a group of disorders unified by defects in type I collagen synthesis. Defects in types 2, 10, and 11collagen have also been identified.

Osteopetrosis is a group of diseases characterized by decreased osteoclast bone resorption that results in skeletal sclerosis. In some cases, the defective resorption is a result of a deficiency in carbonic anhydrase II that is required to excrete hydrogen ions and create an acidic environment.

Disorders such as **rickets and osteomalacia** can result in abnormal matrix mineralization. Rickets is the term used when this disorder occurs in children, while osteomalacia refers to undermineralized bone in adults. Both are typically the result of lack of vitamin D or disturbance in vitamin D metabolism. **Paget disease** is also caused by osteoclast dysfunction. In Paget disease, periods of intense bone resorption (osteolytic stage) are followed by heavy bone formation (osteoblastic stage). Finally, bone cell activity diminishes (burnt-out osteosclerotic stage). The ultimate result is structurally unsound bone characterized by a mosaic, haphazard histologic appearance.

Osteoporosis is the result of reduced bone mass that predisposes bones to fracture. Peak bone mass is achieved during young adulthood and is dependent on a variety of factors including physical activity, diet, and hormones. By the third and fourth decade, skeletal mass begins to diminish, and some degree of age-related bone loss is expected. However, this leads many Americans susceptible to fractures. Vertebral fractures can cause loss of height, deformity, and pain. Femoral neck fractures can lead to prolonged debilitation, pulmonary embolism, and pneumonia. Prevention and treatment, including appropriate exercise, calcium and Vitamin D intake, and pharmacologic agents such as bisphosphonates, play a large role in reducing morbidity and mortality from osteoporosis.

JOINT PATHOLOGY

Introduction

Joints allow for movement while also providing mechanical support. Joints can be divided into two types: synovial and nonsynovial. Synovial joints have a joint space that allows for a wide range of motion. These joints are located between the ends of bones and are strengthened by a fibrous capsule, ligaments, and muscles. The synovial membrane forms the boundary of the joint. The synovial membrane is composed of two cell types and produces synovial fluid. Type A cells are found beneath the surface and engage in phagocytosis under the appropriate conditions. Type B cells are found on the surface. Synovial fluid is a filtrate of plasma containing hyaluronic acid, and its role is to act as a lubricant and provide nutrition for the articular hyaline cartilage. Hyaline cartilage is composed of type 2 collagen, water, proteoglycans, and chondrocytes. Its purpose is to act as a shock absorber. The metabolism of hyaline cartilage is carefully regulated through a balance of degradative enzymes and enzyme inhibitors. Nonsynovial joints are also known as synarthrosis and provide structure and support.

The majority of joint pathology relates to damage to the articular surface that can happen through degenerative mechanisms or as a result of an inflammatory process. The inflammation may be secondary to crystal deposition in or around the joint, infection, or an autoimmune disorder. The end result of these processes **is arthritis.** Less commonly, tumors and tumor-like conditions can affect the joints. A variety of these lesions will also be discussed including degenerative joint disease, inflammatory arthropathy, and gout.

CASE 18-11

A 75-year-old woman presents with painful hip. She underwent total hip replacement. Gross examination revealed a shiny smooth, eburnated articular surface.

Histologic review of the surgical specimen revealed a markedly damaged articular surface with near-complete loss of articular cartilage. Subchondral cysts are noted. These findings are consistent with **degenerative joint disease** (Figure 18-39 left).

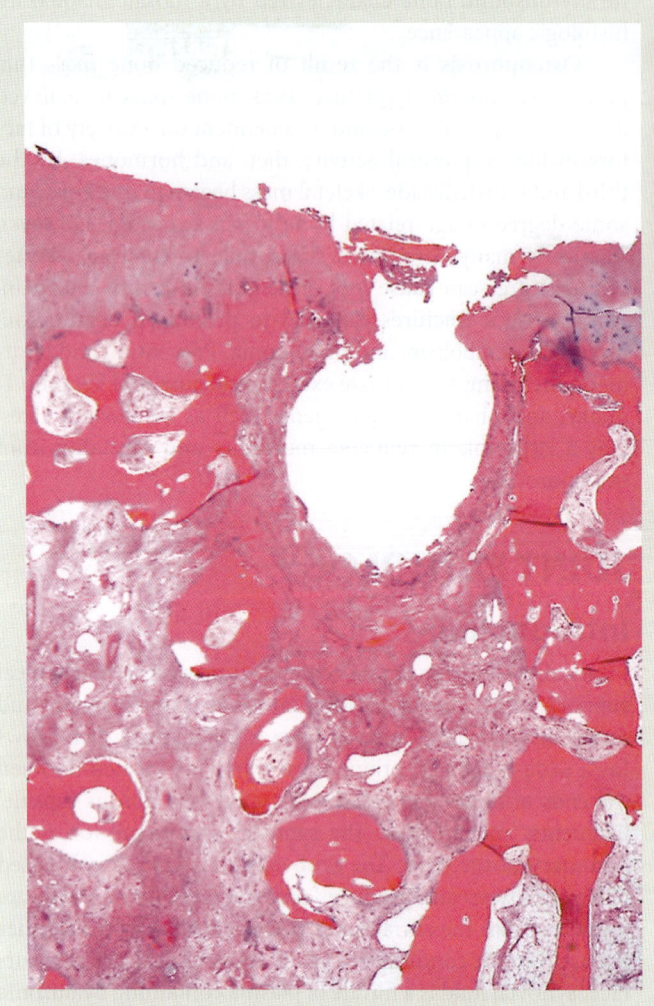

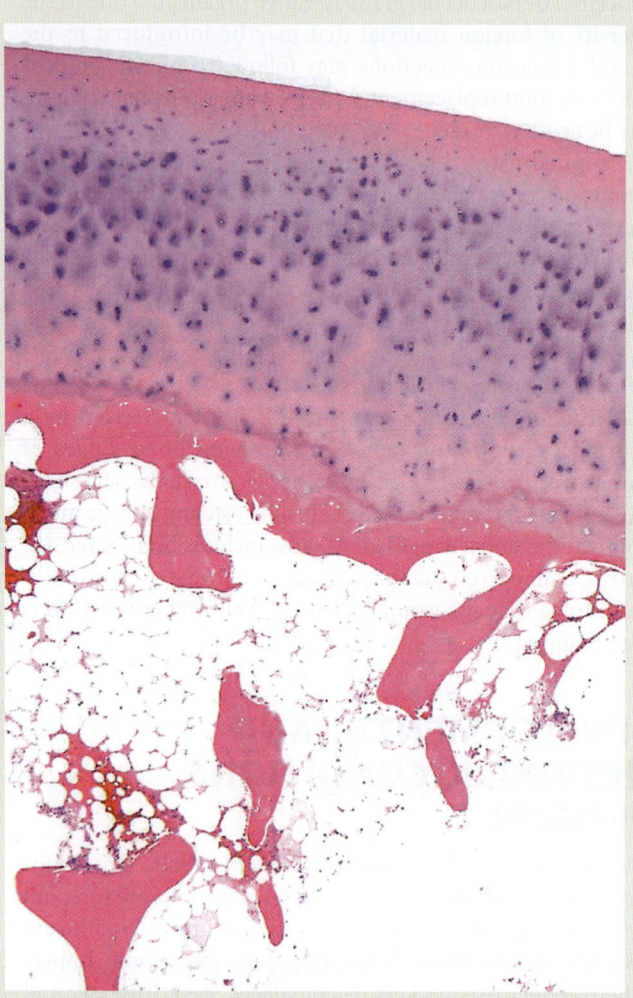

FIGURE 18-39 Osteoarthritic joint. Histologic review (left) revealed a markedly damaged articular surface with near-complete loss of articular cartilage. Subchondral cysts are noted. These findings are consistent with degenerative joint disease [normal articular surface (right) for comparison].

DEGENERATIVE JOINT DISEASE

Osteoarthritis (see Case 18-11) is the most common type of joint disease in developed nations and is characterized by erosion of the articular cartilage. Osteoarthritis is a disease of chondrocytes of the articular cartilage. Normally, these chondrocytes maintain a balance between matrix synthesis and breakdown. In osteoarthritis, this balance is disrupted. Many factors play a role in the development of osteoarthritis including age, repeated mechanical trauma, and genetics.

The clinical course is insidious. Incidence increases with age, and weight-bearing joints like the knees and hip are most commonly affected. Patients usually present with pain that worsens with use, stiffness, crepitus, and decreased range of motion. Gross examination of early disease reveals a granular articular surface as the cartilage is damaged, cracked, and degraded. In later stages, the articular cartilage may be absent entirely. In these cases, friction smoothes and polishes the underlying bone producing a polished ivory (eburnated) appearance. Histologic examination also is variable, and there is little correlation between pathologic findings and clinical severity. The articular surface shows damage including vertical clefting, osteophytes, and degenerative cysts (Figure 18-39).

Inflammatory Arthritis

While **osteoarthritis** is predominantly a noninflammatory condition that leads to joint damage, there are other conditions that lead to joint destruction through inflammatory mediators. These conditions may be infectious or noninfectious.

Rheumatoid arthritis is an example of a chronic inflammatory condition that affects many tissues and organs including joints. Women between the ages of 40 and 70 are most commonly affected. Fingers and knees are common sites. Patients usually present with swollen, hot, and tender joints. Systemic symptoms may also be present including fatigue and weight loss. Autoimmune mechanisms are thought to play a role in the pathogenesis of this disease, and the disease is thought to be triggered by exposure of a genetically susceptible host to an unknown arthritogenic antigen. Activation of lymphocytes leads to release of inflammatory mediators and cytokines that causes joint destruction. Histologic examination of the synovium reveals synovial hyperplasia, a marked lymphoplasmacytic infiltrate, and fibrinous exudate. As mentioned, this inflammatory process leads to destruction of the articular surface.

Microorganisms can enter joints during hematogenous dissemination or direct inoculation to cause infectious arthritis. **Infectious arthritis** may cause rapid and permanent destruction of a joint making early detection and appropriate treatment critical. The most common bacterial organisms include gonococcus, staphylococcus, streptococcus, *Haemophilus influenzae,* and gram-negative bacilli. Risk factors include IV drug use, joint trauma, and immune deficiencies. Individuals with sickle cell disease have a unique susceptibility to Salmonella infection. Patients usually present with sudden onset of a hot, painful joint with fever, and elevated sedimentation rate. A variety of other organisms may also result in infectious arthritis including mycobacteria and viruses.

Metabolic Diseases

Gout is characterized by the crystallization of urates within and around the joints, leading to the formation of gouty tophi. Knees, ankles, and toes are most commonly affected, and the first metatarsophalangeal joint is the most common site for acute attacks. Patients usually present with monoarticular arthritis with swelling, pain, and sometimes low-grade fever.

Uric acid is the end-product of purine metabolism. While all patients with gout have hyperuricemia, not everyone with hyperuricemia develops gout. Many factors such as age, genetics, alcohol use, obesity, and drugs all play a role in the development of gout in hyperuricemic patients. Under the right conditions, prolonged hyperuricemia will cause crystals and microtophi of urates to develop within the synovium and joint cartilage. Once the crystals are released into the joint fluid, inflammatory cells are recruited through the release of chemokines. Free radicals, leukotrienes, and destructive lysosomal enzymes damage and destroy the articular surface. Repeated attacks of such acute arthritis lead to severe cartilage damage.

Tophi are the hallmark of gout and consist of aggregates of urate crystals. Individual crystals are negatively birefringent and needle-shaped when viewed under polarized light. Tophi are typically surrounded by intense inflammation including lymphocytes, macrophages, and multinucleated giant cells.

Pseudogout (calcium pyrophosphate deposition disease, chondrocalcinosis) usually occurs in individuals over 50 years of age. Crystals develop in the articular matrix, menisci, and intervertebral disks and appear as purplish deposits microscopically. Individual crystals are generally rhomboid-shaped and weakly birefringent. Pseudogout is generally asymptomatic.

NEOPLASMS OF THE SYNOVIUM

The synovium of tendon sheath, bursa, and joint is best regarded as one anatomic unit that is capable of giving rise to a family of tumors. In order to best understand this group of lesions, it is important to know that different terms exist but usually refer to the same process. While the anatomic location and presentation of these lesions vary, the cellular constituents are the same: multinucleated giants cells, hemosiderin-laden macrophages, foamy histiocytes, and mononuclear cells. Two types of mononuclear cells are present: small lymphocyte-like cells and larger ganglion-like cells with abundant cytoplasm and eccentrically placed nuclei.

Tenosynovial giant cell tumors can be categorized as intra-articular and extra-articular. Extra-articular forms can be further divided into localized and diffuse types. Localized extra-articular tenosynovial giant cell tumors are also known as giant cell tumor of tendon sheath and most commonly present as a finger or hand mass (see Case 18-12). They also occur on the feet and less commonly near large joints. Women are more commonly affected than men. These tumors usually develop slowly and are typically attached to deep structures. Histologic examination reveals a nodular or lobulated mass with a smooth overall contour. The lobules are divided by dense collagenous septa. While the proportions of cell types vary in each tumor, most lesions contain a mixed population of mononuclear cells, giant cells, xanthoma cells, and hemosiderin-laden macrophages. These are benign tumors that may locally recur in up to 20% of cases. Recurrences can be managed with simple re-excision.

Extra-articular tenosynovial giant cell tumors may also exhibit a diffuse growth pattern. These tumors may present near a joint or in soft tissue away from a joint. These tumors are much less common than the localized forms. Histologic review demonstrates sheetlike growth rather than a nodular architecture. Limited studies have shown a significant rate of local recurrence.

CASE 18-12

A 50-year-old man presents with a finger nodule.

Histologic sections show a nodular, circumscribed polymorphous proliferation composed of foamy histiocytes, multinucleated giant cells, hemosiderin-laden macrophages, and mononuclear cells. The clinical and morphologic features are consistent with **the localized extra-articular form of tenosynovial giant cell tumor (giant cell tumor of tendon sheath)** (Figure 18-40).

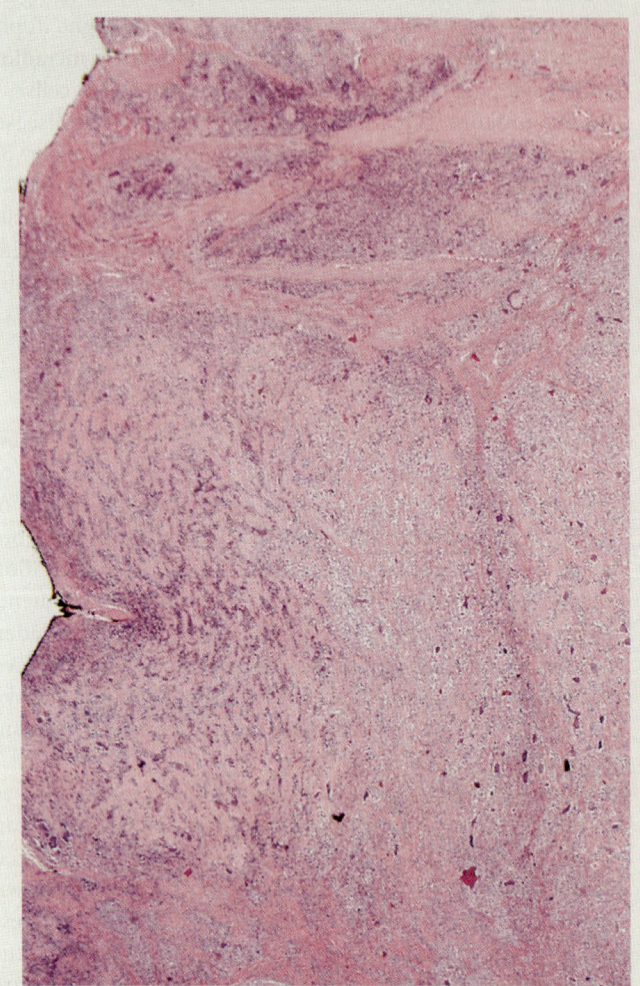

FIGURE 18-40 Tenosynovial giant cell tumor Left low power view shows a lobulated tumor mass with lobules divided by thick collagen fibers (left, low-power view). High power view (right) shows a mononuclear cell population (the neoplastic cell population admixed with multinucleated giant tumor cells).

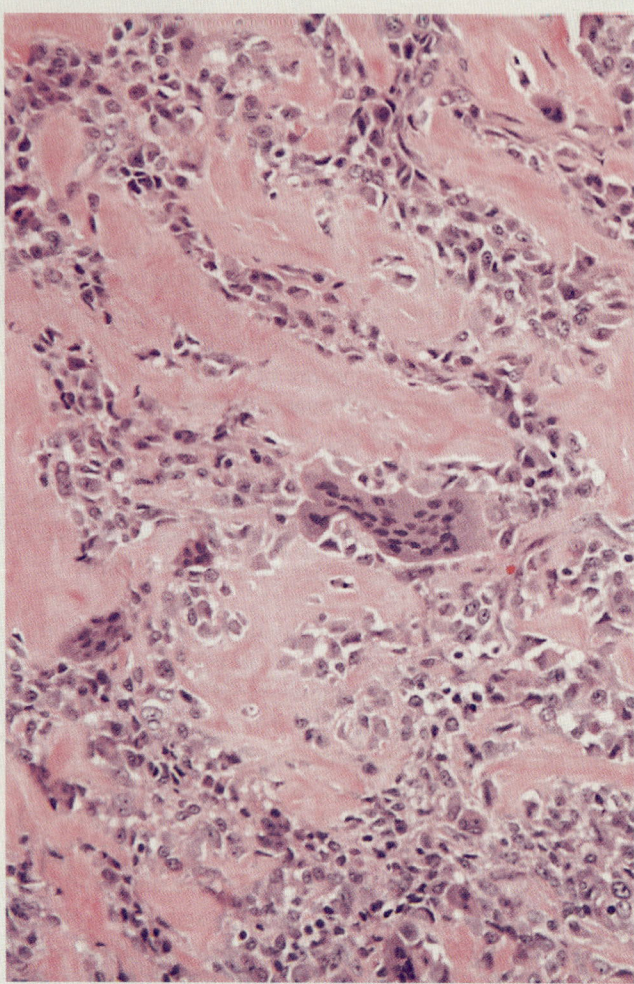

The intra-articular form of tenosynovial giant cell tumor (also known as pigmented villonodular synovitis) most commonly affects larger weight-bearing joints such as the knees and hips. Patients usually present with pain, joint swelling, and limitation of motion. Grossly, these tumors appear as irregular brown papillary projections that cover the entire synovial surface. Microscopically, these tumors are very similar to the extra-articular lesions. Unfortunately, the intra-articular form can be locally aggressive and multiple recurrences are not uncommon (Table 18-7).

TABLE 18-7 Localized versus diffuse tumors of the synovium/tendon sheath.

	Localized	Diffuse
Intra-articular	—	Pigmented villonodular synovitis
Extra-articular	Tenosynovial giant cell tumor, localized type Giant cell tumor of tendon sheath	Tenosynovial giant cell tumor, diffuse type

> **IN TRANSLATION**
>
> While there has been long-standing debate as to whether tenosynovial giant cell tumors proliferations were reactive or neoplastic, recent evidence has shown recurrent translocations of chromosome 1 involving the *CSF1* gene, supporting the theory that these lesion are true neoplasms. Additional work has shown the mononuclear population, although often representing only a minority of the lesional cells, is the neoplastic population.

Synovial chondromatosis is a metaplastic condition in which multiple nodules of cartilage are produced from the articular or tendon synovial sheath membranes. Some of the nodules may become detached and float in the joint. This condition is rare but usually peaks in mid adult life, and males are more commonly involved. Weight-bearing joints such as the knee, hip, and elbow are most commonly affected. Patients usually present with pain, swelling, and limitation of motion. Imaging usually shows multifocal articular and periarticular nodules with stippled or ringlike calcifications. Grossly, the nodules range from less than 1 mm to greater than 1 cm. Microscopic examination reveals multiple, circumscribed nodules of cartilage composed of clusters of chondrocytes with a relatively uniform distribution. Synovial chondromatosis is usually a self-limited condition that eventually reaches a quiescent stage. Treatment usually involves removing the cartilaginous nodules and synovial membrane.

Synovial lipomas may be circumscribed or diffuse (lipoma arborescens). The circumscribed form is rare but grossly and microscopically identical to soft tissue lipoma. Lipoma arborescens is more common and diffusely involves the joint capsule. Grossly, these lesions are composed of multiple papillary excrescences of mature adipose tissue lined by synovial cells.

CHAPTER 19

Neuromuscular Pathology

Eric T. Lee, D.O. and Nizar Chahin, M.D.

QUICK REVIEW
Organization of Skeletal Muscle

Neuromuscular diseases include a wide-ranging variety of pathologies that can produce significant disability for the patient. The history and physical examination are very important in narrowing the differential, and the muscle biopsy provides an additional layer of granularity to assist in making the diagnosis. To understand muscle pathology, one must understand the organization of the skeletal muscle and the histochemical stains that provide the means necessary to distinguish between potential differentials (Figures 19-1 and 19-2).

Fascicles
- Perimysium: Connective tissue surrounding the fascicles
- Endomysium: Connective tissue surrounding the muscle fibers inside the fascicles
- Epimysium: Connective tissue covers the outer surface of the muscle

Muscle Fibers
- Myofibrils: An elongated structure containing cytoskeletal elements allowing the muscle to contract
- Sarcomere: Thick (myosin) and thin filaments (actin, troponin, tropomyosin)
- The striated muscle appearance is created by pattern of alternating dark and light bands

Sarcolemma (Plasma Membrane)
- Sarcoplasma: Specialized cytoplasm of a muscle cell
- Nuclei and mitochondria are located just beneath the sarcolemma
- Sarcoplasmic reticulum extends between the myofibrils

WHAT TO DO
Evaluation of Myopathies

To appropriately work up a myopathy, the following elements should be included:

- Detailed history, including related family medical conditions
- Detailed neurological examination especially of the different muscle groups to determine the distribution of weakness
- Laboratory testing: CK, liver function tests, ESR, CRP, ANA (antinuclear antigen), anti-double stranded DNA antibody, ENA (extractable nuclear antigens), rheumatoid factor, complement (C3, C4), myositis profile
- Genetic testing
- Electrophysiological studies
- Muscle biopsy

Muscle Biopsy

A muscle biopsy includes several investigational components including the following features:

- Routine histochemical analysis
- Immunostaining
- Biochemical analysis
- Genetic analysis

Muscle Fiber Types

Muscle fibers can be divided based on specific characteristics and can be found in different concentrations in different muscles throughout the body. Muscles form a mosaic or checkerboard pattern of different fiber types.

- Type 1: Slow-twitch, oxidative
- Type 2A: Fast-twitch, oxidative-glycolytic
- Type 2B: Fast-twitch, glycolytic
- Type 2C: Undifferentiated

Type 1 fibers have the following properties:

- Loaded with mitochondria
- Depend on cellular respiration for ATP
- Fatty acids are the main energy source
- Resistant to fatigue
- Rich in myoglobin (red meat)
- Activated by small diameter, slow conducting motor neurons
- Slow twitch fibers

- Muscles used in activities requiring endurance

Type 2 fibers have the following properties:

- Few mitochondria
- Rich in glycogen
- Depend on creatine phosphate and glycolysis for ATP production
- Low in myoglobin (white meat)
- Activated by large diameter fast conducting motor neurons
- Fast twitch fibers
- Rapid and forceful movement

Muscle Staining (Figures 19-3 to 19-5)

A. Hematoxylin & eosin (H&E): Enables visualization of the general structure including fiber size, position of nuclei, fibrosis, inflammation, evidence for necrosis, and invasion by macrophages (myophagocytosis)
B. Gomori trichrome: Stains mitochondria, nemaline rods, and membranous whorls of rimmed vacuoles red; type 1 fibers are darker
C. Nicotinamide adenine dinucleotide (NADH): Enables separation of fiber types based on density of mitochondria, reveals distribution of mitochondria, and can show myofibrillar disruption; type 1 fibers are darker (Figures 19-6 to 19-8).
D. Adenosine triphosphatase (ATPase) 4.3: Reveals the distribution and involvement of the different fiber types and their subtypes. At this pH type 1 fibers stain darker
E. Adenosine triphosphatase (ATPase) 9.6: Same as 4.3. At this pH type 2 fibers stain darker
F. Periodic acid-Schiff (PAS): Heavily stains those fibers with excessive glycogen; fibers with loss of glycogen are white. The example shown is McArdle disease.
G. Myophosphorylase: Absence of this enzyme in muscle fibers occurs in McArdle disease (myophosphorylase deficiency)
H. Congo red: Reveals the presence of β-amyloid as seen in inclusion body myositis as discussed below

MUSCLE PATHOLOGY

Neuromuscular diseases demonstrate a wide variety of pathology with regard to muscle biopsies. Each muscle sample provides different clues based on the different stains mentioned above that guide the investigator and help narrow the differential. These clues for the investigator include

- Fiber shape and size: Muscles fibers can become, for example, more rounded in muscular dystrophies and angulated in neurogenic pathologies
- Atrophy patterns: Atrophy of particular muscle types can produce a pattern called group atrophy affecting both type 1 and 2 fibers that is often seen in neurogenic pathologies. In dermatomyositis, a specific pattern is seen that is perifascicular atrophy as shown later
- Denervation and reinnervation: When denervated muscle becomes reinnervated the checkerboard pattern is disrupted. Sprouts of adjacent motor fibers reinnervate the denervated muscle causing an enlarged motor unit composed of an increased number of fibers. These fibers are of the same type and produce fiber-type grouping that suggests reinnervation is occurring
- Sarcolemmal nuclei position: In normal muscle the nuclei are placed peripherally, but in myopathic muscle there is an increase in the central position of the nuclei (Figures 19-9 and 19-10)
- Muscle fiber necrosis and regeneration (Figures 19-9 and 19-10): Muscle fiber necrosis represents an injury to all organelles of the fiber or to a segment of the fiber. Necrotic fibers are faintly stained and can be invaded by macrophages (myophagocytosis). Simple necrosis is seen with myopathies, such as autoimmune necrotizing myopathy. Regenerating fibers often have a bluish tinge and enlarged nuclei. When a muscle fiber is damaged a satellite cell, which is located on the periphery of the muscle fiber and contains one nucleus, which fills most of the cell volume, fuses with the injured fiber with donation of the nucleus.
- Fibrosis and adipose tissue: The endomysial or perimysial connective tissue may proliferate leading to a clear separation of muscle fibers. It is commonly seen in Duchenne and Becker muscular dystrophy. Excess adipose tissue may accompany fibrosis that is commonly seen in some congenital muscular dystrophies such as central core disease.
- Changes in fiber architecture and structural abnormalities: many different architecture patterns can be seen. For example, in central core disease the core zone lacks mitochondria and oxidative enzyme activity that is in contrast to the normal peripheral zone.
- Deficiency of enzymes: This can be seen in pathologies such as myophosphorylase deficiency as described above.
- Accumulation of glycogen: This pathology can be seen in disorders like acid maltase deficiency (Pompe disease) in which there is a deficiency of α-1,4-glucosidase that hydrolyzes chains of glycogen to glucose.

Neurogenic changes in muscle biopsy include:

- Small, angulated muscle fibers (adults) of both fiber type (1 and 2)
- Small, round muscle fibers (infants)
- Target fibers
- Fiber type grouping

Myopathic changes on muscle biopsy include:

- Muscle fiber size variability
- Endomysial fibrosis

NEUROMUSCULAR PATHOLOGY 529

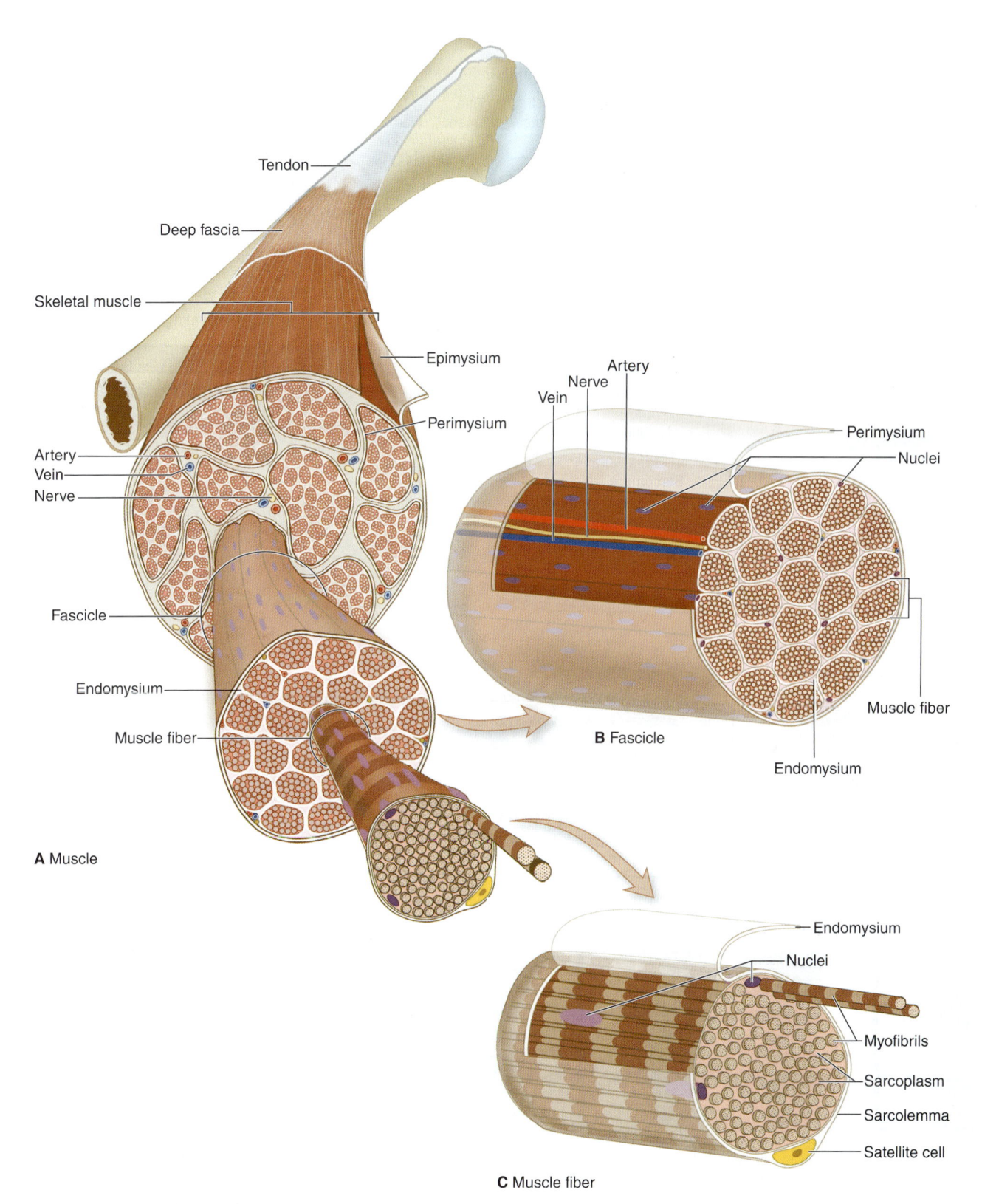

FIGURE 19-1 Organization of skeletal muscle. **(A)** An entire skeletal muscle is enclosed within a dense connective tissue layer called the **epimysium** continuous with the tendon binding it to bone. **(B)** Each fascicle of muscle fibers is wrapped in another connective tissue layer called the **perimysium**. **(C)** Individual muscle fibers (elongated multinuclear cells) are surrounded by a very delicate layer called the **endomysium**, which includes an external lamina produced by the muscle fiber (and enclosing the satellite cells) and ECM produced by fibroblasts. (From Mescher AI, Junqueira's Basic Histology, 12th ed. McGraw Hill Lange New York 2010, Chapter 10, Figure 10-3, page 170.)

FIGURE 19-2 Structure of a myofibril: a series of sarcomeres. (A) Diagram indicates that each muscle fiber contains several parallel bundles called myofibrils. (B) Each myofibril consists of a long series of sarcomeres that contain thick and thin filaments and are separated from one another by Z discs. (C) Thin filaments are actin filaments with one end bound to α-**actinin**, the major protein of the Z disc. Thick filaments are bundles of myosin, which span the entire A band and are bound to proteins of the M line and to the Z disc across the I bands by a very large protein called **titin**, which has spring-like domains. (D) The molecular organization of the sarcomeres has bands of greater and lesser protein density, resulting in staining differences that produce the dark and light-staining bands seen by light microscopy and TEM. (From Mescher AI, Junqueira's Basic Histology, 12th ed. McGraw Hill Lange New York 2010, Chapter 10 Figure 10-8, page 173.)

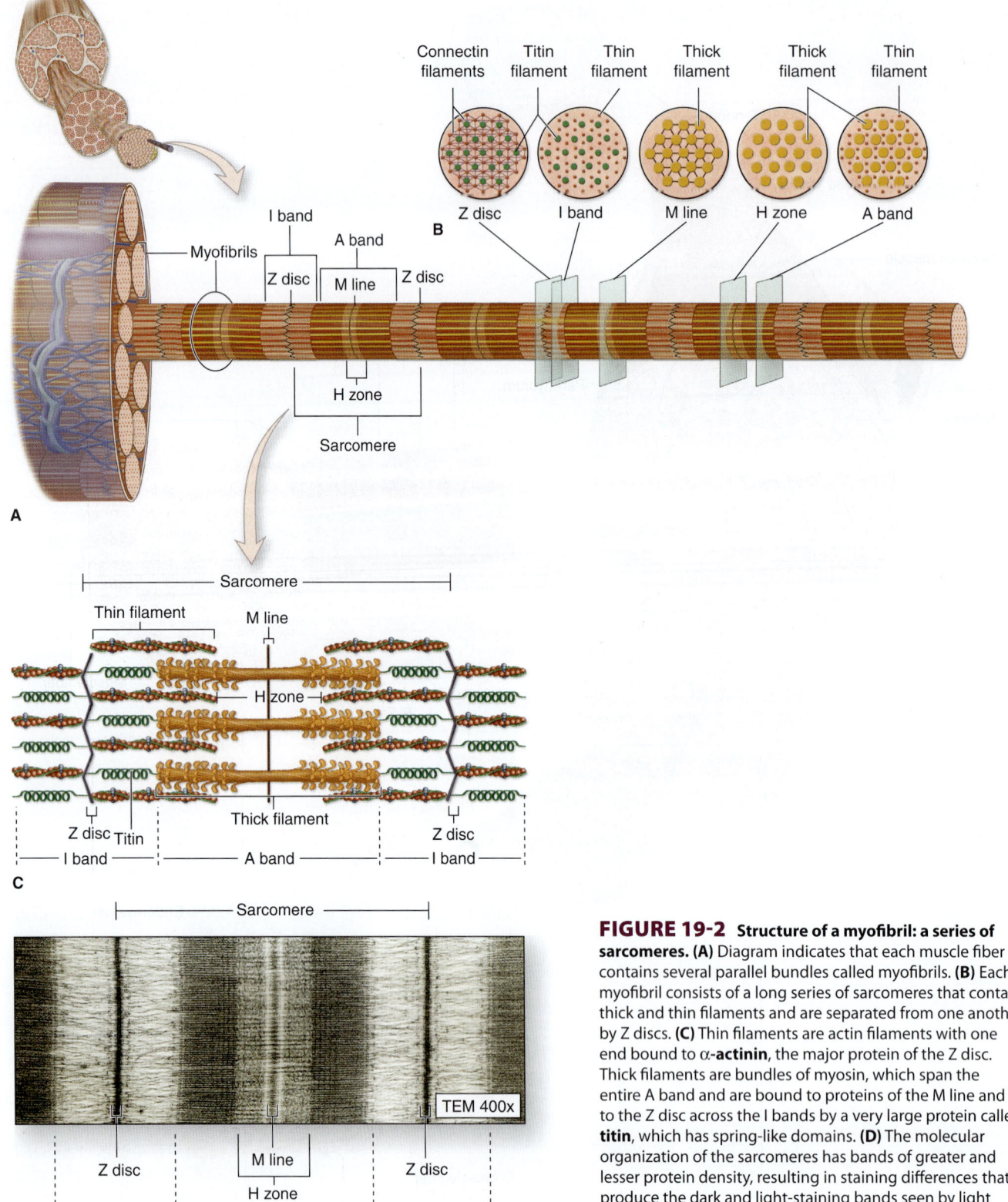

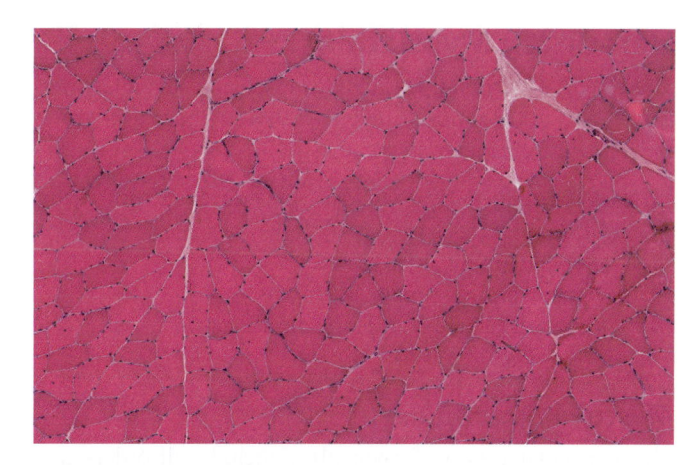

FIGURE 19-3 Hematoxylin & eosin (H&E) stain of skeletal muscle in cross-section.

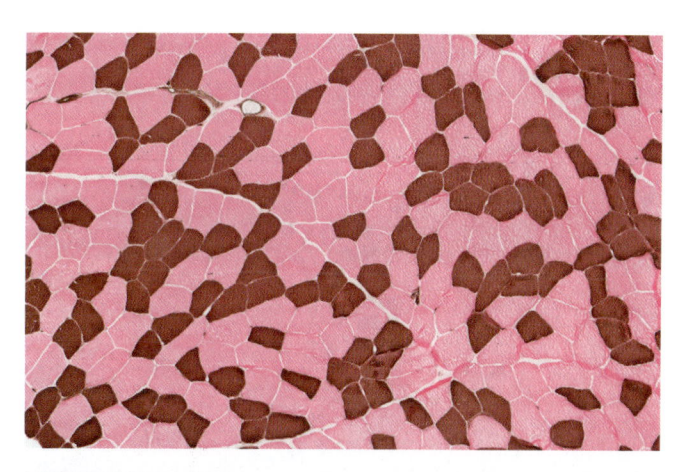

FIGURE 19-6 Adenosine triphosphatase 4.3 stain of skeletal muscle in cross-section.

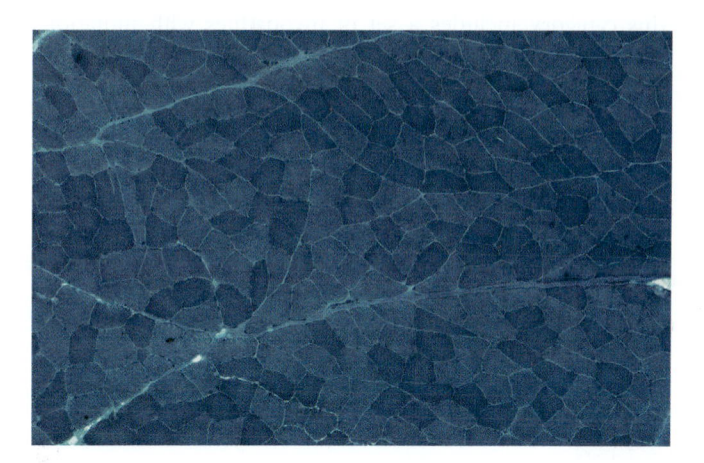

FIGURE 19-4 Gomori trichrome stain in cross-section.

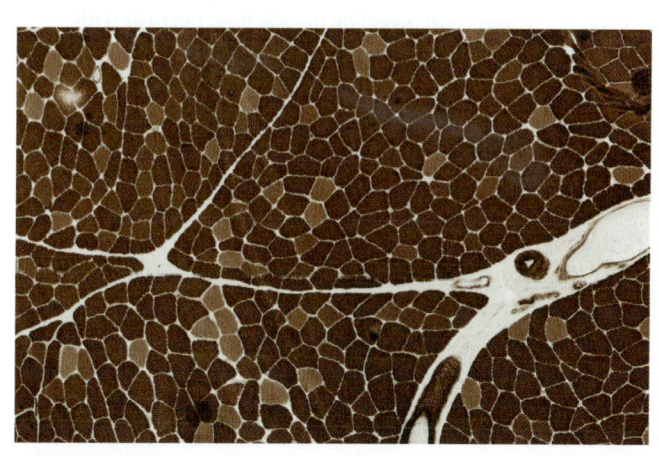

FIGURE 19-7 Adenosine triphosphatase 9.6 stain of skeletal muscle in cross-section.

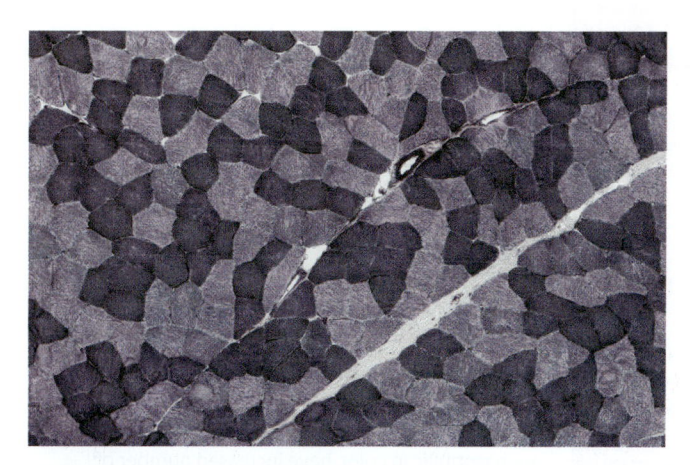

FIGURE 19-5 Nicotinamide adenine dinucleotide stain of skeletal muscle in cross-section.

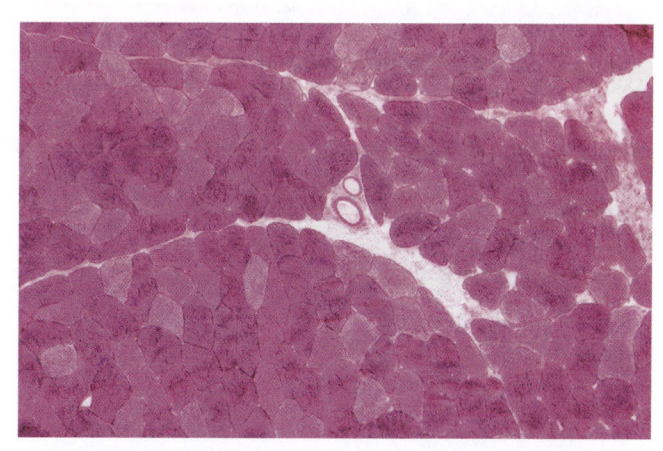

FIGURE 19-8 Periodic acid-Schiff (PAS) stain of skeletal muscle in cross-section.

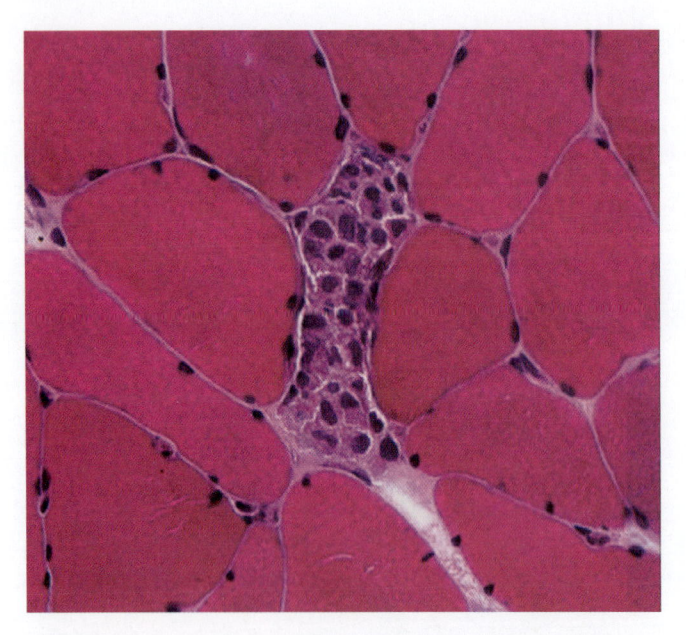

FIGURE 19-9 Hematoxylin & eosin (H&E) stain of skeletal muscle in cross-section revealing muscle fiber necrosis with myophagocytosis.

- Increased central nuclei (>3% of muscle fibers)
- Segmental necrosis of muscle fibers, often with myophagocytosis
- Regeneration
- Ring fibers
- Fatty infiltration and replacement
- Myocyte hypertrophy
- Fiber splitting

Hereditary Myopathies

The hereditary myopathies include muscular, congenital, metabolic, and mitochondrial myopathies. They have as a group the following characteristics:

1. Skeletal deformities: scoliosis, hyperlordosis, pes cavus, contractures
2. Calf hypertrophy
3. Very slow progression of symptoms
4. Early onset (usually) and long duration

Muscular Dystrophies

This particular group of myopathies includes disorders that have a defect in the muscle membrane proteins, for example, Duchenne and Becker muscular dystrophy, and limb-girdle muscular dystrophy.

Congenital Myopathies

This category includes a set of myopathies with mutations in the sarcomere proteins that are most often recognized at birth or in early childhood, but some may have an adult onset. There is often hypotonia present to the degree the young child is called floppy. The muscle weakness tends to be nonprogressive, but there can be diaphragmatic weakness and respiratory insufficiency. The muscle weakness tends to be proximal in the girdle distribution. A common feature is the long myopathic face with some degree of weakness present hypertrophy and atrophy of muscle fibers often seen without necrosis or regeneration. Centrally placed nuclei can be seen with myotubular and centronuclear myopathies seen in this group.

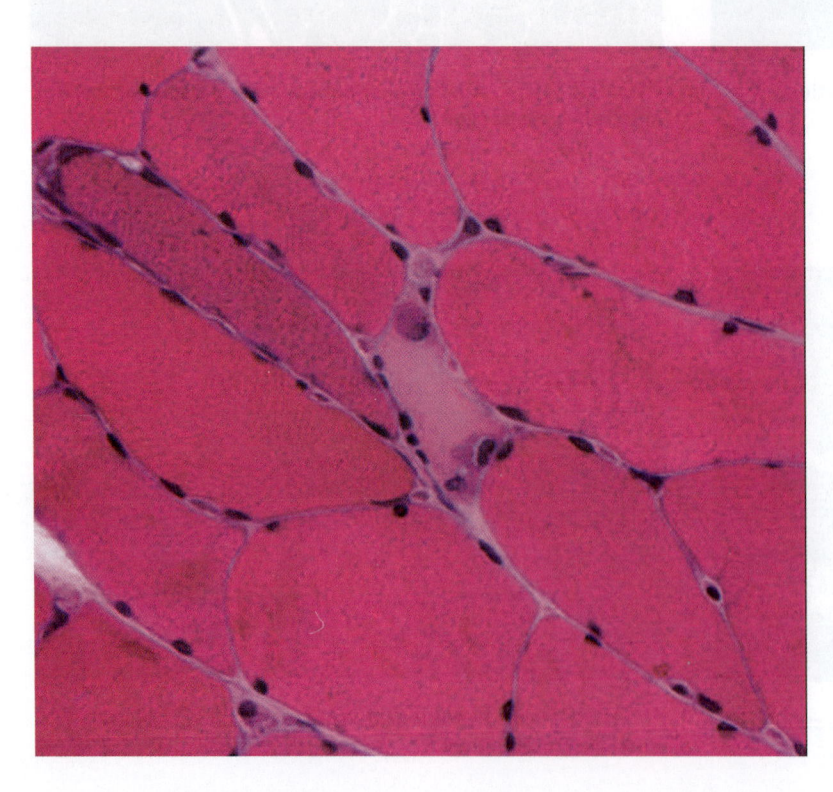

FIGURE 19-10 Hematoxylin & eosin (H&E) stain of skeletal muscle in cross-section. Regenerating fibers are basophilic in color, have increased number of subsarcolemmal nuclei, and contain large, dark, and prominent nucleoli.

CASE 19-1

A 3-year-old boy who was the product of normal vaginal delivery and with normal developmental milestone until recently presented with the inability to run. He had difficulty getting up from a low sitting position or climbing stairs (Gower maneuver). On examination, he was found to have symmetric proximal muscle weakness with marked calf hypertrophy. He had a CK level of 10,019 U/L. Results of a muscle biopsy are shown in Figures 19-11 and 19-12.

Case Discussion

Duchenne muscular dystrophy (DMD) is a hereditary myopathy with X-linked inheritance that affects boys between 2 and 3 years of age. Most of the mutations are deletions. Becker muscular dystrophy (BMD) affects boys between 5–15 years of age and is a milder form than DMD. Both DMD and BMD patients carry deletions in the dystrophin gene. Dystrophin stabilizes the muscle membrane glycoprotein complex and protects the cell from degradation. DMD is a result of base pair deletion that disrupts the reading frame causing premature truncation, leading to a nonfunctional protein and a severe disease phenotype. In contrast, BMD is also a result of base pair deletion, but it does not disrupt the reading frame allowing internally deleted dystrophins to retain part of their functionality. Both disorders have the possible consequence of developing cardiomyopathy.

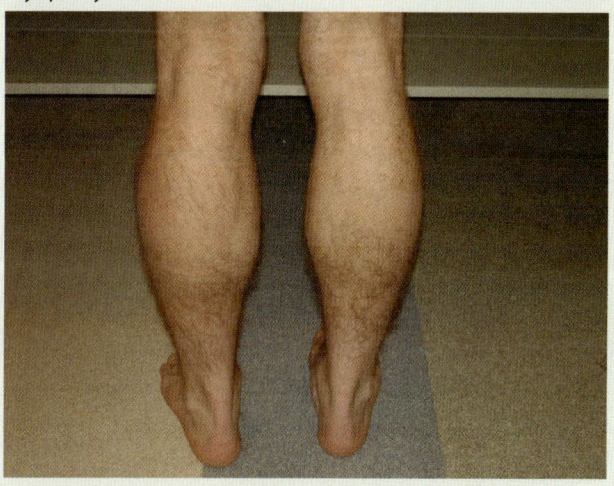

FIGURE 19-11 Calf hypertrophy found in a patient with Duchenne muscular dystrophy.

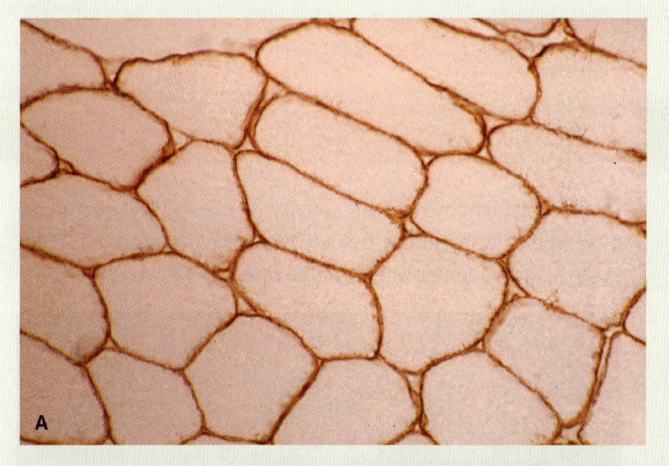

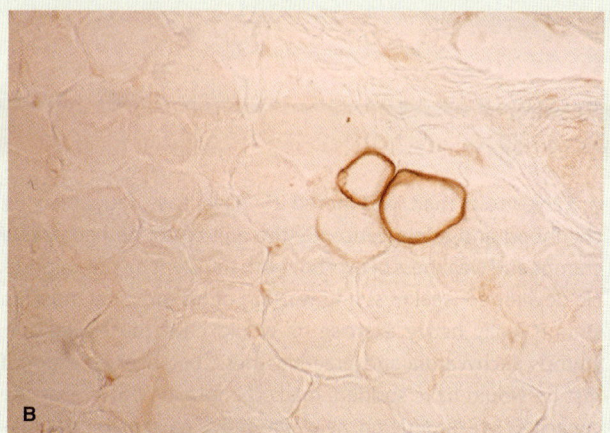

FIGURE 19-12 (A) Normal staining for dystrophin. (B) Almost complete absence of dystrophin staining in the patient's muscle biopsy.

Metabolic Myopathies

This category includes a wide range of glycogenosis and disorders of fatty acid metabolism. The primary source of energy for muscle is glycogen and disorders to the glycogen breakdown pathways can produce myopathies causing muscle fatigue, cramps, and rhabdomyolysis. On muscle biopsy, there is an excessive amount of glycogen that may occur in vacuoles. Examples for this category include **Pompe disease** (acid maltase deficiency), Cori disease (debrancher enzyme deficiency), **McArdle disease** (myophosphorylase deficiency), and **carnitine palmitoyl transferase deficiency**.

Mitochondrial Myopathies

The mitochondrial disorders are a vast array of diseases that can present with often more than one of the following neurological manifestations: global developmental delays, autism spectrum disorder, seizures, migraine headache, dementia, movement disorders such as myoclonus, stroke and stroke-like episodes, and neuropsychiatric symptoms. Other systems are often involved such as cardiovascular, ophthalmologic and gastroenterologic. The primary mitochondrial disorders may follow patterns of maternal inheritance as found in mtDNA mutations or classical Mendelian inheritance as found in nDNA mutations.

CASE 19-2

A 5-year-old female was noted to be a floppy infant at birth with a high arched palate, micrognathia, finger contractures, and joint hypermobility. Later, as a toddler she was noted to have weakness of ankle dorsiflexion, knee flexion, and the trunk. She had a nasal quality to her voice and had some respiratory weakness. A muscle biopsy was performed. Gomori trichrome stain demonstrated clusters of blue staining rods at the periphery of most fibers (Figure 19-13).

Case Discussion

Nemaline rod myopathy has several variants that have been identified. This patient has a nemaline rod myopathy type 2 that is the typical recessive form. The muscle biopsy reveals nebulin present with subsarcolemmal rods revealed by Z disk aberrations. Nebulin is a large protein that is thought to bind and stabilize actin filaments while acting as a template for thin filament assembly.

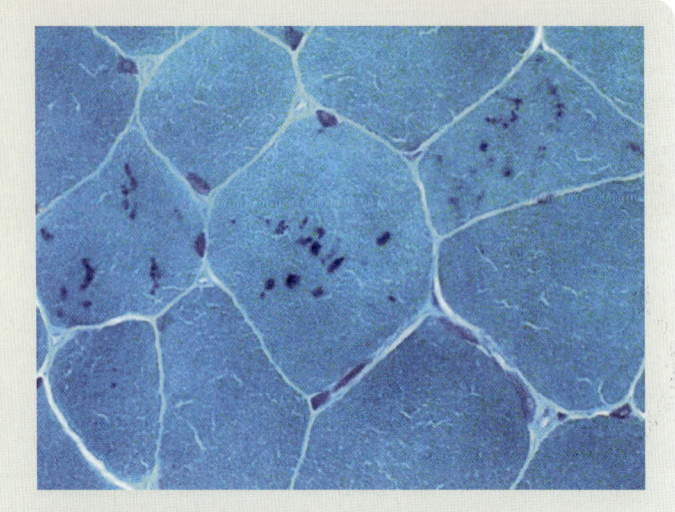

FIGURE 19-13 Nemaline rod myopathy, Gomori trichrome (GT) stain. Dark blue structures are seen only with this stain. They contain Z disk material, including α-actinin and tropomyosin. (From Congenital Myopathies, Author: Glenn Lopate, MD; Chief Editor: Amy Kao, MD, http://emedicine.medscape.com/article/1175852)

CASE 19-3

A 52-year-old man was noted to have easy fatigability in childhood and adolescence. By the age of 20, he had severe cramps and weakness of exertion with transient myoglobinuria. He developed weakness and wasting of his proximal muscles. During really heavy exercise he would have muscle fatigue, cramps, tachycardia and breathlessness, but after a period of rest he would have sudden, marked improvement in exercise capacity. On examination, he was noted to have marked hypertrophy of the deltoid, biceps, and calves. He had mild proximal muscle weakness and was noted to have a CK of up to 2500. He had an EMG that showed myopathic changes (Figure 19-14).

Case Discussion

McArdle disease (myophosphorylase deficiency) is also called glycogen storage disease type V and is a myopathy associated with exercise induced pain and myoglobinuria (rhabdomyolysis). It is a disorder with a defect of glycogen metabolism specifically of the phosphorylase enzyme causing abnormal accumulation of glycogen in muscle fibers. Many McArdle disease patients like this one experience a second wind phenomenon in which exercise tolerance improves after a short rest. The second wind probably results from a switch in metabolic pathway from the glycolytic pathway to oxidative phosphorylation. With immunohistochemistry, the activity of phosphorylase can be observed from a patient tissue with complete absence of enzyme activity seen only in McArdle disease.

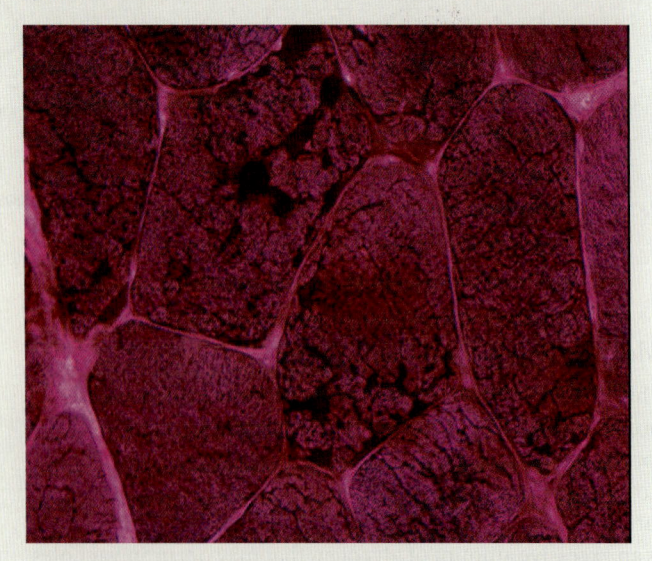

FIGURE 19-14 Periodic acid-Schiff (PAS) stain showing the presence of subsarcolemmal vacuoles or blebs that contain PAS-positive glycogen granules.

CASE 19-4

A 25-year-old female who was a product of a normal pregnancy with normal motor development developed exercise intolerance and fatigue in early childhood. She has bilateral eye ptosis, an inability to move her eyes, and a limb-girdle pattern of muscle weakness. Her symptoms were slowly progressing and she has no bulbar symptoms. Her mother had mild bilateral eye ptosis and exercise intolerance. On examination, the patient has bilateral ptosis, weakness in eye abduction and adduction and mild bilateral facial, mild neck flexor, and limb-girdle muscle weakness. Her CK levels ranged up to 2000, lactate and pyruvate were elevated. A biopsy was obtained from the left biceps muscle as shown in **Figures 19-15** to **19-17**.

Case Discussion

Kearns-Sayre Syndrome is a hereditary mitochondrial myopathy that occurs by large-scale deletion of the mitochondrial genome producing the triad of retinitis pigmentosa, progressive external ophthalmoplegia, and heart block. There are characteristically elevated levels of lactate and pyruvate found in the plasma and CSF as in this patient. Ragged red fibers are identified on Gomori trichrome stain, which signify prominent peripheral accumulations of abnormal mitochondria involving primarily type 1 fibers. The SDH, which is encoded in the cell nucleus, stain also shows mitochondrial aggregates that intensely stain in the periphery. COX negativity as shown by the white areas reveals those fibers with mitochondria carrying a mutation in cytochrome oxidase that is located in the mitochondrial genome.

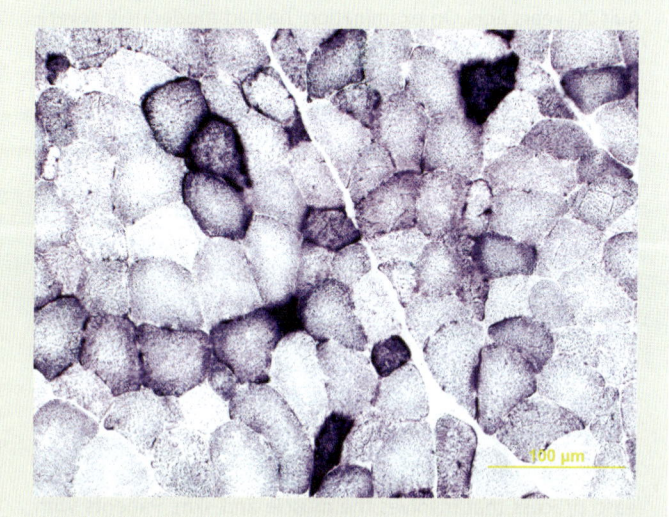

FIGURE 19-16 Succinate dehydrogenase staining showing ragged blue fibers that are intensely reactive granules.

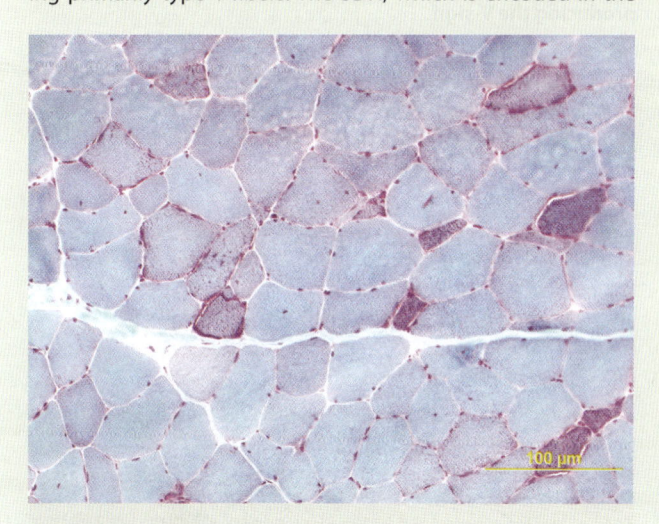

FIGURE 19-15 Ragged red fibers are identified on Gomori trichrome stain.

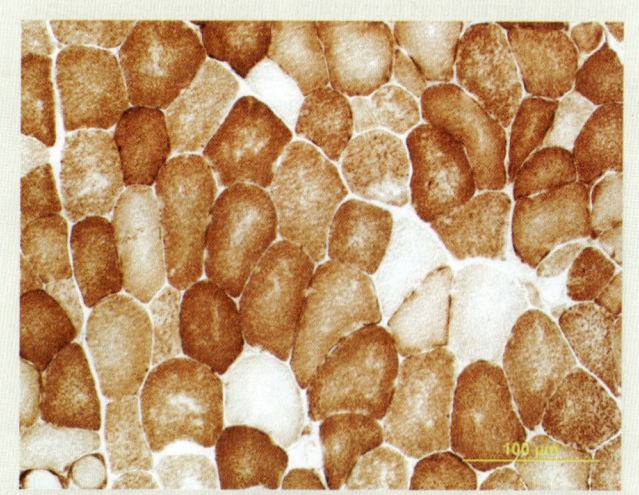

FIGURE 19-17 Cytochrome oxidase negative fibers are shown in white.

Acquired Myopathies

The acquired myopathies include inflammatory, endocrine, and toxic myopathies. It also includes myopathy associated with monoclonal gammopathy. They have as a group the following characteristics:

1. Acute to subacute onset of symptoms
2. Later age of onset
3. Rapid progression of symptoms

Inflammatory Myopathies

The inflammatory myopathies include disorders with inflammation in the muscles, necrosis, and regeneration as found in polymyositis and dermatomyositis and disorders with mixed inflammatory and degenerative components as found in inclusion body myositis. This diverse group also includes myopathies of bacterial, parasitic, viral, and toxic origin. There are many possible underlying causes that could include a connective tissue disorder with the presence of inflammatory markers or malignancy.

CASE 19-5

A 45-year-old man presented with a 7-month history of rapidly progressive, proximal more than distal muscle weakness. Two months after the onset of weakness, he noticed a lump at the angle of his left neck. Five months later he noticed his face was getting red. He used to smoke a 1 and half pack for 15 years and quit 20 years ago. On examination, he had moderately severe proximal more than distal muscle weakness, normal tendon reflexes and sensory exam, skin changes, and a hard, immobile, nontender mass at the angle of the left jaw. He had the following positive labs: CK 6295 U/L, AST 391 U/L, ALT 267 U/L, ANA speckled type, titer >1:640. He had the following negative labs: ENA, dsDNA, rheumatoid factor, paraneoplastic panel, and myositis profile. He had a normal colonoscopy and serum PSA. He underwent a CT chest, abdomen, and pelvis with contrast that was negative, except for an enhancing mass in the neck, which leads to radical dissection of squamous cell carcinoma (Figure 19-18 and 19-19).

Case Discussion

Dermatomyositis is an acquired, inflammatory myopathic disease process that involves the muscle and skin. Patients with this disease like the case presentation have proximal muscle weakness with elevated CK most of the time. There are characteristic skin findings that include a heliotrope rash, which is a violaceous discoloration of the upper eyelids, and Gottron sign, which is seen in Figure 19-17 and erythema and prominent hyperpigmentation seen in Figure 19-19. Figure 19-20 demonstrates the characteristic histopathology associated with dermatomyositis including perimysial and perivascular inflammation. With this condition, there is an association with malignancy in 25–40%, especially in people over 50 years of age. Once the diagnosis is made, it is necessary to screen for malignancy.

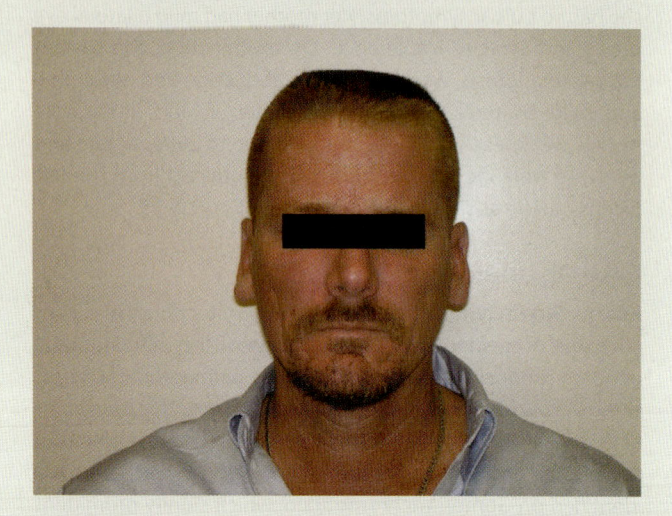

FIGURE 19-19 Erythema and prominent hyperpigmentation involving the face and upper chest producing the V-sign.

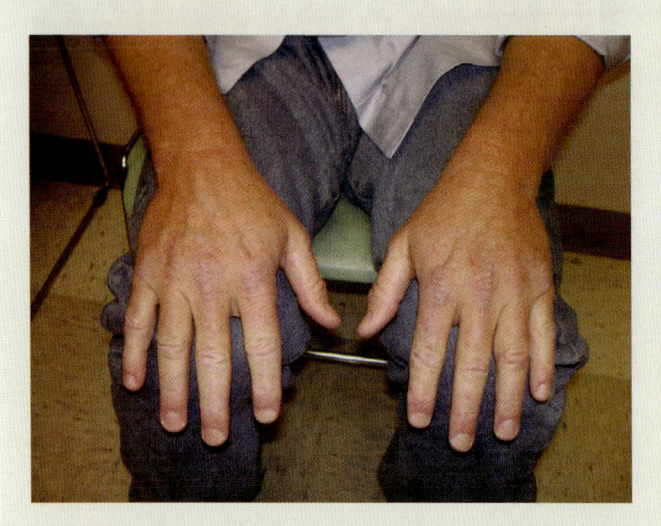

FIGURE 19-18 Violaceous raised papules overlying the metacarpal and interphalangeal joints.

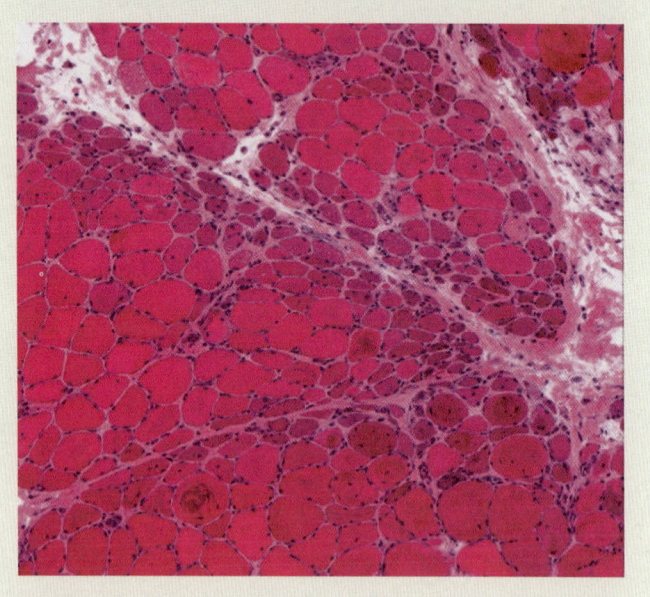

FIGURE 19-20 Hematoxylin & eosin (H&E) stain showing perifasicular atrophy and perimysial and perivascular inflammation.

CASE 19-6

A 71-year-old man presented with a 2-year history of falls and progressive muscle weakness. He had a difficult time getting up from a low position and lifting his arms **(Figure 19-21** to **19-24)**. He had difficulty holding a golf club, opening jars, and turning doorknobs. On examination, he had proximal more than distal muscle weakness with absent tendon reflexes and a normal sensory exam with a normal CK.

Case Discussion

Inclusion body myositis is the most common acquired inflammatory myopathy after the age of fifty. It is found more often in males than females. The distribution is unique in that it has selective involvement of finger flexors and quadriceps muscles. The histopathology reveals a mixed inflammatory and degenerative disease of the muscle with endomysial CD8+ T cells surrounding and invading non-necrotic muscle fibers. There is an accumulation of Alzheimer characteristic proteins such as amyloid-β and phosphorylated tau that are identified by Congo red staining.

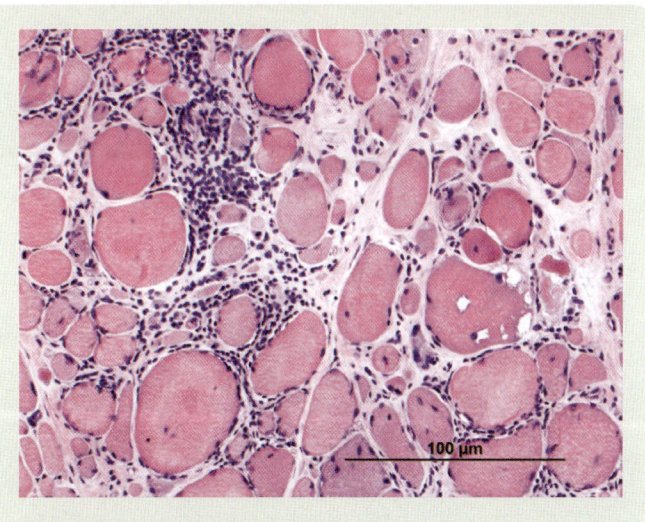

FIGURE 19-22 Hematoxylin & eosin (H&E) stain showing endomysial inflammation and fibers with rimmed vacuoles.

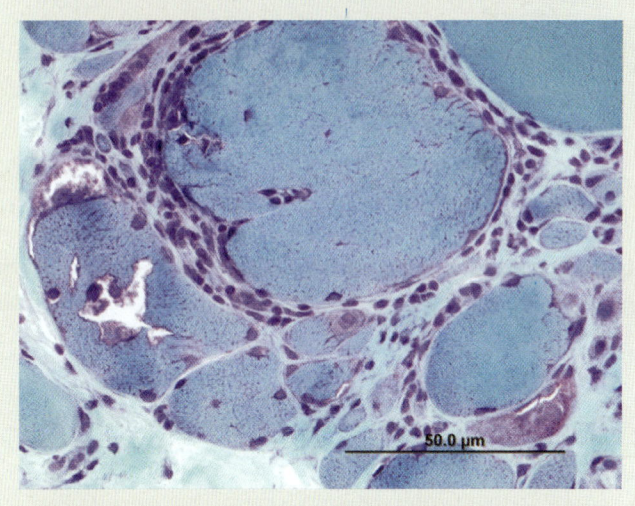

FIGURE 19-23 Gomori trichrome stain showing fibers with vacuoles rimmed by basophilic granules.

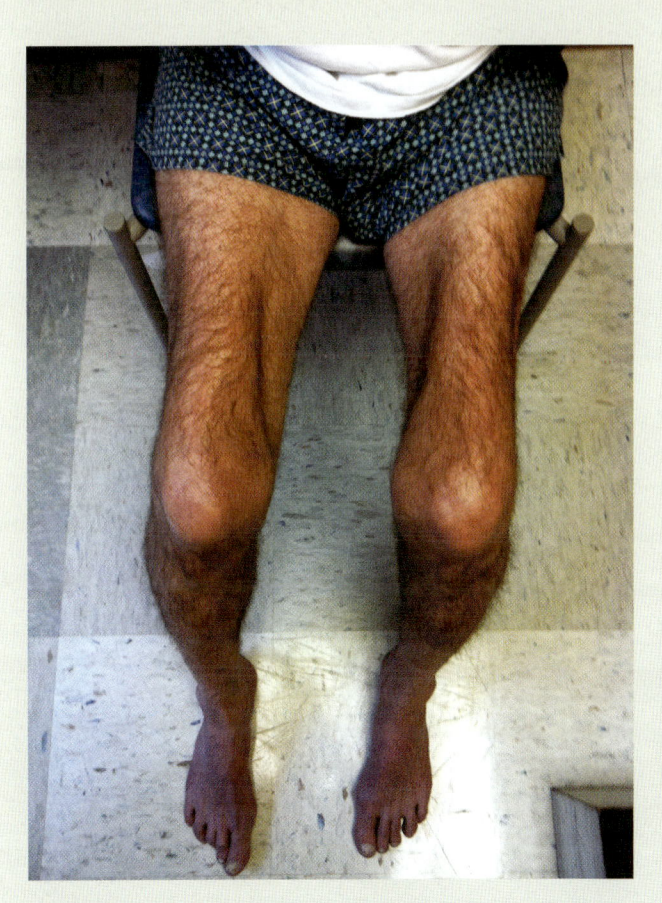

FIGURE 19-21 Image demonstrates severe atrophy of the quadriceps muscles in a patient with inclusion body myositis.

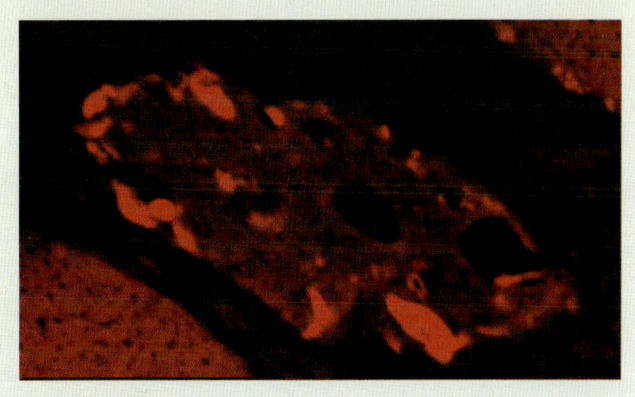

FIGURE 19-24 Congo red staining showing discrete areas of congophilia reflecting the presence of β-amyloid deposits.

CHAPTER 20

Pathology of the Skin

Jayson R. Miedema, Christopher Sayed, and Daniel C. Zedek

INTRODUCTORY CASE (BULLOUS PEMPHIGOID)

A 77-year-old woman presents to a local emergency room after developing numerous blisters over her trunk and extremities. She reports that the evening prior she developed an intensely pruritic red rash, and the next morning she was alarmed when she woke and noticed large, painful blisters erupting within the rash. Examination shows numerous tense bullae with erythematous, indurated borders over the trunk and extremities. A dermatologist is called for consultation and performs a punch biopsy from the edge of one of the large blisters. Clinical image and results of hematoxylin and eosin (H&E) staining are shown in **Figure 20-1A–C**.

Microscopic examination is most notable for a split at the dermoepidermal junction. While this finding can be seen in other blistering disorders, it is perhaps most characteristic of bullous pemphigoid. Bullous pemphigoid is an autoimmune blistering disorder caused by formation of pathogenic antibodies to a component of hemidesmosomes, specifically bullous pemphigoid antigen 2, which is necessary for binding of the superficial component of the skin, the epidermis, to the deeper component, the dermis. An accompanying inflammatory infiltrate with prominent eosinophils is also highly indicative of bullous pemphigoid. As discussed in the cases below, further diagnostic studies using immunofluorescence can often help cinch the diagnosis.

PART 1: INTRODUCTION

The skin is the largest organ in the body and serves as its external covering, separating our sometimes fragile interior from the dangers of our environment. It provides a barrier that protects the body from both physical and environmental threats. It also acts as the primary defensive layer of the immune system by preventing infectious organisms from entering the body. Additionally, the skin plays a significant role in thermoregulation and is important in preventing overheating or overcooling of the body.

In medicine, the skin is involved in a vast number of pathological conditions. While there is a large number of conditions that primarily and exclusively manifest in the skin, our external surface can also give us diagnostic clues to pathology taking place elsewhere in the body. Because there are such a large number of conditions affecting the skin, it is sometimes useful to think of the conditions that affect the skin in groups. These may include inflammatory, immune-mediated, neoplastic, and infectious processes. Study of the skin is not the sole realm of the dermatologist as almost every field or subfield in medicine requires at least a basic understanding of dermatopathologic conditions, and it is often the case that certain specialties and subspecialties require an even more in-depth knowledge. For example, an ear, nose, and throat specialist may become an expert regarding *basal cell* and *squamous cell carcinoma*, while the gynecologist may develop an important familiarity with *lichen planus*, *lichen sclerosus*, and certain types of adnexal tumors affecting the female genital area. Similarly, a gastroenterologist may develop an expertise with a disorder such as *dermatitis herpetiformis*, which often occurs with the common disorder of gastrointestinal distress, *celiac disease*.

Here we hope to provide a basic, practical foundation in dermatopathology on which a student can build as they become further specialized. This will serve them in communicating with colleagues from their own specialties and others. Of course, it is not possible for us to discuss each of the protean number of diseases exhaustively. We have thus chosen to highlight diseases for which professionals from most if not all fields require knowledge. Different texts on the subject have divided dermatopathology content in different ways and many disease processes could fit into multiple groups. For simplicity, we have divided the following content into groups based on conditions and prototypes in order to provide an introductory knowledge. We first begin with a general discussion of skin anatomy and histology to serve as a basis for the subsequent sections.

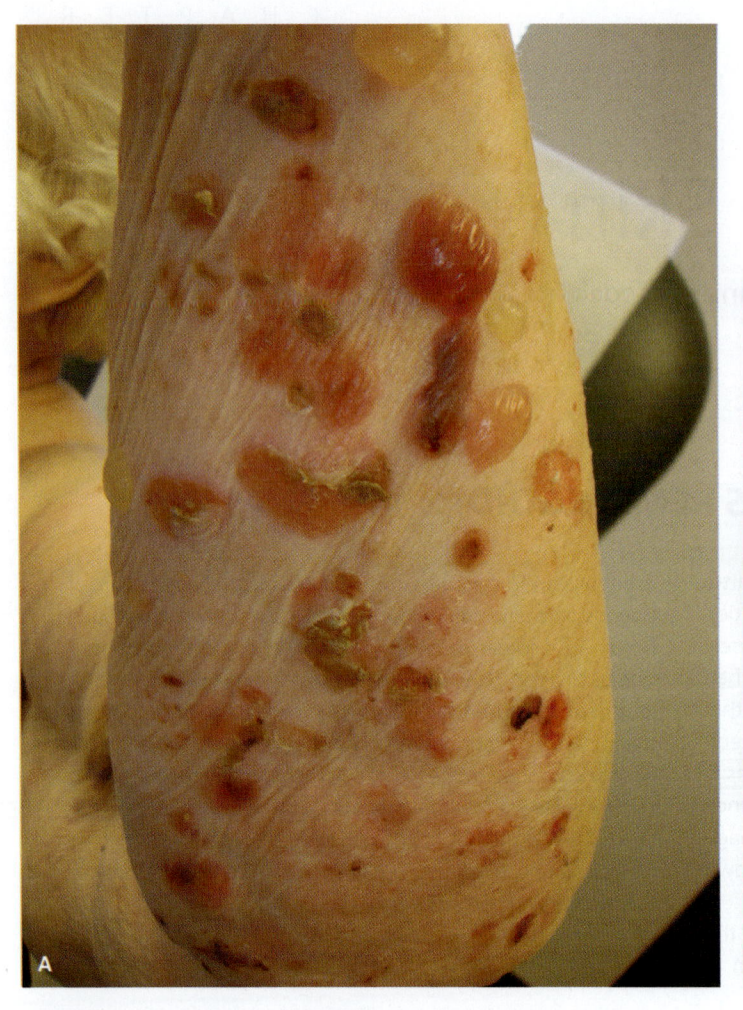

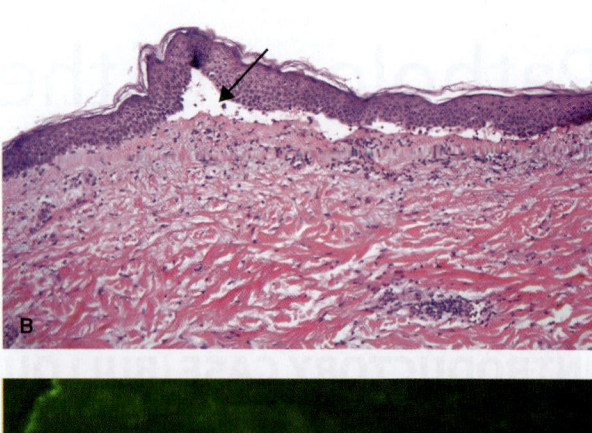

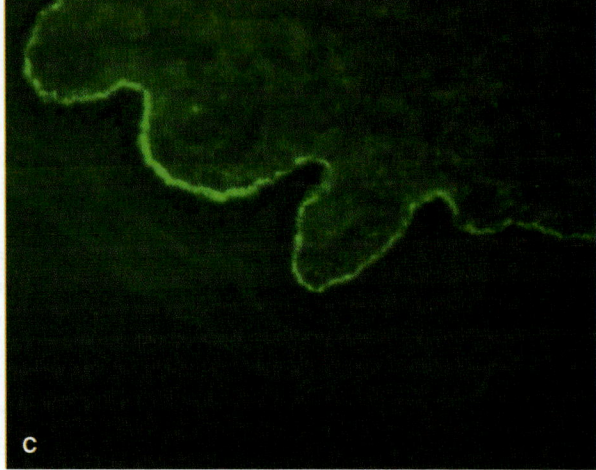

FIGURE 20-1 Bullous pemphigoid. **(A)** Tense bullae overlying an erythematous base in bullous pemphigoid. Photograph Courtesy of Dr. Luis Diaz, UNC Dermatology. **(B)** Hematoxylin and eosin stained biopsy with split at dermal–epidermal junction (arrow). **(C)** Direct immunofluorescence demonstrating linear staining of IgG at the basement membrane zone. Image used with permission of Dr. Luis Diaz and Dr. Donna Culton, UNC Dermatology.

SKIN STRUCTURE

QUICK REVIEW

The superficial or external surfaces of the body are generally divided into three zones. These are, from superficial to deep, the *epidermis, dermis, and subcutis*. The epidermis is the overlying squamous layer and is analogous to epithelial linings that cover other body surfaces, including the mucosal surfaces of the airways, the epithelium overlying the gastrointestinal tract, and the epithelial surfaces in the reproductive and urinary organs. The epidermis is commonly divided into different layers that become useful in describing histological findings. The deepest of these layers is the *basal layer (stratum basale)* that lines the epidermal side of the dermoepidermal junction, and includes mostly cuboidal-appearing cells called *basal cells (aka basal keratinocytes)*. The basal layer is the site of mitosis or proliferation of skin cells. These cells can sometimes appear slightly more basophilic or blue than more superficial cells, and are connected to the dermis by structures called *hemidesmosomes*. The basal layer is also home to a second cell type known as *melanocytes*. Melanocytes are responsible for *melanin* pigment production and for the transfer of melanin to keratinocytes, where most of the melanin is stored. Melanin pigment helps to protect the skin from the sun (an increase in the amount of melanin in darker skin individuals is the main reason why they burn less readily). Along with the cells of the basal layer, the melanocytes line the deepest layer of the epidermis and occur in a ratio of basal cell to melanocyte of approximately 1:10.

The majority of cells along the basal layer are known as *keratinocytes* and as they age will mature superficially in the epidermis. They have intercellular connections between cells, known as *desmosomes*, which become microscopically apparent superficial to the basal layer. It is for this reason that the next layer of the epidermis is known as the *spinous layer (stratum spinosum; the desmosomes give a spinous appearance)*. The desmosomes are responsible for holding keratinocytes together and resisting shearing forces. Just superficial to the spinous layer the cytoplasm of the keratinocytes undergoes slight horizontal elongation and takes on a more granular appearance due to the appearance of purple *keratohyalin granules*. It is for this reason that cells in this layer are known as *granulocytes*, which populate the *granular layer (stratum granulosum)*. Exaggeration or attenuation of this layer is an important diagnostic feature in some conditions.

In the most superficial layer of the epidermis, the horizontal elongation of keratinocytes continues and is accompanied by a loss of their nuclei. They also become even less eosinophilic (less pink) and take on a "cleared out" appearance. This layer is called the *cornified layer (stratum corneum)*. This is the most superficial layer and is an important clue not only to the presence of certain types of skin conditions but also to their age. Pathologically, cells of the most superficial layer can take on a more basophilic, less oval appearance, and retain their nuclei. This is known as *parakeratosis* and is often a clue that not only is disease present, but also that it has been occurring for at least several weeks. Remember that the epidermis develops from superficial to deep and you will understand why evidence of parakeratosis in the superficial layers means that the pathological insult has affected even the "oldest" cells, since cells from the basal layer take 14 days to migrate to the cornified layer, and then an additional 14 days to detach from the epidermis entirely.

Other cell types are also found in the epidermis including antigen presenting or dendritic cells, tactile cells, and cells involved in sensorium.

The whole of the epidermis takes on an undulating texture at low microscopic power and these undulations are known as *rete ridges*. Changes in the lengths of these rete ridges as well as changes in their appearance can also serve as important diagnostic clues. It is also worth pointing out that not all skin is the same over all body surfaces. For example, skin in "special sites" may have unique appearances and may cause diagnostic difficulties in some cases, especially involving melanocytic lesions. *Acral* skin or skin on the palms and soles is known to have well-pronounced rete ridges and a thickened cornified layer.

The *dermis* is the layer of connective tissue and supporting structures that is directly beneath or deep to the epidermis. It is composed of collagen fascicles and elastic fibers that provide the tensile and elastic properties of the skin. The dermis at the level of the rete ridges is known as the *papillary dermis*, while the dermis deep to the rete is known as the *reticular dermis*. Changes in the appearance of these collagen fascicles can also provide important clues to the nature of certain diseases. The dermis also is home to the glands of the skin, specifically three types: *sebaceous, eccrine,* and *apocrine*. These glands function in sweat and oil production as well as temperature regulation and are closely related to hair follicles in origin and function. They are closely related to *hair follicles*. Small *arrector pili* muscles attach to the hair follicles and are responsible for "goose bumps" when they contract and raise the hair. Along with sensory nerves, there are also small *superficial and deep vascular layers* of the dermis that provide important blood supply to the dermis as well as the epidermis (the epidermis itself is avascular).

Deep to the dermis is the *subcutis*, which is composed mostly of fat, blood vessels, nerves, and connective tissue (**Figure 20-2**).

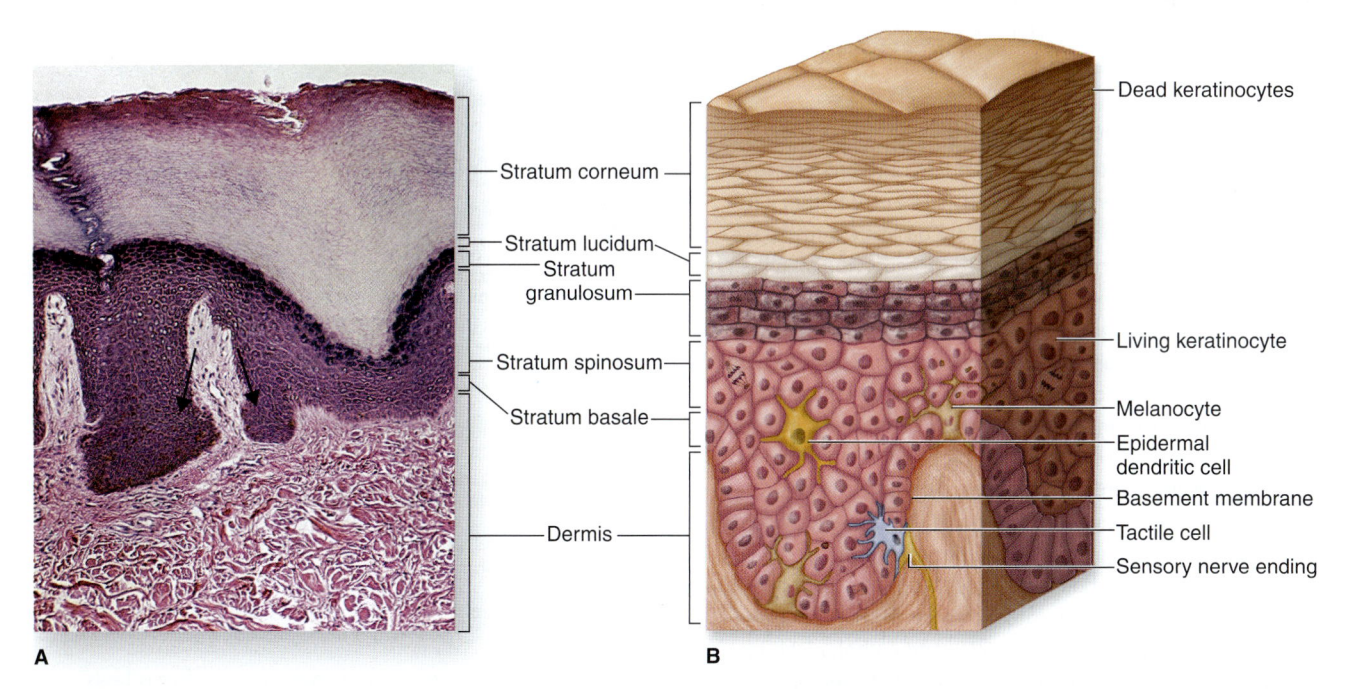

FIGURE 20-2 Skin structure. (**A**) Hematoxylin and eosin section of normal skin with prominent rete ridge undulations (arrow). (**B**) Layers and cell types of the epidermis and their relationship to the dermis. (Reproduced with permission from McKinley M, O'Loughlin VD. Human Anatomy, 2nd ed. New York: McGraw-Hill; 2008.)

> **WHAT TO DO**
> **The Curse of History**
> There are thousands of rashes. Physicians have been looking at skin for centuries, and for most of that time rashes were named and grouped based on clinical appearance. This yielded a burgeoning nomenclature laden with peculiar Greek and Latin names unrelated to pathogenesis. As an example, consider some of the "erythemas:" erythema multiforme, a dermatitis triggered by herpes virus (among other immune triggers) in which distant sites in the epidermis are attacked immunologically; erythema annulare centrifugum, a dermatitis with lesions resembling hives; and erythema nodosum (EN), a panniculitis (inflammation of the subcutaneous fat). The only thing these dermatoses have in common is redness. As with all bad medical nomenclature, the nomenclature of dermatology is firmly entrenched and will remain inviolate.
>
> Why are there so many rashes and skin problems?
> *You can see your skin, but you cannot see your liver*. Therefore, even the most subtle permutations of skin redness and scaliness can be analyzed by both patients and physicians, but inflammation in the liver and most other organ systems remains occult unless organ dysfunction or failure occurs. The skin has an incredibly delicate and complex neural network, with the capability to produce symptoms such as itching and burning. These symptoms motivate the patient and doctor to classify, diagnose, and treat even minor skin diseases. In other (less innervated) organ systems, minor disorders may remain asymptomatic and occult.
>
> *Your skin is in constant contact with the environment*. Much like the bowel, the skin is exposed to a steady stream of insults from our often-noxious surroundings, which results in countless episodes and variations in immune responses. Other organ systems have a more filtered, and thus safer view of the world.
>
> **Biopsy Types and Processing**
> A quick word regarding specimen biopsy and processing is in order for the understanding of the student, whether a future clinician or pathologist. There are basically three types of biopsies that are commonly used for removing small lesions or sampling extensive lesions: these are the *shave*, *punch*, and *excisional* biopsies. The type of biopsy chosen often is dependent on the clinical impression. If the clinician suspects that the lesion is a superficial process, a shave biopsy is typically performed. For deeper processes involving the dermis or even subcutis, a punch biopsy is often required. For larger lesions, an excisional biopsy, where the clinician narrowly removes the whole lesion, is the best method of sampling. Since diagnosis of a skin disease often depends on tissue sampling, choice of proper biopsy becomes very important and can sometimes be an art form. Proper and sufficient feedback between clinician and pathologist is important to ensure the tissue is being sampled adequately.

PHYSICAL DESCRIPTIONS FOR PRIMARY SKIN LESIONS

Histological diagnoses of dermatological specimens are rarely made without clinical context and history in mind. Important items for consideration are timing, distribution, and appearance. Primary skin lesions are those that arise as the direct result of a disease process without distortion from outside factors. In order to minimize confusion, clinicians tend to use specific terms. Some important terms are listed in Tables 20-1 to 20-3.

PART 2: PERTINENT DERMATOLOGICAL CONDITIONS AND CASE PRESENTATIONS

Skin Cysts

Follicular Cysts

There are several different types of cysts observed in the skin. Features used to classify cysts include the type of epithelium making up the cyst wall, the contents of the cyst, and the types of cells or structures surrounding the cyst. While a detailed discussion of every type of skin cyst is beyond the scope of this text, we do highlight the most common cyst types. The

TABLE 20-1 Physical descriptions for primary and secondary skin lesions.

Primary lesions demonstrate the natural presentation of a skin lesion that is unadulterated by outside forces.
Macule – <1 cm flat area of discoloration
Patch – >1 cm flat area of discoloration
Papule – <1 cm, elevated, palpable skin lesion
Plaque – >1 cm, elevated, palpable skin lesion
Nodule – A rounded, palpable skin lesion of roughly equal diameter and depth
Vesicle – A fluid-filled space (blister), <1 cm in diameter
Bulla – A fluid-filled space (blister), >1 cm in diameter
Pustule – A pus-filled space
Secondary lesions are those that result from primary lesions following influence from extraneous factors or the passage of time. These include the lesions below:
Scale – Thin fragments of keratinized stratum corneum
Crust – Layer formed from dried serous, purulent, or sanguineous exudate
Excoriation – Disruption in the skin as a result of scratching
Fissure – Linear clefts through the epidermis +/– the dermis, result of thick, inelastic skin
Erosion – Loss of epidermis; heals without scar. Often the remnant of a ruptured bulla
Ulcer – Loss of both epidermis and a portion of the dermis, heals with scar

TABLE 20-2 Important histological terms.

Acanthosis	Thickening of the epidermis
Acantholysis	Loss of cohesion between keratinocytes of the epidermis
Basket weave	Term given to typical appearing keratin layer
Dysplasia	Cellular changes that may be indicative of a premalignant or malignant process
Parakeratosis	The presence of nuclei in the cornified layer
Verrucous	Having a warty architecture
Infiltrative	Jagged aggregates of cells invading underlying tissue, often implying a more aggressive phenotype
Circumscribed	Well demarcated

TABLE 20-3 Common special stains and immunostains.

S100 protein, HMB-45, Melan A	Commonly used to stain melanoma
AE1/AE3, cytokeratin, p63	Commonly used to identify cells of squamous differentiation
CD45	Identifies most hematopoietic cells
CD68	Commonly used to identify macrophages (histiocytes)
CD31/34	Used to identify cells of vascular origin
PAS (periodic acid-Schiff)/diastase	Stains a variety of entities including fungi and glucose; diastase sensitivity indicates presence of glucose
CD1a	Stains Langerhans cells
Ki-67	Used as a proliferation marker, increased staining with high proliferation rate
GMS (Gomori-Grocott methenamine silver stain)	Used to stain fungi

infundibular follicular, commonly known as an *epidermal inclusion cyst*, is by far the most common type of cyst in the skin. It can occur anywhere, but has a predilection for the head and neck. It is typified histologically by a cyst wall resembling the surface epidermis with a granular layer and a cyst space filled with lamellated keratin. These are also referred to as *epidermoid cysts* or colloquially as "sebaceous cysts" although they do not have anything to do with the sebaceous glands. Milia are small epidermoid cysts (1–3 mm), which are often seen in newborns on the face, upper trunk, and extremities. They can also be seen after scarring processes.

In contrast, the *pilar cyst* (*trichilemmal cyst*) is characterized by compact pink keratin surrounded by squamous epithelium lacking a granular layer. It is usually seen as a cyst on the scalp. A related lesion, the *pilomatricoma*, is benign and occurs in the head and necks of children (Figure 20-3A, B, C).

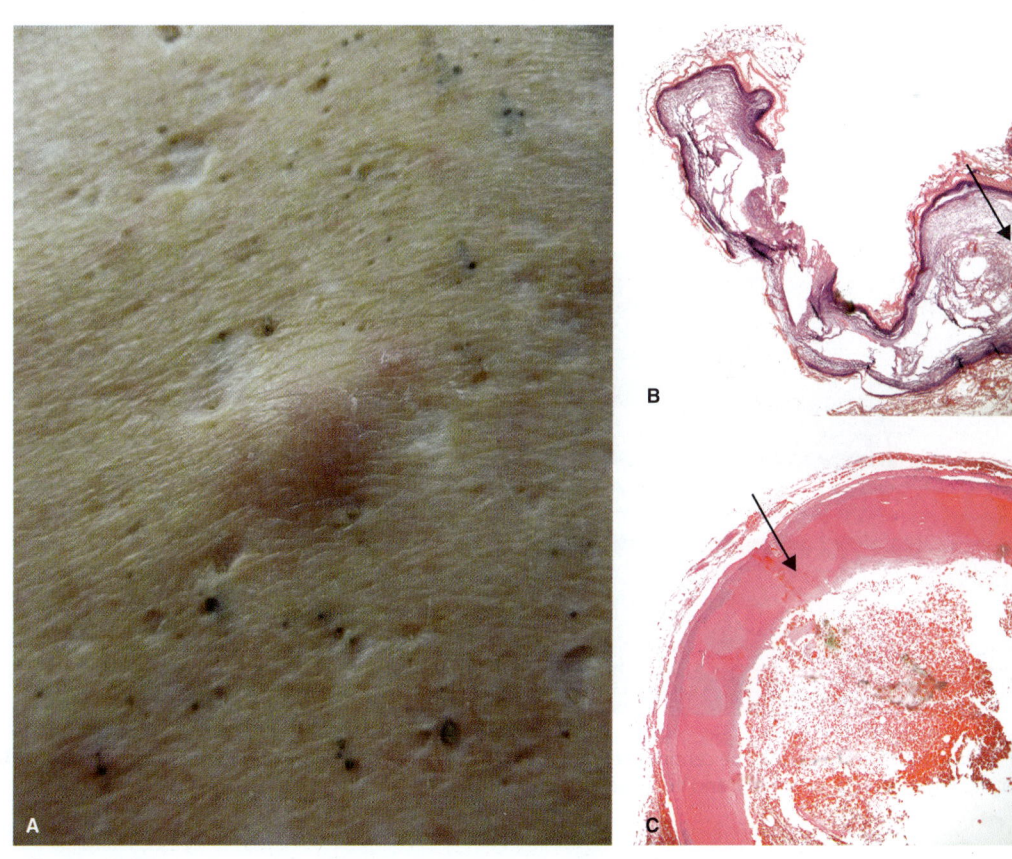

FIGURE 20-3 Follicular cysts. **(A)** Clinical presentation of follicular cysts. **(B)** Note the prominent lamellated keratin (arrow) of the epidermal inclusion cyst. **(C)** In contrast, the pilar cyst is characterized by compact pink keratin (arrow).

EPIDERMAL LESIONS AND TUMORS

An *actinic keratosis* is considered a premalignant lesion, typically arising with increasing age and sunlight exposure (Figure 20-4). These are common on sun-exposed areas of older individuals with fair skin types. These lesions are considered to be precancerous (an intermediate to squamous cell carcinoma); however, the overwhelming majority will never progress to cancer. Histologically, these lesions are typified by atypical keratinocytes present within the basal portion of the epidermis. Full-thickness atypia, by definition, warrants the diagnosis of squamous cell carcinoma in situ (*Bowen disease*).

Seborrheic keratosis is one of the most common tumors of the skin and frequently appears as an incidental finding in older patients. The most common presentation is a waxy, "stuck on" tan-brown papule or small plaque (Figure 20-5), although occasionally they take on a skin-colored or slightly erythematous appearance. They commonly occur on the head, neck, and trunk, with a propensity for areas of friction such as under bra straps or waistbands. Although seborrheic keratoses have no malignant potential, they are often biopsied when confused with other pigmented lesions, or when pruritus or other symptoms arise.

CASE 20-1

A 72-year-old woman presents with a subtle scaly papule on her forehead, just above the eye. It is painless and is shown in Figure 20-4.

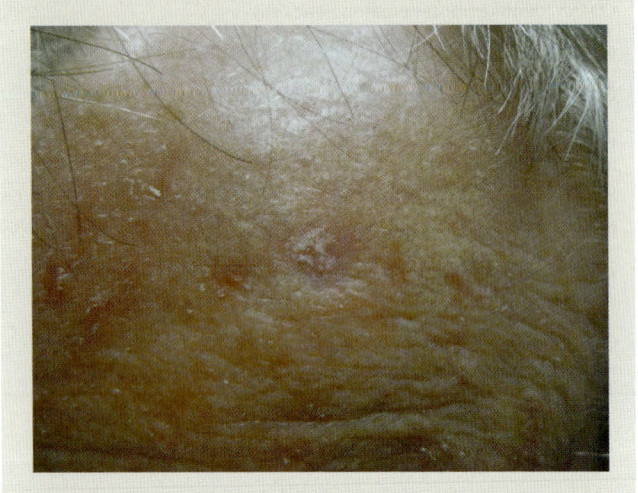

FIGURE 20-4 Actinic keratosis. Female presenting with scaly papule on forehead consistent with an actinic keratosis.

CASE 20-2

A 65-year-old man presents with a 1 cm brown waxy lesion on his forehead. The lesion has a "stuck on" appearance. The specimen is processed and histology is shown in Figure 20-5A, B.

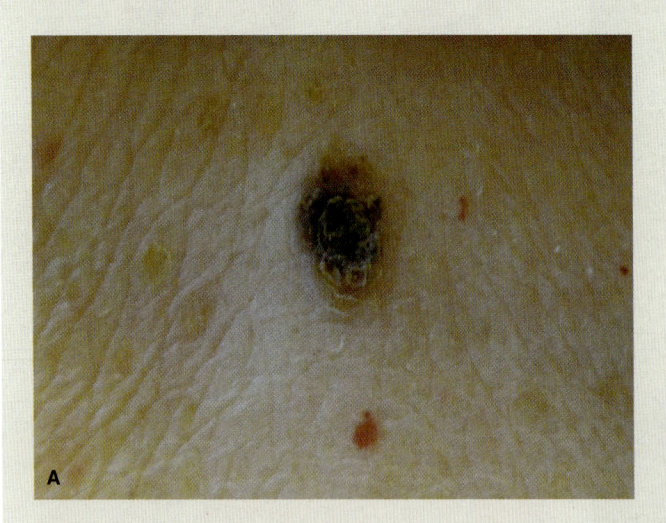

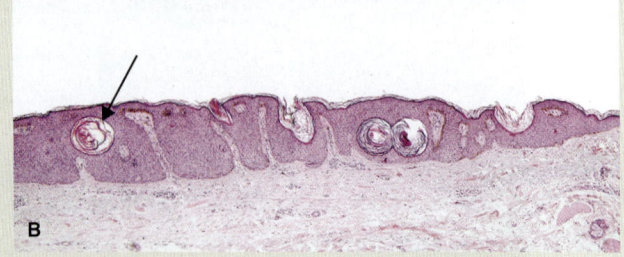

FIGURE 20-5 Seborrheic keratosis. (A) One centimeter lesion with waxy "stuck on" appearance of a seborrheic keratosis. **(B)** Acanthosis without significant atypia, symmetry, and horn pseudocysts (arrow).

CASE 20-3

A 65-year-old man presents with a pink, shiny papule on his cheek. There is central ulceration of this lesion and telangiectasias. His dermatologist performs a shave biopsy and the light microscopic examination is shown in **Figure 20-6A, B.**

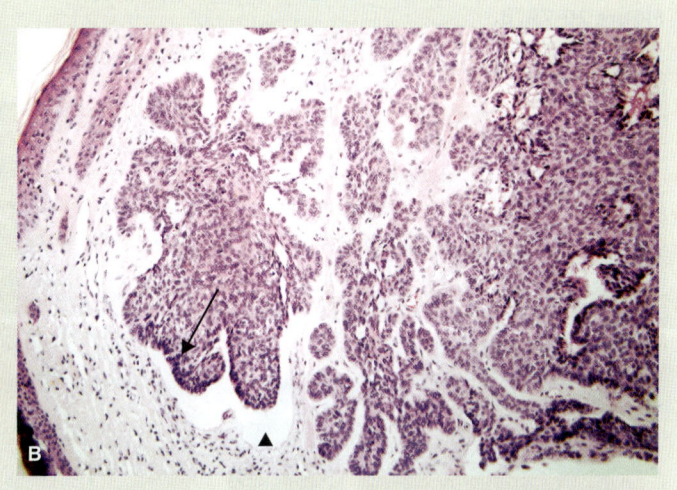

FIGURE 20-6 Basal cell carcinoma. **(A)** Pink, shiny papule with telangiectasias (arrow) consistent with basal cell carcinoma. **(B)** Blue (basophilic) cells with peripheral palisading (arrow) and clefting (arrowhead).

The appearance of seborrheic keratosis on microscopic examination is somewhat variable, but all cases have in common lack of significant atypia, mitotic figures, cellular pleomorphism, or other characteristics suggestive of more aggressive lesions. Seborrheic keratosis often demonstrates thickening of the epidermis (acanthosis), with a flat, symmetrical base, and horn pseudocysts (called pseudo because they presumably connect to the surface, hence not true cysts).

BASAL CELL CARCINOMA

Basal cell carcinoma is the most common skin tumor in man and occurs most commonly in the areas of the head and neck, but can occur anywhere on the body. Tumors that go untreated for years can directly invade underlying or adjacent structures; however, most that have been treated early do not cause significant problems. Only extremely rare incidences of metastatic disease have been reported. Incidence increases with age and sun exposure, and the vast majority is found in patients with fair skin. Histologically, several classic features typify these lesions. One is a striking basophilia or blue appearance to the tumor cells themselves, and there is often an increase in mitotic rate or necrosis within collections of tumor cells. There is a lining up of the basal cells around the periphery of cellular collections, an appearance commonly referred to as "peripheral palisading." There is also "clefting" between palisades of tumor cells and the surrounding stroma. This is a separation and contraction of tumor cells from the surrounding stroma during processing and can be an important clue in differentiating this lesion from other similar lesions.

The *nevoid basal cell carcinoma syndrome* (*Gorlin syndrome*) is a rare autosomal dominant condition in which patients are predisposed to the development of basal cell carcinomas, especially at an early age, as well as odontogenic keratocysts, abnormal facies, congenital malformations, and systemic malignancy to name a few. This is thought to be due to a mutation in the *protein patched homolog 1 tumor suppressor protein* (PTCH) located on chromosome 9q.

SQUAMOUS CELL CARCINOMA

The second most common tumor of the skin is *squamous cell carcinoma*. This tumor can occur in many different locations throughout the body. Cutaneous squamous cell carcinoma occurs more commonly in sun-exposed Caucasian skin and has an increasing incidence with age. This tumor originates from abnormally developing keratinocytes and is typified by atypical keratinocytes, frequently with increased nuclear pleomorphism, abnormal keratinization, frequent mitotic figures, and irregular architecture. This lesion exists in an in situ form, meaning that all of the abnormal tumor cells are limited to the epidermis.

Squamous cell carcinoma with an invasive component, in contrast, is identified by abnormal tumor cells that invade into and through the basement membrane. These tumors are easily confused with other less-threatening entities,

CASE 20-4

A 61-year-old man presents with a 0.5 cm ulcerated and irregular papule on his ear. Histological examination reveals the following Figure 20-7A, B.

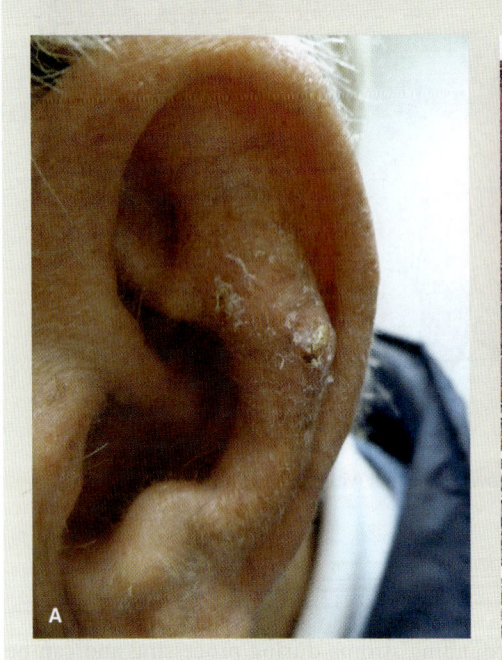

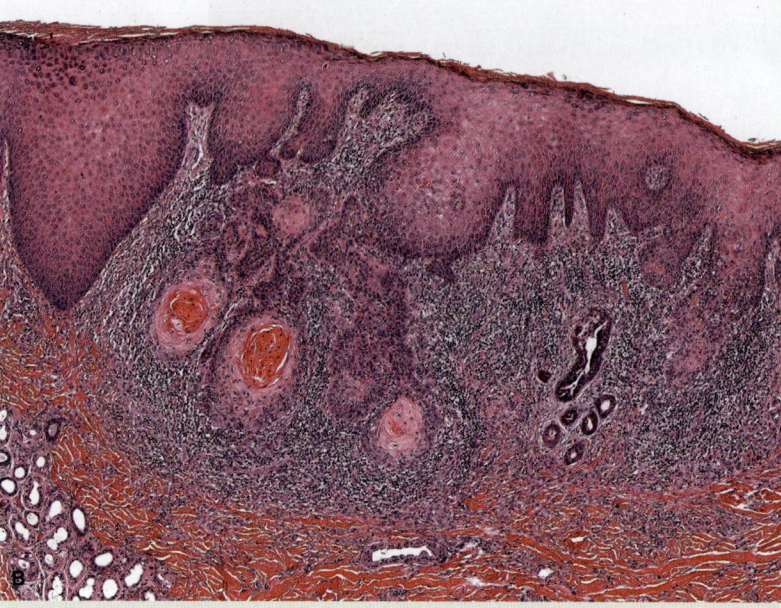

FIGURE 20-7 Squamous cell carcinoma. **(A)** Squamous cell carcinoma presenting on the external ear. **(B)** Atypical squamous cells invading into the dermis. (Image courtesy of Dr. John Woosley UNC Pathology.)

especially on limited sampling. Similar to basal cell carcinoma, these lesions can often exist for some time without causing problems for the patient, but local destruction can result. Metastasis is possible in thick lesions. Patients who are immunosuppressed, particularly patients who have a received a transplant, are at particularly high risk of developing many squamous cell carcinomas. Certain lesions predispose to the development of squamous cell carcinoma including actinic keratosis, lichen sclerosus, scars, sites of irradiation, and burns. Patients with *epidermodysplasia verruciformis*, an autosomal recessive skin disorder resulting in an abnormal susceptibility to human papillomavirus (HPV, see below) infection, are also at higher risk, as well as patients with *xeroderma pigmentosum*, an autosomal recessive disorder of DNA repair.

KERATOACANTHOMA

Keratoacanthoma is a neoplasm that commonly occurs on the face of Caucasians. Clinically, this tumor is a keratinized papule that arises and grows quickly over the course of weeks to a few months, and spontaneous regression usually, but not invariably, also occurs over this same timeframe. Given the marked keratinization that is evident both grossly and histologically, some experts think of the tumor as "keratinizing itself to death." Histologically, this tumor is typified by a central cup-shaped architecture filled with a keratin "plug." Lesional cells at the base of and surrounding the central keratin "plug" often exhibit abundant eosinophilic (pink) cytoplasm and can demonstrate some cytologic atypia. Because predicting the course of the lesion histologically is difficult, some prefer the term *squamous cell carcinoma, keratoacanthoma type* (Figure 20-8A, B).

A Note About Solar/Ultraviolet Light Damage

Not only do the tanning (mostly UVA) and burning (mostly UVB) rays of the sun cause actinic keratosis, basal cell carcinoma, and squamous cell carcinoma that manifest when humans are older, they also cause wrinkles that are manifest when humans are relatively young. Even though you and your patients may have already received a significant dose of UV light, it is never too late to begin a healthy relationship with the sun. Tanning salons boast they are safe since they only use UVA spectrum

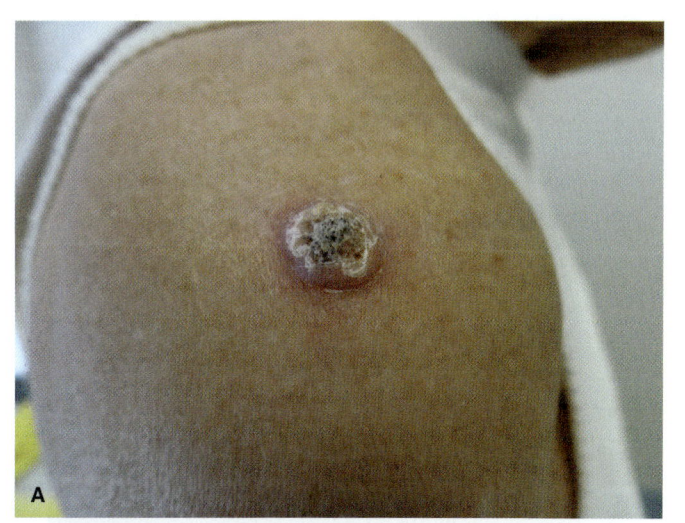

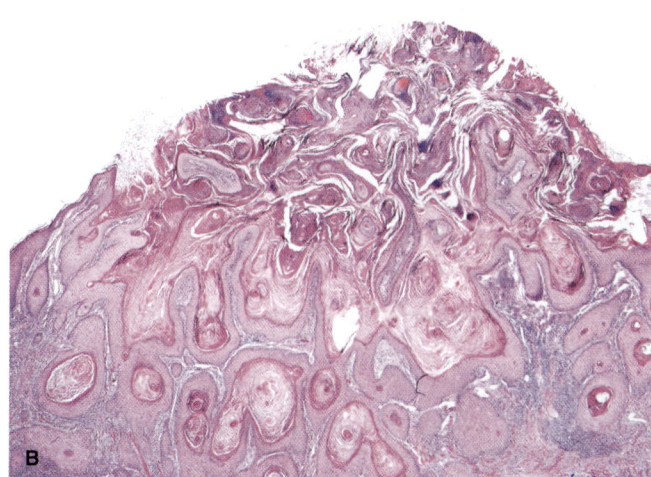

FIGURE 20-8 **Keratoacanthoma.** **(A)** Keratoacanthomas arise quickly and often spontaneously regress. **(B)** Keratoacanthoma demonstrates extreme keratinization.

lamps, but these not only cause skin aging but are also linked to increased risk of all skin cancers, including melanoma. Avoid sunburn. Wear sunscreen on a daily basis and use a sunscreen that blocks both UVA and UVB. Wear a hat. Wear sunglasses. While squamous and basal cell carcinomas have traditionally been afflictions of elderly patients, it is becoming more commonly seen in patients in their 20s and 30s with extensive UV exposure history.

PIGMENTED LESIONS

Lesions that arise from the pigment-producing cells of the skin, melanocytes, are known as melanocytic lesions. It is convenient for pathologists to classify lesions involving these cell groups as "pigmented," although certainly other types of lesions can demonstrate pigment as well. Like lesions arising from any cell type in the body, many benign proliferations of melanocytes exist. A malignant proliferation of melanocytes is called melanoma and is one of the most deadly of all human neoplasms, especially if not detected and treated at an early stage. The most common and significant melanocytic lesions are discussed below.

Freckle (Ephelide)/Melanotic Macule

These are very common lesions that occur most frequently on the face, chest, and shoulders as well as the hands and arms. They occur as multiple red/tan macules scattered over the affected area and are usually 2–3 mm in diameter or less. Histologically, melanocytes in these lesions are generally not increased as it is actually an increased amount of melanin pigmentation in keratinocytes that causes the clinical appearance. Unlike lentigos, which are discussed below, ephelides often fade in the absence of UV exposure and return on future exposure (**Figure 20-9**).

Melasma

Similar to freckles, melasma is a common condition that affects the face and is characterized by irregular and confluent hyperpigmentation. Also like freckles, it is characterized histologically by an increase in melanin pigmentation of keratinocytes. It is most frequently seen during pregnancy, is accentuated by UV exposure, and has been associated with oral contraceptives.

FIGURE 20-9 **Ephelides.** Ephelides (freckles) are common macules.

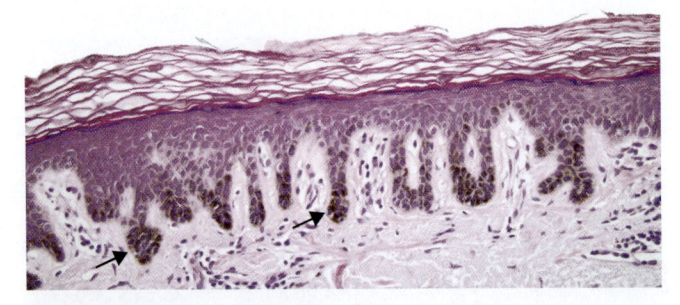

FIGURE 20-10 **Solar lentigo.** "Club like" rete ridges (arrows) of solar lentigo.

Solar Lentigo

These are common lesions of the elderly, which develop in sun-damaged skin of the arms, hands, and face. They occur clinically as hyperpigmentation in the form of a tan or brown macules or patches. Histologically, they are characterized by elongated and rounded, "club like" rete ridges with prominent excess pigment at the base along with solar elastosis (Figure 20-10).

Lentigo Simplex

These are small (less than 5 mm) hyperpigmented macules that can occur anywhere on the body and are often congenital or arise at young age. These lesions are asymptomatic but can be related to a number of syndromes. Histologically, these lesions are characterized by an increase in normal melanocytes along the dermoepidermal junction and an increase in melanin pigment (Figure 20-11).

Melanocytic Nevus

The patient in case 20-12 has what is known as a *conventional nevus*, a type of melanocytic lesion. Melanocytic lesions are those that develop from melanocytes, the cells that produce melanin, especially in response to solar stimulation, and reside in the basal layer of the epidermis. The cells can and often do

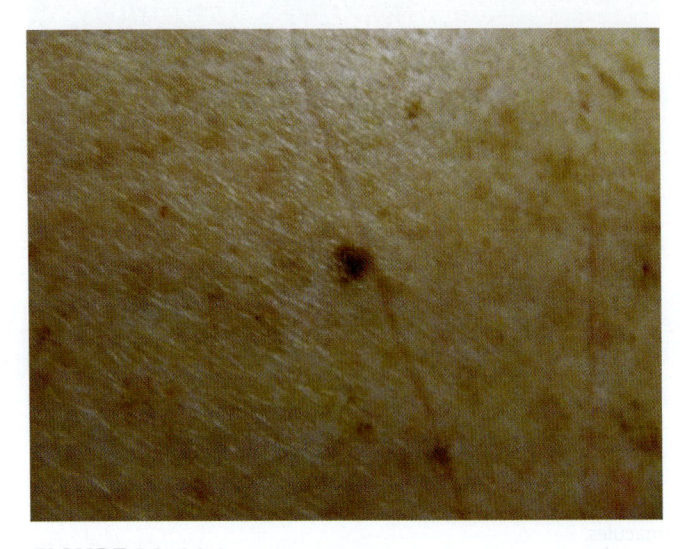

FIGURE 20-11 **Lentigo simplex.** Hyperpigmented macule of lentigo simplex.

CASE 20-5

A 34-year-old woman presents with a red-brown nodule on her trunk. It is regular in size, color and shape, but she asks to have it removed for cosmetic reasons. Clinical examination and light microscopy are shown in Figure 20-12.

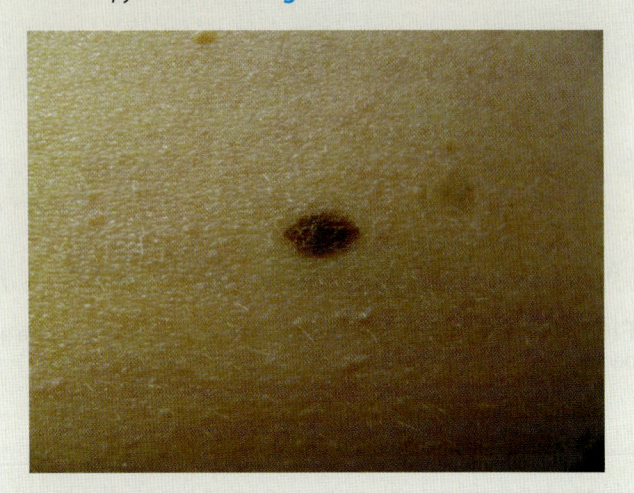

FIGURE 20-12 **Melanocytic nevus.** Red brown, symmetrical nodule on trunk consistent with a melanocytic nevus.

undergo proliferation, both in benign fashion as *nevi* or moles and, more rarely, in malignant fashion in the form of *melanoma*. Melanoma is a significant cause of morbidity and mortality in the Western world with increasing incidence. Early detection, diagnosis, and treatment are essential to proper care. Skin color is a major factor in predisposition to this disease, with fair-skinned people experiencing the highest incidence. The presence and number of acquired and *dysplastic melanocytic nevi* (a specific type of nevi) are also major factor. For the pathologist, diagnosing these lesions is a very important, difficult, and at times a dangerous area of practice – a missed diagnosis of melanoma is the single most common reason for filing a malpractice complaint against a pathologist.

There are many different types of benign nevi and these have been classified in different ways. The important thing to remember about all of these lesions is that they are benign; there is no such thing as a malignant nevus. Differentiating these lesions from malignant melanoma (a redundancy, there is no such thing as "benign melanoma") is what does matter to the clinician and to the patient. To this end there are several features, both architectural (i.e., involving the overall shape of the lesion microscopically) and cytological (i.e., involving how the individual cells appear), which help us to differentiate the two.

Nevi are often divided according to their location in the epidermis and dermis. For example, a *junctional melanocytic nevus* is one in which the melanocytes reside along the dermoepidermal junction. A *compound nevus* is one with melanocytes at both the dermoepidermal junction and within the dermis, and a *dermal nevus* is one with melanocytes only in the dermis. The widely held belief is that nevi tend to develop along the dermoepidermal junction, and slowly migrate toward the dermis as they evolve from junctional to compound and finally to dermal nevi. Clinically, this correlates with evolution from a pigmented macule to a pigmented papule, and finally to a skin-colored papule.

A particular subtype of melanocytic nevus known as the *congenital melanocytic nevus* is typified by a generally larger size than those of conventional nevi with very bland appearing cells often arranged in nests that extend more deeply in the dermis. It is common for the cells of a congenital melanocytic nevus to track down adnexal structures.

A *halo nevus* is another type of melanocytic nevus, which is typified clinically as a nevus surrounded by a "halo" of skin that is of lighter color than the surrounding skin as well as the center. Histologically, these lesions are generally seen as melanocytic proliferations, which often have a quite significant lymphocytic infiltrate both surrounding and intermixed with the melanocytic cells. A *blue nevus* is made up of spindled melanocytes that involve the dermis, but not the epidermis, and generally have a prominent amount of melanin, giving the clinical appearance of a blue or slate gray lesion.

Melanoma

Melanocytic lesions with malignant potential are known as melanoma. Melanoma is suspected clinically by the observation of the ABCDEs of melanoma. These are *A*symmetry, *B*order irregularities, *C*olor heterogeneity, *D*iameter greater than 6 mm, and *E*volution of the lesion (changes with time).

As is the case with nevi, there are also several different subtypes of melanoma. All of these subtypes have features in common, both architecturally (asymmetry, invasiveness, spread into the epidermis, nerves and blood vessels) and cytologically (prominent mitotic figures, cellular pleomorphism, prominent nucleoli, hyperchromaticism, etc.). The most common subtypes of melanoma are *superficial spreading, lentigo maligna melanoma, nodular melanoma, and desmoplastic melanoma*. Superficial spreading melanoma is typified as having a growth phase that is often nested and runs along the dermoepidermal junction with atypical cells and irregular architecture. Lentigo maligna melanoma tends to include single cells that grow irregularly along the dermoepidermal junction. Nodular melanoma tends to grow downward or deep as opposed to horizontally, without much of component along the dermoepidermal junction. Desmoplastic melanoma occurs when melanocytes arise within a fibrosing reaction in the dermis, which can make it difficult to recognize clinically and microscopically. Another important, and often clinically challenging variation, is the *amelanotic melanoma*, which makes up nearly 10% of all melanomas. Since these produce minimal to no pigment, they are usually pink or tan papules that lack the color variation and asymmetry that typically trigger clinical suspicion.

CASE 20-6

A 45-year-old woman presents with a dark, asymmetrical lesion on her leg. She has noticed that the lesion has become more irregular and larger over time. She also gives a history of multiple sunburns during childhood (Figure 20-13A, B).

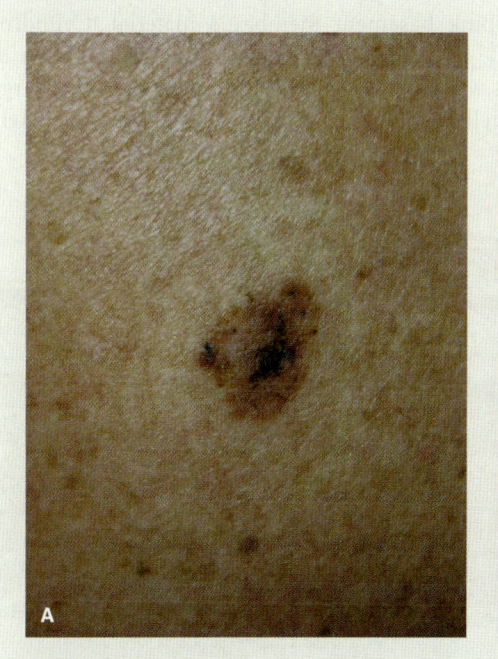

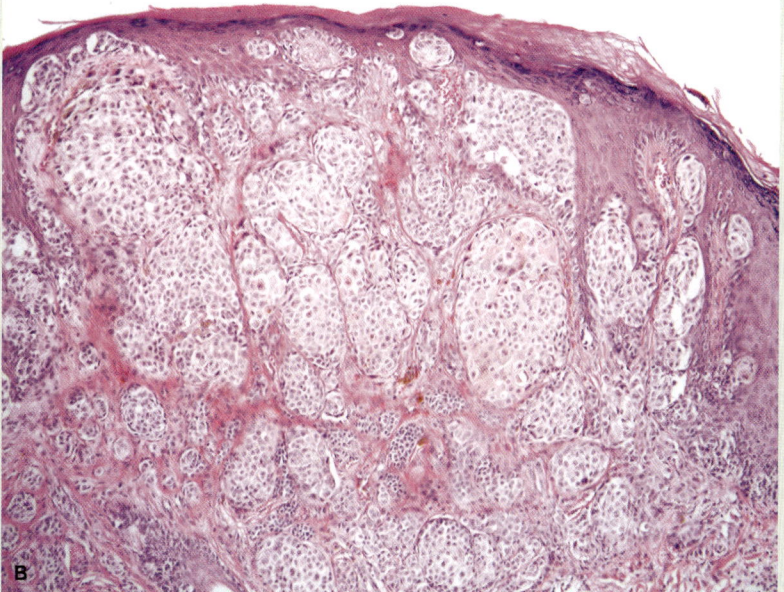

FIGURE 20-13 Melanoma. **(A)** Dark, asymmetrical, irregular lesion. **(B)** Biopsy exhibits striking architectural asymmetry, cytological atypia, and spreading of neoplastic cells into the epidermis (epidermotropism) thereby confirming the diagnosis of melanoma.

Some, but not all, types of melanoma are associated with UV exposure. Some have emphasized the number of major burn episodes in youth as being associated with a positive predictive value of developing melanoma. Needless to say, epidemiological studies of this sort are not always easy to interpret. Important prognostic indicators in patients with localized melanoma are tumor thickness, mitotic rate, and ulceration.

Exciting new work is being done regarding distinct genetic alterations involved in melanoma. BRAF mutations for example are now serving as therapy targets in appropriately selected tumors. It is hoped that identification of additional mutations in the future will help to further guide drug therapy.

The treatment of melanoma consists mainly of surgical intervention at this time. The greatest depth of invasion measured, in millimeters, from the top of the granular layer into the dermis or subcutis is the *Breslow depth*, and it is the number one prognostic factor for patients with melanoma. This depth dictates the need for further staging with imaging, width of surgical margins, indication for sentinel lymph node biopsy, and further therapy. For individuals in which surgery has failed or surgical intervention is not an option, the prognosis is unfavorable. Lack of effective therapeutic options has left survival rates in metastatic disease both poor and static for decades, but exciting new biologically active drugs are showing promise in clinical trials.

ADNEXAL (APPENDAGEAL) TUMORS

Adnexal tumors are those that arise from the hair follicle or from related glands. These tumors occur with less frequency than epidermal tumors, but must be kept in the differential of more common lesions. As dermatopathology has evolved, dozens of entities have been classified. Here, we highlight some of the more pertinent tumors most clinicians should be aware of.

Poroma

Poroma is a relatively uncommon tumor on the scalp or sole that is easily misdiagnosed as seborrheic keratosis. Clinically, it is a friable papule. Histologically, it is composed of benign-appearing poroid cells (small, pink, cuboidal), sometimes with clearing. Small sweat ducts are often present. Its cousins are the closely related lesions of *nodular hidradenoma, hidroacanthoma simplex, nodular hidradenoma,* and *dermal duct tumor*. These lesions behave in a benign fashion (Figure 20-14).

Syringoma

This lesion usually presents as multiple, small, skin-colored papules underneath the lower eyelid. Syringomas are characterized histologically by small "tadpole" shaped ducts in an eosinophilic (pink), sclerotic stroma. They can be easy to confuse histologically with other more-threatening lesions (basal cell carcinoma, microcystic adnexal carcinoma) so it is important to have a good sample to evaluate (Figure 20-15).

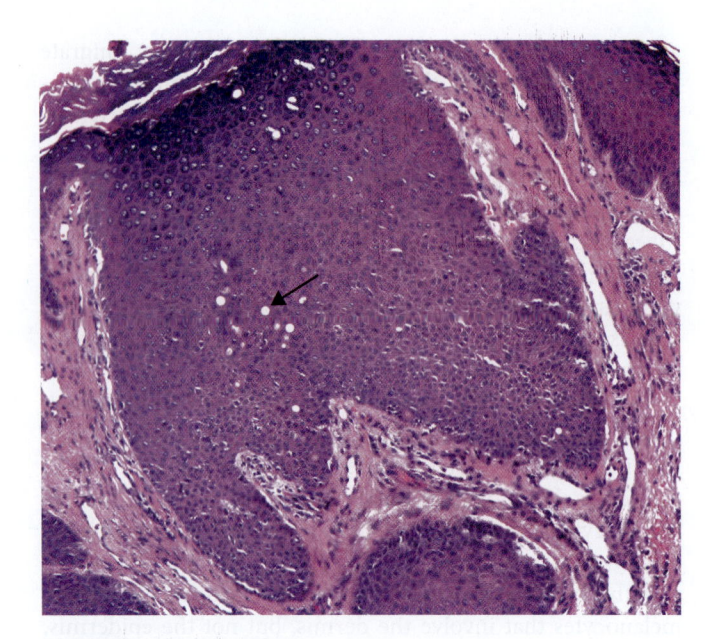

FIGURE 20-14 Poroma. Note the small sweat ducts present in the lesion (arrow).

Cylindroma/Spiradenoma

These closely related lesions have some of the more characteristic histological findings in dermatopathology. *Spiradenomas* are more often sporadic and occur as single large lesions whereas *cylindroma* tends to occur in clusters. Histologically, they are characterized by very basophilic cells intermixed with globules of pink basement membrane material. Cylindromas are made up of a "jigsaw puzzle" -like configuration of small islands, while spiradenomas form a single or few large nodules of cells with identical appearance. They are likely

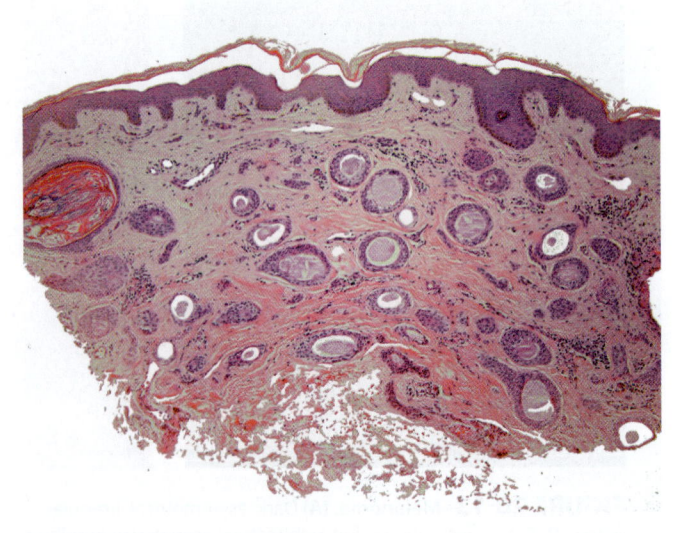

FIGURE 20-15 Syringoma. Syringoma is characterized by tadpole shaped ducts in a pink (eosinophilic) stroma.

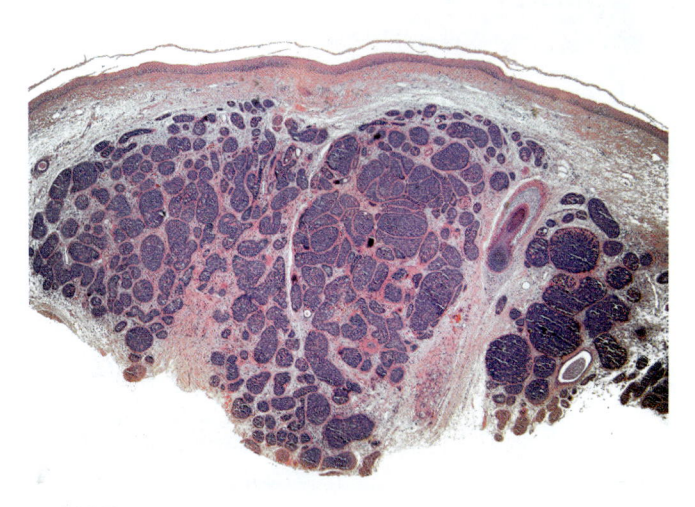

FIGURE 20-16 Cylindroma. Cylindroma is characterized by basophilic islands that fit together like a jigsaw puzzle.

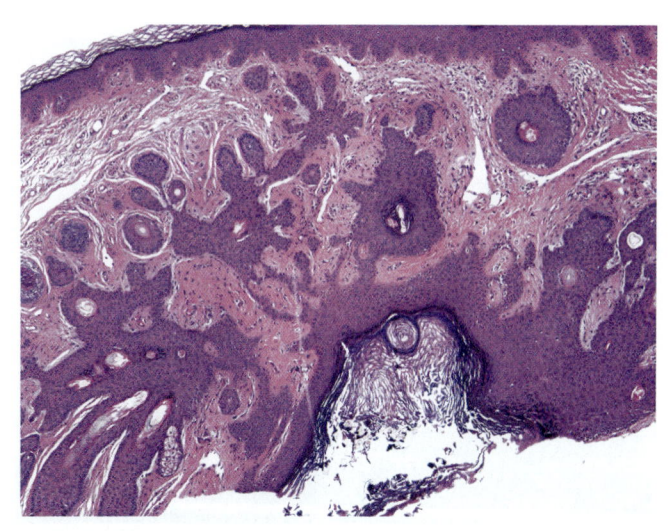

FIGURE 20-17 Trichofolliculoma. Trichofolliculoma is composed of a large central follicle with numerous surrounding smaller follicles.

variations of the same process and are frequently found together. Clinically, they are rare and associated with syndromes such as Brooke–Spiegler syndrome in which they are found in large numbers on the scalp and forehead – this has resulted in the common moniker of "turban tumors" (**Figure 20-16**).

Microcystic Adnexal Carcinoma

This is a somewhat rare entity that occurs most frequently on the lips and cheeks and may be subtle clinically. On histological examination, this lesion may appear similar to the syringoma or to a morpheaform basal cell carcinoma, but key features, which help to differentiate microcystic adnexal carcinoma, are that it is deeply invasive, lacks symmetry, and may exhibit perineural extension.

Trichofolliculoma

Trichofolliculoma is characterized by a papule with a thin hair shaft or small tuft of hair extruding from it. They are characterized histologically by a central dilated hair follicle that contains many small hair shafts. There are multiple small follicles that "empty" into this large central follicular infundibulum, each containing a small hair fiber (**Figure 20-17**).

Trichilemmoma

Trichilemmoma, can be solitary but is also associated with *Cowden syndrome*. Cowden syndrome, or *multiple hamartoma syndrome*, is an autosomal recessive inherited tumor syndrome. Patients are at risk not only of trichilemmoma but also other types of neoplasms as well. Cowden syndrome is caused by a mutation in the *tumor suppressor gene phosphatase and tensin homolog* (PTEN). Trichilemmomas are composed of lobules of clear cells at the epidermis along with a peripherally palisading border of cells. Below the cells of the lesion, there is a thickened "glassy" pink basement membrane.

Sebaceous Hyperplasia

Sebaceous hyperplasia results from an increased number of benign sebaceous glands in a localized area, usually on the face or forehead. These lesions are not threatening but may be confused clinically for basal cell carcinoma, and are often of cosmetic concern to patients (**Figure 20-18A, B**).

Sebaceous Carcinoma

Sebaceous carcinoma is characterized histologically by a proliferation of pleomorphic, hyperchromatic, and atypical cells that, unlike sebaceous hyperplasia, have the potential to metastasize and cause significant morbidity and mortality. They typically occur on the eyelids and ocular conjunctiva. Mitotic figures are common and invasion and infiltration may be noted into surrounding structures. This tumor (along with another lesion, the *sebaceous adenoma*) is associated with *Muir–Torre* syndrome. Muir–Torre is an inherited cancer syndrome, thought by some to be part of *Lynch syndrome* or *hereditary nonpolyposis colorectal cancer*. These patients are at increased risk of skin and other tumors because of inherited mutations in DNA mismatch repair, leading to microsatellite instability.

SOFT TISSUE LESIONS AND NEOPLASMS

Hemangioma

Benign vascular neoplasms come in a variety of flavors. The vast majority of vascular lesions are benign; however, both intermediate and malignant forms exist (see section on angiosarcoma, below). Benign hemangiomas are often congenital in children or may be acquired in older populations. They are subclassified histologically and can be composed of predominately arteries, veins, capillaries, or a mixture of vascular types. A *microvenular hemangioma* is characterized

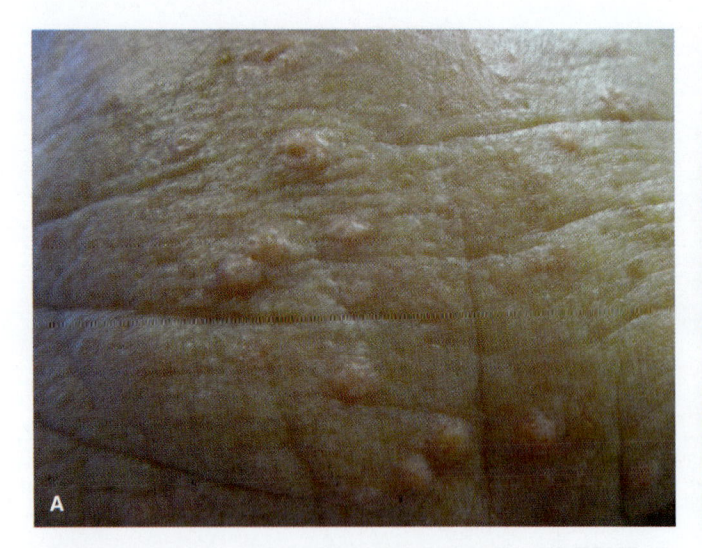

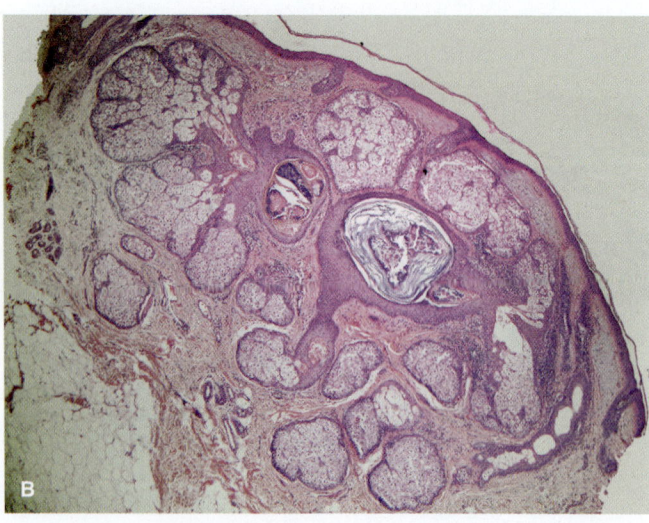

FIGURE 20-18 Sebaceous hyperplasia. **(A)** Papules of sebaceous hyperplasia are common on the face and forehead. **(B)** Sebaceous hyperplasia is characterized by and increased number of normal-appearing sebaceous glands.

by numerous small vascular channels. *Cherry angiomas* are common small, reddish-purple papules that can develop at any age. A *port-wine stain* is a capillary malformation of the head and neck and can be found in patients with *Sturge–Weber syndrome*. *Pyogenic granuloma* (PG) refers to a lesion that is neither purulent nor granulomatous and is also called *lobular capillary hemangioma*. PG presents as an ulcerated, reddish papule, frequently on the hand or foot, and often there is a history of recent bleeding. PG is a vascular proliferation that occasionally develops at the site of an injury, and is thought to represent either an abnormal wound healing reaction or a benign neoplasm. Microscopically, PG consists of aggregations of thin-walled blood vessels that may have accompanying inflammation and ulceration **(Figure 20-19A, B, C)**.

Xanthoma

Xanthomas usually present as small yellow-red papules, and are often multiple. They are related to abnormal accumulation of lipid in the skin and there are a variety of types. They occur typically on the buttocks and extensor surfaces of the extremities and are occasionally associated with hereditary conditions such as lipoprotein lipase deficiency. More commonly, they are seen in conjunction with secondary causes including obesity, hypothyroidism, pancreatitis, or excessive alcohol intake. Histologically, these lesions are characterized by the accumulation of lipid within the cytoplasm of histiocytes, known as foam cells or lipid cells. *Eruptive xanthoma* occurs on the buttock and thighs and is common after rapid lipid increase. *Xanthelasmas* are xanthomatous lesions that occur around the eye **(Figure 20-20A, B)**.

Neurofibroma

These lesions can occur sporadically (and commonly) as solitary lesions or as multiple lesions in patients with neurofibromatosis (*von Recklinghausen disease*), often as flesh-colored nodules or tumors. Neurofibromatosis is an autosomal dominant genetic disorder caused by a genetic defect in the gene coding for *neurofibromin* on chromosome 17. Multiple and associated with neurofibromatosis, neurofibromas can be very disfiguring. They are characterized histologically by oval or wavy nuclei in the dermis without epidermal involvement that, when taken in aggregate, may give a "school of fish" appearance. These cells are small and without significant pleomorphism, mitotic figures, or atypia. When found in neurofibromatosis, they appear in conjunction with other findings of this syndrome including axillary freckling, *café-au-lait* macules (flat, well demarcated patches resembling in color that of coffee with milk.), and *Lisch* nodules (hamartomas of the iris), among other findings **(Figure 20-21A, B)**.

Primary Cutaneous Neuroendocrine Carcinoma (Merkel Cell Carcinoma)

Merkel cell carcinoma is a rapidly growing neoplasm, usually found on the head and neck of adults, which portends a poor prognosis. Merkel cells are involved in sensory functions in the skin, although the connection between these cells as the site of origin of Merkel cell carcinoma has been a source of some debate. Recently, Merkel cell carcinoma has been linked to a *polyomavirus* known as *Merkel cell virus*. This lesion presents most commonly on the face and neck and metastasis occurs quickly. Histologically, cells are basophilic, small, and atypical, and mitotic figures are prominent. Special stains help to rule out other items on the differential, including lymphoma. CK20 positivity is the most characteristic immunohistochemical feature **(Figure 20-22)**.

Dermatofibroma

Dermatofibroma is the most common neoplasm of fibrocystic lineage, and typically presents as a firm hyperpigmented papule or nodule on the extremity. Since dermatofibromas sometimes develop at sites of trauma or after insect bites, some

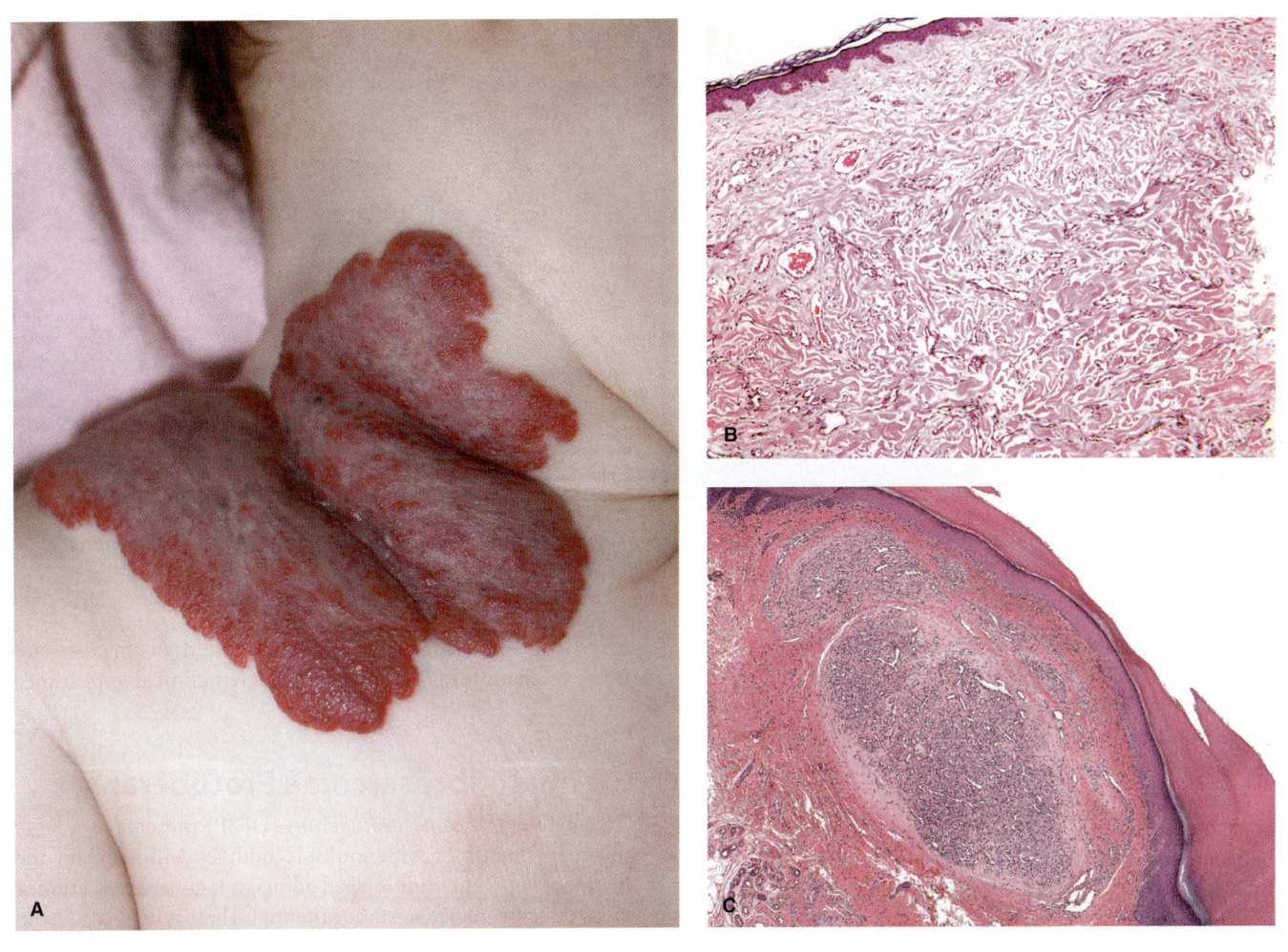

FIGURE 20-19 Hemangioma. (A) Hemangiomas are common in young children. (Image used with permission from Dr. Dean Morrell, UNC Dermatology.) **(B)** Microvenular hemangioma is characterized by numerous small benign vascular channels. **(C)** Pyogenic granuloma is characterized by thin-walled blood vessels in a cellular background.

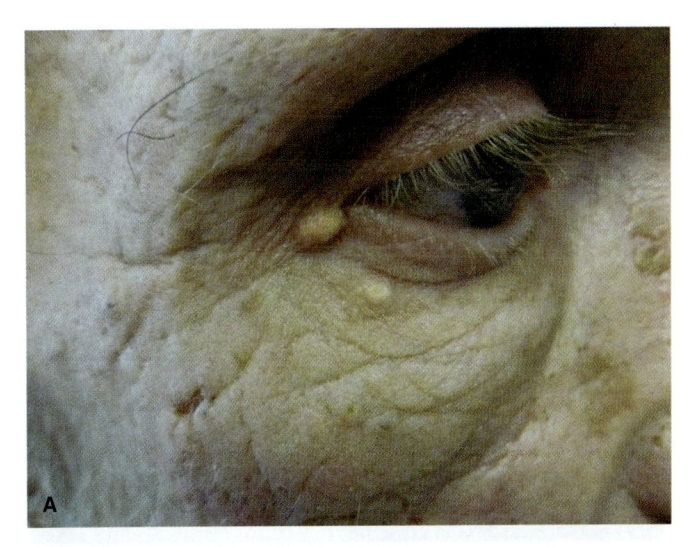

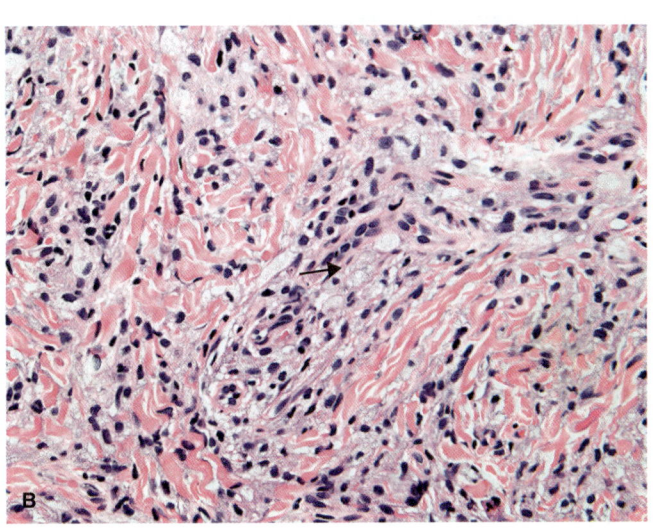

FIGURE 20-20 Xanthelsma. (A) Xanthelasma presents as a yellow papule on the eyelid. **(B)** Xanthomatous lesions are characterized by numerous foamy macrophages (histiocytes, examples at arrow), often the result of lipid accumulation.

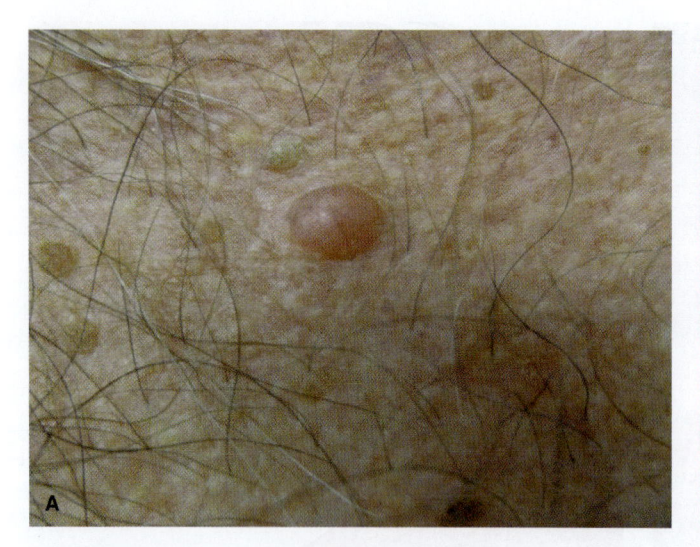

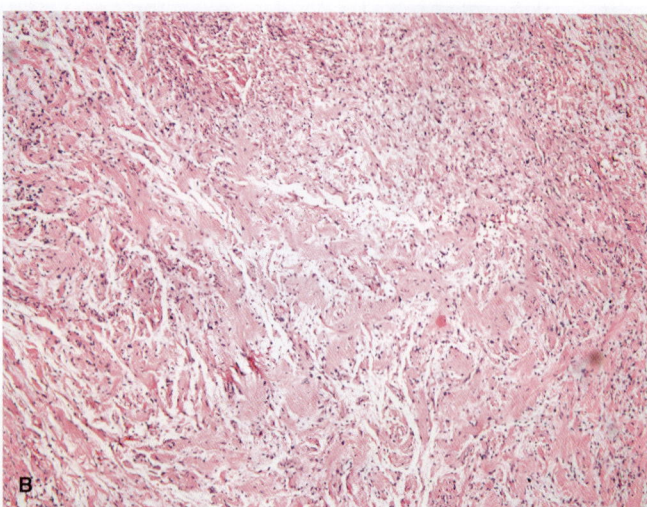

FIGURE 20-21 **Neurofibroma. (A)** Neurofibroma can be solitary or multiple and present as a flesh-colored nodule. **(B)** Neurofibroma is characterized by wavy spindle cells in a pink stroma.

authorities have considered dermatofibroma as a reactive, inflammatory condition, but the lesions generally persist, and thus display the biological behavior of a benign neoplasm. Classically, these lesions are associated with leg shaving in females. Dermatofibromas are often hyperpigmented. Microscopically, the neoplasm consists of a nodular proliferation of spindled and dendritic cells, usually positioned between markedly thickened collagen bundles. The cells are believed to actively secrete either cytokines or growth factors that induce hyperplasia and hyperpigmentation of the overlying epidermis. The induced epidermal changes are the explanation for the hyperpigmented clinical appearance **(Figure 20-23)**.

Dermatofibrosarcoma Protuberans

Dermatofibrosarcoma protuberans (DFSP) presents as a large plaque, sometimes with multiple nodules within it, on the trunk of young to middle-aged adults. It is considered a tumor with intermediate metastatic potential. There is no relationship to sun exposure, unlike other more common skin neoplasms (basal cell carcinoma, squamous cell carcinoma, melanoma, etc.) Unlike dermatofibroma, this tumor can infiltrate fat and can be locally aggressive and even metastasize over time. This infiltration of fat is often observed histologically as a "honeycomb pattern" **(Figure 20-24)**.

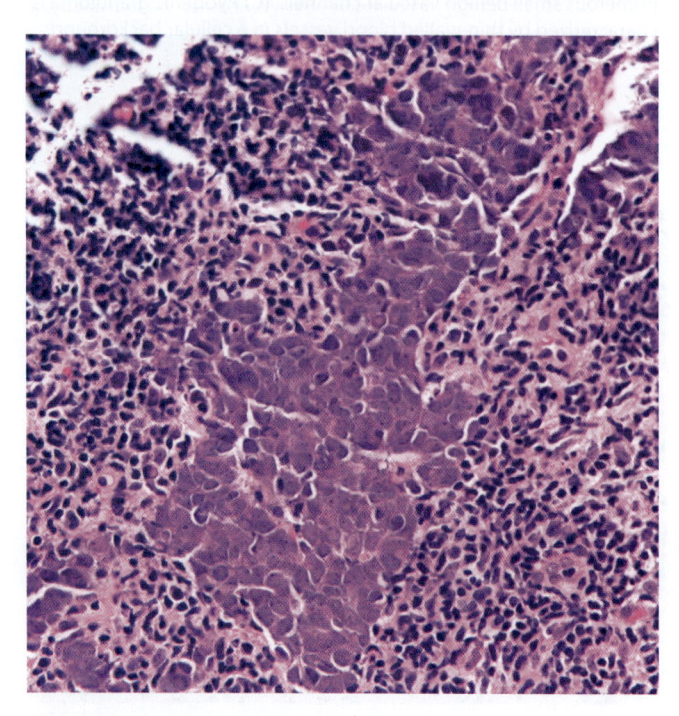

FIGURE 20-22 **Merkel cell carcinoma.** Here surrounded by lymphocytes, demonstrates small, crowded, hyperchromatic, atypical cells on histology and lends a poor prognosis.

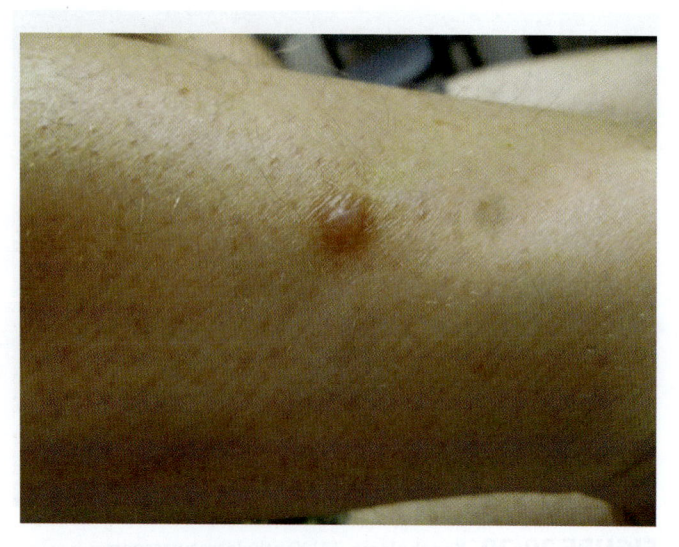

FIGURE 20-23 **Dermatofibroma.** The lesion presents as a firm hyperpigmented nodule.

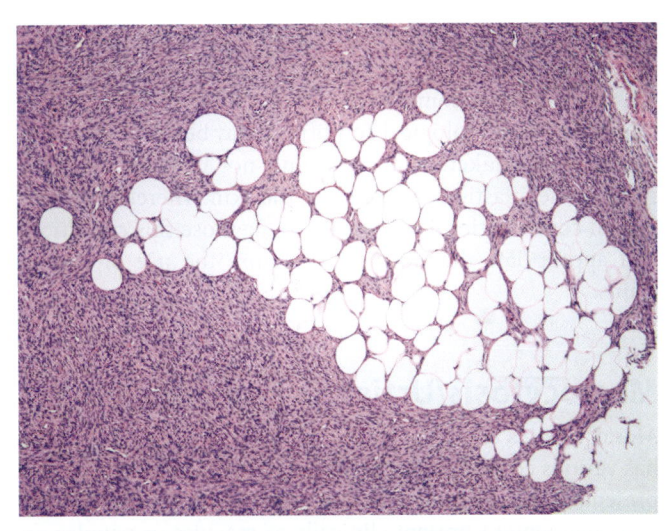

FIGURE 20-24 Dermatofibrosarcoma protuberans (DFSP). Fat trapping, "honeycombing," is a helpful clue toward making the diagnosis of dermatofibrosarcoma protuberans (DFSP).

Angiosarcoma

Most benign tumors of the skin have a malignant histological counterpart. As a whole, the malignant counterparts tend to be much more rare than their benign "cousins." *Angiosarcomas* often present in older patients, especially on the scalp. They can also occur in the setting of previous radiation treatment. Histologically, there is irregular proliferation of vasculature and endothelial cells with marked atypia. It is particularly associated with chronic lymphedema and radiation therapy, and prognosis is uniformly poor **(Figure 20-25A, B)**.

Kaposi Sarcoma

Kaposi sarcoma is an important vascular tumor that underwent a dramatic surge in incidence with the AIDS epidemic. While it can exist in a non-AIDS associated form, in the United States it most often occurs in association with AIDS and is seen in cells infected with *human herpes virus 8* (HHV 8).

NEOPLASMS OF IMMUNE ORIGIN

Neoplasms of immune cells are relatively rare in the skin but all clinicians should be aware of them as diagnostic possibilities. While these entities may be suspected clinically, the diagnosis is often cinched histologically, often with the aid of immunohistochemistry. With the advent and increasing usage of new investigational techniques, especially in regard to molecular pathology, the field of hematopathology will certainly be evolving. This is equally true for hematopoietic neoplasms involving the skin.

Mycosis Fungoides/Cutaneous T-Cell Lymphoma

Mycosis fungoides is, by far, the most common type of primary cutaneous lymphoma and is a diagnosis that can only be made after carefully correlating both the clinical and histological findings. It is the prototype of the cutaneous T-cell lymphomas. T-cell lymphomas are much more common in the skin than B cell lymphomas. Lesions of mycosis fungoides are slow growing and tend to progress from a patch to a plaque to a tumor stage based on the gross shape of the tumor. There is a male predominance and patients tend to be older. Lesions are most common on the trunk or thighs.

Histologically, there is a band-like infiltrate of lymphocytes beneath the dermoepidermal junction with extension of lymphocytes into the overlying epidermis (epidermotropism) as well as small collections of atypical lymphocytes in the epidermis (called Pautrier microabscesses) **(Figure 20-26)**. Immunohistochemical staining aids in the diagnosis including

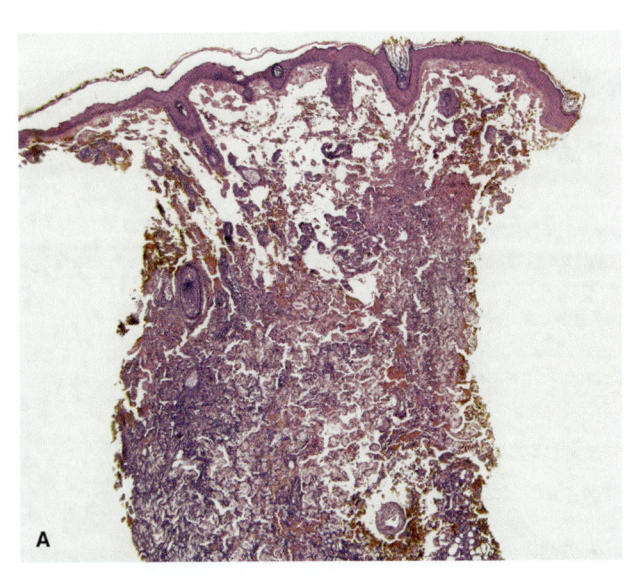

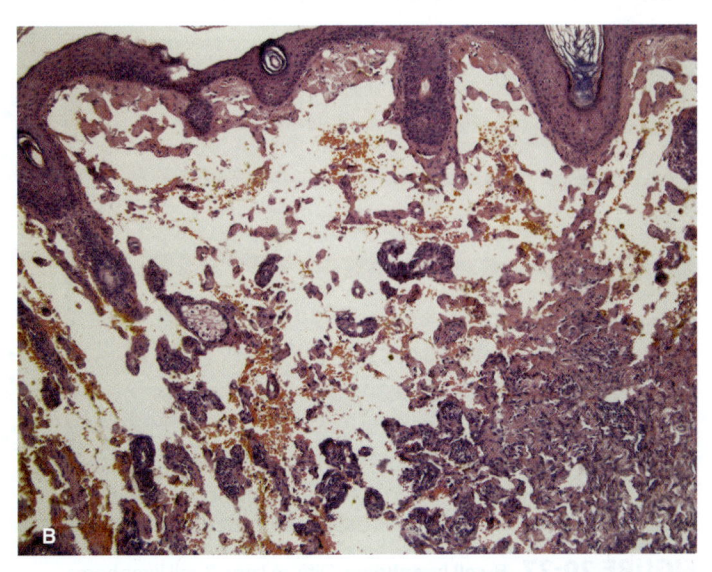

FIGURE 20-25 Angiosarcoma. **(A)** The dermis has been largely replaced by highly atypical cells in this patient with angiosarcoma. **(B)** Malignant cells form bizarre vascular channels. The prognosis of angiosarcoma is poor.

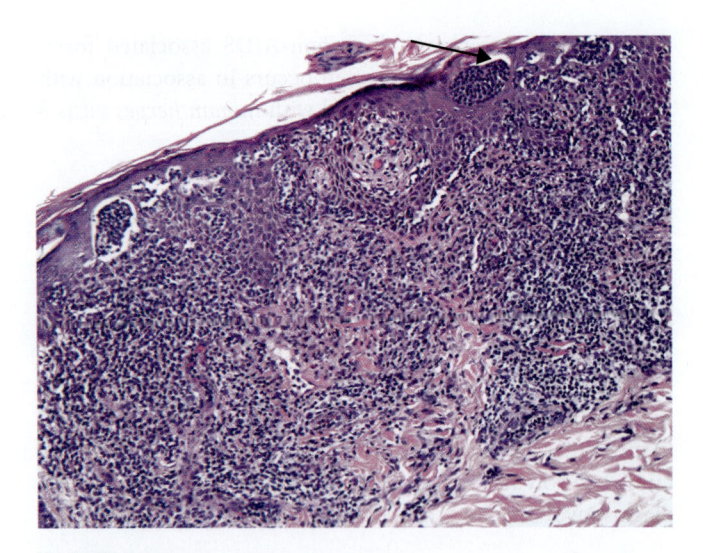

FIGURE 20-26 **Mycosis fungoides.** Atypical lymphocytes invade the epidermis both singly and in groups (Pautrier microabscesses, example at arrow) in mycosis fungoides.

loss of pan-T-cell markers like CD7. *Clonal T-cell gene rearrangements* are also helpful.

B-Cell Lymphoma

Numerous lymphomas not only occur in other places in the body but can also present primarily or secondarily in the skin. These include marginal zone lymphoma, diffuse large B-cell lymphoma, mantle cell lymphoma, and follicle center lymphoma. Histological and immunohistochemical findings for each of these diseases are dependent on the specific disease. While these are relatively uncommon, it is prudent to keep them as a diagnostic consideration (Figure 20-27).

Leukemia Cutis

Leukemia cutis is the term given to cutaneous infiltrate of a systemic leukemia. Leukemic deposits in the skin are very rarely encountered; however, when they do occur they occur late in the disease course and portend a poor prognosis. This occurs most commonly in acute myeloid leukemia. A number of dermatological conditions may be encountered in patients with leukemia, and certainly not all of them are the result of neoplastic cells invading the skin. Therefore, histological confirmation is necessary to diagnose this condition, and appropriate diagnosis may require the use of special stains.

Mastocytosis/Urticaria Pigmentosa

Mastocytosis is an abnormal proliferation of mast cells, which has various clinical presentations, but which most commonly presents in the form of *urticaria pigmentosa*. Lesions of urticaria pigmentosa present clinically as macules or papules on the trunk, and often demonstrate the *Darier sign* (urtication with stroking). Most childhood cases of urticaria pigmentosa have a good prognosis with resolution by puberty. In adults, systemic involvement becomes more prevalent. In addition to urticaria pigmentosa, solitary lesions can present anywhere in the body as *mastocytomas*.

Histologically, "fried egg" appearing cells may aggregate into collections as in urticaria pigmentosa or mastocytoma, or may be more sparsely situated around blood vessels, as is the case in the variant known as *telangiectasia macularis eruptiva perstans*. Cells tend to involve the upper third of the dermis (Figure 20-28). Mast cells stain with CD117 (c-kit).

Langerhans Cell Histiocytosis (Histiocytosis X)

Langerhans cells are dendritic antigen presenting cells involved in processing and presenting foreign antigens to lymphoid cells. *Langerhans cell histiocytosis* is a disease that

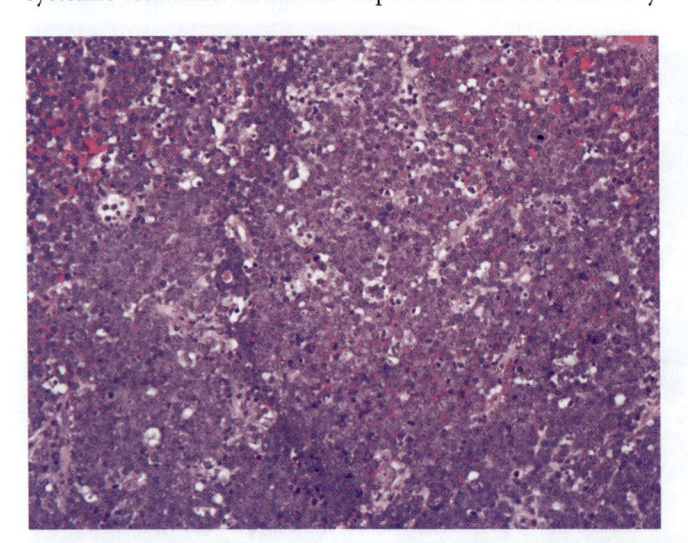

FIGURE 20-27 **B-cell lymphoma.** Diffuse large B cell lymphoma is characterized by sheets of large, irregular B cells with significant atypia, and numerous mitotic figures.

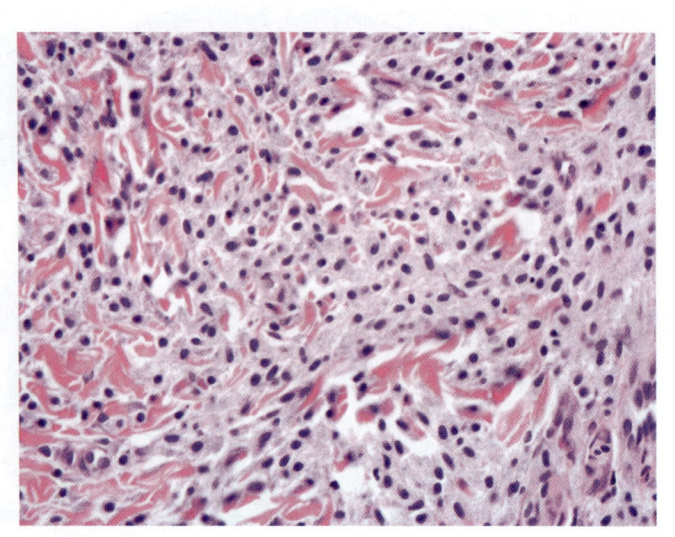

FIGURE 20-28 **Mastocytosis.** Mast cells infiltrating the dermis in mastocytosis have a fried egg appearance.

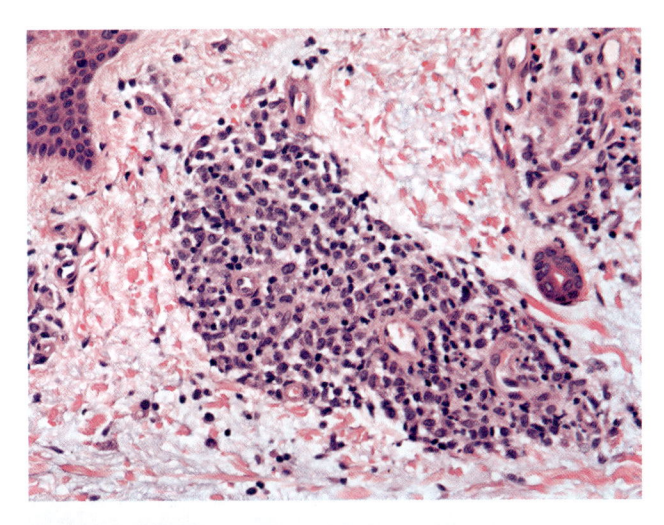

FIGURE 20-29 Langerhans cells histiocytosis. The lesion is characterized by reniform or "kidney shaped" cells.

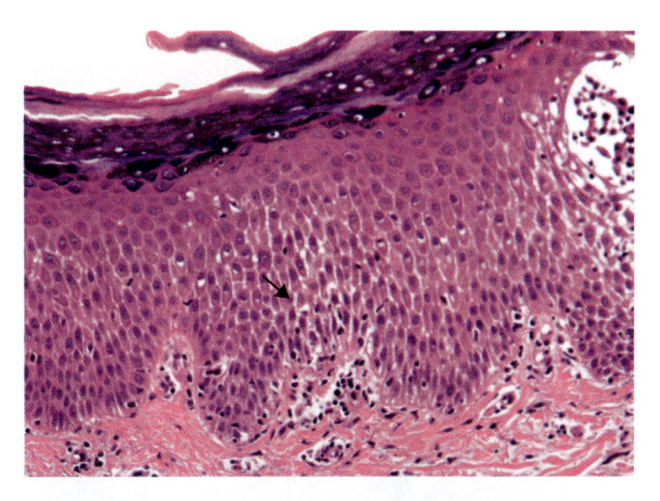

FIGURE 20-30 Spongiotic dermatitis demonstrates spongiosis of the epidermis with vesicle formation. Note expansion of the spaces between keratinocytes at arrow.

is classified into three entities based on clinical findings: *Letterer–Siwe disease, Hand–Schuller–Christian disease,* and *eosinophilic granuloma,* which sometimes have significant overlap. Other organ systems may also be involved. Children are most commonly affected and generally have a good prognosis. The histological appearance is one of *reniform* or *cerebroid* histiocytic Langerhans cells, generally in the dermis and often surrounded by eosinophils **(Figure 20-29)**. Electron microscopic appearance is classic for tennis racket-shaped *Birbeck granules,* although in modern clinical practice electron microscopy is rarely performed. Langerhans cells tend to be CD1a and S100 protein positive. The disease may resolve spontaneously, but in some cases systemic involvement may prove fatal.

MAJOR INFLAMMATORY REACTION PATTERNS AND PROTOTYPES

Several conditions are commonly included in this category. *Atopic dermatitis* or *eczema* is the prototype lesion of spongiotic dermatitis and occurs on the face, neck, and antecubital areas in people predisposed to allergies. *Allergic contact dermatitis* arises in areas of skin in contact with a specific inciting agent resulting in a delayed hypersensitivity reaction (type IV or cell-mediated reaction). Common inciting agents are nickel (on belts and jewelry), fragrances, rubber additives, and latex. These diseases, along with several others, share the features of "spongiotic dermatitis," namely expansion and swelling of the spaces between keratinocytes, often accompanied by an inflammatory infiltrate in the dermis. Seborrheic dermatitis (dandruff) is another condition that manifests with spongiosis clinically. As is the case regarding many inflammatory skin conditions, histology is used to support clinical diagnoses rather than to make the diagnosis directly **(Figure 20-30)**.

The prototype lesion of the *psoriasiform* reaction pattern is that of *psoriasis vulgaris.* Psoriasis is a disease that manifests clinically by sharply demarcated erythematous plaques with a thick silvery scale. Lesions occur most commonly on the scalp, elbows, knees, trunk, and buttock. Nail changes are also common, and psoriasis may be associated with a destructive arthritis. The disease is known to relapse and remit with time, and severity of histological changes varies with time. The histological picture is that of elongation of the epidermal rete ridges with thinning of the epidermis immediately above the dermal papillae. There is often hyperkeratosis with parakeratosis and neutrophils in the cornified layer (*Munro microabscesses*) **(Figure 20-31A, B)**.

This woman in case 18-8 suffers from *lichen planus,* which demonstrates an *interface reaction pattern*. Lichen planus is known clinically by the five "p's," commonly used to describe the clinical presentation and appearance. These are planar, pruritic (itchy), purple, papules, and plaques. These lesions are especially common on the wrists, hands, and legs and have been associated with *hepatitis C*. Involvement of oral mucosa or genitals is also common. The interface reaction pattern is characterized by lymphocytic infiltrate immediately below the dermoepidermal junction causing vacuolar alteration and scattered dyskeratotic keratinocytes. This pattern is commonly seen in numerous skin diseases, of which *lichen planus* is the prototype. Other histological characteristics of lichen planus include acanthosis or thickening of the epidermal layer with a characteristic "saw-toothed" appearance to the rete ridges and a band-like lymphocytic infiltrate (a *lichenoid* infiltrate). Because there are several types of lesions that may give a similar histological picture, the combination of both clinical and histological appearance is often needed to make the correct diagnosis. Variants of lichen planus include *lichen planopilaris*, which involves the hair follicles, and *lichen nitidus*, which presents as tiny papules and is more common in children.

Other conditions that histologically display the interface reaction pattern include *erythema multiforme, Stevens–Johnson*

CASE 20-7

A 45-year-old woman presents with multiple well-demarcated, scaly silver-white plaques on her scalp, neck, and arms. Clinical image and biopsy results are shown below.

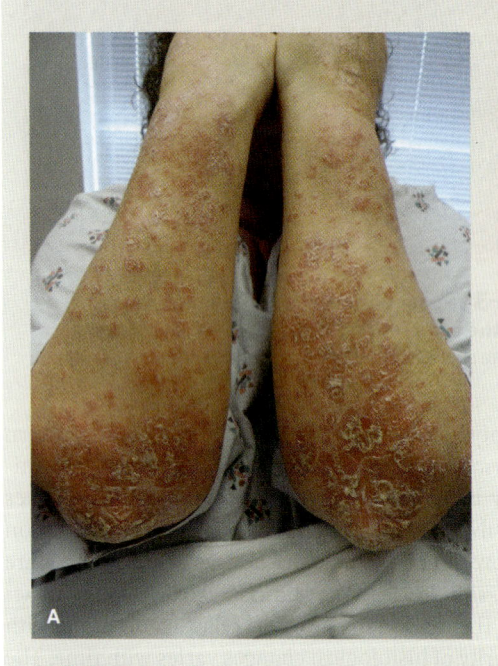

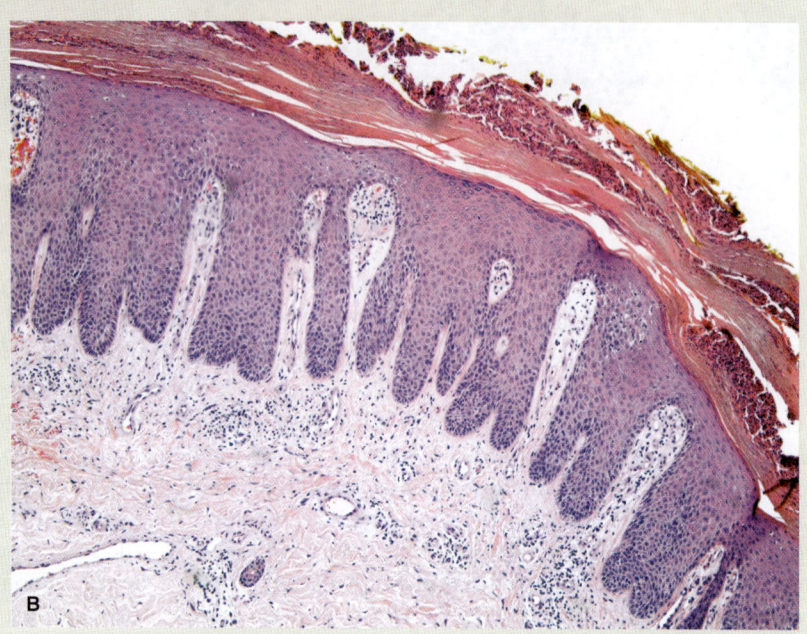

FIGURE 20-31 **Psoriasis. (A)** Scaly silver plaques of psoriasis. **(B)** Psoriasis is characterized by symmetrical epidermal hyperplasia.

CASE 20-8

A 38-year-old woman presents with multiple papules on the flexural surfaces of her wrists. These are pink/purple and are very itchy. These have been present for several months. A clinical picture is given below, along with the histological image from her punch biopsy (Figure 20-32A, B).

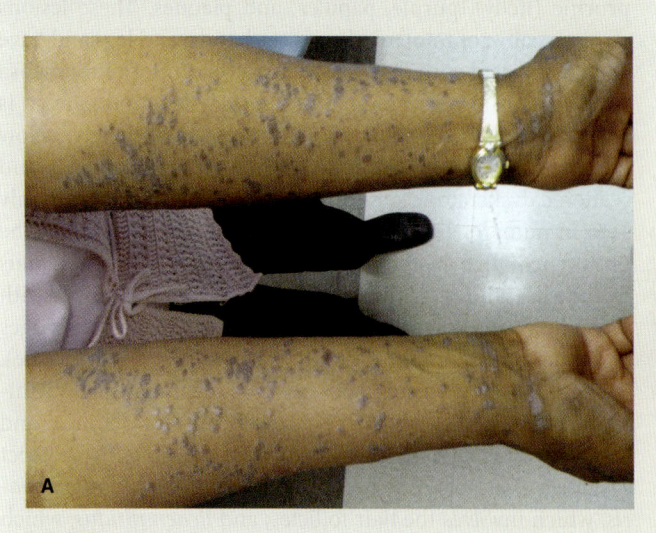

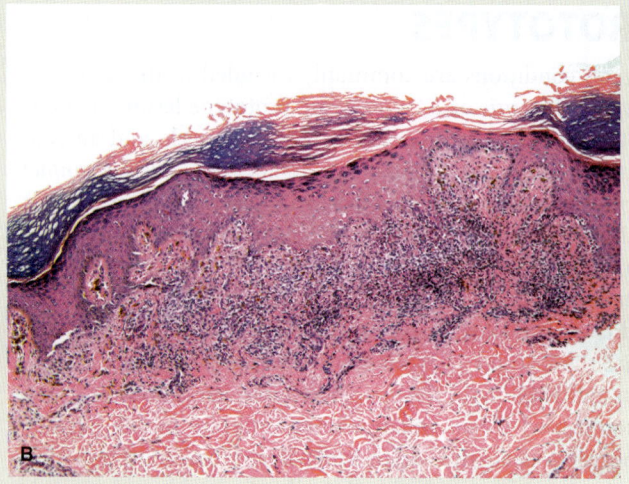

FIGURE 20-32 **Lichen planus. (A)** Purple papules of lichen planus. **(B)** A subepidermal lymphocytic infiltrate with a saw tooth pattern to the rete ridges characteristic of lichen planus.

syndrome, *and* toxic epidermal necrolysis. Erythema multiforme is an inflammatory reaction thought to be related to infections by viruses (most often herpes simplex), drugs, or other infectious agents. Genetic susceptibility may play a role. The classic clinical presentation is that of small erythematous targetoid lesions, especially on the hands and feet. Stevens–Johnson syndrome and toxic epidermal necrolysis may have similar histological presentations, but are more extensive clinically and can be life threatening.

Skin reactions caused by drugs can take on almost any form, both clinically and histologically, but often manifest with a pattern of interface dermatitis.

Lichen Sclerosis

Lichen sclerosis is a relatively common condition presenting on the vulva and perineum of females but can appear in other areas as well. Clinically, they present as white plaques with the appearance of scarring, and can result in pruritus and discomfort. The histological trademarks are those of an atrophic epidermis with subepidermal hyalinized collagen. Lichen sclerosis increases the risk of squamous cell carcinoma and may lead to functional morbidity as well (closure of the vaginal aperture, etc.). The male correlate is known as *balanitis xerotica obliterans* (Figure 20-33A, B).

Vesiculobullous (Bullous Pemphigoid)

A variety of blistering (*vesiculobullous*) disorders exist, the most common of these are *bullous pemphigoid* and *pemphigus vulgaris*. Bullous pemphigoid is an autoimmune disorder that tends to occur in older patients and presents as tense bullae. It is associated with certain HLA types and is associated with other types of autoimmune diseases. It is caused by IgG autoantibodies that attack bullous pemphigoid antigen 2 in the hemidesmosomes of the basement membrane.

Pemphigus vulgaris is an autoimmune disease with a pathophysiological mechanism similar to that of bullous pemphigoid. Unlike *bullous pemphigoid*, however, autoantibodies are directed against keratinocyte cell surface molecules desmoglein 1 and 3. This causes the histological picture of keratinocyte acantholysis or separation of keratinocytes from one another in the epidermis itself.

Both pemphigus vulgaris and bullous pemphigoid (along with other diseases) can be confirmed using immunofluorescent techniques. Bullous pemphigoid demonstrates linear deposition of IgG and C3 at the dermoepidermal junction, while pemphigus vulgaris demonstrates a net-like deposition of IgG within the intercellular spaces of the epidermis.

We highlight a third type of vesiculobullous disease that is of special interest because of its association with *celiac disease*, a hypersensitivity reaction to gluten protein found in many founds containing wheat. This vesiculobullous disease is dermatitis herpetiformis and presents as an intensely pruritic vesicular rash over extensor surfaces. The vast majority of cases are related to gluten sensitivity and a gluten-free diet is considered to be a first-line therapy. Histological examination classically reveals a subepidermal blister with neutrophils in the dermal papillae (Figure 20-34).

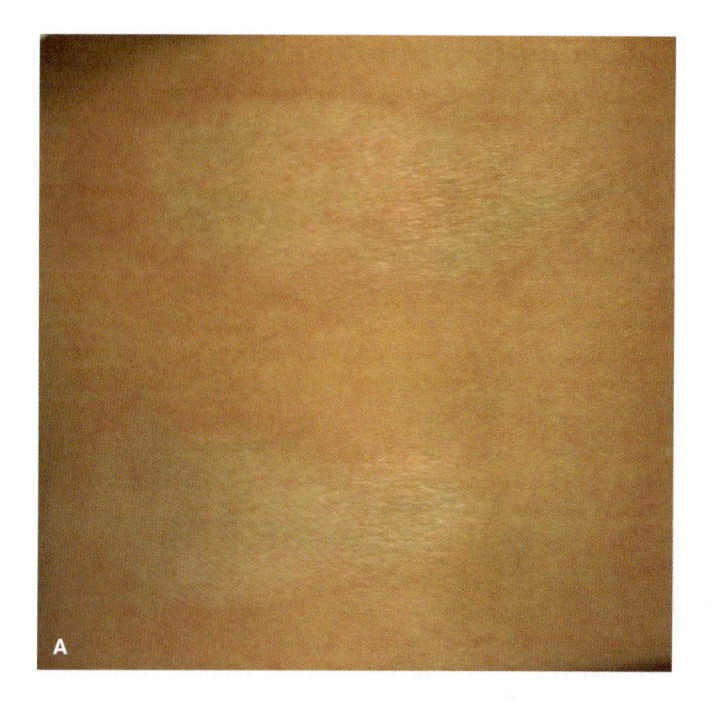

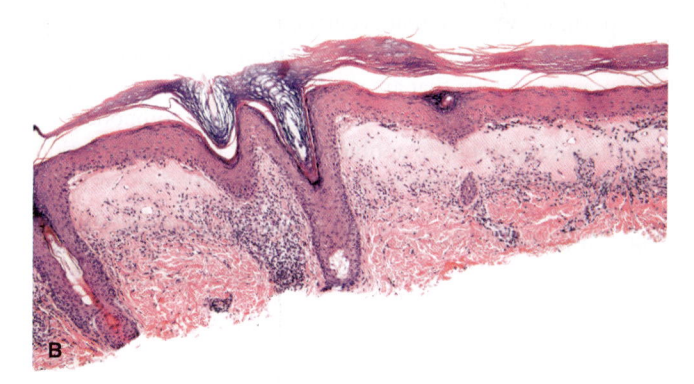

FIGURE 20-33 Lichen sclerosis. (A) Lichen sclerosis is characterized by white plaques, usually on the vulva and perineum, but can occur in other areas. (Image used with permission from Dr. Dean Morrell, UNC Dermatology.) (B) There is prominent hyalinization of the subepidermal collagen in lichen sclerosis.

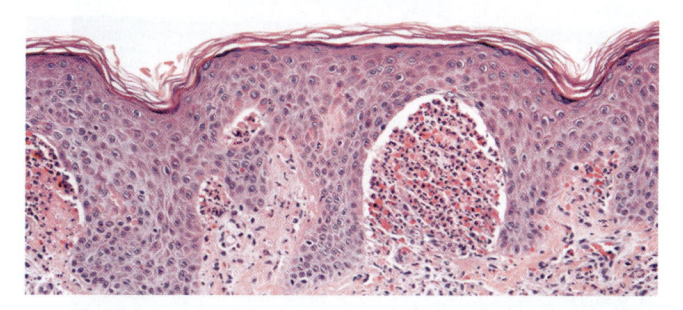

FIGURE 20-34 Dermatitis herpetiformis. The condition is related to celiac disease and shows subepidermal blisters with collections of intrapapillary neutrophils.

Folliculitis (Suppurative Folliculitis)

Folliculitis is the medical term for "zit." There are infectious and inflammatory causes of inflamed hair follicles. The prototypes are *suppurative folliculitis* and *acne vulgaris*. *Suppurative folliculitis* is a follicular infection generally caused by bacteria such as staphylococci. Patients often present with red papules and pustules, often itchy, on the trunk, thigh, face, and scalp. A short course of oral antibiotics is usually curative, although some scalp folliculitis is resistant to therapy. Microscopically, a hair follicle is filled with and surrounded by a mixture of inflammatory cells, and neutrophils are often abundant. In acne, there are two fundamental pathogenic processes. The hair follicles keratinize abnormally, and thus have a tendency to get "clogged" (a process known as comedo formation), and the clogged follicles are subsequently prone to becoming inflamed, which is the basis for the papules and pustules seen clinically.

Both pathogenic mechanisms are treatable. The abnormal keratinization is usually treated using vitamin A derivatives known as retinoids. The topical retinoid of choice is tretinoin (Retin-A), and the systemic retinoid most commonly employed in severe cases is *isotretinoin* (Accutane). It is important to realize that accutane is highly teratogenic; in the United States, females must have monthly physician visits with pregnancy tests that are registered in a national database prior to drug dispensation. The inflammatory component of acne usually responds to antibiotics, either through alteration in follicular flora, an anti-inflammatory mechanism, or both. It is the inflammatory response to acne that triggers scarring, and thus treatment of acne is important. Acne can be exacerbated by hormonal influences, which is why acne is so common during puberty.

Granulomatous Dermatitis (Granuloma Annulare)

The prototypic skin lesion of the granulomatous reaction pattern is that of *granuloma annulare*, a benign condition that tends to affect young people, especially on the hands, feet, and elbows. It is typically of limited duration (sometimes lasts up to several years), largely asymptomatic, and responds poorly to topical and systemic therapies. Clinical findings are that of tan or erythematous annular (ring-shaped) papules and plaques. The histological findings of this disease include loosely formed granulomas surrounding central collagen degeneration and mucin deposition (Figure 20-35A, B).

Sarcoidosis

Sarcoidosis is an immune-mediated systemic condition that most commonly presents among young to middle-aged African American females. While not all patients have skin involvement, in some the disease is exclusively confined to the skin. Skin lesions can occur with or without pulmonary involvement, but hilar lymphadenopathy is classic and is seen in the majority of patients. Sarcoidosis is generally a clinical diagnosis that can often be confirmed histologically. Clinical findings include elevated calcium level, elevated *angiotensin-converting enzyme (ACE) level* (ACE), *elevated antinuclear antibody (ANA) titer*, and characteristic radiographic findings. Clinical course is variable and ranges from a self-limiting disease in some to a terminal process in others. On histological examination, granulomas are composed of epithelioid histiocytes, generally without necrosis (noncaseating), and are characteristically discrete. Microscopically, the classic "sarcoidal" granuloma is characterized by the absence of a surrounding infiltrate of lymphocytes around a collection of epithelioid histiocytes (Figure 20-36A, B). Sarcoidosis is frequently associated with erythema nodosum.

Rheumatoid Nodules

Subcutaneous nodules present in patients with rheumatoid arthritis are called rheumatoid nodules. These nodules often present at sites of trauma and are common over the elbows and fingers (especially the knuckles) and can cause significant

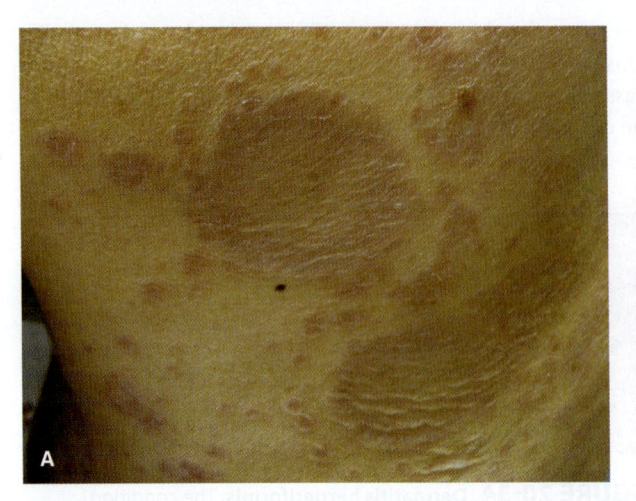

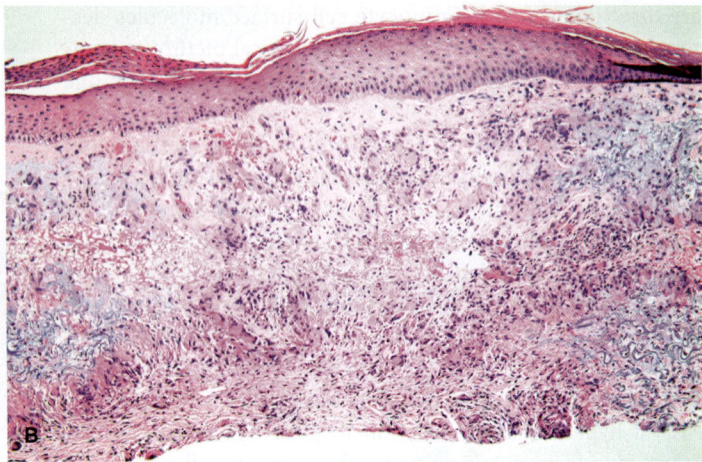

FIGURE 20-35 Granuloma annulare. **(A)** Annular-shaped plaques of granuloma annulare. **(B)** Granuloma annulare is characterized by loosely formed granulomas in the dermis.

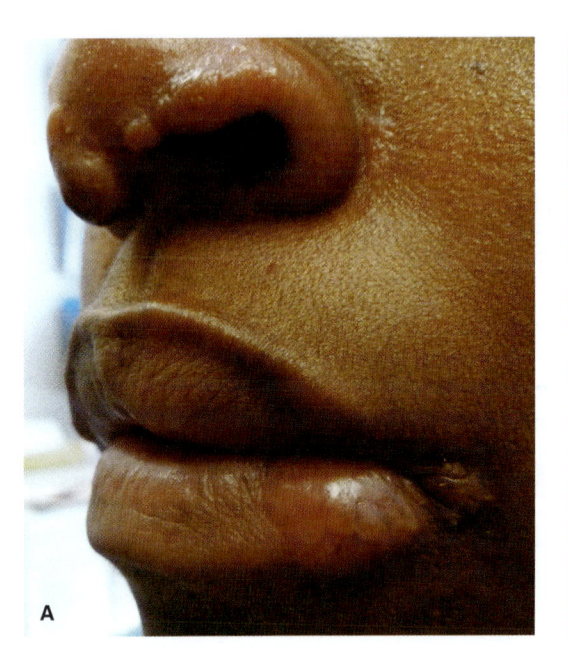

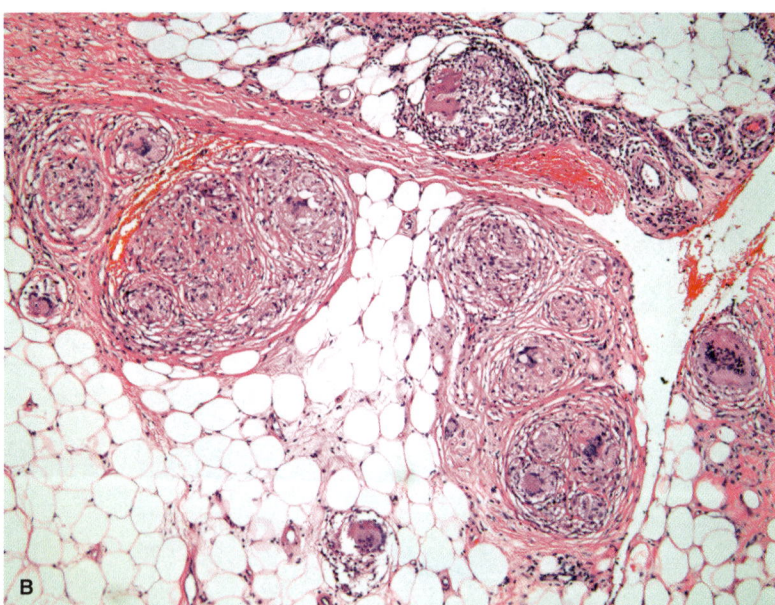

FIGURE 20-36 Sarcoidosis. **(A)** Irregular nodules of sarcoidosis. **(B)** Well-defined granulomas of sarcoidosis in subcutaneous fat.

debilitation and morbidity. Clinical symptoms of rheumatoid arthritis include joint pain and swelling. Histological examination demonstrates loose, palisading granulomas surrounding an intensely eosinophilic degenerative center. Neutrophils and fibrosis are also common features.

Foreign Bodies and Foreign Body Granulomas

Granulomas are formed in an attempt to isolate and remove foreign objects and it can be surprising how frequently foreign bodies are encountered during the practice of pathology. These include a wide range of items including wood splinters, sutures, injected material, tattoos, or remnants of medical intervention. Foreign bodies of numerous types can elicit a sometimes dramatic response. On light microscopy, certain foreign bodies, such as plant matter in splinters, exhibit a characteristic appearance. The degree of inflammatory reaction that each foreign body elicits is dependent on both the type of foreign body and the host's immune system. Granulomas are commonly formed as reaction to the rupture of cysts or follicles, or in response to tattoos or medications injected into the dermis and subcutis (Figure 20-37A, B, C).

Sclerosing Disorders (Morphea/Scleroderma)

Scleroderma is a diffuse skin disease that demonstrates thickening and stiffening of connective tissue in the dermis and subcutis that also has systemic manifestations. Scleroderma can affect other organs outside the skin and also has a variation known as CREST syndrome (calcinosis, Raynaud phenomenon, esophageal dysmotility, sclerodactyly, telangiectasia). Patients often have elevated levels of autoimmune antibodies, particularly ANA, anti-Scl-70, and anti-RNP. *Morphea* presents with similar findings histologically, but manifests as single or multiple discrete plaques affecting only focal areas. Punch biopsies of both conditions often demonstrate a "square" appearance overall with thickened eosinophilic dermal collagen bundles (Figure 20-38).

Panniculitis (Erythema Nodosum)

Panniculitis refers to inflammation of the subcutaneous fat, which consists of *lobules* of adipocytes separated and supported by fibrous *septa*, and thus inflammatory reactions are divided into lobular panniculitis and septal panniculitis based on the zone in which the inflammation predominates. Based on the distribution of inflammation and the composition of the infiltrate, the panniculitides can be further classified. The prototypical panniculitis is a septal panniculitis, erythema nodosum (EN). Patients with EN develop red, indurated, warm, deep nodules, and plaques, most commonly on the lower extremities. Recent infections and medications (especially oral contraceptives) are the most common triggers. There is also an association with *inflammatory bowel disease* (IBD) and *sarcoidosis*. Immune complexes and vasculitis have long been thought to play a pathogenic role, but the precise pathogenesis remains uncertain. Under the microscope, EN displays inflammation in the subcutaneous fat in a predominantly septal distribution (Figure 20-39).

INFECTIOUS SKIN DISEASES

Fungal Infections (Dermatophyte)

Numerous types of fungal infections can be encountered in the skin. Dermatophyte (tinea) infections are superficial fungal infections that are most frequently caused by organisms

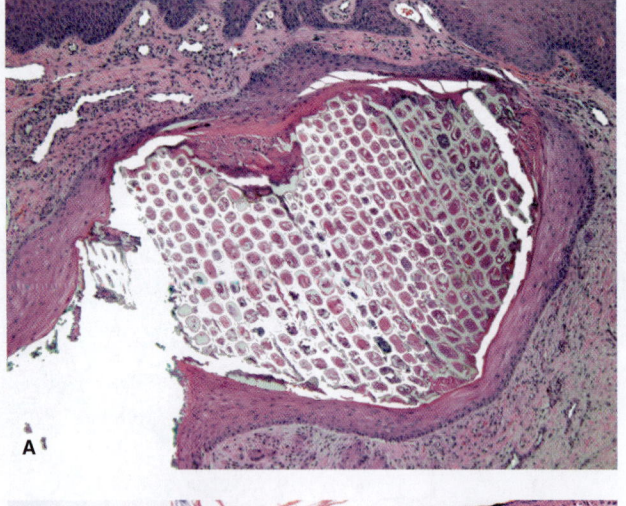

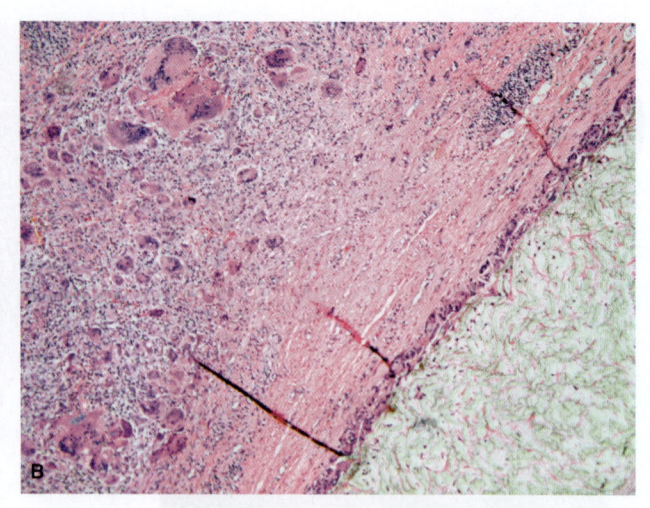

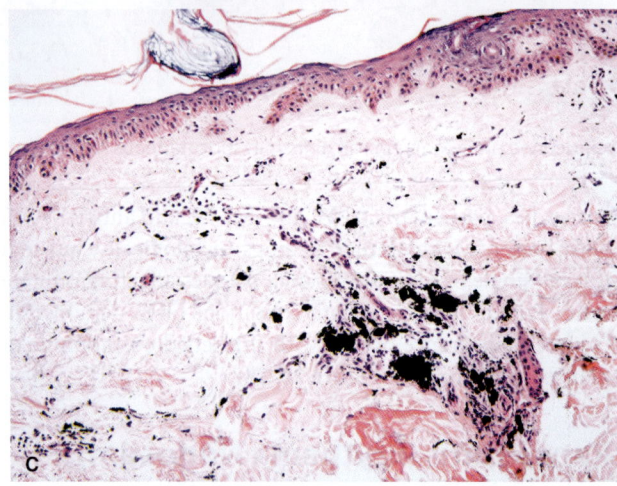

FIGURE 20-37 Foreign body reaction. (A) Wood Splinter. **(B)** Vascular stent (only a portion shown, bottom right) with abundant foreign body giant cell reaction. **(C)** Tattoo with minimal inflammatory reaction.

from the genera *Trichophyton, Epidermophyton,* and *Microsporum.* The clinical condition is often named after the body part affected (tinea corporis-body; tinea faciale-face, tinea pedis-foot, etc.), and lesions are often scaly, sometimes annular plaques. In immunosuppressed patients (AIDS, diabetes, chronic steroid use, etc.), more invasive fungal infections may be encountered. These include infections caused by *Aspergillus, Mucor, Cryptococcus, Coccidioides,* and *Histoplasma* among many others. *Candida* infections can affect the vagina in normal individuals, but may be exacerbated in the

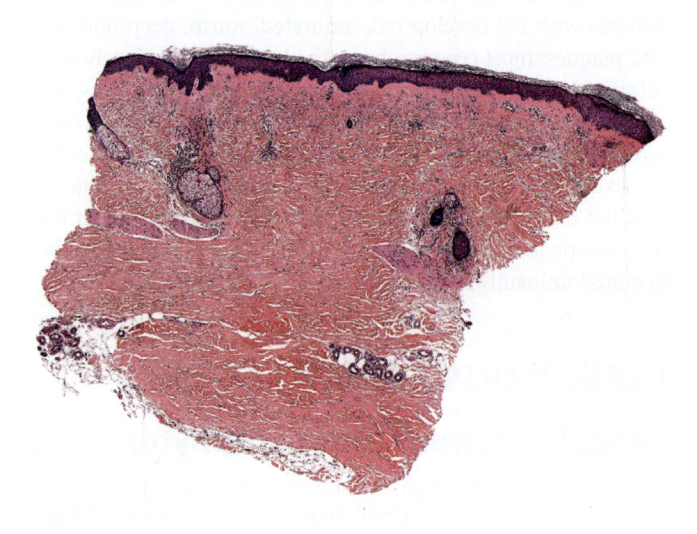

FIGURE 20-38 Morphea/scleroderma. Square appearance of morphea/scleroderma with thick collagen bundles.

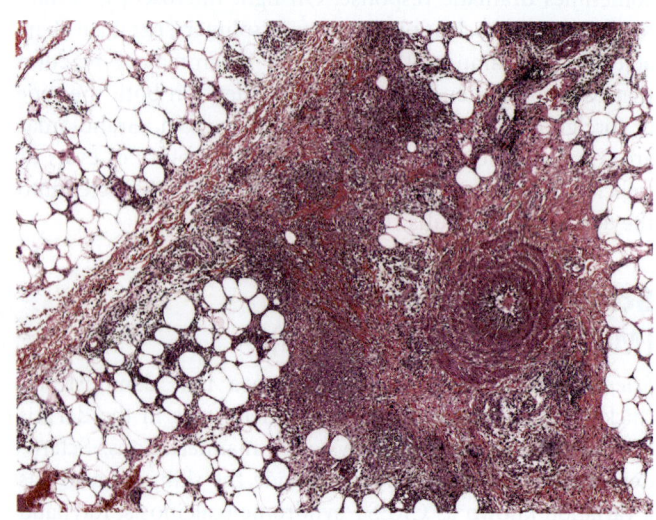

FIGURE 20-39 Erythema nodosum. The lesion is characterized by inflammation and fibrosis (especially in older lesions) in a septal distribution.

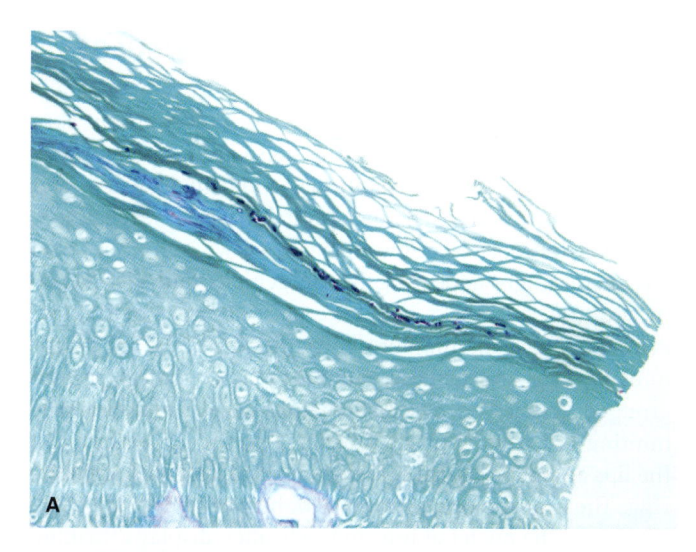

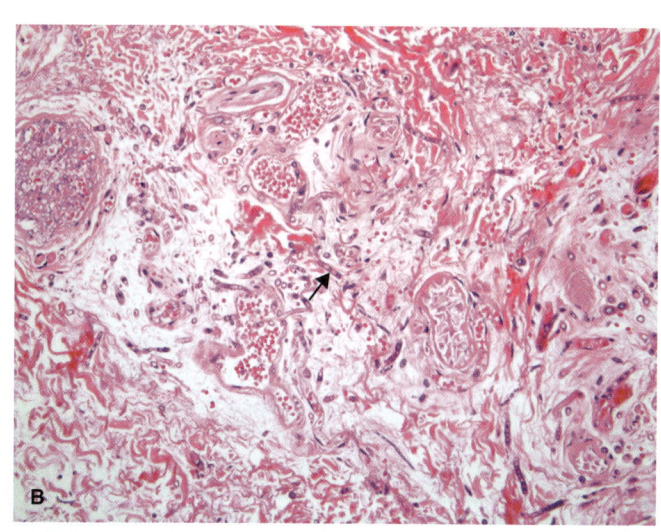

FIGURE 20-40 Fungal infection. **(A)** Periodic acid-Schiff (PAS) stain is often used to highlight fungal organisms (pink), seen in the stratum corneum. **(B)** Numerous fungal organisms (example at arrow) are identified in the dermis of this immunocompromised patient with invasive aspergillosis.

immunosuppressed state. Histochemical stains like *Grocott methenamine silver* (GMS) and *periodic acid-Schiff* (PAS) stains are often used to highlight organisms (Figure 20-40A, B).

Bacterial Infections (Impetigo/Erysipelas)

Impetigo is the colonization of the superficial epidermis by bacteria, often Staphylococcal or Streptococcal species. This is manifested clinically by red, well-demarcated tender plaques. In the case of staphylococcal impetigo, a classic honey-colored crust, bullae, and vesicles are commonly seen. Bacteria can often be visualized histologically on H&E staining or with a Gram stain. *Erysipelas* is a sharply demarcated superficial dermal bacterial infection, most often caused by beta-hemolytic group A streptococci (*Streptococcus pyogenes*). *Cellulitis* is the term given to bacterial infections involving the dermis and subcutis.

Viral Infections

CASE 20-9

A 53-year-old man presents with a hyperkeratotic white/gray papule on the knuckle of his second finger. Clinical image and biopsy are shown in Figure 20-41A, B.

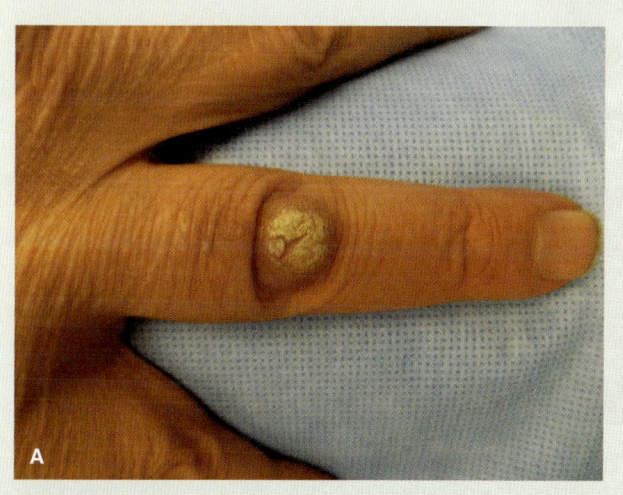

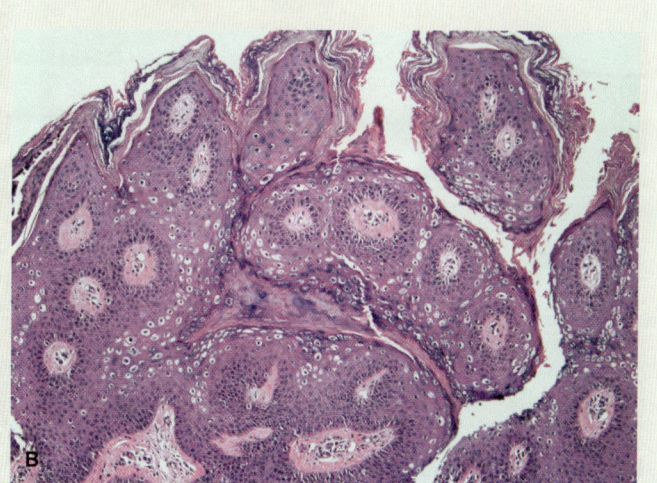

FIGURE 20-41 Verruca vulgaris. **(A)** Hyperkeratotic white/gray papule of verruca vulgaris. **(B)** Verrucous architecture and prominent koilocytic changes (keratinocytes with perinuclear clearing).

Verruca Vulgaris

Verruca (warts) are proliferations of keratinocytes that can appear on any area of the body, but commonly occurs on the hands and fingers. These tumors are very common. There are many different types of warts including the verruca vulgaris or "common wart," the plantar wart located on the plantar surface of the skin, verruca plana ("flat wart"), as well as *condyloma acuminatum*, also known as a venereal or genital wart. These lesions are related to HPV, and specific locations are sometimes related to specific HPV strains. For example, HPV-1 is related to the plantar wart, while HPV-2 is related to the common wart. HPV-6 and 11 are related to condyloma acuminatum. The histological picture of these lesions can range from subtle to striking and usually consists of papillomatous or verrucous changes to the epidermis (sharp undulations both superficially and deeply), koilocytic changes (keratinocytes with perinuclear clearing), and often hypergranulosis and hyperkeratosis. These lesions can be notoriously difficult to treat and often recur.

From a public health standpoint, exciting advances have been made in the prevention of condyloma acuminatum (genital warts), in the form of a vaccine that protects against infection by the most common strains of HPV, including 6 and 11. More importantly, this vaccine also protects against HPV strains that cause cervical cancer, particularly 16 and 18. Time will tell to what degree the widespread implication of these vaccines will affect screening, incidence, and prevalence of cervical cancer and genital warts.

Conditions Caused by Herpes Viruses

The herpes viruses are a group of large, enveloped DNA viruses that cause several different types of common skin conditions. The most common of these are herpes simplex types I and II that are traditionally known to cause oral (*herpes simplex labialis*) and genital herpes, respectively, although these associations seem to be weakening as type I is increasingly appearing in the genitals and vice versa. In addition, outbreaks may take place in areas of trauma. Primary infections may present with constitutional symptoms of fever and malaise. Herpes infection causes painful grouped vesicles on an erythematous base, which are self-limiting but frequently recur after a period of latency. On the lips and genitals, these lesions tend to heal without scarring. The morphological findings of herpes viruses are characteristic. The nuclei of infected cells often display a striking "steel-gray" change with nuclear molding. Multinucleated giant cells may be present.

Other variations include *herpetic whitlow*, which often presents on the fingers (classically of dentists), and *herpes gladiatorum* on the trunk or limbs of wrestlers. Trauma is also rarely associated with infection. *Eczema herpeticum* (Kaposi varicelliform eruption) occurs in persons with atopic dermatitis, and can be widespread and life threatening with systemic dissemination. Rarely, herpes infection can result in central nervous system infection, classically associated with temporal lobe involvement. All types of herpes infection can be treated with *acyclovir* to reduce the replication of

CASE 20-10

A 6-year-old man presents with multiple papules, erosions, and vesicles on an erythematous base on his lower and upper lips. These lesions are causing him pain. Clinical image and light microscopy are shown in **Figure 20-42A, B**.

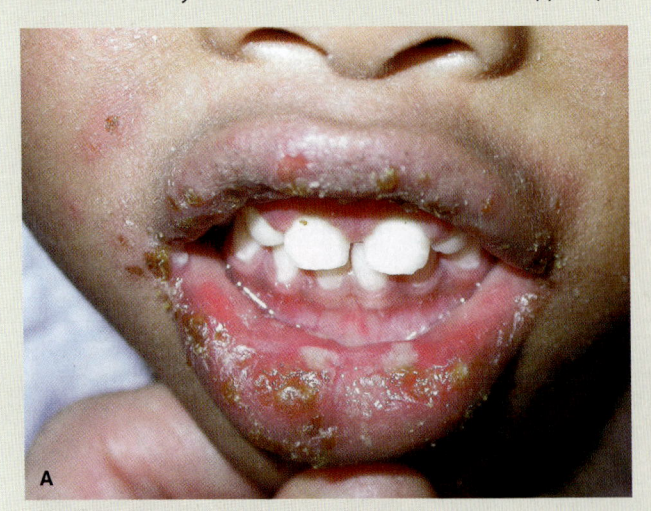

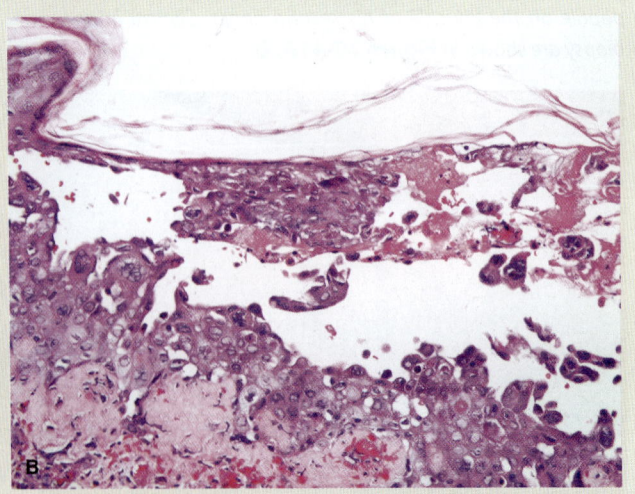

FIGURE 20-42 Herpes simplex. **(A)** Oral herpes simplex labialis. (Image used with permission from Dr. Dean Morrell, UNC Dermatology.) **(B)** Herpes infection often results in blister formation and is characterized by multinucleated giant cells and cells with characteristic viral cytopathic effect.

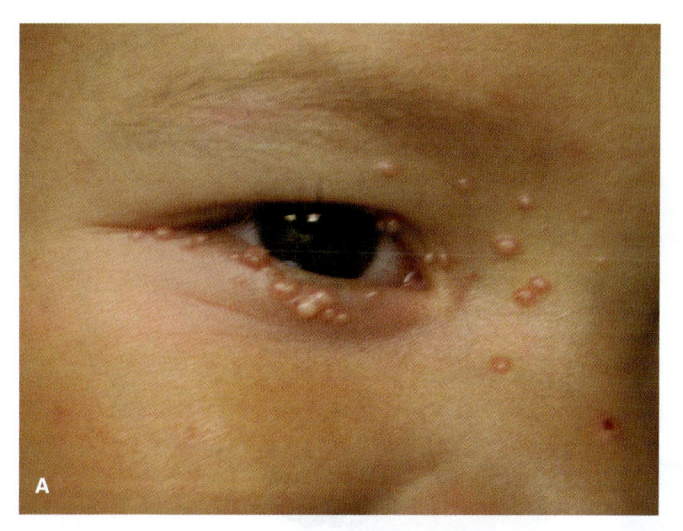

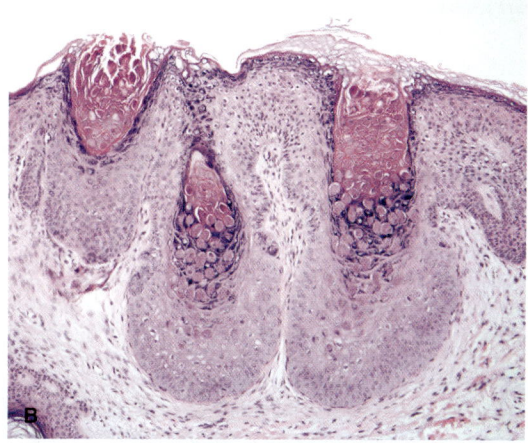

FIGURE 20-43 Molluscum contagiosum. **(A)** Small pearly papules of molluscum contagiosum in a young boy. (Image used with permission from Dr. Dean Morrell, UNC Dermatology.) **(B)** Molluscum contagiosum with molluscum bodies.

the virus, reduce the size of lesions, and minimize morbidity. For patients with frequent recurrences, prophylactic acyclovir (or its longer acting form, *valacyclov*ir) is often indicated (Figure 20-42A, B).

Varicella Zoster Virus/ Shingles/Chicken Pox

Another group of diseases are caused by a different type of herpes virus, known as *varicella zoster virus* (herpes type III). Primary infection with this virus is responsible for the *chicken pox,* which was much more common in children prior to the widespread use of the varicella vaccine. Clinically, this presents as numerous, widespread, individual vesicles on an erythematous base with the appearance of "dew on a rose petal." This is meant to indicate the drop-like appearance of the vesicle and surrounding base of erythema. The virus can then lay dormant in the dorsal nerve roots and reactivate years later, especially in the elderly and immunocompromised, in the form of *herpes zoster* or *shingles*. This is a self-limiting infection that often occurs on the chest or back in a dermatomal distribution or around the eye (*herpes zoster ophthalmicus*) in a trigeminal distribution. This can lead to chronic, severe, and difficult to manage pain and neuropathy known as *postherpetic neuralgia* in some individuals.

Molluscum Contagiosum

Molluscum contagiosum is caused by a poxvirus and is commonly spread in children via direct contact or in adults where it is often a sexually transmitted infection. Lesions of molluscum present as small pearly papules with central umbilication. Histologically, these lesions show characteristic molluscum bodies (*Henderson-Patterson bodies*). Like common warts, these are typically self-limited over the course of months to years, and treatment is indicated to prevent spread and occasional inflammation or pruritus (Figure 20-43A, B).

Arthropod-Associated Lesions (Scabies)

Scabies is a common infection caused by the transmission of the extremely contagious mite, *Sarcoptes scabiei* var. *hominis.* Because transmission is often human-to-human through body contact, this condition is common in school children, but also in people living in close quarters or resident homes. It is associated with low socioeconomic status and overcrowding, but all populations are vulnerable. Transmission may also occur through sexual contact. Patients are symptomatic because of a hypersensitivity reaction that takes place once the mite burrows beneath the skin. Scabetic burrows are commonly seen between the digits, on the flexor surfaces of the elbows and wrists, and on the abdomen (especially along the waistline) and are intensely pruritic. Histologically, it is often possible to see the organism, ova, or feces (scybala) in the stratum corneum (Figure 20-44).

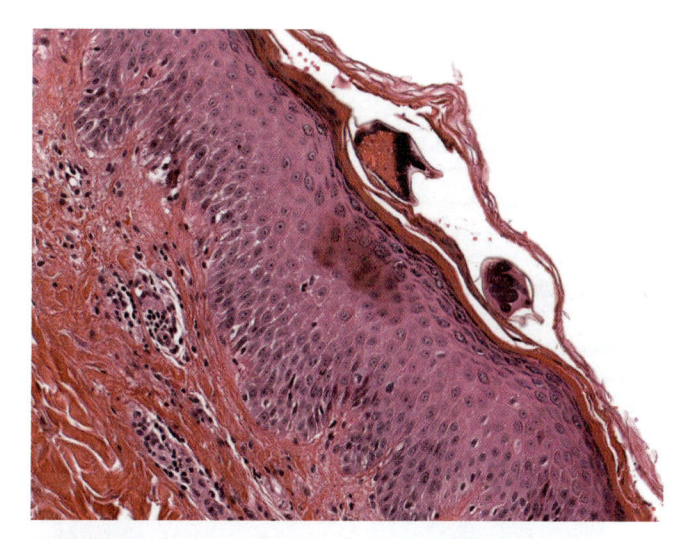

FIGURE 20-44 Scabies. The diagnosis of scabies is often made clinically but can be confirmed through the demonstration of the organism (in the stratum corneum) on microscopy. The curly, eosinophilic chitin in the exoskeleton is prominent.

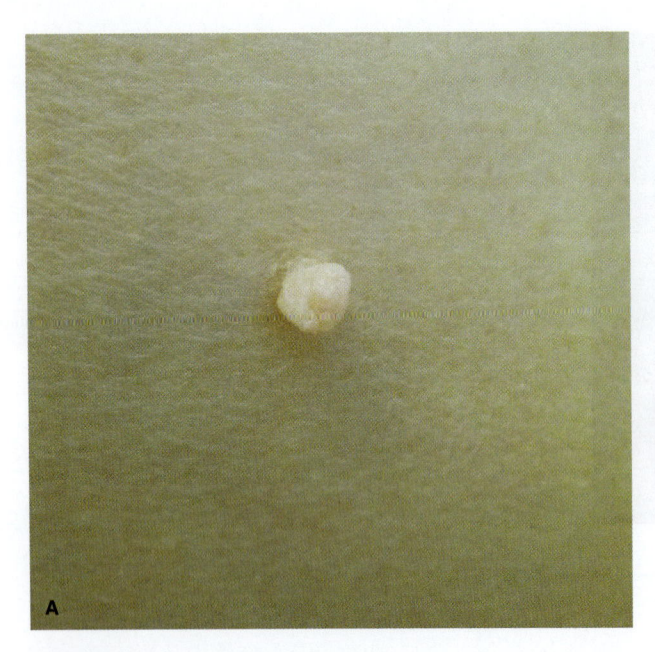

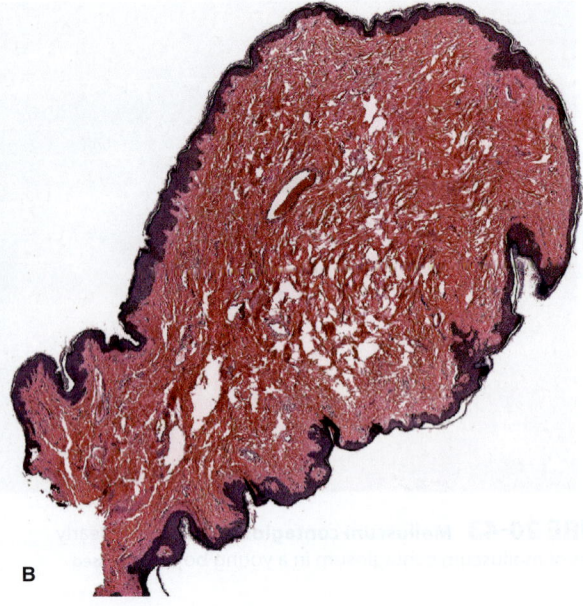

FIGURE 20-45 **Fibroepithelial polyp. (A)** Fibroepithelial polyp. **(B)** Fibroepithelial polyps (skin tags) are common and cytologically bland with characteristic pedunculated architecture.

Fibroepithelial Polyp

A *fibroepithelial polyp* (also known as a *skin tag* or *acrochordon*) is a very common benign lesion that typically occurs in overweight females, but can appear on many middle-aged or older patients. Clinically, they are small, often skin colored, and often pedunculated lesions. They can occur almost anywhere, but commonly occur around the axillae, neck, and groin. Histologically, they are typified by connective tissue surrounded by bland squamous epithelium with a papillated architecture. Acrochordons may be increased in number in patients with *Birt–Hogg–Dube* syndrome, an autosomal dominant inherited syndrome that places patients at risk of certain types of cancers, particularly renal cancer **(Figure 20-45A, B)**.

Secondary (Metastatic) Neoplasms of the Skin

It is important to recognize that not all lesions that have features of malignancy in the skin or subcutis are primary to the skin. While rare, a number of tumors can cause metastasis to the skin. When these occur they tend to occur later in the disease process; however, they can rarely be the initial finding so one must always be vigilant. Among tumors known to metastasize to the skin from distant locations are lung cancer, breast cancer, renal cell carcinoma, gastrointestinal cancers, and melanoma. Special stains can often help clarify ambiguities **(Figure 20-46A, B)**.

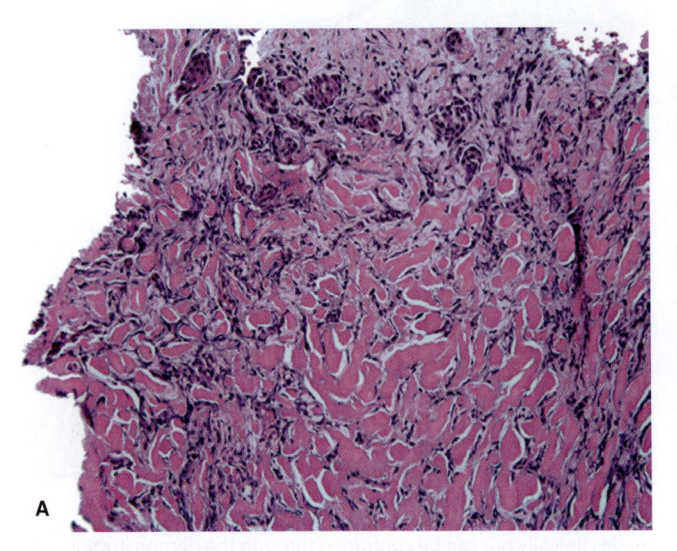

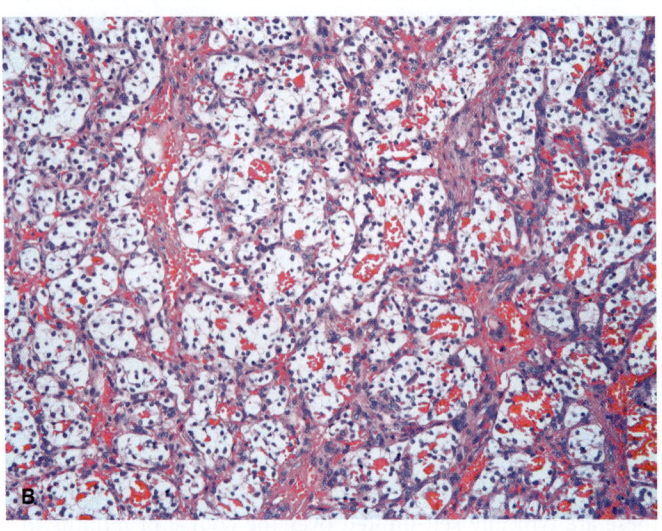

FIGURE 20-46 **Secondary neoplasm. (A)** Metastatic breast cancer has a characteristic infiltrative pattern between collagen bundles. **(B)** The metastatic cells of clear cell renal cell carcinoma have a characteristic clear cell appearance with numerous blood vessels and hemorrhage.

CHAPTER 21

Pathology of the Nervous System

Diane Armao and Thomas Bouldin

INTRODUCTION: THE CENTRAL NERVOUS SYSTEM

The central nervous system (CNS) comprises the brain and spinal cord and is the most complex organ system in the human body. The CNS differs from other organ systems in the variety of functions that it provides and in the localization of these functions to specialized areas of the CNS. The localization of specialized functions means that a relatively small, focal lesion in the CNS can produce a profound deficit, for example, loss of speech. This localization also results in the various populations of neurons within the CNS having unique capabilities and also unique vulnerabilities to disease. For example, Parkinson disease (PD) preferentially affects the neurons of the substantia nigra in the brain stem, while Alzheimer disease (AD) preferentially affects the neurons of the cerebral cortex.

CNS HISTOLOGY AND COMMON CELLULAR RESPONSES TO INJURY

QUICK REVIEW

Neurons (Figure 21-1) are the principal cell type within the nervous system. Acute neuronal injury is most often due to ischemia, but there are many other causes, including trauma, infections, toxic/metabolic diseases, and genetic diseases. Neurons undergoing acute cell death often show red (eosinophilic) cytoplasm and pyknotic nuclei histologically and are referred to as *red neurons* (Figure 21-2). Neurons may also undergo programmed cell death (apoptosis). Central chromatolysis refers to the changes that occur in the neuronal cell body (usually a lower motor neuron) when its axon is injured (axonal reaction). This axonal reaction is characterized by enlargement of the neuronal cell body, displacement of the neuron's nucleus to the periphery of the cell body, and disappearance of the more centrally located Nissl bodies (stacks of rough endoplasmic reticulum). The more peripherally located Nissl bodies remain, hence the term central chromatolysis.

Astrocytes are a type of glial cell that provide numerous support functions for neurons. Astrocytes are somewhat analogous to fibroblasts elsewhere in the body, in that astrocytes react to injury by forming glial filaments (scar tissue). In contrast to the extracellular collagen fibers produced by fibroblasts, glial filaments are intracytoplasmic. The glial filaments immunostain for glial fibrillary acidic protein (GFAP) and highlight the star-shaped astrocytes (Figure 21-3). *Gliosis* (reactive astrocytosis)—the reaction of astrocytes to a brain injury—occurs in many pathologic contexts (e.g., ischemia,

FIGURE 21-1 Neurons in cerebral cortex.

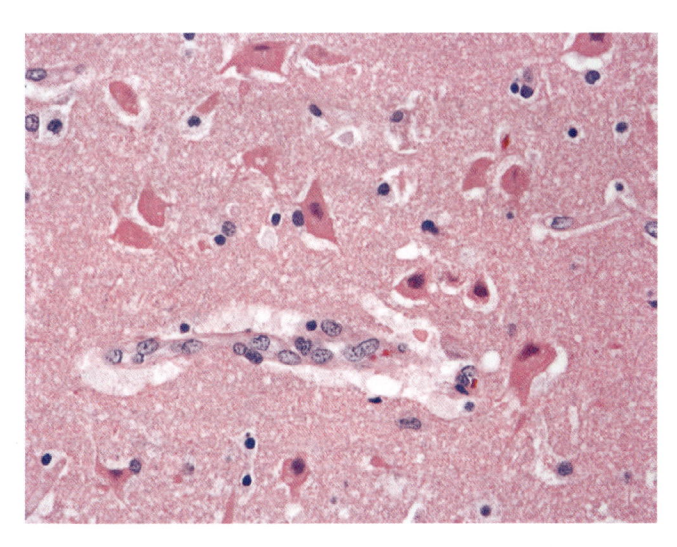

FIGURE 21-2 Red neurons.

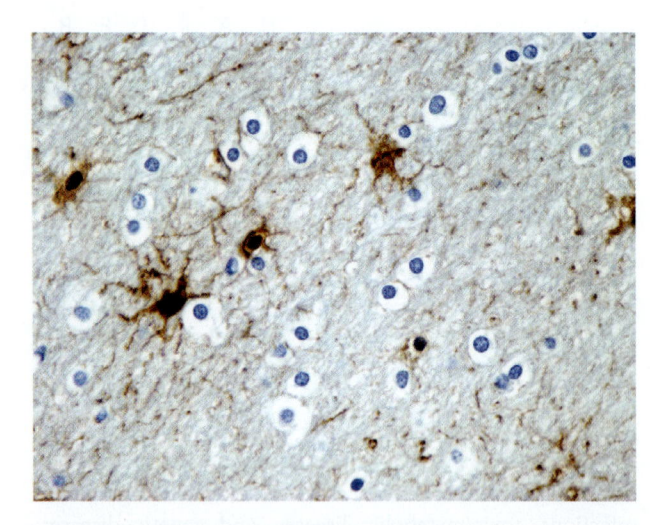

FIGURE 21-3 GFAP-positive (brown-staining) astrocytes and oligodendrocytes with perinuclear halos in cerebral white matter.

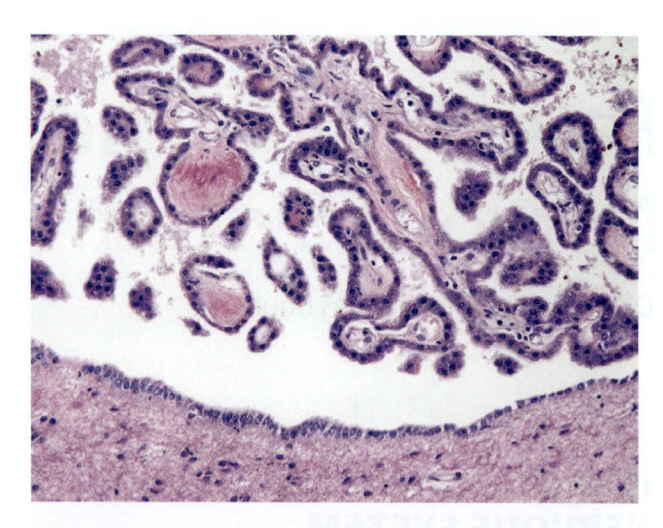

FIGURE 21-5 Choroid plexus epithelium covers the fibrovascular papillae above, and ependymal cells line the ventricular wall below.

trauma, infection, neurodegenerative diseases, demyelinating diseases). Normally, the cytoplasm of an astrocyte is inconspicuous, so that the astrocytic nuclei appear to have no cytoplasm. However, after a brain injury, astrocytes proliferate and develop large amounts of perinuclear cytoplasm as they synthesize glial filaments. These reactive astrocytes are known as hypertrophic or "gemistocytic" astrocytes. After an injury, reactive astrocytosis becomes evident histologically after 4 days, well established after 7–10 days, and maximal at 2–3 weeks. Alzheimer type II glia are astrocytes with enlarged, pale nuclei, and inconspicuous cytoplasm that develop during hyperammonemic states, such as those associated with acute liver failure or a portosystemic shunt secondary to hepatic cirrhosis. This "metabolic astrocytosis" reflects the major role of astrocytes in the detoxification of ammonium ion in the CNS.

Oligodendrocytes (Figure 21-3) are a type of glial cell that myelinate axons in the CNS. Direct injury of the myelin sheath or its oligodendrocyte may result in breakdown of the myelin sheath. If the myelin breakdown is associated with preservation of the underlying axon, the process is referred to as *demyelination*. Degeneration of the underlying axon always leads to breakdown of the axon's myelin sheath.

Ependymal cells are a type of glial cell that line the ventricles of the brain (Figure 21-4) and the central canal of the spinal cord. Unlike astrocytes, ependymal cells do not proliferate in response to a brain injury.

The epithelial cells of the *choroid plexus* closely resemble ependymal cells and cover the fibrovascular papillae of the choroid plexus (Figure 21-5). Choroid-plexus tissue is found in the lateral, third, and fourth ventricles and produces the cerebrospinal fluid (CSF).

Microglia (Figure 21-6) are phagocytic cells and function as the macrophages of the CNS. The brain contains several different macrophage/monocyte populations, including resident brain macrophages (microglia) and perivascular macrophages. All of these macrophage/monocyte cells are

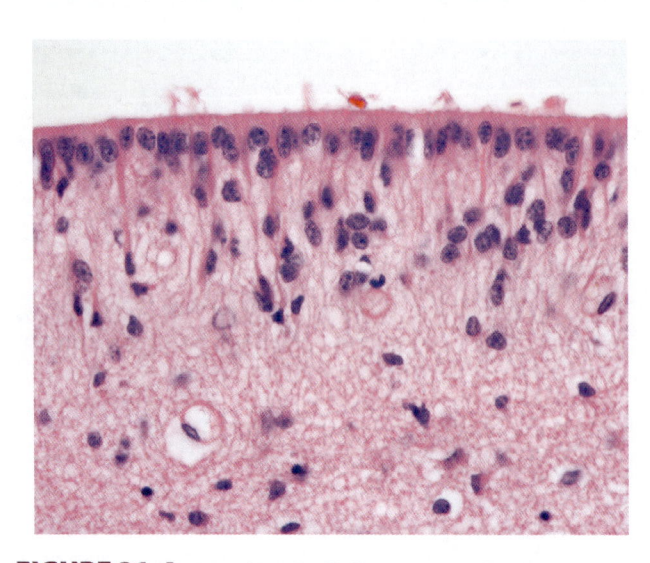

FIGURE 21-4 Ependymal cells lining ventricle of brain.

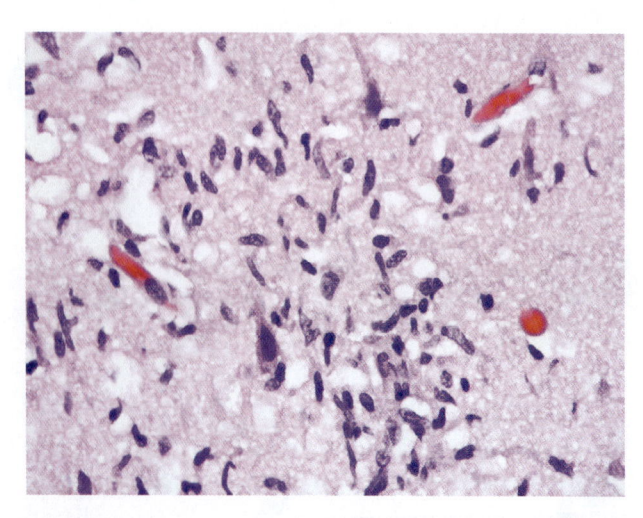

FIGURE 21-6 Cluster of microglial cells (microglial nodule) in brain.

of bone marrow origin and have roles in phagocytosis of debris and in immune surveillance. The resident microglia handle the cleanup of minor debris, but the cleanup of larger amounts of necrotic debris requires the recruitment of blood-borne monocytes/macrophages to the area. Activated macrophages within the brain typically have spindle-shaped nuclei (rod cells). As the macrophages ingest debris, they become the lipid-filled macrophages (foam cells) often found around areas of brain necrosis. Small clusters of microglial cells within the brain parenchyma (*microglial nodules*) are a distinctive, but not pathognomonic, feature of viral and rickettsial encephalitis. The multinucleated giant cells that characterize HIV-associated encephalitis are also of macrophage origin.

Common Responses of the Brain to Injury

Increased Intracranial Pressure

Intracranial pressure (ICP) is the pressure inside the cranium and is normally 1–15 mmHg. The skull serves as a rigid vault enclosing a fixed volume of brain, blood, and CSF. Any increase in volume of one component means that one or both of the other components must be reduced in volume (Monro–Kellie hypothesis). Cerebral perfusion pressure (CPP) is the mean arterial pressure minus the mean ICP. Thus, as the ICP increases, the CPP decreases. There are multiple causes of increased ICP (Table 21-1), with *mass lesions* being the most common cause. Increased ICP is evidenced clinically by headache, nausea, vomiting, and papilledema (swelling of the optic disc). The elevated ICP also causes enlargement of the head and a tense or bulging anterior fontanel in young children in whom the cranial sutures have not yet fused.

Major complications of a mass lesion and raised ICP are brain ischemia and brain herniation (Figure 21-7). Brain ischemia occurs when the raised ICP approaches systemic arterial blood pressure, thereby causing decreased cerebral perfusion and brain ischemia. Brain herniation occurs when there is a displacement or shift of brain tissue from one intracranial compartment to another. The major forms of brain herniation are subfalcine, transtentorial, and tonsillar. A *subfalcine herniation* (Figure 21-8) occurs when the cingulate gyrus herniates horizontally under the falx cerebri. *Transtentorial (uncal, central diencephalic) herniation* (Figure 21-9) occurs

TABLE 21-1 Common causes of increased intracranial pressure.

- Mass lesion (intracranial hematoma, neoplasm, abscess, etc.)
- Hydrocephalus
- Diffuse brain edema from global brain ischemia, traumatic brain injury, acute encephalitis, bacterial leptomeningitis, and other causes
- Obstruction of a major dural venous sinus
- Idiopathic intracranial hypertension (pseudotumor cerebri)

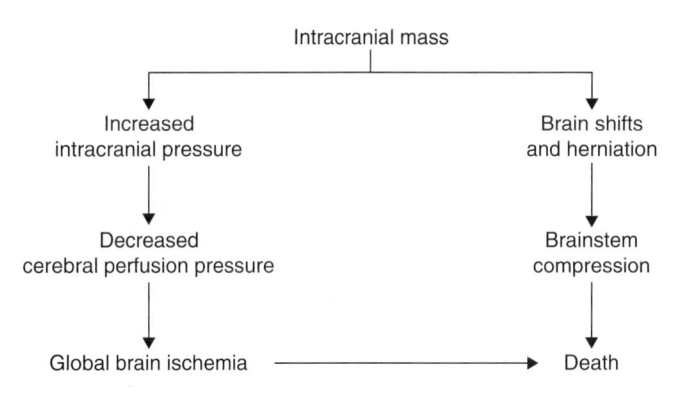

FIGURE 21-7 Complications of increased intracranial pressure.

when the medial aspect (uncus) of one temporal lobe or the lower diencephalon herniates downward through the tentorial incisura. The herniating uncus compresses the ipsilateral third cranial nerve and midbrain, leading to dilatation of the ipsilateral pupil, contralateral hemiparesis, impairment of upper brain stem functions, and midbrain hemorrhages. *Tonsillar herniation* (Figure 21-10) occurs when the cerebellar tonsils herniate downward through the foramen magnum because of a mass in the posterior fossa. The herniating tonsils compress the medulla, causing apnea and death.

Brain Edema

The term edema refers to an abnormal accumulation of fluid in tissue spaces. Brain edema accompanies many disease processes. The edema causes brain swelling and magnifies any mass effect caused by the underlying pathologic process. Brain edema thus contributes to an increase in the ICP and to the

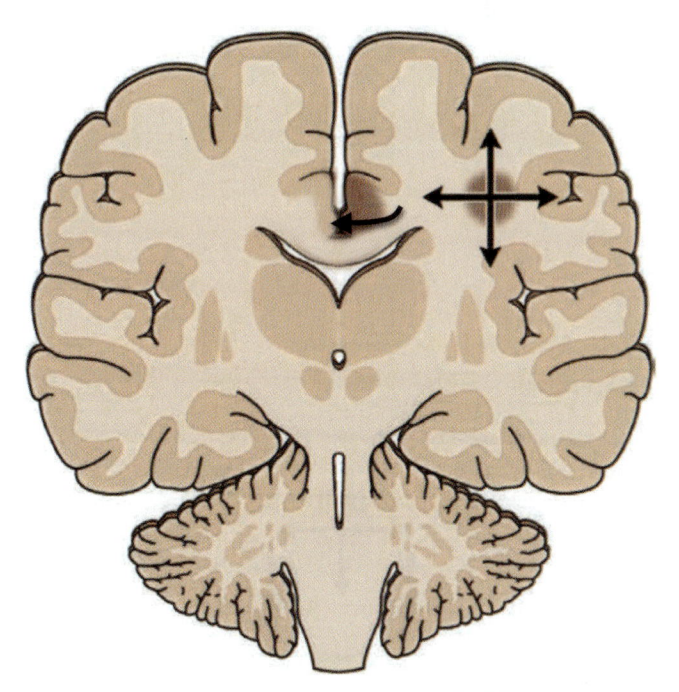

FIGURE 21-8 Subfalcian herniation associated with hemispheric mass lesion and lateral brain shift.

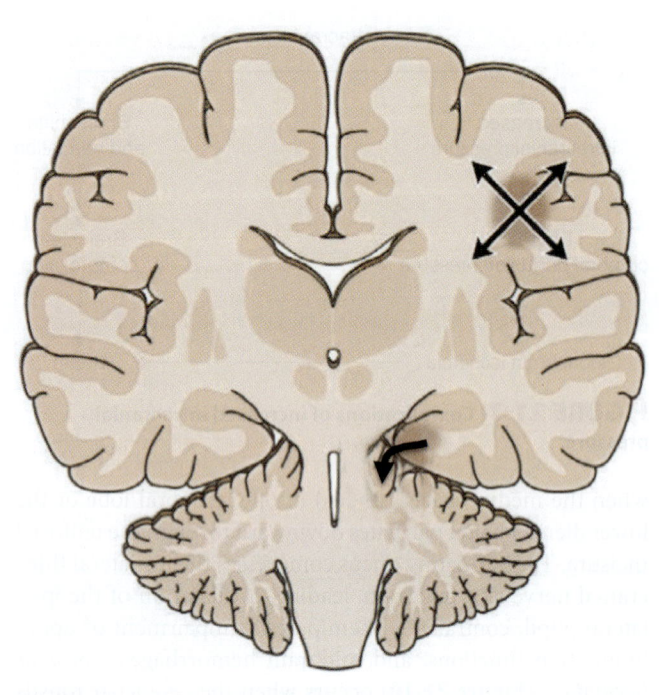

FIGURE 21-9 Uncal herniation associated with hemispheric mass lesion and downward transtentorial brain shift.

possibility of a brain herniation. Brain edema is classified as vasogenic, cytotoxic, or interstitial.

Vasogenic brain edema—extracellular edema due to increased permeability of the blood–brain barrier (BBB). The BBB is an anatomical and physiologic barrier that helps maintain a controlled extracellular environment around the neurons and glial cells of the CNS. The barrier is located at the level of the brain capillaries and regulates the movement of molecules into the extracellular space of the brain. The BBB helps prevent the entry of blood-borne infectious agents and toxins into the brain but also may impede the delivery of antibiotics and chemotherapeutic agents to the CNS. Many disease processes are associated with breakdown of the BBB. The increased capillary permeability leads to greater passage of osmotic particles into the brain's extracellular space and results in an extracellular accumulation of water (vasogenic brain edema). Vasogenic edema is found primarily in the white matter. The integrity of the BBB is a useful marker of disease and can be assessed radiologically by administering an intravenous contrast agent prior to the radiologic study. When the BBB has been compromised by a pathologic process, the contrast agent will leak out of the brain capillaries into surrounding brain tissue and can be seen in the radiologic images.

Cytotoxic (cellular) brain edema—intracellular edema (hydropic cellular swelling) due to an osmotic imbalance between the cell and the extracellular fluid. There is no expansion of the extracellular space. The cell may swell because of loss of control of ion movements across its cell membrane (e.g., with cerebral ischemia, the cell does not have sufficient energy for its ion pumps) or because of an increased imbalance between intracellular and extracellular osmolarity (e.g., acute water intoxication). Cellular edema is found primarily in the gray matter and is most commonly associated with acute ischemic brain injury. Radiographically, cytotoxic edema is not associated with a positive contrast study, since there is no breakdown of the BBB.

Interstitial (hydrocephalic) brain edema—extracellular edema arising from the transependymal flow of CSF. The transependymal movement of CSF is due to increased CSF pressure, which is caused by an obstruction of CSF pathways. The obstruction of normal CSF flow also causes ventricular dilatation (hydrocephalus). The transependymal edema is in the periventricular white matter surrounding the dilated ventricles and can be seen radiologically.

Combined forms of brain edema are common. For example, the brain edema associated with ischemia is a combination of cytotoxic edema and vasogenic edema. The cytotoxic edema develops almost immediately after the onset of the brain ischemia, while the vasogenic edema develops hours to days later.

Hydrocephalus

Hydrocephalus literally means increased water (CSF) in the head. Hydrocephalus is traditionally defined as enlarged ventricles (*ventriculomegaly*) due to the obstruction of the bulk flow of CSF (**Figure 21-11**). Normally, the total volume of CSF is around 150 mL, of which about 25 mL are within ventricular system and the remainder in the craniospinal subarachnoid space. Approximately 500 mL of CSF are produced each day. The CSF has multiple functions, including providing buoyancy for the brain, maintaining a highly regulated extracellular fluid compartment for the cells of the brain and spinal cord, and providing a buffer so that changes in the volume of

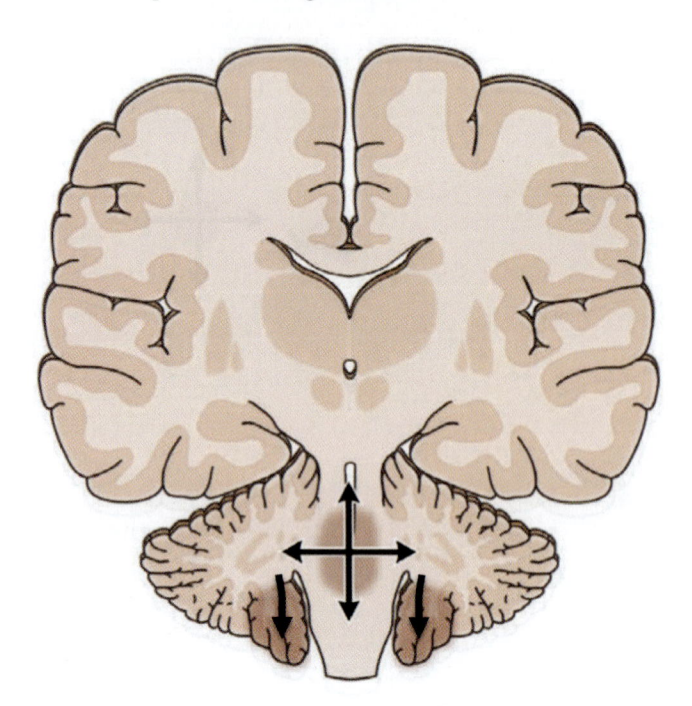

FIGURE 21-10 Tonsillar herniation associated with infratentorial mass lesion.

PATHOLOGY OF THE NERVOUS SYSTEM 571

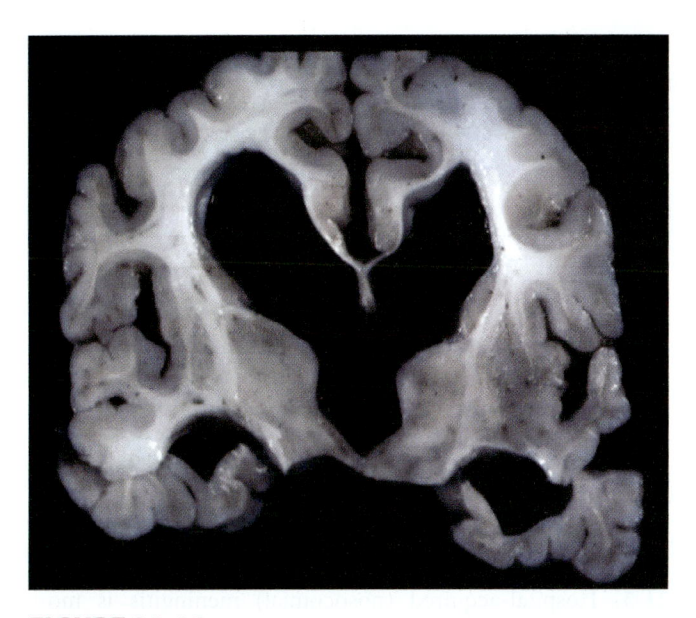

FIGURE 21-11 Hydrocephalus with striking enlargement of lateral and third ventricles and atrophy of cerebral white matter.

the other intracranial components (i.e., brain and blood) can occur within the intracranial cavity.

Hydrocephalus may be classified as *noncommunicating hydrocephalus* if the obstruction of CSF flow is within the ventricular system (e.g., stenosis of the cerebral aqueduct between the third and fourth ventricles) or as *communicating hydrocephalus* if the obstruction is within the subarachnoid space or arachnoid villi (e.g., complication of subarachnoid hemorrhage, SAH). Hydrocephalus may be acute or chronic in onset and may be present at birth (congenital hydrocephalus) or acquired later in life.

Obstruction of CSF flow in adults leads to hydrocephalus and clinically to signs and symptoms of increased ICP—headache, nausea, vomiting, and papilledema. In young children, who have an expandable cranium because their sutures have not yet fused, the obstruction of CSF flow leads to hydrocephalus and a progressively increasing head circumference. In both adults and children, the ventricles enlarge at the expense of the periventricular white matter, so that hydrocephalus can produce considerable neurologic deficits over time.

CASE PRESENTATION: Mass Lesion

A 40-year-old woman with a history of HTN presents to the local ED with symptoms of nausea, vomiting, vertigo, weakness in the legs and a headache localized to the "back of her head" progressing over the past 24 hrs. An MRI was performed (left panel) (**Figure 21-12**).

MRI discloses an acute left-sided cerebellar infarct with tonsillar herniation, obstructive hydrocephalus, and cerebral edema. (Right panel) Medical illustration, worth 1000 words.

In this case, an emergency resection of involved cerebellum with placement of a shunt was a life-saving measure.

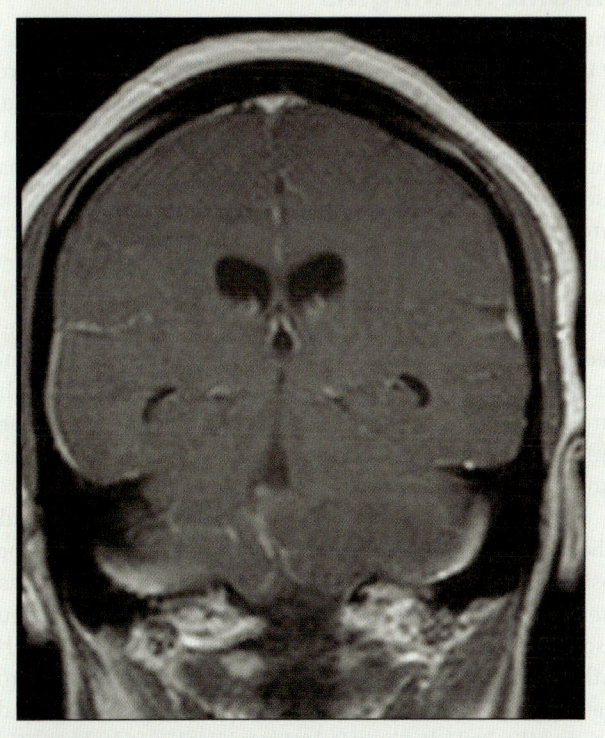

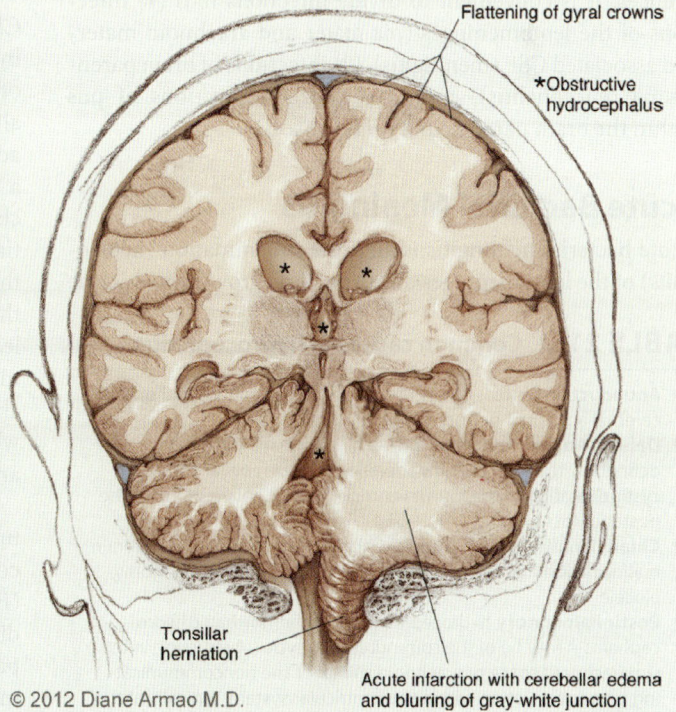

FIGURE 21-12 Mass lesion. (Copyright 2012, Diane Armao, MD, Departments of Radiology and Pathology and Laboratory Medicine, University of North Carolina, Chapel Hill, NC.)

> **HUNTING FOR ZEBRAS**
>
> Curiously, ventriculomegaly develops in some adults who have no obvious increase in CSF pressure and no demonstrable obstruction of CSF flow. These patients are thought to have a chronic communicating hydrocephalus due to periodic increases in the ICP. This syndrome, termed *normal pressure hydrocephalus* (NPH), is evidenced clinically by the triad of dementia, gait ataxia, and urinary incontinence. Placement of a CSF shunt may be beneficial in patients with NPH.

Ventricular enlargement may also be a consequence of brain atrophy. Ventriculomegaly secondary to brain atrophy (*hydrocephalus ex vacuo*) is not related to a blockage of CSF flow, is not associated with increased ICP, and does not benefit from placement of a CSF shunt.

There are many causes of hydrocephalus (Table 21-2). In infants and young children, hydrocephalus is often due to a congenital malformation, such as a congenitally malformed cerebral aqueduct. Inflammation, hemorrhage, or neoplasm within the ventricular system or subarachnoid space may cause obstruction of CSF flow and hydrocephalus in both children and adults.

INFECTIONS

The nervous system is susceptible to many infectious agents, including bacteria, viruses, fungi, amebae, and parasites. CNS infections are oftentimes life threatening with serious consequences. It is convenient to divide infections into (1) infections of the leptomeninges (pia mater and arachnoid mater) and associated CSF (meningitis), (2) infections of brain parenchyma (encephalitis), and (3) localized collections of pus within the brain parenchyma (brain abscess).

Acute Bacterial Meningitis

Acute bacterial meningitis is an acute inflammation (neutrophils) of the leptomeninges due to bacteria growing within the

TABLE 21-2 Common causes of hydrocephalus.

- **Aqueductal stenosis**—may result from a congenitally malformed cerebral aqueduct or from an acquired stenosis
- **Dandy–Walker malformation**—a hindbrain malformation defined by the triad of (1) hypoplasia of the cerebellar vermis, (2) cystic dilatation of the fourth ventricle, and (3) enlargement of the posterior fossa
- **Chiari II malformation** (Arnold-Chiari malformation)—a hindbrain malformation that is closely associated with lumbar meningomyelocele
- **Postinflammatory** hydrocephalus or posthemorrhagic hydrocephalus—may be of the communicating type (obstruction in the subarachnoid space or arachnoid villi) or of the noncommunicating type (obstruction within the ventricular system, typically at the cerebral aqueduct)
- **Tumors**—may obstruct flow of CSF within ventricular system or within the subarachnoid space

TABLE 21-3 Usual causes of acute bacterial meningitis.

- Neonate—Group B streptococcus, *Listeria monocytogenes*, and enteric bacilli
- Child—*Streptococcus pneumoniae* and *Neisseria meningitidis*
- Adult—*Streptococcus pneumoniae* and *Neisseria meningitidis*

CSF. Clinical features of headache, fever, stiff neck, and altered mental status have their onset over hours to days. The bacteria often reach the CSF through the bloodstream. Sometimes, the bacterial infection spreads to the meninges from a parameningeal infection in the sinuses or skull. Head trauma, especially penetrating injuries, and neurosurgical procedures, such as a ventriculoperitoneal shunt, are also potential causes of infection. Age is an important factor in determining the type of bacterial infection in community-acquired meningitis (Table 21-3). Hospital-acquired (nosocomial) meningitis is most often due to gram-negative rods. Clinicopathologic correlates of acute bacterial meningitis include stiff neck and headache from meningeal inflammation and mental status changes and seizures from toxins in the pus within the CSF. These toxins are also responsible for brain edema and its associated mass effect. The acute inflammatory process may involve blood vessels and cranial nerves in the subarachnoid space, resulting in brain infarcts and cranial nerve palsies. The pus or postinflammatory meningeal fibrosis may also obstruct CSF flow and lead to a communicating hydrocephalus.

Chronic Meningitis

Chronic meningitis may complicate infections characterized by chronic or granulomatous inflammation. Clinical features of chronic meningitis include headache, fever, stiff neck, and altered mental status. Although purulent meningitis has an acute (hours to days) clinical course, chronic meningitis has a subacute (weeks) to chronic (months) clinical course. The chronic or granulomatous inflammatory infiltrates preferentially involve the leptomeninges at the base of the brain and the associated structures (blood vessels and cranial nerves) in the basal subarachnoid space. Inflammation of blood vessels leads to thrombosis and consequent brain infarcts; inflammation of cranial nerves leads to cranial nerve palsies. The chronic inflammatory process also causes meningeal fibrosis, which may obstruct CSF flow within the subarachnoid space and produce a communicating hydrocephalus.

Diseases associated with chronic meningitis include tuberculosis, syphilis, some fungal infections (e.g., cryptococcosis, coccidioidomycosis, blastomycosis), and Lyme disease (*Borrelia burgdorferi*). Sarcoidosis, while not an infectious disease, also causes chronic granulomatous meningitis. The pathogenesis of CNS tuberculosis is illustrated diagrammatically in **Figure 21-13**. CNS complications of longstanding syphilis include chronic leptomeningitis and obliterative arteritis (meningovascular syphilis), chronic encephalitis with neuronal loss (paretic dementia), and chronic inflammation of

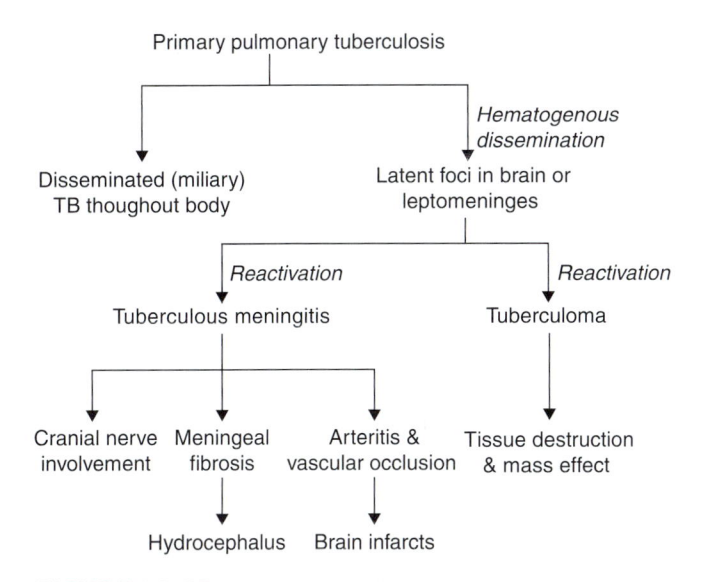

FIGURE 21-13 Pathogenesis of CNS tuberculosis.

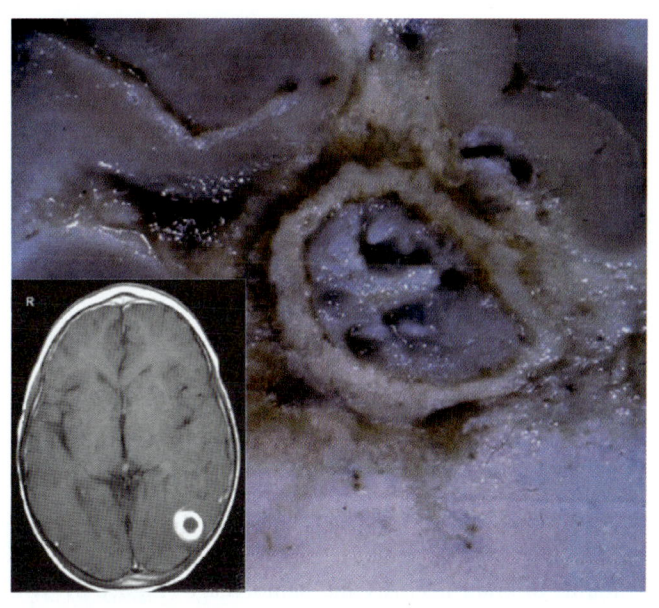

FIGURE 21-14 Bacterial brain abscess. A pus-filled abscess cavity is surrounded by a thick, vascularized, fibrous capsule at the junction of cortex and white matter. The thick fibrovascular capsule brightly enhances in the brain MRI (inset).

the dorsal roots and ganglia with loss of dorsal-root ganglion cells and degeneration of the posterior columns of the spinal cord (tabes dorsalis).

Brain Abscess

A brain abscess is a localized collection of pus within the brain parenchyma (Figure 21-14). The pus is walled off from the surrounding brain tissue by a layer of highly vascularized fibrous tissue (granulation tissue). The surrounding brain is edematous and has a reactive gliosis. As the abscess enlarges, it usually tracks centripetally through the white matter toward the ventricular system. This centripetal spread is thought to be due to the white matter having relatively less vascularity than the gray matter.

The pathogenesis of a brain abscess often involves bacteremia from a distant focus of infection. Bacteremia-associated brain abscesses are frequently multiple and often begin at the junction between cortex and white matter. Direct extension of a parameningeal infection (e.g., sinusitis, mastoiditis) is another cause of brain abscess. Penetrating head trauma is a potential, but uncommon, cause of brain abscess. Brain abscesses often contain a mix of aerobic and anaerobic bacteria; less commonly, fungi are responsible.

A brain abscess causes tissue destruction, with resultant neurologic defects, and mass effect, with increased ICP and risk of herniation. An abscess may rupture into the ventricular system, causing ventriculitis and usually leading to death.

Viral Meningitis

Viral infections of the CNS may cause a meningitis or encephalitis (Figure 21-15). If the virus selectively infects cells of the leptomeninges, the inflamed meninges (meningitis) are

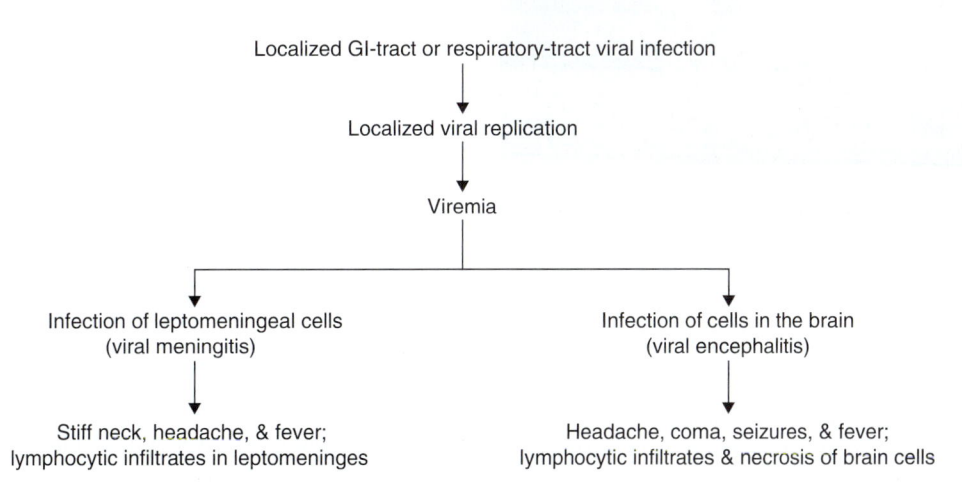

FIGURE 21-15 Pathogenesis of viral meningitis and viral encephalitis.

associated with headache and a stiff neck. Viral meningitis is characterized histologically by lymphocytic infiltrates in the leptomeninges. Enteroviruses are the most common cause of viral meningitis. Other common causes include arboviruses, HIV, HSV-2, mumps virus, and lymphocytic choriomeningitis virus. The infectious agent is often not cultured in cases of lymphocytic meningitis, so that the disease is sometimes referred to as an "aseptic" meningitis. Viral meningitis is usually a benign, self-limited disease.

Viral Encephalitis

In viral encephalitis, the virus selectively infects cells of the brain (Figure 21-15). The inflamed brain (encephalitis) is associated with an altered mental state, neurologic dysfunction, and often seizures. Viral encephalitis is characterized histologically by microglial nodules and perivascular lymphocytic infiltrates within the brain tissue and variable amounts of brain necrosis and hemorrhage (Figure 21-16).

TABLE 21-4 Viral tropism in CNS infections.

- HSV-1—encephalitis preferentially involving temporal and inferior frontal lobes
- Poliovirus—anterior horn cells (poliomyelitis)
- JC virus—oligodendrocytes (progressive multifocal leukoencephalopathy)
- Rabies virus—hippocampus and cerebellum
- Varicella–Zoster virus—dorsal root ganglia
- Lymphocytic choriomeningitis virus—leptomeninges

Common causes of viral encephalitis include HSV-1, Varicella–Zoster virus, arboviruses (e.g., Eastern & Western equine encephalitis), enteroviruses (including poliovirus), measles virus, and mumps virus. Some viruses are associated with intranuclear [e.g., HSV-1, progressive multifocal leukoencephalopathy (PML), CMV] or intracytoplasmic (e.g., CMV, rabies) viral inclusions. Some viruses typically show a characteristic involvement of certain cell types or areas of the CNS (Table 21-4).

The pathogenesis of viral encephalitis involves viral entry into the CNS via two main routes—bloodstream or axons. Many viruses use a viremia to gain access to the CNS. These hematogenously disseminated viral infections, which include the enteroviruses and arboviruses, first proliferate locally in the respiratory tract, GI tract, or skin, then disseminate hematogenously (viremia) to the CNS.

Rabies virus and herpesviruses gain entry to the CNS via axons. In the case of rabies virus, the virus first proliferates locally in the region of the wound (bite), and then travels centripetally along peripheral nerves via retrograde axonal transport to the spinal cord and brain.

HIV encephalitis is the result of direct infection of the CNS by HIV, causing a subacute encephalitis with multinucleated giant cells. The subacute encephalitis is characterized by perivascular chronic inflammation, foci of reactive gliosis, and scattered microglial nodules. Also present and virtually pathognomonic are multinucleated giant cells, which are derived from macrophages and contain HIV antigens. There may also be areas of pallor and gliosis of the cerebral white matter (HIV leukoencephalopathy). In infants and children, HIV encephalitis may also be accompanied by calcification of small cerebral blood vessels.

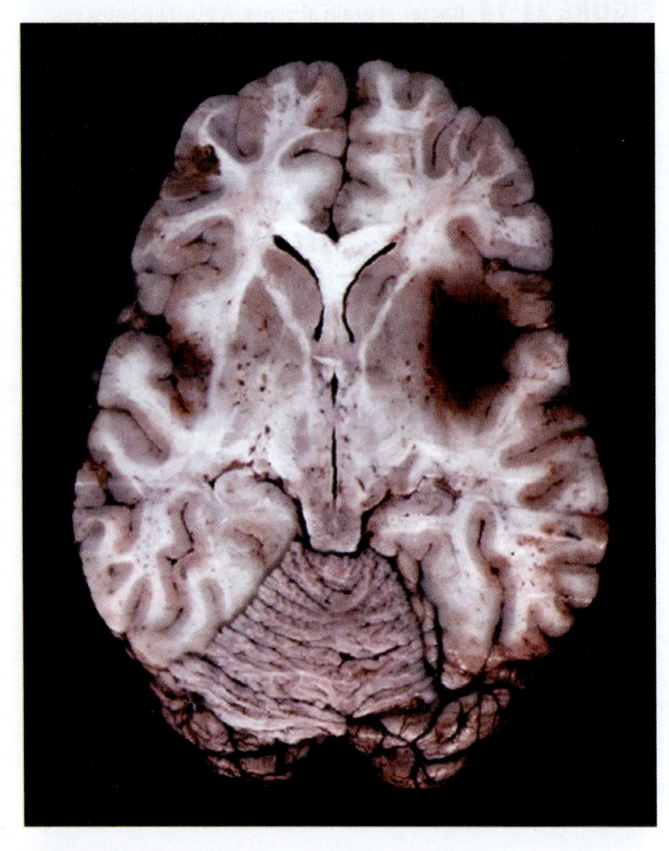

FIGURE 21-16 **HSV-1 encephalitis is the most commonly occurring sporadic viral encephalitis.** This young adult presented with confusion and later developed seizures and coma and died. The horizontally cut postmortem brain specimen shows the characteristic predilection of HSV-1 for the temporal lobe. Note that HSV-1 encephalitis is very destructive, causing necrosis and hemorrhage in the brain. Microscopically, the brain necrosis is accompanied by perivascular lymphocytic infiltrates, microglial nodules, and intranuclear viral inclusions. Viral leptomeningitis, in contrast, does not show inflammation and necrosis of brain tissue and has a benign clinical course.

Fungal Infections of the CNS

Fungal infections account for an increasing proportion of CNS infections due to the widespread use of immunosuppressive therapy, the increase in the relative numbers of aging individuals, and AIDS. Common clinical presentations are a chronic granulomatous meningitis, brain abscess, or fungal arteritis with brain infarcts. Cryptococcosis, blastomycosis, coccidioidomycosis, and histoplasmosis most often present as a chronic meningitis. Aspergillosis often presents as a fungal arteritis with brain infarcts.

Parasitic Infections of the CNS

HUNTING FOR ZEBRAS

The CNS may be involved in a variety of parasitic diseases, including cysticercosis, toxoplasmosis, and amebiasis. Cysticercosis is becoming an increasingly important cause of seizures in adults in the United States. The pig tapeworm (*Taenia solium*) is found in humans, the definitive host. As humans shed tapeworm eggs, pigs may become infected (intermediate host) due to their eating food contaminated with human feces. The ingested eggs become larvae in the pig GI tract and then spread hematogenously to muscles and other tissues, where they become encysted. When humans eat undercooked pork, the encysted larvae get into to the human GI tract and evolve into tapeworms, completing the lifecycle. If humans become infected by other humans (fecal–oral transmission), the newly infected human becomes the intermediate host and develops the encysted forms (cysticercosis). Diagnostic studies may reveal one to many parasitic cysts in the brain, spinal cord, leptomeninges, or ventricles in neurocysticercosis.

CASE PRESENTATION: Acute Bacterial Leptomeningitis

A 54-year-old man had a 3-day history of fever, severe headache, rigors, and cough. At a drugstore health clinic, 2 days prior, he was advised to rest, drink fluids, and take acetaminophen. However, his symptoms worsened and he was found unresponsive in bed. Emergency medical services efforts were unsuccessful and he died. Postmortem findings in the leptomeninges are shown in **Figure 21-17**.

The white dura mater (top of figure) is reflected back to reveal a gray exudate (pus) tracking along blood vessels and lying on the brain surface beneath the shiny leptomeninges. The patient died from acute bacterial leptomeningitis.

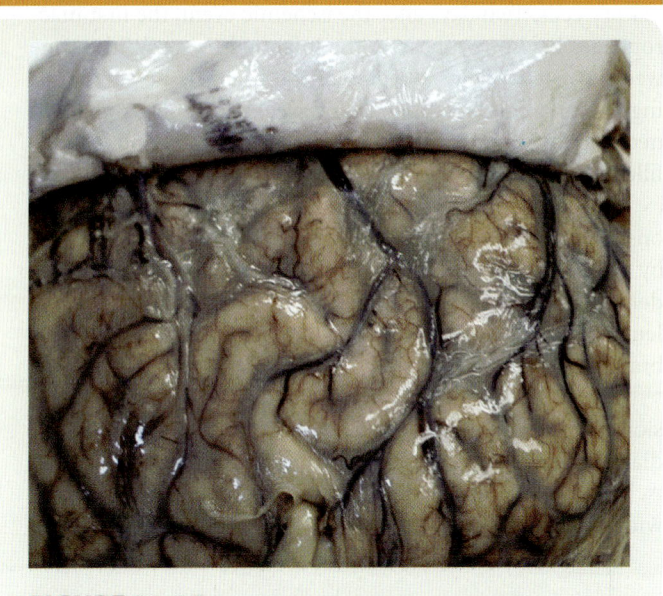

FIGURE 21-17 Acute bacterial leptomeningitis.

CEREBROVASCULAR DISEASE

Cerebrovascular disease is a leading cause of morbidity and the fourth leading cause of mortality in the United States. Stroke is a clinical term describing a neurologic deficit that is sudden in onset and lasts for more than 24 hours. The pathologic process causing a stroke is an infarct in the brain or a hemorrhage in the brain or subarachnoid space.

Brain Infarct (Ischemic Stroke)

A brain infarct is an area of coagulative necrosis caused by a decrease or cessation of blood flow to the area (ischemic stroke). Brain infarcts are responsible for 85% of strokes. Occlusion of an artery by a thrombus (thrombotic stroke) or embolus (embolic stroke) causes a localized area of brain ischemia and is the most common cause of a brain infarct (**Figure 21-18; Table 21-5**).

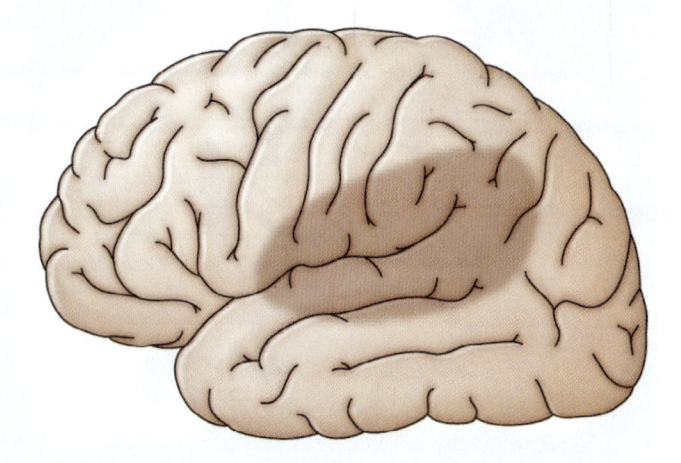

FIGURE 21-18 Cortical infarct due to occlusion of a large artery. Such infarcts are usually due to atherothrombosis or an embolus in a major artery.

TABLE 21-5 Causes of arterial occlusion and brain ischemia.

- Atherosclerosis
- Thrombosis (atherothrombosis, hypercoagulable states)
- Embolism (cardiogenic, artery-to-artery, air, fat, neoplastic cells, foreign material)
- Arteritis (systemic arteritis or primary angiitis of CNS)
- Arterial dissection
- Fibromuscular dysplasia
- Moyamoya disease
- CADASIL (cerebral autosomal dominant arteriopathy with subcortical infarcts & leukoencephalopathy)

There is a consistent pattern to the gross and microscopic changes in an infarct. One day after the ischemic event, the infarcted brain is discolored and swollen and microscopic examination reveals red neurons and an influx of acute inflammatory cells. Two days after the ischemic event, the first macrophages begin to appear in the infarcted tissue. Within one week, a reactive gliosis begins in the brain tissue surrounding the infarct. Over the ensuing weeks to months, the soft necrotic debris in the infarct is slowly resorbed and a fluid-filled cavity develops (Figure 21-19).

The local destruction of brain tissue may lead to the abrupt onset of a neurologic deficit. The type of deficit is determined by the location of the infarct. Multiple brain infarcts may cause dementia (*multi-infarct dementia*). The acute infarct is swollen, due to cytotoxic and vasogenic edema, and may cause brain herniation.

In contrast to local brain ischemia, which is due to occlusion of an artery or vein, global brain ischemia is due to a cardiac arrest or severe systemic hypotension. The global brain ischemia associated with cardiac arrest may result in very widespread injury to the brain (*global ischemic encephalopathy*)

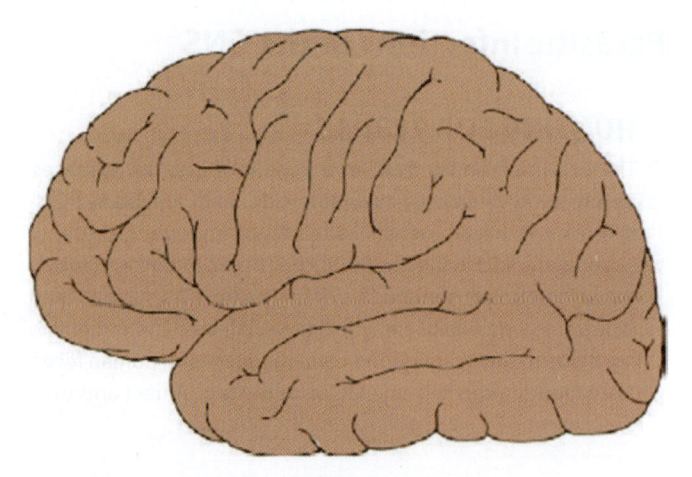

FIGURE 21-20 Global ischemic injury (global ischemic encephalopathy) due to prolonged cardiac arrest or severe hypotension.

(Figure 21-20). The brain injury associated with systemic hypotension is typically concentrated in the border zones (watershed areas) between vascular distributions (*watershed infarcts*) (Figure 21-21).

Brain Hemorrhage

Brain hemorrhage (intracerebral hemorrhage, hemorrhagic stroke) accounts for 10% of strokes. There are multiple causes of spontaneous (nontraumatic) intracerebral hemorrhage (Table 21-6). Chronic hypertension (hypertensive intracerebral hemorrhage) is the most common cause, accounting for about 50% of cases.

The usual sites for brain hemorrhage are the basal ganglia, thalamus, cerebral (lobar) white matter, pons, and cerebellum

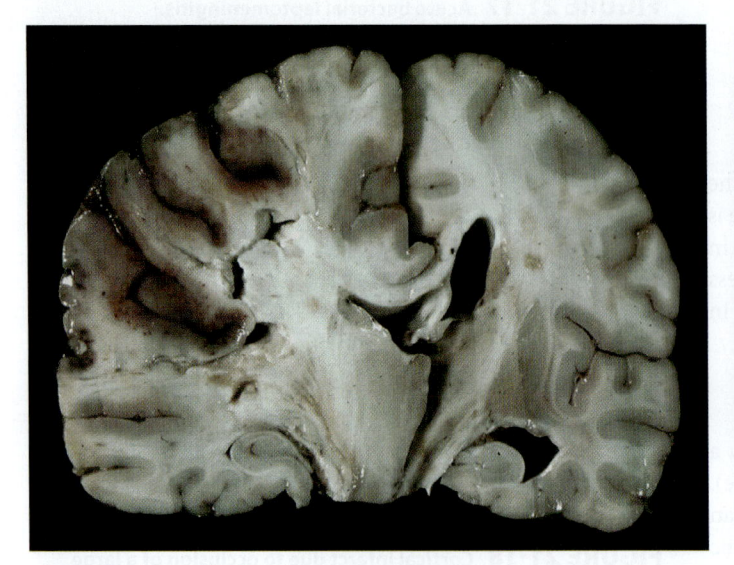

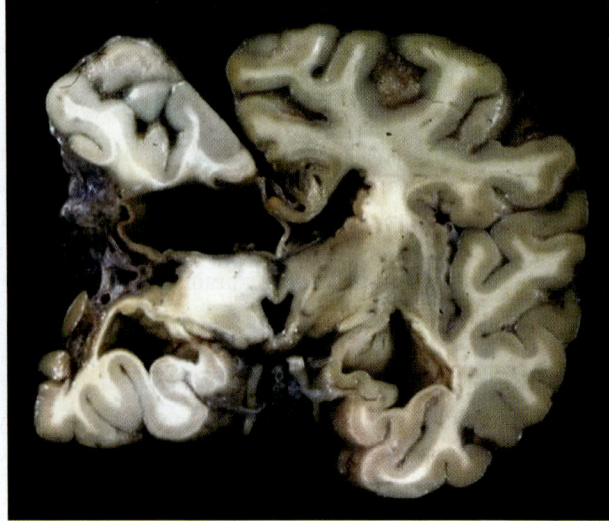

FIGURE 21-19 (Left panel) Acute infarct in distribution of left middle cerebral artery (MCA). The infarcted brain is swollen due to edema and shows prominent mass effect, including herniation of the left cingulate gyrus. (Right panel) Remote infarct in distribution of left MCA. The infarct has undergone cavitation, due to removal of the necrotic brain tissue. The old infarct is no longer a mass lesion.

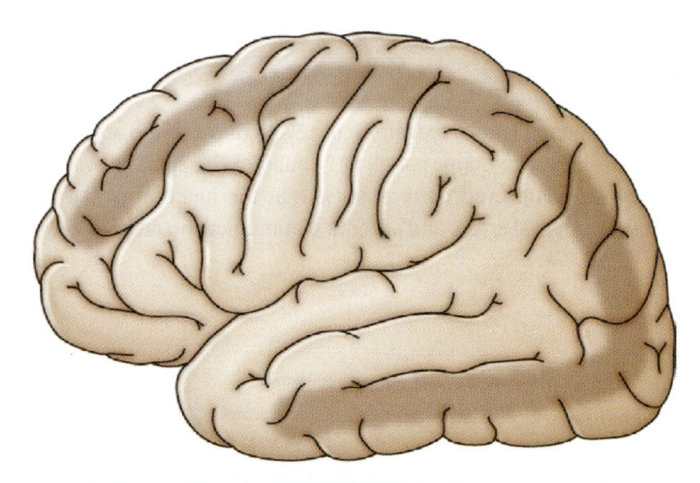

FIGURE 21-21 "Watershed" (border-zone) infarct occurs in the border zone between two arterial distributions. Watershed infarcts are usually due to systemic hypotension.

(Figure 21-22). From a clinical standpoint, there are significant consequences of spontaneous intracerebral hemorrhage, including local brain destruction, mass effect, and extension of the hemorrhage to the ventricular system (Figure 21-23). Large brain hemorrhages are lethal. Small brain hemorrhages are resorbed over time, leaving behind a hemosiderin-stained cavity in the brain.

The cause of hypertensive intracerebral hemorrhage is thought to be small-vessel arteriosclerosis, which leads to weakening of the arterial walls. It has been speculated that rupture of microaneurysms (Charcot–Bouchard aneurysms), which may develop on these arteriosclerotic arteries, is responsible for the intracerebral hemorrhage.

Subarachnoid Hemorrhage (SAH)

Acute SAH is the cause of 5% of strokes. Most cases of acute SAH are due to rupture of a berry (saccular) aneurysm (aneurysmal SAH). A berry aneurysm is a saccular-shaped outpouching on one of the large intracranial arteries of the circle of Willis in the subarachnoid space at the base of the brain. The aneurysms arise at bifurcation points and are multiple in 20% of cases. Most aneurysms (85%) are on the anterior (internal carotid artery) circulation, with the remaining 15% on the posterior (vertebrobasilar) circulation. The prevalence of aneurysms is 2% in adults; they are almost never found in children. Most aneurysms do not rupture, so that the annual risk of rupture is less than 1%. The mean age at rupture is 50. The risk of rupture increases with increasing size of the aneurysm.

Berry aneurysms are typically sporadic, but there is a higher incidence in persons with autosomal dominant polycystic kidney disease or a family history of aneurysms. Berry aneurysms are also associated with brain arteriovenous malformations (AVMs) and with coarctation of the aorta. Risk factors for aneurysmal rupture include hypertension, cigarette smoking, cocaine use, heavy alcohol consumption, female sex, and family history of SAH.

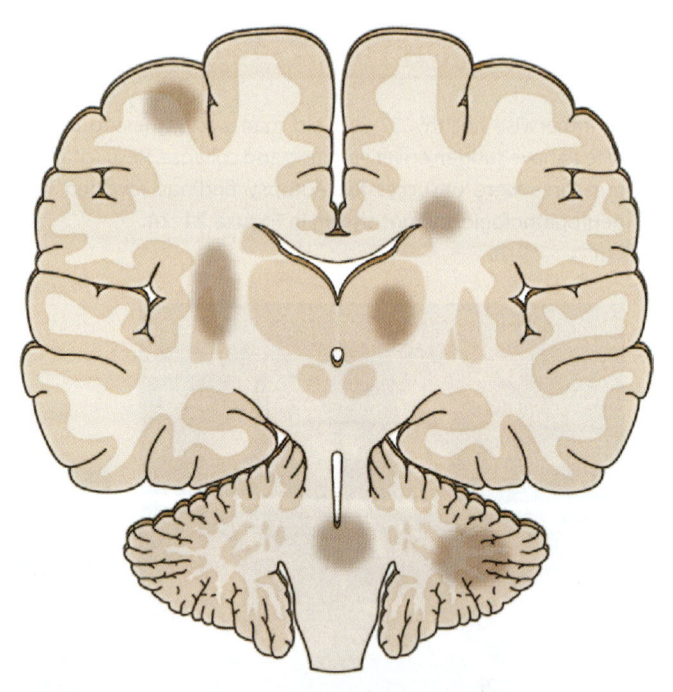

FIGURE 21-22 Sites of brain hemorrhage: putamen, caudate nucleus, thalamus, cerebral white matter, pons, and cerebellum.

TABLE 21-6 Causes of brain hemorrhage.

- Chronic systemic hypertension
- Cerebral amyloid angiopathy (occurs in older persons and in Alzheimer disease)
- Anticoagulants, coagulopathies, blood dyscrasias, thrombolytic agents, thrombocytopenia
- Ruptured vascular malformation (arteriovenous malformation, cavernoma) or ruptured berry aneurysm
- Hemorrhage within a primary or metastatic neoplasm in the brain
- Drug abuse (amphetamines, cocaine, etc.)

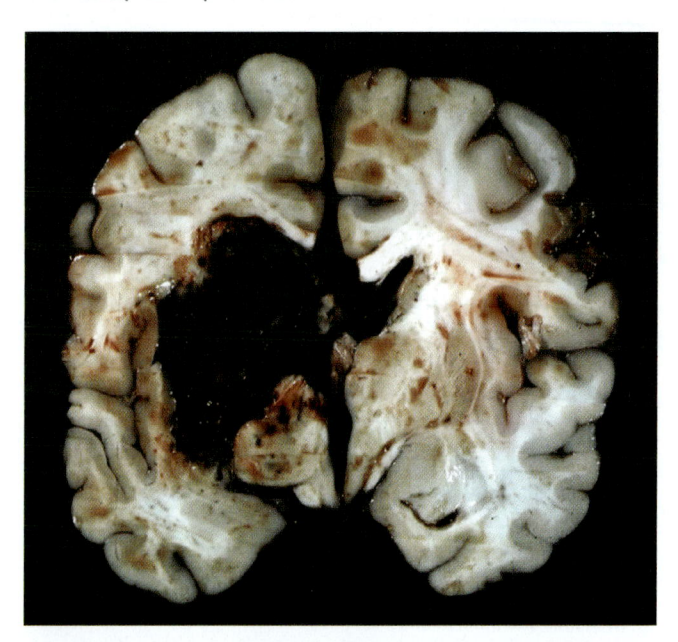

FIGURE 21-23 Brain hemorrhage originating in the putamen and extending into ventricle.

CASE PRESENTATION: Aneurysmal Subarachnoid Hemorrhage

An otherwise healthy, 37-year-old man was witnessed by his wife to have sudden onset vomiting and collapse. Resuscitation measures were unsuccessful. Autopsy findings revealed the neuropathologic findings shown in **Figure 21-24**.

(Left panel) There is severe, acute SAH concentrated at the base of the brain. (Right panel) Dissection of the circle of Willis reveals a ruptured berry aneurysm at the junction of the anterior cerebral artery and anterior communicating artery.

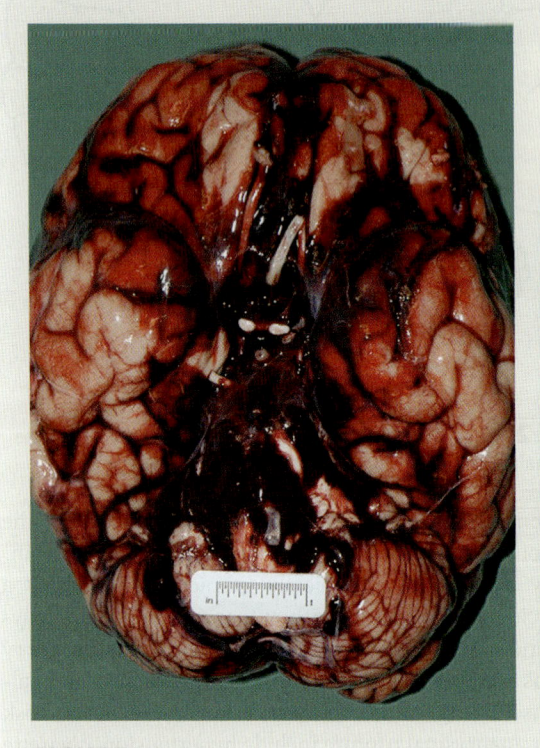

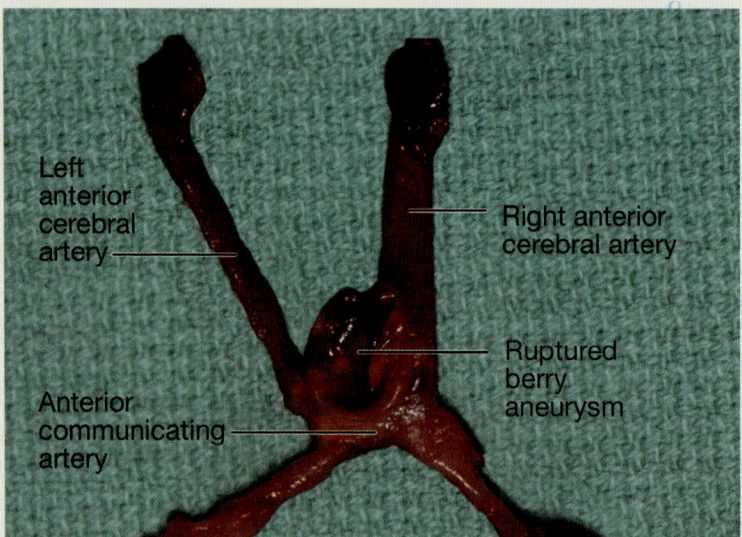

FIGURE 21-24 Aneurysmal subarachnoid hemorrhage.

Aneurysmal SAH is a very severe form of stroke—a third of the patients die and another third are significantly impaired neurologically. The consequences of aneurysmal SAH are listed in **Table 21-7**.

Most cases of clinically significant SAH are due to rupture of a saccular aneurysm. SAH may also be associated with a ruptured cerebral AVM. Head trauma is a frequent cause of SAH, but the hemorrhage is moderate in degree and rarely clinically significant.

TABLE 21-7 Consequences of subarachnoid hemorrhage.

- Subarachnoid hemorrhage at base of brain
- Raised intracranial pressure
- Rebleeding may occur during the first 4 weeks after rupture
- Arterial vasospasm may occur 3–14 days after rupture due to the blood in the subarachnoid space. The vasospasm leads to cerebral ischemia and brain infarcts
- Hydrocephalus may develop, either acutely from the blood in the CSF pathways or more chronically from meningeal fibrosis

BRAIN TUMORS
Overview

Brain tumors may be classified as primary or secondary. *Primary tumors* arise from the glial cells and neurons of the CNS, arachnoid cells of the craniospinal leptomeninges, Schwann cells of the craniospinal nerves, and other sources. The most common types of primary intracranial tumor are glioma, meningioma, pituitary adenoma, and vestibular schwannoma. *Secondary tumors* arise elsewhere in the body and spread to the CNS through hematogenous dissemination (metastasis) or by direct extension from adjacent structures.

Histologic classification and grading of primary brain tumors provide critical information for predicting biologic behavior and prognosis and in determining appropriate therapy. The histologic classification of primary nervous-system tumors is based on the phenotypic expression of the neoplastic cells **(Table 21-8)**. Histologic features of anaplasia (loss of differentiation) within a neoplasm include enlarged, darkly staining nuclei, cellular pleomorphism, mitotic activity, foci

TABLE 21-8 Histologic classification of tumors of the nervous system.

Differentiation of Tumor Cells	Histologic Classification
Glial	Astrocytoma and glioblastoma
	Oligodendroglioma
	Ependymoma
Embryonal	Medulloblastoma
Arachnoid cell	Meningioma
Schwann cell	Schwannoma and neurofibroma
	Malignant peripheral nerve sheath tumor (MPNST)
Miscellaneous	Pituitary adenoma
	Lymphoma
	Hemangioblastoma
	Craniopharyngioma
	Germ-cell neoplasms

WHAT WE DO

Tumors are graded, based on their biologic behavior and prognosis. The World Health Organization (WHO) classification of brain tumors assigns one of four grades (I–IV) to each histologic type of tumor. In general, grade I tumors are slow-growing, potentially curable tumors if surgically excised; grade II tumors are low-grade malignancies with survival times of 5–10 years following treatment; grade III tumors are high-grade malignancies with survival times of 2–5 years following treatment; and grade IV tumors are high-grade malignancies with survival times of less than 1 year unless appropriately treated.

Brain tumors are often difficult to completely excise because of their infiltrative nature or location and become increasingly large mass lesions (**Figure 21-25**). Hence, even low-grade tumors may be lethal due to mass effect. Unlike cancers arising in other organs, brain tumors rarely metastasize outside the CNS.

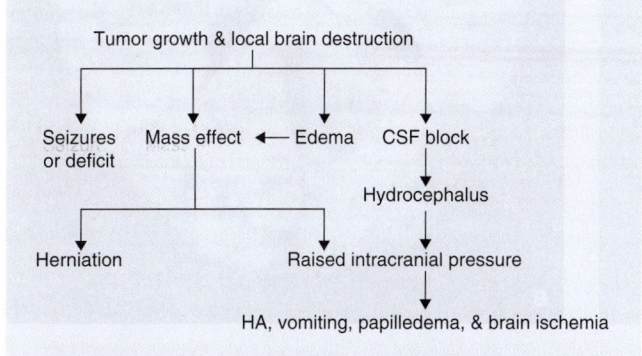

FIGURE 21-25 Consequences of a brain tumor.

of tumor necrosis, and microvascular proliferation. The proliferating microvessels lack a BBB and produce a contrast-enhancing lesion radiographically.

Gliomas

Diffuse astrocytoma is an infiltrating glioma that is classified as WHO grade II or grade III, based on degree of anaplasia. These tumors are most commonly found in the cerebral hemisphere of an adult, but may occur at any age and in any location within the brain or spinal cord. Grade II diffuse astrocytomas typically evolve over time to grade III tumors (*anaplastic astrocytoma*) or grade IV tumors (*glioblastoma*).

Glioblastoma is the most malignant type of astrocytoma and the most common glioma (**Figure 21-26**). Age of onset is typically around 55. The cerebral hemisphere is the favored location (**Figure 21-27**). Histologically, glioblastoma shows features of an astrocytoma with nuclear atypia, mitotic figures, tumor necrosis, and microvascular proliferation.

Pilocytic astrocytoma is a slowly growing, relatively circumscribed WHO grade I glioma that typically arises in children and young adults and may occur in the brain or spinal cord. The tumor contains distinctive, eosinophilic, cigar-shaped structures (*Rosenthal fibers*). Unlike the diffuse astrocytoma the pilocytic astrocytoma rarely evolves into a higher grade neoplasm.

Oligodendroglioma is an infiltrating glioma of the cerebral hemisphere of adults. The characteristic histopathologic features are intratumoral microcalcifications and perinuclear halos. These tumors are classified as WHO grade II or grade III.

Ependymoma is a relatively circumscribed glioma that occurs in children and adults. The brain around the fourth ventricle, spinal cord, and cerebral hemisphere are favored sites. An ependymoma is characterized histologically by a relatively uniform population of neoplastic cells that sometimes form rosettes around blood vessels (perivascular pseudorosette) or structures mimicking the central canal of the spinal cord (ependymal rosette). These neoplasms are classified as WHO grade II or grade III.

Medulloblastoma

The *medulloblastoma* arises only in the cerebellum and occurs in children and young adults. This embryonal neoplasm is composed of monotonous sheets of small round cells that sometimes form neuroblastic (Homer Wright) rosettes. The medulloblastoma shows significant potential for metastasis through the CSF. These tumors are highly malignant (WHO grade IV) but very responsive to therapy.

Meningioma

Meningiomas arise from the cells of the leptomeninges and are extra-axial, that is, external to the brain and spinal cord. The meningioma is a neoplasm of adults and occurs more frequently in women (**Figure 21-28**). Meningiomas typically

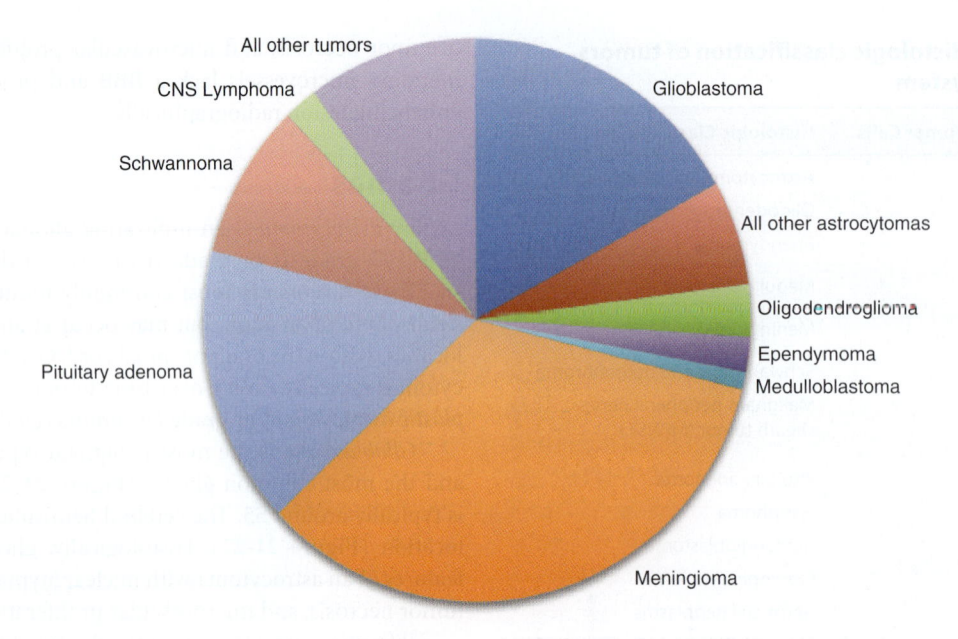

FIGURE 21-26 Relative incidence of primary brain tumors.

arise over the cerebral convexities, parasagittal area, sphenoid wing, parasellar area, and along the spinal meninges. Multiple meningiomas sometimes occur and may be associated with neurofibromatosis type 2. Meningiomas invade the dura mater and sometimes the overlying skull, but they only rarely invade the underlying brain. Histologically, the neoplastic cells vary from oval- to spindle-shaped and sometimes forming cellular whorls. Foci of calcification (psammoma bodies) are frequently present. Most meningiomas are classified as WHO grade I or grade II.

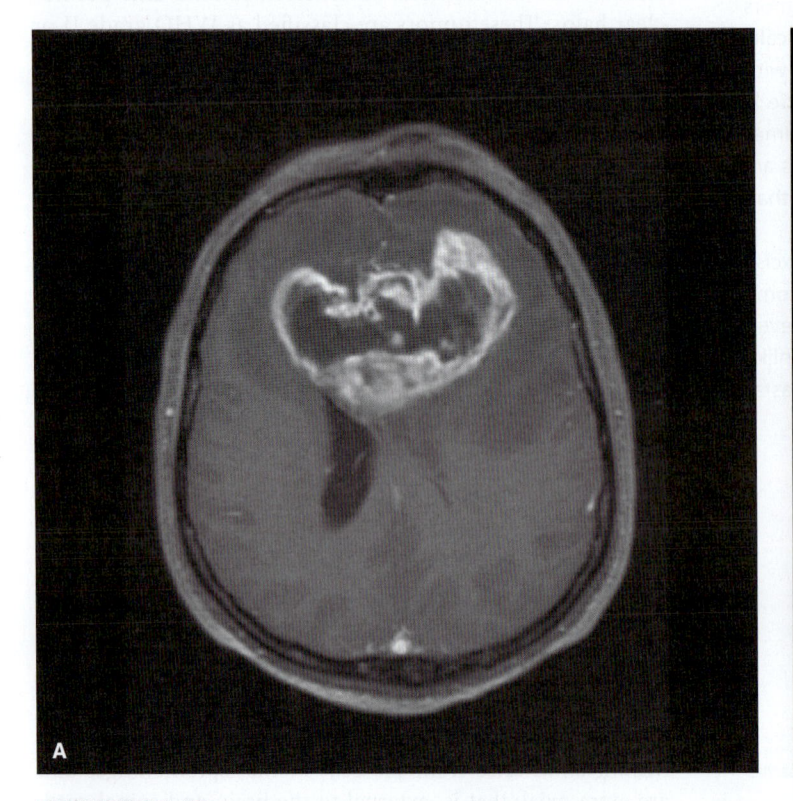

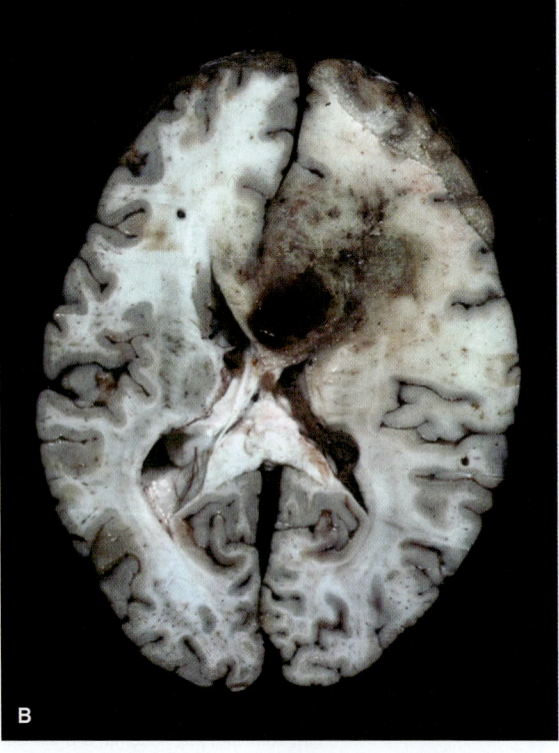

FIGURE 21-27 **Glioblastoma.** Brain MRI **(A)** reveals that this glioblastoma crosses the corpus callosum and involves both hemispheres ("butterfly glioma"). Postmortem specimen **(B)** shows the necrosis and hemorrhage typical of these high-grade gliomas. The glioblastoma's infiltrative nature precludes a complete surgical excision and contributes to its poor prognosis.

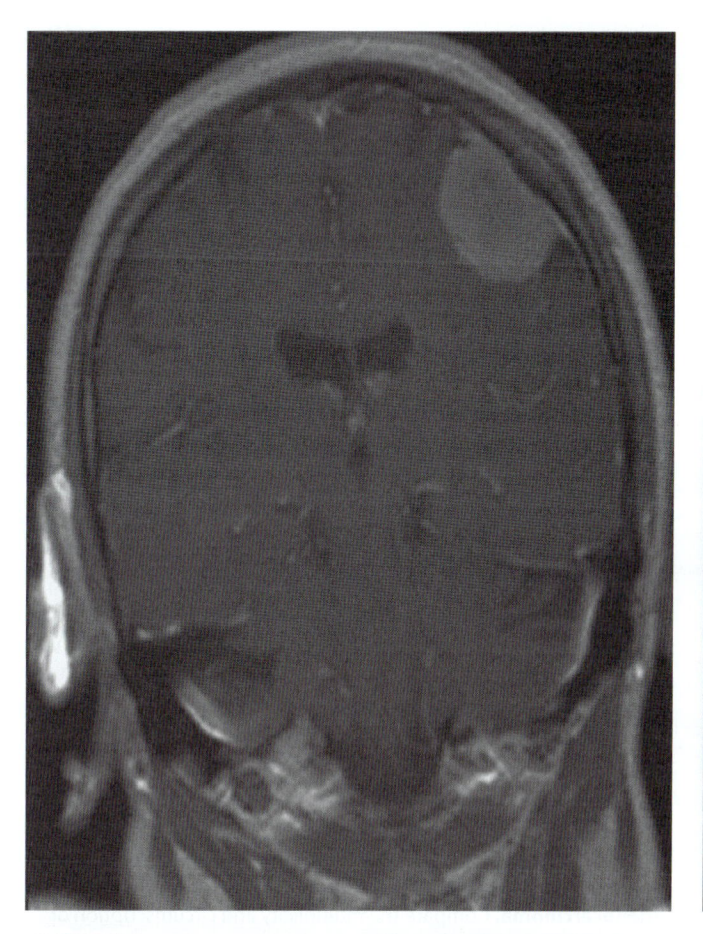

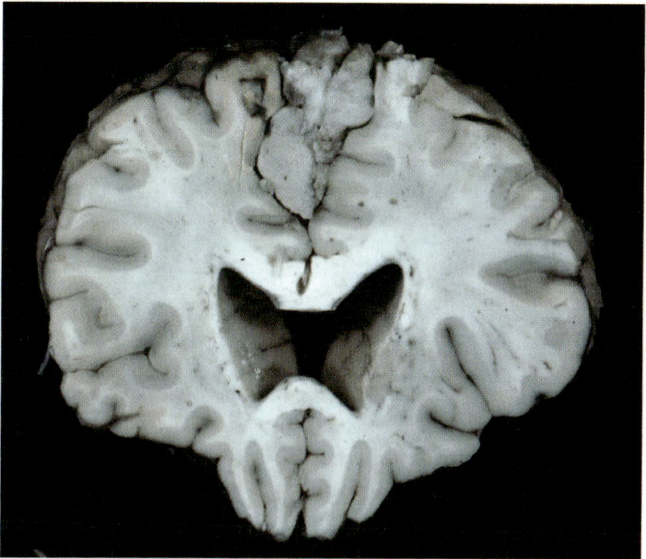

FIGURE 21-28 Common sites of meningioma. (Left panel) A meningioma arises from the dura mater over the convexity of the brain. (Right panel) A meningioma arises in the midline from the falx cerebri. Meningiomas are extra-axial and usually do not infiltrate underlying brain. These tumors rarely metastasize and can often be completely excised, giving them a good prognosis.

Schwannoma

Schwannomas arise on cranial nerves, spinal roots, or peripheral nerves of the trunk or extremities. Intracranial schwannomas usually arise on eighth cranial nerve, usually the vestibular branch, at the cerebellopontine angle. Spinal schwannomas usually arise on posterior (sensory) nerve roots and may extend through the intervertebral foramen to form a dumbbell-shaped tumor. The schwannoma is encapsulated and grows slowly and is classified as WHO grade I. Bilateral eighth-nerve schwannomas are a defining feature of neurofibromatosis type 2. Microscopically, the schwannoma is a benign-appearing spindle-cell neoplasm with compact areas (Antoni A pattern) and loose, vacuolated areas (Antoni B pattern). Palisades of nuclei (Verocay bodies) are also common in schwannomas.

Primary CNS Lymphoma

Lymphoma within the brain may be primary or secondary. *Primary CNS lymphoma* (PCNSL) is a tumor of adults, especially those with immunosuppression, and mainly involves the brain parenchyma. PCNSL arising in immunosuppressed patients shows a strong association with Ebstein–Barr virus (EBV). PCNSL is primarily a diffuse large B cell lymphoma. A characteristic histologic feature of PCNSL is its angiocentric pattern. PCNSL has a poor prognosis, especially in immunosuppressed patients.

Colloid Cyst

Usually presenting in adults aged 20–50 years, the *colloid cyst* is found only in the third ventricle. The cyst, which is attached to the roof of the ventricle, may intermittently block the interventricular foramen, causing an acute block of CSF flow and acute hydrocephalus. The cyst is composed of a thin, collagenous wall lined by a single cell layer of benign columnar epithelium.

Brain Metastases

Metastases are the most common type of brain tumor. In some autopsy series, about 25% of patients dying with carcinoma will show brain metastases. Remarkably, brain metastases are very circumscribed and do not diffusely infiltrate the surrounding brain (Figure 21-30). The metastasis causes local brain destruction, with resultant loss of neurologic function, and may cause seizures. A metastasis, whether intra-axial or

CASE PRESENTATION: Schwannoma of the Eighth Cranial Nerve

The patient is a 45-year-old woman with a history of migraine headache. For the past 2 months, she has been experiencing symptoms of vertigo, tinnitus, and mild subjective hearing loss. Brain MRI is shown in **Figure 21-29**.

An extra-axial, high-signal-intensity tumor is located at the cerebellopontine angle and is arising from cranial nerve VIII. The tumor was completely surgically excised and pathologic evaluation revealed a schwannoma.

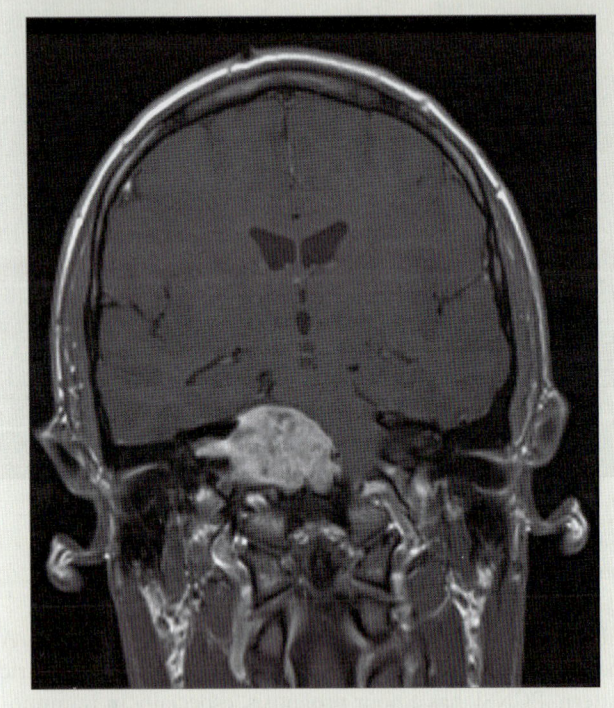

FIGURE 21-29 Schwannoma of the eighth cranial nerve arising in the cerebellopontine angle.

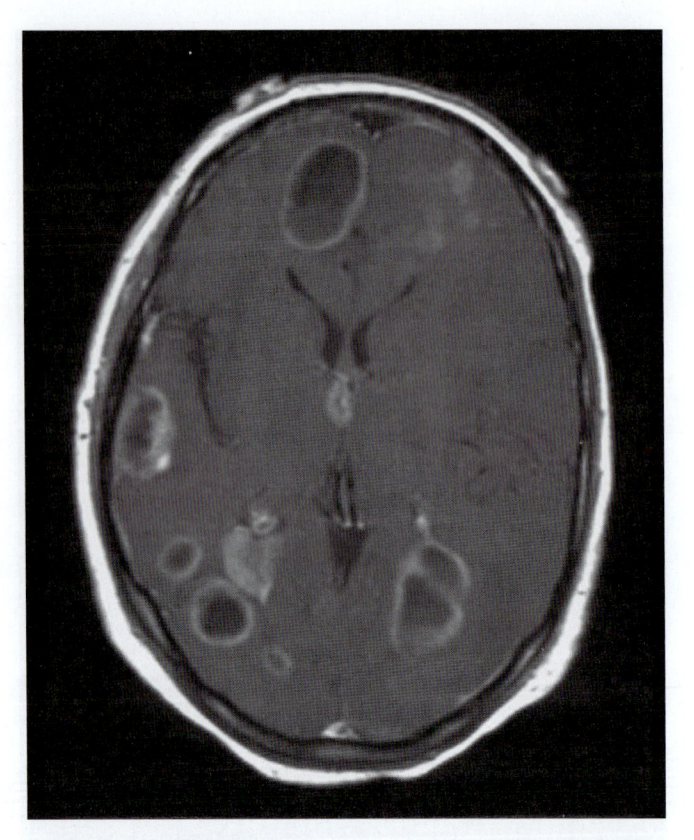

FIGURE 21-30 Note the multiple, discrete, well-defined metastases in the brain of this patient with a history of lung adenocarcinoma. Compare the multiplicity and circumscription of these metastases with the solitary, but highly infiltrative nature of glioblastoma (Figure 21-27).

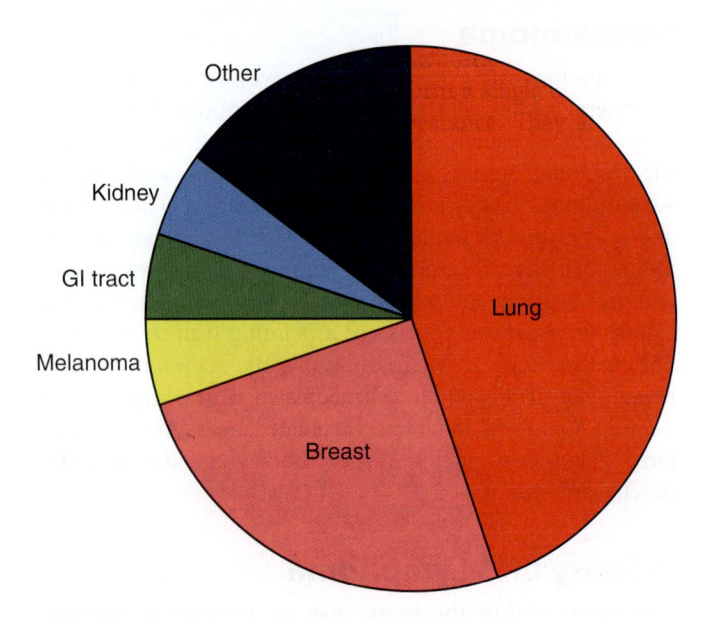

FIGURE 21-31 A chart of the relative frequency of primary neoplasms metastatic to the brain shows the predominance of lung and breast primaries.

extra-axial, is also a mass lesion. The neoplasms most commonly metastasizing to the brain are lung carcinoma, breast carcinoma, and melanoma **(Figure 21-31)**. Brain metastases are most common in the cerebral hemispheres, often at the junction between gray matter and white matter, and may be single or multiple.

DEMYELINATING DISEASES

Demyelination refers to a process in which there is a selective loss of myelin from the intact axon. The demyelinating disorders are a prime example of selective vulnerability in the nervous system, with the oligodendrocyte/myelin unit being selectively injured and the axon relatively spared. Demyelinating diseases are of diverse etiology and include both inherited and acquired diseases. The loss of myelin prevents the axon from effectively conducting nerve impulses and leads to loss of function. There is no significant remyelination of demyelinated axons in the CNS and thus no significant return of function in these axons. This contrasts sharply with the PNS, where remyelination of demyelinated axons and return of function normally occurs.

Multiple Sclerosis

Multiple sclerosis (MS) is the most common, chronic neurologic disease affecting young adults in the United States. The disease occurs between 15 and 50 years of age, with the average age of onset at 30. The etiology and pathogenesis of MS are not known. It is currently viewed as an autoimmune-mediated disorder influenced by complex environmental and hereditary factors. Diagnosis of MS is a clinical one and is based on neurologic symptoms, MRI abnormalities, and the detection of oligoclonal bands of immunoglobulins in the CSF. As with all of the demyelinating diseases, MS typically targets the white matter of the CNS. Most cases of MS present as the relapsing-remitting form (RRMS), characterized by intermittent attacks of neurologic dysfunction followed by periods of remission with partial to complete recovery. Signs and symptoms of MS include visual disturbances, paralysis, ataxia, and motor and sensory disturbances at all levels of the CNS.

The principal pathologic lesion of MS is the plaque, which can occur anywhere in the CNS but is most frequent in the periventricular white matter (Figure 21-32), optic nerves and anterior visual pathways, brain stem, and ascending and descending white matter tracts of the spinal cord. It is important to understand that, by definition, the lesions of MS are disseminated in space (more than one lesion in the CNS) and in time (lesions of different ages). The typical plaque is sharply circumscribed, firm, and gray. Microscopically, plaques show loss of myelin, relative preservation of axons, and reactive gliosis. "Active" plaques additionally show macrophages containing myelin breakdown products and perivascular lymphocytic infiltrates. Loss of oligodendrocytes is common and may be seen in both actively demyelinating plaques and in chronic plaques. Some degree of axonal injury is expected in MS lesions and is considered to contribute significantly to the neurologic dysfunction caused by MS.

Acute Disseminated Encephalomyelitis

Acute disseminated encephalomyelitis (ADEM) is a monophasic, autoimmune-mediated demyelinating disease involving the white matter of the CNS. The pathogenesis is unknown. ADEM more commonly affects children and young adults and typically occurs within 4 weeks after an upper respiratory viral illness or vaccination. Patients acutely develop headache, vomiting, and fever followed by weakness, ataxia, visual and sensory loss, mental status changes, and seizures. The clinical course of ADEM is short, and many patients make a full recovery.

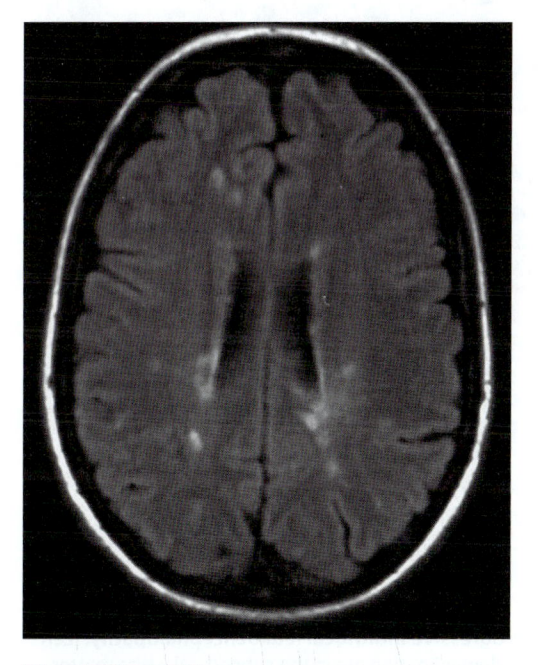

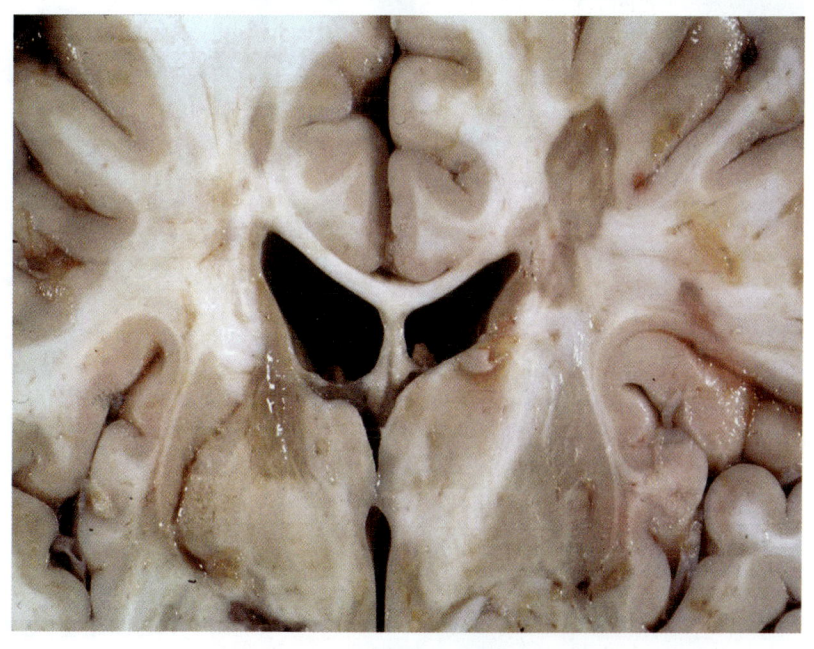

FIGURE 21-32 **Multiple sclerosis.** With brain MRI (left panel), plaques of multiple sclerosis appear as multiple small foci of high-signal intensity in the periventricular white matter of the cerebrum. Coronal section of brain (right panel) shows multiple gray-tan, demyelinated plaques in the periventricular white matter. The axons are relatively preserved in these demyelinated plaques.

ADEM is characterized histologically by perivenous demyelination in the white matter of the brain and spinal cord. The myelin loss is accompanied by relative sparing of axons and an infiltrate of lymphocytes and macrophages.

Progressive Multifocal Leukoencephalopathy

PML is a demyelinating disease of the CNS. The demyelination is the result of infection of oligodendrocytes by the JC strain of papovavirus. The disease typically occurs in immunocompromised patients, especially AIDS patients. The clinical manifestations of PML include a several-month course of progressive visual, motor and sensory symptoms, and profound personality changes. The disease has a short clinical course and is often fatal within 6 months.

The brain shows multiple, punctate, gray areas in the subcortical white matter in the early phase. The lesions may later coalesce to form larger, necrotic, cavitating lesions involving white matter and adjacent cortex (Figure 21-33). Microscopically, the myelin loss is accompanied by relative preservation of axons, viral inclusions within the nuclei of oligodendrocytes, and large, bizarre astrocytes.

Radiation Necrosis of White Matter

Radiation therapy for brain tumors may sometimes be complicated by delayed necrosis of the irradiated brain tissue. *Radiation necrosis* (radionecrosis) is limited to the white matter and typically develops months to years after the radiotherapy. The affected white matter shows areas of coagulative necrosis, similar to that found in a brain infarct. Small and medium-sized blood vessels in the irradiated area show fibrosis and hyalinization of their walls. Some vessel walls may also show fibrinoid necrosis. The brain necrosis is likely related to the associated vascular damage and resulting brain ischemia. The radionecrosis may mimic very closely recurrent brain tumor on imaging studies.

The Leukodystrophies

The *leukodystrophies* are a heterogeneous group of inherited diseases characterized by perturbation in the formation or maintenance of the myelin sheath and caused by a defect in one of the genes involved in myelin metabolism. As opposed to MS or PML, where the myelin loss is asymmetric and multifocal, a leukodystrophy shows extensive, symmetric regions of confluent demyelination. There is often a characteristic

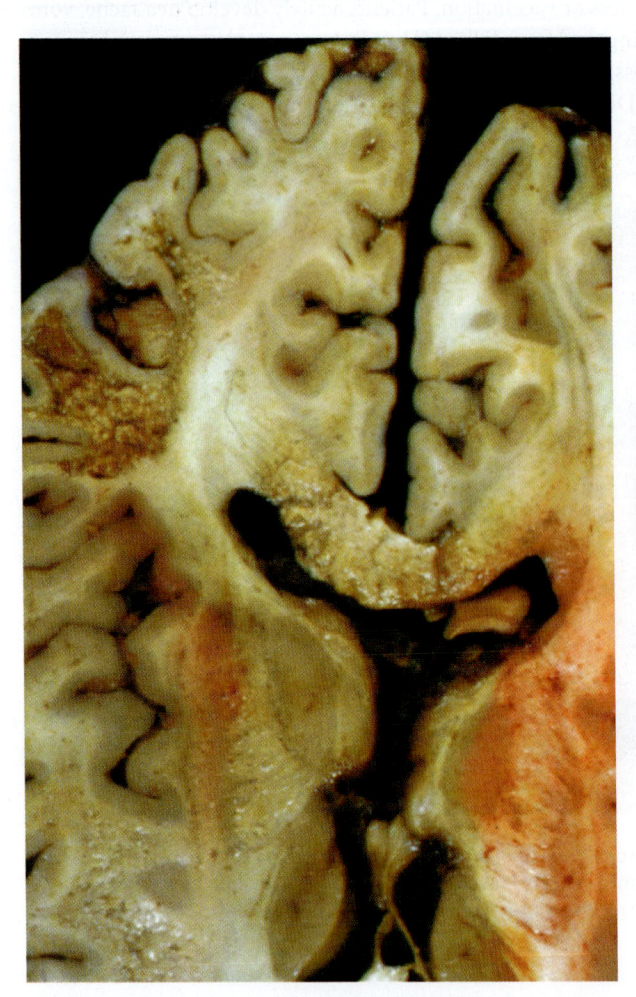

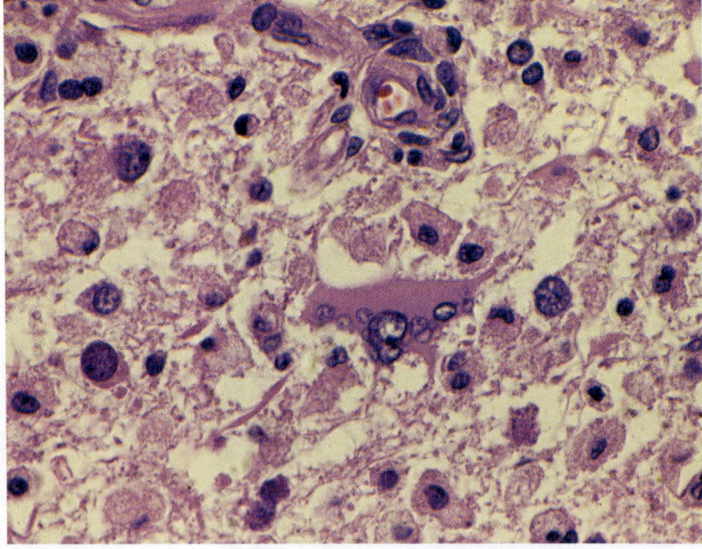

FIGURE 21-33 Progressive multifocal leukoencephalopathy. (Left panel) Large regions of demyelination are in the subcortical white matter, corpus callosum, and internal capsule. (Right panel) Histologic section shows an enlarged, multinucleated, bizarre astrocyte in the center of a field of demyelination. (Courtesy of Kinuko Suzuki, MD, Tokyo Metropolitan Institute of Gerontology; retired faculty, Department of Pathology and Laboratory Medicine, University of North Carolina, Chapel Hill, NC.)

CASE PRESENTATION: Radiation Necrosis of Brain

The patient is a 65-year-old man with a past medical history significant for lung adenocarcinoma with a single brain metastasis in the left temporal lobe, treated 1 year ago with radiation therapy to the CNS. He presents to the Emergency Department(ED) with seizures. The differential diagnosis includes recurrent tumor versus radiation necrosis. Combined magnetic resonance spectroscopy (MRS, left panel) for analysis of metabolites and brain MRI (right panel) is performed (Figure 21-34).

Based on the MRS analysis of the metabolites in the brain lesion, the patient was given a diagnosis of radiation necrosis.

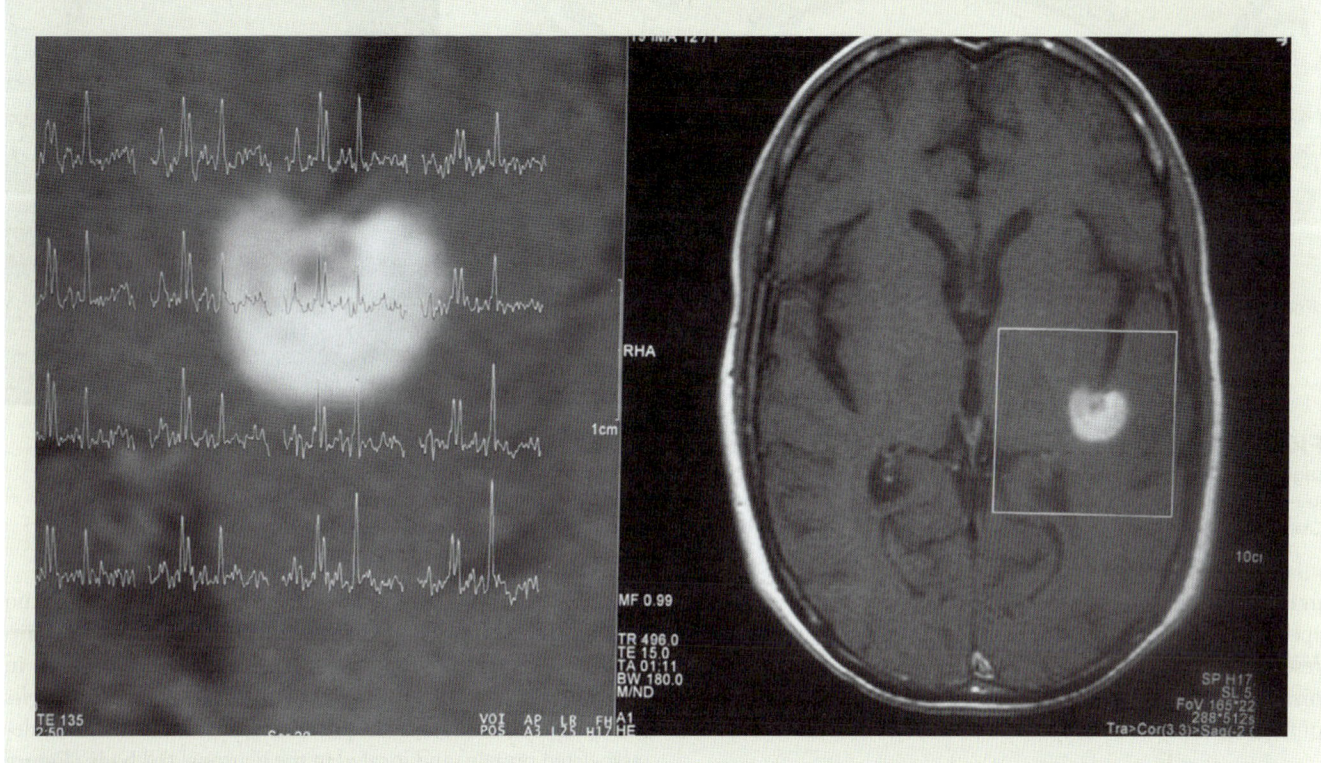

FIGURE 21-34 Radiation necrosis of brain. (Courtesy of Lester Kwock, PhD, Department of Radiology, University of North Carolina, Chapel Hill, NC.)

---

sparing of a thin strip of myelinated fibers coursing just beneath the cortex (short arcuate fibers or subcortical U-fibers) in the leukodystrophies (Figure 21-35).

Adrenoleukodystrophy (ALD) is an X-linked inherited disorder affecting myelin in the CNS and PNS and characterized by demyelination and adrenal insufficiency. The metabolic defect leads to an accumulation of saturated, very-long-chain fatty acids in tissues and body fluids. ALD occurs in children between the ages of 3 and 10 years and shows bilateral, symmetric, confluent demyelination that is most pronounced in the parieto-occipital lobes of the brain. The PNS also shows demyelination. Histologically, the lesions show demyelination, perivascular lymphocytic infiltrates, and macrophages filled with abnormal storage material.

Krabbe disease (*globoid-cell leukodystrophy*) is an autosomal recessive, rapidly progressive demyelinating disorder of infancy caused by a deficiency of galactocerebroside β-galactosidase. The demyelination involves the CNS and PNS. Microscopically, the affected white matter of the brain shows severe loss of myelin associated with perivascular clusters of large macrophages stuffed with undigested galactocerebroside (globoid cells).

NEURODEGENERATIVE DISEASES

Neurodegenerative diseases are distinguished by the progressive dysfunction and death of neurons. In the neurodegenerative diseases, the primary abnormality is a selective degeneration of certain populations of neurons in the CNS. The clinical presentation of each disease is dictated by the particular function of the population of neurons involved. Thus, diseases characterized by degeneration of neurons of the cerebral cortex (e.g., AD) are associated with cognitive impairment and dementia; diseases characterized by degeneration of neurons in the basal ganglia (e.g., Huntington disease, HD) are associated with involuntary movements; and diseases characterized by degeneration of upper and lower motor neurons (e.g., amyotrophic lateral sclerosis, ALS) are associated with loss of voluntary movement. In many diseases, the neuronal degeneration is accompanied by accumulation of abnormal protein within affected neurons or

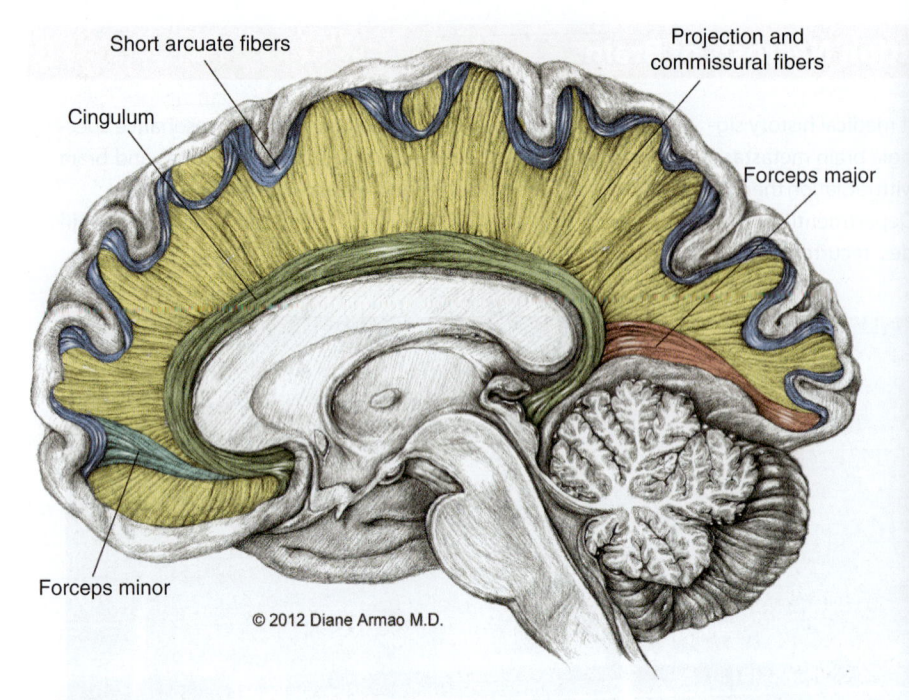

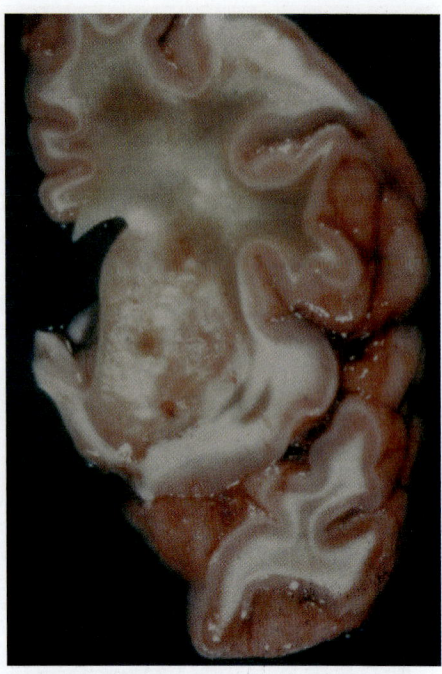

FIGURE 21-35 (Left panel) Short arcuate fibers (U fibers) in sagittal section of brain. (Copyright 2012, Diane Armao, MD, Departments of Radiology and Pathology and Laboratory Medicine, University of North Carolina, Chapel Hill, NC.) (Right panel) Leukodystrophy. Coronal section of brain shows large regions of demyelination with sparing of the short arcuate fibers. (Courtesy of Kinuko Suzuki, MD, Tokyo Metropolitan Institute of Gerontology; retired faculty, Department of Pathology and Laboratory Medicine, University of North Carolina, Chapel Hill, NC.)

in the extracellular space. Most neurodegenerative diseases are sporadic; a few have Mendelian inheritance. Although ongoing research continues to provide valuable insights into the mechanisms of neurodegenerative diseases, the precise pathogenesis of the various neurodegenerative diseases is unknown.

Alzheimer Disease

Alzheimer disease (AD) is a progressive neurodegenerative disease characterized by progressive loss of memory and judgment and changes in personality. AD is the most common cause of dementia in adults and is responsible for 50–75% of cases of dementia in patients over age 65.

AD is characterized primarily by a degeneration of the neurons in the cerebral cortex and hippocampus. The affected brain shows prominent cerebral cortical atrophy with shrinkage of the gyri and widening of the sulci, most pronounced in the fronto-temporal regions. There is prominent hydrocephalus ex vacuo due to the cerebral atrophy (**Figure 21-36**). Microscopic examination of the cerebral cortex reveals neurofibrillary tangles in neurons and senile plaques in the neuropil. *Neurofibrillary tangles* are composed of abnormally phosphorylated tau, a microtubule-associated protein, and located in the neuronal cell body (**Figure 21-37**). *Senile plaques* are extracellular deposits of β-amyloid protein in the neuropil. The plaques are surrounded by tau-filled neuronal processes (**Figure 21-38**). The β-amyloid protein is also deposited in the walls of leptomeningeal and cortical blood vessels (*cerebral amyloid angiopathy*) (**Figure 21-39**). Cerebral amyloid angiopathy is a risk factor for intracerebral hemorrhage.

Parkinson Disease

Recognized since ancient times by resting tremor, truncal rigidity, and bradykinesia, *idiopathic* PD is a common movement disorder. The mean onset of PD is 61 years of age, and the average disease duration is 13 years. The pathogenesis of this sporadically occurring disease is unknown. Rare familial forms do occur and have been linked to several different genes.

Adverse drug effects and other disease processes can also produce tremor, rigidity, and bradykinesia, and thus a Parkinson-like picture clinically. Among the diseases associated with the parkinsonism syndrome are certain psychiatric medications (e.g., phenothiazines) and designer drugs (MPTP), post-encephalitic parkinsonism, infarcts of the substantia nigra, and certain other neurodegenerative diseases.

PD is a neurodegenerative disease characterized mainly by degeneration and loss of the darkly pigmented, neuromelanin-

IN TRANSLATION

The etiology and pathogenesis of AD are unknown. However, there are some clues, such as the observation that most adults with Down syndrome develop the pathologic changes of AD by age 40. Most cases are sporadic, but a small percent of cases are familial and the genes have been identified, including the β-amyloid precursor protein gene and the presenilin-1 and presenilin-2 genes. Inheritance of the apolipoprotein E ε4 allele is an established risk factor.

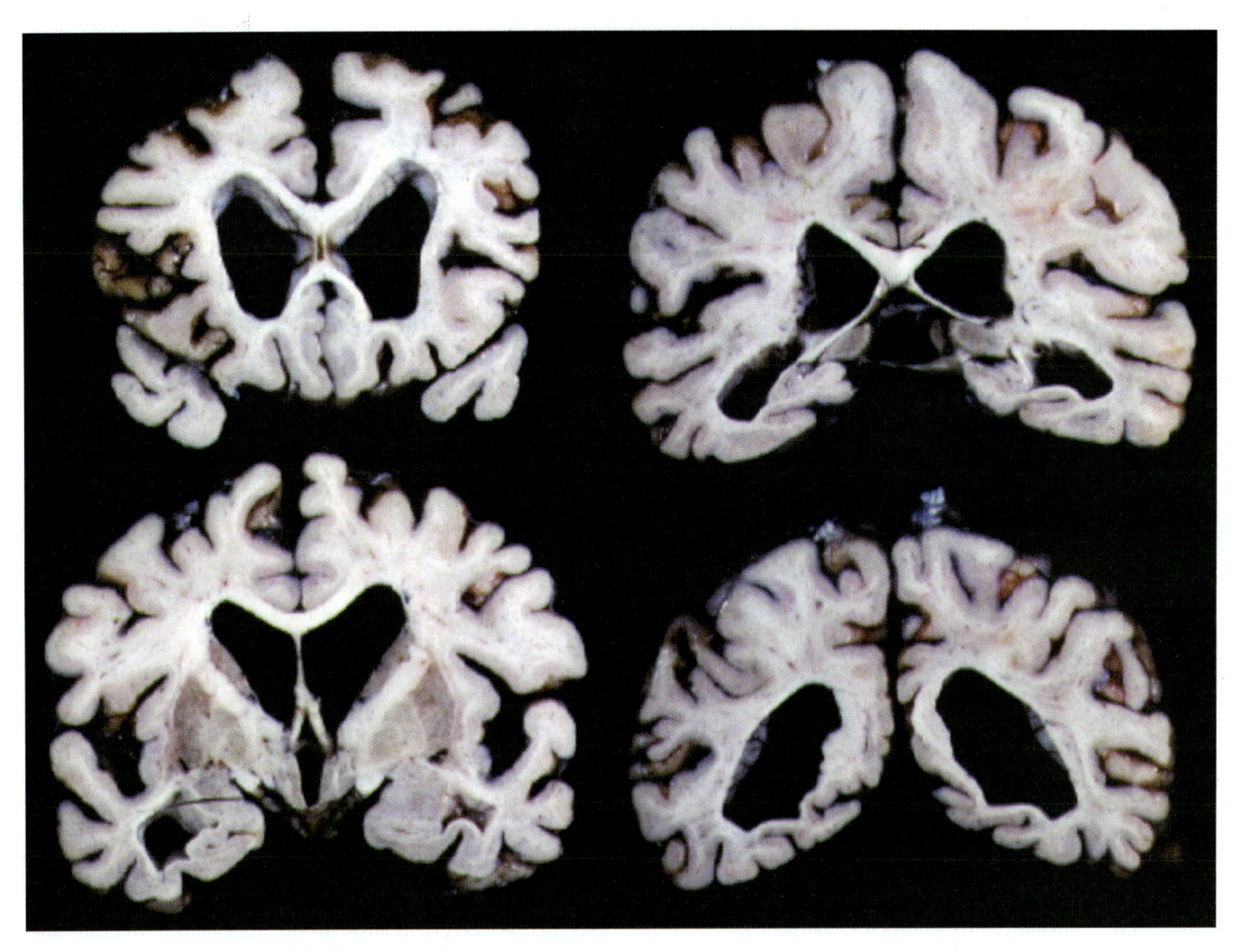

FIGURE 21-36 **Alzheimer disease showing pronounced cortical atrophy and secondary hydrocephalus ex vacuo.** (Courtesy of Kinuko Suzuki, MD, Tokyo Metropolitan Institute of Gerontology; retired faculty, Department of Pathology and Laboratory Medicine, University of North Carolina, Chapel Hill, NC.)

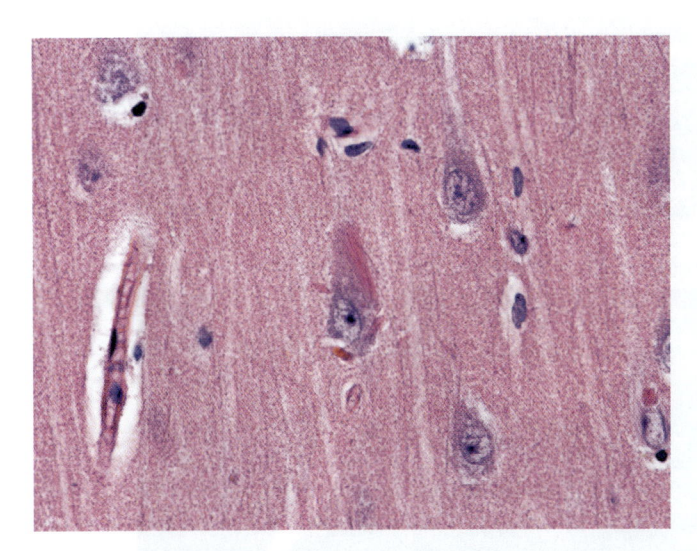

FIGURE 21-37 **Neurofibrillary tangle (NFT).** A bright red, elongated NFT partially fills the cell body of a large neuron (center of field) in the cerebral cortex of a patient with Alzheimer disease.

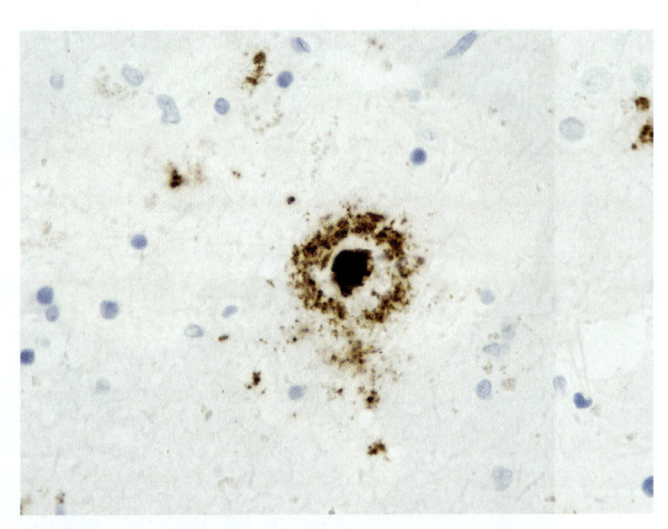

FIGURE 21-38 **Senile plaque.** A brown-staining senile plaque with a central core of beta-amyloid protein is in the cerebral cortex of a patient with Alzheimer disease.

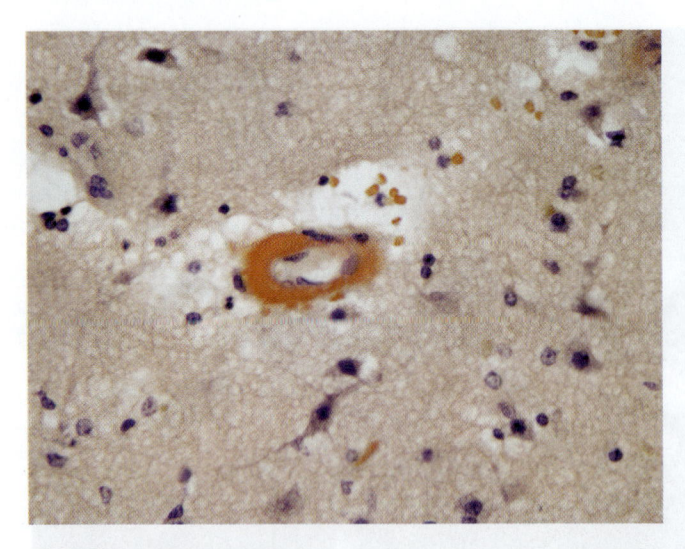

FIGURE 21-39 Orange-staining beta-amyloid protein infiltrates wall of blood vessel in cerebral cortex in cerebral amyloid angiopathy.

containing neurons of the substantia nigra in the midbrain. The loss of pigmented cells is so profound that it can be detected grossly by the pronounced pallor of the substantia nigra (Figure 21-40). The loss of neurons in the substantia nigra leads to depletion of the neurotransmitter, dopamine, and produces the clinical picture of parkinsonism.

Microscopic examination of the midbrain reveals loss of pigmented neurons in the substantia nigra. Remaining neurons often contain *Lewy bodies*, which are eosinophilic, proteinaceous, intracytoplasmic inclusions composed primarily of α-synuclein. Lewy bodies are characteristic of PD, but they can be seen in other neurodegenerative diseases, such as dementia with Lewy bodies and multiple system atrophy. Neurodegenerative diseases characterized by intracytoplasmic accumulations of α-synuclein are referred to as α-*synucleinopathies*.

Huntington Disease

First described in 1872 by George Huntington, a recent medical school graduate, HD is characterized by autosomal dominant inheritance, chorea, dementia, and death 15–20 years after onset. The HD gene is located on chromosome 4 and encodes for a novel protein, huntingtin. The genetic alteration consists of an expansion of a trinucleotide (CAG) repeat. The incidence of HD is approximately 1 in 20,000. Disease onset usually occurs around 20–50 years of age. The chorea is characterized by excessive, uncontrolled, nonrhythmic and rapid movements, and is caused by the neuronal loss in the basal ganglia. The dementia is caused by neuronal loss in the cerebral cortex.

The brain shows moderate atrophy of the cerebral cortex and striking atrophy of the caudate nucleus and putamen as a consequence of the neuronal loss (Figure 21-41). There is a compensatory enlargement of the frontal horns of the lateral ventricles due to the atrophy of the caudate nuclei. Histologic examination of the brain reveals loss of the smaller neurons in the caudate nucleus and putamen, as well as neuronal loss throughout the cerebral cortex. The neuronal loss is accompanied by a reactive gliosis.

Amyotrophic Lateral Sclerosis (Motor Neuron Disease)

Amyotrophic lateral sclerosis (ALS) is a neurodegenerative disease that preferentially involves the upper motor neurons and lower motor neurons of the CNS. Degeneration of upper motor neurons results in degeneration of the anterior and lateral

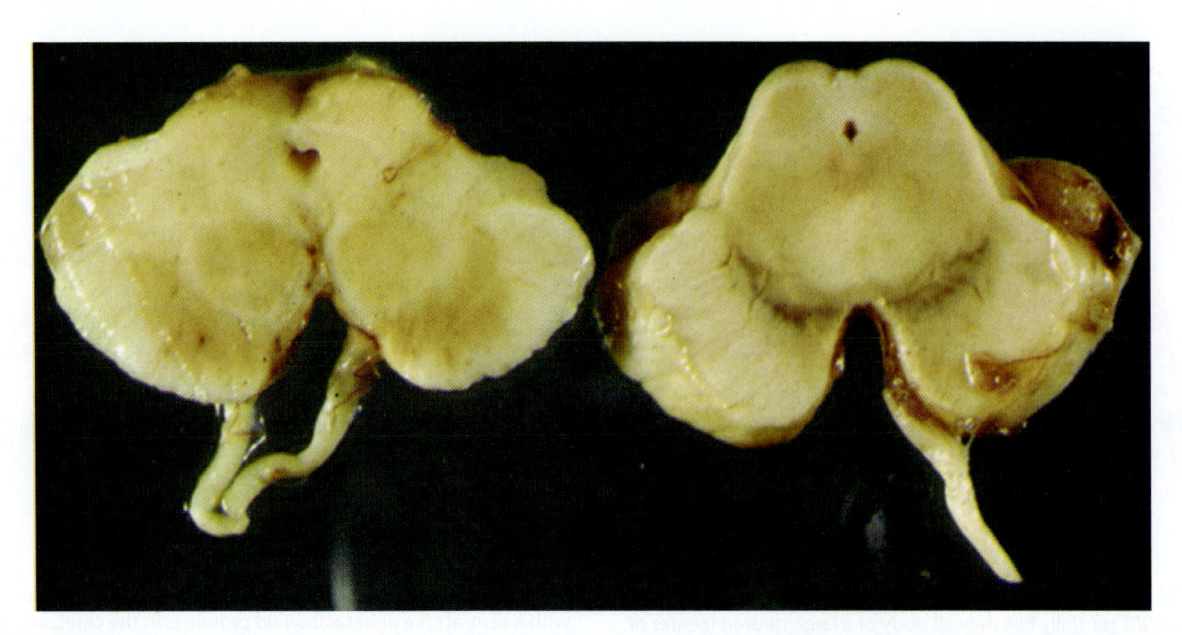

FIGURE 21-40 (Left panel) Pronounced loss of pigmentation of the substantia nigra in the midbrain in Parkinson disease. (Right panel) Normal substantia nigra. (Courtesy of Kinuko Suzuki, MD, Tokyo Metropolitan Institute of Gerontology; retired faculty, Department of Pathology and Laboratory Medicine, University of North Carolina, Chapel Hill, NC.)

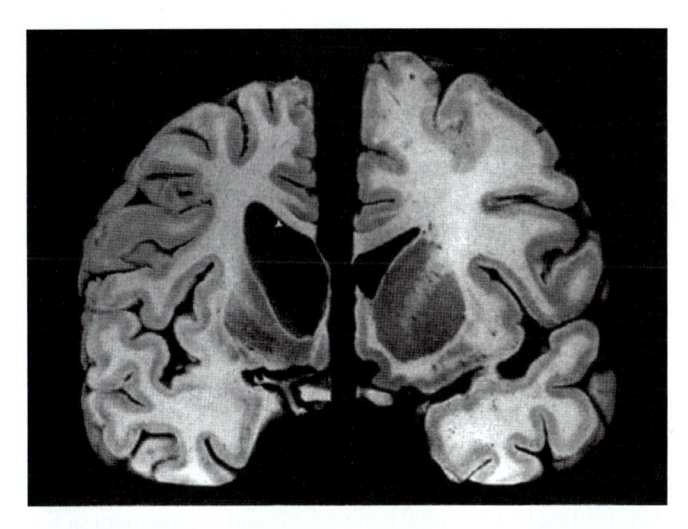

FIGURE 21-41 Left hemispheric section shows severe atrophy of the caudate nucleus and putamen and associated hydrocephalus ex vacuo in Huntington disease. Right hemispheric section shows caudate nucleus and putamen in normal adult brain. (Courtesy of Kinuko Suzuki, MD, Tokyo Metropolitan Institute of Gerontology; retired faculty, Department of Pathology and Laboratory Medicine, University of North Carolina, Chapel Hill, NC.)

TRAUMATIC HEAD INJURY

Trauma is a major cause of death and head trauma is contributing factor in a third of these trauma-related deaths. Head trauma may lead to wounds of the scalp, skull fractures, intracranial hematomas, focal brain lesions, and diffuse brain injury. In addition, head trauma may lead to secondary brain injury due to the effects of mass lesions, raised ICP, brain edema, brain ischemia, or infection.

Traumatic brain injury may be due to impact forces or to inertial (acceleration or deceleration) forces that cause brain movement within the skull. Impact forces, such as those associated with a focal, nonpenetrating, blunt-force head injury produce a contact injury and focal brain injury. Acceleration/deceleration forces, such as those associated with a motor-vehicle accident, produce mechanical strain manifested as stretching or shearing of axons and blood vessels and lead to diffuse brain injury. Nonpenetrating head trauma (closed head injury) from a blunt-force injury (contact injury) or acceleration/deceleration injury is more common that penetrating head trauma (missile head trauma).

Epidural Hematoma

An *epidural (extradural) hematoma* is an extra-axial (external to the brain) accumulation of blood between the calvaria (skull cap) and the underlying dura mater. An epidural hematoma is usually associated with a skull fracture and tearing of the middle meningeal artery (Figure 21-43). From a clinical standpoint, the patient may have a lucid interval after the head trauma and then develop neurologic deterioration leading to coma (talk and die syndrome). The hematoma acts as a rapidly enlarging mass lesion and may cause brain shifts and herniation. Epidural hematomas have a better prognosis than subdural hematomas, since the skull absorbs some of the energy and the brain is relatively spared. Approximately 10% of patients with an epidural hematoma die as a direct result of the hematoma.

Subdural Hematoma

A *subdural hematoma* is usually due to tearing of a bridging vein by acceleration/deceleration forces. The bridging veins

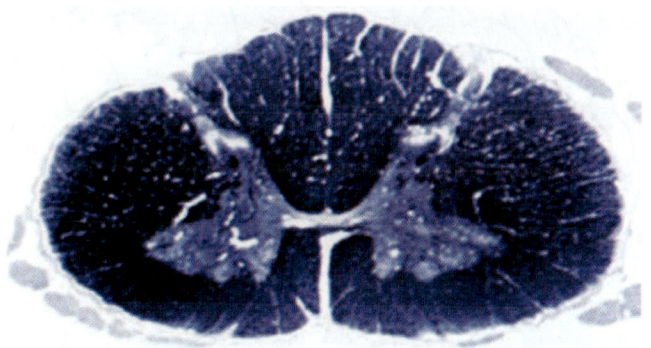

corticospinal tracks, and degeneration of lower motor neurons results in denervation of skeletal muscle (denervation atrophy). ALS is a progressive disease process marked by muscle wasting and weakness, with patients eventually dying from impairment of their respiratory muscles. Despite profound loss of motor function, intellectual capacity usually remains intact. Although familial cases occur, the vast majority of cases are sporadic. Mutations in the superoxide dismutase (SOD1) gene on chromosome 21q are present in a portion of the familial cases.

The defining histologic feature of ALS is loss of motor neurons in three sites: (1) motor cortex of the cerebrum; (2) brain stem motor nuclei, especially the hypoglossal nucleus; and (3) anterior horn cells of the spinal cord (Figure 21-42). Affected neurons often have intracytoplasmic inclusions containing, ubiquitinated proteins. A striking additional microscopic feature is degeneration of the lateral and anterior corticospinal tracts in the spinal cord.

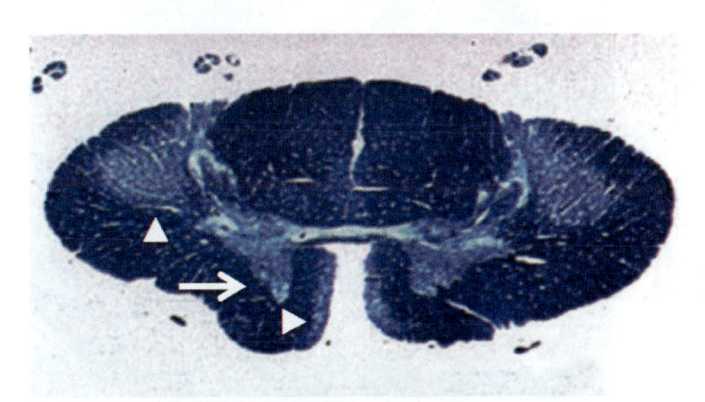

FIGURE 21-42 (Left panel) Cervical spinal cord in amyotrophic lateral sclerosis shows dramatic atrophy of gray matter in anterior horns (arrow) due to loss of motor neurons. The pale-staining areas in the lateral and anterior columns (arrowheads) of the spinal cord reflect the great loss of myelinated axons in the lateral and anterior corticospinal tracts. (Right panel) Normal cervical spinal cord. (Courtesy of Kinuko Suzuki, MD, Tokyo Metropolitan Institute of Gerontology; retired faculty, Department of Pathology and Laboratory Medicine, University of North Carolina, Chapel Hill, NC.)

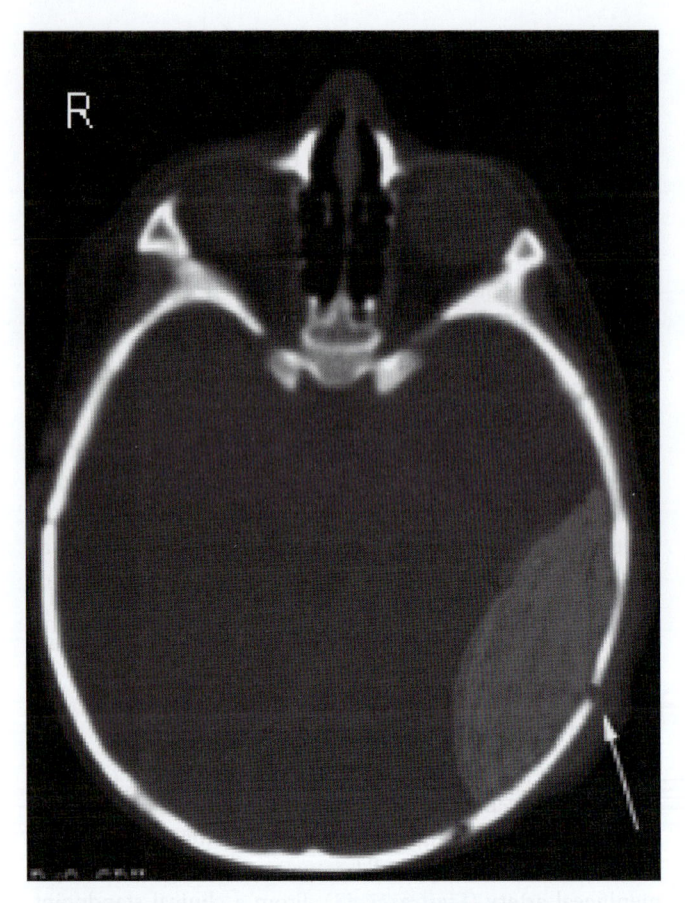

FIGURE 21-43 CT scan shows an epidural hematoma between skull and dura mater. Note fracture (arrow) in the overlying skull, which lacerated the middle meningeal artery.

extend between the arachnoid mater and the dura mater and drain into the dural sinuses. The hematoma acts as an enlarging mass lesion and may lead to brain shifts and herniation. The hematoma may present acutely or chronically. *Acute subdural hematomas* are often associated with substantial underlying brain injuries, including brain contusions and diffuse axonal injury (DAI). Subdural hematomas are more common than epidural hematomas and have a higher mortality rate due to the associated underlying brain injuries.

Tearing of a bridging vein can also lead to a *chronic subdural hematoma*. Chronic subdural hematomas are more commonly found in elderly or alcoholic patients, who have some degree of brain atrophy. The atrophying brain puts extra tension on the bridging veins and makes them more susceptible to tearing. From a clinical standpoint, it is important to note that chronic subdural hematomas are often the result of trivial or forgotten head trauma. Over the course of a few weeks the subdural hematoma undergoes organization and becomes encased by a fibrovascular membrane composed of granulation tissue. As organization proceeds, very small new blood vessels grow into the blood clot. These thin-walled vessels are prone to rupture, leading to additional hemorrhage and enlargement of the subdural hematoma. Chronic subdural hematomas are typically found over the convexities of the cerebral hemispheres, may be bilateral, and may act as mass lesions.

Brain Contusions and Lacerations

A *contusion* is a superficial cortical hemorrhage (bruise). Contusions occur on the crests of gyri that have had a forceful impact with the inner table of the skull. If the force is great, there may be lacerations of the pia mater and underlying brain parenchyma. Microscopically, a contusion is characterized by foci of hemorrhage within the cortex of the brain and a variable amount of brain necrosis (contusion necrosis).

Favored sites for contusions are the frontal and temporal poles, inferior surfaces of the frontal and temporal lobes (Figure 21-44), and cortex above and below Sylvian fissures. Contusions of the occipital lobes and cerebellum are rare unless associated with an overlying skull fractures. The crests of gyri are characteristically involved in brain contusions. In contrast, small cortical infarcts preferentially involve the deeper, perisulcal cortex. Remote contusions are evidenced by

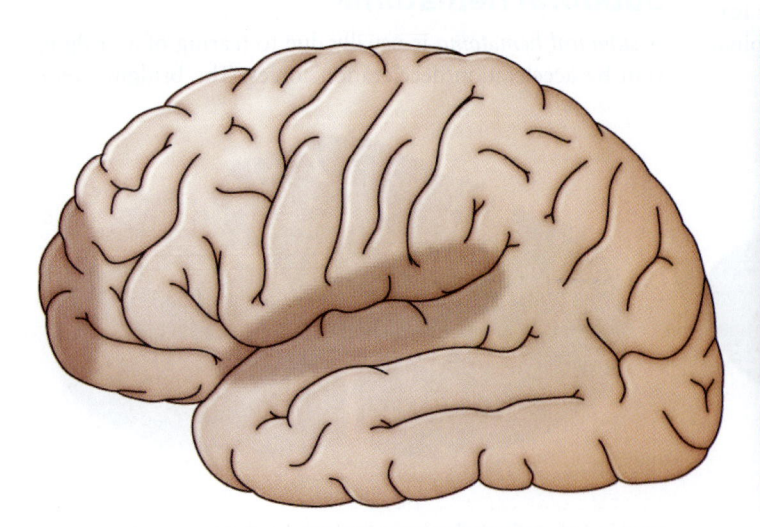

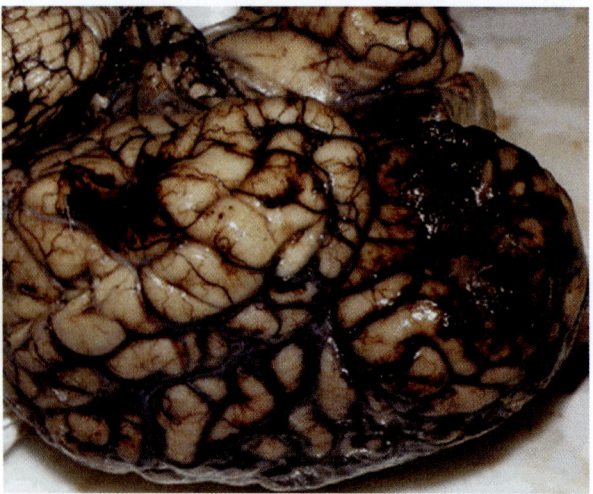

FIGURE 21-44 (Left panel) Schematic diagram showing common sites for brain contusions in the frontal and temporal lobes and around the Sylvian fissure. (Right panel) Lateral view of the brain with acute contusional injury affecting frontal and temporal lobes.

yellow-brown, hemosiderin-stained areas of cortical atrophy. A contusion occurring directly beneath the site of head impact is referred to as a *coup* contusion, while a one occurring at a site opposite the impact is a *contrecoup* contusion. In general, coup contusions are associated with the stationary head being hit by a moving object, whereas contrecoup contusions are associated with the moving head hitting a stationary object.

Intracerebral Hematoma

Intraparenchymal brain hemorrhage indicates severe head injury and suggests that shearing forces have led to diffuse vascular injury. More superficially located intracerebral hemorrhages are usually associated with overlying contusions and are more common in the frontal and temporal lobes. Deeper brain hemorrhages involving the basal ganglia and thalamus are commonly associated with DAI and diffuse vascular injury.

Diffuse Axonal Injury (DAI, Traumatic Axonal Injury)

Diffuse axonal injury (DAI) is the term given to the widespread disruption of axons attributable to shear strains and stretching forces occurring during an acceleration/deceleration injury. Patients who have sustained severe DAI are typically unconscious from the moment of injury, do not experience a lucid period, and remain comatose or severely neurologically disabled until death. DAI is the most common cause of coma in the absence of an intracranial hematoma and the most common cause of severe disability after head injury. Milder degrees of DAI are probably responsible for *concussion*, which is defined as a disturbance in brain function caused by a direct or indirect force to the head. It is important to understand that concussion is a clinical diagnosis and relates to a functional change rather than a morphologic change in the brain.

The gross pathology of DAI and diffuse vascular injury includes focal hemorrhages in the corpus callosum (Figure 21-45) and dorsolateral quadrants of the rostral brain stem (region of the superior cerebellar peduncles). Microscopically, the damaged axons develop axonal swellings.

Complications of Traumatic Head Injury

Epidural, subdural, and intracerebral hematomas are mass lesions and can cause increased ICP, brain shifts, and brain herniation. Vasogenic edema occurs with brain contusions and intracerebral hematomas and may contribute significantly to the mass effect (Figure 21-46). Vasogenic edema also occurs with DAI and leads to raised ICP and the possibility of global brain ischemia secondary to decreased CPP. Trauma may also lead to systemic hypotension, cardiorespiratory arrest, or status epilepticus, which may also contribute to ischemic brain damage.

Other complications of traumatic head injury include infection, as meningitis may occur as a complication of an open fracture and brain abscess may occur with a penetrating injury. Repetitive brain injury may be associated with *chronic traumatic encephalopathy*, a progressive neurodegenerative disease with neurofibrillary tangles.

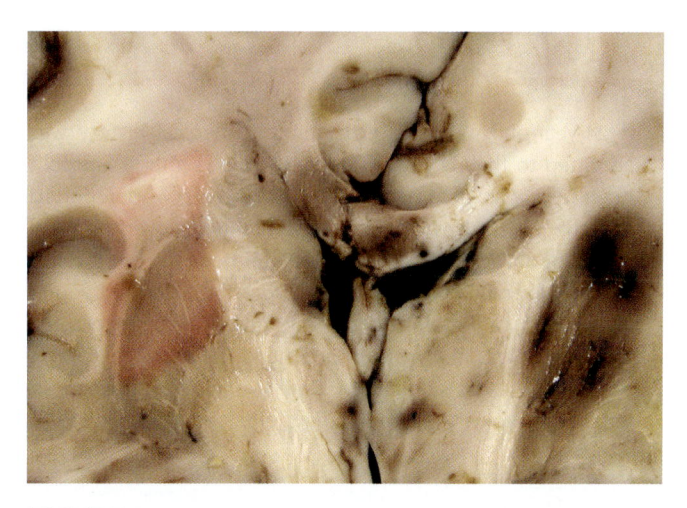

FIGURE 21-45 Diffuse axonal injury and diffuse vascular injury are evidenced by small hemorrhages in the corpus callosum and basal ganglia.

Nonaccidental Head Injury (NAHI, Shaken Baby Syndrome, Abusive Head Trauma)

QUICK REVIEW

Each year in the United States, over 79,000 children are victims of physical abuse and some 2000 children die from abuse. These numbers are almost certainly an underestimate,

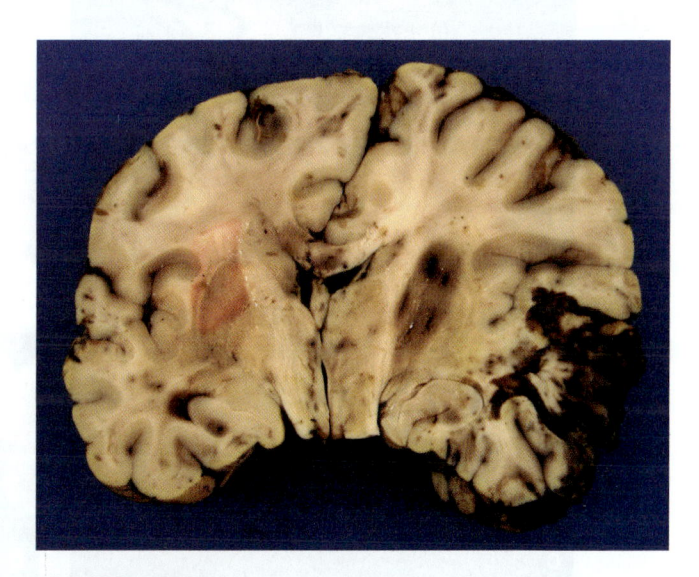

FIGURE 21-46 (same case as in Figure 21-45) The severe traumatic brain injury is associated with contusions of the temporal lobe and prominent vasogenic brain edema. The mass effect of the contusions and brain edema has resulted in subfalcian (cingulate gyrus) herniation.

CASE PRESENTATION: Acute Subdural Hematoma

A 24-year-old man with no significant medical history was admitted to the ED with acute head trauma after a barroom brawl. He was accompanied by his friends who reported that the patient had been struck several times over the head with a pool stick, and shortly thereafter began acting "weird." Physical examination in the ED revealed a lethargic young male, who was intermittently responsive to commands. As the patient was in transport for a head CT, acute neurologic deterioration was signified by rapidly diminishing alertness, left-sided pupillary dilatation, and left-sided hemiplegia. An emergency craniotomy was performed. Despite all medical efforts, the patient died in the neurosurgery recovery area. The postmortem findings are shown in Figure 21-47.

This case provides an excellent example of clinical–pathologic correlation. The patient's left-sided pupillary dilation relates to the herniating left uncus compressing the left oculomotor (III) nerve. In addition, the patient's left-sided paralysis relates to the left-to-right shift of the midbrain compressing the right cerebral peduncle against the free edge of the tentorium.

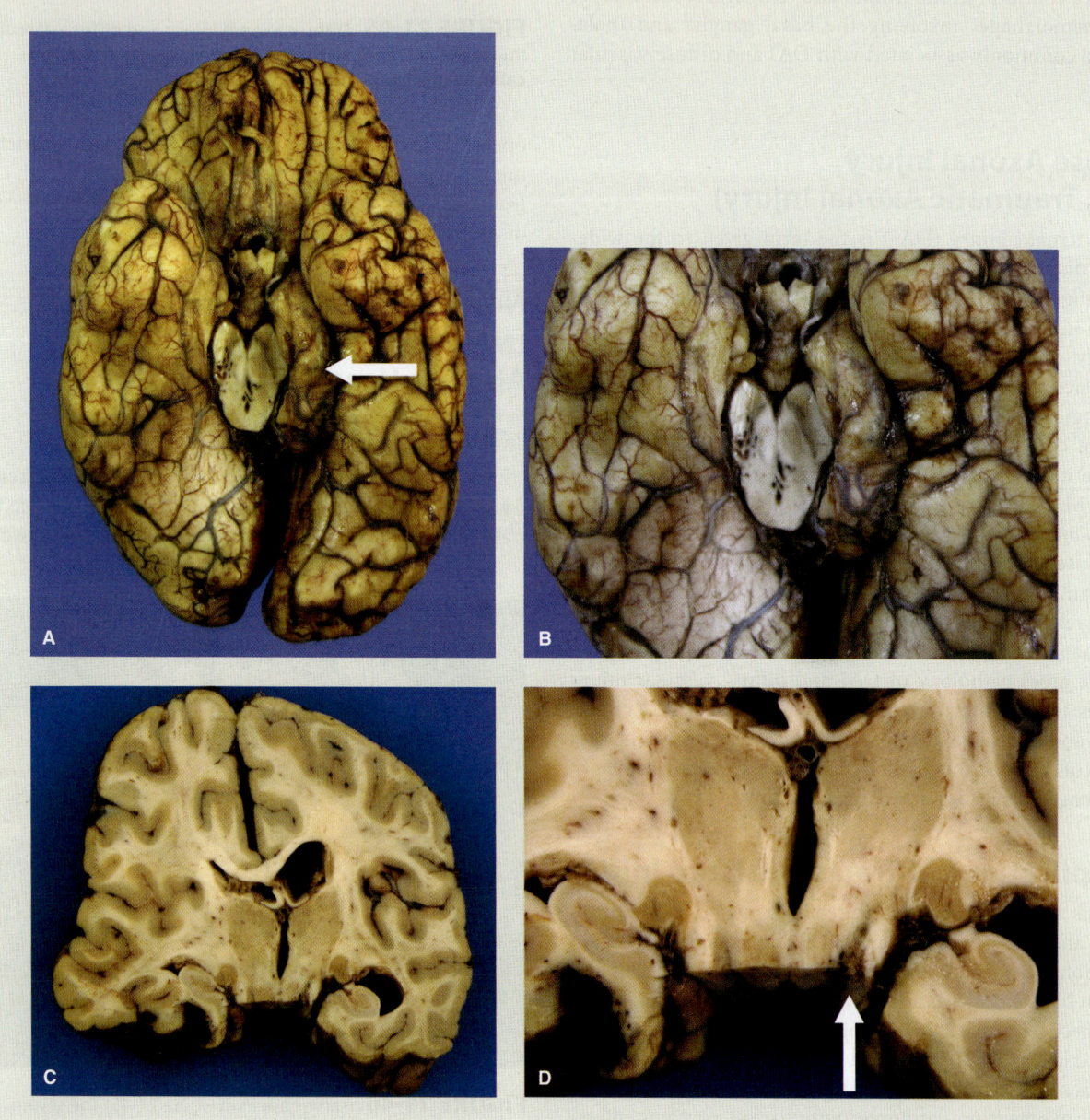

FIGURE 21-47 Acute subdural hematoma. **(A)** Note severe brain swelling with left-sided uncal and parahippocampal-gyrus herniation (arrow). **(B)** Close-up showing the herniation and secondary midbrain hemorrhages. **(C)** Coronal section showing compression of the brain caused by a left-sided subdural hematoma. The mass has caused a left-to-right midline shift, left subfalcine herniation, and left uncal herniation. **(D)** The left uncal herniation and resultant left-to-right midbrain shift caused necrosis and hemorrhage in the midbrain's right cerebral peduncle (arrow).

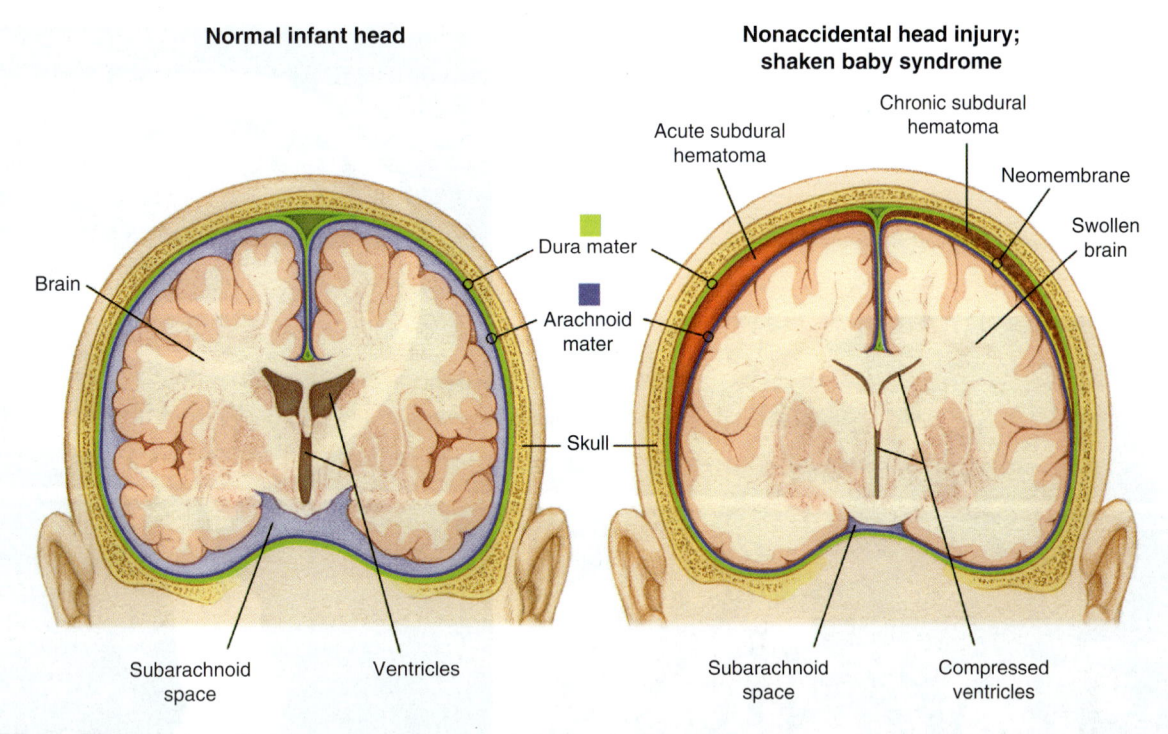

FIGURE 21-48 (Left) Normal infant head. (Right) Pathologic findings in shaken baby syndrome. (Copyright 2009, Lauren Keswick, MS, Medical Illustration, *Medicalartstudio.com*.)

since cases go unreported or unrecognized. The most recent American Academy of Pediatrics and American College of Radiology practice guidelines recommend that all clinicians should maintain a low threshold for performing CT and MRI of the head in all cases of suspected child abuse.

The clinical findings of shaken baby syndrome (SBS) include acute subdural hemorrhage, acute encephalopathy, and multiple retinal hemorrhages in a child less than 2 years of age. The pathology of SBS consists of the triad of acute subdural hemorrhage, diffusely swollen brain, and multiple retinal hemorrhages **(Figure 21-48)**.

There is controversy over the pathogenesis of the traumatic brain injury. Some experts believe that shaking alone can cause this syndrome and prefer the term SBS **(Figure 21-49)**. Other authorities believe that the shaking injury must always be accompanied by a focal blunt force (impact) injury

FIGURE 21-49 Shaken baby syndrome. (Copyright 2009, Lauren Keswick, MS, Medical Illustration, *Medicalartstudio.com*.)

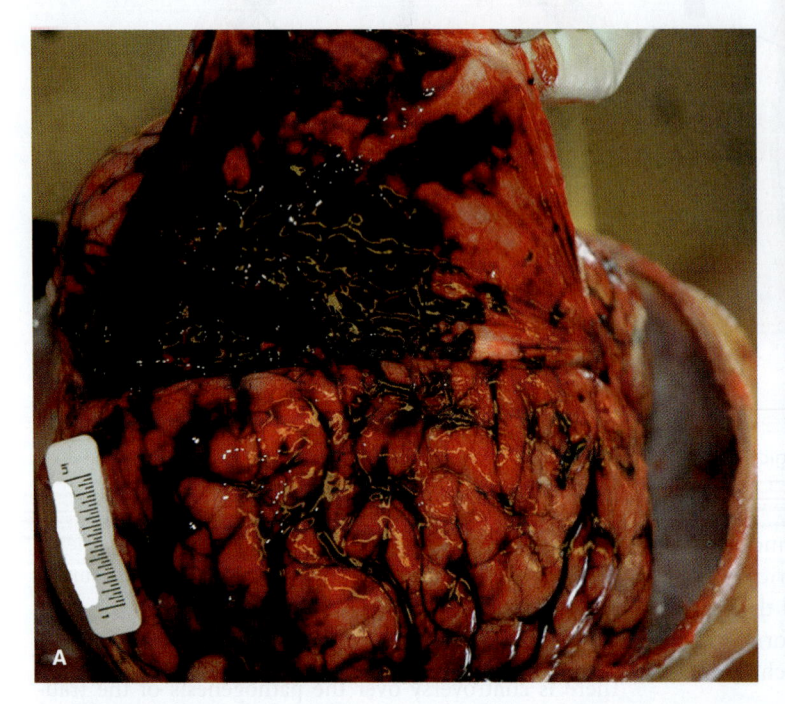

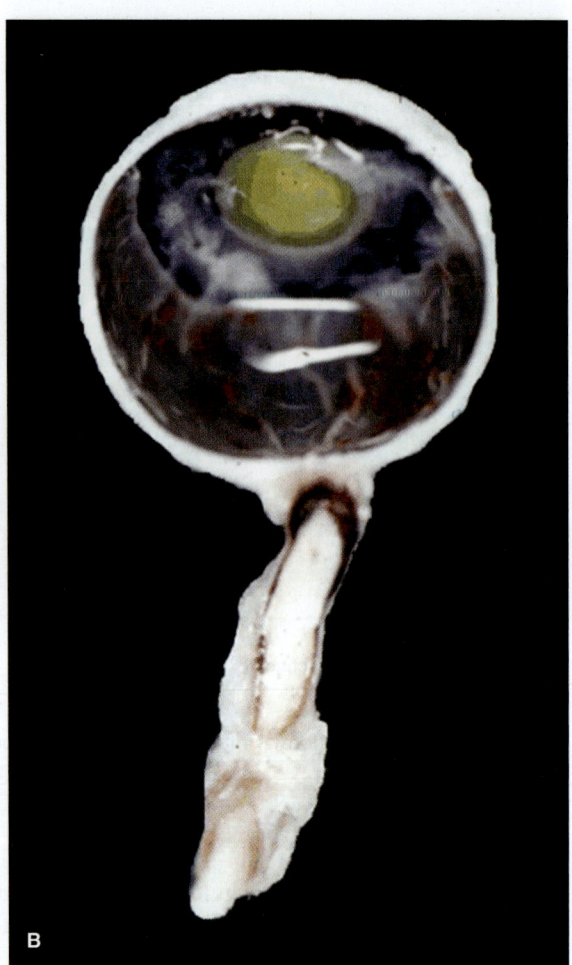

FIGURE 21-50 Acute subdural hematoma **(A)** and retinal hemorrhages **(B)** characterize the shaken baby syndrome. (Courtesy of Bill Holloman and Clay Nichols, MD, Office of the Chief Medical Examiner, University of North Carolina, Chapel Hill, NC.)

to produce the characteristic lesions and prefer the designation of shaking impact syndrome. There is also controversy concerning the underlying cause of the brain injury and encephalopathy. Some authorities believe that DAI, a consequence of acceleration/deceleration forces, is responsible for the encephalopathy. Other authorities believe that diffuse brain ischemia is the principal cause of the encephalopathy. In any event, it is the brain damage, not the acute subdural hematoma, which is responsible for the acute encephalopathy and death of the infant (**Figure 21-50**).

CASE PRESENTATION: Shaken Baby Syndrome

A 6-month-old infant was brought to the ED by the mother's boyfriend who contended that the baby "was not acting right." Upon questioning, the boyfriend stated that, earlier in the day, while the mother was at work, the infant "rolled off the changing table." After feeding the baby, the caretaker stated that he "put the infant down for his nap." Several hours later the boyfriend found the infant nonresponsive. In the ER, the infant was obtunded with no external signs of trauma. A head CT was ordered and showed brain swelling with diffuse hypoxic-ischemic injury and acute subdural hemorrhage. Despite medical intervention, the infant expired 12 hours later in the neonatal intensive care unit. Neuropathologic evaluation revealed the findings shown in Figure 21-50.

Reflection of the dura mater revealed acute subdural hemorrhage and diffuse brain edema (A) and hemisection of an eye showed acute retinal hemorrhages (B). In some cases of SBS, one also finds evidence of chronic subdural hemorrhage, which reflects previous episodes of head trauma.

Index

Note: Page numbers followed by 't' and 'f' indicate tables and figures, respectively.

A

AAA. See Abdominal aortic aneurysm (AAA)
α2-antiplasmin, 83
ABC. See Aneurysmal bone cyst (ABC)
Abdominal aortic aneurysm (AAA), 177
ABPA. See Allergic bronchopulmonary aspergillosis (ABPA)
Abrasions, 98, 99f
Absolute neutrophil count (ANC), 360
Abusers administering drugs, 109
Acetaminophen toxicity, 110
Achondroplasia, 507
Acid-fast bacillus (AFB), 393
Acquired myopathies, 521
Acquired stenosis, 205
Acral myxoinflammatory fibroblastic sarcoma, 492
Acromegaly, 392
ACTH. See Adrenocorticotropin hormone (ACTH)
Activated partial thromboplastin time (aPTT), 58
Activation transcription factor 2 (ATF-2), 27
Active colitis, 260, 261f
Active surveillance, 348
Acute antibody-mediated rejection, 325–326
Acute appendicitis, 268–269, 269f
Acute bacterial leptomeningitis, 561f
Acute bacterial meningitis, 558
Acute cell-mediated rejection, 324–325
Acute cholecystitis, 285
Acute coronary syndrome, 178–179
Acute disseminated encephalomyelitis (ADEM), 569–570
Acute hemorrhagic gastritis, 246, 248
Acute inflammation
 cellular phase of, 47
  diapedesis and, 61
  endothelial cell–neutrophil interactions, 62–63, 62f
  LAD syndromes and, 63–64
  PAMPs and DAMPs, 61
  paracellular migration and, 61
 definition of, 47
 resolution of, 70
 time course and degree of persistence, 47
 vascular phase of, 47
  AA derivatives, 52, 54f
  basophils, 51, 53f
  chemokines, 61
  complement system, 58, 59f, 60–61
  histamine and mast cells, 50–51, 51f
  leukotirenes, 56–57, 56f
  nitric oxide, 57–58
  physical and cardinal signs, 48–49
  plasma contact system, 58, 58f
  platelet-activating factor, 57, 57f
  platelets, 52, 54f
  prostanoids, 52–56
  tissue edema, 49–50

Acute kidney injury (AKI), 321
Acute leukemias, 370–376, 371t
 of ambiguous lineage, 376
Acute mastitis, 422
Acute monocytic leukemia, 372, 374
Acute myeloid leukemias (AML), 372, 375
Acute pancreatitis, 291, 291f
Acute pericarditis, 215–216
Acute phase reactants, 70–71
Acute postinfectious glomerulonephritis, 310–311, 311f
Acute promyelocytic leukemia (APL), 372, 373
Acute prostatitis, 344
Acute rheumatic fever, 207–208
Acute subdural hematomas, 576, 579f
Acute suppurative thyroiditis, 410
Acute tubulointerstitial nephritis, 322–323, 323f
AD. See Alzheimer disease (AD)
Adaptive immunity, 43
Addiction to illicit drugs, 109
ADEM. See Acute disseminated encephalomyelitis (ADEM)
Adenocarcinoma in situ (AIS), 452, 453f
 of cervix, 452, 453f
Adenocarcinomas, 32, 220, 245, 246f, 250–251, 251f, 257, 258f, 333
Adenoid cystic carcinoma, 221
Adenomatous polyps, 265–266, 266f
Adenovirus, 229, 229f
ADH. See Antidiuretic hormone (ADH)
Adipose tissue, 469, 470f
Adrenal cortex, 396, 397f
Adrenal medulla, 403–404
Adrenocorticotropin hormone (ACTH), 394
Adrenoleukodystrophy (ALD), 571
Adult lung
 anatomy, 217
 physiology, 217–218
Adult respiratory distress syndrome (ARDS), 234
AFB. See Acid-fast bacillus (AFB)
Aging
 cellular senescence and telomere decay, 85–86
 definition of, 85
 factors in
  DNA damage, 86–89, 88f
  endogenous mutagens, 89
 and nutrition, 90–91
AHO. See Albright hereditary osteodystrophy (AHO)
AITD. See Autoimmune thyroid diseases (AITD)
AKI. See Acute kidney injury (AKI)
Albright hereditary osteodystrophy (AHO), 416
Alcoholic liver disease (ALD), 276, 277f
Alcohols toxicity, 110–111
ALD. See Adrenoleukodystrophy (ALD); Alcoholic liver disease (ALD)

Aldosterone, 396, 398
ALH. See Atypical lobular hyperplasia (ALH)
Allergic bronchopulmonary aspergillosis (ABPA), 226
Alpha 1-antitrypsin deficiency, 280, 280f
Alpha-defensins, 68
Alpha-fetoprotein (AFP), 337, 338
Alport syndrome, 315
ALS. See Amyotrophic lateral sclerosis (ALS)
Alveolar ducts, 217
Alveolar rhabdomyosarcomas, 486–487
Alzheimer disease, 14
Alzheimer disease (AD), 572, 573f
AMA. See Antimitochondrial antibodies (AMA)
Amyloidosis, 303
Amyloid precursor protein (APP), 14
Amyotrophic lateral sclerosis (ALS), 574–575
Anaphylactoid purpura, 163
Anaphylotoxins, 60
Anaplastic thyroid carcinoma (ATC), 414
Anasarca, 299
ANC. See Absolute neutrophil count (ANC)
ANCA. See Antineutrophil cytoplasmic autoantibody (ANCA)
ANCA glomerulonephritis, 313–314, 314f
 eosinophilic granulomatosis with polyangiitis, 314
 granulomatosis with polyangiitis, 314
 microscopic polyangiitis, 314
 renal limited, 314
Androgen-independent prostate, 349
Anemias, 357–359, 358t
 causes, 358t
 Copper-deficiency, 360
 iron-deficiency, 358, 358f
 refractory, 359, 359f
Aneurysmal bone cyst (ABC), 505
Angelman syndrome, 15
Angelman syndrome gene (UBE3A), 15
Angina pectoris, 23
 preinfarction, 179
 prinzmetal or variant, 179
 stable or typical, 178–179
 unstable or crescendo, 179
Angiogenesis, 71
Angiolipomas, 471
Angiomyoma, 482
Angiosarcoma, 392, 477f, 478–479, 541, 541f
Anterior (adenohypophysis), 387
Anthracotic pigment in lung, 33, 34f
Antidiuretic hormone (ADH), 394
Anti-GBM glomerulonephritis, 312–313
Anti-inflammatories, 42
Antimitochondrial antibodies (AMA), 279
Antineutrophil cytoplasmic autoantibody (ANCA), 157, 305
Antithrombin (AT), 84
Anxiolytics, adverse effects of, 109–110

595

Aortic dissection
  classification
  complications, 155
  DeBakey classification, 153–154
  histology, 154, 155f
  pathology, 154
  Sanford classification, 153
  surgical treatment, 155
  symptoms, 153
Aortitis
  noninfectious, 155
  Takayasu disease, 155–156, 156f
Apoptosis, 43
  molecular mechanisms of, 40, 42f
    caspases, 41
    extrinsic pathway, 41
    granzyme B (CTl) pathway, 41, 42
    intrinsic pathway, 41
  vs. necrosis, 34, 40
  suppression of, 43
Apoptotic bodies, 41f
APP. See Amyloid precursor protein (APP)
Appendix
  anatomy, 268
  diseases
    acute appendicitis, 268–269, 269f
    goblet cell carcinoids, 269
    neoplasms, 269
    neuroendocrine tumors, 269–270
    pseudomyxoma peritonei, 269
  histology, 268
Arachidonic acid (AA) derivatives, 52, 54f
ARDS. See Adult respiratory distress syndrome (ARDS)
Arrhythmogenic right ventricular cardiomyopathy (ARVC), 201
Arsenic exposure, 112
Arterial occlusion and brain ischemia, 562t
Arteries, 147–149
Arterioles, 149
Arteriolosclerosis, 166
Arteriovenous fistula, 150
Arteriovenous malformation (AVM), 150–151, 152f
Arthritis, 507
Arthropod-associated lesions (scabies), 551, 551f
ARVC. See Arrhythmogenic right ventricular cardiomyopathy (ARVC)
ASCAD. See Atherosclerotic CAD (ASCAD)
ASCHD. See Atherosclerotic coronary heart disease (ASCHD)
ASCVD. See Atherosclerotic cardiovascular disease (ASCVD)
ASD. See Atrial septal defect (ASD)
Aspergilloma, 226
Aspergillus, 226
Asphyxia, 104–105
  blood circulation, compromise of, 104
  breathing, compromise of, 104
  cellular respiration, compromise of, 105
  drowning, 105
  oxygen-deficient environments, 105
  pathological findings in, 105
Asphyxiation, 110
Asthma, 229–230
Astrocytes and oligodendrocytes, 553–554, 553f
Asymptomatic hematuria, 305

ATC. See Anaplastic thyroid carcinoma (ATC)
Atheroembolization, 320, 320f
Atheromas, 170
  initiation and formation phase, 170
Atherosclerosis, 23, 170, 320
Atherosclerotic CAD (ASCAD), 178
Atherosclerotic cardiovascular disease (ASCVD), 178
Atherosclerotic coronary heart disease (ASCHD), 178
Atherosclerotic (or atherothrombotic) lesions, 171–173
Atherosclerotic plaque. See atheromas
Atherothrombosis, 170
Athlete "pumping iron," 25
Atrial septal defect (ASD), 189, 191–192
  caval, 192
  ostium secundum, 192
Atrioventricular (AV) node, 180, 180f
Atrioventricular valves, 180
Atrogin1, 30
Atrophic gastritis, 248–249, 249f
Atrophy
  and autophagy, 30
  definition of, 25, 28
  factors in development of, 28f
  molecular mechanisms of, 28–30, 29f
  pathological, 28
  physiological, 28
Atypical carcinoid tumors, 221
Atypical fibrous histiocytoma, 481
Atypical hyperplasias, 428, 429f
Atypical lipomatous tumor (ALT), 472, 472t, 473f
Atypical lobular hyperplasia (ALH), 428
Autocrine, 385
Autoimmune gastritis, 249
Autoimmune hepatitis, 277, 277f
Autoimmune hypoparathyroidism, 416
Autoimmune thyroid diseases (AITD), 409
Autophagolysosomes, 33
Autophagy, and atrophy, 30
Autopsy
  pathologists, 121
  pathology, 122
Autosomal dominant disorders, 11
  inheritance patterns associated with, 11f
Autosomal recessive disorders, 11–12
  inheritance patterns associated with, 11f
Autosomes, in cytogenetic disorders, 13
Autosplenectomy, 390
Avascular necrosis, 505
AVM. See Arteriovenous malformation (AVM)
Avulsions, 99
Azurocidin, 68

B
BAC. See Bronchioloalveolar carcinomas (BAC)
Bacterial pneumonias, 225–226
Bactericidal permeability increasing (BPI) protein, 68
BAD. See Bicuspid aortic disease (BAD)
Balanitis, 340
Balanitis xerotica obliterans, 340, 340f, 545
Barrett esophagus (BE), 31, 244, 244f

Barrett metaplasia, molecular mechanisms of, 32–33
Basal cell carcinoma, 531
Basal cells, 526
Basal plasmacytosis, 260
Basophils, 51, 53f
B-cell lymphoma, 542, 542f
BCR–ABL1, 131, 134
BE. See Barrett esophagus (BE)
Beckwith–Wiedemann syndrome, 15
Beer drinker's cardiomyopathy, 201
Behçet disease, 164–165
Benign adipocytic tumors, 471–472
Benign bone-forming tumors, 497
Benign epithelial lesions
  columnar cell lesions, 425, 427
  fibrocystic change, 424, 424f, 425f
  papillary lesions, 427–428
  radial scar/complex sclerosing lesion, 427
  sclerosing adenosis, 425
Benign fibrous histiocytoma, 481, 481f
Benign neoplasms, 280
Benign peripheral nerve tumors, 488–490
Benign proliferative lesions, 331–332
Benign prostatic hyperplasia (BPH), 344–345
Benign vascular tumors, 477–478
  vs. malignant vascular lesions, 477t
Berry aneurysm, 149–150, 151f
Beta-amyloid protein, 574f
Beta-human choriogonadotropin (β-HCG), 337, 338
Bicuspid aortic disease (BAD), 155
Bile canaliculi, 273
Bile duct adenocarcinoma, 285
Biomechanical stress sensors, 27
Bladder cancer, 332
Bleeding disorders, 82t
Blood vessels, 147, 147f
  arteries, 147–149
  capillary system, 149
  lymphatics, 149
  pulmonary vasculature, 149
Bloom syndrome, 18
Blunt injury, 98–99
  abrasions, 98, 99f
  avulsions, 99
  bruises, 98, 98f
  fractures, 99
  lacerations, 98, 99f
B lymphoblastic leukemia (B-ALL), 372, 376
Bone and joint pathology
  bone organization, 495
  histology, 495–496, 495f
  lesions of bone, 496
Borrelia burgdorferi, 200
Botryoid-type rhabdomyosarcoma, 486
Bowel wall, at site of injury, 97f
Bowen disease, 341
BPH. See Benign prostatic hyperplasia (BPH)
Bradykinin (BK), 58, 58f
Brain abscess, 559
Brain atrophy in neurodegenerative disease, 29, 29f
Brain contusions, 576–577
Brain death, 21–22
Brain edema, 555–556
Brain hemorrhage, 562–563, 563f, 563t

Brain infarct, 561–562, 562f
Brain metastases, 567–568, 568f
Breast, indurated lesion on, 38f
Breast cancer predisposition syndromes, 430–433
Breast pathology
　anatomy, 419, 420f
　benign breast disease
　　atypical hyperplasias, 428–429
　　epithelial lesions, 424–428
　　fibroepithelial lesions, 429–430
　　gynecomastia, 430
　　inflammatory lesions, 421–424
　carcinoma
　　assessing tumor biology, 439–440
　　definitions, 430
　　ductal carcinoma in situ, 433–434, 433f
　　epidemiology, 430
　　invasive mammary carcinomas, 435
　　lobular carcinoma in situ, 434–435
　　microinvasive carcinoma, 435
　　paget disease, 434
　　predictive factors, 439–440
　　prognostic factors, 438, 439t
　　risk factors, 430–433, 431t
　clinical evaluation, 420, 422t
　clinical symptoms, 420–421, 422t
　histology, 419
　introduction, 419
Bronchiectasis, 226, 231
Bronchioles, 217
Bronchioloalveolar carcinomas (BAC), 220
Bronchopneumonia, 226
Brown tumor, 417
Bruises, 98, 98f
　abdominal, 97f
　"tramline," 98f
Brunn buds, 331
Brunn nests, 331
Burkitt lymphoma, 397, 397f
Burns, 114–115, 115f
　electrical, 117f
　first-degree, 114
　second-degree, 114
　third-degree, 114–115
　water temperature effects on skin, 115f

C

Cachexia, 28
Caenorhabditis elegans, 7
Calcific aortic stenosis, 20–206
Calcineurin signaling, 27
Calcitonin, 405
Calcium concentration, and necrosis, 36
Calcium sensing receptor (CaSR), 416
Calf hypertrophy, 519f
Caliectasis, 322
Call-Exner bodies, 442
Calpain activation, 36
Campylobacter, 261
Campylobacter-like organism (CLO) testing, 246
Cancer
　associated with faulty DNA repair mechanisms, 17
　DNA hypermethylation in, 18
　DNA hypomethylation in, 18
　epigenetics of, 18–19
　　genetics interplay with, 19
　familial. *See* Familial cancer
　histone modifications in, 19
　nonfamilial, 17
Cancer susceptibility genes, 16–17
　CDK4 gene, 16
　CDKN2A gene, 16
　inherited mutations in, 16–17
　Rb1 gene, 16–17
Candida albicans, 444, 444f
Candida esophagitis, 242–243, 243f
Capillary hemangioma, 151, 152f
Capillary system, 149
Carbon monoxide exposure, 112
Carcinoid heart disease, 213
Carcinosarcoma, 458
Cardiac hypertrophy
　factors in development of, 28f
　molecular mechanisms of
　　clinical significance, 26
　　initial signals of, 27
　　signaling pathways, 27–28, 28f
Cardiac myocytes
　coagulative necrosis of, 23, 23f
　infiltration of infarct, 24, 24f
　normal and hypertrophic, 23f
Cardiac myxoma, 213–214
Cardiac rhabdomyoma, 486
Cardiac sarcomas, 214–215
Cardiac tamponade, 215
Cardiogenic shock, 183
Cardiovascular system, 147
Cartilaginous tumors, 497–500
Caseating granulomatous necrosis, 38
Caseous necrosis, 40, 40f
CaSR. *See* Calcium sensing receptor (CaSR)
Casts, 37
Cathelicidins (hCAP-18), 68
Cationic peptides, 68
Caval ASDs, 192
Cavernous hemangioma, 151, 152f
CBG. *See* Cortisol-binding globulin (CBG)
CD. *See* Celiac disease (CD)
CDK4 gene, 16
CDKN2A gene, 16
Celiac disease (CD), 254, 255, 255f
Cell death, 21–22
　and inflammation, 42–43
　mechanisms of, 42
　　apoptosis. *See* Apoptosis
　　necroptosis. *See* Necroptosis
　　necrosis. *See* Necrosis
　　pyroptosis. *See* Pyroptosis
　significance of, 42–43
Cell injury
　mechanisms of, 33–36
　and necrosis. *See* Necrosis
　overview, 21–22
　reversible, 22–33
　tissue ischemia, 33
Cell swelling, 33, 34f
Cellular senescence and telomere decay, 85–86
Central dogma, of molecular biology, 1–2, 2f
Ceroid (lipofuscin), 30, 33
Cervical intraepithelial neoplasia 1 (CIN 1), 450f, 451
Cervical intraepithelial neoplasia 2 (CIN 2), 451, 451f
Cervical intraepithelial neoplasia 2 (CIN 3), 451, 452f
Cervical metaplasia, 32, 32f
Cervix, formation of transformation zone in, 32, 32f
C1 esterase inhibitor (C1NH), 60
CF. *See* Cystic fibrosis (CF)
CFTR gene, 134
Chaperone-mediated autophagy, 30
Charcot-Leyden crystals, 230
Chargaff rule, 3
Chemical injury, 94, 108–113
　air pollutants and, 112
　carbon monoxide, exposure to, 111
　cyanide salts, exposure to, 111–112
　drugs and medications, 108–112
　　abusers administering drugs, 109
　　acetaminophen, 110
　　addiction to illicit drugs, 109
　　alcohols, 110–111
　　anxiolytics, 109–110
　　cocaine, 109
　　erythema multiforme associated with, 108
　　hallucinogens, 110
　　inhalants, 110
　　methamphetamine, 109
　　narcotic analgesics, 109
　　stimulants, 109
　heavy metals, exposure to, 112
　insecticides, exposure to, 112
　occupational chemical exposure, 112
　substance exposure, 112
　testing for toxic agents in, 113
　tobacco use and, 111
　toxins of natural origin and, 112–113
Chemokine, 61
　synthesis and release, 51
Cherry angiomas, 477
"Chicken-wire" pattern, 500
Chief cells, 415, 416f
Childbirth, uterine involution following, 29, 29f
cHL. *See* Classical hodgkin lymphoma (cHL)
Chlamydia, 161
Cholangiocarcinoma, 282–283, 283f
Cholecystitis, 284
Cholelithiasis, 284
Cholestasis, 278, 278f
Cholesterol stones, 284, 285f
Chondroblastoma, 500
Chondrosarcoma, 497, 498, 499, 499f
Chop injury, 99
Chordae tendineae, 180
Chordoma, 505
Choriocarcinoma, 338–339, 468, 468f
Chorionic villi, 465
Choroid plexus epithelium, 554, 554f
Chromosomal deletion, 6
Chronic active colitis, 261
Chronic cholecystitis, 285, 285f
Chronic colitis, 260–261, 261f
Chronic gastritis, 248
Chronic granulomatous disease (CGD), 68, 226
　and NADPH oxidase, 69–70
Chronic granulomatous inflammation, 71, 72

Chronic inflammation, 43, 73f
  characterization of, 71
  definition of, 47
  and granulomas, 47
  macrophages in, 72–74
  persistent response, 71–72
  time course and degree of persistence, 47
Chronic lymphocytic leukemia, 365, 366
Chronic meningitis, 558–559
Chronic myelogenous leukemia (CML), 362–363, 364
Chronic myelomonocytic leukemia (CMML), 67
Chronic pancreatitis, 291–292, 292f
Chronic passive congestion, 273, 274
Chronic prostatitis, 343, 343f, 344
Chronic rejection, 326
Churg–Strauss syndrome (CSS), 162, 314
Cigarette smoking, 174–175
Circumflex artery, 182
Cirrhosis, 75, 75f, 273, 274f
Classical hodgkin lymphoma (cHL), 386–388
Clerical error, 124
Clinical Laboratory Improvement Act of 1988 (CLIA), 138
Clostridium difficile enterocolitis, 261–262, 262f
Clostridium perfringens, 93
Clostridium tetani, 93
CML. *See* Chronic myelogenous leukemia (CML)
CMML. *See* Chronic myelomonocytic leukemia (CMML)
CMV. *See* Cytomegalovirus (CMV)
Coagulation cascade, 80–81, 81f
  endothelium role in regulation of, 84, 85
  extrinsic pathway, 80
  intrinsic pathway, 58, 80–81
Coagulation disorders, 82t
  and bleeding disorders, 82t
  DIC, 81–82
  hemophilia A and B, 82
  vitamin K deficiency, 81
Coagulation factor deficiencies, 82t
Coagulative necrosis and hemorrhage, 38, 39f
Coarctation of aorta, 197–199
Cocaine toxicity, 109
Cockayne syndrome group B (CSB), 89
Cognitive error, 124
Colloid, 405
Colloid cyst, 567
Colon
  anatomy, 258–259, 259f
  colorectal carcinogenesis
    adenocarcinoma, 267, 268f
  diseases
    active colitis, 260, 262f
    chronic colitis, 260–261, 261f
    Clostridium difficile enterocolitis, 261–262, 262f
    Crohn disease, 264–265, 264f
    developmental disorders, 260
    diverticular disease, 262–263
    Hirschsprung disease, 260, 260f
    infectious colitis, 261, 262f
    inflammatory bowel disease, 263
    inflammatory disorders, 260
    ischemic colitis, 262–263f
    ulcerative colitis, 263–264
  histology, 258–259

  polyps and neoplasms
    adenomatous polyps, 265–266, 266f
    hamartomatous polyps, 265, 266f
    inflammatory polyps, 265
    precursor lesions, 265
    serrated polyps, 267, 267f
  Colorectal adenocarcinoma, 267–268, 268f
  Columnar cell lesions, 425, 426f, 427
Combined hepatocellular–cholangiocarcinoma, 283
Combined pituitary hormone deficiency (CPHD), 390
Comedo formation, 546
Complement deficiencies, 60–61
Complement system
  activation pathways, 58–60, 59f
  functions of, 58
  products activity, 60
  regulation of, 60
Complicated plaques, 173
Condyloma acuminatum, 341, 341f
Condyloma lata, 341
Congenital adrenal hyperplasia, 403
Congenital aortic stenosis, 199
Congenital aortic valve stenosis, 199
Congenital atresia, 334
Congenital heart disease
  cardiac septation defects, 189
  noncyanotic congenital heart disease
    atrial septal defect, 191–192
    patent foramen ovale, 191
    truncus arteriosus, 196
    ventricular septal defect, 190–191, 191f
  obstructive congenital anomalies, 196
    coarctation of aorta, 197–199
    congenital aortic stenosis, 199
    congenital aortic valve stenosis, 199
    supravalvar aortic stenosis, 199–200
  terminology and concepts, 190
Congenitally abnormal aortic valve disease, 155
Congenitally bicuspid aortic valve, 206
Congenital megaureter, 334
Congenital melanocytic nevus, 535
Congenital myopathies, 518
Congenital vascular anomalies
  arteriovenous malformation, 150–151
  berry aneurysm, 149–150, 151f
Congestive cardiomyopathy, 200
Congo red staining, 523f
Connective tissue framework, 379
Constrictive pericarditis, 216
Contusions, 98
Core biopsies, 420
Cornified layer (stratum corneum), 527
Coronary arteries, 177–178
Coronary atherosclerosis, smoking and, 111
Cortex, 379
Cortical infarct, 561f
Corticotropin-releasing hormone (CRH), 394
Cortisol, 398
Cortisol-binding globulin (CBG), 398
COX isoforms, 53
CpG islands, 7
  containing genes, 7f
CPHD. *See* Combined pituitary hormone deficiency (CPHD)
Craniopharyngiomas, 395

Crescent, 308
CREST syndrome, 401
Cretinism, 409
CRH. *See* Corticotropin-releasing hormone (CRH)
Crista supraventricularis, 190
Crohn disease, 256, 264–265, 264f-265f
Cryopyrinopathies, 46
Crypt abscess, 260
Cryptitis, 260
Cryptococcus, 226
Cryptorchidism, 336
Crystals of Reinke, 340
CSS. *See* Churg–Strauss syndrome (CSS)
CST6. *See* Cystatin *(CST6)*
Cullen sign, 291
Curschmann spirals, 230, 230f
Cushing syndrome
  definition, 400
  diagnosis, 401
  etiological categories, 400–401
Cyanide exposure, 111–112
Cyanosis, 190
Cyclic neutropenia, 362
Cystatin *(CST6)*, 7
Cystic fibrosis (CF), 230–231, 231f
Cystic medial necrosis, 154, 154f
Cystinosis, 326
Cystitis, 330–331, 330f
Cystitis cystica, 331
Cystitis glandularis, 331
Cytogenetic disorders, 13
Cytokeratins, 32, 124
Cytokine-mediated signaling, 27
Cytokines, 51
  and ubiquitin-proteasomal degradative pathway, 30
Cytomegalovirus (CMV), 228–229, 229f, 243f, 244, 262f
Cytopathologists, 122
Cytopathology, 122
Cytoplasmic receptors, 45–46

D
DAD. *See* Diffuse alveolar damage (DAD)
DAI. *See* Diffuse axonal injury (DAI)
Danger-associated molecular pattern (DAMP), 34
DCIS. *See* Ductal carcinoma in situ (DCIS)
DCM. *See* Dilated cardiomyopathy (DCM)
DDD. *See* Dense deposit disease (DDD)
Dead space, 218
Death, medical determination of, 21–22
DeBakey dissection scheme, 153–154, 154f
Decay accelerating factor (DAF), 60
Dedifferentiated chondrosarcoma, 500
Dedifferentiated liposarcoma, 173, 173f
Deep fibromatosis, 479–480
Deep venous thrombi (DVT), 238
Degenerative joint disease, 508–509
Dehydroepiandrosterone (DHEA), 399
Demyelinating diseases, 568–569
  acute disseminated encephalomyelitis, 569–570
  leukodystrophies, 570–571
  multiple sclerosis, 569
  progressive multifocal leukoencephalopathy, 570, 570f
  radiation necrosis, 570

Demyelination. *See* Nervous system, pathology
Denervation atrophy of skeletal muscle, 26
Dense deposit disease (DDD), 312, 313*f*
Deoxyribonucleic acid (DNA)
    building blocks of, 3*f*
    chemical nature of, 2–3
    complementary strands of nucleotides, 130*f*
    function of, 4–5
        genetic recombination, 5
        replication, 4–5
        transcription RNA, 5
    as source of genetic information, 1
    structure of, 3–4
DeQuervain thyroiditis, 410–411, 410*f*
Dermatofibroma, 538–540, 540*f*
Dermatofibrosarcoma protuberans (DFSP), 540, 541*f*
Dermatomyositis, 522
Dermatophyte, 547–549, 549*f*
Desmoplastic small round cell tumor (DSRCT), 494, 495*f*
Desmosomes, 201, 526
Desquamative interstitial pneumonitis (DIP), 233, 234–235
Developmental diseases, 14–15
    chromosomal abnormalities and, 15
    deformations, 14
    disruptions, 14
    epigenetic mechanisms and, 15
    gene alterations and, 15
    major forms of, 14
    malformations, 14
DGS. *See* DiGeorge syndrome (DGS)
Diabetes insipidus, 396
Diabetes mellitus, 174, 292
    gestational, 293
    type 1, 293
    type 2, 293
Diabetic glomerulosclerosis, 299, 303, 303*f*
Diabetic nephropathy, 303
Diagnostic anatomic pathology
    current practice of, 122–124
        clinical presentation, 122
        errors in, 124
        hematoxylin and eosin stain in, 123
        immunohistochemical techniques, 123–124
        pathological diagnosis, 122–123
        prognosis, 123
        radiographical presentation, 122
        techniques in tissue analysis, 123
    future practice of, 125–127
        computer-based prognosis and prediction, 127
        individual identity determination, 125
        integrated testing, 125
        rapid cytogenetics, 125
        rapid nucleic acid sequence, 125–127
        RNA abundance screening, 125–127
        serum biomarkers, 127
        smaller diagnostic biopsies with larger clinical significance, 125
    overview, 121–122
Diethylstilbestrol (DES), 113
Diffuse alveolar damage (DAD), 47, 48*f*, 234
Diffuse axonal injury (DAI), 577, 577*f*
Diffuse large B-cell lymphoma (DLBCL), 379, 385, 386*f*, 386
    case study, 386
    vs. PTCL, 385–386
    vs. reactive immunoblastic proliferation, 385
Diffuse subarachnoid hemorrhage, 150
DiGeorge syndrome (DGS), 416
Dilated cardiomyopathy (DCM), 200–202, 200*f*
DIP. *See* Desquamative interstitial pneumonitis (DIP)
Disease. *See also* Developmental diseases; Specific diseases
    history of, 21–22
    host reaction to, 21
Dissecting aortic aneurysm, 152
Disseminated intravascular coagulation (DIC), 81–82
Diverticular disease, 262–263, 263*f*DLBCL. *See* Diffuse large B-cell lymphoma (DLBCL)
DMD. *See* Duchenne muscular dystrophy (DMD)
DNA damage mechanism
    DNA alkylation, 88–89
    germ line mutational events, 86, 88
    hydrolysis and hydrolytic deamination, 89
    oxidative, 88
    somatic mutational events, 88
DNA hypermethylation, 18
DNA hypomethylation, 18
DNA methylation, 7–9, 8*f*
    CpG islands, 7, 7*f*
    DNA methyltransferase enzymes, 7–8
    genomic imprinting, 9
    regulation of transcription, 8–9, 8*f*
DNA methyltransferase (DNMT) enzymes, 7–8
DNA mutation, 5–6
    chromosomal alterations, 5–6
    nucleotide sequence alterations, 6
    silent mutation, 6
    somatic *vs.* germ-line mutation, 6
DNA sequencing, 132–134
DNMT1, 7–8, 8*f*
DNMT3a, 8
DNMT3b, 8
DNMT enzymes. *See* DNA methyltransferase (DNMT) enzymes
Down syndrome, 13
Drosophila, 190
Drowning, 105
DSRCT. *See* Desmoplastic small round cell tumor (DSRCT)
Duchenne muscular dystrophy (DMD), 12, 519
Ductal carcinoma in situ (DCIS), 433–434, 434*f*
Duct ectasia, 423*f*, 424
Dupuytren contracture, 479
DVT. *See* Deep venous thrombi (DVT)
Dysphagia, 31
Dysplasia, 24, 27*f*, 33

E

EBV. *See* Epstein–Barr virus (EBV)
EBVSMT. *See* Epstein–Barr virus-associated smooth muscle tumor (EBVSMT)
EC. *See* Endothelial cells (ECs)
Eclampsia, 466–467
    and preeclampsia, 317, 317*f*
Ectopic pregnancy, 442, 442*f*
EGFR exon 21, 126*f*
Eicosanoid synthesis, 55*f*
Eisenmenger syndrome, 190
Elastic arteries, 148–149
Electrical injury, 117–118, 117*f*
    generated electricity injury, 117
    mechanism of, 117–118
    static electricity injury, 117
Electron transport chain, damage to, 35–36
Embryonal carcinoma, 338, 338*f*
Embryonal rhabdomyosarcoma, 334, 448, 485, 485*f*, 486
EMF. *See* Endomyocardial fibrosis (EMF)
Emphysema, 236–237
Encapsulated PTC, 413
Enchondromas, 497, 498–499
Endocardium, 179
Endocrine, 385
Endocrine gland hyperplasia, 25*f*
Endocrine system, 386*f*
    adrenal cortical hyperfunction
        congenital adrenal hyperplasia, 403
        cushing syndrome, 400–401
        medulla, 403–404
        pheochromocytoma, 404–405
        primary hyperaldosteronism (PH), 401–403
    adrenal glands
        adrenal cortex, 396, 397*f*
        hormones, 397–398, 397*t*
    adrenal hormones
        aldosterone, 398
        cortisol, 398
        dehydroepiandrosterone, 399
    adrenal insufficiency
        diagnosis, 400
        etiology, 399–400
    hormone transport, 385–387, 387*t*
    hypothalamic–pituitary axis, 387–389
    parathyroid, 414–416
        hyperparathyroidism, 416–417
        hypoparathyroidism, 414–415
    posterior pituitary, 395
        diabetes insipidus, 396
        SIADH, 396
    principles, 385
    regulation and rhythms, 387
    thyroid
        benign diseases, 408–410
        congenital abnormalities, 407–408
        follicular cell-derived neoplastic diseases, 411–414
        function testing, 405–407
        hormone, 407
        neuroendocrine cell-derived neoplastic diseases, 414
        thyroiditis, 410–411
    trophic hormones of anterior pituitary
        adrenocorticotropin hormone, 394
        follicle-stimulating hormone, 394
        growth hormone, 389–393
        human chorionic gonadotropin, 394–395
        luteinizing hormone, 394
        prolactin, 393–394
        thyroid-stimulating hormone, 394–395
    tumors affecting pituitary function
        craniopharyngiomas, 395
        malignant pituitary tumors, 395
        pituitary adenomas pathogenesis, 395

Endometrial carcinoma
  type I, 457–458
  type II, 458
Endometrial hyperplasia, 456, 457f–458f, 457t
Endometrial stromal tumors, 459, 459f
Endometrioid, 458
Endomyocardial fibrosis (EMF), 203
Endomysium, 513, 515f
Endothelial cells (ECs), 147, 149
  activation, 50
  damage, 50
  and neutrophil interactions, 62–63, 62f
  role in coagulation regulation, 84, 85
Endothelins, 386f
Endotheliosis, 317
Endothelium, 170
Entamoeba histolytica, 261
Environmental thermal injury, 115–116
  heat exhaustion, 116
  heatstroke, 115
  hyperthermia, 115
  hypothermia, 116
Enzymatic fat necrosis, 38, 40, 40f
EoE. *See* Eosinophilic esophagitis (EoE)
Eosinophilic esophagitis (EoE), 241–242, 243f
Eosinophilic granulomatosis with polyangiitis, 162, 162f
Ependymal cells, 554, 554f
Epicardial coronary arteries, 182
Epicardium, 179
Epidermal inclusion cyst, 529
Epidermal response to mechanical stress, 28f
Epididymitis, 336
Epidural hematoma, 575
Epimysium, 513, 515f
Epispadias, 340
Epithelial follicular cells, 405
Epithelial tumors, 461–462, 463t
Epithelioid histiocyte, 227
Epstein–Barr virus (EBV), 228
Epstein–Barr virus-associated smooth muscle tumor (EBVSMT), 483f, 484
Errors in pathology practice, 124
Erythema marginatum, 207
Erythema multiforme, associated medications, 108
Erythemas, 528
  and prominent hyperpigmentation, 522f
Erythroplasia of Queyrat, 341
ES. *See* Ewing sarcoma (ES)
Escherichia coli, 113, 261
Esophagus
  anatomy, 241, 242f
  esophagitis
    eosinophilic, 241–242
    reflux, 241
  infectious esophagitis
    Candida, 242–243, 243f
    cytomegalovirus, 243f, 244
    herpesvirus, 244, 244f
  neoplasms and precancerous disease
    adenocarcinoma, 245, 246f
    Barrett esophagus, 244, 244f
    benign, 244
    malignant, 244
    squamous cell carcinoma, 244–245, 245f
  pathology
    developmental abnormalities, 241, 242f
    region of, 31, 31f
ESR1. See Estrogen receptor 1 *(ESR1)*
Estrogen receptor 1 *(ESR1),* 7
Ethanol toxicity, 110–111
Ewing sarcoma (ES), 502–504, 503f
EWSR1 gene, 133f
"Excited delirium," 109
External genitalia, 340–341
Extracardiac rhabdomyoma, 186
Extrinsic pathway, 41
  of apoptosis, 41
  of coagulation cascade, 80
Exudation, mechanism of, 49, 49f

F
Fabry disease, 326
Factor XII (FXII), 58
False lumen, 152, 155
Familial adenomatous polyposis (FAP), 17, 412
Familial cancer
  gastric, 17
  inherited mutation of susceptibility genes in, 16–17
  of pancreas, 17
  of prostate, 17
  Rb1 gene function in, 16–17
Familial cancer syndromes, 16
Familial cold autoinflammatory syndrome (FCAS), 46
Familial disease
  Alzheimer disease, 14
  epigenetic mechanisms in, 13–14
  Parkinson disease, 14
Familial glucocorticoid deficiency, 400
Familial hyperaldosteronism (FH) Type I., 402
Familial hypocalciuric hypercalcemia (FHH), 417
Familial hypoparathyroidism, 417
Familial melanoma, 16
Fanconi syndrome, 324
FAP. *See* Familial adenomatous polyposis (FAP)
Fat necrosis, 423f, 424, 469, 471f
Fatty change in liver, 33, 34f
Fatty liver disease, 276
Fatty streaks, 171, 171f
Female reproductive tract
  adult anatomy, 443, 444f
  cervix, 449f
    benign findings, 449–450
    HPV-related cervical carcinogenesis, molecular biology, 452
    malignant neoplasms, 450–451
    premalignant, 450
    squamous cell lesions, 451t
  embryology, 442
  fallopian tubes, 459–461
  infections, 443–444
  introduction, 441–442
  ovary
    germ cell tumors, 462–464
    metastatic tumors, 465
    nonneoplastic lesions, 461
    sex cord/stromal tumors, 464–465
    surface epithelial tumors, 461–462, 462f
    tumors, 461, 461f
  placental and gestational disease
    gestational trophoblastic disease, 467
    infections, 466
    multiple gestations, 467
    placental attachment disorders, 467
    preeclampsia/eclampsia, 466–467
  uterine corpus
    benign changes of uterus, 454
    carcinoma of uterus, 456
    endometriosis, 454
    hormone therapy/dysregulation, 453–454
    hyperplasia, 456
    menstrual cycle, 453, 453f
    mesenchymal (stromal) lesions, 459
    Type I endometrial carcinoma, 457–458
    Type II endometrial carcinoma, 458–459
  vagina
    benign lesions and malformations, 447
    malignant neoplasms, 447
    premalignant, 447
  vulva
    anatomy, 444
    dermatologic diseases/benign tumors, 445–446
    developmental anomalies, 444–445
    malignant tumors, 446–447
    premalignant tumors, 446–447
Ferruginous bodies, 236
Fetal genes, 27
FH. *See* Follicular hyperplasia (FH)
FHH. *See* Familial hypocalciuric hypercalcemia (FHH)
Fibrin degradation products (FDPs), 83
Fibrinolysis
  disorders of, 83
  role in maintaining hemostasis, 82
Fibrinolytic system
  for clot degradation, 82
  regulatory proteins, 83
Fibroadenoma, 429, 429f
Fibroblast growth factor (FGF), 27
Fibroblastic lesions, 479
Fibrocystic change, 424, 424f, 425f
Fibroepithelial lesions
  fibroadenoma, 429, 429f
  phyllodes tumors, 429–430, 430f
Fibroepithelial polyp, 552, 552f
Fibrohistiocytic lesions, 480–481
Fibrolamellar variant of HCC, 282, 282f
Fibroma/Thecoma, 463f, 464
Fibromatoses, 479–480
Fibro-osseous lesions, 500–505
Fibrosarcoma, 481
Fibrosis, 24, 75
Fibrous cap, 173
Fibrous dysplasia, 500–501, 502f
Fibrous pericardium, 215
Field effect (urothelial malignancy), 332
Fine-needle aspiration (FNA), 408
First-degree burns, 114
FISH. *See* Fluorescence in situ hybridization (FISH)
Fitz-Hugh–Curtis syndrome, 443
FL. *See* Follicular lymphoma (FL)
Floppy, 518
Fluorescence in situ hybridization (FISH), 473
  for chromosomal alterations, 5–16

for Ewing sarcoma, 133f
for localizing specific DNA sequences, 134
FMR1, 14
FNA. *See* Fine-needle aspiration (FNA)
Foam cells, 538
Focal nodular hyperplasia (FNH), 280, 280f
Focal segmental glomerulosclerosis (FSGS), 299, 301–302, 302f, 302t
Follicles, 405
Follicle-stimulating hormone (FSH), 394
Follicular adenomas, 412, 412f
Follicular carcinoma, 412
Follicular cysts, 528–529, 529f
Follicular hyperplasia (FH), 379, 388–389
Follicular lymphoma (FL), 381, 382, 383f
Follicular thyroid carcinoma (FTC), 413, 413f
Follicular variant of papillary thyroid carcinoma (FVPTC), 413
Folliculitis (suppurative folliculitis), 546
Force injuries, 43
Foreign bodies and foreign body granulomas, 547, 548f
FoxO transcription factors, 27
  negative and positive regulation of, 90, 91f
Fractures, 99, 505, 506f
Fragile X syndrome, 14
Framingham study, 173–175
Freckle (ephelide)/melanotic macule, 533, 533f
FSGS. *See* Focal segmental glomerulosclerosis (FSGS)
FTC. *See* Follicular thyroid carcinoma (FTC)
FVPTC. *See* Follicular variant of papillary thyroid carcinoma (FVPTC)

G
Gallbladder and extrahepatic biliary tract
  anatomy, 283–284, 284f
  diseases of
    acute cholecystitis, 285
    cholecystitis, 284
    cholelithiasis, 284
    cholesterol stones, 284, 285f
    chronic cholecystitis, 285
    pigment stones, 284
  histology, 283–284, 284f
  masses
    bile duct adenocarcinoma, 285
    gallbladder carcinoma, 285, 285f
Gallbladder carcinoma, 285, 285f
Ganglioneuroma, 404
Gastric ulcers 249–250, 250f
Gastroesophageal junction (GE), 241
Gastroesophageal reflux disease (GERD), 31
  and Barrett metaplasia, 32
Gastrointestinal stromal tumor (GIST), 251–252, 252f
GATA4, 189
GCPR activation, 50
GE. *See* Gastroesophageal junction (GE)
Gene expression
  methylation-dependent epigenetic regulation of, 8f
  post-transcriptional regulation of, 10
Generated electricity injury, 117
Genetic diseases, 10–14
  cytogenetic disorders, 13

familial disease, 13–14
major forms of, 10
polygenic disorders, 12
single gene disorders, 11–12
  autosomal dominant disorders, 11, 11f
  autosomal recessive disorders, 11–12, 11f
  mitochondrial disorders, 12
  X-linked disorders, 12
Genetic recombination, 5
Germ cell tumors, 462, 464t
Germ-line mutation *vs.* somatic mutation, 6
Gestational trophoblastic, 467
GHRH. *See* Growth hormone releasing hormone (GHRH)
Giant-cell arteritis, 157–159, 159f
Giant condyloma of Buschke and Lowenstein, 341
Giardia lamblia, 256
Giardiasis, 256
Gigantism, 392
GIST. *See* Gastrointestinal stromal tumor (GIST)
Gleason grading system, 348
Gliomas, 565, 566f
Global ischemic injury, 562f
Glomerular disease, 298, 298f
Glomerulitis, 325
Glomerulonephritis, 299
Glucocorticoids, 36, 396
Glycogen storage disease type V, 520
GMS. *See* Gomori methenamine silver (GMS)
Goblet cell carcinoids, 270
Gomori methenamine silver (GMS), 393
Gomori trichrome (GT) stain, 520f, 523
Goodpasture syndrome, 312
Gout, 509
GPA. *See* Granulomatosis with polyangiitis (GPA)
G protein-coupled response (GPCR) signaling, 27
Granular cell tumor, 491, 491f
Granulation tissue, 76f
Granulocytes, 527
Granulomas, 74, 74f, 227
  and chronic inflammation, 47
Granulomatosis with polyangiitis (GPA), 238
Granulomatous dermatitis (granuloma annulare), 546, 546f
Granulomatous mastitis, 419f, 421–422
Granulomatous prostatitis, 344
Granulomatous thyroiditis, 410–411
Granulosa cell tumor, 441f, 442, 464
Granzyme B (CTl) pathway, 41, 42
Graves disease, 409, 409f
Grey Turner sign, 291
Growth hormone (GH), 389–393
  deficiency, 389–390
  hypopituitarism, 389–391
  stimulating tests examples, 392t
Growth hormone releasing hormone (GHRH), 389
Gynecomastia, 430

H
Hairy cell leukemia, 390
Hallucinogens, mind-altering effects of, 110
Hamartomatous polyps, 265, 266f
Hashimoto thyroiditis (HT), 409, 411, 411f
HAV. *See* Hepatitis A (HAV)

HBB (beta globin) gene, 134
HBV. *See* Hepatitis B (HBV)
HCC. *See* Hepatocellular carcinoma (HCC)
hCG. *See* human chorionic gonadotropin (hCG)
HCIE. *See* Health-care associated infective endocarditis (HCIE)
HCM. *See* Hypertrophic cardiomyopathy (HCM)
HDI. *See* Hypothalamic diabetes insipidus (HDI)
HDL. *See* High-density lipids (HDLs)
Health-care associated infective endocarditis (HCIE), 209
Heat exhaustion, 116
Heat shock protein genes, 27
Heatstroke, 115
Heavy metal exposure, 112
Helicobacter gastritis, 248, 249f
Helicobacter pylori, 246
Hemangioendothelioma *vs.* angiosarcoma, 392
Hemangiomas, 280–281, 281f, 391, 476, 476f, 477, 537–538, 539f
Hematocele, 341
Hematopathology
  erythroid cells disorders
    anemias, 357–359, 358t
    polycythemias, 359, 359t
  overview, 357
  platelets disorders
    thrombocytopenias, 367–369
    thrombocytoses, 369–370
  primary bone marrow disorders
    acute leukemias, 370–372
    plasma cell dyscrasias, 377–379
  primary lymph node disorders, 379–388
    classical hodgkin lymphoma, 386–388
    DLBCL, 385
    follicular hyperplasia *vs.* follicular lymphoma, 380
    follicular lymphoma, 381
    nodular lymphocyte-predominant hodgkin lymphoma, 381–385
  spleen disorders
    red pulp, 389–391
    white pulp, 388–389
  thymic hyperplasia, 393–397
  tumorlike lesions
    inflammatory pseudotumor, 392–393
  white blood cells disorders
    lymphocytoses, 363–367
    monocytoses, 367
    neutropenia, 360–362, 361t
    neutrophilia, 362–363
Hematoxylin and eosin (H&E) stain, 123, 522f, 523f
  biopsy, 526f
  of brain biopsy, 126f
Hemidesmosomes, 526
Hemochromatosis, 279, 279f
Hemolytic uremic syndrome (HUS), 317, 318–320, 318t, 319f
Hemophilia A and B, 82
Hemorrhagic disorders, diagnosis of, 84t
Hemosiderosis, 33, 34f
Hemostasis
  evaluation of, 84
  and inflammation, interplay between, 78
  primary. *See* Primary hemostasis
  secondary. *See* Secondary hemostasis

Henoch–Schönlein purpura, 310
Heparan sulfate, 84
Hepatic ducts, 271
Hepatic lobules, 271, 272, 273f
Hepatitis A (HAV), 274–275
Hepatitis B (HBV), 275, 275t
Hepatitis C (HCV), 275–276, 276f
Hepatitis D, 276
Hepatitis E, 276
Hepatoblastomas, 283
Hepatocellular adenomas, 281, 281f
Hepatocellular carcinoma (HCC), 275, 281–282
Hepatosplenic T-cell lymphoma, 390–391, 391f
Hereditary myopathies
   congenital myopathies, 518
   metabolic myopathies, 519
   mitochondrial myopathies, 519
   muscular dystrophies, 518
Hereditary nephritis, 314–316
Hereditary nonpolyposis colon cancer (HNPCC), 17
Herpes simplex virus (HPV), 229, 229f
Herpes viruses, 550–551, 550f
Herpesvirus esophagitis (HSV), 244, 244f
HES. *See* Hypereosinophilic syndrome (HES)
HFE C282Y mutation, 129
High-density lipids (HDLs), 174
High-grade squamous intraepithelial lesion (HSIL), 451t
High-mobility group box 1 (HMGB1) protein, 43
High molecular weight cytokeratin (HWCK), 343
High molecular weight kininogen (HMWK), 58
Hilar cells, 443
Hirschsprung disease, 260, 260f
Histamine, 50
Histone acetylation, 10
Histone code, 9, 9f
Histone H3 lysine 4 (H3K4), 19
Histone H3 lysine 27 (H3K27), 19
Histone H3 lysine 9 (H3K9) methylation, 19
Histone methylation, 10
Histone methyltransferase (HMT), 19
Histone modifications, 9–10
   in cancer, 19
Histone phosphorylation, 10
Histone proteins, 9–10
Histoplasma, 226–227
H4K20 methylation, 19
HL. *See* Hodgkin lymphomas (HL)
HMT. *See* Histone methyltransferase (HMT)
HNPCC. *See* Hereditary nonpolyposis colon cancer (HNPCC)
Hodgkin lymphomas (HL), 379
Homeobox transcription factor expression, 32–33
Homozygous hypercholesterolemia, 174
Hormonal control, 387
Hormonal variations, and hyperplasia, 26
Hormones, 385
   injury and, 113
Host response to injury, 21
   pathogen recognition receptors. *See* Pathogen recognition receptors
   sterile/force injury, 43–44
   triggers of inflammation, 43

Hox gene function, in developmental disease, 15
HPV. *See* Herpes simplex virus (HPV)
HSV. *See* Herpesvirus esophagitis (HSV)
HT. *See* Hashimoto thyroiditis (HT)
Human chorionic gonadotropin (hCG), 394–395
Human epigenome, 7–10
   DNA methylation, 7–9, 8f
      CpG islands, 7, 7f
      DNA methyltransferase enzymes, 7–8
      genomic imprinting, 9
      regulation of transcription, 8–9, 8f
   histone acetylation, 10
   histone code, 9, 9f
   histone methylation, 10
   histone modifications, 9–10
   histone phosphorylation, 10
   histone proteins, 9–10
   post-transcriptional regulation of gene expression, 10
Human genome, 1–6
   central dogma of molecular biology, 1–2
   chemical nature of DNA, 2–3
   DNA as source of genetic information, 1
   DNA damaging agents, 5
   DNA function, 4–5
   DNA mutation, 5–6
      chromosomal alterations, 5–6
      nucleotide sequence alterations, 6
      somatic *vs.* germ-line mutation, 6
   organization of, 4
   sequence of, 4
   structure of DNA, 3–4
Huntington disease, 574, 575f
HUS. *See* Hemolytic uremic syndrome (HUS)
Hutchinson–Gilford Progeria (HGP), 89–90, 90f
HWCK. *See* High molecular weight cytokeratin (HWCK)
Hyaline membrane disease, 234
Hybridization, 129
Hydatidiform moles, 467–468, 468t
Hydrocele, 341
Hydrocephalus, 556–558, 557f
Hydronephrosis, 344
Hydropic swelling, 33, 34f
Hydroureter, 344
HYPB, 19
Hyperacute rejection, 325–326
Hyperbilirubinemia, 278
Hypereosinophilic syndrome (HES), 203
Hyperlipidemia, 174Hyperoxaluria, 326
Hyperparathyroidism (HyperPT), 415, 416
Hyperplasia
   anoxic stress in, 26
   associated with disease, 26
   definition of, 25
   endocrine gland, 25f
   of exercised skeletal muscle, 25
   and hormonal variations, 26
   and hypertrophy, 25
   molecular mechanisms of, 26–28
Hyperplastic polyps, 267, 267f
Hyperplastic thyroid gland, 25f
HyperPT. *See* Hyperparathyroidism (HyperPT)
Hypersensitivity pneumonia/extrinsic allergic alveolitis, 233
Hypersensitivity tubulointerstitial nephritis, 323
Hypersensitivity vasculitis, 162–163, 163f

Hypertensive arterionephrosclerosis, 316–317
Hyperthermia, 115
Hyperthyroidism, 409
Hypertrophic cardiac myocytes, 23, 23f
Hypertrophic cardiomyopathy (HCM), 201–203
Hypertrophic obstructive cardiomyopathy (HCM), 202
Hypertrophy
   associated with disease, 26
   definition of, 25
   molecular mechanisms of, 26–28
Hypoparathyroidism, 415
Hypophysis, 387
Hypopituitarism, 389–391, 391t
   in adults, 391
   in children, 391
Hypoplastic left heart syndrome, 189, 197
HypoPT. *See* Primary hypoparathyroidism (HypoPT)
Hypospadias, 340
Hypothalamic diabetes insipidus (HDI), 396
Hypothermia, 116
Hypothyroidism, 408–409, 408f

I

Iatrogenic injury, 119. *See also* Physical injury
ICR. *See* Imprinting control region (ICR)
Idiopathic cardiomyopathy, 200
Idiopathic hyperaldosteronism (IHA), 402
Idiopathic hypertrophic subaortic stenosis, 201–202
Idiopathic RCM, 203
Idiopathic reactive FH, 388
IgA nephropathy, 308–310, 309f
IgA vasculitis, 308–310
IGF2, 9
IGF2R, 9
IgG4-related systemic diseases (IgG4-RSD), 411
IGHD. *See* Isolated growth hormone deficiency (IGHD)
IHA. *See* Idiopathic hyperaldosteronism (IHA)
Immunohistochemistry, 123–124
Impetigo/erysipelas, 549
Imprinting control region (ICR), 9
Incised wounds, 99, 101f
Inclusion body myositis, 523
Infectious arthritis, 509
Infectious colitis, 261, 262f
Infectious diseases, 21
Infective endocarditis (IE)
   classification, 209
   clinical features, 210
   prognosis, 210
   risk factors, 209–210
Infiltration of infarct, 24, 24f
Infiltrative RCM, 203
Inflammasome
   activation, 47
   Nalp1 (NLRP1) and cryopyrin (NLRP3), 46
   and nod-like receptors, 45–46
   PRR signaling, 46, 46f
Inflammation, 34, 40
   acute. *See* Acute inflammation
   and cell death, 42–43
   chronic. *See* Chronic inflammation
   factors triggering, 47

and hemostasis, interplay between, 78
as host response to injury, 43
macrophages role in, 47
patterns in tissue, 47, 48f
Inflammatory arthritis, 509
Inflammatory disorders, 246
Inflammatory lesions
  acute mastitis, 422
  duct ectasia, 423f, 424
  fat necrosis, 423f, 424
  granulomatous mastitis, 421–422
  lymphocytic/fibrous mastopathy, 422, 424
  subareolar abscess (periductal mastitis), 422
Inflammatory myopathies, 521
Inflammatory polyps, 265
Inflammatory pseudotumor, 392–393
Infundibular follicular, 529
Inhalants, adverse effects of, 110
Injurious agents, 33
Injury, 93–96. See also specific injuries
  acute, 93
  complexity of, 105
  electrical forces and, 94
  emergency department visits for, 94t
  external factors for, 94
  ionizing radiation and, 94
  patterned, 94
  repeated, 94
  scalding, 115, 116f
  unintentional, 95
Innate immunity, initiation of, 43
Inner zona reticularis, 396
INS, 9
Insecticides exposure, 112
In situ hybridization, 131, 133f
Insulin-like growth factor1 (IGF1) pathway, 90
Insulitis, 293
Intercalated discs, 179
Interpretive error, 124
Interstitium, 217
Intestinal columnar metaplasia, 30–31
Intracellular accumulations, abnormal, 33, 34f
Intracerebral hemorrhage, 100
Intracranial pressure (ICP), 554, 554f, 555, 555t
Intramural arteries, 182
Intramuscular hemangioma, 477–478
Intramuscular lipomas, 471, 471f, 472
Intramuscular myxoma, 492
Intraparenchymal brain hemorrhage, 577
Intratubular germ cell neoplasia, 337
Intravenous drug abuse (IVDA), 209
Intravenous leiomyomatosis (IVL), 459, 459f
Intrinsic pathway
  of apoptosis, 41
  of coagulation, 58, 80–81
Invasive aspergillosis, 226
Invasive carcinomas, 333
Invasive ductal adenocarcinoma, 294–295, 295f
Invasive mammary carcinomas, 435–438, 437f, 439t
Invasive squamous cell carcinoma, 218, 218f, 341
Ionizing radiation, 118
Iron-deficiency anemia, 358, 358f
Irreversible coma, 21–22
Irreversible injury, 22, 33, 39f
  mechanisms of, 34
  visual clues associated with, 37

Ischemia, 177–178
Ischemic AKI, 321–322, 322f
Ischemic cardiomyopathy, 188
Ischemic cell death, 34
Ischemic colitis, 262, 263f
Ischemic heart disease, 178, 188
Islets of Langerhans, 289f, 290
Isolated growth hormone deficiency (IGHD), 390
Isopropanol toxicity, 110
Isthmus, 443
IVDA. See Intravenous drug abuse (IVDA)
IVDA endocarditis, 209

J
Janus kinases (JK), 27
Joint pathology, 507

K
Kaposi sarcoma, 541
Kawasaki disease (KD), 160–161, 161f
KD. See Kawasaki disease (KD)
Kearns-Sayre Syndrome, 521
Keloids, 77, 77f
Keratinocytes, 526
Keratoacanthoma, 532, 533f
Kimmelstiel–Wilson nodules, 303
Kinetic energy, in physical injury, 96–97
Klinefelter syndrome, 13
Koilocytes, 450
Krabbe disease, 571
Krukenberg tumor, 465
Kufor-Rakeb disease, 14
Kwashiorkor, 28

L
Laboratory medicine, 137
  case study, 137
  clinical laboratory and, 138–139
  clinical performance of tests, 143–144
    analytical vs. biological variation, 143–144
    biological variation, 144
    sensitivity, specificity, predictive value, 143–144
  dealing with unexpected results, 144
  disciplines, 138t
  role in patient care, 137f
  test result interpretation, 141–142, 142f
    clinical decision limits, 142
    reference ranges, 141–142
  total testing process, 139–141, 139f
    analytic phase, 140–141
    postanalytical phase, 141
    preanalytical phase, 139–140
    specimen types and use in, 140t
  value of laboratory testing, 144–144
Lacerations, 98, 99f, 100f, 576–577, 576f
Lacteals, 243
Lactic dehydrogenase (LDH), 338
Langerhans cell histiocytosis (LCH), 233, 504–505, 504f, 542–543, 543f
Large cell neuroendocrine carcinoma, 221
Large cell undifferentiated carcinoma (LCUC), 220, 221f

Laryngeal squamous papillomatosis, 229
LCH. See Langerhans cell histiocytosis (LCH)
LCIS. See Lobular carcinoma in situ (LCIS)
LCUC. See Large cell undifferentiated carcinoma (LCUC)
LDH. See Lactic dehydrogenase (LDH)
LDL. See Low-density lipid (LDL)
Lead exposure, 112
Left main artery, 182
Left ventricular hypertrophy, 23
Leiomyomas, 459, 459f
Leiomyomatosis peritonealis disseminata, 482
Leiomyosarcoma, 459, 459f, 482–484
Lentigo simplex, 534, 534f
LES. See Lower esophageal sphincter (LES)
Lesch–Nyhan syndrome, 12
Leukemia cutis, 542
Leukocyte adhesion deficiency (LAD) syndromes, 63–64
Leukodystrophies, 570–571, 572f
Leukotirenes (LTs), 51
  autocrine and paracrine effects of, 56
  cyst-LT, 57
  LTB_4, 56
  synthesis of, 56, 56f
Leydig cell tumors, 339–340, 340f
Libman–Sacks endocarditis, 211
Lichen sclerosis, 545, 545f
Life expectancy, 85
Li-Fraumeni syndrome, 16
Ligature marks, in suicidal hanging, 105f
Light chain cast nephropathy and tubulopathy, 323–324
Limiting plate, 271
Lipiduria, 299
Lipoblasts, 469
Lipomas, 471
Lipomatous neoplasms, cytogenetic findings in, 474t
Lipomatous tumors
  adipose tissue histology, 469–471
  rules, 469–470
Liquefactive necrosis, 38, 39f
Liver
  anatomy, 271, 272f
  biliary tract disease
    bilirubin metabolism and jaundice, 277–278
    primary biliary cirrhosis, 279
    primary sclerosing cholangitis, 278, 278f
  diseases
    cirrhosis, 273, 274f
    liver failure, 273
  drug- and toxin-induced liver injury, 277, 278f
  fatty change in, 33, 34f
  functions of, 271
  histology, 271–273
  infectious hepatitis disorders
    Hepatitis A, 274
    Hepatitis B, 275
    Hepatitis C, 275–276
    Hepatitis D, 276
    Hepatitis E, 276
    viral hepatitis, 274–275
  masses
    benign neoplasms, 280
    cholangiocarcinoma, 282–283, 283f

Liver *(Continued)*
  combined hepatocellular–cholangiocarcinoma, 283
  fibrolamellar variant of HCC, 282, 282*f*
  focal nodular hyperplasia, 280, 280*f*
  hemangiomas, 280, 281, 281*f*
  hepatoblastomas, 283
  hepatocellular adenomas, 281, 281*f*
  hepatocellular carcinoma, 281–282, 282*f*
  malignant neoplasms, 281
  metastatic cancer, 283, 283*f*
  mimickers of neoplasia, 280
  nodular regenerative hyperplasia, 280
  metabolic disorders
    alpha 1-antitrypsin deficiency, 280, 280*f*
    hemochromatosis, 279, 279*f*
    Wilson disease, 280
  noninfectious hepatitis disorders
    alcoholic liver disease, 276
    autoimmune hepatitis, 277, 277*f*
    fatty liver disease, 276
    nonalcoholic fatty liver disease, 276–277, 277*f*
  transplantation, 283
  vascular disorders
    chronic passive congestion, 273, 274*f*
    portal hypertension, 274
Liver failure, 273, 273*f*
Lobar pneumonia, 226
Lobular capillary hemangiomas, 477, 538
Lobular carcinoma in situ (LCIS), 434–435, 435*f*
Loeffler endomyocarditis, 203
Low-density lipid (LDL), 174
Lower esophageal sphincter (LES), 241
Lower urinary tract, 329, 329*f*
  and male GU development, 329–330
Lower urinary tract symptoms (LUTS), 344
Low-grade noninvasive papillary lesions, 333
Lung
  adenocarcinoma of, 220, 220*f*
  airway diseases
    asthma, 229–230
    cystic fibrosis, 230–231
    emphysema, 236–237
    primary ciliary dyskinesia, 231–232
  alveolar and adjacent interstitial diseases
    desquamative interstitial pneumonia, 234–235
    diffuse alveolar damage, 234
    pneumoconiosis, 235–236
    usual interstitial pneumonia, 235
  anatomy, 217–218
  anthracotic pigment in, 33, 34*f*
  inflammatory events in, 47, 48*f*
  neoplasms, 218–219
    non-small cell lung carcinomas, 219–221
    small cell lung carcinomas, 222–223, 223*f*
  peribronchovascular diseases
    hypersensitivity pneumonia/extrinsic allergic alveolitis, 233
    langerhans cell histiocytosis, 233
    sarcoidosis, 232–233
  physiology, 217–218
  and pleural infections
    bacterial pneumonias, 225–226
    fungi, 226–227
    mycobacteria, 227–228

mycoplasma pneumonia, 226
    viruses, 228–229
  vascular diseases
    pulmonary artery hypertension, 238
    pulmonary thromboemboli, 238
    vasculitis, 238–239
Lupus glomerulonephritis, 305–308
Luteinizing hormone (LH), 394
LUTS. *See* Lower urinary tract symptoms (LUTS)
Lymphatics, 149
Lymphocytic/fibrous mastopathy, 422, 424
Lymphocytic thyroiditis, 410
Lymphocytoses, 363–367
  causes, 365*t*
  infection with EBV, 365
Lysozyme, 68

M
Macroadenomas, 392
Macrophage
  in chronic inflammation, 72–74
  and neutrophil apoptosis, 73–74
  phagosome maturation, 67
  role in inflammation, 47
Macula adherens, 201
MAHA. *See* Microangiopathic hemolytic anemia (MAHA)
Malakoplakia, 330–331
Male infertility
  post-testicular causes, 336
  pretesticular causes, 335
  testicular causes, 335–336
Malformations, 14
Malignant adipocytic tumors, 472–473
Malignant bone-forming tumors, 497
Malignant fibrous histiocytoma (MFH), 481
Malignant mesothelioma, 223–225, 223*f*, 224*f*
Malignant neoplasms, 281, 412–414
Malignant peripheral nerve sheath tumors (MPNST), 481, 490–492
Malignant pituitary tumors, 395
Malignant tumors, 244
Malignant vascular tumors, 478–479
MALT. *See* Mucosa-associated lymphoid tissue (MALT)
Manual strangulation, 106*f*
Marasmus, 28
Marfan syndrome, 155
Marginal-zone B-cell lymphoma, 252, 252*f*
MAS. *See* McCune–Albright syndrome (MAS)
Mast cells, 51*f*
  function of, 52*f*
  stimuli activating, 51
  synthesis of, 50
Mastocytosis/urticaria pigmentosa, 542, 542*f*
Mature carcinoid tumor, 221, 221*f*
McArdle disease, 520
McCune–Albright syndrome (MAS), 395
MDM2 gene amplification, 473
Mechanical stress, epidermal response to, 28*f*
Meckel diverticulum, 252–254, 254*f*
Medical renal disease
  acute tubular epithelial injury, 321–322
  glomerular disease syndromes
    acute postinfectious glomerulonephritis, 310–311, 311*f*

amyloidosis, 303
    ANCA glomerulonephritis, 312–314, 314*f*
    anti-GBM glomerulonephritis, 312–313
    asymptomatic hematuria, 305
    atheroembolization, 320
    atherosclerosis, 320
    diabetic glomerulosclerosis, 303, 303*f*
    eclampsia and preeclampsia, 317, 317*f*
    focal segmental glomerulosclerosis, 301–302
    hemolytic uremic syndrome, 318–320
    hereditary nephritis, 314–316
    hypertensive arterionephrosclerosis, 316–317
    IgA nephropathy, 308–310, 309*f*
    IgA vasculitis, 308–310
    lupus glomerulonephritis, 305–308
    membranoproliferative glomerulonephritis, 311–312, 312*f*
    membranous glomerulopathy, 301
    minimal-change glomerulopathy, 301
    monoclonal immunoglobulin deposition disease, 303–305
    nephritic syndrome, 305
    nephrotic syndrome, 299, 299*t*, 301*t*
    thin basement membrane lesion, 314–316
    thrombotic microangiopathies, 317
    thrombotic thrombocytopenic purpura, 317–318
    tubular and interstitial disease, 320–321, 321*f*
  introduction, 297
  renal transplant pathology
    acute antibody-mediated rejection, 325–326
    acute cell-mediated rejection, 324–325
    chronic rejection, 326
    hyperacute rejection, 325–326
    renal transplant disease not caused by rejection, 326–327
  role of nephropathologists, 297
  tubulointerstitial nephritis
    acute, 322–323, 323*f*
    hypersensitivity, 323
    light chain cast nephropathy and tubulopathy, 323–324
  vs. urologic disease, 297
  vascular disease, 298, 298*f*
Medicine
  laboratory. *See* Laboratory medicine
  pathocentric view of, 22*f*
Medicolegal death investigation systems, 95
Mediterranean fever (FMF), 47
Medium-sized arteries, 149
Medullary carcinoma, 412
Medullary cords, 379
Medullary thyroid carcinoma (MTC), 414
Medulloblastoma, 565
Megakaryocytes, 78*f*
Meigs syndrome, 464
Melanocytes, 526
Melanocytic lesions, 533
Melanocytic nevus, 534–535, 534*f*
Melanoma, 533, 535–536
Melasma, 533
Membrane attack complex (MAC), 58
Membranoproliferative glomerulonephritis (MPGN), 311–312, 312*f*
Membranous glomerulopathy, 299, 301

MEN1. *See* Multiple endocrine neoplasia syndrome type 1 (MEN1)
Menin, 395
Meningioma, 565–566, 567*f*
Mercury exposure, 112
Merkel cell carcinoma, 538, 540*f*
Merkel cell virus, 538
Mesangiolysis, 319
Mesenteric fat wrapping, 264
Mesenteric tear, 97*f*
Metabolic diseases, 509
Metabolic myopathies, 519
Metaplasia, 26*f*
  change of ciliated columnar epithelium, 30, 32
  definition of, 25, 30
  intestinal columnar, 30–31
  molecular mechanisms of, 32–33
Metastatic cancer, 283, 283*f*
Metastatic disease, 496
Metastatic prostate cancer, 350
Methamphetamine toxicity, 109
Methanol toxicity, 110
Methyl-CpG-binding (MBD) proteins, 8–9, 8*f*
MFH. *See* Malignant fibrous histiocytoma (MFH)
MGUS. *See* Monoclonal gammopathy of undetermined significance (MGUS)
Michaelis–Gutmann bodies, 331
Microalbuminuria, 303
Microangiopathic hemolytic anemia (MAHA), 317
Microglia, 554–555, 554*f*
Microinvasive carcinoma, 435
MicroRNA (miRNA), 2
Microsatellite instability, 268
Microscopic polyangiitis (MPA), 160
Mimickers of neoplasia, 280
Minimal-change glomerulopathy, 299, 301, 302*f*
miRNA. *See* MicroRNA (miRNA)
Missense mutation, 6
Mitochondrial damage, and reactive oxygen species, 36, 36*f*
Mitochondrial disorders, 12
Mitochondrial myopathies, 519
Mitogen-activated protein kinase (MAPK) cascades, 27
Mitral valve annulus, calcification of, 212–213
Mitral valve prolapse, 211–212
Mitral valve stenosis, 206–209
Mixed hyperplastic/adenomatous polyps, 267
MLH1 gene, 19
Molecular biology, central dogma of, 1–2, 2*f*
Molecular pathology, 129–136
  case study, 129
  laboratory procedures, 130–135
    DNA sequencing, 132–134
    microarray technology for gene expression profiling, 134–135, 135*f*
    polymerase chain reaction, 130–131, 131*f*, 132*f*
    in situ hybridization, 131, 133*f*
    steps in validating, 136*t*
  molecular technologies and, 129
    medical applications of, 129–130
    specimen preparation, 130
  pathologist's role, 135–136
  the practice of, 129

Molluscum contagiosum, 551, 551*f*
Mönckeberg medial calcific stenosis, 170, 170*f*
Monoclonal gammopathy of undetermined significance (MGUS), 379, 379*f*
Monoclonal immunoglobulin deposition disease, 303–305
Monocytopenia, 365, 367
Monocytoses, 367
Mononuclear cells, 72*f*
MPA. *See* Microscopic polyangiitis (MPA)
MPGN. *See* Membranoproliferative glomerulonephritis (MPGN)
MPNST. *See* Malignant peripheral nerve sheath tumors (MPNST)
MRFIT. *See* Multiple Risk Factor Intervention Trial (MRFIT)
MS. *See* Multiple sclerosis (MS)
MTC. *See* Medullary thyroid carcinoma (MTC)
mTOR protein, 27, 29–30
Mucocutaneous lymph node syndrome, 160
Mucoepidermoid carcinoma, 221
Mucosa-associated lymphoid tissue (MALT), 246
Muir–Torre syndrome, 17
Multifocal atrophic gastritis, 249
Multiorgan failure syndromes, 42
Multiple endocrine neoplasia syndrome type 1 (MEN1), 395
Multiple Risk Factor Intervention Trial (MRFIT), 173, 175
Multiple sclerosis (MS), 569, 569*f*
Mummification, 22
Mural thrombus, 186, 186*f*
Muscle pathology
  myopathic changes, 514
  neurogenic changes, 514
Muscular dystrophies, 518
Muscular septum, 190
MYB. See Myeloblastosis viral oncogene *(MYB)*
Mycobacterium avium, 261
Mycobacterium tuberculosis, 227–228, 261
Mycoplasma pneumonia, 226
Mycosis fungoides/cutaneous T-cell lymphoma, 541–542, 542*f*
Myeloblastosis viral oncogene *(MYB)*, 7
Myocardial infarctions
  classification, 182
  early complications
    cardiac dysrhythmias, 183–184
    mural thrombus, 186
    myocardial rupture, 184–186
    pericarditis, 186
    pump dysfunction, 183
  late complications
    ventricular aneurysm, 187
  location of, 182
  morphology, 182–183
  outcome of, 182
  treatment, 187–188
Myocardial ischemia, 178, 179
Myocardial rupture, 184–186
Myocardium, 179
Myocyte enhancer factor-2 (MEF-2), 27
Myofibrils, 484*f*
Myofibroblastic lesions, 479
Myofibroblasts, 479
Myositis ossificans, 32

Myostatin, 30
Myxofibrosarcoma, 478, 478*f*, 480
Myxoid liposarcoma, 473, 474*f*

N

NADPH oxidase system
  assembly of, 68, 69*f*
  molecular products of, 69
  oxidative killing, defects in mechanism of, 69–70
  role in host defense, 68
NAFLD. *See* Nonalcoholic fatty liver disease (NAFLD)
NAHI. *See* Nonaccidental head injury (NAHI)
Narcotic analgesics, toxic effects of, 109
National Cholesterol Education Program, 142
Native valve endocarditis (NVE), 209
NBT. *See* Nitroblue tetrazolium chloride (NBT)
NBTE. *See* Nonbacterial thrombotic endocarditis (NBTE)
Necroptosis, 34
Necrosis, 23
  vs. apoptosis, 34, 40
  and cell injury
    reversible and irreversible, 36–37
  definition of, 34
  molecular mechanisms of, 35–36, 35*f*
  and pyroptosis, 35
  types of, 37–40
Nemaline rod myopathy, 520
Neonatal severe hyperparathyroidism (NSHPT), 417
Neoplastic diseases, 15–19
  classification of, 15
  epigenetics of cancer, 18–19
  gene mutation in, 17–18
  genetic predisposition of, 15–17
    cancer associated with faulty DNA repair mechanisms, 17
    cancer susceptibility, 17
    chromosomal instability, 17
    familial cancer syndromes, 16
    inherited mutations in cancer susceptibility genes, 16–17
  nonfamilial, 17
    abnormal DNA repair mechanisms in, 18
    gene mutations in, 17–18
Nephritic syndrome, 305
Nephrogenic metaplasia (nephrogenic adenoma), 331
Nephrologists, 297
Nephropathologists, 297
Nephrotic syndrome, 299, 299*t*, 301*t*
Nephrotoxic acute tubular necrosis, 37
Nephrotoxic AKI, 321, 322*f*
Nervous system, pathology
  brain tumors
    brain metastases, 567–568, 568*f*
    colloid cyst, 567
    consequences, 565*f*
    gliomas, 565, 566*f*
    histologic classification, 565*t*
    medulloblastoma, 565
    meningioma, 565–566, 567*f*
    primary CNS lymphoma (PCNSL), 567
    schwannoma, 567

Nervous system, pathology (Continued)
  central nervous system (CNS)
    astrocytes and oligodendrocytes, 553–554, 553f
    brain edema, 555–556
    choroid plexus epithelium, 554, 554f
    ependymal cells, 554, 554f
    hydrocephalus, 556–558, 557f
    intracranial pressure (ICP), 554, 554f, 555, 555t
    mass lesion, 557, 557f
    microglia, 554–555, 554f
    neurons, 553, 553f
    red neurons, 553, 553f
  cerebrovascular disease
    acute bacterial leptomeningitis, 561f
    arterial occlusion and brain ischemia, 562t
    brain hemorrhage, 562–563, 563f, 563t
    brain infarct, 561–562, 562f
    cortical infarct, 561f
    global ischemic injury, 562f
    SAH, 563–564, 564f, 564t
  demyelination, 568
    acute disseminated encephalomyelitis (ADEM), 569–570
    adrenoleukodystrophy (ALD), 571
    Krabbe disease, 571
    leukodystrophies, 570–571, 572f
    multiple sclerosis, 569, 569f
    progressive multifocal leukoencephalopathy (PML), 570, 570f
    radiation necrosis, 570
  infections
    acute bacterial meningitis, 558
    brain abscess, 559
    chronic meningitis, 558–559
    fungal infections of CNS, 560
    parasitic infections of CNS, 561
    viral encephalitis, 560
    viral meningitis, 559–560
Neuroblastoma, 404
Neurodegenerative diseases, 571–572
  Alzheimer disease, 572
  amyotrophic lateral sclerosis, 574–575
  brain atrophy in, 29, 29f
  Huntington disease, 574
  Parkinson disease, 572, 574
Neuroendocrine tumors, 257–258, 258f, 269–270, 269f
Neurofibrillary tangles (NFT), 573f
Neurofibromas, 490, 538, 540f
Neurohypophyseal, 396
Neuromuscular pathology
  acquired myopathies, 521
  hereditary myopathies, 518–519
  muscle biopsy, 513
  muscle fiber types, 513–514
  muscle pathology, 514
  muscle staining, 514, 517f–518f
  myofibril, 513, 516f
  myopathies evaluation, 513
  skeletal muscle, organization, 513, 515f
Neurons, 553, 553f
Neutropenia, 360–362
  causes, 361t
  cyclic, 362
  drug therapy, 362

Neutrophilia, 362–363, 363f
  causes, 363t
  chronic myelogenous leukemia, 362–363
Neutrophils, 183
  apoptosis, 70
    and macrophages, 73–74
  chemotaxis, 64–65, 64f
  and endothelial cell, interactions between, 62–63, 62f
  extracellular traps, 70
  nets, generation of, 71
  pathogen inactivation by
    NADPH oxidase, 68–69, 69f
    neutrophil granules and host defense, 67–68
  phagocytosis, 65–66, 66f
  phagosome maturation, 67
  polarization, 65, 65f
  transmigration of, 63, 63f
Nevus flammeus, 151
NFT. See Neurofibrillary tangles (NFT)
NHL. See Non-Hodgkin lymphomas (NHL)
Nitric oxide (NO), 57–58
  basal levels of, 49
Nitric oxide synthase 3 (NOS3), 49
Nitroblue tetrazolium chloride (NBT), 183
Nkx2-5, 189
NLPHL. See Nodular lymphocyte-predominant hodgkin lymphoma (NLPHL)
Nod-like receptors (NLRs)
  CARD and PYD domains of, 45
  and inflammasome, 45–46
  NOD domain of, 45
Nodular fasciitis, 479
Nodular goiter, 408, 408f
Nodular lymphocyte-predominant hodgkin lymphoma (NLPHL), 381–385, 382t
Nodular regenerative hyperplasia, 280
Nonaccidental head injury (NAHI), 577–580
Nonalcoholic fatty liver disease (NAFLD), 276–277, 277f
Nonbacterial thrombotic endocarditis (NBTE), 211
Nonfamilial cancers, 17
Non-Hodgkin lymphomas (NHL), 379
Noninfectious aortitis, 155
Nonionizing electromagnetic radiation injury, 119
Non-neoplastic testicular lesions, 336
Nonossifying fibroma, 501–502
Nonseminomatous germ cell tumors, 338
Nonsense mutation, 6
Non-small cell lung carcinomas (NSCLC), 219–221
Non-ST elevation myocardial infarction (non-STEMI), 182
non-STEMI. See Non-ST elevation myocardial infarction (non-STEMI)
Nonsteroidal anti-inflammatory drugs (NSAIDs), 53, 54
Normal heart, 179–182, 180f
Nosocomial infective endocarditis, 209
NSCLC. See Non-small cell lung carcinomas (NSCLC)
NSD1, 19
NSHPT. See Neonatal severe hyperparathyroidism (NSHPT)

Nuclear factor of activated T cells (NFATs), 27
Nuclear transcription factor, and Barrett metaplasia, 32–33
Nutrition, and aging, 90–91
NVE. See Native valve endocarditis (NVE)

O

Obliterative endarteritis, 283
Occupational chemical exposure, 112
Occupational injuries, 105–107, 116f–117f
Oncosis, 35
Oral contraceptives (OC), 113
Orchitis, 336
Osler–Weber–Rendu disease, 152, 152f
Osteitis fibrosa cystica (OFC), 417, 417f
Osteoarthritis, 508–509
Osteoblastoma, 497
Osteochondroma, 499–500
Osteofibrous dysplasia, 501
Osteogenesis imperfecta, 507
Osteoid osteoma, 497
Osteomalacia, 507
Osteomyelitis, 505–507
Osteopetrosis, 507
Osteoporosis, 507
Osteosarcoma, 497, 498, 498f
Ostium primum, 192
Ostium secundum, 192
Outlet VSDs, 190
Oxidative stress, 36
Oxyphil cells, 415
Oxytocin, 395–396

P

Paget disease, 434, 507
Palmar fibromatosis, 479
PAN. See Polyarteritis nodosa (PAN)
Pancarditis, 207
Pancreas
  anatomy, 287, 288f
  diabetes mellitus, 292
    gestational, 293
    type 1, 293
    type 2, 293
  diseases, 290
    acute pancreatitis, 291
    chronic pancreatitis, 291–292, 292f
    pseudocyst, 291, 292f
  ductal system, 287, 290f
  histology, 287, 289f, 289t
  hormones, 289t
  neoplasms, 293, 293t
    invasive ductal adenocarcinoma, 294–295, 294f
    well-differentiated pancreatic endocrine, 295–296, 295t
Pancreatic ductal system, 287, 290f
Panhypopituitarism, 390
Panniculitis, 547, 548f
Papaver somniferum, 109
Papillary carcinomas, 411, 412
Papillary dermis, 527
Papillary endothelial hyperplasia, 478
Papillary lesions, 427–428

Papillary microcarcinomas, 413
Papillary thyroid carcinoma (PTC), 412–413, 413f
Paracortex, 379
Paracrine, 385
Paradoxical embolism, 191
Parafollicular, 405
Paraganglioma, 404
Parakeratosis, 527
Paraneoplastic neutrophilia, 363
Paraprotein, 377
Parathyroid glands (PT), 414–416, 415f
    hyperparathyroidism, 416–417
        familial, 417
            osteitis fibrosa cystica, 417, 417f
        hypoparathyroidism
            autoimmune, 416
            primary hypoparathyroidism (HypoPT), 416
            pseudohypoparathyroidism, 416
Parathyroid hormone (PTH), 415
Parkinson disease, 14, 572, 574
15 Parkinson disease loci (PARK1-15), 14
Pars distalis, 387
Pars intermedia, 387
Pars tuberalis, 387
Partial atrioventricular canal defect, 192
PAS. See Periodic acid-Schiff (PAS)
Patent foramen ovale (PFO), 191
Pathogen-associated molecular patterns (PAMPs), 44
Pathogen recognition receptors (PRRs)
    cytoplasmic receptors, 45–46
    families of, 45f
    toll-like receptors (TLRs)
        localization and signaling pathways of, 44, 44f
        PAMP specificity of, 45
Patterned injury, 94
Pautrier microabscesses, 541
PBC. See Primary biliary cirrhosis (PBC)
PCD. See Plasma cell dyscrasias (PCD); Primary ciliary dyskinesia (PCD)
PCOS. See Polycystic ovarian syndrome (PCOS)
PD. See Peptic duodenitis (PD)
PDGFRA. See Platelet-derived growth factor receptor alpha genes (PDGFRA)
PE. See Pulmonary thromboemboli (PE)
Peliosis, 281, 392
Penetrating injury, 99–102
    closeness of weapon and, 102
    distant weapon and, 102
    entry bullet wounds, 101, 102f
    exit bullet wounds, 101–102, 102f
    gunshot wounds, 100–101
    range of fire and, 102
    stab wounds, 99–100
    weapon contact and, 102
Peptic duodenitis (PD), 255–256, 256f
Peptide hormones, 387
Pericardial tamponade, 155
Pericarditis, 186
Perimembranous VSDs, 190Perimysium, 513, 515f
Periodic acid-Schiff (PAS), 393, 520f
Periorbital ecchymosis, 100f
Peripheral nerve, 488
Peripheral T-cell lymphoma, not otherwise specified (PTCL, NOS), 385–386

Peritonitis, 97f
Periurethral glands, 444
Perivascular cell tumors (PEComas), 492
Peyronie disease, 340
PFO. See Patent foramen ovale (PFO)
PH. See Primary hyperaldosteronism (PH)
Phagocytosis, 65–66, 66f
Phagosome maturation, 67
Pheochromocytomas, 404–405, 404f
Phopholipase activation, 36
Phosphoinositide 3 kinase (PI3K)/Akt pathway, 27
Phospholipase C beta activation, 50
PHP. See Pseudohypoparathyroidism (PHP)
PHP type 1a, 416
Phyllodes tumors, 429–430, 430f
Physical injury, 94
    blunt injury, 98–99
    factors influencing, 96–97
    penetrating injury, 99–102
    pressure injury, 102–104
    quantity of force in, 96–97
        area over force applied, 96
        body area(s) affected by, 96
        fitness of individual and, 96–97
        time interval during force applied, 96
        tissue resistance to, 96
    sharp injury, 99
Physical trauma
    histopathology of, 97–98
    mechanisms of, 98–107
        asphyxia, 104–105
        blunt injury, 98–99
        occupational injuries, 105–107, 116f–117f
        penetrating injury, 99–102
        pressure injury, 102–104
        sharp injury, 99
Pigmented villonodular synovitis, 510
Pigment stones, 284
PIN. See Prostatic intraepithelial neoplasia (PIN)
Pituicytes, 389
Pituitary adenomas, 392–393, 393f
    pathogenesis, 395
Pituitary apoplexy, 392
Pituitary hormones, 389t
Pituitary lag, 409
Plasma cell dyscrasias (PCD), 377–379
Plasma cell myeloma, 380
Plasma contact system, 58, 58f
Plasma kallikrein (PK), 58
Plasminogen, 82
    deficiency, 83
Plasminogen activator inhibitor-1 (PAI-1), 83
Platelet-activating factor (PAF), 51, 57, 57f
Platelet-derived growth factor receptor alpha genes (PDGFRA), 251
Platelet function analysis (PFA), 80
Platelets, 54f
    function, defects in, 80
    function of, 52
    granules, 78–79
    production, defects in, 79
Pleomorphic rhabdomyosarcoma, 487
Plethora, 401
Pleural neoplasms, malignant mesothelioma, 223–225
Plexiform neurofibroma, 490
Plexiform vascular lesions, 238

Pneumoconiosis, 235–236
Pneumocystis, 227
Point of care testing (POCT), 138,
Polyarteritis nodosa (PAN), 159–160, 160f
Polycystic ovarian syndrome (PCOS), 461, 461f
Polycythemias, 359, 359t
Polycythemia vera (PV), 361
Polygenic disorders, 12
Polyglandular autoimmune syndromes, 399
Polymerase chain reaction (PCR), 130–131, 131f
    clinical utility of, 131
    meltcurve analysis, 130–131, 133f
    multiplex, 130
    quantitative, 130
    real-time, 130, 132f
    reverse transcription, 130
Polymorphonuclear leukocytes (PMNs), 24
Polymyalgia rheumatica, 158
Polyneuropathy, organomegaly, endocrinopathy, monoclonal gammopathy, and skin changes syndrome (POEMS), 379
Polyps, 265
Polyuria, 396
POMC. See Proopiomelanocortin (POMC)
Poorly differentiated thyroid carcinoma, 412, 414
Portal hypertension, 274
Port-wine stain, 151
Positron emission tomography (PET), 122
Posterior (neurohypophysis), 387
Posterior interventricular artery, 178
Postherpetic neuralgia, 551
Postpartum thyroiditis, 410
Postpubertal cervix, formation of transformation zone in, 32, 32f
Post-transplant lymphoproliferative disorders (PTLD), 229
p53 pathway, 43
PPCI. See Primary percutaneous coronary intervention (PPCI)
Preanalytical error, 124
Precursor lesions, 265
Preeclampsia, 466
Preinfarction angina, 179
Pressure injury, 102–104
    atmospheric pressure and
        decreased, 103–104
        elevated, 103
    explosion and, 102–103
Primary biliary cirrhosis (PBC), 279, 279f
Primary ciliary dyskinesia (PCD), 226, 231–232
Primary CNS lymphoma (PCNSL), 567
Primary hemostasis, 78–80
    and secondary hemostasis, defects in, 83t
Primary hyperaldosteronism (PH), 401–403
Primary hypoparathyroidism (HypoPT), 416
Primary percutaneous coronary intervention (PPCI), 187
Primary sclerosing cholangitis (PSC), 278, 278f
Primary splenic marginal zone lymphoma, 389
Progerias, 89
Progeroid syndromes
    genetic lesions responsible for, 89
    Hutchinson–Gilford Progeria (HGP), 89–90, 90f
    Werner syndrome, 90
Progressive ischemic cardiovascular disease, 24
Progressive multifocal leukoencephalopathy (PML), 570, 570f

Prolactin (PRL), 393–394
Prolactinomas, 392
Proopiomelanocortin (POMC), 394
Prostacyclin, 170
Prostaglandins (PG), 51
    formation, biological effects, and tissue source of, 55f
    paracrine and autocrine roles of, 54
    prostacyclin (PGI$_2$), 54
    prostaglandin D$_2$ (PGD$_2$), 54, 56
    prostaglandin E$_2$ (PGE$_2$), 53, 54
    prostaglandin F$_2\alpha$ (PGF$_2\alpha$), 56
    prostaglandin H$_2$, 54, 56
Prostanoids, 52–56
Prostate
    anatomy, 33–35
    diseases
        benign prostatic hyperplasia, 344–345
            prostate carcinoma, 346–350
            prostatitis, 344
    histology, 33–35
    physiology, 33–35
Prostate carcinoma, 346–350
    needle biopsy diagnosis, 346
Prostatic acid phosphatase (PSAP), 343
Prostatic intraepithelial neoplasia (PIN), 347
Prostatic-specific antigen (PSA), 343
Prostatitis, 344
Prosthetic heart valves, 213
Prosthetic valve endocarditis (PVE), 209
Protease-activated receptors (PARs), 78
Proteolytic enzymes, 68
PSA. *See* Prostatic-specific antigen (PSA)
PSAP. *See* Prostatic acid phosphatase (PSAP)
PSA screening, 347–348
PSC. *See* Primary sclerosing cholangitis (PSC)
Pseudocyst, 291, 292f
Pseudogout, 509
Pseudohypoparathyroidism (PHP), 416
Pseudomembranes, 262
Pseudomonas aeruginosa, 507
Pseudomyxoma peritonei, 269
Psoriasis, scaly silver plaques, 543, 544f
PT. *See* Parathyroid glands (PT)
PTC. *See* Papillary thyroid carcinoma (PTC)
PTCL, NOS. *See* Peripheral T-cell lymphoma, not otherwise specified (PTCL, NOS)
PTH. *See* Parathyroid hormone (PTH)
PTLD. *See* Post-transplant lymphoproliferative disorders (PTLD)
Pulmonary artery hypertension, 238
Pulmonary hypertension, 191
Pulmonary thromboemboli (PE), 238
Pulmonary vasculature, 149
PV. *See* Polycythemia vera (PV)
PVE. *See* Prosthetic valve endocarditis (PVE)
Pyelonephritis, 37
Pyloric stenosis, 246
Pyogenic granulomas, 477
Pyroptosis, 35
Pyrosequencing, 134

R

Radial scar/complex sclerosing lesion, 427
Radiation injury, 118–119
    acute and chronic effects of radiation, 118–119
    environmental radiation in, 118
    radiation dosage and, 118f
    radiation therapy and, 119
    radon and, 118
    sources of radiation exposure, 118t
Radiation necrosis, 570, 571f
Radiation vasculitis, 165
Ragged red fibers, 521f
Rapidly progressive glomerulonephritis (RPGN), 299
RBILD. *See* Respiratory bronchiolitis and interstitial lung disease (RBILD)
RCM. *See* Restrictive cardiomyopathy (RCM)
Reactive fibroblastic lesions, 479
Reactive gastropathy, 250, 250f
Reactive oxygen species and mitochondrial damage, 36, 36f
Red neurons, 553, 553f
Red pulp spleen disorders, 389–391, 390t
Reepithelialized surgical wound, 77f
Reflux esophagitis, 241, 242f
Refractory anemia, 359, 359f
Renal amyloidosis, 299
Renal infarct, 39f
Renal ischemia, 35
Renal pelvis and ureter
    congenital disorders, 334
    obstruction, 334
    tumors, 334
Renovascular hypertension, 320
Reperfusion injury, 36
Respiratory bronchiolitis and interstitial lung disease (RBILD), 233, 235, 235f
Response-to-injury theory, 170
Restrictive cardiomyopathy (RCM), 203
Rete ridges, 527
Reticular dermis, 527
Retinoids, 546
Reverse transcription PCR (rtPCR), 130
Reversible cell injury, 33, 39f
    biochemical and molecular analysis, 22
    case study, 23, 23f
    coagulative necrosis, 23–24, 23f
    infiltration of infarct, 24, 24f
    visual clues associated with, 37
Rhabdomyomas, 486
Rhabdomyosarcoma, 486, 486t
Rheumatic valvular heart disease
    acute rheumatic fever, 206–207
    definition, 206
    diagnosis, 207
    pathogenesis, 207
    symptoms, 208–209
Rheumatoid arthritis, 509
Rheumatoid nodules, 546–547
Rickets, 507
Right coronary artery, 182
RPGN. *See* Rapidly progressive glomerulonephritis (RPGN)
rtPCR. *See* Reverse transcription PCR (rtPCR)

S

Saccharomyces cerevisiae, 7
Saccular aneurysm, 149
S-adenosylhomocysteine (SAH), 19
S-adenosylmethionine (SAM), 19
SAH. *See* S-adenosylhomocysteine (SAH); Subarachnoid hemorrhage (SAH)
Salmonella, 261
SAM. *See* S-adenosylmethionine (SAM)
Sampling error, 124
Sarcoidosis, 232–233, 232f 546, 547f
Sarcomas, 333
Sarcomatoid carcinomas, 221
SAS. *See* Subaortic stenosis (SAS)
SBS. *See* Shaken baby syndrome (SBS)
Scalding injury, 115, 116f
SCD. *See* Sudden cardiac death (SCD)
Schistosomiasis, 331
Schwannomas, 488–489, 489f, 567
SCLC. *See* Small cell lung carcinomas (SCLC)
Sclerosing adenosis, 425, 426f
Sclerosing disorders (morphea/scleroderma), 547, 548f
Scrapes, 98
Secondary adrenal insufficiency, 400
Secondary cardiac tumors, 215
Secondary hemostasis, 80–81
Secondary hyperaldosteronism, 402
Secondary (metastatic) neoplasms, 552, 552f
Secondary polycythemia, 360
Secondary syphilis, 341
Second-degree burns, 114
Semilunar valves, 180
Seminomas, 338, 338f
Serous pericardium, 215
Serprocidins, 68
Serrated polyps, 267, 267f
Sertoli cells (SC), 335
Sertoli cell tumors, 340, 340f
Sertoli–Leydig cell tumor, 464, 465f
Sessile serrated adenomas, 267, 267f
Sex chromosomes, in cytogenetic disorders, 13
Sex cord/stromal tumors, 464–465
SFT. *See* Solitary fibroma tumors (SFT)
Shaken baby syndrome (SBS), 579, 579f–580f
Sharp injury, 99
Sheehan syndrome, 391
Shigella, 261
Shunt, 190
Shunting, 218
SIADH. *See* Syndrome of inappropriate ADH secretion (SIADH)
Sickle cell anemia, 390
Silent mutation, 6
Single cigarette, 175
Single gene disorders, 11–12
    autosomal dominant disorders, 11, 11f
    autosomal recessive disorders, 11–12, 11f
    mitochondrial disorders, 12
    X-linked disorders, 12
Single-nucleotide polymorphism (SNP), 4
Sinoatrial (SA) node, 181, 180f
Sinuses, 379
Sinus venosus ASD, 192
Sipple syndrome, 404
Skeletal muscle
    benign tumors, 486
    denervation atrophy of, 26
    histology, 484, 484f
    neoplasms, 485–486
Skene glands, 444
Skin

adnexal (apendageal) tumors
　microcystic adnexal carcinoma, 537
　poroma, 536, 536f
　sebaceous carcinoma, 537
　sebaceous hyperplasia, 537, 537f, 538f
　syringoma, 536–537, 537f
　trichilemmoma, 537
　trichofolliculoma, 537, 537f
basal cell carcinoma, 531
cornified layer, 527
epidermal lesions and tumors, 530–531, 531f
erythemas, 528
follicular cysts, 528–529, 529f
hematoxylin and eosin stained biopsy, 526f
infectious diseases
　arthropod-associated lesions (scabies), 551, 551f
　dermatophyte, 547–549, 549f
　fibroepithelial polyp, 552, 552f
　herpes viruses, 550–551, 550f
　impetigo/erysipelas, 549
　molluscum contagiosum, 551, 551f
　secondary (metastatic) neoplasms, 552, 552f
　varicella zoster virus, 551
　verruca vulgaris, 550
keratinocytes, 526
keratoacanthoma, 532, 533f
major inflammatory reaction patterns and prototypes, 543
　folliculitis (suppurative folliculitis), 546
　foreign bodies and foreign body granulomas, 547, 548f
　granulomatous dermatitis (granuloma annulare), 546, 546f
　lichen sclerosis, 545, 545f
　panniculitis, 547, 548f
　psoriasis., scaly silver plaques, 543, 544f
　rheumatoid nodules, 546–547
　sarcoidosis, 546, 547f
　sclerosing disorders (morphea/scleroderma), 547, 548f
　vesiculobullous (bullous pemphigoid), 545, 545f
melanocytes, 526
parakeratosis, 527
pigmented lesions
　freckle (ephelide)/melanotic macule, 533, 533f
　lentigo simplex, 534, 534f
　melanocytic nevus, 534–535, 534f
　melanoma, 535–536
　melasma, 533
　solar lentigo, 534, 534f
primary and secondary lesions, 528, 528t
rete ridges, 527
soft tissue lesions and neoplasms
　angiosarcoma, 541, 541f
　B-cell lymphoma, 542, 542f
　dermatofibroma, 538–540, 540f
　dermatofibrosarcoma protuberans (DFSP), 540, 541f
　hemangioma, 537–538, 539f
　kaposi sarcoma, 541
　langerhans cell histiocytosis, 542–543, 543f
　leukemia cutis, 542
　mastocytosis/urticaria pigmentosa, 542, 542f

　Merkel cell carcinoma, 538, 540f
　mycosis fungoides/cutaneous T-cell lymphoma, 541–542, 542f
　neurofibroma, 538, 540f
　xanthoma, 538, 539f
　squamous cell carcinoma, 531–532, 532f
　stains and immunostains, 529t
　structure, 527f
　tense bullae, 526f
SLE. See Systemic lupus erythematosus (SLE)
Small arteries, 149
Small cell lung carcinomas (SCLC), 222–223, 223f
Small intestine
　anatomy, 252
　developmental disorders
　　Meckel diverticulum, 252–254
　histology, 252, 253f
　infectious diseases
　　whipple disease, 256–257, 257f
　inflammatory
　　Crohn disease, 256
　　peptic duodenitis, 255–256, 256f
　malabsorption
　　celiac disease, 254–255
　　tropical sprue, 255
　neoplasms
　　adenocarcinomas, 257, 258f
　　neuroendocrine tumors, 257–258, 258f
SMARCB1, 19
Smoker's macrophages, 235, 235f
Smooth muscles
　histology, 481–482, 481f
　malignant tumors, 482–484
　neoplasms, 482
SNP. See Single-nucleotide polymorphism (SNP)
SNRPN, 9
Soft tissue tumors of uncertain differentiation, 492–495
Solar lentigo, 534, 534f
Solitary fibroma tumors (SFT), 492, 494f
Solitary osteochondroma, 500
Somatic death, 21
　denition of, 21
　and injury, 22
Somatic mutation vs. germ-line mutation, 6
Somatotropin-release inhibiting factor (SRIF), 389
Somatropin, 113
Sotos syndrome, 19
Spermatocele, 341
Spider telangiectasia, 152
Spindle cell/pleomorphic lipoma, 471–472, 472f
Spindle cell/Sclerosing rhabdomyosarcoma, 487
Spinous layer, 526
Splenic white pulp, 388
Squamous cell carcinoma, 219–220, 219f, 244–245, 245f, 333, 341, 531–532, 532f
Squamous cell lesions, 450
Squamous metaplasia, 331
SRIF. See Somatotropin-release inhibiting factor (SRIF)
Staphylococcus, 161, 210
Staphylococcus aureus, 210, 422, 506
Static electricity injury, 117
Stein–Leventhal syndrome, 461

ST elevation myocardial infarcts (STEMI), 182
STEMI. See ST elevation myocardial infarcts (STEMI)
Stimulants toxicity, 109
Stomach
　anatomy, 245–246, 247f
　diseases
　　acute hemorrhagic gastritis, 246, 248
　　atrophic gastritis, 248–249
　　autoimmune gastritis, 249
　　chronic gastritis, 248
　　developmental disorders, 246
　　gastric ulcers, 249–250, 250f
　　Helicobacter gastritis, 248
　　inflammatory disorders, 246
　　multifocal atrophic gastritis, 249
　　pyloric stenosis, 246
　　reactive gastropathy, 250, 250f
　gastric neoplasms
　　adenocarcinoma, 250–251, 251f
　　gastrointestinal stromal tumor, 251–252, 252f
　　marginal-zone B-cell lymphoma, 252, 252f
　histology, 245–246, 248f
Strangulation, manual, 106f
Strawberry hemangioma, 151
Streptococcus, 161, 210
Streptococcus bovis, 211
Streptococcus viridans, 211
Struma ovarii, 464
Sturge–Weber syndrome, 151
Subacute thyroiditis, 410–411
Subaortic stenosis (SAS), 199
Subarachnoid hemorrhage (SAH), 563–564, 564f, 564t
Subareolar abscess (periductal mastitis), 422
Subcutaneous nodules, 207
Subdural hematoma, 575–576
Subendocardial infarct, 182
Subendocardial layer, 179
Succinate dehydrogenase staining, 521f
Sudden cardiac death (SCD), 188–189
Superficial fibromatosis, 479
Superficial or cutaneous leiomyoma, 482
Supravalvar aortic stenosis (SVAS), 199
Surgical pathologists, 121
Surgical pathology, 122
SUV4-20H enzyme, 19
SVAS. See Supravalvar aortic stenosis (SVAS)
Sydenham chorea, 207
Synarthrosis, 507
Syndrome of inappropriate ADH secretion (SIADH), 396
Synovial chondromatosis, 511
Synovial lipomas, 511
Synovial sarcoma, 493
Synpharyngitic, 310
α-synuclein, 14
Syphilis, 340–341
Syphilitic aortitis, 156, 156f
Systemic hypertension, 165
　for atherosclerosis, 173
Systemic inflammatory response syndrome (SIRS), 60
Systemic lupus erythematosus (SLE), 238
Systemic progrowth factors, 29–30

T

Takayasu disease, 155–156, 156f
Tall-cell variant PTC, 413
Tamm–Horsfall protein, 305
"Target of rapamycin" (mTOR) pathway, 90
Tbx5, 189
T-cell prolymphocytic leukemia, 365, 366
TDLU. See Terminal-duct lobular units (TDLU)
Tear, 98
    mesenteric, 97f
Telangiectasia macularis eruptiva perstans, 542
Telomere decay, 85–86
Temporal arteritis, 157
Teniae coli, 259
Tenosynovial giant cell tumors, 509–510, 510f
Tense bullae, 526f
Teratomas, 339
Terminal-duct lobular units (TDLU), 419, 420f
Testis
    anatomy, 334
    diseases
        gonadal stromal/sex cord tumors, 339–340
        male infertility, 335–336
        non-neoplastic testicular lesions, 336
        testicular tumors, 337–339
    histology, 334, 335f
    torsion of, 336
Tetralogy of Fallot (TOF), 190
Thermal injury, 94, 114–115
    burns, 114–115, 115f
        first-degree, 114
        second-degree, 114
        third-degree, 114–115
        water temperature effects on skin, 115f
    environmental, 115–116
        heat exhaustion, 116
        heatstroke, 115
        hyperthermia, 115
        hypothermia, 116
    scalding, 115, 116f
Thermus aquaticus (Taq), 130
Thin basement membrane lesion, 314–316
Third-degree burns, 114–115
Thrombin, 78
Thrombin activatable fibrinolytic inhibitor (TAFI), 83
Thromboangiitis obliterans (TAO), 163–164, 164f
Thrombocytopenias, 367–369
    causes, 369t
    due to peripheral destruction, 79t
    ITP, 369
Thrombocytoses, 369–370
    causes, 369t
    iron deficiency, 370
Thromboembolism, 186
Thrombopoietin (TPO), 78
Thrombotic microangiopathies, 317
Thrombotic thrombocytopenic purpura (TTP), 79, 80, 317–318Thymic carcinoma, 393, 395f
Thymic hyperplasia, 393
Thymoma, 393, 396
Thyroglobulin, 405
Thyroid
    benign diseases
        endemic and hypofunctioning goiters, 409
        graves disease, 409, 409f
        hyperthyroidism, 409
        hypothyroidism, 408–409
        nodular goiter, 408
        thyroid autoantibody detection in AITD, 410
        toxic multinodular goiter, 409
    congenital abnormalities, 407–408
    definition, 405
    follicular cell-derived neoplastic diseases, 411
        follicular adenomas, 412, 412f
        malignant neoplasms, 412–414
    function testing, 405–407
    histological features, 405
    hormone, 407
    thyroiditis
        acute suppurative, 410
        chronic autoimmune, 411
        subacute, 410–411
Thyroid autoantibody detection in AITD, 410
Thyroidization, 322
Thyroid-stimulating hormone (TSH), 394–395
Tissue edema, mechanism of, 49–50, 49f
Tissue factor (TF), 80
Tissue ischemia, 33–34
Tissue repair
    and parenchymal regeneration, 75
    stages of
        hemostatic phase, 75–76
        inflammatory phase, 76
        proliferative phase, 76–77
        remodeling phase, 77
T lymphoblastic leukemia (T-ALL), 378
T-lymphoblastic lymphoma, 396–397
TNF-related apoptosis inducing ligand (TRAIL), 43
TNG. See Toxic multinodular goiter (TNG)
Tobacco use, adverse effects of, 111
TOF. See Tetralogy of Fallot (TOF)
Toxemia of pregnancy, 317
Toxic multinodular goiter (TNG), 409
"Tramline" bruises, 98f
Transdifferentiation, 32
Transforming growth factor (TGF), 27
Transmural infarcts, 182
Transudation, mechanism of, 49, 49f
Traumatic head injury
    brain contusions, 576–577
    complications, 577, 577f
    diffuse axonal injury, 577
    epidural hematoma, 575
    intraparenchymal brain hemorrhage, 577
    lacerations, 576–577
    Nonaccidental head injury, 577–580
Traumatic neuroma, 488
Treatment-induced RCM, 203
"Trench foot," 116
Treponema pallidum, 156, 340
3,4,3'-triiodothyronine (T3), 405
Triphenyltetrazolium chloride (TTC), 183
Tropheryma whipplei, 256
Tropical sprue (TS), 255
Truncus arteriosus, 196, 197f
Trypanosoma cruzi, 200
TS. See Tropical sprue (TS)
TSH. See Thyroid-stimulating hormone (TSH)
TTC. See Triphenyltetrazolium chloride (TTC)
TTP. See Thrombotic thrombocytopenic purpura (TTP)
Tubular and interstitial disease, 320–321, 321f
Tubulitis, 322
Tubulopathy, 304
Tunica adventitia, 475
Turcot syndrome, 17
Turner syndrome, 13
Twin–twin transfusion system, 467

U

UBE3A. See Angelman syndrome gene (*UBE3A*)
Ubiquitin ligases (ULs), 30
UIP. See Usual interstitial pneumonia (UIP)
Ulcerative colitis, 263, 264f
Ureter, 334
    duplication, 334, 334f
Ureteric valves, 334
Urinary bladder
    benign proliferative lesions, 331–332
    chronic obstruction, 332
    congenital anomalies
        diverticula, 330
        exstrophy, 330
        urachal remnants, 330
    cystitis, 330–331, 330f
    tumors, 332–334
Urokinase plasminogen activator (uPA), 83
Urolithiasis, 322
Urothelial carcinoma in situ, 333, 333f
Urothelial (transitional cell) neoplasms, 333
Urothelium, 330
Usual interstitial pneumonia (UIP), 235
Uterine involution following childbirth, 29, 29f
Uterine leiomyoma, 459f
Uterus, benign changes
    adenomyosis, 454
    infections, 454
    pregnancy, 454

V

Varicella zoster virus, 551
Varicocele, 341
Vascular disease, 298, 298f
Vascular ectasias, 151–152
Vascular response to injury and disease
    fibrin deposition, 77
    fibroblasts, 77
    primary hemostasis, 78–80
    secondary hemostasis, 80–81
Vascular system
    arteriosclerosis
        acute coronary syndrome, 178–179
        atherosclerotic (or atherothrombotic) lesions, 171–173
        complications, 177
        coronary artery, 177–178
        epidemiology, 173
        risk factors, 173–174
        types, 169
    blood vessels, embryology of, 147–149, 148f
    cardiac tumors
        cardiac myxoma, 213–214
        secondary, 215

cardiomyopathies
    arrhythmogenic right ventricular, 201
    definition, 200
    dilated, 200–201
    hypertrophic, 201–203
    restrictive, 203
chronic ischemic heart disease, 188
    classification, 182
    early complications, 183–186
    late complications, 187
    location of, 182
    morphology, 182–183
    outcome of, 182
    treatment, 187–189
congenital heart disease
    cardiac septation defects, 189
    noncyanotic congenital heart disease, 190–194
    obstructive congenital anomalies, 196–200
    terminology and concepts, 190
diseases
    aortic dissection, 152–155
    Behçet disease, 164–165
    capillary hemangioma, 151
    congenital vascular anomalies, 149–151
    eosinophilic granulomatosis with polyangiitis, 162, 162*f*
    giant-cell arteritis, 157–159, 159*f*
    hypersensitivity vasculitis, 162–163, 163*f*
    Kawasaki disease, 160–161, 161*f*
    noninfectious aortitis, 155
    polyarteritis nodosa, 157–160, 160*f*
    radiation vasculitis, 165
    syphilitic aortitis, 156
    Takayasu disease, 155–156, 156*f*
    thromboangiitis obliterans, 163–164, 164*f*
    vascular ectasias, 151–152
    Wegener granulomatosis, 161, 162*f*
hypertensive disease
    etiology, 166
    pathologic changes, 166

pericardial diseases
    acute pericarditis, 215–216
    constrictive pericarditis, 216
sudden cardiac death, 188–189
valvular heart disease
    calcific aortic stenosis, 205–206
    clinical symptoms, 206
    congenitally bicuspid aortic valve, 206
    definition, 203–204
    mitral valve stenosis, 206–207
    valvular insufficiency, 209–213
Vascular tumors, 474–476
Vasculitis, 157, 157*f*, 238–239
    nomenclature, 158*t*
Ventricular aneurysm, 187
Ventricular septal defect (VSD), 185, 190–191, 191*f*
    membranous septum, 190
    muscular septum, 190
    outlet, 190
Verruca vulgaris, 550
Verrucous carcinoma, 341
Vesiculobullous (bullous pemphigoid), 545, 545*f*
VHL syndrome, 404
VIN. *See* Vulvar intraepithelial neoplasia (VIN)
Violaceous raised papules, 522*f*
Viral encephalitis, 560
Viral hepatitis, 266
Viral meningitis, 559–560
Visceral layer, 215
von Recklinghausen syndrome, 404
von Willebrand disease (vWD), 80
von Willebrand factor (vWF), 317
VSD. *See* Ventricular septal defect (VSD)
Vulnerable plaques, 178
Vulvar intraepithelial neoplasia (VIN), 446, 446*f*

W

Wegener granulomatosis, 161, 162*f*, 314
Well-differentiated liposarcoma (WDL), 472

Well-differentiated pancreatic endocrine neoplasms, 295–296, 295*t*
    nonfunctioning *vs.* functioning tumors, 295
Werner syndrome (WS), 90
Whipple disease, 256–257, 257*f*
White pulp spleen disorders, 388–389
Wilson disease, 280
Workplace injuries. *See* Occupational injuries
Wounds
    close range chest, 103*f*
    entry bullet, 101, 102*f*
    exit bullet, 101–102, 102*f*
    gunshot, 100–101
    host reaction to, 21
    incised, 99, 101*f*
    stab, 99–100
Wound track, 103*f*
WT1, 9

X

Xanthogranulomatous pyelonephritis, 322
Xanthoma cells, 322, 538, 539*f*
45X karyotypy, 13
X-linked disorders, 12
X-linked recessive inheritance, 12
46XX karyotypy, 13
47XXY karyotypy, 13
46XY karyotypy, 13

Y

Years of potential life lost (YPPL), 94*t*
Yolk sac tumor, 338, 339*f*, 465, 465*f*

Z

Zellballen, 404
Zona fasciculata, 396
Zona glomerulosa, 396